NYHUS AND CONDON'S
HERNIA

NYHUS AND CONDON'S
HERNIA

FIFTH EDITION

Editors

ROBERT J. FITZGIBBONS, JR., M.D.

Department of Surgery
Creighton University
Omaha, Nebraska

A. GERSON GREENBURG, M.D., PH.D.

Department of Surgery
Brown Medical School
and
Department of Surgery
The Miriam Hospital
Providence, Rhode Island

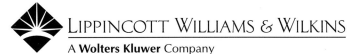

LIPPINCOTT WILLIAMS & WILKINS
A **Wolters Kluwer** Company
Philadelphia · Baltimore · New York · London
Buenos Aires · Hong Kong · Sydney · Tokyo

Acquisitions Editor: Lisa McAllister
Managing Editor: Susan Rhyner
Developmental Editor: Joanne Bersin
Production Editor: Jonathan Geffner
Manufacturing Manager: Colin J. Warnock
Cover Designer: Christine Jenny
Compositor: Lippincott Williams & Wilkins Desktop Division
Printer: Maple Press

© 2002 by LIPPINCOTT WILLIAMS & WILKINS
530 Walnut Street
Philadelphia, PA 19106 USA
LWW.com

Library of Congress Cataloging-in-Publication Data

Nyhus and Condon's hernia / edited by Robert J. Fitzgibbons, Jr. and A. Gerson Greenburg.—5th ed.
        p. ; cm.
    Rev. ed. of: Hernia / edited by Lloyd M. Nyhus, Robert E. Condon. 4th ed. c1995.
    Includes bibliographical references and index.
    ISBN 0-7817-1962-3
    1. Hernia. I. Title: Hernia. II. Fitzgibbons, Robert J., 1949– III. Greenburg, A. Gerson. IV. Nyhus, Lloyd M. (Lloyd Milton), 1923–
    [DNLM: 1. Hernia. WI 950 N9938 2001]
    RD621 .H47 2001
    617.5′59—dc21
                                                                                    2001029558

Care has been taken to confirm the accuracy of the information presented and to describe generally accepted practices. However, the authors, editors, and publisher are not responsible for errors or omissions or for any consequences from application of the information in this book and make no warranty, expressed or implied, with respect to the currency, completeness, or accuracy of the contents of the publication. Application of this information in a particular situation remains the professional responsibility of the practitioner.

The authors, editors, and publisher have exerted every effort to ensure that drug selection and dosage set forth in this text are in accordance with current recommendations and practice at the time of publication. However, in view of ongoing research, changes in government regulations, and the constant flow of information relating to drug therapy and drug reactions, the reader is urged to check the package insert for each drug for any change in indications and dosage and for added warnings and precautions. This is particularly important when the recommended agent is a new or infrequently employed drug.

Some drugs and medical devices presented in this publication have Food and Drug Administration (FDA) clearance for limited use in restricted research settings. It is the responsibility of the health care provider to ascertain the FDA status of each drug or device planned for use in their clinical practice.

10 9 8 7 6 5 4 3 2 1

CONTENTS

PART III: LAPAROSCOPIC AND ENDOSCOPIC GROIN HERNIA REPAIRS

PART IV: COMPLICATIONS OF GROIN HERNIA

PART V: VENTRAL INCISIONAL HERNIAS

PART VI: PEDIATRIC HERNIAS

CONTRIBUTING AUTHORS

John J. Aiken, M.D. Assistant Professor, Division of Pediatric Surgery, Medical College of Wisconsin; Assistant Professor and Section Chief, Division of Pediatric Surgery, Children's Hospital of Wisconsin, Milwaukee, Wisconsin

Joseph F. Amaral, M.D. Professor, Department of Surgery, Brown University School of Medicine; President and CEO, Rhode Island Hospital, Providence, Rhode Island

Parviz K. Amid, M.D. Department of Surgery, Harbor UCLA and Harbor UCLA Research and Education Institute, Torrance, California; Department of Surgery, Cedars-Sinai and Harbor UCLA Medical Centers; and Lichtenstein Hernia Institute, Los Angeles, California

Maurice E. Arregui, M.D. Program Director, Fellowship in Laparoscopy, Endoscopy and Ultrasound, Department of Surgery, St. Vincent Hospital and Health Care Center, Indianapolis, Indiana

Keith W. Ashcraft, M.D. Emeritus Professor of Surgery, University of Missouri at Kansas City; Surgeon-in-Chief (Retired), Children's Mercy Hospital, Kansas City, Missouri

Robert Bendavid, M.D. Elisha Hospital, Mount Carmel, Haifa, Israel

David Bennett, M.D. Consultant Surgeon, Department of Surgery, Derriford Hospital, Plymouth, Devon, United Kingdom

Reinhard Bittner Department of Surgery, ULM University; Chief, Department of Surgery (General/Visceral), Marienhospital Stuttgart, Stuttgart, Germany

Torben Callesen M.D. Associate Professor, University of Copenhagen; Consultant, Anesthetics Department, Rigshospitalet, Copenhagen, Denmark

James E. Carter M.D., Ph.D. Associate Clinical Professor, Department of Obstetrics and Gynecology, University of California–Irvine, College of Medicine, Orange, California; Medical Director, Women's Health Center of South Orange County Inc., Mission Viejo, California

Gene L. Colborn, Ph.D. Professor and Chairman, Department of Anatomical Sciences, Ross University School of Medicine, Commonwealth of Dominica, West Indies

Hugh P. Cowdin, Jr., M.D. Clinical Assistant Professor, Department of Anesthesia, Brown University; Staff Anesthesiologist, Department of Anesthesia, The Miriam Hospital, Providence, Rhode Island

David L. Crawford, M.D. Assistant Clinical Professor, Department of Surgery, University of Illinois at Chicago, College of Medicine at Peoria, Peoria, Illinois

Johann Cunningham, M.D. Trauma Fellow/Clinical Lecturer, University of British Columbia; Attending Staff, Trauma Services, Vancouver General Hospital, Vancouver, British Columbia, Canada

James R. DeBord, M.D. Clinical Professor, Department of Surgery, University of Illinois College of Medicine at Peoria; Peoria Surgical Group, Ltd., Peoria, Illinois

Demetrios Demetriades, M.D., Ph.D. Professor, Department of Surgery, University of Southern California School of Medicine; Director, Department of Surgery, Division of Trauma and Critical Care, LAC+USC Medical Center, Los Angeles, California

José A. Díaz-Elizondo, M.D. Professor, Department of General Surgery, Instituto Tecnológico y de Estudios Superiores de Monterrey; Department of General Surgery, Hospital San José–Tec de Monterrey, Monterrey, Mexico

Dorothy D. Dunlop Research Associate Professor, Institute for Health Services, Department of Research and Policy Studies, Northwestern University, Evanston, Illinois

Charles J. Filipi, M.D. Professor, Department of Surgery, Creighton University, Omaha, Nebraska

Eva Fischer, M.D. Associate Professor, Department of Surgery, Joan and Sanford Weill Medical College of Cornell University; Attending Surgeon, Department of Surgery, New York Presbyterian Hospital, New York, New York

Robert J. Fitzgibbons, Jr., M.D. Harry E. Stuckenhoff Professor of Surgery, Chief, Division of General Surgery, Department of Surgery, Creighton University, Omaha, Nebraska

Jean B. Flament, M.D. First Class Professor, Department of Surgery, Reims University; Chief, Department of General Surgery, Hopital Robert Debre, Reims, France

Neil R. Floch, M.D. Assistant Attending Surgeon, Department of Surgery, Norwalk Hospital, Floch Surgical Associates, Norwalk, Connecticut

Morris E. Franklin, Jr. M.D. Texas Endosurgery Institute and Surgery Department, University of Texas at San Antonio, San Antonio, Texas

Donald E. Fry, M.D. University of New Mexico School of Medicine, Albuquerque, New Mexico

Glenn C. Gardner, M.D. Resident, Department of Surgery, Creighton University, Omaha, Nebraska

W. Peter Geis, M.D. Department of Surgery, St. Peter's University Hospital, New Brunswick, New Jersey

James Gibbs, Ph.D. Research Assistant Professor, Institute for Health Services Research and Policy Studies, Northwest University, Evanston, Illinois; Research Health Scientist, Cooperative Studies Program Coordinating Center (151K), Edward Hines, Jr. VA Hospital, Hines, Illinois

Arthur I. Gilbert, M.D. Associate Professor, Department of Surgery, University of Miami; Surgery Director, Hernia Institute of Florida, Miami, Florida

G. Kevin Gillian, M.D. Chief, Division of General Surgery, Southern Maryland Hospital Center, Clinton, Maryland

Finn Gottrup, M.D. Dr. Med Sci. Professor, Copenhagen Wound Healing Center, University of Copenhagen; Chief, Copenhagen Wound Healing Center, Bispebjerg Hospital, Copenhagen, Denmark

Michael F. Graham M.D. Hernia Institute of Florida, South Miami, Florida

A. Gerson Greenburg, M.D., Ph.D. Professor, Department of Surgery, Brown Medical School; Surgeon-in-Chief, Department of Surgery, The Miriam Hospital, Providence, Rhode Island

Antonio Guarnieri, M.D. Chief, Department of Surgery, Clinica Guarnieri, Rome, Italy

Francesco Guarnieri, M.D. Chief, Department of Surgery, Clinica Guarnieri, Rome, Italy

Staffan Haapaniemi, M.D. Department of Surgery, University of Linköping; Department of Surgery, University Hospital, Linköping, Sweden

William G. Henderson, Ph.D. Director, VA Cooperative Studies Program Coordinating Center, VA Hospital, Hines, Illinois

León Herszage, M.D. Associate Professor, Department of Surgery, Salvador University; Chief of Abdominal Wall Surgery, Department of General Surgery, Hospital I. Pirovano, Buenos Aires, Argentina

Ronald A. Hinder, M.D. Professor and Chair, Department of Surgery, Mayo Clinic, Jacksonville, Florida

Kathleen C. Hittner, M.D. Clinical Professor, Department of Surgery–Anesthesiology, Brown University; President, CEO, and Anesthesiologist, Department of Anesthesiology, The Miriam Hospital, Providence, Rhode Island

Leif A. Israelsson, M.D., Ph.D. Associate Professor, Department of Surgery, Umeå University, Umeå, Sweden; Surgeon Consultant, Department of Surgery, Sundsvall Hospital, Sundsvall, Sweden

Marc Jansen, M.D. Scientific Assistant, Department of Surgery, Rhenish Westphalian Technical University; Assistant, Department of Surgery, University Hospital, Aachen, Germany

Olga Jonasson, M.D. Professor, Department of Surgery, University of Illinois; American College of Surgeons, Chicago, Illinois

Lars N. Jorgensen, M.D. Associate Professor, Department of Surgical Gastroenterology, University of Copenhagen; Associate Professor, Department of Surgical Gastroenterology, Bispebjerg Hospital, Copenhagen, Denmark

Henrik Kehlet, M.D., Ph.D. Professor and Chief Surgeon, Department of Surgical Gastroenterology 435, Hvidovre University Hospital, Hvidovre, Denmark

Uwe Klinge, M.D. Consultant, Department of Surgery, Rhenish Westphalian Technical University Hospital Aachen, Aachen, Germany

Bernd Klosterhalfen, M.D. Consultant, Department of Surgery, Rhenish Westphalian Technical University Hospital Aachen, Aachen, Germany

Barbara Kraft, M.D. Senior Resident, Department of Surgery (General/Visceral), Marienhospital Stuttgart, Stuttgart, Germany

Klaus Kraft, M.D. Senior Resident, Department of Surgery (General/Visceral), Marienhospital Stuttgart, Stuttgart, Germany

Bernd Kuckuk, M.D. Senior Resident, Department of Surgery (General/Visceral), Marienhospital Stuttgart, Stuttgart, Germany

Robert D. Kugel, M.D. Hernia Treatment Center Northeast, Olympia, Washington

Arlet G. Kurkchubasche, M.D. Assistant Professor, Department of Surgery, Brown University Medical School; Attending Surgeon, Department of Pediatric Surgery, Rhode Island Hospital/Hasbro Children's Hospital, Providence, Rhode Island

Matthias Kux, M.D. Associate Professor, Department of Surgery, University of Vienna; Chief, Department of Surgery, St. Joseph Hospital, Vienna, Austria

Bernhard J. Liebl, M.D. Vice Chairman, Department of Surgery (General/Visceral), Marienhospital Stuttgart, Stuttgart, Germany

Eugene C. Mangiante, M.D. Professor, Department of Surgery, University of Tennessee; Chief, Department of Surgery, VAMC, Memphis, Tennessee

Robert E. Marsh, M.D. Department of Surgery, Creighton University, Omaha, Nebraska

J. Stephen Marshall, M.D. Assistant Professor, Department of Surgery, University of Illinois at Peoria; Staff Surgeon, Department of Surgery, OSF–St. Francis Medical Center, Peoria, Illinois

David A. McCluskey III, M.D. Resident, Department of Surgery and Centers for Surgical Anatomy & Technique, Emory University School of Medicine, Atlanta, Georgia

Mohammed Ashraf Memon, M.B.B.S., D.C.H. Department of Surgery, Queen's Medical Center, Nottingham, United Kingdom

James A. Murray, M.D. Assistant Professor, Department of Surgery, University of Southern California–Keck School of Medicine; Assistant Professor, Division of Trauma, LAC+USC Medical Center, Los Angeles, California

Ulrike Muschaweck, M.D. Chief Surgeon, Department of Hernia Surgery, Arabella-Klinik, Munich, Germany

David A. Napoliello, M.D. Surgeon, Surgical Associates of Venice and Englewood, Venice, Florida

Leigh A. Neumayer, M.D., M.S. Associate Professor, Department of Surgery, University of Utah; Staff Surgeon, Department of Surgery, Salt Lake City VA Medical Center, Salt Lake City, Utah

Enrico Nicolò, M.D. Assistant Clinical Professor, Department of Surgery, University of Pittsburgh Medical Center, UPMC McKeesport, McKeesport, Pennsylvania

Erik Nilsson, M.D., Ph.D. Associate Professor, Department of Surgery, Linköping University, Sweden; Consultant Surgeon, Department of Surgery, Motala Hospital, Motala, Sweden

Lloyd M. Nyhus, M.D. Warren H. Cole Professor and Head Emeritus, Department of Surgery, University of Illinois College of Medicine at Chicago; Surgeon-in-Chief Emeritus, University of Illinois Hospital, Chicago, Illinois

Jean P. Palot, M.D. Second Class Professor, Department of Surgery, Reims University; Department of Surgery, Hôpital Robert Debré, Reims, France

Konstantino Papadakis, M.D. Assistant Professor of Surgery, Department of Surgery, University of Tennessee; Attending Physician, Department of Surgery, East Tennessee Children's Hospital, Knoxville, Tennessee

José F. Patiño, M.D. Honorary Professor, Department of Surgery, National University of Colombia; Honorary Chairman, Department of Surgery, Santa Fe of Bogotá Foundation, Bogotá, Colombia

Russell K. Pearl, M.D., M.S. (Surg.), Associate Professor of Surgery and Biomedical Visualization, Department of Surgery, University of Illinois at Chicago; Attending Surgeon, Division of Colon and Rectal Surgery, Cook County Hospital, Chicago, Illinois

Galen Perdikis, M.D. Senior Associate Consultant, Department of Plastic Surgery, Mayo Clinic, Jacksonville, Florida

Edward H. Phillips, M.D. Clinical Associate Professor, Department of Surgery, University of Southern California School of Medicine; Director, Endoscopic Surgery, Chair, Minimally Invasive Surgery, Department of Surgery, Cedars–Sinai Medical Center, Los Angeles, California

Thomas H. Quinn, Ph.D. Professor of Anatomy, Department of Biomedical Sciences, Creighton's School of Medicine, Omaha, Nebraska

Raymond C. Read, M.D., Ph.D., M.A., M.S. Professor, Department of Surgery, University of Arkansas Medical School; Chief of Surgery, Department of General Thoracic Surgery, Central Arkansas Veterans Medical Center, Little Rock, Arkansas

Domenic J. Reda, Ph.D. Associate Director, Cooperative Studies Program Coordinating Center, Edward Hines, Jr. VA Hospital, Hines, Illinois

Alan T. Richards, M.B., B.Ch. Associate Professor, Residency Program Director, Department of Surgery, Creighton University School of Medicine; Staff Surgeon, Department of Surgery, Saint Joseph Hospital, Omaha, Nebraska

Robb H. Rutledge, M.D. Clinical Professor, Department of Surgery, University of Texas Southern Medical School, Dallas, Texas; Consulting Surgeon, Department of Surgery, John Peter Smith Hospital, Fort Worth, Texas

Volker Schumpelick, M.D. Head, Department of Surgery, Rhenish Westphalian Technical University Hospital Aachen, Aachen, Germany

Kuldeep Singh, M.D. Director, Minimally Invasive Sugery, Department of Surgery, St. Agnes Healthcare, Baltimore, Maryland

John E. Skandalakis, M.D., Ph.D. Director, Centers for Surgical Anatomy and Technique, Chris Carlos Distinguished Professor (Emeritus) of Surgical Anatomy and Technique, Emory University School of Medicine; Senior Attending Surgeon, Department of Surgery, Piedmont Hospital, Atlanta, Georgia

Lee J. Skandalakis, M.D. Clinical Professor, Centers for Surgical Anatomy & Technique, Emory University School of Medicine; Director of Surgical Education, Department of Surgery, Piedmont Hospital, Atlanta, Georgia

Julia H. Sone, M.D. Associate Professor, Department of Surgery, Rush–Presbyterian St. Luke's Medical Center; Chairman, Section of Surgical Endoscopy, Department of Surgery, Cook County Hospital, Chicago, Illinois

Lars T. Sorensen, M.D. Research Fellow, University of Copenhagen; Research Fellow, Copenhagen Wound Healing Center & Department of Surgical Gastroenterology, Bispebjerg Hospital, Copenhagen, Denmark

James R. Starling, M.D. Department of Surgery, University of Wisconsin–Madison, University of Wisconsin Hospital and Clinics, Madison, Wisconsin

Lawrence E. Stern, M.D. Senior Resident in General Surgery, Department of Surgery, University of Cincinnati College of Medicine; Research Fellow, Division of Pediatric Surgery, Children's Hospital Medical Center, Cincinnati, Ohio

René E. Stoppa, M.D. Emeritus Professor, Department of Surgery, University de Picardie Jules Verne; Honorary Chief, Department of Surgery, Centre Hospitalier Universitaire, Amiens, France

Francisco Tercero, M.D. Department of Surgery, Creighton University, Omaha, Nebraska

Arnaldo F. Trabucco, M.D. Chief, Department of Surgery, Division of Urologic Surgery, Trabucco Institute, Rego Park, New York

Ermanno E. Trabucco, M.D. Director, Department of Surgery, Trabucco Hernia Institute, Long Island City, New York

Thomas F. Tracy, Jr., M.S., M.D. Professor of Surgery and Pediatrics, Department of Surgery, Brown University School of Medicine; Pediatric Surgeon-in-Chief, Department of Pediatric Surgery, Rhode Island Hospital/Hasbro Children's Hospital, Providence, Rhode Island

Andrew S. Triebwasser, M.D. Clinical Assistant Professor, Department of Anesthesiology, Brown University; Staff Anesthesiologist, Department of Anesthesiology, Rhode Island Hospital, Providence, Rhode Island

Son Ngog Truong, M.D. Professor, Department of Surgery, Rhenish Westphalian Technical University; Head of Surgical Endoscopy and Sonography, Department of Surgery, University Hospital, Aachen, Germany

Guy R. Voeller, M.D. Associate Professor, Department of Surgery, University of Tennessee–Memphis; Midsouth Center for Minimally Invasive Surgery, Memphis, Tennessee

George E. Wantz, M.D.* Clinical Professor, Department of Surgery, Joan and Sanford Weill Medical College of Cornell University; Attending Surgeon, Department of Surgery, New York Presbyterian Hospital, New York, New York

Brad W. Warner, M.D. Professor, Department of Surgery, University of Cincinnati; Attending Surgeon, Division of Pediatric Surgery, Children's Hospital Medical Center, Cincinnati, Ohio

Ronald K. Woods, M.D., Ph.D. Surgery Fellow, Division of Cardiothoracic Surgery, University of Washington, Seattle, Washington

Alene J. Wright, M.D. Resident, Department of Surgery, Creighton University School of Medicine, Omaha, Nebraska

Robert M. Zollinger, Jr. M.D. Professor, Vice Chairman, Department of Surgery, Case Western Reserve University School of Medicine; Department of Surgery, University Hospitals of Cleveland, Cleveland, Ohio

---

* Deceased

PREFACE

It is particularly exciting to have the privilege of producing this Fifth Edition of *Hernia*, now titled *Nyhus and Condon's Hernia*, as there recently have been so many important changes in hernia surgery. Although these changes are most evident for the treatment of groin hernias, many of the newer principles have spilled over into the broader field of hernias of the abdominal wall, including incisional, umbilical, diaphragmatic, and the less common ones.

The first half of the 20th century was dominated by the Bassini-type inguinal hernia repairs and their variants, which included the Marcy, McVay, Halstead, Andrews, Ferguson, and Shouldice repairs. These repairs have in common suture lines under some degree of tension because a prosthetic is not used to bridge the hernia defects. Although the results of these nonprosthetic operations seemed more than acceptable for decades, it has now become apparent that these repairs are more painful than was generally acknowledged and that the recurrence rate is much higher than most surgeons performing these operations ever suspected.

In this Fifth Edition of *Nyhus and Condon's Hernia*, treatment strategies are outlined that would have been considered heretical only a few years ago. The changes in surgeon's attitudes are the result of four general concepts that have affected the way surgeons practice their craft. These include: (a) the widespread acceptance of the "tension-free" principle; (b) routine use of prosthetic materials; (c) the realization that the preperitoneal space can be used for hernia repair; and (d) therapeutic laparoscopy.

"The subject of hernia has always fascinated the surgeon. This has never been more apparent than today. Seemingly impregnable bastions of ignorance in the area of inguinal hernia are under attack. The facets of sliding hiatal hernia under discussion are legion. Many old areas of controversy have recently been reopened to discussion and study and new knowledge seem to appear on the horizon daily." Incredibly, this quote does not come from the Fifth Edition but from Drs. Nyhus and Harkins, 37 years ago in the preface of the First Edition of *Hernia*. While new knowledge has infused the subject and with its application, new and ongoing controversy has emerged.

Included in this edition are contributions that address a new paradigm in hernia surgery. The differences of opinion drive the intellectual curiosity that both raises and addresses important questions. In the process, new information is generated that can be applied directly to patient care. Many chapters have been revised and new ones added, because the knowledge base has literally exploded. The volume is comprehensive, limited only by the fact that new information based on current research appears quite rapidly. What is missing is a body of well-done sufficiently large, randomized prospective studies, and trials designed to address specific issues. Scantly represented in the literature of today, these studies are essential if we are ever to get a handle on the issues and address them in a scientific manner. To that end, we have included a detailed model of how to approach clinical trials with the hope of stimulating readers to pursue this avenue of research. As in previous editions, we have endeavored to include current and appropriate information to help surgeons everywhere treat patients effectively and efficiently.

Robert J. Fitzgibbons, Jr., M.D.
A. Gerson Greenburg, M.D., Ph.D.

ACKNOWLEDGMENTS

We particularly express our appreciation to Drs. Nyhus and Condon for the confidence they have demonstrated in passing to us the stewardship of this important publication. It is our most sincere hope that we have attained the level of quality achieved in the previous editions of *Hernia*. Thanks go to Lisa McAllister, Susan Rhyner, and Joanne Bersin of Lippincott Williams & Wilkins in Philadelphia. Their support, guidance, and counsel helped to deliver the final product. Spencer Phippen has created clear and useful illustrations, a much-needed element for this subject. A special thanks is owed to Nancy Coelho in Providence and Sheila Cherney in Omaha, whose untiring efforts in support of this undertaking are genuinely appreciated.

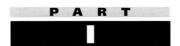

PART
I

ETIOLOGY, HISTORY, AND ANATOMY OF HERNIAS

1

WHY DO HUMAN BEINGS DEVELOP GROIN HERNIAS?

RAYMOND C. READ

Most abdominal herniation arises in the groin (from the Latin word *inguen*), so named because it is the transition zone between the abdomen and thigh. All groin hernias emerge through the myopectineal orifice of Fruchaud, the opening in the lower abdominal wall, bounded by the transversus abdominis arch and the superior pubic ramus. It allows the passage of blood vessels, nerves, lymphatics, muscles, tendons, fasciae, and the vas deferens in and out of the hind limb and scrotum. The upper and lower halves are divided by the inguinal ligament. Inguinal protrusions present anteriorly; femoral, posteriorly.

Historically, hernial causation was attributed to a mechanical disparity between visceral pressure and the resistance of the musculature. Cooper (4) (1804) not only identified the transversalis fascia, but also pointed out it was the last barrier to groin herniation. He listed factors that increase intraabdominal pressure: cough, obesity, constipation, pregnancy, ascites, and unusual exertion, e.g., heavy lifting. Now, we would add, with an increasingly aged population, prostatism. Claims were made in the 1960s on similar grounds that inguinal herniation could presage asymptomatic cancer of the colon, especially the sigmoid. However, later studies could not confirm such a relationship since diagnostic barium enemas and sigmoidoscopy did not demonstrate neoplasia. Strength of the abdominal wall was considered to be diminished by congenital deficiency, debility, or aging. Rupture of the peritoneum or abdominal musculature (Galen) was disproved as a factor by dissection and the fact that trauma, unless massive, did not result in herniation.

INGUINAL HERNIATION

Anatomy

During most of the 19th century, repair of these hernias differed little from that described 2,000 years earlier in Rome

R. C. Read: Department of Surgery, University of Arkansas Medical School; Department of Thoracic Surgery, Central Arkansas Veterans Medical Center, Little Rock, Arkansas.

by Celsus. The main indications remained pain, incarceration, and strangulation unresponsive to taxis. An inguinoscrotal incision was made in and beyond the external inguinal ring, the peritoneal sac dissected free from the spermatic cord, pulled down, ligated high, and allowed to retract. The pillars of the external ring were then stitched around the cord with deep sutures, obliterating the distal inguinal canal. However, despite surgical stagnation, anatomy blossomed into a golden age, laying the groundwork for Bassini (1889), the father of modern herniology. An underlying assumption was that the tissues lining the inguinal rings were normal and would stay so.

The frequency of protrusions in the groin was attributed to the absence of the posterior rectus sheath below the arcuate line and gravitational stress brought about by the erect posture. Prior to Cooper's discovery of the transversalis fascia, protection against inguinal herniation was considered to depend on reflex contraction of the abdominal musculature in response to coughing, straining, and lifting. The shutter is produced by descent of the transversus arch and "conjoint" tendon towards the inguinal ligament, in front of the internal abdominal ring. Contraction of the transversus abdominis muscle also tenses the crura of the internal ring, derived from its transversalis fascia. At the same time, the anterior wall of the canal, made up of external oblique aponeurosis, presses on the internal inguinal ring and the floor of the inguinal canal, counterbalancing intraabdominal forces pushing outward. The inguinal ligament is pulled upward by the same contraction, moving craniad to narrow the inguinal canal. As muscular power diminishes with age or disease, i.e., neuropathy, wasting, etc., these protective mechanisms fail, leaving the transversalis fascia at risk.

Persistence of the Processus Vaginalis: A Congenital Influence

Since groin hernias are common in infants, especially boys, and then are almost always indirect, i.e., into the spermatic cord, a developmental defect connected with the descent of the testis was suspected early. John Hunter, in the late 18th century, showed that some hernial sacs, even in adults, encircled the testis, as in fetal life. Cloquet (3) (1819) observed that the processus vaginalis does not always close at birth. In the adult, most inguinal hernias are still indirect, and their peritoneal sacs, as in the neonate, are invested by all the layers of the spermatic cord. His findings have been repeatedly confirmed, with Hughson (1925) reporting that, at autopsy, 15% to 30% of men without a history of inguinal herniation retained a patent processus vaginalis.

Russell (14), an Australian pediatric surgeon, in 1906 advanced the saccular theory regarding the formation of hernia. He carried it to an extreme, suggesting it was the basis for all abdominal herniation,

> "which rejects the view that hernia can ever be acquired in the pathological sense . . . the presence of a developmental diverticulum is a necessary antecedent in every case. . . . We may have an open funicular peritoneum with perfectly formed muscles. We may have congenitally weak muscles with a perfectly closed funicular peritoneum, and we may have them separately or together in infinitely variable gradations."

The introduction of continuous ambulatory peritoneal dialysis for renal failure has demonstrated, as did ascites, that a persistent processus vaginalis or canal of Nuck, if subjected to increased intraabdominal pressure over a period of time, will dilate to produce a hydrocele or hernia. Carcinomatosis, decompensated liver, or heart disease can therefore present as recent onset herniation. Histologic examination of such hernial sacs is warranted, but not in the routine. Herniorrhaphy should be attempted only after efforts have been made to control ascites. Otherwise, recurrence rates of 10% to 15% may ensue. Peritonitis may similarly evoke inguinal hernias, but then incarceration or strangulation is suspected because of tenderness. The discovery of pus mandates exploratory laparotomy.

Buoyed by the saccular hypothesis, a number of surgeons between the World Wars attempted repair of indirect herniation in adults, as in children, by simple excision of the sac. The results in the former were disastrous. This experience, plus the autopsy evidence showing that the presence of a patent processus vaginalis does not necessarily lead to inguinal herniation, indicated that additional factors must be brought to bear in order to produce indirect inguinal herniation.

A Fascial Factor

Harrison (6), who trained at Johns Hopkins and became a missionary surgeon in Saudi Arabia, was the first, in 1922, to seriously question the saccular theory of Russell. "When we consider the dozens and hundreds of men who first show a hernia at 50 or 60, after their active lives are over, the hypothesis becomes improbable to say the least. However, the main objection to the theory is that even if true, it

gives no useful guidance. In and of itself, the persistence of a more or less elongated narrow processus vaginalis should not predispose to a future hernia if all elements of strength present in the wall of the abdomen were also present in the wall of the processus... the muscles, however, appeared to be normal... the natural conclusion is that the cause of an indirect hernia, as of a direct hernia, is the failure of the transversalis fascia to withstand the intra-abdominal pressure to which it is subjected."

Two years later, Sir Arthur Keith (8) dealt another blow to the saccular concept, stating, "There is one other matter that deserves further consideration. We are so apt to look on tendons, fascial structures, and connective tissues as dead, passive structures [*which they are to anatomists dissecting cadavers!*]. They are certainly alive and the fact that hernias are so often multiple in middle-aged and old people leads me to suspect that a pathological change in the connective tissues of the belly wall may render certain individuals particularly liable to hernia." And further, "It is most important that surgeons should form a just and true opinion concerning the manner in which hernias arise. If they occur only in those who have hernial sacs already formed during fetal life, then we must either excise the sacs at birth or stand by and do nothing but trust to luck. But if the occurrence of hernia is due to circumstances over which we have control, then the prevention of hernia is a matter worthy of our serious study."

Andrews (1), who in 1924 had observed at herniorrhaphy normal-looking muscles but an atrophied conjoint tendon, emphasized the importance of fascial supports. Little attention was given to these pioneers. Thus, in their 1967 textbook, Zimmerman and Anson continued to state that inguinal herniation developed as a result of a congenital predisposition. Indirect hernias were ascribed to the presence of a preformed sac; direct herniation was explained by the congenital absence of the lowermost fibers of the internal oblique muscle, leaving the transverse layer of the inguinal canal floor unsupported. It was not until 1964 that the first evidence pointing to connective tissue abnormality as a possible cause of herniation in humans was presented. Wirtschafter and Bentley (20) cited an increased incidence of hernia in patients suffering from lathyrism and were able to induce a similar phenomenon in animals using lathyrogens.

Metabolic Factors

My own interest in the etiology of inguinal herniation was stimulated by intraoperative findings made in the late 1960s. We (13) were modifying the McEvedy–Nyhus posterior preperitoneal approach for the repair of groin hernias. The rectus sheath, some centimeters cephalad to the defects, appeared thinner than normal and felt greasy. Samples of constant size weighed significantly less (12) than those taken from matched controls operated on for conditions other than herniation. Patients with direct or bilateral hernias showed more attenuation than those with indirect defects. Atrophy was unrelated to age or muscle mass. Hydroxyproline content, and therefore collagen, which makes up 80% of the rectus sheath, was strikingly decreased (16). The collagen showed altered salt precipitability and impaired hydroxylation with a decreased amount of mature, insoluble, thick (polymeric) forms (17). Cultured fibroblasts proliferated less and had reduced uptake of radioactive proline. On electron microscopy, collagen fibrils showed irregular periodicity and variable width, with some intracellular fibrillar positioning (18). These changes in ultrastructure were later confirmed in the transversalis fascia by Peacock (1974), Berliner (1978), Nikolov and Beltshev (1990), and Pans et al. (11) (1997). The latter concluded, "The collagen framework was modified, mainly in the direct hernia group, associated with increased vascularity and cellularity. Similar changes were observed on the nonherniated sides, suggesting that connective tissue pathology plays a role in the genesis of groin hernias."

Since our own studies were made in the anterior rectus sheath, from which the transversalis fascia is derived, the objection that the connective tissue changes observed result from the protrusion itself is negated. The exacerbation of this pathology in direct herniation suggests that patency of the processus vaginalis allows inguinal herniation with less fascial damage than that required for direct hernias. The increase in bilaterality, seen with the latter lesions, is further evidence of the widespread nature of the fascial disorder.

Cigarette Smoking and Proteolysis

The connective tissue changes we had observed were systemic—skin, lung, and pericardial biopsies showing similar damage. Lathyrism was ruled out because collagen cross-linking was unaffected. The common denominator in our patient population was that they were all veterans of World War II who had become addicted to nicotine as a result of cigarettes being sent up with the rations. They were presenting in late middle age with a surprisingly high incidence of primary inguinal herniation, almost half having direct or bilateral defects. Most had smoked heavily for 40 years or more, many having already suffered the consequences of emphysema, lung cancer, accelerated atherosclerosis, etc.

Since the connective tissue changes in the groin and elsewhere resemble those previously described in the lungs and skin (wrinkles) of patients with pulmonary emphysema known to be caused by smoking, we attributed our findings to "metastatic emphysema" (2). This hypothesis envisaged smoke not only damaging the lungs, but also spilling over to cause a systemic effect, thereby affecting the abdominal wall. This lesion allowed herniation through a locus minoris resistentiae, the inguinal canal. The conclusion was that long-term excessive exposure to tobacco smoke was a risk factor for groin herniation.

To ascertain the detailed mechanisms involved, we first considered what is known about how smoking damages the lungs. Prior to 1962, clinicians speculated that destruction of alveoli in emphysema resulted from mechanical factors—cough, shouting, wind instruments, etc. However, then reports of predisposition to the disease from inherited deficiency of α_1-antitrypsin, along with the production of emphysema in rats by intratracheal installation of proteolytic enzymes, led to the now accepted hypothesis of a protease–antiprotease imbalance. Smoking, the most common cause of pulmonary emphysema, evokes a neutrophil–macrophage response. Priming of these white cells and their 5- to 10-fold concentration in the lungs, with release of elastase and collagenase, destroys the parenchyma. Further, oxidants produced from combustion of tobacco damage antiprotease defenses.

To explain the systemic effects on connective tissue, in particular those observed in the groin, we envisaged that the chronic inflammatory response in the lungs affected the circulating blood. Uninhibited proteolytic activity, large numbers of activated neutrophils and macrophages, along with products of tobacco combustion, caused peripheral collagenolysis and inhibited repair. The process, metastatic emphysema, is analogous to the distant damage seen in the lungs and skin of patients with acute pancreatitis or visceral ischemia.

Supporting Data for the Hypothesis (Metastatic Emphysema)

Our patients, many of whom had pulmonary emphysema, did demonstrate leukocytosis with elevated circulating elastase and a reduced antiproteolytic inhibitory capacity. Neutrophils were primed with an increase in their zymogen granules. These changes were more marked in patients with direct or bilateral herniation. In 1987, Weitz and colleagues (19) provided independent support for our hypothesis when they "unequivocally recovered the fingerprints of free, active neutrophil elastase (increased fivefold)" from the plasma of cigarette smokers by measuring a specific fibrinopeptide cleavage product of fibrinogen identified by radioimmune assay. They concluded, "Our findings raise the possibility that the systemic complications of cigarette smoking may be the result of uncontrolled neutrophil elastase activity."

The following year, the use of tobacco was reported to be significantly more common in patients presenting with groin herniation, especially women. Scott (1998) found that cigarette smoking was twice as common in patients operated upon for recurrent inguinal herniation compared to those undergoing primary repair. The most elegant prospective demonstration that cigarette smoking specifically impedes collagen synthesis is that of Jorgensen et al. (7) in 1998. A plastic wound-healing model was implanted subcutaneously into the upper arm of 37 young male and female volunteers. Deposition of total protein and mature collagen was measured. Nonsmokers produced twice as much hydroxyproline in granulation tissue as did their counterparts who smoked an average of 20 cigarettes a day. Other amino acids were unaffected.

Aneurysm

This, another abdominal protrusion, was also blamed on mechanical factors turbulence, hypertension, and aging. Nevertheless, in 1968, cigarette smoking was shown to be a risk factor. In 1980, Swanson and Busuttil invoked a metabolic mechanism, endogenous white-cell-derived collagenase and elastase. Two years later, my colleagues and I found inguinal herniation to be twice as common in patients with aortic aneurysm compared to those with Leriche's syndrome (12). The former demonstrated leukocytosis and a reduced antiproteolytic capacity. Our findings were later confirmed by Lehnert and Wadouh (9). The formation, expansion, and rupture of intracerebral aneurysms have also been correlated with cigarette smoking rather than a congenital etiology. The incidence of these lesions increases eightfold in patients suffering from α_1-antitrypsin deficiency, another cause of systemic protease–antiprotease imbalance.

Genetic Influences

There is a familial tendency to groin herniation. A quarter of these patients give a history of similar hernias in their parents and grandparents (Watson, 1938). A study of 280 families with congenital indirect inguinal hernias in China indicated that transmission was autosomal dominant with incomplete penetrance of a preferential paternal factor. The hernia usually occurred on the right side, consistent with later descent of the testis on that side. Such herniation, which is more common with prematurity, has been ascribed to a delay in maturation. Inguinal defects may be multiple, familial, or part of various connective tissue disorders, osteogenesis imperfecta, Marfan's or Ehlers–Danlos syndrome, congenital elastolysis (cutis laxa), or more commonly, hip dislocation of childhood. Recently (1997), autosomal dominant polycystic kidney disease, which is known to involve an abnormality of basement membrane, or extracellular matrix production, has been added to the list. Up to 43% of adults with this abnormality develop herniation. Most of the congenital conditions described above have been shown to arise from genetic mutations (10).

In 1992, Deak et al. (5) demonstrated abnormal synthesis (collagen gene expression) in cultured skin fibroblasts taken from two patients with multiple aneurysms, suggesting sporadic mutation. The following year, this group studied nine men 17 to 67 years of age, with either indirect or direct inguinal herniation. Few smoked, some had a famil-

ial history, and one third demonstrated joint hypermobility. Isotopically labeled skin fibroblasts secreted twice as much type III collagen (one of the two common among the 29 different forms) as controls. The altered ratio with the usually predominant type I collagen led to a decrease in insoluble, thick (polymeric) fibrils, confirming our original observations. Thus, the proportion of collagen types regulates fibrillogenesis, fibril diameter, and bundle architecture. According to the authors, "An increase in type III collagen (a metabolic abnormality of production) may predispose certain individuals to the development of inguinal herniation." A similar condition, genitourinary prolapse in women, had been shown earlier (1990) to be similarly associated with hypermobility, suggesting an underlying connective tissue disorder. In 1996, collagen deficiency with increased cross-linking and decreased solubility associated with collagenolysis was identified in this condition.

Trauma: Spontaneous or Iatrogenic

It is remarkable how strong the abdominal wall is. It takes massive trauma to cause inguinal herniation. Aponeuroses are then detached from their insertions into the pubis. A similar result can follow fractures or osteotomies. Symphysiotomies, especially for prostatic surgery, if not properly repaired, cause distraction of the rectus tendon insertion and suprapubic or parapubic herniation, sometimes diagnosed as primary direct inguinal defects. Previous appendectomy may be followed by right inguinal herniation, as first described by Hoguet in 1911. However, the classic McBurney incision rarely produces such sequelae. Apparently, the more cosmetic unilateral Pfannenstiel approach has been incriminated because of damage to the iliohypogastric nerve. Certainly, flank herniation has been described secondary to diabetic neuropathy.

Physical Exertion

Historically, the etiology of groin herniation has been strongly related to manual work—strains of lifting and strong muscular or athletic exertion. An enormous legal and insurance industry has developed to support claims in this regard. More and more evidence is now accumulating that casts doubt on the legal foundation for such compensation. Weightlifters do not have an abnormal incidence of groin herniation, and their intraabdominal pressure does not increase significantly in the erect posture. A single strenuous event preceded the appearance of inguinal herniation in only 7% of men questioned after presentation (15). Groin pain in athletes has been correlated with tearing of the conjoint or rectus tendon at their insertions. The new evidence regarding the importance of metabolic and genetic factors, along with the important role of cigarette smoking, needs to be better understood by medicolegal authorities.

FEMORAL HERNIATION

Unlike inguinal herniation, this protrusion is rare in infancy and childhood; therefore, its etiology is probably not congenital, despite earlier claims to the contrary. These hernias usually appear in middle age, suggesting that weakening of the tissues plays a role. It is more common in multiparous women. The reason seems to be that the femoral ring is larger and more oval in women, and the inguinal ligament appears to be weaker and the iliopsoas muscle smaller. Earlier, claims were made that the pelvis is broader and Gimbernat's ligament narrower, but recent studies have not supported this explanation. Pregnancy may well stretch the musculature at the brim of the pelvis and the "conjoint tendon" attachment may also be narrower in women. Finally, femoral herniation is seen after a previous Bassini-type sutured repair of inguinal herniation. This sequela emphasizes the fact that femoral protrusions pass beneath the inguinal ligament, which, as McVay pointed out, is poorly attached and can be elevated if used for fixation. There is some evidence that normally the femoral canal is filled with extraperitoneal fat and lymphatics, including Cloquet's node. Loss of this tissue with emaciation may, as with obturator herniation, lead to peritoneal protrusion in elderly women.

REFERENCES

1. Andrews E. A method of herniotomy utilizing only white fascia. *Ann Surg* 1924;80:225–238.
2. Cannon DJ, Read RC. Metastatic emphysema: a mechanism for acquiring inguinal herniation. *Ann Surg* 1981;194:270–278.
3. Cloquet J. *Recherches sur les causes et l'anatomie des hernies abdominales.* Paris: Mequignon–Marvis, 1819.
4. Cooper AP. *The anatomy and surgical treatment of inguinal and congenital hernia.* London: Longman, 1804.
5. Deak SB, Ricotta JJ, Mariani TJ, et al. *Abnormalities in the biosynthesis of type III procollagen in cultured skin fibroblasts from two patients with multiple aneurysms.* Matrix, Stuttgart: Gustav Fischer Verlag, 1992;12:92–100.
6. Harrison PW. Inguinal hernia: a study of the principles involved in the surgical treatment. *Arch Surg* 1922;4:680–689.
7. Jorgensen LN, Kallehave F, Christensen E, et al. Less collagen production in smokers. *Surgery* 1998;123:450–455.
8. Keith A. On the origin and nature of hernia. *Br J Surg* 1924;11:455–475.
9. Lehnert B, Wadouh F. High coincidence of inguinal hernias and abdominal aortic aneurysms. *Ann Vasc Surg* 1992;67:134–137.
10. Morris-Stiff G, Coles G, Moore R, et al. Abdominal wall hernia in autosomal dominant polycystic kidney disease. *Brit J Surg* 1997;84:615–617.
11. Pans A., Pierard GE, Albert A, et al. Adult groin hernias: new insight into their biomechanical characteristics. *Eur J Clin Invest* 1997;27:1–6.
12. Read RC. Attenuation of the rectus sheath in inguinal herniation. *Am J Surg* 1970;120:610–614.
13. Read RC. Preperitoneal exposure of inguinal herniation. *Am J Surg* 1968;116:653–658.
14. Russell RH. The saccular theory of hernia and the radical operation. *Lancet* 1906;3:1197–1203.
15. Smith GD, Lewis PA, Crosby DL. Inguinal hernia and a single strenuous event. *Ann R Coll Surg Engl* 1996;78:367–368.
16. Wagh PV, Leverich AP, Read RC, et al. Direct inguinal herniation in men: a disease of collagen. *J Surg Res* 1974;17:425–433.
17. Wagh PV, Read RC. Collagen deficiency in rectus sheath of patients with inguinal herniation. *Proc Soc Exp Biol Med* 1971;37:382–384.
18. Wagh PV, Read RC. Defective collagen-synthesis in inguinal herniation. *Am J Surg* 1972;124:819–822.
19. Weitz JI, Crowley KA, Landman SL, et al. Increased neutrophil elastase activity in cigarette smokers. *Ann Intern Med* 1987;107:680–682.
20. Wirtschafter ZT, Bentley JP. Hernias as a collagen maturation defect. *Ann Surg* 1964;160:852.

EDITOR'S COMMENT

Indeed, why do humans develop groin hernias? Dr. Read has provided us with a singularly useful compilation and analysis of data supporting the existence of a metabolic or biochemical basis for this common clinical problem. In classical fashion, he has presented an almost irrefutable argument that there is a defect, however triggered, common to all groin hernia patients. Given the recently completed Human Genome Project, with its clearly implied but as-yet-unrealized potential for genetic manipulation as a means of disease management, there may be yet another approach to the management of groin hernia on the distant horizon. When that day arrives, much of the discussion regarding the surgical management of groin hernia will become moot, and texts like this one will be relegated to historic archives, a source of information about the past. Appreciating the biochemical abnormalities and the mechanisms by which they exert an influence on the tissues of the groin will be important for future therapies. Dr. Read's contributions have demonstrated that this can be a productive field of academic endeavor.

Others have expanded upon many of the concepts he has proposed, and the details are beginning to unfold (Chapter 2). Early discussions of the cause of groin hernia attributed it to the evolution of humans from quadrupeds to bipeds. This change in posture, stance, and gait would clearly be associated with changes in the anatomy of the muscles and fascia of the abdominal wall and the groin in particular. By logical extension, if this were true, then all humans would have groin hernias, or at the very least, the potential to develop one. While it was an interesting idea and plausible argument when first proposed, the evolutionary theory is now relegated to history.

Attention next focuses on embryology and the role of the patent processus vaginalis as the offending culprit. The literature on this subject is quite extensive and very confusing, implicating the persistent patency of the processus as a cause of groin hernia. This theory could explain, at best, some of the indirect inguinal hernias but fails to explain the other types of groin hernia.

Failure or compromise of the "shutter mechanism," an interesting physiologic phenomenon of the internal ring, has been implicated in the etiology of groin hernia. Some underlying anatomic and/or metabolic abnormality may contribute to the functional impairment; here again, if there is failure of the mechanism, indirect herniation is the more likely result, and that is not observed in large studies.

The role of increased intraabdominal pressure as a cause of groin hernia has been promulgated since the time of Cooper (2). This process may be associated with groin hernia because it effects a repeated mechanical stress on the abdominal wall. The abdominal wall, subjected to repeated injury in a sense, deteriorates because the scar tissue formed in the healing process, if there ever is healing, with or without an underlying metabolic defect, will be less strong and less resilient than the original tissue.

Dr. Read has presented an excellent and persuasive argument for a systemic collagen defect being causally related to the formation of groin hernias. Surprisingly little basic science research effort has been directed to this issue considering the high incidence of the diagnosis in most populations. However, the era of molecular biology has been extended to the mundane area of groin herniation, and there are well done basic science efforts that have started to unravel the mysteries. Bellon and colleagues (1) have demonstrated an overexpression of metalloproteinases in cultured, isolated fibroblasts grown from the tissues of young patients with direct inguinal hernias. This evidence is highly suggestive of a genetically defined defect playing a role and minimizes the role of acquired or environmentally induced factors as primarily responsible for the hernias. Of course, in combination with a potent environmental factor like smoking, the impact on tissues of the groin could be devastating. Overexpression of enzymes in this family and the particular enzymes in question has been noted in aneurysms as well, a point that Read has made clear.

Further corroboration of a genetically defined biochemical abnormality of fascia in patients with groin hernia can be found in the recent work of Pans et al. (3). In this study, well-defined fascia samples from patients with groin hernias and controls were obtained. Subjected to stringent biochemical assays, the fascia from patients with groin hernia had an increased quantity of extractable collagen compared to the controls. There were no differences detected in the types of collagen or their relative ratios between the patients and the controls. Pans concluded that some "molecular alteration in collagen may be involved in the genesis of groin hernias." Why this defect appears preferentially in the inguinal region remains a mystery.

The more we learn about the basic underlying mechanisms of groin hernia, the closer the horizon of the future becomes. I sense we have entered a new, very productive and most exciting era of basic science research with respect to groin hernia. The future is full of untold possibilities once we harness the knowledge learned and turn it into therapy.

A.G.G.

REFERENCES

1. Bellon JM, Bajo AG, Honduvilla N, et al. Fibroblasts from the transversalis fascia of young patients with direct inguinal hernias show constitutive MMP-2 overexpression. *Ann Surg* 2001;233:287–291.
2. Cooper A. *The anatomy and surgical treatment of inguinal hernia.* London: T. Cox, 1804.
3. Pans A, Albert A, Lapiere CM, et al. Biochemical study of collagen in adult groin hernias. *J Surg Res* 2001;95:107–113.

Nyhus and Condon's Hernia, Fifth Edition, edited by Robert J. Fitzgibbons, Jr. and A. Gerson Greenburg. Lippincott Williams & Wilkins, Philadelphia © 2002.

BIOCHEMICAL ASPECTS OF ABDOMINAL WALL HERNIA FORMATION AND RECURRENCE

LARS T. SORENSEN
LARS N. JORGENSEN
FINN GOTTRUP

Much evidence suggests that hernia formation and recurrence depends in part on a systemic predisposition due to an abnormal metabolism of the connective tissue and in part on other risk factors, surgical as well as nonsurgical. However, the pathophysiologic mechanisms for hernia formation and recurrence have yet to be fully defined. The aim of this chapter is to give an overview of the biochemical mechanisms that may be involved in hernia formation and recurrence. The main focus will be pointed at possible pathophysiologic aspects of collagen metabolism and other biomechanical connective tissue features.

NONSURGICAL FACTORS ASSOCIATED WITH ABDOMINAL WALL HERNIA FORMATION AND RECURRENCE

Connective Tissue Disorders and Other Diseases

A higher prevalence of inguinal hernia is well known among patients suffering from congenital connective tissue disorders like osteogenesis imperfecta, cutis laxa, and Ehlers–Danlos, Hurler–Hunter, and Marfan's syndromes. In children with congenital hip dislocation, inguinal hernia occurs five times more often in girls and three times more often in boys compared to children without this disease

L. T. **Sorensen:** Department of Surgical Gastroenterology, University of Copenhagen; Department of Surgical Gastroenterology, Bispebjerg Hospital, Copenhagen, Denmark.

L. N. **Jorgensen:** Department of Surgical Gastroenterology, University of Copenhagen; Department of Surgical Gastroenterology, Bispebjerg Hospital, Copenhagen, Denmark.

F. **Gottrup:** Copenhagen Wound Healing Center, University of Copenhagen; Copenhagen Wound Healing Center, Bispebjerg Hospital, Copenhagen, Denmark.

(38). Some reports indicate that patients with indirect inguinal hernia tend to have hypermobile joints, presumably due to a lower type I:type III collagen ratio compared with patients without joint hypermobility (17).

A patent processus vaginalis is a well-known congenital factor for indirect inguinal herniation. Epidemiologic evidence has shown that 20% of men pass into adulthood with a patent processus vaginalis, but less than 50% develop clinical herniation (15,29). In addition, indirect inguinal hernia may appear first in a man over 40 years of age (29). These observations are not clearly explained by failure of the processus vaginalis to obliterate during fetal life. Therefore, other factors may play a role in the development of an indirect hernia, such as structural abnormalities of the internal ring, acquired attenuation of transversalis fascia, or abnormal muscle function accompanying the congenital defect (29).

Increased destruction of connective tissue, especially elastin, is believed to be an important pathogenic factor for the abdominal aortic aneurysmal disease. Several studies have demonstrated a significantly higher prevalence of ventral incisional hernia and inguinal hernia among patients undergoing open reconstruction for abdominal aortic aneurysm than patients with aortoiliac occlusive disease (3,35). Also a higher prevalence of recurrent hernia has been found (18). These findings support the view that there is a common causative defect in connective tissue metabolism in abdominal aortic aneurysmal disease as well as abdominal wall hernia formation and recurrence (12,21).

Other Nonsurgical Factors

In smokers with inguinal hernia, especially the direct type, significantly higher blood levels of elastin-degrading activity have been measured, as well as a significant lower serum α_1-antitrypsin capacity (13). The authors hypothesized that smoking may induce a systemic imbalance in levels of protease and antiprotease, which alters the architecture of the connective tissue of the groin. A similar imbalance has also been found in smokers with abdominal aortic aneurysm (12). Recent evidence from our group suggests that smokers accumulate less collagen in surgical test-wounds than nonsmokers (Fig. 2.1) (19). Impaired collagen biosynthesis in smokers may be due to tissue hypoxia induced by nicotine and carbon monoxide, indicating reduced biomechanical properties in the connective tissue of smokers. However, results from epidemiologic studies are not consistent as to whether smoking is a causative factor for hernia formation. Bielecki and Pulawski found a significant higher prevalence of smokers among patients with inguinal hernia (11). Others, however, have not been able to confirm this finding (14,16). In a recent study of patients undergoing hernia repair, we found a significant twofold higher risk of recurrence 2 years after hernia repair among smokers compared to nonsmokers after adjusting for other risk factors (34).

The prevalence of inguinal hernia rises significantly with patient age (2). Recent experimental evidence shows that the activity of collagen-degrading enzymes is higher in older patients, presumably due to a reduced inhibition of collagenase (8).

If the strength of the collagen fibers in the fascia transversalis is not optimal, the ability to withstand intraabdominal pressure is reduced. Prolonged stretching and pressure of the fascia transversalis caused by chronically raised intraabdominal pressure is considered an additional facilitating factor for groin hernia formation (1,10). This condition may be secondary to obstructive pulmonary disease, varicose veins, hemorrhoids, ascites, hyperplasia of the prostate, constipation, or pregnancy. Heavy workload and lifting of heavy objects repeatedly over long periods of time have also been found to be associated with development of inguinal hernia (14,16). Furthermore, indirect hernia has been found to be associated with patient height, suggesting that taller patients tend to develop indirect inguinal hernia presumably due to increased intraabdominal pressure (14,16).

BIOCHEMICAL ASPECTS OF ABDOMINAL WALL HERNIA FORMATION

Connective Tissue Pathology

Attenuation of the anterior rectus abdominis sheath has been demonstrated in biopsies from patients with both indirect and direct inguinal hernias compared to patients undergoing other surgical procedures than hernia repair (31). Additional studies showed that patients with direct hernia had significantly less mean collagen content of anterior rectus sheath tissue compared to patients with indirect hernia as well as controls (40).

Major structural changes have also been found in biopsies of the transversalis fascia of patients undergoing repair for primary or recurrent unilateral indirect hernia (29). In this study, more than half of the patients had attenuation of the endopelvic fascia of the asymptomatic side, suggesting a metabolic abnormality of connective tissues in the area of the internal ring.

A recent study has confirmed the hypothesis that connective tissue pathology is involved in hernia genesis (27). In this study, a series of biomechanical tests were performed on biopsies from the transversalis fascia and the rectus abdominis sheath in 63 patients with groin hernia and 30 controls. The biopsies from the *transversalis fascia* from patients with direct hernia showed significantly higher levels of biologic elasticity and maximal distention compared with controls. Elasticity and distention measurements of the *transversalis fascia* from patients with indirect hernia were intermediate. In either group, no difference in elasticity or maximal distention was found in the *anterior rectus sheaths*. Interestingly, there was a significant difference between the contralateral nonherniated fascia and the fascia of the controls independent of the hernia type. These findings suggest that the fascia of the asymptomatic side already present pathologic features at the time of surgery. Furthermore, they support the proposition that biomechanical alterations of the fascia cause herniation rather than being a result of such.

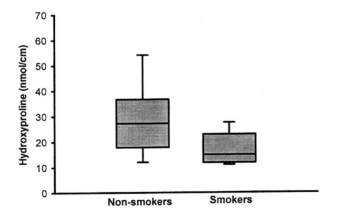

FIGURE 2.1. Amount of hydroxyproline accumulated in expanded polytetrafluoroethylene tubing according to group volunteers. Median, interquartile range (*boxes*) and range (*bars*) are shown; *p*<0.01 for comparisons between groups, Mann–Whitney test. (From Jorgensen LN, Kallehave F, Christensen E, et al. Less collagen production in smokers. *Surgery* 1998;123: 450–455, with permission.)

Collagen Synthesis and Proliferation

The development of biomechanical strength in wound tissue depends on several complicated steps in the formation of mature collagen. In short, proliferating fibroblasts produce and secrete procollagen, which converts extracellularly to tropocollagen. These long triple-helix molecules contain high concentrations of lysine and proline. In the presence of oxygen, vitamin C, and Fe^{++}, a hydroxylation process converts these amino acids to hydroxylysine and hydroxyproline. This produces strong cross links between several aligned tropocollagen molecules making up collagen fibrils and fibers in the wound cleft. After the proliferation phase of healing, the maturation phase involves equilibration between formation and degradation of collagen. Collagen fibers are reoriented and redistributed, leaving them more compact, thickened, and parallel to one another. The tensile strength of the wound in almost all types of tissue increases rapidly on the fifth day after wounding and continues to increase up to 1 year after wounding.

In several studies, high levels of soluble collagen have been observed in biopsies from patients with inguinal hernia (39–41). This may be due to retarded cell proliferation and cellular biosynthesis, which has been shown in cultures of fibroblasts obtained from biopsies of patients with hernia (41). This finding has been confirmed by another study, which has demonstrated a significant decrease in cell proliferation rates in fibroblast cultures harvested from the internal oblique muscle and the cremasteric muscle of hernia patients compared to controls (6). Both studies found that incorporation of radioactively labeled proline (^{14}C) in the tissue from cultured fibroblasts was significantly depressed in hernia patients, suggesting a lower rate of matrix synthesis.

Ultrastructure and Stability of Collagen

An abnormality of collagen ultrastructure in rectus sheath biopsies from patients with direct inguinal hernia has been suggested by electron microscopic studies (39). Contrary to patients with indirect hernia and controls, the diameters of collagen fibrils from patients with direct hernia were quite variable, as well as smaller in size and periodicity. Neither the collagen measurements nor the ultrastructural findings of the rectus sheath biopsies showed any association with muscular status or patient age. Interestingly, the changes observed in the rectus sheath biopsies from patients with direct hernia have also been found in other tissues such as the pericardium (42). This supports the view of a systemic connective tissue disorder.

In wound healing, collagen type I and type III are two of the major fibrillar collagens. Type III collagen dominates the early phases of wound healing, while type I is the most abundant component of the later scar tissue. Often the type I:type III collagen ratio is altered in patients with an abnormal collagen metabolism. High levels of type III collagen relative to type I collagen may result in nonpolymeric soluble collagen because the associative properties of collagen I are diminished. Bellón et al. found no difference in collagen fibril diameter in the transversalis fascia between patients with direct and indirect hernia, nor was there any difference in the type I:type III collagen ratio (10). However, Friedman et al. found a significantly lower type I:type III procollagen ratio, as well as a significant increase of recovery of α1(III) procollagen mRNA when analyzing secreted material from skin fibroblasts obtained from hernia patients compared to controls (Figs. 2.2 and 2.3) (17). The authors hypothesized that nonpolymerized collagen relatively rich in type III collagen may not be sufficient as a biomechani-

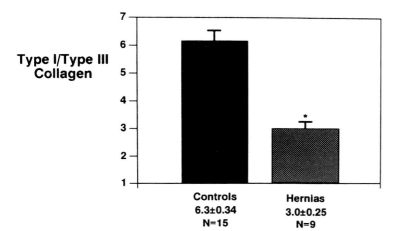

FIGURE 2.2. Type I:type III collagen ratios in fibroblast cultures from control patients and from patients with inguinal hernias. All data expressed as mean ± S.E.M. *$p<0.001$ as compared to controls. (From Friedman DW, Boyd CD, Norton P, et al. Increases in type III collagen gene expression and protein synthesis in patients with inguinal hernias. *Ann Surg* 1993;218:754–760, with permission.)

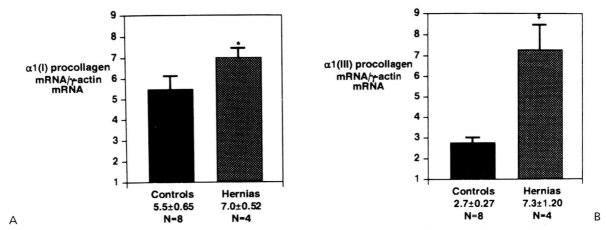

FIGURE 2.3. Steady-state levels of α1(I) **(A)** procollagen mRNA and α1(III) **(B)** procollagen mRNA in fibroblasts from control patients and from patients with inguinal hernias. All data expressed as mean ± S.E.M. *p=NS, ‡p<0.0004. (From Friedman DW, Boyd CD, Norton P, et al. Increases in type III collagen gene expression and protein synthesis in patients with inguinal hernias. *Ann Surg* 1993;218:754–760, with permission.)

cal barrier in the abdominal wall and may predispose some individuals to formation of hernia or perhaps recurrence after primary repair.

Tensile strength of wound is highly dependent of stable collagen molecules. Hydroxylation of proline and lysine plays an important role in stabilizing collagen as this process produces inter- and intramolecular cross-linking and glycosylation of collagen (27). Significantly lower levels of proline and lysine hydroxylation seem to be present in fascia samples from direct hernia patients compared to those from indirect hernia patients (10,39). This finding suggests that the stability of the collagen within the transversus abdominis aponeurosis is compromised in patients with direct hernia.

The importance of the collagen integrity for the prevention of hernia formation has been demonstrated in studies using animal models. In rats, the lathyrogenic agent β-aminoproprionitrile (BAPN) blocks the enzyme lysyl oxidase, which reduces hydroxylysine and impairs cross link formation between collagen molecules (15). The effect of this agent is more extractable collagen resulting in significantly less tensile strength. In a study by Wirtschafter and Bentley, 50% of young male rats (30 days old) got a hernia after eating the seeds of *Lathyrus odoratus* versus none of the older rats (88 days old) (43). This finding suggested that lathyrus-induced hernia formation was due to failure in aggregation or aging of newly formed collagen molecules rather than to breakdown of mature fibers. In another study of male rats, systemic treatment with BAPN and transection of the internal ring resulted in herniation in 90% of the animals, compared to 6% to 10% treated with BAPN alone and compared to 20% who only underwent transection of the internal ring

(15). In most animals in this study, both an anatomic defect and an abnormality of collagen cross-linking were needed to produce herniation.

BIOCHEMICAL ASPECTS OF WOUND HEALING AFTER HERNIA REPAIR

Collagenolysis and Proteases

In the transversus abdominis fascia, significantly higher levels of metalloproteinase II (MMP-2) have been found in biopsies from patients with direct inguinal hernia compared to patients with indirect hernia. As MMP-2 is an enzyme that degrades types IV, V, VII, X, and XI collagens, gelatin, elastin, fibronectin, and other matrix components, this finding may reflect proteolysis of connective tissue as a possible mechanism for formation and recurrence of direct inguinal hernia (10).

In wound healing, MMP-2 is important during the prolonged phase of matrix remodeling, whereas MMP-9, which is primarily derived from neutrophils, plays an important role in early repair processes (4). In a recent study of hernia wound healing, we assessed a possible association between wound fluid collagenases (MMP-2 and MMP-9) and the amount of collagen deposited in an implanted expanded polytetrafluoroethylene (ePTFE) fiber within the surgical wound (5). High levels of MMP-9 were found 24 hours after surgery with a significant decline 48 hours after surgery, reflecting the inflammatory activity of polymorphonuclear leucocytes and monocyte–macrophages (5). The concentration of MMP-9 after the first postoperative day was negatively associated with the amount of collagen deposited in the implanted

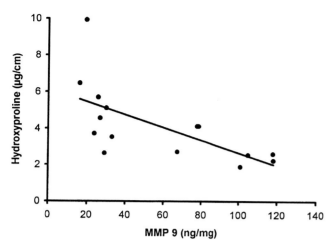

FIGURE 2.4. Relationship between deposited collagen on post-operative day 10 (measured as micrograms of hydroxyproline per centimeter length of expanded polytetrafluoroethylene tube) and matrix metalloproteinase 9 (*MMP 9*) concentration in wound fluid at 24 hours in each of the 15 patients (Spearman *r* = [–0.08], *p*<0.01). (From Agren MS, Jorgensen LN, Andersen M, et al. Matrix metalloproteinase 9 level predicts optimal collagen deposition during early wound repair in humans. *Br J Surg* 1998;85:68–71, with permission.)

ePTFE fiber after 10 days, indicating that the concentration of MMP-9 may be a predictor of healing in this type of wound (Fig. 2.4). However, it is unknown whether concentrations of MMPs and cytokines in wound fluid reflect those of the extracellular compartment of the transversalis fascia. In a study of collagenase activity in biopsies from the internal oblique muscle, Ajabnoor and co-workers did not find any detectable differences in the rates of collagen breakdown between patients with and without hernia (6).

In experimental studies, matrix metalloproteinases impede healing as assessed by anastomotic dehiscence of rat colon (33). Witte and co-workers recently showed in a rat model that the application of an MMP inhibitor (GM6001) results in a significant rise in wound mechanical strength even though collagen deposition did not increase (44). This response may be due to lower collagen turnover or an increase of maturation and cross-linking of the collagen.

In surgical patients with diseases other than hernia, an association between high persistent postoperative levels of MMP-9 and compromised healing has been found (36). Similar findings have been obtained in human chronic wounds and in skin biopsies from elderly patients, which have yielded increased concentration and activity of proteases such as MMP-2 and MMP-9 (7,36,45). Furthermore, reduced levels of the tissue inhibitor of matrix metalloproteinases have been found in the elderly (8). These

findings may explain why both direct and indirect inguinal herniation is associated with high patient age.

Synthetic Mesh or Autologous Tissue as Promoters of Wound Healing

Synthetic mesh material used in hernia repair induces a foreign body reaction with intense inflammatory response and secondary fibrillogenesis and connective tissue deposition. However, the tissue response depends on the implanted mesh material (26). For example, the structure of polypropylene allows penetration of newly formed vessels and a total integration with reparative tissue, whereas the ePTFE mesh is embedded sandwich-like by orderly connective tissue on the internal and external surface (9). All types of mesh material, however, provide a scaffold for the reparative processes, creating a firm fibrotic scar plate.

Transplantation of autologous tissue such as the anterior rectus sheath or the fascia lata has been shown to accelerate the synthesis and deposition of collagen for at least 2 years (28). It has been argued that the use of autologous tissue may not be a perfect solution in hernia repair, as this tissue may express a similar generalized defect in fibrillogenesis. It is therefore believed that synthetic material is to be preferred.

In experimental studies, the implantation of type I collagen sponges seeded with fibroblasts or coated with the basic fibroblast growth factor raised the collagen deposition and the tensile strength of dermal wounds (23). Future clinical studies are needed to show the applicability of similar material with stimulatory effect on collagen synthesis and deposition in hernia repair.

Wound Tension as a Promoter of Wound Healing

Experimental studies have demonstrated that the tensile strength of skin wounds in rabbits and rats is significantly higher when they are closed under limited tension (30,37). Although wounds closed under tension are more likely to dehisce during the early phases of healing, the tensile strength increases as the closing tension of the wound increases (Fig. 2.5) (25). Histologic sections comparing wound closed with and without tension have revealed a better orientation of fibers and fibroblasts in the direction of the tension (37). Others have found a higher fibroblast activity and collagen deposition in wounds closed under tension during the first 2 weeks of healing, as well as a higher degree of organization and cross-linking between the collagen fibers in the later phases of wound healing (30).

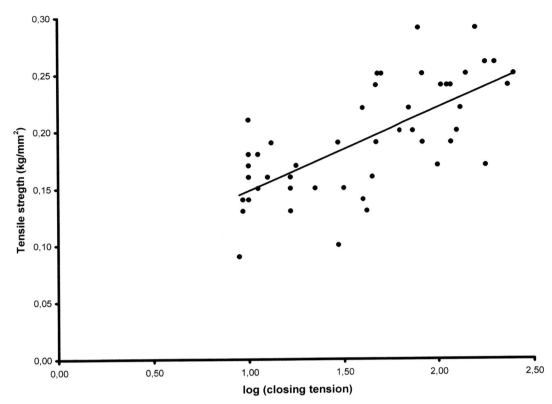

FIGURE 2.5. Log10 closing tension versus tensile strength. (From Morin G, Rand M, Burgess LPA, et al. Wound healing: relationship of wound closing tension to tensile strength in rats. *Laryngoscope* 1989;99:783–788, with permission.)

BIOCHEMICAL ASPECTS OF RECURRENT AND INCISIONAL WALL HERNIA

To our knowledge, no studies have examined biochemical aspects of recurrent abdominal wall hernia. Likewise, only little objective data exist on the healing process of the abdominal wall in patients operated on for recurrent groin or abdominal incisional hernia. It seems logical that abnormalities in production and degrading of connective tissue, which apparently play a role in hernia formation, may play a similar role in hernia recurrence.

The conventional repair of inguinal hernia is known to have a relatively high recurrence rate of around 10% to 15% (22). In this method of repair, the transversus abdominis fascia is forcibly stretched down and sutured to the inguinal ligament, creating an immense tension on the suture line (32). Furthermore, the combined high suture-line tension and intraabdominal pressure load induces a stress, which increases the vulnerability of wounds to suture-line necrosis and separation (1). It has been suggested that hernia repair performed under tension increases the risk of recurrence. If this hypothesis is true, one should expect the majority of hernias to recur within the first months after repair. It is generally assumed that technical

failures due to surgery are the main reason for hernia recurrence within the first 6 to 9 months postoperatively, but inguinal hernias may recur as long as 15 years following the initial surgery (17,29). In addition, there is experimental evidence to suggest that a hernioplasty closed under tension without tissue tearing by the sutures may result in higher tissue tensile strength.

Although hernia repair using mesh is associated with a much higher success rate, recurrence has been observed in the mesh-recipient tissue interface (10). The firmness of the anchoring of the mesh therefore seems important, as the recipient tissue may express the same connective tissue abnormalities that lead to herniation in the first place. A recent experimental study has demonstrated that the amount of connective tissue formation induced by the mesh material is associated with a decrease in abdominal wall mobility (20). The compound scar plate and decreased mobility of the abdominal wall surrounding the herniated site seem to create a mechanical barrier that may be the major important factor in preventing hernia recurrence (24).

There is still too little knowledge on how to classify hernia patients into different categories of risk for compromised healing. Future studies are needed to characterize biochemical and biomechanical features of the fascia transversalis or aponeurotic tissue obtained from patients with recurrent abdominal wall hernia. In addition, tensiometric studies should be applied to test the mechanical stability and anchoring of synthetic mesh material. If simple and relevant assays on collagen metabolism become available in the future, the choice of hernia repair method should then be influenced by the wound-healing potential of each individual patient.

SUMMARY

In the literature, there is strong evidence for an association between abnormal metabolism of connective tissue and the development of groin hernia. Clinical studies have shown a higher prevalence of inguinal hernia in patients with connective tissue disorders and other nonsurgical factors associated with defective connective tissue metabolism. Biochemical, morphologic, and biomechanical differences have been found in the connective tissue in patients with hernia, especially direct hernia, when compared to controls. Studies on cell cultures and biopsies suggest a diminished synthesis of matrix and defects in ultrastructure and stability of collagen. Predominance of nonpolymerized collagen may constitute an insufficient biomechanical barrier in the abdominal wall, predisposing to hernia formation or recurrence. Specific proteases that are related to different stages in the healing process play a major role in the turnover of collagen, and this may be associated with later recurrence.

Finally, the importance of surgical technique has been discussed. Experimental studies have shown that controlled wound-closing tension has a beneficial effect on the healing process. A guided fibrotic response induced by synthetic mesh material has proven efficient in providing a firm scar plate and localized immobility of the abdominal wall. Without mesh implantation, the tissue may express the same abnormalities that presumably resulted in primary herniation. Future studies are needed in hernia repair to determine the potential of pharmaceutical stimulation of the healing process with growth factors (e.g., basic fibroblast growth factor and platelet-derived growth factor) or inhibitors of proteinases.

CONCLUSION

A defective connective tissue metabolism resulting in reduced quality and amount of collagen is an important factor for hernia formation. In hernia recurrence, insufficient surgical technique may not be the only explanation for recurrence, but more likely it is a combination of an ongoing defect in connective tissue metabolism and pathophysiologic factors associated with the surgical technique applied.

REFERENCES

1. Abrahamson J. Etiology and pathophysiology of primary and recurrent groin hernia formation. *Surg Clin North Am* 1998;78: 953–972.
2. Abrahamson JH, Gofin J, Hopp C, et al. The epidemiology of inguinal hernia. *J Epidemiol Community Health* 1978;32:59–67.
3. Adye B, Luna G. Incidence of abdominal wall hernia in aortic surgery. *Am J Surg* 1998;175:400–402.
4. Agren MS. Gelatinase activity during wound healing. *Br J Dermatol* 1994;131:634–40.
5. Agren MS, Jorgensen LN, Andersen M, et al. Matrix metalloproteinase 9 level predicts optimal collagen deposition during early wound repair in humans. *Br J Surg* 1998;85:68–71.
6. Ajabnoor MA, Mokhtar AM, Rafee AA, et al. Defective collagen metabolism in Saudi patients with hernia. *Ann Clin Biochem* 1992;29:430–436.
7. Ashcroft GS, Horan MA, Herrick SE, et al. Age-related differences in the temporal and spatial regulation of matrix metalloproteinases (MMPs) in normal skin and acute cutaneous wounds of healthy humans. *Cell Tissue Res* 1997;290:581–591.
8. Ashcroft GS, Herrick SE, Tarnuzzer RW, et al. Human ageing impairs injury-induced in vivo expression of tissue inhibitor of matrix metalloproteinases (TIMP)-1 and -2 proteins and mRNA. *J Pathol* 1997;183:169–176.
9. Bellón JM, Bujan J, Contreras L, et al. Integration of biomaterials implanted into abdominal wall: process of scar formation and macrophage response. *Biomaterials* 1995;16:381–387.
10. Bellón JM, Buján J, Honduvilla NG, et al. Study of biochemical substrate and role of metalloproteinases in fascia transversalis from hernial processes. *Eur J Clin Invest* 1997;27:510–516.
11. Bielecki K, Pulawski R. Is cigarette smoking a causative factor in the development of inguinal hernia? *Pol Tyg Lek* 1988;43: 974–976.
12. Cannon DJ, Casteel L, Read RC. Abdominal aortic aneurysm, Leriche's syndrome, inguinal herniation, and smoking. *Arch Surg* 1984;119:387–389.
13. Cannon DJ, Read RC. Metastatic emphysema: a mechanism for acquiring inguinal herniation. *Ann Surg* 1981;194:270–278.
14. Carbonell JF, Sanchez JLA, Peris RT, et al. *Eur J Surg* 1993;159: 481–486.
15. Conner WT, Peacock EE Jr. Some studies on the etiology of inguinal hernia. *Am J Surg* 1973;126:732–735.
16. Flich J, Alfonso JL, Delgado F, et al. Inguinal hernia and certain risk factors. *Eur J Epidemiol* 1992;8:277–282.
17. Friedman DW, Boyd CD, Norton P, et al. Increases in type III collagen gene expression and protein synthesis in patients with inguinal hernias. *Ann Surg* 1993;218:754–760.
18. Hall KA, Peters B, Smyth SH, et al. Abdominal wall hernias in patients with abdominal aortic aneurysmal versus aortoiliac occlusive disease. *Am J Surg* 1995;170:572–576.
19. Jorgensen LN, Kallehave F, Christensen E, et al. Less collagen production in smokers. *Surgery* 1998;123:450–455.
20. Klosterhalfen B, Klinge U, Schumpelick V. Functional and morphological evaluation of different polypropylene-mesh modifications for abdominal wall repair. *Biomaterials* 1998;19: 2235–2246.
21. Lehnert B, Wadouh F. High coincidence of inguinal hernias and abdominal aortic aneurysms. *Ann Vasc Surg* 1992;6: 134–137.
22. Lichtenstein IL, Shulman AG, Amid PK. The cause, prevention, and treatment of recurrent groin hernia. *Surg Clin North Am* 1993;73:529–544.
23. Marks MG, Doillon C, Silver FH. Effects of fibroblasts and basic fibroblast growth factor on facilitation of dermal wound healing

by type I collagen matrices. *J Biomed Mater Res* 1991;25: 683–696.

24. McArdle G. Is inguinal hernia a defect in human evolution and would this insight improve concepts for methods of surgical repair? *Clin Anat* 1997;10:47–55.

25. Morin G, Rand M, Burgess LPA, et al. Wound healing: relationship of wound closing tension to tensile strength in rats. *Laryngoscope* 1989;99:783–788.

26. Pans A, Pierard GE. A comparison of intraperitoneal prostheses for the repair of abdominal muscular wall defects in rats. *Eur Surg Res* 1992;24:54–60.

27. Pans A, Pierard GE, Albert A, et al. Adult groin hernias: new insight into their biomechanical characteristics. *Eur J Clin Invest* 1997;27:863–868.

28. Peacock EE Jr. Subcutaneous extraperitoneal repair of ventral hernias: a biological basis for fascial transplantation. *Ann Surg* 1975;181:722–727.

29. Peacock EE Jr, Madden JW. Studies on the biology and treatment of recurrent inguinal hernia: II. Morphological changes. *Ann Surg* 1974;179:567–571.

30. Pickett BP, Burgess LP, Livermore GH, et al. Tensile strength versus healing time for wounds closed under tension. *Arch Otolaryngol Head Neck Surg* 1996;122:565–568.

31. Read RC. Attenuation of the rectus sheath in inguinal herniation. *Am J Surg* 1970;120:610–614.

32. Read RC, McLeod PC Jr. Influence of relaxing incision on suture tension in Bassini's and McVay's repair. *Arch Surg* 1981;116: 440–445.

33. Savage FJ, Lacombe DLP, Hembry RM, et al. Effect of colonic obstruction on the distribution of matrix metalloproteinases during anastomotic healing. *Br J Surg* 1998;85:72–75.

34. Sorensen LT, Friis E, Vennits B, et al. Smoking is a risk factor for recurrence of groin hernia. *World J Surg (in press)*.

35. Stevick CA, Long JB, Jamashbi B, et al. Ventral hernia following abdominal aortic reconstruction. *Am Surg* 1998;54:287–289.

36. Tarlton JF, Vickery CJ, Leaper DJ, et al. Postsurgical wound progression monitored by temporal changes in the expression of matrix metalloproteinase-9. *Br J Dermatol* 1997;137: 506–516.

37. Thorngate S, Ferguson DJ. Effect of tension on healing of aponeurotic wounds. *Surgery* 1958;44:619–624.

38. Uden A, Lindhagen T. Inguinal hernia in patients with congenital dislocation of the hip. A sign of general connective tissue disorder. *Acta Orthop Scand* 1988;59:667–668.

39. Wagh PV, Leverich AP, Sun CN, et al. Direct inguinal herniation in men: a disease of collagen. *J Surg Res* 1974;17:425–433.

40. Wagh PV, Read RC. Collagen deficiency in rectus sheath of patients with inguinal herniation. *Proc Soc Exp Biol Med* 1971; 137:382–384.

41. Wagh PV, Read RC. Defective collagen synthesis in inguinal herniation. *Am J Surg* 1972;124:819–822.

42. White HJ, Sun CN, Read RC. Inguinal hernia: a true collagen disease. *Lab Invest* 1977;36:359.

43. Wirtschafter ZT, Bentley JP. Hernias as a collagen maturation defect. *Ann Surg* 1969;160:852–859.

44. Witte MB, Thornton FJ, Kiyama T, et al. Metalloproteinase inhibitors and wound healing: a novel enhancer of wound strength. *Surgery* 1998;124:464–470.

45. Yager DR, Zhang L-Y, Liang H-X, et al. Wound fluids from human pressure ulcers contain elevated matrix metalloproteinase levels and activity compared to surgical wound fluids. *J Invest Dermatol* 1996;107:743–748.

3

A HISTORY OF THE TREATMENT OF HERNIA

JOSÉ F. PATIÑO

Since the dawn of surgical history, hernias have been a subject of interest, and their treatment has evolved through distinct stages (10,54,57). The history of hernia is the history of surgery.

In the past two editions of this textbook, erudite reviews were presented of the history of hernia and its treatment. Read (57) and others (3,10,51,52,54) also have dealt with this topic, which has fascinated surgeons of all latitudes through the years of recorded medical history. In an excellent historic treatise by Zimmerman and Veith (67), the operation for hernia surges as a paramount indicator of the progress of surgical technique.

On November 17, 1892, William S. Halsted of The Johns Hopkins School of Medicine read his classic paper, "The Cure of Inguinal Hernia in the Male" (23) at the Annual Meeting of the MedicoChirurgical Faculty of Maryland in Easton, Maryland. The paper begins as follows:

> Shuh said, "If no other field were offered to the surgeon for his activity than herniotomy, it would be worth while to become a surgeon and to devote an entire life to this service." Quite as well, certainly, might this be said of operations for the radical cure of hernia. There is, perhaps, no operation which, by the profession at large, would be more appreciated than a perfectly safe . . . cure for rupture.

No other entity permits the study of the origin and evolution of surgical theory and technique as does inguinal hernia. The described details of the operation constitute a superb parameter of the scientific knowledge of anatomy and the quality of the art and science of surgery as it existed and was practiced in the different ages.

In reviewing the historic evolution in chronologic sequence, this chapter highlights the milestones in the development of the surgical therapy of hernia through quotations from the original texts by the surgeon–authors to underlay the importance of the major contributions.

J. F. Patiño: National University of Colombia; Department of Surgery, Santa Fe Foundation of Bogotá, Bogotá, Colombia.

ANCIENT TIMES

The *Edwin Smith Surgical Papyrus,* the oldest scientific text that deals with surgery, written during the Egyptian Old Kingdom (3000–2500 B.C.) and copied in the ensuing centuries (the extant copy dates from circa 1700 B.C.), has no reference to hernia.

The earliest recorded reference to hernias appears in the *Egyptian Papyrus of Ebers* (circa 1552 B.C.). According to the monumental illustrated history of medicine by Lyons and Petrucelli (31) this papyrus contains observations on hernias: "When you judge a swelling on the surface of a belly . . . what comes out . . . caused by coughing."

GRAECO–ROMAN MEDICINE

The foundations of Western civilization, culture, and science lie in the philosophic tradition of the Ionian nature philosophers and the intellectual splendor of classical Greece.

Hippocrates (460–377 B.C.), "the father of medicine," and Aristotle (384–324 B.C.), "the philosopher" and the first real theoretic and physical scientist, had the greatest influence on the development of scientific medicine, a discipline that attained distinction in Alexandria in the Hellenistic era (310–250 B.C.).

Amazingly, the *Corpus Hippocraticum* (25), the collected writings—more than 70 books—by Hippocrates and his followers, mentions hernia only in passing, although the surgical writings contain detailed anatomic descriptions and indicate refined surgical techniques. The book, *On the Surgery,* contains superb descriptions of the operating room, the people that intervene, the lighting, the instruments, the positioning of the patient, and the techniques of bandaging and dressing. Yet hernia, an easily diagnosed disease entity, is cited in the Hippocratic text only in the section on the effect of different kinds of water: "The children are specially liable to rupture (hernia) and the men to varicose veins and ulcers of the legs" (25). As stated by Zimmerman and Veith

(67), the omission of hernia and of bladder stone (a specific injunction against cutting for bladder stone is made in the "Oath") from the Hippocratic texts is puzzling and may be due to the loss of the original texts.

A great medical school flourished in the legendary Museum (from *mouseion,* meaning "sanctuary dedicated to the muses") of Alexandria, the Egyptian city founded by Alexander the Great (356–323 B.C.). The Museum of Alexandria was the home of the largest library of antiquity, and surgery was performed there with a high level of sophistication following the Hippocratic precepts. The outstanding medical figures in Alexandria were Herophilus of Chalcedon (circa 300 B.C.), recognized as the founder of anatomy, and Erasistratus of Keos (circa 330–250 B.C.), known as the father of physiology—both acknowledged as accomplished surgeons who practiced the ligature of vessels for hemostasis in operations for hernia, lithotomy, plastic repairs, and tracheotomy, reputedly under anesthesia induced by the administration of the juice of mandragora (67). The practice of surgery in Alexandria during the Hellenistic era was much more rational than the barbaric practices that prevailed in Europe in the Middle Ages and early Renaissance.

The Roman culture spans from the first century B.C. to about A.D. 500. In the first century B.C. and the first century A.D., the Roman encyclopedists flourished, among them Aulus Cornelius Celsus (?–A.D. 50) and Gaius Plinius Secundus (Pliny the Elder, A.D. 23–79), the most famous Roman authors on medicine who were nonphysicians. Celsus, who transmitted in his writings much of what we know of Alexandrian surgery, was a disciple of Asclepiades of Prusa, the Bithynian physician who practiced in Rome. The works of Asclepiades are lost, but he and his texts are referred to by Celsus, Galen, Oribasius, and many others (28).

As an ardent follower of Hippocrates, Celsus was the first to introduce Greek and Alexandrian medicine to Rome, for which he has been called the *Latin Hippocrates*; he is also known as the *Cicero of Medicine* for his fine literary style (35). His *De Medicina* (12), together with the *Corpus Hippocraticum* and the works of Galen (A.D. 131–201), constitute the greatest legacy of Graeco–Roman medicine.

Among Celsus' descriptions of surgical procedures is that of the operation for the treatment of hernia, preceded by a review of the anatomy and clinical presentation of "those lesions which are apt to arise in the genital parts around the testicles . . . the nature of the said region must be briefly described first."

Celsus' detailed description of the hernia operation constitutes a magnificent record of fine surgery in the Alexandrian tradition, performed with hemostasis by ligature of the vessels and careful efforts to preserve the testicle:

> When these lesions have been recognized their treatment must be discussed . . . . I shall now speak of those cases demanding the knife . . . . Now the laying open is to be done boldly, until the outer tunic, that of the scrotum itself, is cut through, and the middle tunic reached. When an incision has been made, an

opening presents leading deeper. Into this the index finger of the left hand is introduced, in order that by separation of the intervening little membranes the hernial sac may be freed . . . many blood vessels are met with; the smaller ones can be summarily divided; but larger ones, to avoid dangerous bleeding, must be first tied with rather long flax thread . . . lower down, however, not all is to be removed: for at the base of the testicle there is intimate conexion with the inner tunic, where excision is not possible without extreme danger . . . the testicle having been thus cleared is to be gently returned through the incision along with the veins and arteries and its cord . . . .

Heliodorus lived in the Graeco–Roman period at the beginning of the second century A.D.; he practiced as physician and surgeon during the reign of Trajan (A.D. 98–117). Referring to the radical cure of hernia, Leonardo (28) brings forth the following quotation: "We ligature the larger vessels, but as for the smaller ones we catch them with hooks and twist them many times, thus closing their mouths."

According to Read (57), the concept of rupture comes from Galen of Pergamum (A.D. 129–199), the most prominent physician of the Graeco–Roman period. Galen traveled extensively and visited Alexandria, where the tradition of the surgical teachings and research by Herophilus and Erasistratus persisted, with "personal inspection" (i.e., *autopsia,* or human autopsy) as a major component of instruction. In Pergamum and in Rome, Galen was surgeon to the gladiators; he wrote extensively on surgical matters, with important observations on local pathology. Galen thought that herniation was produced by rupture of the peritoneum and overstretching of the overlying fascia and muscles. He recommended operation, which consisted of the ligature of the sac and cord with amputation of the testicle, something that represented a regression after the Alexandrian practice of preserving the testicle.

THE MIDDLE AGES

The notable technical advances of Alexandrian and Graeco–Roman surgery were largely lost during the Dark Ages, the age of Faith and Scholasticism, the period spanning from A.D. 476 (fall of the Roman Empire) to the fifteenth century (Renaissance). Scientific and cultured idiom was Latin. The first universities were founded in Europe in the twelfth and thirteenth centuries, and in them the formal teaching of medicine was started. Surgery was not a learned trade, being only concerned with fractures and the crude treatment of wounds of war. Compared with what was practiced in Alexandria during the Hellenistic period, surgery in the Middle Ages, as performed by barbers, cutters, and incisors—people usually ignorant and often illiterate—was characterized by primitivism and regressive trends. Hemostasis was not done through ligature of vessels but rather by the dreadful cautery, and the use of any type of anesthesia was absent.

Paul of Aegina (Paulus Aegineta, seventh century A.D.) (1) was an important physician encyclopedist of the Byzantine period, which followed the downfall of the Roman Empire in the fifth century A.D. His work, which includes one book totally dedicated to surgery—intended as a compendium of Greek and Roman medicine—became an important source for Arabic medicine in the ensuing centuries. His meticulous and accurate description of the operation for hernia, however, also constitutes a regression from the classical surgeons of Alexandria and the Roman Celsus since it includes the routine sacrifice of the testicle.

Albucasis, Abul Qasim al-Zahrawi, the great Moorish surgeon who lived between the years A.D. 1013 (some authors place the date of his birth in the year 936) and 1106, produced the first rational, complete, and illustrated treatise, *On Surgery and Instruments* (2), in which he described many original operative procedures and instruments of his own design. This great book, whose "purpose was to revive the art of surgery as taught by the 'the Ancients,' the content of which term ranges from Hippocrates to Paulus Aegineta, whose lifetimes were separated by some eleven hundred years," was translated into Latin by Gerard of Cremona and published in Toledo, Spain, in the second half of the twelfth century under the title *Liber Alsaharavi de Cirurgia*; it then appeared in Venice together with Guy de Chauliac's *Cyrurgia Parva* in 1497.

With Pliny's *Historia Naturalis,* Albucasis' *On Surgery and Instruments* was among the first medical books printed in Venice in the second half of the fifteenth century, just a few years after Gutenberg's Bible (1454). Albucasis' treatise had enormous influence on European surgeons in the ensuing centuries. Albucasis was probably born in a royal city near Cordova, Spain, where he practiced and taught. Cordova was a center of learning and culture, with a large library and several hospitals.

In the 1973 beautiful bilingual edition (Arabic and English texts) of Albucasis' text by Spink and Lewis and the Wellcome Institute of the History of Medicine (2), one can read a detailed description of ruptures:

On the cauterization of hernia.

> When a rupture occurs in the groin, and part of the intestine and omentum comes down into the scrotum, being the onset of the disease, forbid the patient to take food for one day and have him use laxatives to empty the bowel. Then let him lie on his back in front of you and bid him hold his breath till the intestine or omentum comes out; then put it back with your finger. Then below the hernia over the pubic bone, mark a semicircle whose extremities point upward. Then heat a cautery of this type (illustration). When it is white hot and emits sparks then return the intestine or omentum into his abdominal cavity, and have an assistant put his hand over the place to prevent the exit of the intestine. You should first have parted his legs and put a pillow under him; let another assistant sit on his legs and another on his chest, holding his hands. Then apply the cautery to the mark, keeping the cautery upright, and hold it till it reaches the bone . . . . You must take

the greatest care that the intestine does not come out while you are cauterizing, lest you burn it and it result in death or grave injury to the patient (pp 134–136).

On the treatment of intestinal hernia.

This hernia is due to a split occurring in the membrane stretched from the hypogastrium over the belly in the region of the groin. Through this opening the bowel descends upon one of the testes; this opening is due to the membrane's splitting or stretching. And these two kinds occur from a number of causes: from a blow or jumping or shouting, or lifting a heavy weight, or a similar cause . . . it is a slow and chronic development and does not happen on a sudden . . . . The treatment of the varieties of this disease with the knife is dangerous; so be cautious of rushing at it. . . . The incision should be sufficiently large to allow the testicle to be drawn out. Then dissect away the tissues that lie beneath the skin of the scrotum so that the hard tunica albuginea be exposed all round . . . . Feel with your finger that there be no part of the intestine that has got twisted within the tough white membrane; and should you find any push it back into the abdomen. Then take a needle with a stout tenfold thread and enter the end of the membrane which lies beneath the skin of the testicles alongside the rupture; then cut the end of the loop thread to make four sutures and arrange one over the other in the form of a cross; and with these ligate the membrane of which we have spoken with a strong ligature on each side; then twist the ends of the thread and lie them with a strong knot to prevent anything from reaching the nutrient vessels of the testicles, lest an abscess occur thereby; and make also another ligature outside the first one, rather less than two fingers' breadth from it; and after making these two ligatures leave a finger's breadth of the membrane that is beneath the skin of the testicles and cut the rest way round, and with it remove the testis.

On the treatment of the rupture that occurs in the groin.

Sometimes there occurs a rupture in the groin . . . no part of the intestine descends into the scrotum. It arises from a stretching of the membrane (i.e. the peritoneum) in the groin . . . . Its treatment by the cautery is as I have already described. Sometimes also is treated with the knife in this manner: . . . make an incision three fingers wide, transversally across the swelling of the rupture which projects. Then perforate the subcutaneous tissues so as to expose the white membrane (i.e. the deep fascia) that lies under the skin alongside the rupture. Take a probe and place it upon the projecting part of the fascia and push it back into the depths of the abdomen. Then sew together the two swollen portions of the membrane over the end of the probe and suture the one to the other . . . . On no account make the incision into the fascia nor touch the testis nor anything else, as I taught on the subject of treating the intestinal hernia (p 448).

Albucasis also writes on the umbilical hernia, the "protruding navel," and describes the operation after a differential diagnosis to exclude other causes of protrusion.

The medical school at Salerno, in southern Italy, is recognized as "the first stirring in the reawakening of medicine in Western Europe." The "flowering of the civitas Hippocratica, as Salerno came to be known," which started in the ninth century but expanded greatly in the twelfth century, was due to its lay organization and to the wise rules that introduced the first system of examination for doctors, including surgeons, and the first regulations concerning medical education and licensure for practice. Salernitian surgery, including the operation for hernia, was highly developed and produced important surgical texts that had profound influence on surgical practice over the ensuing two centuries (67).

William of Salicet (circa 1210–77) represents an innovator in surgery. Regarding hernia, in his *Cyrurgia,* translated into French by Paul Pifteau in 1898 (53), he writes: "And if you were to be assured of this manner of opening, then permit the testicle to redescend to its place, and do not dream in any fashion of extirpating it, as do some stupid and ignorant doctors who know nothing . . . ." He is the first author since Celsus, in the first century B.C., to reject mutilation of the testicle as an essential part of the operation for the cure of hernia (67).

THE RENAISSANCE

The outstanding medical figure of the Renaissance era (fifteenth to midseventeenth centuries) is Ambroise Paré

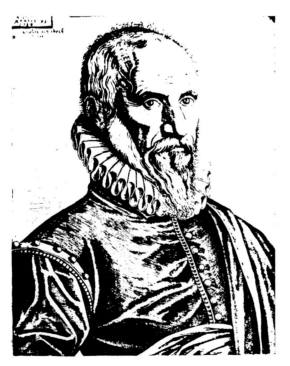

FIGURE 3.1. Ambroise Paré (1510–90) at age 75. Illustration is from an engraving by Horbeck in the British Museum and is reproduced in *Selections from the Works of Ambroise Paré: With a Short Biography and Explanatory and Biographical Notes,* by Dorothea Waley Singer (New York: William Wood & Co, 1924). The book is in the personal library of J.F. Patiño.

(1510–90; Fig. 3.1), who studied anatomy and surgery at the Hotel Dieu of Paris and who is largely responsible, with John Hunter (1728–93), for the development of modern surgery. One of Paré's greatest contributions was the ligature of vessels, which supplanted the method of hemostasis by the use of hot oil or cautery.

Paré elevated the surgeon's profession from an ill-reputed handicraft to a respected art. An entire chapter on hernias appears in Paré's *The Apologie and Treatise* (50):

Of hernia. Of the tumors of the groins and codds, called Herniae, that is rupture.

> The ancient Phisitions have made many kinds of Ruptures, yet indeed there are only three to be called by that name that is, the Intestinalis, or that of the guts, the Zirbalis, or that of the kall, and that which is mixed of them both . . . . And we must cure it by Chirurgery after this manner, following . . . then presently make an incision in the upper part of the codde, not touching the substance of the guts . . . . We must put it into place of the incision, and put it under the production of the Peritoneum being cut together with the codde, all the length of the production; that so with a sharp knife we may divide the process of the Peritoneum, according to that cavity separated from the guts there contained . . . . When you have made an indifferent incision, the guts must be gently put up into the belly with your fingers, and then so much of the cut Peritoneum must be sowed up, as shall seem sufficient, that by that passage made more straight, nothing may fall into the Codde, after it is cicatrized.

When the rupture cannot be cured as described, "by reason of the great solution of the continuity of the relaxt, or broken *Peritoneum,*" Paré advises the use of the Golden Ligature, or the Punctus Aureus, the golden thread or golden tie. He gives a detailed description of the technique and illustrates the instruments, including a "croked needle, having an eye not farre from the point, through which you may put the golden wyre." Well known are Paré's illustrations of diverse trusses for the control of hernias (Fig. 3.2). He severely condemned the itinerant herniotomists who produced castration (28).

Pierre Franco (circa 1500–65), a provincial French surgeon, has been placed as a middleman between a barber–surgeon and an itinerant cutter. Because of his devotion to elevating the status of operative surgery and his important innovations, he also is considered by some to be the premier surgeon of the sixteenth century. Franco was deeply interested in the surgical treatment of hernia. His *Traité des Hernies* was published by E. Nicaise in Lyon in 1561. With its detailed descriptions of the radical operation, which included an original technique that left unharmed the spermatic vessels and testis, as well as an operation for strangulated hernia, this treatise is a major contribution to surgery.

Kaspar Stromayr was a cutter, or incisor, of hernia in Germany in the sixteenth century. His *Practica Copiosa* (63a), a beautifully and profusely illustrated German manuscript dated July 4, 1559, deals principally with hernia and establishes for the first time the distinction between indirect

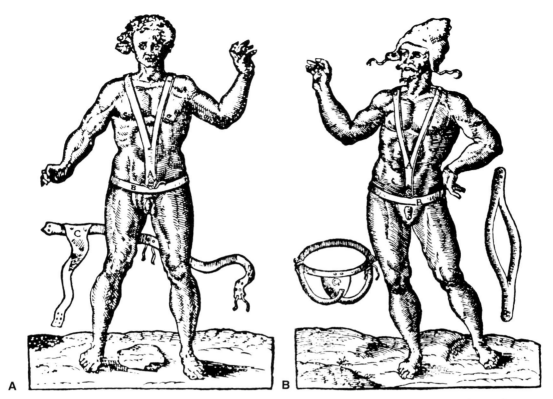

FIGURE 3.2. A and **B:** Trusses illustrated in the chapter on "Herniae, That is, Ruptures," in *Apologie and Treatise of Ambroise Paré: Containing the Voyages Made into Divers Places With Many of His Writings Upon Surgery.* From a 1951 edition of the book, in the personal library of J.F. Patiño, a gift of Professor Gustaf E. Linskog, Yale University, Christmas of 1957.

and direct hernias (Fig. 3.3). Removal of the testis was sanctioned in operations for hernias of the indirect type but not for the other forms.

THE POSTRENAISSANCE ERA

Antonio Scarpa (1752–1832), author of the *Treatise on Hernias,* which was published in an English translation by Wishart in Edinburgh in 1814, studied at the University of Padua, where his mentor was the renowned pathologist Giovanni Battista Morgagni. In his treatise, Scarpa described accurately, based on autopsy studies, the sliding hernia.

The most distinguished pupil of John Hunter was Astley Paston Cooper of Norfolk (1768–1841), whose great interests resided in the study of hernia, the breast, and arterial surgery. His contributions to anatomy and physiology were

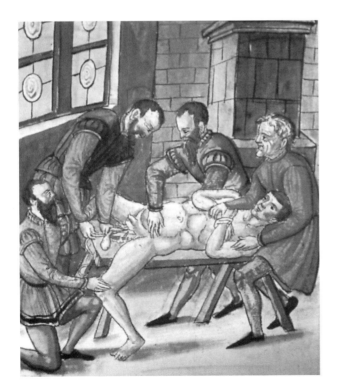

FIGURE 3.3. Operation for hernia, as illustrated in *Practica Copiosa,* by Kaspar Stromayr, written in 1559. The author himself may have been the illustrator. According to A.G. Carmichel and R.M. Ratzan, the manuscript was not discovered until 1909. This illustration appears in their book *Medicine: A Treasury of Art and Literature* (New York: Hugh Lauter Levin Associates, 1991).

enormous. In his *Treatise on Hernia,* published in London in 1804 and 1807, and in *The Anatomy and Surgical Treatment of Abdominal Hernia,* published in Philadelphia in 1844, Cooper described for the first time the superior pubic ligament, which now bears his name, and the fascia transversalis, with full recognition of its role in the pathogenesis of hernias:

> When the lower portions of the internal oblique and transversalis muscles are raised from their subjacent attachments, a layer of fascia is found to be interposed between them and the peritoneum, through which the spermatic vessels emerge from the abdomen. This fascia, which I have ventured to name fascia transversalis, varies in density, being strong and unyielding towards the ilium, but weak and more cellular towards the pubes.

August Gottlieb Richter (1742–1812), professor of surgery at the University of Göttingen in 1776, was the founder of the first German surgical journal (1782–1804) and was highly influential in establishing scientific surgery in Germany. His work on hernia, *Abhandlung yon der Brüchen* (1777–79), was considered the best treatise of his time (28).

THE NINETEENTH AND TWENTIETH CENTURIES

Edoardo Bassini (1844–1924; Fig. 3.4) of Pavia revolutionized the treatment of inguinal hernia by the introduction of a technique designed "to restore those conditions in the area of the hernial orifice which exist under normal circumstances" (9). Read (58) published a historic review of Bassini's pioneer work on the centenary of his landmark contribution to inguinal herniorrhaphy.

Bassini's interest in hernia surgery dates back to 1883; he had tried the different methods of correction, which resulted in a high incidence of early failure and the futile need to wear a truss after the operation with the hope of preventing recurrence. He thought that this was due to the inadequacy of a mere ligature of the sac without reconstructing the inguinal canal. Bassini's initial report to the Italian Society of Surgery at Genoa in 1887 (5), which included 38 patients, was followed later in the same year by a presentation to the Italian Medical Association at Pavia (6), which included 72 operations, and in 1888 to the Italian Surgical Society at Naples (7) on 102 repairs. In 1889, Bassini published his celebrated monograph, which contains beautiful illustrations (8). His paper published in Germany in 1890 (9) and later translated into Italian made Bassini's work widely recognized.

Zimmerman and Veith (67) stated that, after Bassini's initial reports on 262 cases with detailed illustrations, "Overnight, hernial surgery of classical antiquity gave way to that of today, and little that is basic has been added despite the myriads of alleged modifications and improvements . . . . The role of Bassini as the creator of modern hernial surgery stands unchallenged."

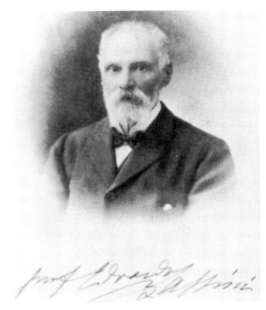

FIGURE 3.4. Edoardo Bassini (1844–1924). (Courtesy of the National Library of Medicine, Bethesda, MD.)

Bassini's repair consists of the high ligation and resection of the sac followed by the reconstruction of the floor (or posterior wall) of the inguinal canal using the conjoined tendon (internal oblique, transversus abdominis) and the fascia transversalis (fascia verticalis Cooperi), a triple layer that is sutured to the shelving border of Poupart's ligament, with the cord covered by the sutured aponeurosis of the external oblique (8).

Many modifications have been introduced to Bassini's repair, and it is performed differently by surgeons around the world. Wantz (65) published an excellent article that contains the full color illustrations appearing in Attilio Catterina's book published in Bologna in 1932 (11). The Shouldice repair is nothing more than a modern revival of the original Bassini procedure (22,58).

In the United States, Marcy (33,34) (1837–1924), a North American disciple of Lister, Halsted (23) (1852–1922), of The Johns Hopkins School of Medicine, and Ferguson (17), of the Chicago College of Physicians and Surgeons (predecessor to the University of Illinois College of Medicine), published techniques similar to Bassini's repair. Summers reviewed in 1946 the classic herniorrhaphies of Bassini, Halsted, Andrews (4), and Ferguson (64).

The matter of the priority in the development of these techniques has been argued over the years. Read (56) refers to Watson, who "in his textbook of 1924 stated that Bassini 'adopted' the operation of Marcy (1837–1924), the Boston surgeon, anatomist and philanthropist, a contemporary of Halsted, described at the International Surgical Congress in London in 1881." Watson continues: ". . . his epoch making technique . . . revolutionized the treatment of hernia and eclipsed the countless methods that had been used with more or less questionable results up to that time." Watson relates: "Marcy told me once that while he was reading his paper he saw Bassini in the audience. He was listening intently, an expression of understanding about him that seemed to change to pleasant conjecture." Marcy himself stated in his book on hernia in 1892, ". . . my own operation described some years previously was practically the same as that designated the Bassini" (34).

Read (56) cites other authors who claim Marcy's priority but concludes that, as stated by Halsted, "Bassini was first," and that "March never accepted Bassini's priority and labored with the help of friends to alter the history of this event, but to no avail."

Marcy was the first to indicate the importance of the high ligation of the hernial sac and closure of the dilated inguinal ring as essential steps in the repair of an inguinal hernia, and the first to describe a transabdominal approach. His two landmark publications date back to 1887 and 1892 (33,34).

An "intraabdominal method of removing inguinal and femoral hernia" was reported by LaRoque (27) in 1932. He described the advantages of the approach: accurate diagnosis, easy dissection, minimal trauma to the cord, and the safe resection of diseased bowel.

William S. Halsted (1852–1922) is the towering figure of modern surgery, and many have discussed the matter of the priority in the design and practice of the operation for the cure of inguinal hernia. The collected *Surgical Papers* (23) of William Stewart Halsted include the papers on the radical cure of inguinal hernia, first presented on November 4, 1889, and ending with "An additional note on the operation for inguinal hernia," dated August 26, 1922. In this note, Halsted refers to the work of Bassini:

> My first cases were reported at a meeting of The Johns Hopkins Hospital Medical Society, November 4, 1889, and were published in the Johns Hopkins Hospital Bulletin for January, 1890. Hence Bassini's brochure anticipated my first report by at least a month or two. Whether my first operation was performed before the appearance of Bassini's pamphlet in Italian I cannot say, for the precise date of the pamphlet is not given. In any event I had not heard of Bassini's operation until his German article appeared—possibly about one year after my first operation; neither was I or any American or German, so far as I know, aware of Bassini's first report until the appearance of the second. Bassini unquestionably has the priority. Our operations differed in several respects, but in the essential features were the same.

In the same note (23), Halsted gives credit to Harvey Cushing, who first performed herniorrhaphies under local anesthesia.

The 1903 paper by Halsted on hernia published in the *Johns Hopkins Hospital Bulletin* has the famed Max Brödel's magnificent drawings, and in the text Halsted refers to the increasing use of rubber gloves by Bloodgood, his resident. Rubber gloves were introduced by Halsted in 1890. In this paper, Halsted first reported the modern relaxing incision over the rectus fascia (Fig. 3.5).

A widely accepted procedure is the Cooper's ligament repair. The technique was described in 1898 by Georg Lotheissen (30) (1868–1935) in Vienna, but was popularized by Chester McVay (1911–87) after his landmark article (39), with Anson as coauthor, published in 1949. In 1958 and 1974, McVay presented the basic anatomic concept of the repair using Cooper's ligament (36,38).

CONTEMPORARY TIMES

The basic principles of hernia repair were laid down in the late nineteenth century. Since then, important modifications have been added to the classic Bassini repair, and for

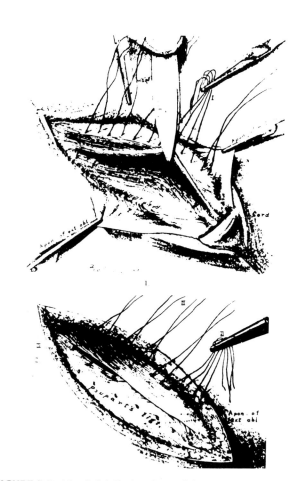

FIGURE 3.5. Max Brödel's drawings of the Halsted operation for the cure of hernia (plate XXII, 1 and 2). "The lower flap of the cremaster muscle and its fascia is drawn up under the mobilized internal oblique muscle and held in this position by very fine silk stitches . . . . The internal oblique muscle, mobilized, and possibly further released by incising the anterior sheath of the rectus muscle, is stitched (the conjoined tendon also) to Poupart's ligament in the Bassini–Halsted manner." (From Halsted WS. The cure of the more difficult as well as the simpler inguinal ruptures. *Johns Hopkins Hosp Bull* 1903;14:208–214.)

some of the favored new procedures, local anesthesia can be advantageously used.

Local anesthesia for the repair of hernias was reported by Harvey Cushing (15,16) at the turn of the century. He used block anesthesia produced by cocaine infiltration, a method that Halsted had been largely responsible for introducing (19). Two major techniques that have proved to be effective are usually done under local anesthesia: the Canadian Shouldice repair and the tension-free prosthetic hernioplasty.

According to Wantz (66), the so-called Canadian repair was developed in the 1950s by Shouldice, Obney, and Ryan, but it was first described in the surgical literature in the late 1960s (41,61). Typically, the procedure is performed under local anesthesia, and it has generated a renewed interest in local anesthesia.

The concept of the tension-free repair was introduced by Lichtenstein and colleagues (29) in 1989, who reported 1,000 consecutive prosthetic hernioplasties followed for 1 to more than 5 years without recurrences. The prosthetic hernioplasty consists of the reconstruction of the floor of the inguinal canal by means of a synthetic mesh.

Condon (14) described the anterior iliopubic tract repair using the traditional anterior approach through the inguinal canal, a method that evolved from the use of the iliopubic tract in operations done by the preperitoneal, or posterior, approach.

In the third edition of this book (45), Nyhus commented: "I am convinced that all recurrent groin hernias must be approached posteriorly and the fascial repair buttressed by prosthetic material." The preperitoneal approach has been well described by Nyhus et al. (42,44,46,48,49) and is the preferred technique for many surgeons in the treatment of all recurrent and complicated hernias.

According to Nyhus (42,44), apparently it was Thomas Annandale of Edinburgh who first presented the concept of the preperitoneal approach in 1876; Annandale did not perform a fascial repair. Meade (40) traces it back to 1743. Bates (9a), of Seattle, advanced the preperitoneal approach concept. Cheatle (13), in 1920, perhaps based on the influence of earlier English procedures (57), described an operation for the radical cure of inguinal and femoral hernias through a median abdominal section, without entering the peritoneal cavity. In 1921, Cheatle reported on the use of Pfannenstiel's incision, but advised against the use of this approach for direct hernias (57). According to Read (57), the preperitoneal approach laid dormant until rediscovered by Henry (24) in 1936; in 1942, Jennings and Anson (26) revived it in the United States. Read (55) and McVay (37) are among the authors who have reported on this approach, but it was Nyhus (44) who established it firmly as a sound operation based on detailed anatomic and clinical studies:

> My associates and I were perplexed about the failure of the method to flourish. In 1955 we began a clinical investigation in a deliberate attempt to explore the potential of the approach

and to provide a large clinical group in which a long-term follow-up study could be accomplished and reported. During the ensuing years our technique for the repair of indirect and direct inguinal and femoral hernias evolved.

In several publications (42–49), Nyhus and associates confirmed their conviction about the merits of this approach, especially when dealing with major herniations, recurrent hernias, and femoral hernias. The detailed description of the technique, which involves repair through the preperitoneal approach, has appeared in the former editions of this textbook as well as in a recent monograph (47). In the 1959 paper (49), Nyhus and colleagues used for the first time a synthetic mesh (Ivalon) to buttress the posterior wall repair.

The preperitoneal approach has been favored by French surgeons (59,62,63), who report excellent results with the implantation of Dacron and Mersilene prostheses. The military surgeons Rignault (59) of France and Rosenthal and Walters (60) of the United States also recommend it, together with the use of prosthesis. Malangoni and Condon (32) recommend the preperitoneal approach for incarcerated and strangulated hernias.

The studies by Nyhus and associates and the reported results since 1959 have made this approach the preferred one for many contemporary surgeons. Our group in Bogotá prefers the preperitoneal approach and repair, and because of Nyhus' leadership and pioneer work, we have proposed that it be known as the *Nyhus operation* (51,52).

The dramatic surge of laparoscopic surgery has led to the use of the new technology for the performance of a variety of operations, including the repair of inguinal hernias. In the early 1980s and 1990, Ger et al. (20,21) reported on a transabdominal approach for hernia repair, on the performance of a repair with staples applied under laparoscopic guidance, and on experimental studies in animals. Recent reports, such as those of Filipi and colleagues (18) of Creighton University (Omaha), describe well the attractive technique, which so far has not convincingly demonstrated superiority over the conventional extraperitoneal operations, especially the important and effective preperitoneal approach. Laparoscopic herniorrhaphy is still considered a procedure in the developmental stage.

REFERENCES

1. Aegineta P. *Paulus Aegineta on surgery: the seven books of Paulus Aegineta.* Translated from the Greek by Francis Adams with a Commentary embracing a complete view of the knowledge possessed by the Greeks, Romans, and Arabians on all subjects connected with medicine and surgery. London: Printed for the Sydenheim Society. (Special edition by The Classics of Surgery Library. Birmingham, AL: 1985.)
2. Albucasis. *On surgery and instruments.* A definitive edition of the Arabic text with English translation and commentary by MS Spink and GL Lewis. London: The Wellcome Institute of the History of Medicine, and Oxford: The University Press, 1973.

3. Andrade Perez E. Desarrollo histórico de la herniorrafia inguinal. *Rev Colomb Cirugía* 1988;3:182.
4. Andrews EW. Major and minor technique of Bassini's operation, as performed by himself. *Med Rec* 1899;56:622.
5. Bassini E. Sulla cura radicale dell'ernia inguinale. *Arch Soc Ital Chir* 1887;4:380.
6. Bassini E. Nuovo metodo per la cura radicale dell'ernia inguinale. *Atti Congr Med Ital* 1887;2:179.
7. Bassini E. Sopra 100 casi di cura radicale dell'ernia inguinale operata col metodo dell'autore. *Arch ed Atti Soc Ital Chir* 1888;5:315.
8. Bassini E. *Nuovo metodo per la cura radicale dell'ernia inguinale.* Padua: Prosperini, 1889.
9. Bassini E. Uber die behandlung des leistenbruches. *Arch fr klinische chirurgie* 1890;40:441.
9a. Bates UC. New operation for the cure of indirect inguinal hernia. *JAMA* 1913;60:2032.
10. Bendavid R. New techniques in hernia repairs. *World J Surg* 1989;13:522–531.
11. Catterina A. *L'operazione di Bassini per la cura radicale dell' ernia inguinale.* Bologna: L. Cappelli, 1932.
12. Celsus. *De medicina.* With an English translation by WG Spencer. Cambridge, MA: Harvard University Press, 1938.
13. Cheatle GL. An operation for the radical cure of inguinal and femoral hernia. *Br Med J* 1920;2:68.
14. Condon RE. Anterior iliopubic tract repair. In: Nyhus LM, Condon RE, eds. *Hernia,* 3rd ed. Philadelphia: JB Lippincott, 1989:137–153.
15. Cushing H. Cocaine anesthesia in the treatment of certain cases of hernia and in operations for thyroid tumors. *Johns Hopkins Hosp Bull* 1898;9:192.
16. Cushing H. The employment of local anesthesia in the radical cure of certain cases of hernia, with a note upon the nervous anatomy of the inguinal region. *Ann Surg* 1900;31:1.
17. Ferguson AH. Oblique inguinal hernia: typical operation for its cure. *JAMA* 1899;33:6.
18. Filipi CJ, Fitzgibbons RJ, Salerno GM, et al. Laparoscopic herniorrhaphy. *Surg Clin North Am* 1992;72:1109–1124.
19. Fulton JF. *Harvey Cushing: a biography.* Springfield, IL: Charles C. Thomas, 1946:141.
20. Ger R. The management of certain abdominal hernias by intra-abdominal closure of the neck of the sac. Preliminary communication. *Ann R Coll Surg Engl* 1982;64:342–344.
21. Ger R, Monroe K, Duvivier R, et al. Management of indirect inguinal hernias by laparoscopic closure of the neck of the sac. *Am J Surg* 1990;159:370–373.
22. Glassow F. The surgical repair of the inguinal and femoral hernias. *Can Med Assoc J* 1973;108:308–313.
23. Halsted WS. *Surgical papers by William Stewart Halsted: the operative treatment of inguinal hernia,* vol 1. Baltimore: Johns Hopkins Press, 1924. (Special edition by The Classics of Surgery Library. Birmingham, AL: 1984.)
24. Henry AK. Operation for femoral hernia by a midline extraperitoneal approach: with a preliminary note on the use of this route for reducible inguinal hernia. *Lancet* 1936;1:531.
25. *Hippocratic writings.* Edited with an introduction by GER Lloyd. New York: Penguin Books, 1983. Chadwick J, Mann WN, translators.
26. Jennings WK, Anson BJ. A new method for repair of indirect inguinal hernia considered in reference to parietal anatomy. *Surg Gynecol Obstet* 1942;74:697.
27. LaRoque GP. The intra-abdominal method of removing inguinal and femoral hernia. *Arch Surg* 1932;24:189.
28. Leonardo RA. *History of surgery.* New York: Froben Press, 1943.
29. Lichtenstein IL, Shulman AG, Amid PK, et al. The tension-free hernioplasty. *Am J Surg* 1989;157:188–193.
30. Lotheissen G. Radikaloperation der Schekelhernien. *Zentralbl Chir* 1898;25:548.
31. Lyons AS, Petrucelli RJ II. *Medicine: an illustrated history.* New York: Harry N. Abrams Publishers, 1987.
32. Malangoni MA, Condon RE. Preperitoneal repair of acute incarcerated and estrangulated hernias of the groin. *Surg Gynecol Obstet* 1986;162:65.
33. Marcy HO. The cure of hernia. *JAMA* 1887;8:589.
34. Marcy HO. *Hernia.* New York: Appleton, 1892.
35. Marti-Ibáñez F. *A pictorial history of medicine.* London: Spring Books, 1962:86.
36. McVay CB. Inguinal and femoral hernioplasty: the evaluation of a basic concept. *Ann Surg* 1958;148:499.
37. McVay CB. Preperitoneal hernioplasty. *Surg Gynecol Obstet* 1966;123:349–350.
38. McVay CB. The anatomical basis for inguinal and femoral hernioplasty. *Surg Gynecol Obstet* 1974;139:931–935.
39. McVay C, Anson BJ. Inguinal and femoral hernioplasty. *Surg Gynecol Obstet* 1949;88:473.
40. Meade RH. The history of the abdominal approach to hernia repair. *Surgery* 1965;57:908.
41. Moran RM, Blick M, Collura M. Double layer of transversalis fascia for repair of inguinal hernia. *Surgery* 1968;63:423–429.
42. Nyhus LM. The preperitoneal approach and iliopubic tract repair of inguinal hernia. In: Nyhus LM, Condon RE, eds. *Hernia,* 2nd ed. Philadelphia: JB Lippincott, 1978.
43. Nyhus LM. The recurrent groin hernia: therapeutic solutions. *World J Surg* 1989;13:541–544.
44. Nyhus LM. The preperitoneal approach and iliopubic tract repair of inguinal hernia. In: Nyhus LM, Condon RE, eds. *Hernia,* 3rd ed. Philadelphia: JB Lippincott, 1989:154–188.
45. Nyhus LM. Editor's comment. In: Nyhus LM, London RE, eds. *Hernia,* 3rd ed. Philadelphia: JB Lippincott, 1989:153.
46. Nyhus LM, Condon RE, Harkins HN. Clinical experiences with preperitoneal hernial repair for all types of hernia of the groin. *Am J Surg* 1960;100:234.
47. Nyhus LM, Klein MS, Rogers FB. Inguinal hernia. *Curr Probl Surg* 1991;28:401–450.
48. Nyhus LM, Pollak R, Bombeck CT, et al. The preperitoneal approach and prosthetic buttress repair for recurrent hernia: the evolution of a technique. *Ann Surg* 1988;208:733–737.
49. Nyhus LM, Stevenson JK, Listerud MB, et al. Preperitoneal herniorrhaphy: a preliminary report in fifty patients. *West J Surg Obstet Gynecol* 1959;67:48.
50. Paré A. *The apologie and treatise: containing the voyages made into divers places with many of his writings upon surgery.* Edited with an introduction by G Keynes. London: Falcon Educational Books, 1951.
51. Patiño JF. Operación de Nyhus: hernioplastia preperitoneal. *Trib Médica (Bogotá)* 1992;86:62.
52. Patiño JF, García-Herreros LG, Zundel N, et al. Hernioplastia preperitoneal con prótesis. *Rev Colomb Cirugía* 1992;7:74.
53. Pifteau P. *Chirurgie de Guillaume de Salicet.* Toulouse: Imprimerie Saint-Cyprien, 1898.
54. Premuda L. The history of inguinal herniorrhaphy. *Int Surg* 1986;71:138–140.
55. Read RC. Preperitoneal exposure of inguinal herniation. *Am J Surg* 1968;116:653–658.
56. Read RC. Marcy's priority in the development of inguinal herniorrhaphy. *Surgery* 1980;88:682–685.
57. Read RC. The development of inguinal herniorrhaphy. *Surg Clin North Am* 1984;64:185–196.
58. Read RC. The centenary of Bassini's contribution to inguinal herniorrhaphy. *Am J Surg* 1987;153:324–326.
59. Rignault DP. Properitoneal prosthetic inguinal hernioplasty

through a Pfannenstiel approach. *Surg Gynecol Obstet* 1986;163: 465–468.

60. Rosenthal D, Walters MJ. Preperitoneal synthetic mesh placement for recurrent hernias of the groin. *Surg Gynecol Obstet* 1986;163:285–286.

61. Shearburn EW, Myers RN. Shouldice repair for inguinal hernia. *Surgery* 1969;66:450–459.

62. Stoppa RE. The treatment of complicated groin and incisional hernias. *World J Surg* 1989;13:545–554.

63. Stoppa RE, Rives JL, Warlaumont CR, et al. The use of Dacron in the repair of hernias of the groin. *Surg Clin North Am* 1984;64:269–285.

63a. Stromayr, K. *Die Handschrift des Schmitt-und Augenarztes*. Lindau in Bodensee, July 4, 1559. Reprinted, Berlin: Idra-Verlagsanstalt Gmbh, 1925.

64. Summers JE. Classical herniorrhaphies of Bassini, Halsted and Ferguson. *Am J Surg* 1947;73:87.

65. Wantz GE. The operation of Bassini as described by Attilio Catterina. *Surg Gynecol Obstet* 1989;168:67–80.

66. Wantz GE. The Canadian repair of inguinal hernia. In: Nyhus LM, Condon RE, eds. *Hernia*, 3rd ed. Philadelphia: JB Lippincott, 1989:236–252.

67. Zimmerman LM, Veith I. *Great ideas in the history of surgery*. Baltimore: Williams & Wilkins, 1961.

SPECIAL COMMENTS

Lloyd M. Nyhus

The distinguished surgeon–historian José Felix Patiño has given us a detailed, precise review of the history of hernia studies from the ancients to the present. I particularly am pleased that he was willing to undertake this task. Patiño preceded me as President of the International Society of Surgery (1989–91), thus giving us the opportunity to work together for the furtherance of the Society and to discuss in depth the many facets of the subject of hernia.

Olch and Harkins, in the first edition of Hernia *(1964), gave an interesting interpretation of events after Bassini. I paraphrase portions of their historic presentation. William S. Halsted (1852–1922) developed an operation similar to Bassini's for the treatment of inguinal hernias. Halsted at this time was Professor of Surgery at The Johns Hopkins School of Medicine. The major difference between Bassini's procedure and the Halsted operation was the transposition of the cord to a position above the external oblique aponeurosis. Minor technical differences included the ligation of superfluous veins about the cord to reduce its size and the sectioning of fibers of the internal oblique muscle and sometimes the transversus abdominis muscle to permit more lateral displacement of the internal ring. This procedure, commonly referred to as the Halsted I procedure* (to differentiate it from the procedure later adopted by Halsted in which the cord was not transposed, the Halsted II procedure)*, was first mentioned in a brief communication to The Johns Hopkins Medical Society in 1889 and published in* The Bulletin of the Johns Hopkins Hospital *("The Radical Cure of Hernia," 1889;1:12). The first detailed description of the procedure was published in a paper, "The Radical Cure of Inguinal Hernia in the Male" (*Bull Johns Hopkins Hosp *1893;4:17). The Halsted II procedure is mentioned in Halsted's article entitled "The Cure of the More Difficult as Well as the Simpler Inguinal Ruptures" (*Bull Johns Hopkins Hosp *1903;14:208).*

*Ravitch (*Surgery *1986;100:59), in a Sherlock Holmes–type article, attempted to prove that Halsted himself had an inguinal hernia treated with a truss. Fortunately, Halsted appears to have had an umbilical hernia, so his name cannot be besmirched by association with the word* truss.

*Also incorporated in the Halsted II procedure was the imbrication of the flaps of the aponeurosis of the external oblique muscle in performing the closure. This principle of imbrication was first adopted and stressed by E. Wyllys Andrews (1856–1927) of Chicago, Professor of Surgery at the Northwestern University Medical School (*Chicago Med Rec *1895;9:67). The Halsted II procedure is also known as the* Ferguson–Andrews operation, *because of the two major surgical techniques involved: leaving the cord in its normal anatomic position, as proposed by Ferguson, and imbrication of the external oblique aponeurosis, as stressed by Andrews. The closure of multiple layers espoused by the Shouldice Clinic of Toronto is this imbrication technique* in extenso.

*The next landmark in inguinal hernia surgery was the use of the iliopectineal ligament (Cooper's ligament, ligamentum pubicum superius) to anchor the medial parietal wall in the repair. This ligament was first used by Georg Lotheissen (1868–1935) of Vienna in 1898 at the suggestion of Narath when he found the inguinal ligament destroyed in a patient with recurrent hernia. He successfully substituted the iliopectineal ligament and repeated the procedure in a series of 12 patients (*Zentralbl Chir *1898;25:548). This innovation was ignored until it was revived by Seelig and Tuholske (*Surg Gynecol Obstet *1914;18:55). The publications of Chester B. McVay and Barry J. Anson (*Surg Gynecol Obstet *1942;74:746; 1949;88:473) led to widespread use of this technique. The contributions of McVay to the repair were so great that it was named the* McVay repair *by Henry Harkins (*Surgery *1942;12:364), and this eponym has been widely adopted.*

*Annandale (*Edinburgh Med J *1876;21:1087) is often quoted in the literature as being the first to use Cooper's ligament in hernial repair. As Koontz showed in his excellent historic analysis of the development of the surgical treatment of femoral hernia (*Surgery *1963;53:551), this is an example of requoting without consulting the original reference. Actually, Annandale used neither Cooper's nor Poupart's ligament in his somewhat esoteric repair of a combined direct–indirect inguinal hernia.*

*The recognition of the importance of the posterior inguinal wall as it relates to both the cause and the treatment of hernia is credited to many authors. One of the strongest presentations in favor of the fascia transversalis as a key factor in the anatomy of hernia was by Harrison (*Arch Surg *1920;4:680). Paul W. Harrison (1883–1962; Fig. 3.6) worked for more than 40 years as a missionary doctor to the people of the Persian Gulf and Saudi Arabia. His early training in the Hunterian laboratory of Harvey Cushing is reflected in the list of other origi-*

nal investigations that were undertaken literally on the sands of the desert: (a) his successful fixation of a femoral fracture with an intramedullary nail of "teak" wood; (b) his early success with the original treatment of aneurysm by cellophane fibrosis; and (c) his development of the concept and clinical trial in 1948 of an aortic Venturi valve in the treatment of ascites.

Another ligament, the iliopubic tract, is important to the full understanding of hernial repair. Depicted by Hesselbach (Neueste anatomischpathologische Untersuchungen über den Ursprung and das Fortschreiten der Leisten and Schenkelbrüche. *Würzburg: Baumgärtner, 1814*) and described by Thomson later during the same century, its use was advocated in the anterior approach by Clark and Hashimoto (Surg Gynecol Obstet *1946;82:480*) and by Griffith (Surg Clin North Am *1959;39:531*). The importance of the iliopubic tract in the preperitoneal approach to repair has been emphasized by Nyhus and associates.

Several good historic articles on hernia are:

Carlson RI. The historical development of the surgical treatment of inguinal hernia. Surgery *1956;39:1031.*

Ravitch MM. The great Boston hernia controversy concerning the permanent cure of reducible hernia or rupture. Bull NY Acad Med *1969;45:767–798.*

Rutkow IM. A selective history of groin herniorrhaphy in the 20th century. Surg Clin North Am *1993;73:395–411.*

Dr. Henry N. Harkins (Fig. 3.7) was a coeditor of the first edition of Hernia. The study of hernia held his interest for almost 3 decades. It is appropriate to comment briefly on his life.

Henry N. Harkins was born in Missoula, Montana, on July 13, 1905. In 1912, the family moved to Chicago, where his father, William Draper Harkins, became the Andrew MacLeish Distinguished Service Professor of Physical Chemistry at the University of Chicago. After graduating from the University of Chicago in 1925 with a major in chemistry and a minor in mathematics, he entered Rush Medical College in 1924, graduated in 1930, and received his medical doctorate after a 2-year rotating internship at Presbyterian Hospital. During this active developmental period in Dr. Harkins' life, he also earned a master of science degree in chemistry in 1926 and a PhD in medicine in 1928, both from the University of Chicago.

Dr. Harkins' surgical residency (1931–36) was completed at the University of Chicago Clinics under the guidance of Dr. Dallas Phemister.

Dr. Harkins spent 4 years as an associate surgeon at the Henry Ford Hospital in Detroit. At Henry Ford, he first became interested in the surgical treatment of varicose veins and hernia, interests that resulted in many original contributions to the medical literature.

In 1943, Dr. Harkins returned to full academic pursuits at The Johns Hopkins University School of Medicine. His relatively short association (1943–47) with Alfred Blalock made a deep impression on Dr. Harkins. In subsequent years, he combined the best of two schools of surgical thought as a guide to the practice of surgery—the Phemister school and the Halsted–Blalock school.

In 1947, Dr. Harkins accepted the position of Chairman of the Department of Surgery at the University of Washington School of Medicine in Seattle. Under his leadership, the department became recognized as one of the finest in the world. In subsequent years, Dr. Harkins' students occupied chairs of surgery at ten universities: Robert E. Condon, the Medical Col-

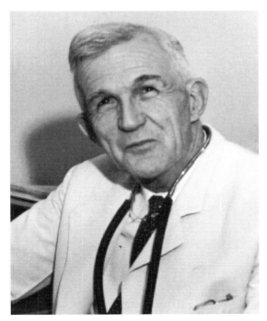

FIGURE 3.6. Paul W. Harrison (1883–1962).

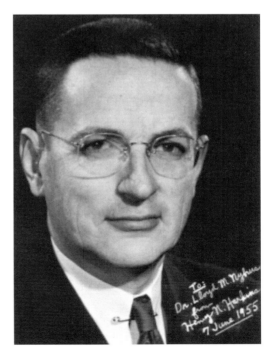

FIGURE 3.7. Henry N. Harkins (1905–1967).

lege of Wisconsin; Keith A. Kelly, Mayo Medical School; Robert W. Barnes, the University of Arkansas; J. Roland Folse, Southern Illinois University; the late John E. Jesseph, Indiana University; Ryoichi Tsuchiya, Nagasaki University, Japan; Jean E. Murat, the University of Tours; Hitoshi Mohri, Yamaguchi University; Teruaki Aoki, Jikei University; and Lloyd M. Nyhus, the University of Illinois.

In 1993, the Henry N. Harkins Chair of Surgery was established at the University of Washington, Seattle, to honor this surgical educator in perpetuity.

Nyhus and Condon's Hernia, Fifth Edition, edited by Robert J. Fitzgibbons, Jr. and A. Gerson Greenburg. Lippincott Williams & Wilkins, Philadelphia © 2002.

4

HISTORIC ASPECTS OF GROIN HERNIA REPAIR

JOHN E. SKANDALAKIS
GENE L. COLBORN
LEE J. SKANDALAKIS
DAVID A. MCCLUSKY III

But if phisitions [physicians] be angry, that I have wryten phisike in englyshe, let theym remembre, that the grekes wrate in greke, the Romanes in latyne. Auicena, and the others in Arabike, whiche were their owne propre and maternal tonges...but those, although they were painimes [pagans] and Jewes, in this parte of charitye they farre surmountid us Christianes, that they wolde not have soo necessary a knowledge as phisicke is, to be hyd frome them, whych wolde be studiouse aboute it.

 —Sir Thomas Elyot (16)

Between the idea
And the reality
Between the motion
And the act
Falls the Shadow
 —Thomas Stearnes Eliot (15)

The history of hernia, one of the most beautiful chapters in the triumphs of anatomy and surgery, is replete with ideas and realities, myths and facts, transmutations and shadows.

The history of hernia *in toto* is as old as the human race. To name all the authors, investigators, and real pioneers of groin anatomy and surgical technique for repair of inguinal and femoral hernia is beyond the scope of this presentation. However, "after centuries of some success and much failure" (60), we note that every period opened avenues for a better understanding.

J. E. Skandalakis and **L.J. Skandalakis:** Centers for Surgical Anatomy & Technique, Emory University School of Medicine; Department of Surgery, Piedmont Hospital, Atlanta, Georgia.

G. L. Colborn: Department of Anatomical Sciences, Ross University School of Medicine, Commonwealth of Dominica, West Indies.

D. A. McClusky III: Department of Surgery, Emory University School of Medicine, Atlanta, Georgia.

ANCIENT AND GRAECO–ROMAN ERAS

In Mesopotamia, the territory between the Euphrates and Tigris rivers (now Iraq), doctors around 4000 B.C. knew about herniotomy (25).

There is a reference in the Ebers medical papyrus (circa 1550–1600 B.C.) that is believed to describe an inguinal hernia:

"VI. Instructions concerning a swelling of the flesh in any limb [part] of the man: If thou examinest a swelling of the flesh in any limb of a man, and thou findest it like the skin of his body, and when it has been rubbed, it goes and comes on account of thy fingers and both [movements] that have arisen in it stop . . ." (14).

The mummy of Pharaoh Merneptah (1215 B.C.) had a large scar on the groin, with the scrotum completely separated from the body (76). When the mummy of Ramses V (1157 B.C.) was examined, it was found to have a scrotal hernia or a hydrocele, or perhaps both (60). Oppenheimer reported that Nestor (believed to be the king of Pylos who took part in the Trojan Wars) perhaps had a hernia (60).

Ancient Hindu surgeons treated hernia by severing the sac and by cautery (76). They employed four techniques of cauterization: the ring, dot, lateral or slanting lines, or rubbing mode (20).

Heliodorus ("Sun's gift") was the surgeon who performed the first hernia operation. He separated the sac from the cord, twisted off the sac, ligated the vessels, but did not touch the testicles and did not reconstruct the posterior wall of the inguinal canal (70).

Aulus Cornelius Celsus (25 B.C. to A.D. 50) was most likely the first medical writer, and not himself a surgeon, although some authors consider him to have been an operator. In the seventh of the eight books that comprise *De Medicina*, he discussed "cures by the hand" (surgery), groin anatomy, and the etiology and pathology of hernias (8):

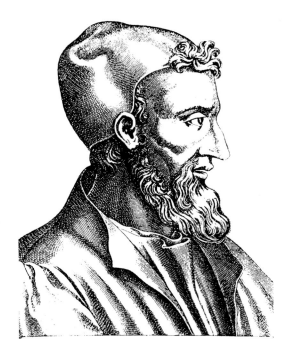

FIGURE 4.1. Galen.

Now sometimes the inguinal region has to be cut into, some-times the scrotum . . . after stretching the scrotum, so that the skin of the groin is rendered tense, the cut is made below the abdominal cavity, where the membranes below are continuous with the abdominal wall. Now the laying open is to be done boldly, until the outer tunic, that of the scrotum itself, is cut through, and the middle tunic reached. When an incision has been made, an opening presents leading deeper. Into this the index finger of the left hand is introduced, in order that by the separation of the intervening little membranes the hernial sac may be freed. Next the assistant grasping the scrotum with his left hand should stretch it upwards, and draw it away as far as possible from the groins, at first including the testicle itself until the surgeon cuts away with the scalpel all the fine membranes which are above the middle tunic if he is unable to separate it with his finger; the testicle is let go in order that it may slip downwards, and show in the wound and then be pushed out by the surgeon's fingers, and laid along with its two tunics upon the abdominal wall. There whatever is diseased is cut round and away . . . . The testicle havi\ng been thus cleared is to be gently returned through the incision along with the veins and arteries and its cord; and it must be seen that blood does not drop down into the scrotum, or a clot remain anywhere. This will be accom-plished if the surgeon takes the precaution of tying the blood vessels; the threads with which the ends of these are tied should hang out of the wound; following upon suppuration they will fall off painlessly. Through the margins of the wound itself two pins are then passed, and over this an agglutinating dressing.

For some peculiar reason, Hippocrates (460–370 B.C.) mentions only inguinal hernias in children. He may have been familiar with hernia cerebri. Chadwick suggests that Hippocrates knew something about pediatric hernia of congenital origin (9).

Attempts to reduce strangulated hernias were made as early as 400 B.C. by Praxagoras of Cos, who practiced taxis (manual replacement) as treatment (80). Praxagoras thought that strangulation was a hardening of the herniated intestinal loop (60). Aretaios of Cappadocia in A.D. 50 described ileus secondary to strangulated hernia (25).

Around A.D. 200, Galen stated that peritoneal rupture is the cause of herniation, a belief that survived for 1,000 years until Guy de Chauliac decided this was not the case. Galen's work dominated medicine for centuries (Fig. 4.1) (25). The respect Galen's teachings commanded is demonstrated by the following anagram: "A Viennese monk called Abraham of Santa Clara (1644–1709) tried to inspire the sick care of his day with the following words: 'The most famous doctor was named Galenus. If one juggles the letters, one gets Angelus, meaning an angel—and that is what every doctor ought to be'" (25). By all means, Galen was great, perhaps one of the greatest physicians for fifteen centuries, but not an angel.

MIDDLE AGES

Oribasius performed herniotomies in the fourth century A.D. Aetius of Amida, sixth century A.D., treated hernia patients with a plaster, a bandage, and a prayer (60).

Paul of Aegina (A.D. ?607 or 625–90), Greece–Alexandria, Egypt performed hernia surgery using double ligation and excision en masse of cord, sac, and testicle. He used the term "enterocele" if the sac contained intestine, "epiplocele" if it contained omentum (from the Greek *epiploon,* meaning omentum), and "hydroenteroepiplocele" if it contained intestine, omentum, and fluid (82). Paul of Aegina described his operation:

> One makes an incision the length of three fingers' width in the inguinal region above the swelling. One separates the skin and the fat and exposes the peritoneum and pushes aside the intestines with the tip of a sound. The bulges of the peri-toneum which are formed on two sides of the sound are united with sutures after the sound is withdrawn; one does not cut the peritoneum or touch the testicles, but one proceeds simply to the treatment of the wound (7).

In the thirteenth century, William of Salicet (1210–77 or 1280?) advocated double ligation and division of the sac, preferring knife to cautery. He said, "All is owed to Nature—the doctor is merely her servant," and recom-mended that the testicle not be removed "as some stupid and ignorant doctors do" (25).

In the fourteenth century, Mondino de Luzzi (Mundi-nus) (1275–1327) described a "radical cure of hernia" in his book on dissection, *Anathomia*. If Mundinus were with us today, he would note that, despite tremendous progress, the ideal cure of hernia still eludes us.

Guido Lanfranchi (Lanfranc) (d. 1315) advocated con-servative treatment for hernias. He performed occasional orchiectomies but was inspired by God to save the testicle

(25). Roland of Parma (1383) recommended the Trende-lenburg position (7).

One of most important contributions of Guy de Chau-liac (1300–68) was rescuing the treatment of hernia from the hands of quacks (Fig. 4.2). He advocated conservative measures. After a regimen that consisted of laxatives, bloodletting, and forbidding foods such as wine, beans, fish, and cheese, he believed the doctor should manually reduce the hernia or let the patient hang by his legs. He then recommended a plaster over the "hernia gate" secured by a band to ensure reduction. The patient was then required to stay in bed for 50 days afterward (25). de Chauliac also operated on hernia using golden thread rather than cauterization (75).

Two statements of de Chauliac, the "Father of Surgery" (75), are immortal: "We are like children sitting on the neck of a giant—who see all that he sees and something besides," and "The same manner that the blinde man worketh in hewynge of a log, so doth a cyrurgen that knoweth not the nathomye" (20).

In his *Chirugia Magna,* de Chauliac is the first to recog-nize inguinal from femoral herniorrhaphy (58). He did not perform surgery, but treated inguinofemoral herniation by cauterization.

In 1412, Gerald of Metz (France) recommended a gold thread around the spermatic cord and the sac, preventing the viscera from traveling downward while permitting good blood supply to the testicles (60). Antonio Benivieni (?1440–1502) described various kinds of hernia in his book *De Abditis Morborum Causis* (The Hidden Causes of Ill-

nesses) (22). Another famous herniotomist was Horace of Norsia, a member of the Norsinin family of Italy, who per-formed 200 herniotomies in 1 year (60).

THE RENAISSANCE

In the sixteenth century, Caspar Stromayr (1559) of Lindan (Lake Leman), Germany produced 186 detailed watercolors to illustrate operations for the cure of hernia, and differen-tiated indirect, direct, and femoral hernias (7). Pierre Franco (1500–61), a Huguenot living in France, improved upon the hernia operation by incising the constricted neck of the sac with the help of a grooved director (22). He first advised orchidectomy, but later spared the testicles during herniotomy. Franco was the first to describe and perform an operation for strangulated hernia (66).

Humble surgeon Ambroise Paré (1510–90) advocated the use of trusses for hernia treatment, but did operate for incarcerated or strangulated hernias (82): "I did him the office of physician, apothecary, surgeon and cook. I dressed him to the end of his cure and God healed him . . . " (55). One night, Paré decided to go to Metz incognito; however, he was recognized by his comrades and "carried through the town in triumph" (Fig. 4.3) (21).

M.G. Purmann (1649–1711) of Silesia stated that if a hernia "could not be held even with the strongest and stur-diest bands at their right place," then surgery is indicated. The testicle and the vas were not to be injured. He did not incise the aponeurosis of the external oblique muscle (68).

Heinrich Callisen's method of handling a constricted hernia was to bleed the patient until he fainted (*ad animi deliquarium*). He believed that with the patient in this con-dition, he could better reduce the hernia (25). Jacques Beaulieu (1651–1714) (Brother John of the nursery rhyme "Frère Jacques") performed more than 2,000 hernia repairs as he traveled from Amsterdam to Rome.

Lorenz Heister (1683–1758) differentiated direct from indirect hernia (58). At the age of 17, Heister observed surgery of the hernia and many other diseases performed by traveling quacks in the market (25):

> In the year 1700, at Easter Market, a boy of nine was brought there with hernia. His parents, unable to get any help from Frankfurt's famous physicians, were now begging for an oper-ation on the child. People of that sort do not try to treat her-nias with bandages since these seldom last longer than the mar-ket and can hardly cure a hernia in such a short time. They have another reason as well: a hernia bandage earns them only ten shillings, whereas an operation costs far more . . . so they always recommend an operation! This migrant doctor took in the patient, gave him a laxative and operated . . .

We are indebted to Heister for the following statement: "It is necessary for a surgeon to have complete, or at least very good, knowledge in anatomy as well as in medicine so that he has enough judgement and understanding to study

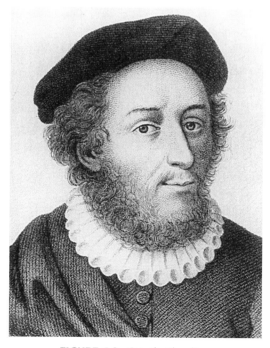

FIGURE 4.2. Guy de Chauliac.

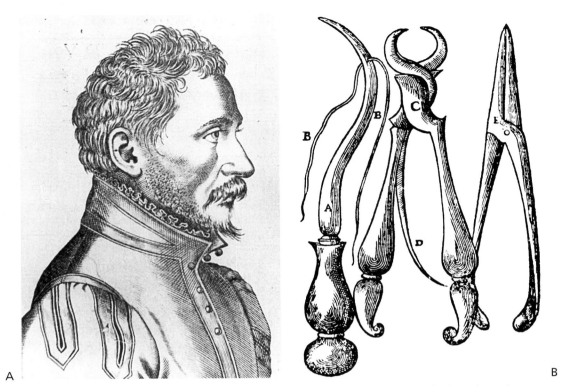

A   B

FIGURE 4.3. A: Ambroise Paré. **B:** The golden thread. (From Paré A. *The apologie and treatise.* New York: Dover, 1968. Keynes G, ed., with permission.)

all the causes and circumstances, and to draw his conclusions from them" (25).

The first account of a transabdominal approach to repair inguinal and femoral hernias was written by Demetrius de Cantemir, Prince of Moldavia, in 1743 after witnessing a hernia repair on his elderly secretary in Constantinople (47). An interesting documentation of hernia surgery in the Ottoman Empire can be seen in Fig. 4.4.

EIGHTEENTH CENTURY

In the eighteenth century, better information about hernial anatomy emerged. In Italy, Antonio Scarpa (1747 or 1752–1832) described the sliding hernia and also improved the technique of hernia repair. He is known for his description of Scarpa's fascia and many other anatomic entities (25,61). In 1754, Albrecht von Haller (1708–77) described congenital hernias (7). Percivall Pott (1714–88) in England correctly described the anatomy of congenital hernias and advised early surgery for constricted hernias (82). Pott's book *Treatise on Ruptures* (1757) described the anatomy and surgery as it was known at that time. According to Flack, he did not mention the preparations and dissections that John Hunter had demonstrated to him a few months earlier (20).

Pieter Camper (1722–89) in Holland reported Camper's fascia and the surgical anatomy of inguinal hernia (22). John

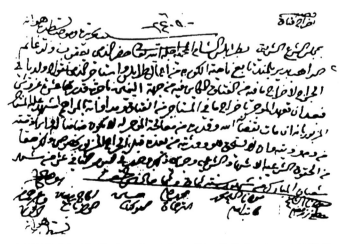

FIGURE 4.4. Medical contract from Tripoli. Date corresponds to November 10, 1677. Partial translation: "Extraction of hernia of the Christian Ya'acoub, son of Ghanim, by the Christian Nichola, son of Yani, on the twelfth day of the month of the Sha'ban, of the year one thousand and eighty eight . . . the Christian Yacoub . . . hired and engaged the Christian surgeon Nichola . . . to extract his (Yacoub's) hernia on the right side for a fee of ten piasters." (From Ajlouni KM. History of informed medical consent [Letter]. *Lancet* 1995;346:980, with permission.)

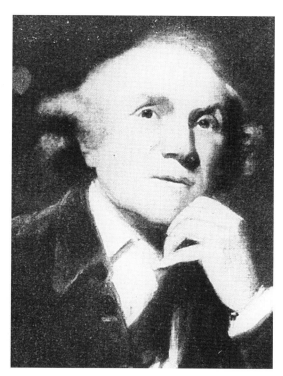

FIGURE 4.5. John Hunter.

Hunter (1728–93) (Fig. 4.5) emphasized the presence of the processus vaginalis and the gubernaculum testis (71). Antonio de Gimbernat (1734–1818) in Portugal divided the ligament named for him to treat strangulation or incarceration of femoral hernia (13). Franz K. Hesselbach (1759–1816) in Germany described Hesselbach's triangle, the home of the direct and external supravesical hernia (Fig. 4.6) (54).

Astley Paston Cooper (1768–1841) is recognized as one of the fathers of modern hernia surgery (Fig. 4.7). He stated, "No disease of the human body, belonging to the province of the surgeon, requires in its treatment a greater combination of accurate anatomical knowledge, with surgical skill, than hernia in all its varieties." Cooper described the ligament of Cooper (pectineal), the cremasteric fascia, and the fascia transversalis (60). He wrote, "the transversalis fascia will be found to consist of two portions, the outer . . . and another structure between [the internal oblique and transversus muscles] and the peritoneum" (11).

NINETEENTH CENTURY

New techniques evolved during the nineteenth century as the understanding of anatomy improved. Bogros (1786–1825) was a French anatomist and surgeon who described a triangular space in the iliac region (6). In 1817, Jules-Germain Cloquet (1780–1883) observed that the processus vaginalis was rarely closed by birth. He also described the iliopubic tract (61). John Gay (1791–1870) described the femoral sheath and femoral canal (40).

There are three persons in the literature with the name of Retzius. Magnus Gustav Retzius was a histologist. Magnus Christian Retzius was an otologist. Anders Adolph Retzius described the retropubic space or cave of Retzius (36). According to Read (63), Retzius in 1858 described "a transversalis fascial lining to his perivesical space."

Bogros published his thesis about the space of Bogros in 1823 (6). In 1858, Retzius (64) wrote about the area known as the space of Retzius. While there is an anatomic relation between both spaces, which are very close neighbors (Bogros'

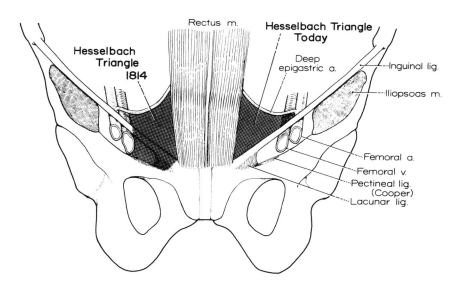

FIGURE 4.6. Left: The triangle described by Hesselbach in 1814. **Right:** The slightly smaller triangle accepted today. (From Skandalakis PN, Skandalakis LJ, Gray SW, et al. Supravesical hernia. In: Nyhus LM, Condon RE, eds. *Hernia*, 4th ed. Philadelphia: JB Lippincott, 1995:400, with permission.)

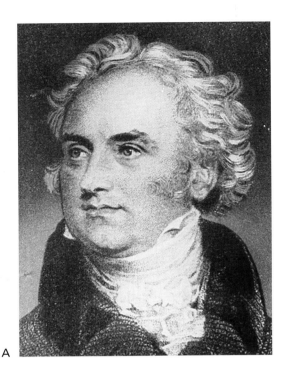

A

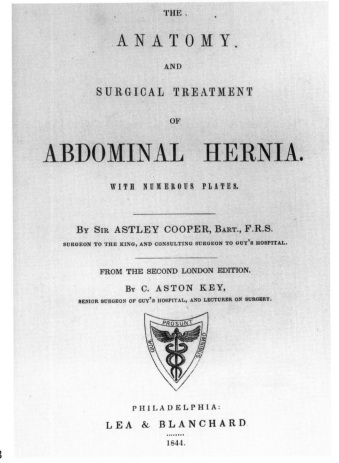

THE

ANATOMY,

AND

SURGICAL TREATMENT

OF

ABDOMINAL HERNIA.

WITH NUMEROUS PLATES.

By Sir ASTLEY COOPER, Bart., F.R.S.

SURGEON TO THE KING, AND CONSULTING SURGEON TO GUY'S HOSPITAL.

FROM THE SECOND LONDON EDITION.

By C. ASTON KEY,

SENIOR SURGEON OF GUY'S HOSPITAL, AND LECTURER ON SURGERY.

PHILADELPHIA:

LEA & BLANCHARD.

1844.

B

FIGURE 4.7. A: Sir Astley Cooper. **B:** Title page of book. (From personal collection of John E. Skandalakis.)

space is an extension of Retzius' space), we do not think that Retzius had any knowledge of the work of Bogros.

Joseph Pancost (1805–82) was credited with "the honor of the discovery of the subcutaneous operation and method of curing hernia, by injection" (79).

While Read (62) credits Thomas Annandale with pioneering modern transperitoneal surgery, we agree with both Koontz (34) and Nyhus (53) that Annandale's operation should not be included in the annals of history of hernia repair.

Georg Lotheissen (1868–1935) of Austria was the first to use Cooper's ligament for repair (52). Just Lucas-Championniere (1843–1913) advised incision of the aponeurosis of the external oblique from the external ring to the arc of the internal ring, and removal of the peritoneal sac (38). Perhaps Lucas-Championniere was the first, or among the first, to perform high ligation of the sac at the deep inguinal ring.

Edoardo Bassini (1844–1924) (Fig. 4.8), the father of modern herniorrhaphy, ligated and resected the sac. We believe that the great Italian was the first to present to the surgical profession this technique for the surgical treatment of inguinal hernia. He recommended approximation with interrupted sutures of the layer of the internal oblique transverse abdominus muscles and transversalis fascia to the shelving border of the inguinal ligament, leaving the cord under the aponeurosis of the external oblique. He advised, "Considering all that is written about the radical treatment of the inguinal hernia up until now, it can be somewhat risky to try to publish more about this subject" (3). All modern modifications of hernia repair spring from the original Bassini repair.

Thorwald (76), in a fictional account of great moments in the history of surgery, gives this thrilling vision of Bassini at work:

> He incised the skin and the hypodermic tissue below the protruding hernia . . . . A new incision opened the inguinal canal and the aponeurosis of the obliquus externus to high above the inner inguinal ring . . . . The hernial sac bulged out, alongside the vas deferens, which had been forced to one side, out of its normal position. Cautiously, Bassini plucked the vas deferens from the hernial sac and raised the latter. He opened it and found a loop of intestine. Carefully, he freed a few adhesions and pushed the intestine back through the ruptured wall into the abdominal cavity. Then he ligated the sac close to the rupture, severed the empty sac, sewed the ligatured spot, and let it likewise drop back into the abdominal cavity.
>
> This is what many surgeons before him had already done in the same or a similar manner. Now the crucial new phase of the operation began. [An assistant] lifted the vas deferens high above the incision. With extremely careful movements Bassini exposed the lower posterior edges of the oblique abdominal muscle. He drew it down, pushed it under the vas deferens, and brought it up to the lower edge of Poupart's ligament. Each phase of the operation made the futilities of earlier surgery seem altogether incredible. Already Bassini was beginning his suture. He used silk thread, and did one button stitch after the other. Close to the pubic bone he took two sutures in the rectus abdominis muscle. Immediately

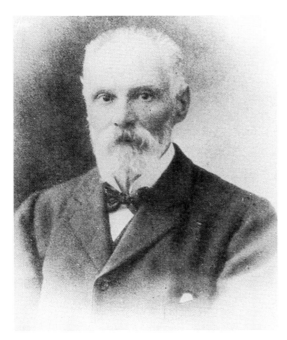

FIGURE 4.8. Edoardo Bassini.

afterward the new abdominal wall lay before us, taut and visibly strong.

Bassini nodded to one of his assistants. The young doctor took a feather and introduced it into the patient's throat. Almost immediately, the patient gagged and began to cough violently. His intestines and all the muscles of the abdomen convulsed. I stared at the sutures in the newly formed abdominal wall. Would they really resist such strain?

My concern was needless. The abdominal wall remained taut and tight until the coughing ceased. Bassini threw us a glance. [The assistant] allowed the vas deferens to slip back. He placed it on the new wall, and over it Bassini sewed the anterior surface of the aponeurosis. Then followed the skin sutures, and a light bandage. Bassini straightened up as the students in the stand applauded wildly.

In 1878, Hutchinson (30) opened the peritoneal cavity for a strangulated inguinal hernia. A decade later, Keetley (32) championed the carefully executed laparotomy:

When it is remembered that since Crompton hit upon the idea of performing laparotomy for the relief of strangulated hernia, no less than four other surgeons have revived the plan, each ignorant at the time of the labors of his predecessors, it will be acknowledged that, should this paper do nothing more than extend the knowledge of and call general attention to the procedure, it will not have been written entirely in vain.

Fenwick (17) commented on Keetley and laparotomy:

The operation is a novel one, and owes its origin to a suggestion of Mr. C.B. Keetley, who pointed out how much easier it is to draw a loop of bowel up than to press it back, piece by piece into the peritoneal cavity.

In 1886, Ward (78) advised a transabdominal approach, echoing Keetley and Fenwick: "What then, surgically

speaking, remains? Laparotomy." In 1887, Maunsell (46) operated on a strangulated femoral hernia by suprapubic laparotomy. He supported an intraperitoneal approach.

William Stewart Halsted (1852–1922) (Fig. 4.9) reported two types of herniorrhaphy that differed in the positioning of the spermatic cord: in Halsted I the cord is under the skin, and in Halsted II it is under the repair. In both types, the repair is similar to Bassini's and consists of creating one layer by suturing the aponeurosis of the external oblique muscle, internal oblique muscle, transversus abdominis muscle, and transversalis fascia to the transversalis fascia, Poupart's ligament, and aponeurotic fiber of the external oblique (52). In 1903, Halsted reported the use of the hinged pedicle graft of anterior rectus sheath as well as the sliding graft (25).

Olch and Harkins (54) presented highly diagrammatic drawings to demonstrate some historic aspects of hernia repair (Fig. 4.10).

Robert Lawson Tait (1845–99) developed a repair of the femoral hernia from within the peritoneal cavity. In 1891, Tait (74), Professor of Gynecology at Queen's College (Birmingham), reported:

. . . I opened the abdomen, removed the tumour, and then attacked the hernia from within.

After undoing the adhesions with great ease, I pulled in what I certainly never could have pushed in. Of course, I might have cut all the omentum away, and thus, in a clumsy manner, have gotten over the difficulty; but had it been an intestinal protrusion, or had there been intestines in the protrusion adherent as the omentum was, this rough and ready

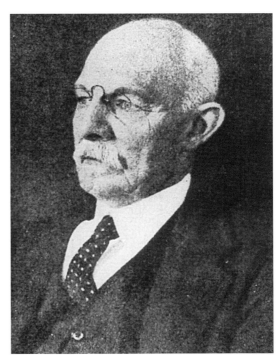

FIGURE 4.9. William Stewart Halsted.

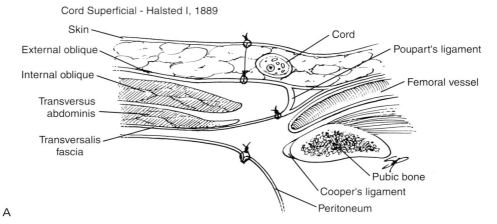

Cord Superficial - Halsted I, 1889

Skin
External oblique
Internal oblique
Transversus abdominis
Transversalis fascia
Cord
Poupart's ligament
Femoral vessel
Pubic bone
Cooper's ligament
Peritoneum

A

Cord Intermediate - Bassini, 1888

Skin
External oblique
Internal oblique
Transversus abdominis
Transversalis fascia
Cord
Poupart's ligament
Femoral vessel
Pubic bone
Cooper's ligament
Peritoneum

B

Cord Intermediate (Imbricated) - Lucas - Championniere, 1892; Andrews 1895

Skin
External oblique
Internal oblique
Transversus abdominis
Transversalis fascia
Cord
Poupart's ligament
Femoral vessel
Pubic bone
Cooper's ligament
Peritoneum

C

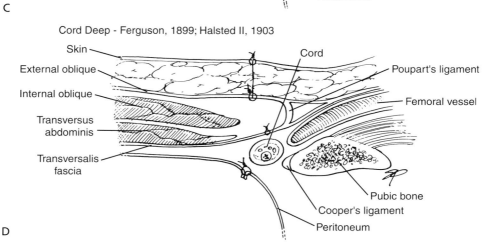

Cord Deep - Ferguson, 1899; Halsted II, 1903

Skin
External oblique
Internal oblique
Transversus abdominis
Transversalis fascia
Cord
Poupart's ligament
Femoral vessel
Pubic bone
Cooper's ligament
Peritoneum

D

Cooper's Ligament Repair - Lotheissen, 1898; McVay 1941

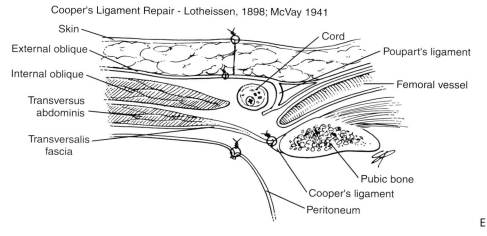

E

Iliopubic Tract Repair for Direct Hernia by the Preperitoneal Approach
NYHUS 1959

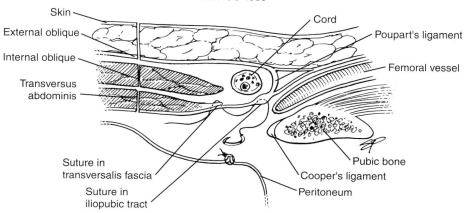

F

Iliopubic Tract Repair for Femoral Hernia by the Preperitoneal Approach
NYHUS 1959

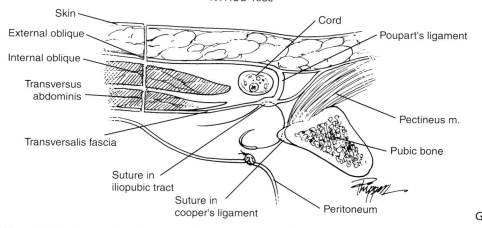

G

FIGURE 4.10. Parasagittal diagrammatic representations of groin hernia repairs. **A:** Cord superficial to the external oblique anastomosis. **B:** Cord in intermediate position between external oblique aponeurosis and fused transversus abdominis aponeurosis and transversalis fascia. **C:** Cord in intermediate position with imbrication between layers of external oblique aponeurosis. **D:** Cord deep to fused transversus abdominis aponeurosis and transversalis fascia. **E:** Cord in intermediate position and fused transversus abdominis aponeurosis and transversalis fascia sutured to Cooper's ligament. **F** and **G:** Direct (**F**) and femoral hernia (**G**). Preperitoneal approach for iliopubic tract repair. (From Olch PD, Harkins HN. Historical survey of the treatment of inguinal hernia. In: Nyhus LM, Harkins HN, eds. *Hernia.* Philadelphia: JB Lippincott, 1964:8, with permission.)

settlement of the case would not have been open to me, and no process known to me could have got intestine back into the abdomen under such circumstances as those before me, save gentle and continuous traction from within. Upon this point I am not speaking from theory but from experience of a considerable number of cases where, in the course of an ovariotomy, I have corrected the displacement of a previously irreducible hernia, and have completely and permanently closed the abnormal tendinous aperture.

Tait stated, "I have the impression that the radical cure of herniae, other than umbilical, will by-and-by, be undertaken by abdominal section."

E.W. Andrews used an imbrication repair for inguinal hernia, reporting the following advantages: "1. A large strong flap of any needed size to fill the internal ring. 2. Triplicate layers of aponeurosis. 3. Interlocking of layers giving broad surfaces of union. 4. Shortening of anterior as well as posterior wall of canal making them mutually supporting and relieving tension on deep structures. 5. Cord amply protected" (1).

In 1899, A.H. Ferguson warned surgeons to "leave the cord alone for it is the sacred highway along which travel vital elements indispensable to the perpetuity of our race" (18).

TWENTIETH CENTURY

In the early part of the twentieth century, several innovators improved upon the treatment of hernia. Henry O. Marcy (1837–1924), an American, performed a procedure that, for all practical purposes, was a closure of the internal ring (44):

> Having divided the external tissues to a sufficient extent, draw up the peritoneal pouch quite sufficient to cause its obliteration upon the inner side and sew it evenly with fine tendon sutures by the so-called shoemaker's stitch. This encloses all the peritoneum and occludes it . . . . Then cut away the redundant pouch and allow the peritoneum to drop back, in order not to include it in the deep suturing of the tendinous structures.

Halsted wrote: "Bassini was first . . . . Marcy never accepted Bassini's priority and labored with the help of friends to alter the history of this event, but to no avail" (26). Marcy's place in medical history has been secured by several advances: reconstruction of the internal ring, antiseptic use of animal sutures, and high ligation of the hernial sac (42,43). His compendious 1892 book is still a storehouse of information (Fig. 4.11) (45).

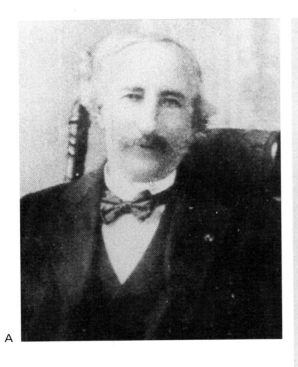

THE

ANATOMY AND SURGICAL TREATMENT

OF

HERNIA

BY

HENRY O. MARCY, A.M., M.D., LL.D.

OF BOSTON

PRESIDENT OF THE AMERICAN MEDICAL ASSOCIATION ; SURGEON TO THE HOSPITAL FOR WOMEN, CAMBRIDGE ;
PRESIDENT OF THE SECTION OF GYNÆCOLOGY, NINTH INTERNATIONAL CONGRESS ;
LATE PRESIDENT OF THE AMERICAN ACADEMY OF MEDICINE ; MEMBER OF THE BRITISH MEDICAL ASSOCIATION ;
MEMBER OF THE MASSACHUSETTS MEDICAL SOCIETY ;
HONORARY MEMBER OF THE NEW YORK STATE MEDICAL ASSOCIATION ; FELLOW OF THE BOSTON GYNÆCOLOGICAL SOCIETY ;
CORRESPONDING MEMBER OF THE MEDICO-CHIRURGICAL SOCIETY OF BOLOGNA, ITALY ;
MEMBER OF THE AMERICAN ASSOCIATION OF OBSTETRICIANS AND GYNÆCOLOGISTS ;
FELLOW OF THE SOUTHERN SURGICAL AND GYNÆCOLOGICAL ASSOCIATION ;
LATE SURGEON UNITED STATES ARMY ; ETC.

*WITH SIXTY-SIX FULL-PAGE HELIOTYPE AND LITHOGRAPHIC PLATES, INCLUDING
EIGHT COLORED PLATES FROM BOUGERY,
AND THIRTY-SEVEN ILLUSTRATIONS IN THE TEXT*

NEW YORK
D. APPLETON AND COMPANY
1892

FIGURE 4.11. A: Henry O. Marcy. **B:** Title page of book. (From personal collection of John E. Skandalakis.)

A

B

LaRoque (35) summarized an era of innovation in 1919:

The importance of standardization of methods in operative surgery is sufficiently obvious to need no emphasis. Within the past 20 years permanent cures of inguinal hernia, following operation at the hands of good surgeons in proper hospitals, have increased to between 90 and 95 per cent of all cases operated upon. These improvements are due largely to more widely diffused comprehension of the purposes to be accomplished by operative treatment and to the standardization of methods of operative procedure. So long, however, as the standard methods of operating for hernia by qualified surgeons shall fail to cure 10 or 1 percent of cases, surgical efficiency is less than 100 per cent perfect and it is desirable to make improvements upon even the standard methods of procedure. After all, standard methods are only the best by test of available methods. No method is better than its results and these are not best if they can be made any better.

In 1920 and 1921, G.L. Cheatle presented articles in the *British Medical Journal* with the respective titles, "An Operation for the Radical Cure of Inguinal and Femoral Hernia" (1920;2:68), and "An Operation for Inguinal Hernia" (1921;2:1025). Cheatle explored both inguinal areas by utilizing a lower midline or Pfannenstiel incision (61). We agree with Read (62) that Cheatle was the first to describe the preperitoneal procedure.

Using a midline incision, Cheatle entered Retzius' space. By a lateral rectus-splitting incision, he retracted the muscle laterally. He closed the internal ring with sutures. In a different operation 1 year later, Cheatle used a Pfannenstiel incision for the exploration of the preperitoneal space and repair of inguinofemoral herniation. At that time, he ligated the sac only. For indirect hernia and femoral hernia, he sutured flap periosteum of pubis to the inguinal ligament.

During the 1920s, J.P. Hoguet converted the direct peritoneal sac into an indirect sac by lateral traction of the peritoneum of the abdominal ring and relocation of the sac laterally to the deep epigastric artery, thus positioning the sac outside Hesselbach's triangle, thereby avoiding a possible urinary bladder injury (56).

A.K. Henry (1886–1962) performed femoral herniorrhaphies by using a pedicle of pectineus fascia. He is one of the pioneers of the midline extraperitoneal approach. In 1936, Henry (27) applied the Cheatle approach. High closure of the sac and fascial repair (flap technique) were the characteristics of Henry's preperitoneal repair: "In a thin patient, as soon as my hand had displaced the peritoneum from beside the bladder, the view obtained of the four relevant structures, Gimbernat's ligament, the hinder edge of Poupart's, the fascia covering the pectineus and the external iliac vein was like that in a specimen prepared for a demonstration" (28). The preperitoneal operation for inguinofemoral herniation was known as the Cheatle–Henry procedure; today it is known as the Nyhus procedure. In 1942, Jennings et al. in the United States treated indirect hernia by suturing the transversalis fascia sling (31).

Musgrove and McCready sutured the inguinal ring to the iliopectineal ligament (50). McEvedy (39) sutured the conjoined tendon (area) to iliopectineal ligament. He expressed reservations about Henry's operation. Hull and Ganey sutured the inguinal ligament to the iliopectineal. They supported the Henry technique (29).

Mikkelsen and Berne (48) modified what they called the Cheatle operation by utilizing transversalis fascia and the aponeurosis of transversus abdominis muscle anchored to the iliopectineal ligament. Mouzas and Diggory (49) modified the McEvedy procedure (femoral herniorrhaphy through the rectus sheath).

The types of prostheses used in repair changed. As Theodore Billroth (1829–94) stated, "If we could artificially produce tissues of the density and toughness of fascia and tendon, the secret of the radical cure of hernia would be discovered" (40). Silver filigree prostheses were first used in 1894. To name a few of the hundreds of investigators, Frances Usher used Marlex in 1958, and Amos Koontz used tantalum gauze in 1962 (34). DeBord (12) wrote an excellent history of prosthetic materials, and classifies them as follows:

Metal prosthetics
  Silver
  Gold
  Tantalum
  Steel
Nonmetallic synthetic prosthetics
  Fortisan fabric
  Polyvinyl sponge
  Nylon
  Silastic
  Teflon
  Carbon fiber
  Polyester (Dacron) mesh
  Polypropylene mesh
  Expanded polytetrafluoroethylene
  Polyglycolic mesh

We enjoy the statement of Zimmerman (81), "Prostheses, whatever their value, cannot replace a full knowledge of the underlying anatomy and pathology of hernia, or substitute for the exercise of the time-honored principles of surgical technique . . . . Prostheses have not proved to be the ultimate solution to the hernia problem . . . " We agree that without both knowledge of surgical anatomy and use of a detailed and accurate technique, the hernia surgeon is nothing more than a glorified technician. As DeBord stated, "Apparently no single 'ideal' operation exists for the permanent cure of hernia, and it is unlikely that a single 'ideal' prosthesis to augment hernia repair will be developed that is universally adaptable" (12).

The etiology of hernia is a subject of much debate. Sir Arthur Keith in 1924 emphasized ". . . the importance of a right understanding of the etiology of the hernia" (33). Keith maintained that inguinal herniation was a result of the erect posture of human beings, which stressed the muscles, aponeuroses, and fascia:

We are so apt to look on tendons, fascial structures and connective tissues as dead passive structures. They are certainly alive, and the fact that hernias are so often multiple in middle-aged and old people leads one to suspect that a pathological change in connective tissues of the belly wall may render certain individuals particularly liable to hernia . . . . If they occur only in those who have hernial sacs already formed during fetal life, then we must either excise the sacs at birth or stand by and do nothing but trust to luck. But if . . . the occurrence of hernia is due to circumstance over which we have control, then the prevention of hernia is a matter worthy of our serious study (33).

R.H. Russell accepted the congenital origin of the hernia, but he maintained, "The final and absolute means of testing the saccular origin of any individual case of hernia is to remove the sac. If . . . the hernia does not recur, then the sac must have been the cause" (61).

The surgeons who made the preperitoneal approach not only well known but also very popular were Nyhus and colleagues in 1960 (51). Since that time, Nyhus has enthusiastically supported preperitoneal repair. We agree with Read's statement, "Nyhus and colleagues deserve credit for making preperitoneal herniorrhaphy popular" (62). Mahorner and Goss (41) repaired herniation following destruction of Poupart's and Cooper's ligaments after repeated operations.

E. Shouldice (1891–1965) of Toronto repaired inguinal hernia by overlapping layers with a continuous suture. Not only did he spare the transversalis fascia, but he also respected both laminae, anterior and posterior. In 1945, he reported his technique (69):

> The two leaves of the split aponeurosis of the external oblique are turned one upwards and the other downwards, thus exposing the inguinal canal and its contents. The outer covering of the spermatic cord (cremasteric and internal spermatic fascia) are incised throughout the length of the wound right down to the sac and the vessels so as to include all the several layers of fascia, and if this is carefully done the layers of fascia can be easily freed through the loose areolar tissue between the sac and vessels and the fascial layers thus exposing the structures of the cord . . . . The coverings of the cord are carefully left in their normal relationship to the posterior wall of the canal (transversalis fascia) and to the inguinal ligament. This is an important step in the operative procedure which ensures that the posterior wall of the canal (transversalis fascia) will not be damaged by separation of these structures . . . . The lower leaf of the cremasteric and internal spermatic fascia is sutured to the conjoined tendon by a suture of silk which passes deep to the upper leaf to reach the conjoined tendon. The upper leaf of the cremasteric and internal spermatic fascia is brought down and sutured to the deep surface of the inguinal ligament by a continuous silk suture . . . . The medial leaf of the external oblique is then sutured to the deep surface of the lateral leaf and in such a position as will place it deep to the lateral leaf. The lateral leaf is folded up overlapping the medial leaf, and its margin is sutured to the surface of the external oblique.

Sachs et al. (68) quotes from the Shouldice Hospital description of this surgery, "The muscles of the abdominal wall are arranged in three distinct layers and we repair the opening, in each layer in turn, by overlapping its margins rather than by stitching them together edge-to-edge . . . . The end result is to reinforce the muscular wall of the abdomen with six rows of suture." Such technique has been masterfully performed at the Shouldice by Bendavid and others, with recurrence rates of less than 1%.

Chester McVay (Fig. 4.12) advised suturing the transverse abdominis arch to Cooper's ligament for repair of inguinal hernias. Lichtenstein presented tension-free mesh hernia repair as follows (37):

> No significant structures have been sacrificed. Crushing or dividing the inferior cremaster bundle containing the genital branch of the genitofemoral nerve is avoided. The muscle fibers and nerve are simply allowed to exit through a separate opening in the repair medial to the internal ring . . . . A sheet of prosthetic mesh measuring about 5 by 10 cm is fashioned. The lower edge is attached by a continuous suture of 000 prolene which secures the mesh medially to the lacunar ligament and then proceeds laterally along Poupart's ligament beyond the internal ring. A slit in the mesh at the internal ring allows emergence of the spermatic cord. The superior edge of the mesh is secured by a similar continuous suture to the rectus sheath and the conjoined muscle and the tendon above . . . . This alone completes the repair without formal reconstruction of the canal floor.

A "sutureless" version of the Lichtenstein technique, traversing the internal ring to place a prosthetic graft between the peritoneum and the transversalis fascia was creatively devised by Gilbert (24). Robbins and Rutkow have

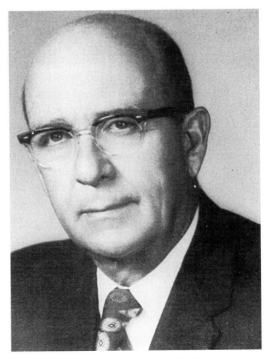

FIGURE 4.12. Chester McVay.

extended the technique with their work on the open mesh plug hernioplasty (66,67). Stoppa, in what he calls a "maximal extension of hernia prosthetic repair" devised a bilateral repair placing a chevron-shaped prosthetic in the retroparietal (preperitoneal) space after using a midline approach (72). This method has been adopted successfully by Wantz to treat recurrent inguinal hernias (77).

I remember once observing (between 1957–60) Dr. Floyd McRay of Piedmont Hospital in Atlanta closing intraabdominally an indirect hernia ring after finishing a right colectomy. The patient had a coincidental inguinal indirect hernia.

LAPAROSCOPIC SURGERY

Laparoscopic repair of inguinal hernias has developed during the past 2 decades. Ger (23) repaired an indirect inguinal hernia laparoscopically in 1982, closing the peritoneal opening of the hernia sac with Michel staple clips using Kocher clamps. Bogojavlensky (5) inserted a plug of polypropylene mesh into the sac of an indirect hernia and closed the internal ring with laparoscopic sutures. In 1990, Popp (59) placed and sutured a dural patch over the defect of an indirect hernia. Arregui (2) introduced TAPP (transabdominal preperitoneal repair) in 1991. Fitzgibbons and colleagues (19) presented IPOM (intraperitoneal mesh repair) using polypropylene mesh.

Phillips and colleagues (57) performed extraperitoneal repair by exposing the myopectineal orifice of Fruchaud and placing polypropylene mesh between the peritoneum and the abdominal wall.

Stoppa et al. (73) stated:

Laparoscopic hernia surgery has spread since 1991, and, despite or perhaps because of its youth, is making a great noise all around the world . . . . The current status of controversy between the supporters of the two approaches is rather tense. In the laparoscopic party one can find "polemists" who defy open surgery, "enthusiastic men" who prophesy that laparoscopic procedures will be tomorrow's surgery, "pseudo ecologists" who stress the mini-invasive approach, when "diplomates" explain that it is only a different approach for the same technique performed inside. Among open surgery defenders, opinion is critical about some controversial aspects of laparoscopic surgery. The incentives for changing are not regularly clear. Excess enthusiasm, professional competition, pressure from the media on surgeons and patients, consumer behavior and/or diversion of normal relations between surgeons and instrument manufacturers all play roles. The cost of mini-invasive access surgery is high, and current instrumentation is imperfect and improvements will further increase cost. Attempts in laparoscopic hernia surgery must be observed with an open mind because hernia surgery is very common, often called "the epitome" of general surgery.

Whatever one's view might be of laparoscopic surgery, the anatomy of laparoscopic repair is no longer anecdotal. Colborn and Skandalakis reported layer by layer and space by space the anatomy of the inguinofemoral area from the peritoneum to the myopectineal orifice of Fruchaud (10).

ENVOI

. . . Pasiphae, Minotaur, Labyrinth, and Ariadne with that beautiful amourous thread branching, guiding in stone darkness. And then, the return of Theseus, Triumphant.
  —Yiannis Ritsos (65)

In 1989, Bendavid (4) exclaimed about the growth of hernia treatment, "Since the epoch-making contribution of Bassini in 1888, no less than 81 inguinal and 79 femoral operative techniques have been described!" A decade later, we must humbly remember that, despite the latest successes in repair, to paraphrase Ritsos, we are in Shadow, awaiting Theseus.

REFERENCES

1. Andrews EW. Imbrication or lap joint method; a plastic operation for hernia. *Chicago Med Rec* 1895;9:67.
2. Arregui ME. Laparoscopic preperitoneal herniorrhaphy. Paper presented at: Annual Meeting of the Society of American Endoscopic Surgeons; 1991; Monterey, CA.
3. Bassini E. Nuovo metodo per la cura radicale dell'ernia inguinale. *Atti Congr Assoc Med Ital* 1887;2:179.
4. Bendavid R. New techniques in hernia repair. *World J Surg* 1989;13:522.
5. Bogojavlensky S. Laparoscopic treatment of inguinal and femoral hernias. Paper presented at: 18th Annual Meeting of the American Association of Gynecological Laparoscopists; 1989; Washington, DC.
6. Bogros AJ. Essai sur l'anatomie chirurgicale de la region iliaque et description d'un nouveau procede pour faire la ligature des arteres epigastrique et iliaque externe [thesis]. Paris: Didot le Jeune, 1823: no. 153.
7. Castiglioni A. *A history of medicine.* New York: Alfred A. Knopf, 1958. Krumbhaar EB, translator.
8. Celsus AC. *De medicina.* Cambridge, MA: Harvard University Press, 1938. Book VII. 19. 1–6. Spencer WG, translator.
9. Chadwick J. *Hippocratic writings.* New York: Penguin, 1983. Mann WN, translator.
10. Colborn GL, Skandalakis JE. Laparoscopic cadaveric anatomy of the inguinal area. *Probl Gen Surg* 1995;12:13.
11. Cooper AP. *The anatomy and surgical treatment of abdominal hernia. In two parts.* London: Longman, 1827.
12. DeBord JR. The historical development of prosthetics in hernia surgery. *Surg Clin North Am* 1998;78:973.
13. de Gimbernat A. *A new method of operating for the femoral hernia.* London: J. Johnson, 1795. Beddoes T, translator.
14. Ebbell B. *The papyrus Ebers: the greatest Egyptian medical document.* London: Oxford University Press, 1937.
15. Eliot TS. The hollow men. In: *Selected poems.* Middlesex: Penguin Books, 1948.
16. Elyot T. *The castel of helthe.* New York: Scholars' Facsimiles & Reprints, 1937.
17. Fenwick EH. Laparotomy as an aid to herniotomy. *Lancet* 1885;2:566.
18. Ferguson AH. Oblique inguinal hernia: typical operation for its radical cure. *JAMA* 1899;38:6.

19. Fitzgibbons RJ Jr, Camps J, Cornet DA, et al. Laparoscopic inguinal herniorrhaphy. Results of a multicenter trial. *Ann Surg* 1995;221:3.
20. Flack IH. *The story of surgery.* New York: Doubleday, Doran & Co Inc, 1939. Harvey Graham, pseudonym.
21. Flack IH. *Surgeons all.* London: Rich & Cowan Ltd, 1939. Harvey Graham, pseudonym.
22. Garrison FH. *An introduction to the history of medicine.* Philadelphia: WB Saunders, 1929.
23. Ger R. The management of certain abdominal hernia by intra-abdominal closure of the neck of the sac. Preliminary communication. *Ann R Coll Surg Engl* 1982;64:342–344.
24. Gilbert AI. Sutureless repair of inguinal hernia. *Am J Surg* 1992; 163:331.
25. Haeger K. *The illustrated history of surgery.* London: Harold Starke, 1988.
26. Halsted WS. The cure of the more difficult as well as the simpler inguinal ruptures. *Bull Hopkins Hosp* 1903;14:208.
27. Henry AK. Operation for femoral hernia by a midline extraperitoneal approach: with a preliminary note on the use of this route for reducible inguinal hernia. *Lancet* 1936;1:531.
28. Henry AK. Quoted in Musgrove JE, McCready FJ. The Henry approach to femoral hernia. *Surgery* 1948;26:608.
29. Hull HC, Ganey JB. The Henry approach to femoral hernia. *Ann Surg* 1953; 137:57.
30. Hutchinson E. Case of strangulated hernia operated on by abdominal section laparotomy. *Ohio Med Surg* 1878;3:499.
31. Jennings WK, Anson BJ, Wright RR. A new method of repair for indirect inguinal hernia considered in reference to parietal anatomy. *Surg Gynecol Obstet* 1942;74:697.
32. Keetley CB. On laparotomy in the treatment of strangulated hernia. *Ann Surg* 1886;3:459.
33. Keith A. On the origin and nature of hernia. *Br J Surg* 1924; 11:455.
34. Koontz A. Historical analysis of femoral hernia. *Surgery* 1963;53:551.
35. LaRoque GP. The permanent cure of inguinal and femoral hernia. A modification of the standard operative procedures. *Surg Gynecol Obstet* 1919;29:507.
36. Last RJ. *Anatomy regional and applied.* Baltimore: Williams & Wilkins, 1972:507.
37. Lichtenstein IL. *Hernia repair without disability,* 2nd ed. St. Louis: Ishiyaku Euroamerica, 1986.
38. Lucas-Championniere J. *Chirurgie operatoire: cure radicale des hernies; avec une etude statistique de deux cent soixante-quinze operations et cinquante figures intercalees dans le texte.* Paris: Rueff et Ciet, 1892.
39. McEvedy BV. Inguinal hernia: the rectus-sheath approach. *West Afr Med J* 1958;7:106.
40. Madden JL. *Abdominal wall hernias.* Philadelphia: WB Saunders, 1989.
41. Mahorner H, Goss CM. Herniation following destruction of Poupart's and Cooper's ligaments: a method of repair. *Ann Surg* 1962;155:741.
42. Marcy HO. A new use of carbolized catgut ligatures. *Boston Med Surg J* 1871;85:315.
43. Marcy HO. The radical cure of hernia by the antiseptic use of the carbolized catgut ligature. *Trans Am Med Assoc* 1878;29:295.
44. Marcy HO. The cure of hernia. *JAMA* 1887;8:589.
45. Marcy HO. *The anatomy and surgical treatment of hernia.* New York: D. Appleton, 1892.
46. Maunsell HW. Advantages of suprapubic laparotomy in strangulated femoral hernia. *N Z Med J* 1887;1:23.
47. Meade RH. The history of the abdominal approach to hernia repair. *Surgery* 1965;57:908.
48. Mikkelsen WP, Berne CJ. Femoral hernioplasty. Suprapubic extraperitoneal (Cheatle–Henry) approach. *Surgery* 1954;35:743.
49. Mouzas GL, Diggory PLC. A modification of the McEvedy repair of femoral hernia. *Lancet* 1956;2:1073.
50. Musgrove JE, McCready FJ. The Henry approach to femoral hernia. *Surgery* 1948;26:608.
51. Nyhus LM, Condon RE, Harkins HN. Clinical experience with preperitoneal hernia repair for all types of hernia of the groin. *Am J Surg* 1960;100:234.
52. Nyhus LM. Editorial comment. In: Nyhus LM, Condon RE, eds. *Hernia,* 2nd ed. Philadelphia: JB Lippincott, 1978:11.
53. Nyhus LM. Editor's comment. Patiño JF. A history of the treatment of hernia. In: Nyhus LM, Condon RE, eds. *Hernia,* 4th ed. Philadelphia: JB Lippincott, 1995:13–15.
54. Olch PD, Harkins HN. Historical survey of the treatment of inguinal hernia. In: Nyhus LM, Harkins HN, eds. *Hernia.* Philadelphia: JB Lippincott, 1964:8.
55. Paré A. *The apologie and treatise.* New York: Dover, 1968. Keynes G, ed.
56. Patiño JF. A history of the treatment of hernia. In: Nyhus LM, Condon RE, eds. *Hernia,* 4th ed. Philadelphia: JB Lippincott, 1995:3–15.
57. Phillips EH, Carroll BJ, Fallas MJ. Laparoscopic preperitoneal inguinal hernia repair without preperitoneal incision. *Surg Endosc* 1993;7:159.
58. Ponka JL. *Hernias of the abdominal wall.* Philadelphia: WB Saunders, 1980.
59. Popp LW. Endoscopic patch repair of inguinal hernia in a female patient. *Surg Endosc* 1990;4:10.
60. Raff J. Hernia healers. *Ann Med Hist* 1932;4:377.
61. Read RC. Historical survey of the treatment of hernia. In: Nyhus LM, Condon RE, eds. *Hernia,* 3rd ed. Philadelphia: JB Lippincott, 1989:3–17.
62. Read RC. Preperitoneal herniorrhaphy. A historical review. *World J Surg* 1989;13:532.
63. Read RC. Conceptual problems regarding hernial rings in the groin. *Probl Gen Surg* 1995;12:27.
64. Retzius AA. Some remarks on the proper design on the semilunar lines of Douglas. *Edinburgh Med J* 1858;3:685.
65. Ritsos Y. *The fourth dimension.* Princeton, NJ: Princeton University Press, 1993. Green P, Bardsley B, translators.
66. Robbins AW, Rutkow IM. The mesh-plug hernioplasty. *Surg Clin North Am* 1993;73:501–63.
67. Rutkow IM. *Surgery: an illustrated history.* St. Louis: Mosby, 1993.
68. Sachs M, Damm M, Encke A. Historical evolution of inguinal hernia repair. *World J Surg* 1997;21:218.
69. Shouldice EE. Surgical treatment of hernia. *Ont Med Rev* 1945;12:43.
70. Skandalakis JE, Gray SW, Skandalakis LJ, et al. Surgical anatomy of the inguinal area. *World J Surg* 1989;13:490.
71. Skandalakis MC, Skandalakis JE. The personal and professional life of John Hunter. *J Med Assoc Ga* 1991;80:445.
72. Stoppa R. The preperitoneal approach and prosthetic repair of groin hernias. In: Nyhus LM, Condon RE, eds. *Hernia,* 4th ed. Philadelphia: JB Lippincott, 1995:188–210.
73. Stoppa R, Wantz GE, Munegato G, et al. *Hernia healers.* Velizy-Villacoublay, France: Arnette, 1998.
74. Tait L. A discussion on treatment of hernia by median abdominal section. *Br Med J* 1891;2:685.
75. Thevenet A. Guy de Chauliac (1300–1370): The "father of surgery". *Ann Vasc Surg* 1993;7:208–212.
76. Thorwald J. *The triumph of surgery.* New York: Pantheon, 1957.
77. Wantz GE. Special comment: personal experience with the Stoppa technique. In: Nyhus LM, Condon RE, eds. *Hernia,* 4th ed. Philadelphia: JB Lippincott, 1995:206–216.

78. Ward E. Abdominal section for displaced hernia. *Lancet* 1886;2:201.

79. Warren JH. *Hernia, strangulated and reducible, with cure by subcutaneous injections together with suggested and improved methods for kelotomy; also an appendix giving a short account of various new surgical instruments.* Boston: CN Thomas, 1881.

80. Watson LF. *Hernia.* St. Louis: CV Mosby, 1924.

81. Zimmerman LM. The use of prosthetic materials in the repair of hernias. *Surg Clin North Am* 1968;48:143.

82. Zimmerman LM, Zimmerman JE. The history of hernia treatment. In: Nyhus LM, Condon RE, eds. *Hernia,* 2nd ed. Philadelphia: JB Lippincott, 1978:4.

Nyhus and Condon's Hernia, Fifth Edition, edited by Robert J. Fitzgibbons, Jr. and A. Gerson Greenburg. Lippincott Williams & Wilkins, Philadelphia © 2002.

5

ANATOMY OF THE GROIN: A VIEW FROM THE SURGEON

MATTHIAS KUX

What can a surgeon's view of today add to our understanding of groin anatomy since that area has been explored and described so extensively by the great surgeon–anatomists of the past? Traditionally, gross anatomy of the groin has been viewed from the aspect of the pathogenesis of groin hernias, and, consequently, with principles of their repair. All modern repair techniques are very effective with regard to recurrence, and the traditional end point recurrence has switched to other outcome measures such as patient comfort, satisfaction, and time to rehabilitation. Several recent studies have shown that up to 10% of patients report moderate to severe pain 2 years postoperatively (4,6,8,14). In one study, 5% of patients assessed their postoperative discomfort as more troublesome than the original hernia, overriding the benefits of the repair that was "successful" with regard to recurrence (8). Problems of male sexuality and fertility following inguinal hernia repair are of even greater concern (7,9,10,20). In this respect, there is not much to be found in the older literature which, on the other hand, abounds with mechanical "pressure" concepts of hernia etiology and repair. As patients and surgeons become more sensitive of unpleasant and litigious sequelae of groin hernia repair, not only techniques but also time-honored concepts behind these techniques may be questioned (e.g., Is hernia caused by "intraperitoneal pressure," or is it caused by a pathology of the extraperitoneal fatty–fascial compartment?). The following view of a surgeon will not resemble the impartial regard of the anatomist. Today, the view of a surgeon will be largely influenced by experience with patients' complaints and the very pragmatic question: How can knowledge of the anatomy be helpful in avoiding complaints following groin hernia repair? This view will be centered on the relation of anatomy to specific repair techniques, including physiology and pathology. It must comprise the

findings from laparoscopy, computed tomography (CT) scans, and the dynamics that are seen during an operation under local anesthesia. Therefore, it must be different from the view that is obtained from a cadaver dissection.

THE UROGENITAL FATTY–FASCIAL COMPARTMENT IN THE GROIN

Anatomists view the groin conceptually as being organized in a laminar arrangement. In schematic parasagittal sections, these layers are illustrated as composing the middle of the groin in flat apposition to each other: skin, oblique and transversus abdominis layers, peritoneum (Fig. 5.1). However, this arrangement is true only in the case of an empty bladder. In a living person, the innermost layer may as well be the wall of the bladder. Numerous bladder injuries during hernia repair bear witness to the fact that a full bladder transforms the Hesselbach triangle into a huge extraperitoneal compartment. When the bladder is filled up with saline during a transabdominal laparoscopic (TAPP) hernia repair the peritoneal protrusion of a direct hernia becomes separated from transversalis fascia by the interposition of the bladder. The preperitoneal space, which is reduced to a flat layer, sometimes even omitted, in schematic parasagittal illustrations, is physiologically deeper than the rest of the abdominal wall. The preperitoneal space not only is neglected in illustrations of the groin, but also is said to have indefinite lateral and posterior margins because it is continuous with the rest of the extraperitoneal and retroperitoneal tissues (5). However, the preperitoneal space represents a well-defined compartment in front of the bladder—the prevesical space. The configuration of the prevesical space can be demonstrated by CT scans of extraperitoneal fluid accumulations (Fig. 5.2). The prevesical space extends laterally to the inferior epigastric artery and posteriorly on both sides of the bladder whereby it assumes the form of a molar tooth on horizontal sections (1). Vertically, it has the form of an inverted V with the apex near the

M. Kux: Department of Surgery, University of Vienna; Department of Surgery, St. Joseph Hospital, Vienna, Austria.

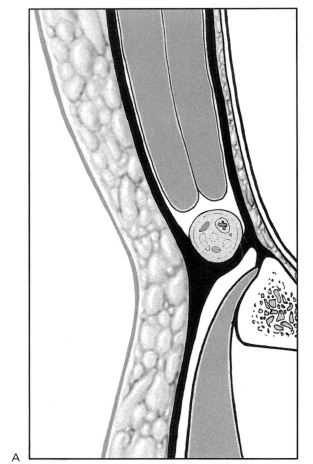
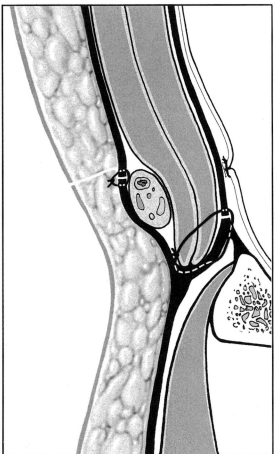

A
B

FIGURE 5.1. Traditional schemes of parasagittal sections. **A:** "Normal groin." Continuity of external oblique aponeurosis at the direct space is seen in women only (Fig. 5.7.) **B:** Schematic presentation of Bassini's repair showing compression of the cord. This laminar arrangement is only found lateral to the inferior epigastric vessels. Transversus abdominis muscle does not extend into the direct space (Fig. 5.5.) The prevesical space is ambiguous. (Adapted from Schumpelick V. *Hernien,* 3rd ed. Stuttgart: Enke Verlag, 1996:68, with permission.)

umbilicus. It is not only by extravesical fluid accumulation, but also by vesical filling that this space can be shown to be real, not "potential" (Fig. 5.2). The distensibility of this space cannot be appreciated at autopsy when connective and soft areolar tissue has lost its elasticity. What anatomists consider to be the weak area of the abdominal wall has to be viewed from inside as a soft cushion and extension reserve for the bladder. The relations depicted in Fig. 5.1 are true only for the abdominal wall lateral to the inferior epigastric vessels, where peritoneum and transversalis fascia are intimately fused without intervening preperitoneal tissues.

A hernia operation that violates the integrity of the prevesical space may have consequences on urinary and sexual function. Infiltration and opacification of the prevesical space and some degree of bladder indentation can be regularly found on postoperative CT scans after sutured and laparoscopic groin hernia repair (Fig. 5.3). A large prosthesis may obliterate the prevesical space, and disturbances of void-

ing, sexuality, and fertility may ensue. One such problem, painful ejaculation following groin hernia repair, is now a well-documented syndrome (2,3,6,8,16). It can be shown that this syndrome may originate from a pathology in the prevesical space: A 35-year-old man was referred to our department because of severe groin pain at and immediately after ejaculation. The pain was suspected to originate from an occult hernia. Instead, a benign leiomyoma was found in front of the bladder and removed (Fig. 5.4). The painful ejaculation syndrome disappeared within 2 weeks postoperatively. One of our patients suffered from painful ejaculation on one side after bilateral hernia repair, which is indicative of a purely somatic origin of that condition.

A highly sensitive, three-dimensional urogenital space is found not only *behind* transversalis fascia, but also *in front* of it! Here, the strongest smooth muscle organ of men, the vas deferens, lies embedded in the groove formed by the internal oblique muscle above and the inguinal ligament

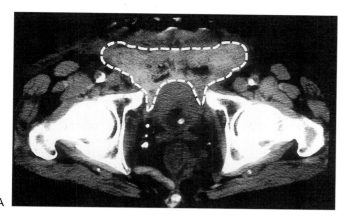

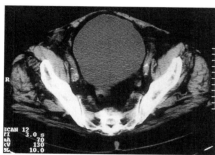

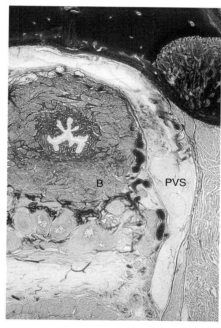

FIGURE 5.2. Prevesical space. **A:** Computed tomography (CT) scan of fluid accumulation in the prevesical space. In the horizontal plane, the filled prevesical space assumes the form of a molar tooth. **B:** CT scan of the bladder, which expands the prevesical space up to the level of the sacroiliac joint. **C:** Fat configuration of the prevesical space in a newborn boy. *B,* bladder; *PVS,* prevesical space. See Color Plate 1. (Courtesy of Prof. Helga Fritsch, Department of Anatomy, University of Innsbruck, Austria.)

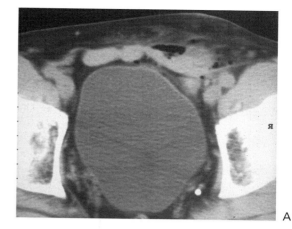

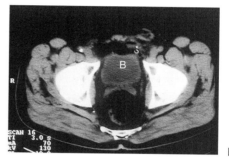

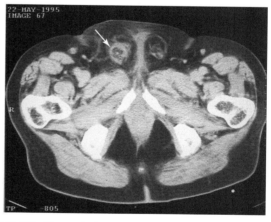

FIGURE 5.3. Urogenital systems after groin hernia repair. **A:** Condensation of the prevesical space and indentation of the bladder after a Shouldice hernia repair. Note that there is muscular continuity over the direct space on the nonoperated side. **B:** Impingement of a prevesical prosthesis on the bladder after a transabdominal laparoscopic (TAPP) repair. *B,* bladder. **C:** Edematous swelling and condensation of the spermatic cord after a Shouldice repair (*arrow*).

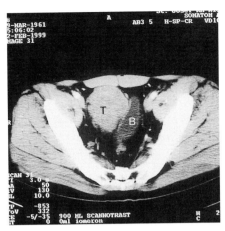

FIGURE 5.4. Prevesical space pathology. Tumorous infiltration of the prevesical space causing painful ejaculation in a 35-year-old man. *B,* bladder; *T,* tumor. Pain was completely relieved by operative removal of the tumor, a benign leiomyoma. Note that the semilunar line is free of muscular elements as opposed to the direct space (Fig. 5.3).

below. Classical suture repair of the Bassini–Shouldice–McVay type results in compression of the cord between the strong new posterior wall and the strong external oblique aponeurosis (Fig. 5.1). Edematous swelling and infiltration of the cord can be regularly demonstrated on postoperative CT scans after groin hernia repair (Fig. 5.3). Viewed from outside, there is one more physiologic correlate for the musculoaponeurotic discontinuity and relative weakness of the direct space: men have an outlet ("inlet") conduit in this area for the ejaculate. No longer is the vas deferens considered a passive conduit: the rich adrenergic innervation, the complexity of the muscle layers, and the metabolically active epithelia suggest a very active role of the vas in sperm transport (19). Surely, passage of the ejaculate at the right moment and at the right pressure is an equally complex and important function as are the other pelvic visceral outlet functions. On either side of the weak area of the groin, a three-dimensional fascia and cushion system accommodates dynamic urogenital systems. If groin hernia surgery attempts to create a "strong posterior wall," it may possibly succeed in preventing recurrence at the price of interfering with the subtle male reproductive physiology. It should be remembered that the vas lies at a great distance from the other cord elements at recurrent hernia repair, testifying to extreme peristaltic activity in the presence of the iatrogenic squeeze (Figs. 5.1 and 5.3). Painful ejaculation may be caused not only by pathology in the prevesical space, but also by scar entrapment of the vas. Painful ejaculation following groin hernia repair has been successfully treated by untethering the vas from scar tissue (3,16). Spermatic granuloma is a well-known sequela of vas deferens injury and surgery and may be etiologically related to postherniorrhaphy perivasal fibrosis (2,3,6,7,9,10,16,19,20).

THE TRANSVERSUS ABDOMINIS LAYER

In the past, surgeon–anatomists have focused their attention on the "wall" function and deficit of the groin at the expense of the urogenital systems in that area. Traditionally, the groin hernia problem has been linked exclusively with the transversus abdominis layer, i.e., the transversus abdominis muscle, its aponeurosis, and transversalis fascia. The transversus layer of the groin is usually presented after "dissection that removed all tissues in the groin, both superficial and deep to the transversus abdominis muscle and aponeurosis, and their associated structures" (5). This layer is then defined as the layer that retains the abdominal contents. Accordingly, the internal oblique muscle and the external oblique aponeurosis have little or nothing to do with the development of a hernia "and will not be discussed in this chapter," as stated by McVay in his contribution to the third edition of this book (13). However, the latter two structures are obviously and by far the strongest and the most consistent structures to be encountered in a groin dissection. When the patient is asked to cough during an operation under local anesthesia, the direct space becomes compressed between the contracting musculoaponeurotic structures of the two oblique layers. At the moment of an acute strain, the direct space is protected by obliteration of the musculoaponeurotic discontinuity, which resembles the effect of a suture repair, as illustrated in Fig. 5.1. The contraction of the external oblique aponeurosis is also felt when the superficial inguinal ring is palpated from outside in the usual way in the upright position.

Under the laparoscope, the innermost layer that can be consistently identified, sutured, or used for creating an artificial cavity is the peritoneum. The transversus abdominis muscle does not extend unto the groin area, and the transversus abdominis aponeurosis becomes discontinuous at the posterior wall of the groin, the intervening spaces being filled only by transversalis fascia. In the living person, trans-

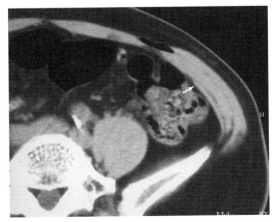

FIGURE 5.5. Computed tomography (CT) anatomy. Muscle-free area of the semilunar zone above the groin. The transversus abdominis muscle does not extend into the groin (*arrow*).

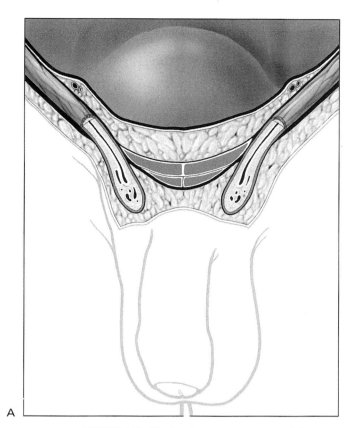
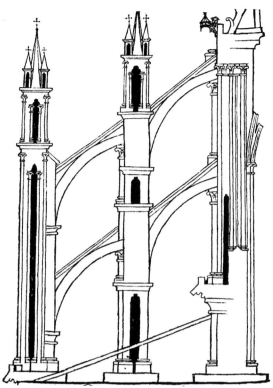

FIGURE 5.6. Nonlaminar arrangement of the groin. **A:** Diagrammatic oblique section through the groin. Holding strength of external oblique aponeurosis is propagated over cremaster muscle and spermatic cord upon transversalis fascia, which separates prevesical space behind from the voluminous cord space in front. **B:** Holding strength of outer lamina is propagated upon inner structures via elements that are called tendons in gothic architectural language (from a medieval design of Reims cathedral).

versalis fascia is, for the most part, a thin, sometimes transparent membrane of little intrinsic strength. This membrane should be able to guard against the development of a direct hernia, since the direct space is said to be covered by transversalis fascia only. Yet, in horizontal CT scans, muscle is regularly present at the direct space (Fig. 5.3). This is in marked contrast to the semilunar zone above the groin, which is regularly free of muscular elements on CT scans (Figs. 5.4 and 5.5). Horizontal anatomic cross sections show the direct space to be covered by cremaster muscle (Fig. 5.6). The spermatic cord and its cremasteric muscular sheath compensate to some extent for the abdominal wall weakness in the groin. Thus, only transversalis fascia may be left of the abdominal wall structures to make up for the transversus abdominis layer.

TRANSVERSALIS FASCIA THEORY

Anatomic and surgical dissection always proceeds in the anteroposterior direction, whereby a single laminar struc-

ture is retained, or created, in the frontal plane. In the area of the direct space, transversalis fascia is a gliding or shearing plane that separates two nonlaminar urogenital spaces from each other. The three-dimensional nonlaminar organization of the medial portion of the groin is well documented on horizontal sections: the voluminous prevesical space is separated by transversalis fascia from the voluminous spermatic cord and cremasteric muscle in front (Fig. 5.6). These spaces are derived from the retroperitoneal urogenital space. Very much like the perirenal space, they are filled with fat, subdivided, and structured by several fascias of which transversalis fascia is but one. Through its fascial framework, the fatty–fascial compartment is integrated into the main supportive structure of the groin, i.e., external oblique aponeurosis and inguinal ligament: there are millions of elderly and young women with a "weak" transversalis fascia but without a direct hernia. It can be seen from Fig. 5.7 that transversalis fascia strength has no importance whatsoever in preventing a direct hernia in women since the direct space is strongly and hermetically guarded by external oblique aponeurosis. The situation is

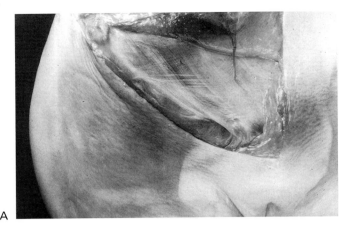

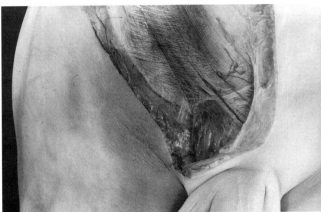

FIGURE 5.7. Gender differences in groin anatomy. **A:** Independently of transversalis fascia strength, direct hernias are rare in women because the direct space is closed hermetically by external oblique aponeurosis. **B:** Holding strength of external oblique aponeurosis is propagated upon inner structures over cord, fat, and fascias. See Color Plate 2. (From Thiel W. *Photographischer atlas der praktischen anatomie I.* Heidelberg: Springer Verlag, 1996:19, with permission.)

different in men inasmuch as the spermatic cord perforates the external oblique aponeurosis. The holding strength of the latter is still propagated onto the structures underneath: cremaster muscle, spermatic cord, transversus abdominis layer and surrounding fat–fascia body, preperitoneal tissues, and peritoneum (Figs. 5.6 and 5.7). This architecture is sufficiently stable to prevent direct hernias in nonobese men under the age of 50. Thereafter, a peak of groin hernia incidence in the 50- to 80-year age group occurs, mainly because of an increase in direct hernias (in men). In this age bracket the tonus and the architecture of the fatty-fascial compartments are compromised through hormonal changes whereby the wear and tear of upright position, ageing, obesity or weight loss become effective within the extraperitoneal compartment. In the author's opinion, transversalis fascia and its strength cannot be considered separately from "all other tissues in the groin, both superficial and deep" to that layer.

EXTRAPERITONEAL ORIGIN OF GROIN HERNIA

What is then the fundamental defect in groin hernias? During fetal development, the defect is caused by an avulsion of the extraperitoneal compartment. This avulsion perforates the muscular abdominal wall at the internal ring, it perforates the external oblique aponeurosis at the superficial ring. A congenital lateral sac in healthy children and young adults has no correlation whatsoever with transversalis fascia strength. In women, the superficial inguinal ring is perfectly guarded by external oblique aponeurosis. Consequently, direct hernias are rare in women. The situation is different in men, wherein the external oblique aponeurosis is perforated and deficient at the superficial ring (Fig. 5.7). Embryologically, the peritoneal processus vaginalis is not formed through a pressure rise or pressure gradient against a laminar fascial containment. The processus vaginalis develops by a process in the extraperitoneal compartment, which involves the peritoneum from outside. The extraperitoneal avulsive process which causes the embryologic processus vaginalis is paralleled by the adult extraperitoneal sliding hernia. Most acquired hernias in elderly adults have an element of so-called lipoma, which is always sliding fat of extraperitoneal origin. The aponeurotic groin hernia defects are not sealed by a drum-like spanned fascia, but are dynamically protected by all lamina and spaces which are integrated into each other by a space architecture (Fig. 5.6). Fat is not only a nuisance to the surgeon and anatomist, and not only grist for the metabolic mill. Fat is a structural, mechanically supportive element of the retro-, sub-, and preperitoneal spaces. In developmental and functional respect, the direct inguinal space is part of the extraperitoneal fatty–fascial compartment. The architecture of this compartment has to allow for retroperitoneal fixation of abdominal organs, for distension and retraction of the bladder, for the transport of urine and sperm.

Transversalis fascia strength has no importance whatsoever in preventing direct hernias in women because the direct space is guarded by external oblique aponeurosis in women. In women, transversalis fascia and external oblique aponeurosis are arranged in a laminar way. Direct hernias in men are not more frequent because men have a "weak transversalis fascia," but because men have a defect in the external oblique aponeurosis (Fig. 5.7). Transversalis fascia separates solid extraperitoneal compartments, not virtual air-chambers (12). With an intact external oblique aponeurosis an indirect hernia bulges the transversalis fascia from outside in and not vice versa (Fig. 5.8). The so-called intraperitoneal pressure can only affect the intestines. The etiologic factor of coughing cannot be an intraperitoneal pressure rise. There is no air and no fluid in the intraperitoneal space that can be compressed to generate a pressure increment. In addition, any theoretical pressure increment caused by a cough impulse is preceded by a direct contrac-

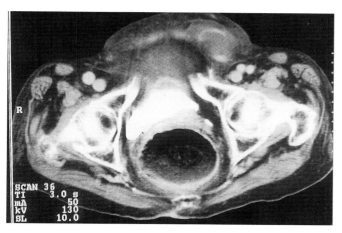

FIGURE 5.8. Indirect hernia in an elderly woman. The prefascial direct space is expanded from outside in, with the hernia backing against external oblique aponeurosis.

tile or tearing force upon the abdominal wall itself. Pressure etiology of inguinal hernia is also linked to obesity, chronic constipation, or prostatic hypertrophy, all of which represent a strain on the extraperitoneal, rather than on the intraperitoneal compartment. Groin hernia may result from a process in this compartment rather than from intra-abdominal pressure.

Quite frequently, the appearance of an acquired hernia is preceded by changes in the body fat mass. Weight loss and malnutrition result in poor fixation and continuous slide of extraretroperitoneal tissues. An increase in fat mass may predilate the obliterated, yet preformed, groin hernial route. The highest intraabdominal pressure is found in pregnancy and is not correlated to groin hernia etiology. The second peak of groin hernia incidence occurs at an older age with less physical stain. The embryologic preperitoneal descent is reopened by force of gravity, not radial expansion.

THE FALLACIES OF THE TRANSVERSUS ABDOMINIS THEORY

There is an important historic root to the transversus abdominis theory. Successful repair of hernias was first accomplished by surgeons who included the transversus abdominis layer in the repair (Bassini, Marcy). Previously, all attempts at hernia repair using the external oblique aponeurosis had failed. In those early days, the hernial sac and the hernial orifice were not dealt with and persisted after manipulations of the superficial ring. Bassini's low recurrence rate of 2.7% served as an argument that "restoration of musculo-aponeurotic continuity in the deep transversus abdominis layer" is needed, and what is done to the more superficial layers is of relatively less importance (5). The success of the Lichtenstein repair is proof to the contrary:

the deep musculoaponeurotic discontinuity is not "restored," and a premuscular sublay patch to the external oblique is highly successful. What had failed in the era before Bassini, namely, tightening of the superficial inguinal ring, is achieved by obliterating the superficial ring, whereby a situation is created similar to that which exists in women (Fig. 5.7). Thirty percent of Bassini's patients were infants and adolescents. It took almost a century until it was established that such a radical "cure" is obsolete in this age group because it may severely impair male sexuality and fertility (7,9,10,20). Clearly, congenital hernias in the children and young adults have no relation to transversalis fascia strength. If a Marcy-type suture of the internal ring is accepted standard in children, why should it not suffice in young adults? A relatively high recurrence rate for the Marcy repair over a life-long follow-up period should not be an argument against it. Recurrence through a "correctly placed" large preperitoneal prosthesis is theoretically inconceivable. Yet, there are considerable early and late recurrence rates for these prostheses. Recurrence does not occur *through* the prosthesis but from the extraperitoneal compartment over the posterolateral edges of the prosthesis. The concept of extraperitoneal origin of groin hernia is supported by the fact that a small prosthesis sublayed to external oblique aponeurosis is at least as effective a repair as a much larger prosthesis sublayed to the transversalis fascia. Thus, the Lichtenstein patch is not in the "wrong" layer, but in the right layer, where the extraperitoneal protrusion emerges (12). The famous "shrinkage" of preperitoneal prostheses is due, at least in part, to a sliding process of the extraperitoneal fatty–fascial compartment. The smaller Lichtenstein prosthesis is held in place better by firm apposition to firm external oblique aponeurosis. Laparoscopically placed preperitoneal prostheses are more prone to a glide and to shrinkage than prostheses placed through the anterior route. The anterior access is always followed by scar obliteration of the access route. Scar obliteration of the access route may be an important effect of all anterior repair techniques. Considering the objections to transversalis fascia theory, the use of preperitoneal prostheses and the deliberate use of the Bassini–Shouldice–McVay repair techniques may be questionable for young adults.

WHICH HERNIA, WHICH REPAIR?

Many schemes for hernia classification and indicatory guidelines have been proposed, and never applied, in the past. These attempts have failed because they were based upon the elusive transversalis fascia theory and the resulting claim for "deep" repair. Surely, most of the deep and radical repair techniques are highly effective with regard to recurrence. However, the urologic and neurologic consequences of these techniques are now becoming apparent. In the younger age group of adults, we do find indirect hernias that resemble closely the congenital infantile hernia: a well-defined peritoneal sac that is blown out like a bulge of an overly inflated balloon. Extra- and retroperitoneal tissues are not present and the content of the sac is always of intraperitoneal origin, mostly ileum. It is the appearance of this infantile hernia that lends itself to the etiology of intraperitoneal pressure. However, an intraperitoneal pressure gradient is inconceivable in intrauterine development. Also, intraperitoneal pressure or a pressure gradient can be expected to be particularly high in the infant who cries a lot. Yet, in the newborn, the open processus vaginalis will mostly retract and obliterate despite the intensive crying pressure of the baby. If it is not cured spontaneously, the open processus vaginalis is readily cured by simple excision of the sac and tightening of the internal ring (Marcy repair).

Again, as with the Bassini-type overtreatment, it may take a very long time until the full consequences of a preperitoneal prosthesis and obliteration of the prevesical space are fully apparent. The originator of the large preperitoneal prosthesis, René Stoppa, has always insisted on an age limit of 50 years before inserting a prosthesis. In a recent article, he listed prostatic hypertrophy, elevated prostate-specific antigen (PSA) levels, bladder polyps, and aortoiliac arteriosclerosis as relative contraindications (17). Thus, the preperitoneal prosthesis may be potentially harmful for both groups, young men in their reproductive age and older men at risk of the aforementioned conditions. An operation that is routine in children, i.e., reduction of the sac and simple tightening of the internal ring, may be appropriate in young adults because it interferes least with urogenital function. It may be appropriate in young adults as in children not to consider a possible direct hernia of later age in the repair technique for a simple indirect hernia at young age.

What about the 50- to 80-year age group, which represents more than half of adult hernia operations today? In acquired hernias in this age group, the extraretroperitoneal origin of groin hernias and their relation to the urogenital fat body are evident: prevesical fat in direct hernias (Fig. 5.2, bottom); retroperitoneal fat in the form of lipoma or fatty infiltration of the cord in indirect hernias; a sliding component of cecum, sigmoid colon, or bladder. In acquired indirect hernias, the direct (prevesical) space becomes involved by enlargement of the deep inguinal ring and displacement of the inferior epigastric vessels. Cremasteric and transversalis fascia are dilated and hypertrophied, and cremasteric muscle is atrophied. This demonstrates the different reaction of fascia and muscle to chronic pressure: scar hypertrophy in fascia, atrophy in muscle. The peritoneal component of an indirect sac may be small compared with extraperitoneal components, or it may be completely absent, particularly in direct hernias. A common denominator of these features is a loss of architectural tone of the fatty–fascial compartment.

In treating a simple groin hernia of the elderly, the employment of local anesthesia is of particular importance. Local anesthesia does not interfere with motor or bladder function, thus avoiding the immobilization, apprehension, and urinary retention that may be associated with general or regional anesthesia. Under local anesthesia, the repair is not subjected to an unphysiologic strain to which it will never be exposed for the rest of the patient's life, (i.e., postnarcotic excitatory phase). Local anesthesia provides postoperative pain relief even after the local anesthetic has worn off (11,18). The combination of local anesthesia and a superficial, interparietal prosthesis of the Lichtenstein type is employed to its greatest advantage in the 50- to 80-year age group. Opponents of prostheses are reminded that the conventional deep suture techniques induce a scar fibrosis similar to a prosthesis. This is very obvious when a recurrence after a Bassini–Shouldice–McVay repair is approached through the same inguinal incision. The preperitoneal approach, open or laparoscopic, carries less risk of testicular complications in repair of a recurrence after a previous inguinal approach. The preperitoneal techniques are favored for this indication.

CONCLUSION

The laminar representation of the groin is misleading since it does not account for the space arrangement of urogenital functions on either side of transversalis fascia. The only laminar structure of holding strength in the groin is external oblique aponeurosis. "Restoration of the deep musculo-aponeurotic layer" is an unphysiologic hernia operation because urogenital physiology requires a soft fat–fascia cushion in the groin. A simple primary hernia repair should not interfere with the deep prevesical space. Distinction between congenital-type hernia of the young and acquired hernia of the elderly is a practical hernia classification and indicatory scheme. Incising an intact inguinal floor and resuturing it with several rows of nonabsorbable material is considered excessive for young adults. Of all sutured techniques, the Marcy repair seems least invasive and most appropriate for the congenital-type hernia in children and young adults. A simple sublay patch under local anesthesia is least invasive for the elderly at the time of the intervention. It also presents the least potential for late complications because it is most superficial and most distant to sensitive deep structures, the prevesical space, and the great vessels. Distinction between congenital-type hernia of the young and acquired hernia of the elderly has the advantage that the less invasive procedure, i.e., the Marcy-type suture, always precedes the Lichtenstein patch. The final decision can then be made according to the intraoperative findings under local anesthesia. The Lichtenstein patch is not in the "wrong" layer, but in the right layer to withstand extraperitoneal sliding forces.

The potential of chronic pain and neuralgia of other than urologic origin is also intimately related to deep abdominal wall structures. Pain has been classified as being of somatic or neurologic origin. Somatic pain most probably arises from sutures in the periosteum and tightness of inguinal ligament (6). Chronic pain of neuropathic origin is most likely to occur, and most frequently seen, after operations that involve the deep structures of the abdominal wall. Incising and suturing the inguinal floor can in itself cause long-lasting pain without direct involvement of a particular nerve. Also, a prosthesis in the preperitoneal space, in particular a three-dimensional plug-like prosthesis, may come into contact with several sensitive nerves. It may cause irritation of scar tissue and pressure of a rigid rim upon a nerve (14). All of this is in support of the main arguments developed in this chapter: The transversalis fascia theory of groin hernia origin and repair should be seriously questioned. A simple hernia repair should *not* interfere with the deep, prevesical space. Of all sutured repair techniques, the Marcy repair is appropriate in the younger age group, in whom no attempt should be made to strengthen the inguinal floor prophylactically. Of all prosthetic techniques, a flat *monolayered* sublay patch to external oblique aponeurosis is sufficient and physiologic because it does not violate the prevesical space. The preperitoneal repair techniques should be reserved for recurrent, femoral, and symptomatic bilateral hernias.

REFERENCES

1. Auh YH, Rubenstein WA, Schneider M, et al. Extraperitoneal paravesical spaces: CT delineation with US correlation. *Radiology* 1986;159:319–328.
2. Bendavid R. Dysejaculation. *Probl Gen Surg* 1995;12:237–238.
3. Butler JD, Hershman MJ, Leach A. Painful ejaculation after inguinal hernia repair. *J R Soc Med* 1998;91:432–433.
4. Callesen T, Kehlet H. Postherniorrhaphy pain. *Anesthesiology* 1997;87:1219–1230.
5. Condon RE. The anatomy of the inguinal region and its relation to groin hernia. In: Nyhus LM, Condon RE, eds. *Hernia,* 4th ed. Philadelphia: JB Lippincott, 1995:16–53; comments 53–72.
6. Cunningham J, Temple WJ, Mitchell P, et al. Cooperative hernia study—pain in the postrepair patient. *Ann Surg* 1996;224:598–602.
7. Friberg J, Fritjofsson A. Inguinal herniorrhaphy and sperm-agglutinating antibodies in infertile men. *Arch Androl* 1979;2:317–322.
8. Gillion JF, Fagniez PL. Chronic pain and cutaneous sensory changes after inguinal hernia repair: comparison between open and laparoscopic techniques. *Hernia* 1999;3:75–80.
9. Homonnai ZT, Fainman N, Paz GF, et al. Testicular function after herniotomy—herniotomy and fertility. *Andrologia* 1980;12:115–120.
10. Imthurn T, Hadziselimovic F, Herzog B. Impaired germ cells in secondary cryptorchid testis after herniotomy. *J Urol* 1995;153:780–781.
11. Kawji R, Feichter A, Fuchsjäger N, et al. Postoperative pain and return to activity after five different types of inguinal herniorrhaphy. *Hernia* 1999;3:31–35.
12. Kux M, Fritsch H. On the extraperitoneal original of hernia. *Hernia* 2000;4:259.
13. McVay CB. Groin hernioplasty: Cooper ligament repair. In: Nyhus LM, Condon RE, eds. *Hernia,* 3rd ed. Philadelphia: JB Lippincott, 1989:119–136.
14. Palot JP, Avisse C, Caillez-Tomasi JP, et al. The mesh plug repair of groin hernias: a three year experience. *Hernia* 1998;2:31–34.
15. Schumpelick V. *Hernien,* 3rd ed. Stuttgart: Enke Verlag, 1996:68.
16. Silich RC, McSherry CK. Spermatic granuloma. An uncommon complication of the tension-free repair. *Surg Endosc* 1996;10:537–539.
17. Stoppa R, Diarra B, Verhaeghe P, et al. Problems in reinterventions after prosthetic repairs of groin hernias. *Chirurgie* 1997;122:369–372; discussion 372–373.
18. Tverskoy M, Cozacov C, Ayache M, et al. Postoperative pain after inguinal herniorrhaphy with different types of anesthesia. *Anesth Analg* 1990;70:29–35.
19. Uzzo RG, Lemack GE, Morissey KP, et al. The effects of mesh bioprosthesis on the spermatic cord structures: a preliminary report in a canine model. *J Urol* 1999;161:1344–1349.
20. Yavetz H, Harash B, Yogev L, et al. Fertility of men following inguinal hernia repair. *Andrologia* 1991;23:443–446.

6

ANATOMY OF THE GROIN: A VIEW FROM THE ANATOMIST

THOMAS H. QUINN

The anterior abdominal wall and the groin have been the subjects of intense interest to surgeons and anatomists for centuries. The large number of persistent eponymous terms associated with this area is testimony to the work of some of them, including Cooper, Poupart, Henle, Gimbernat, Retzius, Bogros, and many others, who have described the pertinent anatomy in great detail. The importance of understanding not only each anatomic nuance, but also the physical properties and interactions of the tissues of the abdominal wall and the groin is evidenced by the number of surgical techniques, both open and laparoscopic, that have been developed, each presumably building on a strength or weakness of its predecessor. It also should be noted that the tissues within the groin are interdependent; the integrity of each layer affects that of adjacent structures. It may be said that groin hernias are not due to the failure of any solitary structure, but rather, weakness develops within a system of tissues.

The body of knowledge that is based on the dissection of the embalmed cadaver—or even an unembalmed cadaver—always has been suspect in the minds of surgeons. It is true that the tissue encountered in the cadaver is not as pliable, elastic, or even somewhat ephemeral, as that found within the living patient. We furthermore cannot gain from the cadaver a full appreciation of the tactile sensations encountered when one incises living tissue. These are important points to consider, but are nevertheless fine points. The cadaver does provide a very firm knowledge of the three-dimensional space involved, as well as the general architectural details of this space. We have endeavored in this chapter to wed the knowledge we have gained from intraoperative experience with that gleaned from cadaver material. A large and constantly growing body of anatomic and surgical literature now exists that thoroughly covers many aspects of the surgical anatomy of the abdominal wall and the groin. We

intend to summarize many of these excellent reports, but our primary intent is to provide a succinct and useful review of this region for surgeons of all levels of seniority performing either open or laparoscopic herniorrhaphy.

Also of primary and intense interest to the surgeon are the courses of vascular and neurologic structures, especially in the preperitoneal space. Many of these structures have not been well studied or previously appreciated, especially by those who primarily have used anterior approaches to herniorrhaphy. Upon close examination of the deep structures, it is readily apparent that major injury can more easily be avoided if the relationship of these structures to readily identified landmarks is carefully noted.

The groin, or inguinal region, is most often defined as the transitional area in which the thigh and the abdomen are joined. Here a portion of the aponeuroses of the abdominal muscles inserts into the inguinal ligament and blends inferiorly with the fascia lata of the thigh. While the definition above adequately characterizes the external anatomy of the inguinal region, it does not define the very complex deep inguinal region. As a consequence, the superficial anterior abdominal wall and the external aspect of the inguinal region will be discussed as a unit, as will the deep aspect of the abdominal wall and the deep inguinal region.

Two major difficulties arise when the anatomy of the groin is discussed, i.e., disparity in terminology, and difficulty establishing a three-dimensional perspective, especially when viewing the groin from the laparoscopic viewpoint. Although, from an anatomist's viewpoint, the most proper terms are those listed in *Terminologia Anatomica* (formerly *Nomina Anatomica*), the everyday usage by surgeons of these formal terms is not common. We have elected, in most instances, to use anglicized terms in general use by contemporary surgeons.

To address the fact that many persons do not have a well-developed three-dimensional concept of the complicated anatomy of the groin, we begin with a brief overview of pelvic reference points. This approach will facilitate the

T. H. Quinn: Department of Biomedical Science, Creighton University School of Medicine, Omaha, Nebraska.

anatomic orientation of other pertinent structures. The subsequent discussion proceeds from the most superficial subcutaneous structures to the peritoneum and its relationships as observed during laparoscopic surgery.

THE PELVIC SKELETON

The pelvic bones include the iliac bones, the pubic bones and the ischial bones, which, with the sacrum, form a complete circle. The pelvis is, of course, the anchor for the majority of the muscular and ligamentous structures we will consider in this chapter. It is nearly as important, however, to think of it as a support for many of the most important structures as they pass through the pelvis. This is especially true of neural and vascular structures, the urinary bladder, and the female pelvic organs.

Even a very cursory overview of the pelvic bones immediately demonstrates that the bones form a funnel shape that is attached to the lumbar vertebral column via the sacrum at approximately a 60-degree angle. The anterosuperior iliac spines and the pubic tubercles would all nearly touch a vertical plane drawn anterior to them. This position allows one to see that the pelvic brim faces anteriorly like a funnel tipped on its side. The posterior, or narrow end, of the funnel faces backward and is ringed by the coccyx, ischial tuberosities, and the superior rami of the pubic bones. When a person stands in the anatomic position, the anterior abdominal wall muscles and their aponeurotic tendons hang sling-like (Fig. 6.1) from the thorax superiorly and from the inguinal ligament, which primarily anchors them to the superior ramus of the pubic bones inferiorly. The pelvic bones are, in the case of the anterior abdominal muscles, merely insertion points. The pubic rami are almost shelf-like in the anatomic position. They support the obturator muscles, the bladder, and the urogenital membrane.

The pelvic inlet or brim (Fig. 6.2) is bounded by the sacral promontory, the arcuate line, the pubic crest (including the pectinate line [pecten pubis], which is the site of the pectineal [Cooper's] ligament), and the pubic symphysis. Although it generally can be stated that the pelvic inlet in women is relatively more rounded (gynecoid), while the male pelvic inlet is more heart-shaped, this is not always the case. It is true, however, that in those women who have a rounded pelvic inlet the distance normally is narrow between the transversus abdominis arch and the superior ramus of the pubis. This partially may account for the extremely low incidence of direct inguinal hernias in women. The relatively large gap between these structures in the male may account for the large number of direct hernias in males. There are many other variables that may predispose the male to direct inguinal hernia, however, that will be dealt with in the sections on abdominal musculature.

The pecten pubis and the pubic symphysis form the lower anterior portion of the pelvic inlet. This roughened ridge

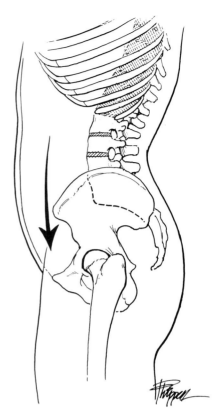

FIGURE 6.1. The relationship of the pelvis to the anterior abdominal wall in the anatomic position. The rectus muscles are suspended sling-like between the lower costal cartilages and the pubic tubercles. The *arrow* indicates the downward force exerted by visceral weight.

(Latin *pectin,* a comb) provides a point of origin for the pectineus muscle. The tendon of origin of this muscle lies just anterior to the pectineal ligament, which is actually not a ligament in the strict sense of the word, but rather, the thickened periosteum of the pecten pubis. At the anterior end of the pectinate portion of the pubic bone is the pubic tubercle. This tubercle is the point at which the pectineal ligament and the inguinal ligament intersect, thereby forming a V shape. The pectineus muscle tendon arises just inferior to this point, and provides a reinforcement to the posterior wall of the inguinal canal. The pubic tubercle also is at least a partial point of origin for the adductor muscles and for the gracilis muscle. The anterosuperior iliac spine is not only a readily palpable subcutaneous landmark, but is also the site of the lateral attachment of the inguinal ligament. The anteroinferior iliac spine is a less important landmark for the surgeon, but it should be remembered that the iliacus portion of the iliopsoas muscle crosses just medial to this structure, and thereby fills a portion of the space deep to the inguinal ligament.

The obturator foramen in the anatomic position faces nearly inferiorly and is interposed between the ischium and the pubis. The foramen and its associated structures carry an appropriate appellation, obturator (Latin *obtura-*

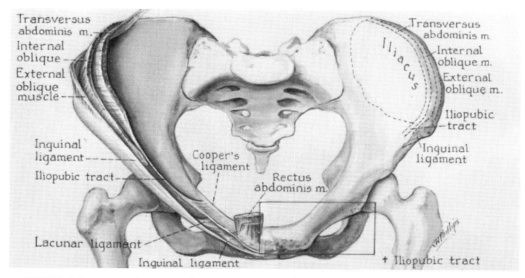

FIGURE 6.2. An anterior view of the pelvic inlet in the anatomic position. Note especially the pectineal (Cooper's) ligament, the inguinal ligament, and the lacunar ligament. The skeletal origins of the three lateral muscles and the rectus abdominis are indicated. The pelvis in the anatomic position is tilted in such a way that the viscera is primarily supported by the abdominal wall.

tor, or cork), since the tough, multilayered obturator membrane and the associated internal and external obturator muscles close off all but the obturator canal at the anterolateral portion of the structure. The canal is often the site of an obturator hernia, which may merely consist of an adventitial plug of subperitoneal fat and preperitoneal connective tissue.

SUPERFICIAL FASCIA OF THE ANTERIOR ABDOMINAL WALL

The anterior abdominal wall is a multilayered distensible encasement for the viscera, which also provides support for the spine and the force necessary to aid respiration, defecation, and urination. A great number of interdependent structures must run through its interior. Failure of any of the layers or the tissues running between them may cause the loss of integrity in the entire system. Even the outermost layer of the wall, the skin, is subject to physical principles as evidenced by Langer's tension lines.

The superficial abdominal fascia above the umbilicus is considered to be a single layer of connective tissue that contains a variable amount of fat. This layer is thicker inferiorly, especially in obese individuals. For descriptive purposes, the superficial fascia is usually described as a distinct fatty layer (Camper's fascia; panniculus adiposus) and a deeper membranous layer (Scarpa's fascia). The superficial layer of fascia is continuous with the outer layer of fascia covering the perineum, the penis, the scrotum, and the thigh. The superficial fatty layer of fascia loses its fat component as it passes into the male external

genitalia. This layer also contains the dartos muscle of the scrotal wall.

The deeper layer of the superficial fascia, or Scarpa's fascia, is thicker and more complex in the inferior abdominal wall than it is superior to the umbilicus. The deep layer of superficial fascia in its inferior reaches contains elastic fibers. It is loosely adherent to the fascia covering the aponeurosis of the external abdominal oblique and, after it crosses the inguinal ligament, to the fascia lata of the thigh. The deep layer of fascia forms the fundiform ligament of the penis, continues onto the penis and the scrotum, and then fuses with the superficial fascia of the perineum.

Hollingshead (7) maintains that the division of the superficial fascia into fatty and membranous layers, as observed in the dissecting laboratory, is probably the result of fixation artifact. He states that the connective tissue of the deeper layers of superficial fascia are simply compressed into a multilaminar fibrous stratum, which mistakenly is thought to be a separate and distinct fibrous layer of the superficial fascia. He further observes that fat is often contained in relatively great abundance in the so-called membranous layer. Based on our dissections and on operative experience, we find that this may indeed be the case, as a distinct cleavage plane between clearly discernable fatty and fibrous layers is often difficult to achieve. It is likely that a subtle gradation from primarily adipose to primarily fibrous tissue exists in the superficial fascia.

The superficial abdominal fascia ultimately is bound to the investing fascia of the external abdominal oblique muscle (the term *fascia innominata*, i.e., no-name fascia, for the investing fascia seems to be a misnomer, since this fascia is, in fact, named). The investing fascia forms a layer that is bound inferiorly to the inguinal ligament and to the pubis. It continues inferiorly onto the thigh, thereby binding the inguinal ligament to the fascia lata of the thigh with which the fascia is continuous. At the external inguinal ring, the investing fascia forms the external spermatic fascia, the outer covering of the spermatic cord. The investing fascia is somewhat thicker at the external inguinal ring, where its intercrural fibers hold the crura of the external ring together.

SUPERFICIAL VESSELS

The anterior abdominal wall is most often solely discussed in terms of muscles and their aponeuroses. The increased use of operative laparoscopic techniques requires the penetration of the anterior wall at multiple sites, with the concomitant complication of hemorrhage within the wall. It is, therefore, imperative to review not only the muscles and fascias of the abdominal wall, but also the courses of major blood vessels.

The superficial vessels of the anterior abdominal wall, i.e., the superficial epigastric, superficial circumflex iliac, and external pudendal vessels, have been the subject of studies prompted by the complication of significant abdominal wall hemorrhage after placement of laparoscopic ports (6,10). The inferior epigastric vessels, of course, are also of concern, but will be discussed in more detail in the section on the deep anterior wall.

The superficial vessels for the most part ramify in the fat of the panniculus adiposus. Perhaps the most graphic visualization of the superficial veins is the caput medusa associated with portal vein occlusion or hepatic cirrhosis. The confluence of the caval system superficial periumbilical veins with the portal system veins running along the ligamentum teres hepatis is well known. The superficial veins also are sometimes visible through the skin of normal individuals or in the transilluminated abdominal wall during laparoscopic surgery. The three major superficial veins are tributaries of the femoral vein, joining it at the saphenous hiatus (Fig. 6.3). The arteries accompanying the veins are branches of the femoral artery. These vessels either emanate from the saphenous hiatus by piercing the cribriform fascia, or pierce the fascia lata. All of the superficial vessels, therefore, must cross the inguinal ligament to course through the fat of the superficial abdominal fascia. The deep circumflex iliac artery is also a branch of the femoral artery, but crosses deep to the inguinal ligament and will be covered in more detail in conjunction with the description of the deep inguinal region.

The peripheral course of the superficial abdominal vessels recently has been the subject of detailed studies employing computed tomography (CT) (9) and Doppler techniques (14). It was determined in female subjects that

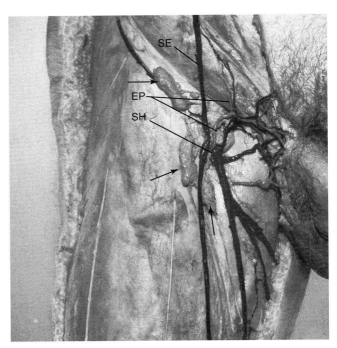

FIGURE 6.3. A dissection of the superficial aspect of the lower anterior abdominal wall and the groin. The saphenous hiatus (*SH*) is the site at which the superficial epigastric (*SE*) and superficial pudendal veins drain into the femoral vein. The external pudendal arteries (*EP*) and the inguinal lymph nodes (*arrows*) are also shown.

the superficial epigastric vessels and the superficial circumflex iliac vessels diverge from each other in such a manner after crossing the inguinal ligament that a trocar piercing the abdomen at a point 5 cm superior to the symphysis pubis and 8 cm from the midline would be placed between the two vessels. Similarly, if a trocar pierces the abdomen at the level of the umbilicus, and a distance of 8 cm from the midline, it also would be located between the two vessels.

Although the superficial external pudendal vessels (Fig. 6.3) primarily are associated with the external genitalia, it is important for the surgeon to review the proximity of both vein and artery to the spermatic cord (or round ligament). The superficial external pudendal artery arises from the medial aspect of the femoral artery, pierces the cribriform fascia, passes beneath the saphenous vein, and winds over the spermatic cord or the round ligament in females at the level of the external inguinal ring. It supplies part of the skin and fascia of the lower abdomen, the anterior scrotum or labia, and penile skin. The superficial external pudendal vein is a tributary of the saphenous vein. It drains part of the scrotum and is joined, usually on one side only, by the superficial dorsal vein of the penis. Even minor intraoperative trauma to these venous structures may result in edema, extravasation, and hematoma in the abdominal, scrotal, and penile skin.

INNERVATION

The skin of the anterior wall is innervated by the anterior and lateral cutaneous branches of the ventral rami of the seventh to the twelfth intercostal nerves and by the ventral rami of the first and second lumbar nerves. The dermatomes of these nerves significantly overlap each other. The nerves gain the anterior and lateral aspects of the abdominal skin by coursing between muscle layers, and ultimately by piercing the sheath of the rectus abdominis (Fig. 6.4). They will, therefore, also be discussed later in this chapter in terms of their relationships with these layers and their role as the motor nerves to the abdominal musculature.

The skin of the lower anterior abdominal wall from the umbilicus to the pubis and part of the external genitalia is supplied by branches of the ventral primary rami of the tenth (level of the umbilicus) through the twelfth thoracic (the subcostal nerve) nerves and the first lumbar nerve. The thoracic nerves have anterior and lateral cutaneous branches. The ventral primary ramus of the first lumbar nerve contributes to the iliohypogastric, ilioinguinal, and genitofemoral nerves (Fig. 6.5). The iliohypogastric nerve has a lateral branch that exits the external oblique muscle just above the iliac crest; it innervates superolateral gluteal skin. Of more importance in the context of hernia repair is the anterior branch of the iliohypogastric nerve, which exits the external oblique aponeurosis just above the external inguinal ring and continues inferiorly to supply the suprapubic skin. Note that the iliohypogastric nerve has some fibers in common with both the subcostal and the ilioinguinal nerves.

The ilioinguinal nerve supplies a portion of the internal oblique muscle and then, without piercing other muscle layers, accompanies the spermatic cord through the external inguinal ring. It supplies the skin of the medial thigh proximal to the inguinal ligament, the root of the penis, and the upper anterior scrotum. In the female, the nerve exits the external inguinal ring and supplies the mons pubis and the labium majus. The genitofemoral nerve emerges from the anterior surface of the psoas major muscle either as a combined genital and femoral nerve, or by two separate branches. The genital branch exits the pelvis through the deep inguinal ring and courses with the spermatic cord, supplying the cremaster muscle, the only muscle innervated or pierced by the genitofemoral nerve. After the nerve's egress from the lateral aspect of the external inguinal ring, it innervates a large area of the anterolateral scrotal skin. The femoral branches of the genitofemoral nerve are derived from both the first and second lumbar nerves. The femoral branches pass under or pierce the inguinal ligament, travel across the thigh lateral to the saphenous hiatus, and then travel a short distance in the femoral sheath, emerging from it to supply the skin over the femoral sheath.

It may be safely stated that the three superficial branches of the lumbar plexus discussed above are the most commonly injured during external herniorrhaphy. It will be seen in subsequent discussion of the deep inguinal region that these nerves also inadvertently may be injured during laparoscopic herniorrhaphy.

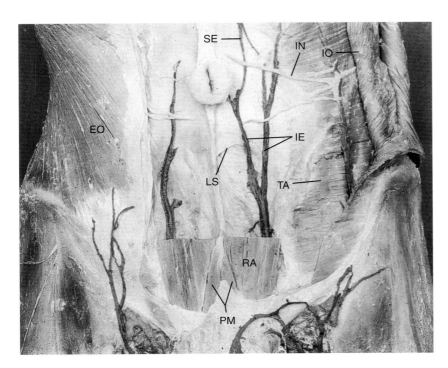

FIGURE 6.4. A dissection of the anterior abdominal wall. The anterior branches of the intercostal nerves (*IN*) are seen coursing between the layers of the lateral abdominal muscle and entering the sheath of the rectus abdominis. The blood supply of the rectus is also seen: superior epigastric artery (*SE*); inferior epigastric artery (*IE*). The midline muscles, rectus abdominis (*RA*), and pyramidalis (*PM*) are seen, as well as the lateral muscles, the transversus abdominis (*TA*), internal oblique (*IO*), and the external oblique (*EO*). *LS*, linea semicircularis.

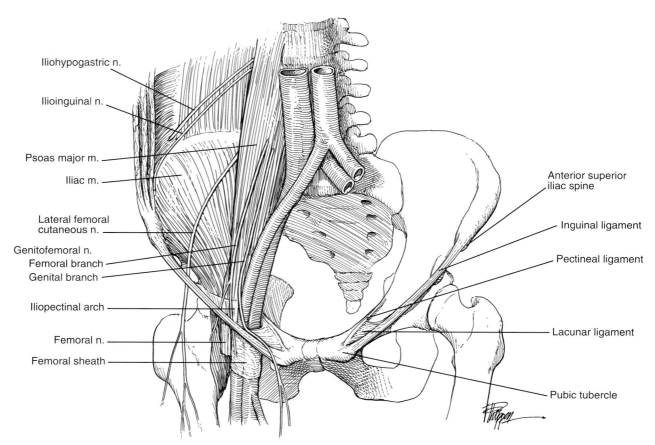

Iliohypogastric n.

Ilioinguinal n.

Psoas major m.

Iliac m.

Lateral femoral cutaneous n.

Genitofemoral n.
Femoral branch
Genital branch

Iliopectinal arch

Femoral n.

Femoral sheath

Anterior superior iliac spine

Inguinal ligament

Pectineal ligament

Lacunar ligament

Pubic tubercle

FIGURE 6.5. The branches of the lumbar plexus. Special notice should be taken of the three superficial nerves of the plexus: genitofemoral, iliohypogastric, and ilioinguinal.

ANTERIOR ABDOMINAL WALL MUSCULATURE AND LIGAMENTS

The muscle bundles and fibrous tissues within each layer of the abdomen are arrayed at an angle to those in the other layers. Each of the layers of muscle is covered by a sheet of investing fascia, which enhances the ability of the muscle bundles to function as a seamless, coherent unit. The apposed investing fascias are loosely adherent to each other between the muscle layers where they collectively are referred to as the interparietal fascia. These fascias are readily separated in the living or in fresh tissue cadaver dissections.

The flat lateral abdominal muscles are inserted via laminated aponeurotic sheets (Fig. 6.6), which further enhance the integrity of the abdominal wall. These lamina contribute to the rectus sheath, which envelops the rectus muscles and ultimately inserts in the midline, thereby forming the linea alba. At a highly variable point inferior to the level of the umbilicus, the aponeurotic fibers all pass anterior to the rectus muscles. The linea semicircularis (line of Douglas) marks this site (Fig. 6.4).

The most superficial of the lateral abdominal muscles is the external abdominal oblique (Fig. 6.7). This muscle arises by small slips from the lower eight ribs. Its upper fibers of origin interdigitate with the serratus anterior, while the latissimus dorsi is associated with the lower fibers of origin. The direction of the muscle fibers changes gradually from nearly vertical posteriorly, to horizontal anterosuperiorly by the xiphoid process, to oblique anteroinferiorly. The extent of the muscular portion of the external oblique is compared with its aponeurotic portion in Fig. 6.6. The muscle fibers that arise posteriorly insert on the anterior half of the iliac crest. The aponeurotic tendon of insertion of the obliquely arranged anteroinferior fibers folds back upon itself to form the inguinal ligament, which is discussed in more detail below.

The aponeurotic fibers of the external abdominal oblique divide into a thick inferomedial crus and a thinner superolateral crus to form the subcutaneous (external) inguinal ring. This so-called ring is actually a triangular aperture that has as its base the crest of the pubis. The apex of the aperture is reinforced superolaterally by the intercrural fibers derived from transversely oriented fibers of the investing fascia of the external oblique muscle. The ring allows the spermatic cord or the round ligament of the uterus to exit the pelvis. The ilioinguinal nerve also leaves the pelvis through the external inguinal ring.

The aponeurosis proper of the external abdominal oblique is the most extensive of the three lateral abdominal

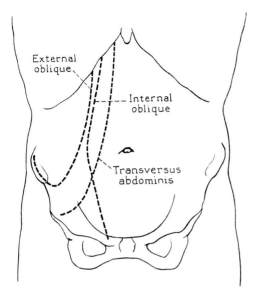

FIGURE 6.6. The approximate lines of transition from muscle to aponeurosis of the three lateral muscles of the anterior abdominal wall. Variations in these proportions are common.

muscles. It only contributes to the anterior rectus sheath, but its fibers are known to cross the linea alba after contributing to it, and to interweave and overlap aponeurotic fibers from the opposite external abdominal oblique aponeurosis (13), thus increasing the strength of the abdominal wall in its lower, more dependent portion.

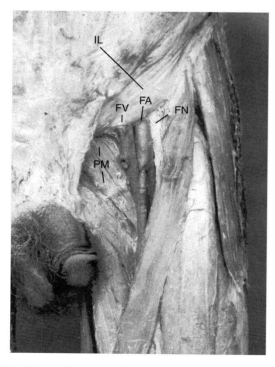

FIGURE 6.7. A dissection of the external abdominal oblique muscle. The inferior insertion of the external abdominal oblique is the inguinal ligament (*IL*). The relationship of the femoral vessels (*FA, FV*) and the femoral nerve (*FN*) to the inguinal ligament and the pectineus muscle (*PM*) can be seen.

LIGAMENTS ASSOCIATED WITH THE ANTERIOR PELVIS

The so-called ligaments of the anterior pelvis (Fig. 6.8) for the most part are not ligaments in the most common use of the term, but rather, they may be tendons of insertion, or in the case of the pectineal (Cooper's) ligament, locally thickened periosteum.

THE INGUINAL LIGAMENT

The inguinal ligament (Fig. 6.8) is not an autonomous cord-like structure, but rather, that portion of the aponeurosis of the external oblique muscle that folds back beneath itself. A more complicated description, however, is called for in order to describe this prominent and useful landmark of the groin. The inguinal ligament is attached at its lateral extreme to the anterosuperior iliac spine. The ligament courses from this point in a graceful inferiorly directed arc toward its primary medial insertion on the pubic tubercle. The inguinal ligament forms a bridge across the iliopsoas muscle, neural, and vascular structures as they pass out of the pelvis. This affords the external abdominal oblique muscle a strong yet distensible anterior insertion where direct attachment to the pelvic brim otherwise is thwarted by the presence of other structures. It should be noted that a continuation and local thickening of the iliac fascia, called the iliopectineal arch, affords an additional lateral attachment for the inguinal ligament. The iliopectineal arch itself anteriorly is attached to the anterosuperior iliac spine, and posteromedially to the iliopubic eminence. The tissue of the arch therefore not only anchors the inguinal ligament, but also divides the space deep to the inguinal ligament into the muscular and vascular compartments (lacunae) containing the iliopsoas muscle and the femoral nerve. The investing fascia of the external abdominal oblique also anchors the inguinal ligament since it passes over it and fuses with it before passing into the thigh, where it blends with the fascia lata.

The fan-shaped medial expansion of the inguinal ligament is called the lacunar ligament; it is so-named because of the depression (Latin *lacuna,* or cavity) formed in the ligament as it spans the area between the inguinal ligament proper and the pectineal ligament. The lacunar ligament forms the most medial part of the floor of the inguinal canal. It does not directly form the medial border of the femoral canal (8), but most often does recurve along the pectinate line, blending in some individuals with the pectinate ligament.

The reflex, or reflected inguinal ligament, when present, is formed by the medial fibers of the external abdominal oblique aponeurosis, which course medially from their attachment to the pectinate line and subsequently join the linea alba. Henle's ligament, here included for the sake of completeness, is a thin ligament found on the opposite (deep) surface of the rectus abdominis muscle that follows a course similar to that of the reflected ligament and is not of major use in groin herniorrhaphy.

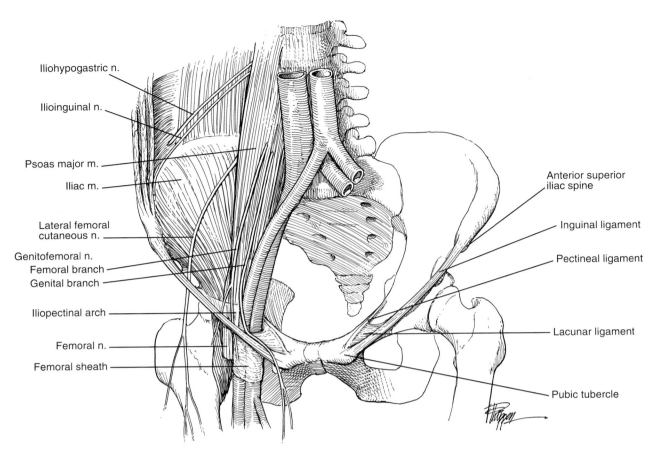

FIGURE 6.8. A view of the principal ligaments of the inguinal region: the inguinal ligament, lacunar ligament, and pectineal (Cooper's) ligament.

THE INTERNAL ABDOMINAL OBLIQUE MUSCLE AND APONEUROSIS

The middle layer of the lateral group of the musculoaponeurotic complex is the internal abdominal oblique muscle. This muscle primarily arises from the iliac fascia along the iliac crest and from a band of iliac fascia fused with the inguinal ligament. The uppermost fibers course obliquely toward the distal ends of the lower three or four ("floating") ribs. The muscle fibers of the internal oblique fan out, following the shape of the iliac crest so that the lowermost fibers are directed inferiorly. These fibers arch over the round ligament or the spermatic cord. Some of the lower muscle bundles in the male join fibers of the transversus abdominis to form the cremaster muscle.

The aponeurosis of the internal oblique (Fig. 6.6) above the level of the umbilicus splits to envelop the rectus abdominis, reforming in the midline to join and interweave with the fibers of the linea alba. Below the level of the umbilicus, the aponeurosis does not split, but rather, runs anterior to the rectus muscle, continues medially as a single sheet, joins the anterior rectus sheath and finally contributes to the linea alba. Note that when viewed from the anterior surface, the aponeurotic portion of the internal oblique curves laterally, most markedly from the midline at the level of the umbilicus.

THE TRANSVERSUS ABDOMINIS MUSCLE AND APONEUROSIS

The transversus abdominis muscle (Fig. 6.4) arises from the iliac fascia along the iliac crest and the inguinal ligament (1) and from the lower six costal cartilages and ribs. The latter fibers also interdigitate with the lateral diaphragmatic fibers. The muscle bundles of the transversus abdominis for the most part run horizontally. The lower medial fibers may, however, continue in a more inferomedial course toward the site of insertion on the crest and pectinate line of the pubis.

The aponeurosis of the transversus abdominis joins the posterior lamina of the internal abdominal oblique, forming above the umbilicus a portion of the posterior rectus sheath. Below the umbilicus, the transversus abdominis aponeurosis is a component of the anterior rectus sheath. The gradual termination of aponeurotic tissue on the posterior aspect of the rectus abdominis forms the arcuate line (of Douglas, Fig. 6.4). The medial aponeurotic fibers of the transversus abdominis insert on the pecten pubis and the crest of the pubis, forming the falx inguinalis. These fibers infrequently (3%) (4), are joined by a portion of the internal oblique aponeurosis; only then is a true conjoined tendon formed.

The arch formed by the termination of the aponeurotic fibers is called the aponeurotic arch (Fig. 6.9A and 6.9B).

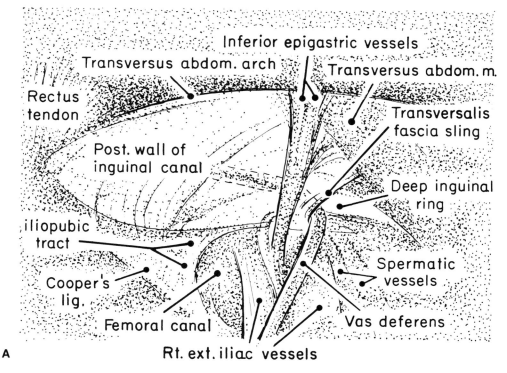

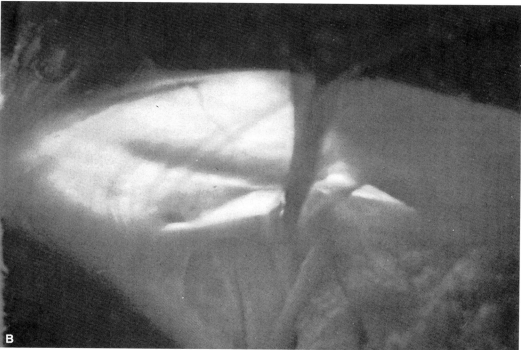

FIGURE 6.9. A drawing and photograph of the transilluminated transversalis muscle and its aponeurosis. **A:** The line drawing identifies many of the important structures in the transversus layer of the groin, shown in part B. **B:** This photograph was taken from within the abdominal cavity on completion of a dissection that removed much of the tissue from the surfaces both superficial and deep to the transversus abdominis muscle and its aponeurosis.

The area beneath the arch varies. A high arch may be a predisposing factor in direct inguinal hernia. The contraction of the transversus abdominis causes the arch to move downward toward the inguinal ligament, thereby constituting a form of shutter mechanism that reinforces the weakest area of the groin when intraabdominal pressure is raised.

FALX INGUINALIS AND THE CONJOINED TENDON

The falx inguinalis (Latin, meaning inguinal sickle) is a variation in the insertion of the transversus abdominis aponeurosis. The fibers of the lower portion of the aponeurosis deflect inferiorly and do not join the rectus sheath. Instead, they form a sickle-shaped thickening of the aponeurosis, which inserts lateral to the rectus sheath. Condon (4) states that this variation is present in only 11% of the bodies that he dissected. Similarly, a true conjoined tendon made up of the inserted fibers of the inferior portion of the aponeuroses of the internal oblique and the transversus abdominis muscles is uncommon (Condon observed 3%). What the surgeon visualizes as "conjoined" tendon is most often solely composed of the fibers of the transversus abdominis aponeurosis, i.e., the falx inguinalis.

RECTUS ABDOMINIS MUSCLE

The rectus abdominis (Fig. 6.10) is a sheathed and segmented strap muscle that arises from the fifth to the seventh costal cartilages and inserts on the pubic symphysis and the pubic crest. The three tendinous intersections that segment the muscle occur just below the xiphoid process, at the umbilicus, and at a point approximately midway between the other two inscriptions. The rectus abdominis muscle is enveloped by a sheath whose anterior component is adherent to the muscle at the tendinous intersections. The muscle laterally is delineated by the semicircular line (linea semicircularis). This line is actually a groove formed by the aponeuroses of the three lateral abdominal muscles. There is normally no muscle in this groove. The line is apparent in thin, well-muscled individuals, but obscured by adipose tissue in an ever-increasing number of individuals.

The small pyramidalis muscle accompanies the rectus abdominis at its origin in a minority of individuals. The pyramidalis arises from the pubic symphysis and by other tendinous fibers on the front of the pubis. It lies within the rectus sheath and tapers to attach to the linea alba, the conjunction of the two rectus sheaths.

THE RECTUS SHEATH

Although the individual aponeuroses that comprise the sheath of the rectus muscle have been discussed separately above, it is helpful now to consider them as a unit. The sheath of rectus abdominis is a complicated lamination of aponeurotic fibers from the three lateral abdominal muscles. The component layers of the rectus sheath vary according to the level of the sheath examined. When a cross section of the rectus abdominis and its sheath are examined

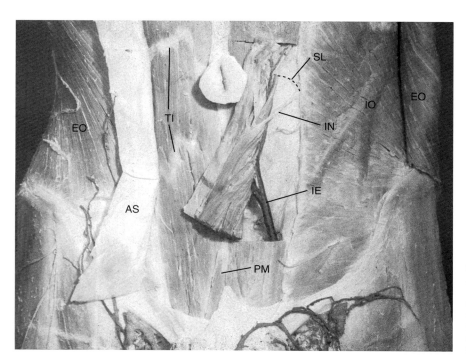

FIGURE 6.10. A dissection of the rectus abdominis muscle. Note the semicircular line (*SL*); tendinous intersections (*TI*); pyramidalis muscle (*PM*); anterior rectus sheath (*AS*); external oblique muscle (*EO*); internal oblique muscle (*IO*); inferior epigastric vessels (*IE*); and some of the intercostal nerves (*IN*) that innervate the rectus abdominis.

immediately inferior to the umbilicus, the anterior sheath is found to be composed of the aponeurosis of the external abdominal oblique, the anterior leaf of the aponeurosis of the internal abdominal oblique, and the aponeurosis of the transversus abdominis. These layers arise at the linea semicircularis and insert in the midline linea alba or join the sheath of the opposite rectus muscle. The linea alba is the midline structure created by the interweaving of the component laminae of the rectus sheath with each other and with those from the opposite rectus sheath. The umbilical ring punctuates it at the level of the disc between the third and fourth lumbar vertebrae. The posterior sheath superior to the umbilicus consists of contributions from the posterior portion of the internal abdominal oblique and the transversus abdominis aponeurosis.

At a variable point inferior to the umbilicus, the anterior sheath is formed by contributions from aponeurotic layers derived from all of the lateral muscles, while none appreciably participate in the formation of the posterior rectus sheath. The macroscopically visible landmark of this transition is the semicircular arcuate line (of Douglas). The tissue intimately covering the posterior aspect of the rectus abdominis at this point is the transversalis fascia (not the aponeurosis of the transversalis muscle).

BLOOD SUPPLY AND INNERVATION OF THE ANTERIOR ABDOMINAL WALL MUSCULATURE

The blood supply of the lateral muscles of the anterior wall primarily is from the lower three or four intercostal arteries (Fig. 6.4), the deep circumflex iliac arteries, and the lumbar arteries. The rectus abdominis has a complicated blood supply derived from the superior epigastric artery (a terminal branch of the internal thoracic), the inferior epigastric artery (a branch of the external iliac), and the lower intercostal arteries. The latter arteries enter the sides of the muscle after traveling between the oblique muscles. The superior and the inferior epigastric arteries enter the rectus sheath and anastomose near the umbilicus. The course of the epigastric arteries will be discussed in more detail in the section on the deep aspect of the anterior wall.

The innervation of the anterior wall muscles is also multiple. The lower intercostal and upper lumbar (T7-12, L1-2) contribute most of the innervation to the lateral muscles, as well as the rectus abdominis and the overlying skin. The nerves pass anteriorly in a plane between the internal abdominal oblique and the transversus abdominis, eventually piercing the lateral aspect of the rectus sheath to innervate the muscle therein. The external oblique muscle receives branches of the intercostal nerves, which penetrate the internal oblique to reach it. The anterior ends of the nerves form part of the cutaneous innervation of the abdominal wall. The first lumbar nerve divides into the ilioinguinal and iliohypogastric nerves. These may divide within the psoas muscle or between the internal oblique and transversus abdominis muscles. The ilioinguinal nerve passes through the external inguinal ring to run with the spermatic cord, while the iliohypogastric nerve pierces the external oblique to innervate the skin above the pubis. The cremaster muscle fibers, which are derived from the internal oblique muscle, are innervated by the genitofemoral nerve (L1-2).

THE ANTERIOR ABDOMINAL WALL AND INGUINAL REGION FROM THE LAPAROSCOPIC VIEWPOINT

The surgeon using laparoscopic techniques must rely heavily on visual cues seen on a television screen rather than on a combination of touch and sight. The luxury of direct palpation and visualization has been replaced by the requisite intervening instrumentation. We have chosen to approach the anatomic structures in this section from deep to superficial, treating the deepest layer, the peritoneum, as the first layer. The basic view from the "inside out" capitalizes on the many easily identified landmarks that must be familiar to anyone who wishes to master minimally invasive herniorrhaphy.

DEEP ASPECT OF THE ANTERIOR ABDOMINAL WALL

The parietal peritoneum consists of a monolayer of mesothelial cells that are supported by a layer of connective tissue, and most often, and perhaps primarily, by the structures that it clings to. The peritoneum is interlaced with blood vessels, which carry on their walls nerves that cause the peritoneum to be sensitive to mechanical, chemical, and thermal stimuli. Since the translucent peritoneum is closely adherent to the posterior abdominal wall structures, many of them can be seen through it. Some structures stand out in relief under the peritoneum, causing the peritoneum to be gathered or thickened to form the so-called peritoneal ligaments (Fig. 6.11). These features are often accentuated by the insufflation of the abdominal cavity during laparoscopic surgery.

Two peritoneal ligaments or peritoneal folds (Fig. 6.11) on each side of the midline form a triangle with its apex at the umbilicus. The base of the triangle is the bladder and the pubic bone. The ligament present in the midline is called the median umbilical ligament. The urachus, the adult remnant of the fetal allantois, is contained within its folds. The urachus may be patent for some distance superior to the bladder. The folds adjacent to it on each side are the medial umbilical ligaments containing the fibrous obliterated portions of the umbilical arteries. The lateral umbil-

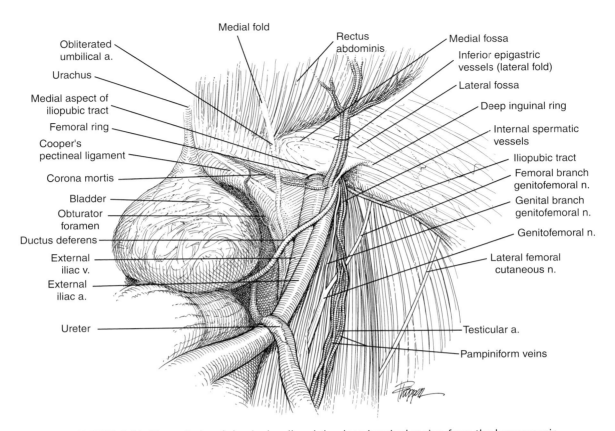

FIGURE 6.11. The anterior abdominal wall and the deep inguinal region from the laparoscopic surgeon's perspective. The three peritoneal folds are the median fold, or urachus, the medial fold, containing the obliterated umbilical artery, and the lateral umbilical fold, containing the inferior epigastric vessels. The deep inguinal ring is also seen, as are the major structures that enter or leave it: the genital branch of the genitofemoral nerve, the pampiniform veins, the ductus deferens, and the testicular artery.

ical ligaments (folds) are created by the underlying inferior epigastric vessels. The vessels course upward from the external iliac vessels toward the arcuate line, at which point they enter the posterior rectus sheath to further supply the rectus muscle and to anastomose with the superior epigastric arteries.

The peritoneum covers only the superoposterior portion of the bladder. A small depression in the peritoneum covering the bladder is called the supravesical fossa. A fold called the transverse vesical fold spanning the area between the two deep inguinal rings may be present. The medial and the lateral umbilical ligaments form the boundaries of the medial fossa. Direct hernias occur in this fossa. The lateral umbilical ligament (epigastric vessels), along with the lateral border of the rectus abdominis muscle, forms the less-well-defined lateral fossa. The lateral border of the fossa is not obvious in the insufflated abdomen. The deep inguinal ring is the principal landmark in the lateral fossa.

The translucency of the peritoneum in most individuals allows the surgeon to observe the darkly colored gonadal vessels, the ductus deferens, or the female round ligament as they course toward the deep inguinal ring.

EXTRAPERITONEAL SPACES, TRANSVERSALIS FASCIA, AND ITS DERIVATIVES

When the peritoneum is opened from within the abdomen, the preperitoneal space is entered. This space is enclosed by the parietal peritoneum posteriorly and the anterior lamina of the transversalis fascia anteriorly. It is now generally accepted that the transversalis fascia can be considered to consist of two laminae. The deep lamina, i.e., the more posterior lamina, is composed of irregularly thickened strands of fibrous tissue intermingled with loculi of adipose tissue. This layer is readily separable from the peritoneum and is often referred to as the preperitoneal fascia. The posterior lamina of the transversalis fascia is anchored inferiorly to the pubic ramus. The anterior lamina of the transversalis fascia is applied to the posterior aspect of the transversus abdominis muscle and its aponeurosis. The area between the parietal peritoneum and the anterior lamina of the transversalis fascia is designated Bogros' space. This space is described by Bendavid (2) and Read (12) as the lateral extension of the retropubic Retzius' space, but others (3) believe that the two spaces are separate. The inferior epigastric vessels and the deep inguinal venous plexus (Fig. 6.12) described by Bendavid (2) are enclosed by the layers of the transversalis fascia. The transversalis fascia is continuous laterally and posteriorly with the endoabdominal and endopelvic fascia and thereby forms with them an extraperitoneal reinforcing layer.

The analogues or derivatives of the transversalis fascia must also be considered. These structures are actually condensations of the transversalis fascia. The most important of these are the crura of the deep inguinal ring, which form the transversalis fascial sling of the deep inguinal ring, the iliopubic tract, part of the pectineal (Cooper's) ligament, and the iliopectineal arch. These derivatives are among the most important to surgeons using laparoscopic techniques since they provide not only dependable landmarks, but also may afford sites for the placement of sutures or staples.

The internal or deep inguinal ring (Figs. 6.11 and 6.13) is formed by the transversalis fascia. The thicker medial aspect of the ring is formed by a redundant portion of the transversalis fascia after the passage of the testicle through the fascia. The lateral portion of the deep ring is attached to the transversus abdominis muscle, which causes the ring to be pulled superolaterally when the muscle contracts. This creates a type of shutter or valve mechanism, which normally guards against indirect hernia formation. The transversalis fascia near the deep ring is the source of the internal spermatic fascia. In addition to the internal spermatic fascia and the testicle, the deep ring transmits the constituents of the spermatic cord: the ductus deferens, genitofemoral nerve, pampiniform plexus of veins, testicular artery, cremaster fibers derived from the internal abdominal oblique muscle, and the external spermatic fascia.

The iliopubic tract (Fig. 6.8) is an aponeurotic band forming the inferior margin of the transversalis fascia, which is mixed with stronger fibers from the transversus abdominis aponeurosis, as recently demonstrated by Page (11) and Gilroy (5) et al. This band of tissue is anchored superolaterally to the medial iliac crest and stretches medially to insert on the pubis. Some of its fibers recurve to blend with the pectineal (Cooper's) ligament. In its course, it provides a reinforcement to the inferior crus of the deep inguinal ring and an inferior extension that becomes the anterior portion of the femoral sheath. The iliopubic tract contributes to the posterior wall of the inguinal canal, where it fuses with the deep fibers of the inguinal ligament. The iliopubic tract has become an important landmark to the surgeon using laparoscopic techniques since it is beneath this ligament that many of the branches of the lumbar plexus (Fig. 6.8) exit the pelvis after running deep to the iliacus fascia (itself a portion of the transversalis fascia). Staples or sutures placed through or inferior to the iliopubic tract may injure the branches of the lumbar plexus.

The pectineal (Cooper's) ligament (Fig. 6.8) is not only one of the most persistent eponymous terms in the anatomic and surgical literature, but also is one of the most useful to the surgeon as a landmark and as a strong anchoring structure for both open and laparoscopic herniorrha-

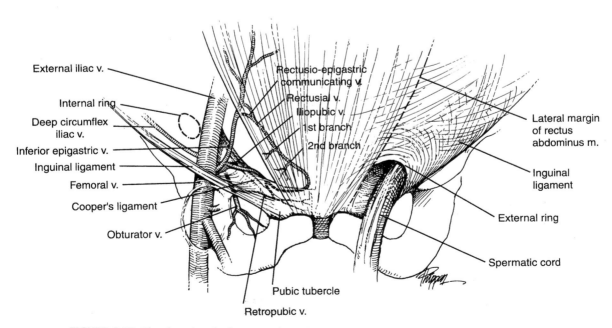

FIGURE 6.12. The deep inguinal venous plexus in Bogros' space. (From Bendavid, R. The space of Bogros and the deep inguinal circulation. *Surg Gynecol Obstet* 1992;174:356–357, with permission.)

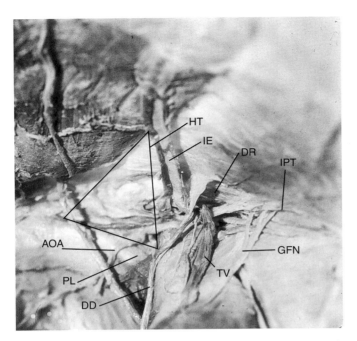

FIGURE 6.13. A dissection of the deep inguinal ring (*DR*) and the structures associated with it. The testicular vessels (*TV*) and the ductus deferens (*DD*) are seen entering the ring, as is the genital branch of the genitofemoral nerve (*GFN*). The ring is made up of two bands of transversalis fascia called crura. The iliopubic tract (*IPT*) can be seen contributing to the inferior crus. The femoral branch of the genitofemoral nerve (*GFN*) courses below it. Its medial border is the rectus abdominis muscle, the inferior border is the pectineal ligament (*PL*), and the lateral border is formed by the inferior epigastric vessels (*IE*). An aberrant obturator artery (*AOA*) can also be seen. The aberrant vessel occurs in approximately 30% of the specimens we have dissected. *HT*, the inguinal (Hesselbach's) triangle.

phy. The ligament proper is actually not a true ligament, i.e., it does not connect two bones, but rather, a blend of thickened fibrous periosteum and the recurved fibers of the iliopubic tract and the inguinal ligament.

The iliopectineal arch (Fig. 6.8) is comprised of the condensed medial fibers of the iliacus fascia, which is a named portion of the transversalis fascia. It forms a band of connective tissue between the lateral neuromuscular compartment containing the iliopsoas muscle, and the femoral and lateral femoral cutaneous nerves and medial compartment containing the femoral vessels. The band of condensed tissue primarily inserts on the pectineal line, but it also contributes to the posterior lamina of the femoral sheath and the floor of the inguinal canal.

The femoral sheath (Fig. 6.14) and its constituent parts are, for the most part, derivatives of the transversalis fascia. The sheath is a fibrous, tubular, downward prolongation of transversalis fascia. Anteriorly and medially, the walls of the sheath are formed by the transversalis fascia that is continuous with the iliopubic tract. Posterolaterally, the sheath is formed by a continuation of the iliopsoas portion of the transversalis fascia. The posteromedial wall of the sheath is derived from the pectineus fascia and the iliopectineal arch. The femoral sheath is divided by septa into a lateral arterial compartment, an intermediate venous compartment, and the medially placed femoral canal. The anterior and posterior walls of the sheath fuse inferiorly with the adventitia of the vessels.

The femoral canal (Fig. 6.14) is found just medial to the femoral vein. The canal contains loose connective tissue and typically a lymph node (Cloquet's). The canal is most likely

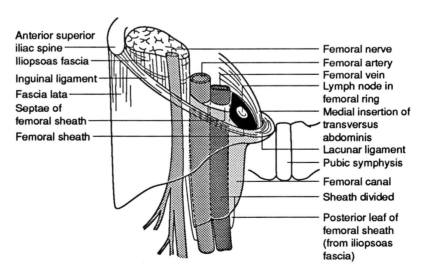

FIGURE 6.14. The femoral sheath and its associated structures. The anterior leaf of the sheath is continuous with the transversalis fascia of the anterior abdominal wall, while the posterior sheath is derived from the iliacus fascia (a portion of the transversalis fascia). Femoral hernias enter the femoral canal, which lies just medial to the femoral vein within its sheath. (From Richards AT, Quinn TH, Fitzgibbons RJ Jr. Abdominal wall hernias. In: Greenfield LJ, Mulholland MW, Oldham KT, et al., eds. *Surgery: scientific principles and practice,* 3rd ed. Philadelphia: Lippincott Williams & Wilkins, 2001:1185–1223, with permission.)

present to allow space for sudden expansion of the femoral vein. The orifice of the femoral canal is a complex crescent moon–shaped structure called the femoral ring. The anterior border of the ring is formed by the iliopubic tract; the medial aspect of the ring is completed by the recurved fibers of the tract as they blend with the pectineal ligament and fascia. The posterior part of the ring is formed by the pectineus fascia and the superior ramus of the pubis. The ring may be sealed by a weak membrane, but this is never adequate prevention against eventration of viscera or connective tissue into the short (2-cm–long) canal.

THE INGUINAL CANAL

The inguinal canal (Fig. 6.15) has been alluded to several times throughout this chapter in terms of its component parts. In order to concisely review the construction of the canal per se, however, it is best to reassemble the canal in one section of the chapter. The inguinal canal envelopes the spermatic cord in males and the round ligament in females. The approximately 4-cm–long canal appears triangular in cross section. The deep inguinal ring is the entrance to the canal (see above), and the external inguinal ring is the exit.

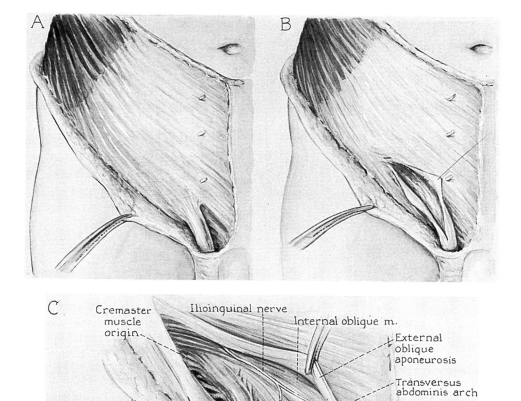

FIGURE 6.15. Three stages in the dissection of the spermatic cord. **A:** The intact external oblique aponeurosis. **B:** The external spermatic fascia (derived from the transversalis fascia) and the superficial investing layer of external oblique fascia (innominate fascia) are opened to reveal more of the spermatic cord. **C:** The external oblique aponeurosis has been widely opened and the spermatic cord mobilized by dissecting many of its cremasteric attachments to the walls of the inguinal canal.

The deep ring previously has been described in detail in this chapter. The external ring is located in the medial third of the anterior wall of the canal. It is actually a small slit-like opening in the aponeurosis of the external abdominal oblique, which provides most of the fibers of the anterior wall. The inguinal ligament is formed by the inferior, rolled-over edge of the external oblique aponeurosis. The ligament, in turn, forms the medial third of the inferior wall of the canal. If it is again stated that the canal has a triangular cross section, the inferior wall can be equated with the base of the triangle. The middle third of the inferior wall is formed by the pectineus muscle and its associated fascia, while the lateral third of the inferior wall is formed by the iliopubic tract and the femoral sheath. The posterior wall or floor of the canal is so called because in the supine position this part of the triangular canal faces the operating table. It is made up of the transversus abdominis aponeurosis and its associated fascia. The medial two thirds of the floor (posterior wall) is also buttressed by the rectus abdominis sheath and the falx inguinalis.

THE INGUINAL (HESSELBACH'S) TRIANGLE

The inguinal triangle (Fig. 6.13) is the weak area through which direct inguinal hernias pass. The boundaries of the triangle are the rectus abdominis and the falx inguinalis medially, the inferior epigastric vessels laterally, and the pectineal (Cooper's) ligament inferiorly. Although the inferior margin has also been described as the inguinal ligament, we use the pectineal ligament because it can be seen from the laparoscopic viewpoint. The weak area beneath the aponeurotic arch of the transversus abdominis allows a direct hernia to push the peritoneum and the transversalis fascia outward and deep or inferior to the spermatic cord.

DEEP INGUINAL AND ABDOMINAL WALL VASCULATURE

The primary blood supply to the lower part of the anterior abdominal wall is from the inferior epigastric artery (Figs. 6.4 and 6.13). It is a branch of the external iliac artery. The inferior epigastric artery may give off a branch called the aberrant obturator artery, which may either replace or accompany the obturator branch of the internal iliac artery into the obturator canal. When both arteries are present, a circle often called the "corona mortis" is formed. This ominous title points to the frequent injury of this vessel. The deep circumflex artery is usually a branch of the inferior epigastric artery. It runs laterally along the iliopubic tract, pierces the iliac fascia, and eventually anastomoses with the deep lumbar arteries. The deep circumflex artery is in some danger of injury during laparoscopic hernia repairs.

REFERENCES

1. Anson BJ, McVay CB. Inguinal hernia. I. The anatomy of the region. *Surg Gynecol Obstet* 1938;66:186–191.
2. Bendavid R. The space of Bogros and the deep inguinal venous circulation. *Surg Gynecol Obstet* 1992;174:355–358.
3. Colborn GL, Skandalakis JE. Laparoscopic inguinal anatomy. *Hernia* 1998;2:179–191.
4. Condon RE. The anatomy of the inguinal region and its relation to groin hernia. In: Nyhus LM, Condon RE, eds. *Hernia,* 4th ed. Philadelphia: JB Lippincott Co, 1995:16–72.
5. Gilroy AM, Marks SC, Lei Q, et al. Anatomical characteristics of the iliopubic tract: implications for repair of inguinal hernias. *Clin Anat* 1992;5:255–263.
6. Green LS, Loughin KR, Kovoussi L. Management of epigastric vessel injury during laparoscopy. *J Endourol* 1992;6:99–101.
7. Hollingshead WH. The abdominal wall and the inguinal region. In: *Anatomy for surgeons,* vol 2. New York: Hoeber–Harper, 1961: 224–227.
8. Hollingshead WH. The abdominal wall and the inguinal region. In: *Anatomy for surgeons,* vol 2. New York: Hoeber–Harper, 1961: 257–258.
9. Hurd WW, Bude RO, DeLancey J, et al. The location of abdominal wall blood vessels in relationship to abdominal landmarks apparent at laparoscopy. *Am J Obstet Gynecol* 1994;171:642–646.
10. Hurd WW, Pearl ML, De Lancey J, et al. Laparoscopic injury of abdominal wall blood vessels: a report of three cases. *Obstet Gynecol* 1993;82:673–676.
11. Page DW, Gilroy A, Marks SC. The iliopubic tract; an essential guide in teaching and performing groin hernia repairs. *Contemp Surg* 1996;49:219–222.
12. Read RC. Anatomy of abdominal herniation: the parietoperitoneal spaces. In: Nyhus LM, Baker RJ, Fisher JE, eds. *Mastery of surgery,* 3rd ed, vol II. Boston: Little, Brown and Company, 1997:1795–1806.
13. Rizk NN. A new description of the anterior abdominal wall in man and animals. *J Anat* 1980;131:373–385.
14. Whitely MS, Laws SA, Wise MH. Use of a hand-held Doppler to avoid abdominal wall vessels in laparoscopic surgery. *Ann R Coll Surg Engl* 1994;76:348–350.

7

CLASSIFICATION OF VENTRAL AND GROIN HERNIAS

ROBERT M. ZOLLINGER, JR.

VENTRAL HERNIAS

Many classifications for groin or inguinal hernias have been proposed over the past 50 years, but none have been published for total classification of all ventral hernias of the abdomen. Using a strict definition of ventral, any hernia of the entire abdomen would qualify—including those of the diaphragm, pelvic floor, and lumbar areas. By common convention, however, ventral hernias are thought of as those occurring in the anterior (ventral) abdominal wall. One possible system to categorize these anterior ventral hernias might be as follows: (a) congenital—present at birth; (b) acquired; (c) incisional; and (d) traumatic. These four groups contain the most commonly seen ventral hernias and many are reviewed in detail elsewhere in this book.

CONGENITAL

Most congenital ventral hernias present at birth are found in or near the midline linea alba and its central opening for the umbilical vessels or cord.

Omphaloceles represent a herniation of the abdominal viscera into the tissues of the umbilical cord. They are variable in size and may contain the majority of the abdominal viscera. An important characteristic is the finding of a hernia sac made of peritoneum, as well as an external layer of amnion. The diagnosis can be made *in utero* with ultrasound imaging, and the infant is usually full term. Omphaloceles are often associated with congenital anomalies or syndromes involving chromosomal defects that

affect the brain, chest, or genitourinary system. A subclassification of omphaloceles has been described by Schuster, wherein the defects are separated into those more or less than 4.0 cm in diameter (19). Those under 2 cm in diameter are thought to occur later in embryologic development and to have a better prognosis.

Gastroschisis typically presents as a small (less than 3.0-cm) defect to the right of the umbilical cord. The mother is usually young and primigravid; and the infant, premature. Visceral malrotation is present, and the majority of the small and large bowel is herniated free without a sac or peritoneal covering. The edematous bowel loops are often adherent. Associated anomalies occur in about 30% of patients. Half involve intestinal atresia or stenosis. After resuscitation, urgent surgery is required.

Umbilical hernias may occur at any age. As a group, umbilical hernias have been subdivided into four categories in the literature, beginning with the umbilical hernias in infants. The other three categories (adult, acquired, and paraumbilical) are discussed later in the acquired, midline hernias section. *Infant umbilical* hernias are the only known hernias that may close spontaneously. This closure usually occurs by the age of 3, especially if the defect is less than 1.5 cm in diameter. Accordingly, infant umbilical hernias are usually observed for 3 years or so before surgery is recommended.

ACQUIRED

A convenient way to categorize acquired ventral hernias is according to their general location—midline, median, or paramedian.

A. *Midline* ventral hernias involve the linea alba. *Diastasis recti* usually occurs in adults and represents a gradual, diffuse thinning of the linea alba. The rectus muscles retract laterally and the midline "bows out" like a keel when the patient sits up or stands. This condition is progressive and

R.M. Zollinger, Jr.: Department of Surgery, Case Western Reserve University School of Medicine; Department of Surgery, University Hospitals of Cleveland, Cleveland, Ohio.

has no complications other than the increasing cosmetic deformity.

Epigastric hernias present through the midline linea alba between the xiphoid and umbilicus. They most commonly occur in adult males who are overweight. This acquired hernia is second in frequency to umbilical hernias among the adult ventral hernias. These hernias tend to have small defects (less than 2.0 cm), and they may not be palpable in an obese patient. The hernia can occur spontaneously, and many are asymptomatic. However, some epigastric hernias make their presence known by intermittent pain from entrapment of preperitoneal fat or the omentum. If the hernia is not palpable, then imaging studies may be helpful in identifying the defect, which some believe relates to the lack of sufficient crisscrossing or decussation of the fascia across the linea alba.

Additional midline hernias include the *adult umbilical* hernia, the *acquired umbilical* hernia, and the *paraumbilical* hernia. These three, along with the *infant* umbilical hernia, constitute the four categories of umbilical hernia mentioned earlier. About 90% of the umbilical hernias in adults occur in women who are often obese or multiparous. Incarceration of preperitoneal fat, or more likely the omentum, is common. The omentum may become adherent to the hernia sac, or it may expand as the patient gains weight. The resultant incarceration can produce pain or gastrointestinal symptoms. The acquired umbilical hernia is a variation on the adult umbilical hernia in that it occurs in the same region, but it is secondary to an abnormally increased intraabdominal pressure such as that found with ascites. The paraumbilical hernia can occur at any age, and it is found immediately above or below the umbilicus. This hernia presents through the linea alba, and as the hernia expands, its lower or upper half distends the umbilical skin. The stretched umbilical skin provides only partial coverage for this hernia as opposed to complete coverage in the typical adult umbilical hernia.

B. *Median* hernias technically could include gastroschises; but in actuality, this category is represented by the supravesical hernias. These hernias occur in the supravesical space above—that is anterior and superior—to the bladder and between the middle umbilical ligament (obliterated urachus) and the two lateral umbilical ligaments (right and left obliterated umbilical arteries). The hernia sac of peritoneum may penetrate in the following directions: (a) anterior to the bladder but behind the pubis (Retzius' space); (b) posterior to the bladder and downward so as to be anterior to the ventral peritoneum that creates the space of Douglas; or (c) lateral to the bladder into the interparietal spaces or the inguinal–femoral canal.

C. *Paramedian* ventral hernias are relatively rare as they reside in the interparietal regions. Spigelian and interparietal hernias are close relatives as both burrow between the abdominal wall layers. *Spigelian* hernias pass through the semilunar (not semicircular) line that identifies the lateral edge of the rectus muscle fascial sheath, where it fuses with the fascia of the lateral abdominal wall muscles. These hernias produce vague nonspecific symptoms, and they may be mistaken for an intraabdominal or abdominal wall mass. Diagnostic imaging with either ultrasound or computed axial tomography (CAT) scans will give the best delineation of the anatomic position and extent of these hernias. The herniation may track laterally into the interparietal spaces or medially either under the rectus muscle (retromuscular space) or under the posterior rectus sheath for what is termed an intravaginal hernia.

Interparietal hernias are created when the herniating peritoneal sac comes anteriorly through the lateral abdominal wall and lies between the various anatomic (parietal) layers. These hernias are often subdivided as follows: (a) preperitoneal—between the peritoneum and the transversalis fascia; (b) interstitial—between transversalis fascia, the transversus muscle, the internal oblique muscle, or the external muscle; and (c) superficial—between the external oblique muscle or its fascia and the skin.

INCISIONAL

Incisional hernias may be subcategorized according to the general anatomic area in which they occur, such as the midline, paramedian, transverse, or special operative sites. Many believe that incisional hernias are a function of the anatomic site and the direction of the preceding incision. Additional features such as suture composition and placement, infection, age, obesity, malnutrition, abnormally increased intraabdominal pressure, steroids, smoking, and chemotherapy all are important in wound nonhealing with subsequent development of an incisional hernia.

Midline incisional hernias are the most common and account for 75% to 80% of these hernias. This frequency may reflect the fact that the midline opening is the most commonly used incision by surgeons. *Paramedian* incisions (through the rectus sheath and muscle) are rarely used today, while *transverse* incisions are frequently used as they provide excellent exposure to the upper abdomen. In the past, many surgeons believed that transverse incisions resulted in stronger closures than did vertical ones (usually paramedian), but it now appears that the modifying factors (infection, malnutrition, etc.) are more important in the solid healing of any incision. *Special operative site* hernias are variations on incisional hernias. These might include the overlapping muscle-splitting incision at McBurney's point used for appendectomies; the ostomy incisions where various abdominal wall muscle groups are split lengthwise to make a round opening for the bowel and stoma; and the port sites used for minimally invasive surgery or for the placement of dialysis catheters. Uncontrolled muscle or fascial splitting results in the loss of a solid intact fascial edge with subsequent herniation of intraabdominal contents that are opposed only by the elasticity of the skin.

TRAUMATIC

Since the classic paper by Cain (2) in 1964, several classification systems for traumatic hernias have been published. Most are defined by the location of the hernia or by the severity of the trauma, inducing force. Cain's criteria for a traumatic hernia were that the hernia appear immediately after the trauma, that the skin be intact, and that a physician observe this phenomenon while signs of trauma were still present. Malangoni and Condon (8) added another criterion: that the hernia must not have a peritoneal sac. Ottero and Fallon (13) proposed a classification consisting of three types: (a) small size, usually in groin, minimal force; (b) small-to-moderate defect, lateral to the rectus muscle, moderate force; and (c) large defect, extensive force. Ganchi and Orgill (4) added autopenetrating from a bone as a new category. Additionally they proposed a classification based upon the mechanism of injury. Their two classes included the following: (a) focal—with direct injury or with autopenetrating injury, versus (b) diffuse with pressure injury (small-to-moderate defect size) and shear injury (high energy or crush with large defect). Neidhardt (10) listed several different categories of abdominal trauma that include these hernias: (a) localized rupture (upper, middle, or lower level) of the anterior abdominal wall; (b) trauma ventral hernias caused by seat belts, especially lap belts; and (c) major extensive traumatic hernias usually associated with bone fractures and visceral rupture. He stated that these injuries have "such extensive muscle tearing that a systematic description cannot be given."

A combination of these various systems is shown in Table 7.1, with three categories for traumatic hernias. The first is *penetrating* occurring after knife or bullet wounds. These can occur anywhere on the abdomen and essentially represent a variation on the special operative site hernias. This category also includes the *autopenetrating* traumatic hernias created by bone fragments. Ventral hernias secondary to *blunt* trauma are quite rare, with less than 100 cases reported in the literature. Most of the authors state that a moderate and diffuse abdominal trauma with sudden rise in intraabdominal pressure is usually decompressed by rupture of the diaphragm. The author proposes that the systems of Ottero and Fallon

TABLE 7.1. VENTRAL HERNIAS

A. Congenital—Present at birth
  1. Omphalocele
  2. Gastroschisis
  3. Umbilical—infant
B. Acquired
  1. Midline
    Diastasis recti
    Epigastric
    Umbilical
      Adult, acquired, paraumbilical
  2. Median
    Supravesical
      Anterior, posterior, lateral
  3. Paramedian
    Spigelian
    Interparietal
C. Incisional
  1. Midline
  2. Paramedian
  3. Transverse
  4. Special operative sites
D. Traumatic
  1. Penetrating, autopenetrating
  2. Blunt
    Focal, minimal injury
    Moderate injury
    Extensive force or shear
  3. Destructive

(13) plus that of Ganchi and Orgill (4) might be combined into three subcategories for blunt traumatic hernias. The first would be those with focal, direct injuries occurring with minimal force. A typical example is the bicycle handlebar into the groin that produces an inguinal or lower-quadrant abdominal wall defect. The second involves compressive energy of moderate force (falls, motor vehicle accidents, lap belts), which results in a lateral abdominal wall decompression such as a spigelian or interparietal hernia. The third group contains the extensive disruptions of the abdominal wall muscles created by extreme force or shear (crush by machinery or being run over by a vehicle). Here Neidhardt states, "the skin appears to float on a bloody fluid where viscera may be palpable"(10).

The last category of traumatic ventral hernias includes those with massive tissue loss or *destruction* such as that found with shotgun blasts or necrotizing fasciitis. The abdominal wall is closed only with skin or bridging prosthetic materials. This type of closure may also be performed to alleviate an "abdominal compartment syndrome," wherein the surgeon accepts the major abdominal wall hernia while planning a staged definitive closure at a later date.

GROIN HERNIAS

Comprehensive reviews by Read (14) and Rutkow and Robbins (15) summarize the historic background, as well as the key events and surgical observations that have created the current *traditional* classification of groin hernias as indirect and direct inguinal or femoral. The majority of surgeons use this simple classification today. However, over the past 40 years, more sophisticated classifications have evolved in an attempt to precisely define inguinal hernias. Better classification systems should allow more uniform comparisons among the diverse techniques used for modern hernia repair, thus allowing surgeons to discover which technique is best for a given type of hernia. In general, these newer classifications have focused on the anatomic location of the defect, the size of the defect, and the loss of functional integrity for various openings or spaces in the inguinal–femoral region.

In the late 1950s, surgeons in North America began reporting large patient series undergoing new operations for inguinal hernias. Harkins (11) in the closing discussion of the presentation by Nyhus on preperitoneal herniorrhaphy, listed four grades in his classification. The presentation itself, however, used the traditional indirect, direct, and femoral categories. Harkins' grade I contained indirect infant hernias, while grade II consisted of the simple indirect hernias in older children and young healthy adults. Grade III hernias were an "intermediate type of hernia (larger indirect inguinal hernias in young adults or small hernias in older patients with strong tissues; also a few small direct inguinal hernias with narrow-necked sacs)." Lastly, grade IV hernias were the advanced types, such as recurrent, femoral, or direct and indirect hernias not specified in the definitions of grades II and III.

Casten (3) in 1967 staged indirect hernias into three categories. Stage I occurred in infants and children with a normally functioning internal ring. These hernias were small. Stage II indirect hernias were characterized by large hernias through a distorted internal ring. Casten grouped together all direct and femoral hernias as stage III. In 1958, McVay and Chapp (9) presented their evaluations of inguinal and femoral hernioplasty for primary and recurrent hernias. They used the traditional classification to categorize their patients in the article, but they also analyzed their results in terms of primary inguinal, recurrent, and combined hernias that contained hernias of any two or all three inguinal–femoral areas. McVay stated that femoral hernias were considered a third variety of inguinal hernia, and he divided indirect hernias into small, medium, and large in his discussion but not in the actual tabulations shown in the paper. In 1970, Halverson and McVay expanded on the earlier observations and they now listed five groups of inguinal hernias (6). The first were the small indirect ones of childhood.

The second were the medium-sized indirect inguinal hernia that had dilation of the internal ring without encroachment or disruption of the lateral aspect of the transversus abdominis in the direct floor area. Thirdly, they combined the very large indirect inguinal hernias with the direct ones as both have destruction of the posterior inguinal floor in the direct area. Femoral hernias were listed as stand-alone different hernias. Halverson and McVay also used the term *combined hernias* to describe any mixture of the three (indirect, direct, or femoral) hernia sites (Table 7.2).

In 1987, Lichtenstein (7) published his data registry form used in over 6,000 cases. He separated direct inguinal hernias into five categories, as follows: (a) the entire direct floor; (b) the lateral half of the direct floor; (c) the medial half of the direct floor; (d) diverticular; and (e) other. Lichtenstein did not use the term *combined hernias*. Instead, he allowed the listing of a principal hernia and a secondary one, thus enabling a description of multiple coexisting (combined) hernias.

Also in the late 1980s, Gilbert (5) created a registry named The Cooperative Hernia Analysis of Types and Surgeries (CHATS), which was used by more than 50 hernia surgeons. This registry contained a classification for five types of inguinal hernia—3 indirect and 2 direct. Type I have a "snug internal ring," whereas type II have a "moderately enlarged internal ring." In type II, the hernia opening is less than two fingerbreadths in width, and the direct floor area is intact. Type III indirect hernias have an enlarged internal ring of "two fingerbreadths or greater." Although not described in his article, Gilbert's diagram shows this type III hernia encroaching into the lateral aspect of the direct floor. Type IV hernias are direct ones that either are very large or involve a disruption of the entire direct floor. The internal ring area is still intact. Type V direct hernias are "diverticular defects of no more than one fingerbreadth in the direct floor" in the presence of an intact internal ring. Rutkow and Robbins expanded this classification in 1993 (Table 7.3) with the addition of a type VI, which they categorized as a "pantaloon or combined indirect and direct" hernia. They also added a type VII femoral hernia. The *Gilbert*

TABLE 7.2. HALVERSON AND MCVAY CLASSIFICATION

Small, indirect
Medium, indirect
Large, indirect, and direct
Femoral
Combined—any mixture of above

TABLE 7.3. GILBERT CLASSIFICATION WITH ADDITIONS OF RUTKOW AND ROBBINS

Indirect	
Small	I
Medium	II
Large	III
Direct	
Entire floor	IV
Diverticular	V
Combined	
Indirect and direct	VI
Femoral	VII

classification with additions by Rutklow and Robbins (16) is shown in Fig. 7.1.

In 1993, Nyhus published in the surgical literature (11) and in the fourth edition of *Hernia* a new classification to "aid in the surgical decision-making best matching the types of hernia with specific operations." A Nyhus type I indirect hernia has an internal ring of "normal size, configuration and structure." These hernias occur in infants or young adults. The hernia sac is contained within the inguinal canal, and the direct floor is intact. Type II indirect hernias are characterized as having an "enlarged and distorted" internal ring without disruption or encroachment into the direct floor of the inguinal canal. In this hernia, the sac can occupy the entire inguinal canal, but it does not extend into the scrotum. Nyhus divided type III hernias into three subcategories. Type III-A contains all direct hernias wherein "the protrusion does not herniate through the internal ring." Type III-B hernias are large indirect ones where the defect has "expanded medially and encroaches on the posterior inguinal wall or direct floor." As these are larger hernias, the sac is often inguinal–scrotal in size. Nyhus also placed sliding hernias in the III-B category as they "always destroy a portion of the inguinal floor." Additionally, this category includes the "pantaloon" hernias, where the separate direct and indirect sacs straddle the epigastric vessels. Nyhus type III-C hernias consist of femoral hernias. All recurrent hernias are listed as type IV, with directs as IV-A, indirects as IV-B, femorals as IV-C, and any combination of these recurrences as IV-D (Table 7.4).

The Nyhus classification system is widely used in the United States and Europe, where Stoppa (20) modified it in 1998. Stoppa added "aggravating factors," which essentially upstage each Nyhus hernia type by one. Thus, a Nyhus type I hernia with aggravating factors becomes a Stoppa type II. These aggravating factors include the "general factors of massive obesity, abdominal distention, collagenosis plus local factors such as voluminous, multiple, or complex hernias." To this were added "complex injuries related to the hernia (its size, degree of sliding, multiplicity, etc.); patient

characteristics; (age, activity, respiratory diseases, dysuria, obesity or constipation); special surgical circumstances (technical difficulties, infection, risks); or any other unfavorable factor which could modify the choice of treatment."

Bendavid (cited in ref. 17) in 1994 proposed a system of classification based on the anatomic area, the size of the hernia defect, and the length of the sac. He named this TSD (*Type, Staging,* and *Dimension*) as shown in Table 7.5. Bendavid used the four anatomic regions in the groin—medial or lateral, and above or below the inguinal ligament—to create four individual types. In this system, the inguinal ligament separates anterior from posterior, while the epigastric vessels demarcate medial from lateral. Type I is anterolateral (indirect); type II, anteromedial (direct); type III, posteromedial (femoral); and type IV, posterolateral (perivascular). The Bendavid stages reflect the degree of the descent for the hernia sac into the scrotum. In stage I, the sac is contained within the inguinal canal; in stage II, the sac has extended outside the external ring but has not entered the scrotum; and in stage III, the sac is clearly scrotal. The dimension criterion measures the diameter of the abdominal wall defect in centimeters. Bendavid further modified his type II anteromedial (direct) hernias with descriptors as to the area involved in the direct floor, e.g., medial, central, lateral, or the entire floor. Additionally, Bendavid included several modifiers after type, such as "R" for recurrent, "S" for slider, "I" for incarcerated, and "N" for necrosis. Alexandre and colleagues (1) published a variation on this classification in 1996. His system produces a TOS (*Type, Orifice, Sac*) classification. The *types* are indirect, direct, femoral, and others. The *orifice* diameter is measured in centimeters, as is the length of the *sac*. Alexandre further allowed modification with the letter "R" for recurrence, "I" for incarceration, and "B" for bilateral.

In 1995, Schumpelick and Arit (18) published what is also known as the *Aachen* classification. In this system, orifice sizing is added to the traditional hernia classification. Schumpelick also made the system more generic, with "L" standing for lateral (indirect); "M," for medial (direct); and "F," for femoral. Rather than listing a precise dimension for each defect, Schumpelick graded them, with grade I being less than 1.5 cm; II being 1.5 to 3 cm; and III being greater than 3 cm. Finally, he added the modifier "C" to describe a combined hernia (Table 7.6). In essence, the Aachen classification adds quantification of the defect size to the traditional classification terms.

In an attempt to bring together the best features of each of the above classifications, the author proposed a *unified* (21) classification that has been modified (Table 7.7). It builds upon the traditional indirect, direct, and femoral anatomic locations, and it relies more on the competence of the internal ring and integrity of the direct floor rather than the actual size of the defect or the length of the hernia sac. As shown in Fig. 7.2, small indirect inguinal hernias (grade

(*text continues on page 79*)

Type 1

Type 2

Type 3

Type 4

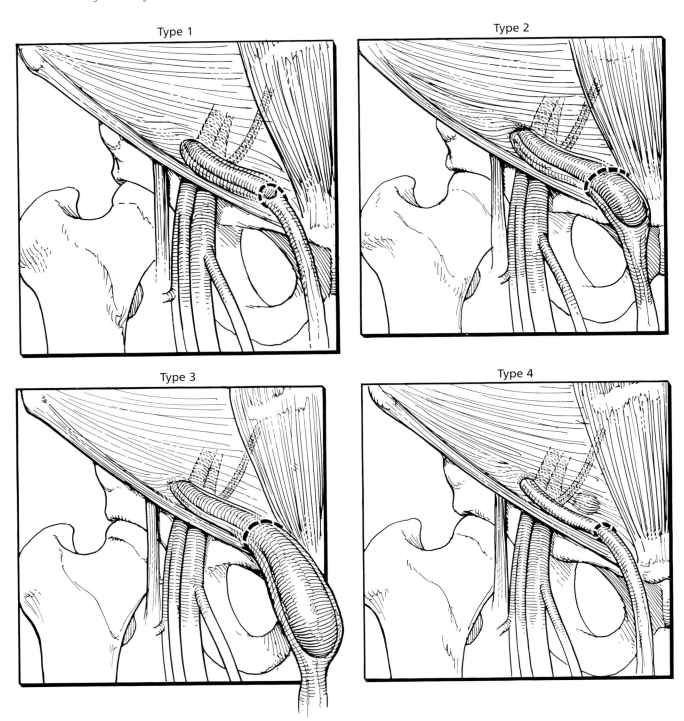

FIGURE 7.1. Gilbert's classification, with additions by Rutkow and Robbins. (Reproduced with permission from Rutkow IM, Robbins AW. Classification systems and groin hernias. Surg Clin North Am 1998;78:1117–1127.)

Type 5

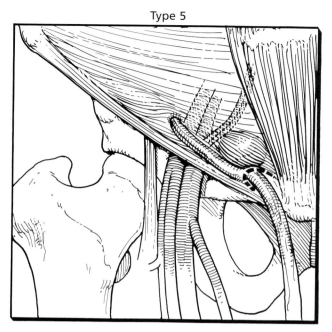

Type 6

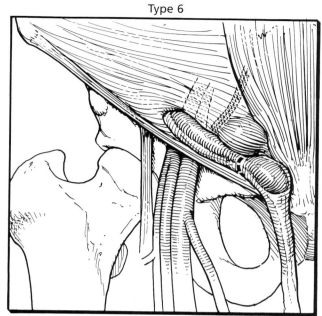

Type 7

FIGURE 7.1. *(continued)*

TABLE 7.4. NYHUS CLASSIFICATION

Type I: Indirect, small
  II: Indirect, medium
  III: A. Direct
      B. Indirect, large
      C. Femoral
   IV. Recurrent
      A. Direct
      B. Indirect
      C. Femoral
      D. Combinations of A, B, C

TABLE 7.5. BENDAVID TSD CLASSIFICATION

Type	Anterolateral (indirect)
	Anteromedial (direct)
	Posteromedial (femoral)
	Posterolateral (perivascular)
Stage	I. Sac in canal
	II. Sac outside external ring
	III. Sac into scrotum
Dimension—orifice maximum in cm	

TABLE 7.6. SCHUMPELICK–AACHEN CLASSIFICATION

L: Lateral (indirect)
M: Medial (direct)
Mc: Medial combined
F: Femoral
Orifice size: grade I <1.5 cm
            II 1.5–3 cm
            III >3 cm

TABLE 7.7. UNIFIED CLASSIFICATION

I	Indirect, small
II	Indirect, medium
III	Indirect, large
IV	Direct, small
V	Direct, medium
VI	Direct, large
VII	Combined–pantaloon
VIII	Femoral
0	Other[a]

[a]Any not classified by number above; femoral + indirect or direct; massive, >8 cm (four fingers) inguinal defect; prevascular.

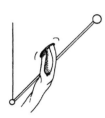
I
INDIRECT SMALL

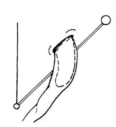
II
INDIRECT MEDIUM

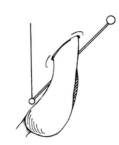
III
INDIRECT LARGE

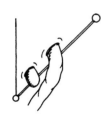
IV
DIRECT SMALL

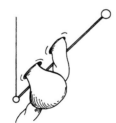
V
DIRECT MEDIUM

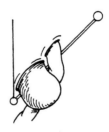
VI
DIRECT LARGE

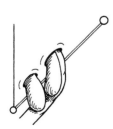
VII
COMBINED

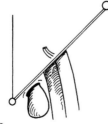
VIII
FEMORAL

0
OTHER
Any Not Classified By Number Above
Femoral + Indirect or Direct
Femoral + Indirect + Direct
Massive >8 cm (4 fingers) Inguinal Defect
Prevascular

FIGURE 7.2. Unified classification—modified.

(text continued from page 75)

I) have an intact internal ring with a small sac that may stay reduced on occasion. These are most often seen in infants and children. The medium indirect hernia (grade II) has an enlarged internal ring—up to 2 fingerbreadths in diameter—and the sac usually is contained in the canal. The large indirect hernias (grade III) have disrupted the internal ring, and the sac usually extends into the scrotum, making this an inguinal–scrotal presentation. The small direct hernias (grade IV) appear as a fifth finger–sized "porthole" in a functional direct floor. The common medium direct hernia (grade V) has a thumb-sized defect that still has an identifiable rim of transversalis floor about its perimeter. The large direct hernias (grade VI) have blown out the entire direct floor. The classic pantaloon hernias with two sacs—both indirect and direct ones—are named combined (grade VII). Femoral hernias (grade VIII) are regarded as a separate entity, and a category of Other (O) is created for the complex hernias not described above, for massive inguinal hernias, or for unusual (prevascular) ones. Lastly, a system of several modifiers was described in this article (12).

In summary, all ventral and groin hernia classifications are somewhat artificial or arbitrary. Only the traditional classification of groin hernias has stood the test of time. It remains for hernia specialists to prove that a more sophisticated set of classifications improves our understanding or operative treatment of hernias.

REFERENCES

1. Alexandre JH, Bouillot JL, Aouad K. *Le Journal de Coelio Chirurgie* 1996;19:53–59.
2. Cain A. Traumatic hernia. *Br J Surg* 1964;51:549–550.
3. Casten DF. Functional anatomy of the groin area as related to the classification and treatment of groin hernias. *Am J Surg* 1967; 114:984–989.
4. Ganchi PA, Orgill DP. Autopenetrating hernia: a novel form of traumatic abdominal wall hernia—case report and review of the literature. *J Trauma* 1996;41:1064–1066.
5. Gilbert AI. An anatomic and functional classification for the diagnosis and treatment of inguinal hernia. *Am J Surg* 1989; 157:331–333.
6. Halverson K, McVay C. Inguinal and femoral hernioplasty. *Arch Surg* 1970;101:127–135.
7. Lichtenstein IL. Herniorrhaphy. *Am J Surg* 1987;153:553–559.
8. Malangoni MA, Condon R. Traumatic abdominal wall hernia. *J Trauma* 1983;23:356–357.
9. McVay CB, Chapp JD. Inguinal and femoral hernioplasty. *Ann Surg* 1958;148:499–512.
10. Neidhardt JPH. Closed trauma of the abdominal wall. In: Chevrel JP, ed. *Hernias and surgery of the abdominal wall*, 2nd ed. Paris: Springer, 1998:106–109.
11. Nyhus LM. Individualization of hernia repair; a new era. *Surgery* 1993;114:1–2.
12. Nyhus LM, Stevenson JK, Listerub MB, et al. Preperitoneal herniorrhaphy. *West J Surg Obstet Gynecol* 1959;67:48–54.
13. Ottero C, Fallon WF. Injury to the abdominal wall musculature: the full spectrum of traumatic hernia. *South Med J* 1988;81: 517–520.
14. Read R. The development of inguinal herniorrhaphy. *Surg Clin North Am* 1984;64:185–196.
15. Rutkow IM, Robbins AW. Classification systems and groin hernias. *Surg Clin North Am* 1998;78:1122–1124.
16. Rutkow IM, Robbins AW. "Tension-free" inguinal herniorrhaphy: a preliminary report on the "mesh plug" technique. *Surgery* 1993;114:3–8.
17. Rutkow IM, Robbins AW. Classification of groin hernias. In: Bendavid R, ed. *Prostheses and abdominal wall hernias*. Austin: RG Landes, 1994:110–112.
18. Schumpelick V, Arit G. *Problems in general surgery.* Philadelphia: Lippincott–Raven Publishers, 1995;12:57–58.
19. Shuster SR. Omphalocoele, hernia of the umbilical cord and gastroschisis. In: Ravich MM, Welch KJ, Benson CD, et al., eds. *Pediatric Surgery*, 3rd ed, vol 2. Chicago: Year Book Medical Publishers, 1979:778.
20. Stoppa R. In: Chevrel JP, ed. *Hernias and surgery of the abdominal wall*. Berlin: Springer, 1998:175–178.
21. Zollinger RM Jr. A unified classification for inguinal hernias. *Hernia* 1999;3:195–200.

EDITOR'S COMMENTS

Dr. Zollinger has nicely summarized the most important classification systems in use around the world today. He has become so familiar with them that he is able to slice out the best of each to propose yet another one. Perhaps this one will rise to the top and supplant the others as it is certainly well thought out. The problem is that just as the number of inguinal herniorrhaphy procedures attests to the fact that the perfect one has yet to be described, so too the number of classification schemes reflects the fact that surgeons are not perfectly happy with any of them. A single classification system for inguinal hernias is especially difficult since the disease can be approached not only with different operations, but also in different anatomic spaces. A system that works well for operations done in the conventional inguinal canal may not be so good for preperitoneal operations.

The primary purpose of a classification system for any disease is to stratify for severity so that reasonable comparisons can be made between various treatment strategies. This classification system is for inguinal hernias since treatment may occur at any point along the broad spectrum of disease severity. Because of this, there are many proposed treatments (operations). Indeed, retrospective studies of inguinal herniorrhaphies are commonly criticized because of obvious disease severity bias. For example, it is ludicrous to compare the results of an inguinal herniorrhaphy performed in young, fit, active-duty military personnel to one conducted in a Veterans Administration facility. A universally accepted inguinal hernia classification system could help to lessen the effect of such biases. In addition, it makes it easier for the surgeon to tailor his/her operation to the hernia to eliminate the "one-size-fits-all" approach.

R.J.F., Jr.

Nyhus and Condon's Hernia, Fifth Edition, edited by Robert J. Fitzgibbons, Jr. and A. Gerson Greenburg. Lippincott Williams & Wilkins, Philadelphia © 2002.

8

DIAGNOSTIC IMAGING IN THE EVALUATION AND MANAGEMENT OF ABDOMINAL WALL HERNIA

SON NGOC TRUONG
MARC JANSEN

Pathologic findings of the abdominal wall and inguinal region are usually readily recognized due to their superficial location. In most cases, the correct diagnosis can be reached on the basis of history, symptoms, and clinical examination. Ultrasound investigations, which are part of our standard routine, merely confirm the clinical findings in the majority of our patients. There are, however, two groups of patients for whom ultrasonography is particularly valuable:

1. Patients, especially obese people, with palpable masses within deep layers of the abdominal wall.
2. Patients with pain and complaints located within the abdominal wall or the inguinal region but without causative clinical findings.

For these patients, various diagnostic imaging tools can be used to help detect pathology and to treat it adequately. In most cases, ultrasound is the method of choice, but in some cases, computed tomography (CT) or magnetic resonance imaging (MRI) may be helpful (2,3,9,10,13,15,21). In this chapter, the following will be discussed: sonography, CT, MRI, and herniography.

SONOGRAPHY OF THE ABDOMINAL WALL

Indications

Sonography is indicated primarily in patients with palpable masses within deep layers of the abdominal wall, and in patients with pain located within the abdominal wall or the inguinal region without any causative clinical findings. In

S. N. Truong: Department of Surgery, Rhenish Westphalian Technical University Aachen; Department of Surgery, University Hospital, Aachen, Germany.
M. Jansen: Department of Surgery, Rhenish Westphalian Technical University Aachen; Department of Surgery, University Hospital, Aachen, Germany.

patients with hernia, a measurement of the defect can be done by sonography.

Technique

For the sonographic examination of the abdominal wall and inguinal region, we use a real time ultrasound with a 5.0-MHz scanner for short focus adjustment and a 7.5-MHz linear scanner for the near region. Additionally, the abdomen of all patients is examined with a 3.5-MHz scanner.

Sonography is performed with the patient in the supine position, and if there are any findings in the inguinal region, further examination is performed in the upright position. The ultrasound scanner is placed above the undeterminable finding or on the site of maximum tenderness on pressure. Compared with the contralateral side, subcutaneous fatty tissue, rectus sheath, muscles, fascias, and vessels are identified. The examination is carried out on at least two planes perpendicular to each other. Under continuous observation of the questionable area, dynamic examinations are performed with Valsalva's maneuver (by coughing or by pressing down on the abdomen).

Sonographic Anatomy of the Abdominal Wall

Although the echographic representation of the anatomy of the abdominal wall and inguinal region is highly variable, depending on the amount of fatty tissue and muscle, there are typical sonographic structures that should be identified in all patients (Fig. 8.1).

The epidermis and dermis are represented by a superficial homogenous echoic layer. Underlying subcutaneous fatty tissue varies considerably between thin and obese individuals. Two kinds of abdominal wall muscles can be identified: the rectus muscle at both sides of the midline and the three flat lateral abdominal muscles. The longitu-

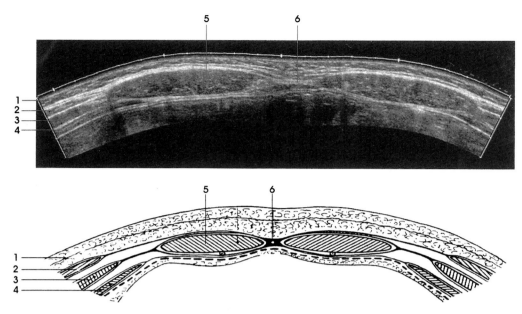

FIGURE 8.1. Normal sonographic anatomy of the abdominal wall above the umbilicus in the midline. *1,* subcutaneous fat; *2,* oblique external muscle; *3,* oblique internal muscle; *4,* transverse muscle; *5,* rectus muscle; *6,* linea alba.

dinally running rectus muscle appears as a hypoechoic and homogenous structure with fine internal, parallel lines of greater echo reflection. It is enveloped by the rectus sheath as a surrounding echogenic line. The anterior lamina of the rectus sheath is formed by fibers of the oblique muscles, while the posterior lamina derives from the aponeurosis of the transverse muscle. In the midline, both rectus sheaths unite to form a thick echogenic aponeurotic layer, the linea alba, extending from the xiphoid to the symphysis pubis.

Below the arcuate line, the semilunar line can be identified; this is the boundary between the body of the rectus muscles and the transverse aponeurosis. This zone is of special interest because it represents a weak area, and the rare spigelian hernia can occur here (Fig. 8.2).

The three flat abdominal muscles in the flanks—the oblique external, oblique internal, and transverse muscles—can be distinguished as three different layers, separated by their thin, highly echogenic aponeuroses (Fig. 8.3). In the inguinal region, the oblique external muscle disappears, and only its aponeurosis can be identified above the oblique internal muscle.

The very thin echogenic line of the peritoneum separates the abdominal wall from the abdominal viscera. It is sometimes difficult to identify this line as a single layer beneath the muscles, especially in young, athletic patients. In obese patients, a hypoechoic heterogeneous zone can often be found between the muscle layers and peritoneum, representing areolar preperitoneal fatty tissue. In the inguinal region the inferior epigastric vessels can be identified by color-coded duplex sonography (Figs. 8.4 and 8.5).

Sonographic Differential Diagnosis of Pathologic Findings

Pre- and postoperative sonographic examinations help us to identify surgical diseases of the abdominal wall and inguinal region. Indications are mainly obesity and complaints with-

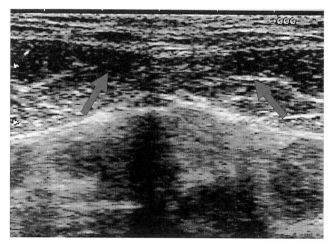

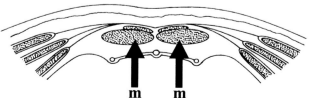

FIGURE 8.2. Normal sonographic anatomy of the abdominal wall below the linea arcuata. *m,* rectus muscle.

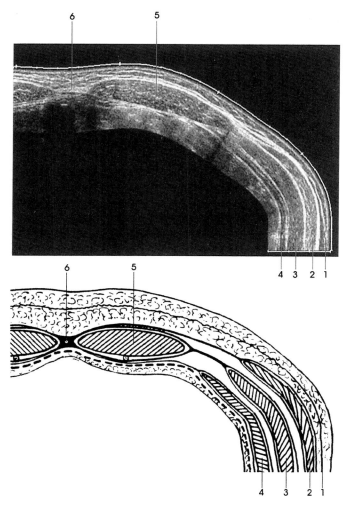

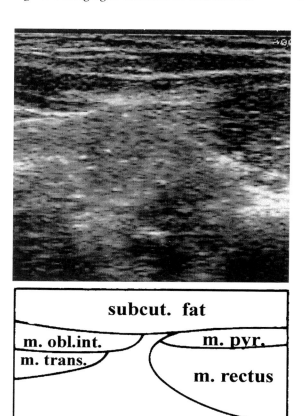

FIGURE 8.3. Normal sonographic anatomy of the abdominal wall above the umbilicus between rectus muscle and lateral abdominal muscles. *1,* subcutaneous fat; *2,* oblique external muscle; *3,* oblique internal muscle; *4,* transverse muscle; *5,* rectus muscle; *6,* linea alba.

FIGURE 8.4. Normal sonographic anatomy of the inguinal region.

out clinical findings in preoperative patients and postoperative examinations for fluid collection.

Preoperative Examinations

Diagnosis of hernia and differential diagnosis are important to lead the surgeon to the correct surgical treatment. It is therefore important to know the sonographic criteria and patterns of the different types of hernia, as well as other undetermined palpable masses of the abdominal wall.

Sonographic Criteria for Hernias

The sonographic image of a hernia is a fascial gap with protruding hernial contents. The hernial contents should be reducible into the peritoneal cavity. The hernial sac should generally reveal an increase in size or a change of location when the patient coughs or presses. In minor hernias, only

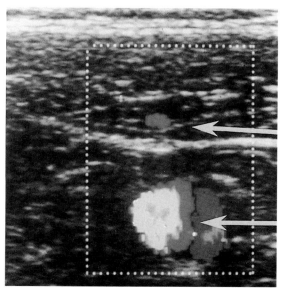

FIGURE 8.5. Typical findings of epigastric artery in the inguinal region. See Color Plate 3.

a small fascial gap or a vaulting is found during dynamic examination. In addition, the hernial contents can be identified by sonography. Intestinal structures are characterized by peristaltic movements and air bubbles, while the omentum appears as a stationary, highly reflective, space-occupying structure (Fig. 8.6).

Epigastric Hernia

For diagnosis of epigastric hernias, the transducer is placed in the epigastric region over the linea alba. The reference structures are the rectus sheath and the linea alba, and the hernia is visualized by a characteristic midline fascial defect (Fig. 8.7).

Inguinal Hernia

Inguinal hernias are found by placing the transducer over the inguinal ligament. The reference structures are the rec-

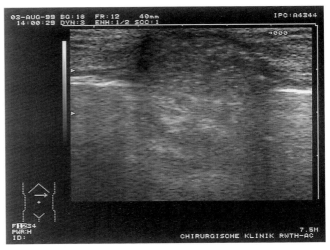

FIGURE 8.7. Sonographic finding of an epigastric hernia.

tus sheath medially and the internal oblique and transverse abdominal muscle laterally. Epigastric vessels are identified by color-coded duplex scan. Although it is difficult to distinguish between direct and indirect hernia, the location of the epigastric vessels might be of help; thus, direct hernias lie medial and indirect hernias lateral to the epigastric vessels (Figs. 8.8 and 8.9).

Femoral Hernia

For femoral hernias, the transducer is placed caudal to the inguinal ligament over the oval fossa. The reference structures are the femoral artery with a constantly filled and pulsating lumen laterally and the femoral vein with a variable volume medial to the artery; this vein expands during Valsalva's maneuver. Between these vessels and the symphysis

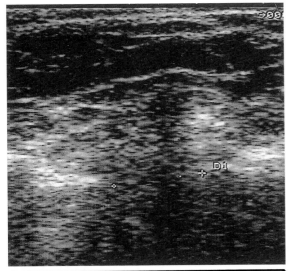

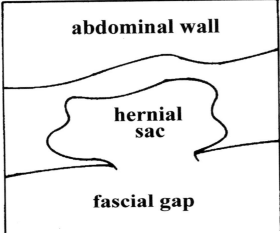

FIGURE 8.6. Typical sonographic finding of a hernia.

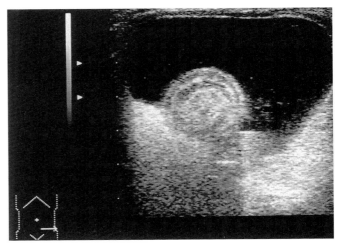

FIGURE 8.8. Sonographic finding of an incarcerated inguinal hernia with small bowel in the hernia sac.

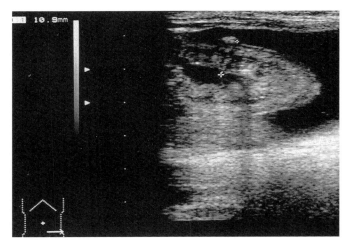

FIGURE 8.9. Sonographic finding of an incarcerated inguinal hernia with ischemic thickening of small bowel.

pubis, femoral hernias demonstrate a low-echo area that bulges caudally during pressing or coughing (Fig. 8.10).

Spigelian Hernia

A spigelian hernia is identified by placing the transducer over the semilunar line. The reference structures are the semilunar line with the lateral abdominal wall muscles as its lateral boundary and the rectus muscle as its medial boundary. A defect in the outline and an anterior bulging of the rectus margin confirm the hernia (Fig. 8.11) (2,13,20).

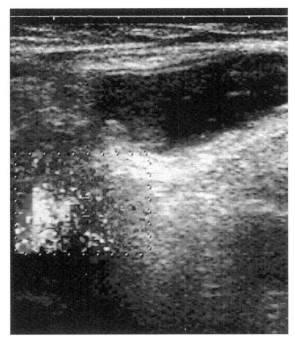

FIGURE 8.10. Sonographic finding of a femoral hernia. See Color Plate 4.

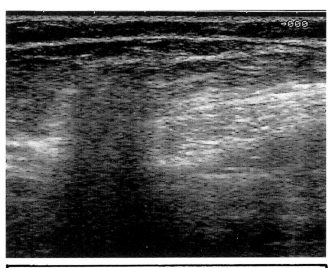

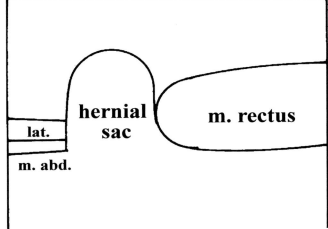

FIGURE 8.11. Sonographic finding of a spigelian hernia. (From Schumpelick V, Kingsnorth AN. *Incisional hernia.* Berlin: Springer–Verlag, 1999, with permission.)

Lumbar Hernia

For lumbar hernias, the transducer is placed over the lumbar and costolumbar triangle. The reference structures are the iliac crest caudally and the inferior costal arch cranially. A hernial orifice below the latissimus dorsi plane is evidence of a superior lumbar hernia. Lateral bulging at the lower insertion of the latissimus muscle indicates an inferior lumbar hernia.

Incisional Hernia

Incisional hernias can occur at nearly any point in the abdominal wall following surgery. They show the typical hernial pattern with a fascial gap and protruding hernial sac. In addition, after mesh repair for hernia, a recurrence can occur at the edge of the mesh (Figs. 8.6 and 8.12).

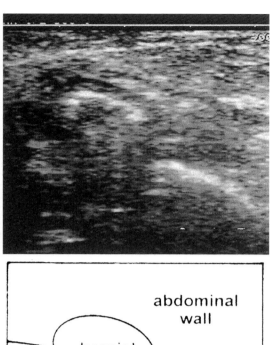

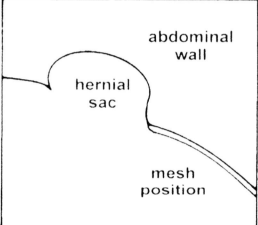

FIGURE 8.12. Sonographic finding of a recurrent incisional hernia.

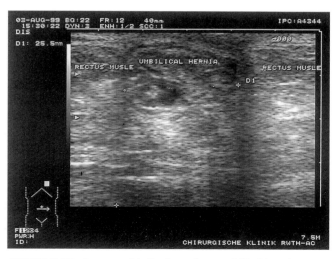

FIGURE 8.13. Sonographic finding of an umbilical hernia.

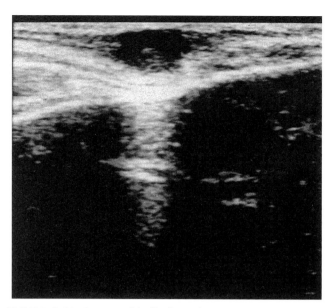

FIGURE 8.14. Sonographic finding of a metastasis within the abdominal wall.

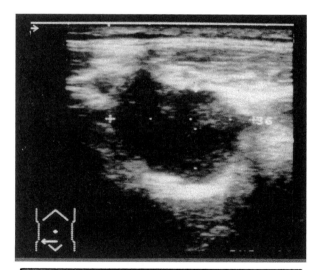

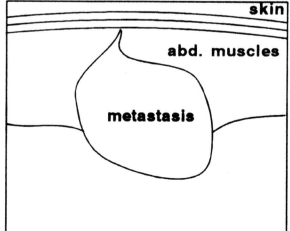

FIGURE 8.15. Sonographic finding of a peritoneal metastasis with infiltration in the abdominal wall.

Umbilical Hernia

Umbilical hernias occur at the umbilicus due to a persistent omphaloenteric duct. The transducer is placed over the umbilicus; the sonographic image shows the fascial gap and the protruding hernial sac (Fig. 8.13).

Further Anomalies

Metastasis

Metastases present sonographically as homogenous, solid, space-occupying structures with plump or polycyclic outlines. Processes in the abdominal wall that are close to the peritoneum can be distinguished from intraabdominal tumors by observing them during inspiration and expiration (Figs. 8.14 and 8.15).

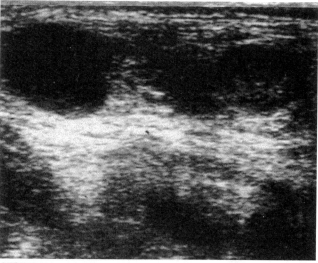

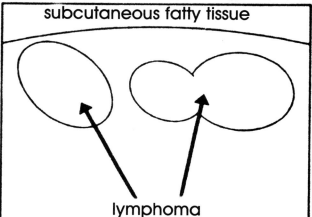

FIGURE 8.17. Typical sonographic finding of a subcutaneous lymphoma. (From Schumpelick V, Kingsnorth AN. *Incisional hernia*. Berlin: Springer–Verlag, 1999, with permission.)

Lipoma

Lipomas present as hypoechoic structures, often with a sharp margin and constant location during dynamic examination (Fig. 8.16).

Lymphoma

Lymphomas are located along the anatomic lymphatic drainage routes. They are homogenous hypoechoic or central hyperechoic space-occupying structures. Lymphomas do not show any connection to deeper structures or the peritoneal cavity. During dynamic examination, they remain constant (Fig. 8.17).

Endometriosis

Endometriosis shows a hypoechoic structure with irregular margins. The sonographic findings are accompanied by a

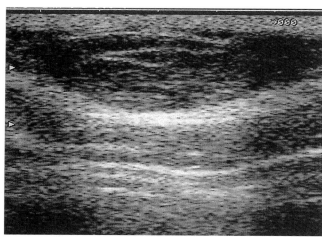

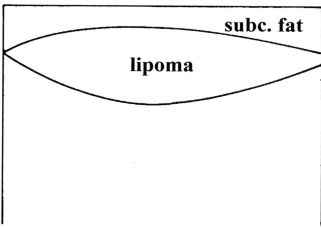

FIGURE 8.16. Sonographic finding of a subcutaneous lipoma. (From Schumpelick V, Kingsnorth AN. *Incisional hernia*. Berlin: Springer–Verlag, 1999, with permission.)

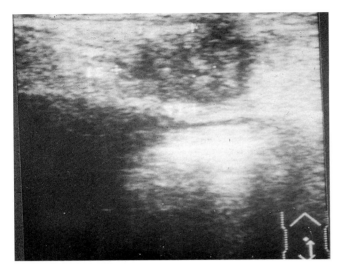

FIGURE 8.18. Sonographic finding of endometriosis.

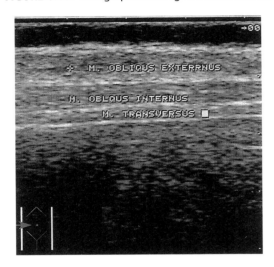

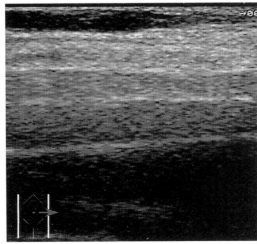

FIGURE 8.19. Sonographic finding of abdominal wall relaxation on the right side (**top**). Compared with the normal left side (**bottom**), the thinner muscle layer without fascial defect on the right side can be demonstrated. (From Schumpelick V, Kingsnorth AN. *Incisional hernia.* Berlin: Springer–Verlag, 1999, with permission.)

typical history of complaints and pain during menstruation (Fig. 8.18).

Abdominal Wall Relaxation

Abdominal wall relaxation following surgery, mainly after retroperitoneal approaches to the kidney, can clinically mimic an incisional hernia. Sonographically, there is no discontinuity of the aponeurosis or fascial gap. All muscle layers of the abdominal wall are present, but they appear thinner in comparison with the unaffected side (Figs. 8.19 and 8.20) (12).

Varicose Nodules

In the transverse plane, varicose nodules of the saphenous vein appear as round, hypoechoic structures in the femoral region. The longitudinal plane reveals a tubular structure with a connection to the femoral vein. Color-coded duplex sonography shows blood flow inside the structure (Fig. 8.21).

Postoperative Investigations

Fluid collection is one of the main indications for sonography, because it presents one of the most common postoperative complications after hernia repair. The indication for fluid aspiration depends on the estimated volume.

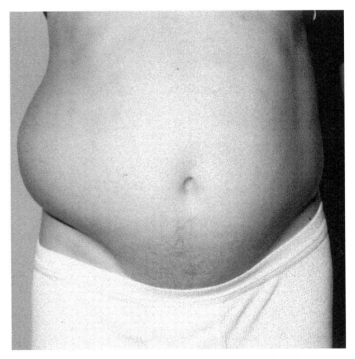

FIGURE 8.20. Patient with abdominal wall relaxation.

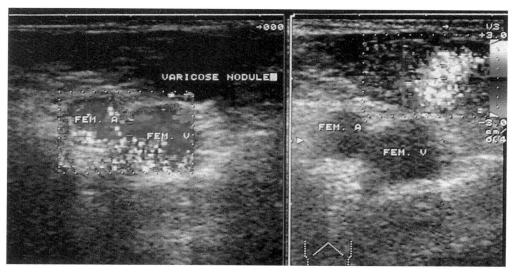

FIGURE 8.21. Sonographic finding of a varicose nodule. The color-coded duplex sonography shows blood flow inside the nodule. See Color Plate 5.

Although it is not easy to determine the type of fluid sonographically, there are sonographic criteria that help us to distinguish between different fluid collections.

Hematoma

Fresh hematomas show a hypoechoic, space-occupying structure with a fine and regular inner echo and distinct margins. Organized hematomas appear as more echogenic structures (Fig. 8.22).

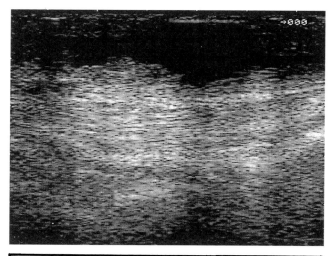

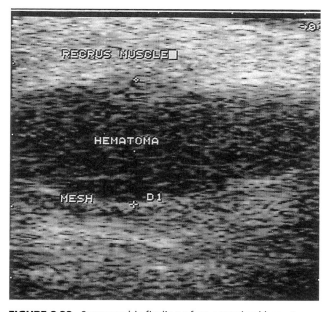

FIGURE 8.22. Sonographic finding of an organized hematoma.

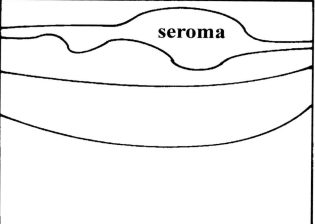

FIGURE 8.23. Sonographic finding of a seroma. (From Schumpelick V, Kingsnorth AN. *Incisional hernia*. Berlin: Springer–Verlag, 1999, with permission.)

Seroma

Seromas present as anechoic structures without inner reflections or sharp margins (Fig. 8.23).

Abscess

An abscess is seen as a hypoechoic process with a heterogeneous structure caused by cell debris and small, plump hyperechoic reflections caused by gas bubbles (Fig. 8.24).

Hematoma of the Rectus Sheath

Further postoperative complications include hematoma of the rectus sheath and wound rupture. Sonography of a hematoma of the rectus sheath shows an increase in the volume of the rectus muscles. The hematoma is situated between the anterior and posterior layer of the rectus sheath (Fig. 8.25).

Wound Rupture (Burst Abdomen)

Postoperative wound rupture or burst abdomen occurs in 0.05% to 3% of patients. Three types of lesions can be distinguished:

- Free, with complete rupture of all layers and viscera protruding out of the abdominal cavity
- Fixed, with complete rupture of all layers, but fixed viscera that remain in the abdominal cavity
- Covered, with rupture of the deeper layers while the cutaneous suture remains intact

The covered burst abdomen is an indication for sonography. The discontinuity of the sutured fascia or aponeurosis is revealed. Seroma or abscess may also be observed (Fig. 8.26).

In diagnosing hernias, there are sometimes difficulties, especially with small hernias or in adipose patients. That is the reason why, in a clinical study by Ponka and Brush (14), only 75% of 216 preoperatively diagnosed femoral hernias were confirmed during surgery. With the use of low-frequency transducers, different pathologic findings of the abdominal wall were, in fact, recognized, and a differential diagnosis was made possible. However, smaller findings failed to be proven sonographically. With the use of a high-frequency 7.5-MHz scanner, it also became possible to detect small fascial defects. The contents of a hernial sac can also be sonographically differentiated. An intestinal loop can be recognized in a cross section by a hyperechoic outer ring, which represents the intestinal wall, and a hypoechoic center when there is fluid in the intestinal lumen. Kerckring's folds of the small intestine are visible in the longitudinal section as long as there is no maximum distention with incarceration. On closer examination, peristaltic movement can possibly be seen. The omentum is

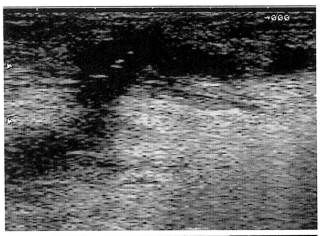

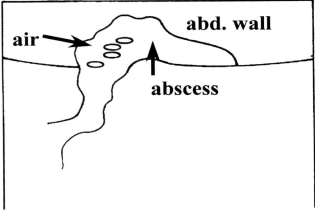

FIGURE 8.24. Sonographic finding of an abscess. (From Schumpelick V, Kingsnorth AN. *Incisional hernia*. Berlin: Springer–Verlag, 1999, with permission.)

shown as an immovable hyperechoic space-occupying process (21).

Urinary bladder (a filled bladder is required during examination) can be identified through a typical hypoechoic zone with consecutive dorsal sound amplification. While a differentiation between tumors with liquid contents (e.g., hematoma, seroma, abscess) and tumors with a solid structure is almost always possible, a distinction among hematomas, seromas, and abscesses is difficult because of the similarity in echogenic structure with deep localization and lack of symptoms.

We studied the specificity and sensitivity of sonography for undetermined pain and palpable masses of unknown origin in 105 patients (21). The correct diagnosis was made sonographically in 89 of 105 patients (84.8%). Sonography showed a sensitivity and specificity of 100% for epigastric hernias. Inguinal hernias were found sonographically with a sensitivity of 82.3% and a specificity of 98.9%. Poor results were found for femoral hernias, with a sensitivity of 72.7%

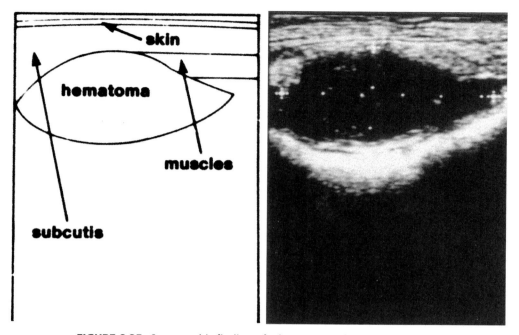

FIGURE 8.25. Sonographic finding of a hematoma of the rectus sheath.

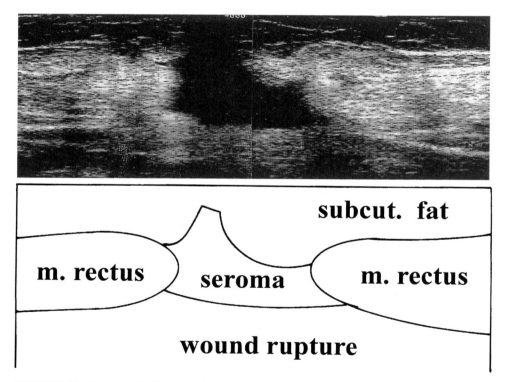

FIGURE 8.26. Sonographic finding of a covered wound rupture with fascial defect and seroma.

TABLE 8.1. SENSITIVITY, SPECIFICITY, AND PREDICTIVE VALUES OF ABDOMINAL WALL SONOGRAPHY

	Sensitivity (%)	Specificity (%)	Predictive Value	
			Pos. Test (%)	Neg. Test (%)
Inguinal hernia	82.3	98.9	93.0	96.6
Hematoma	87.5	97.8	87.5	97.8
Seroma	100.0	97.8	87.5	100.0
Lymphoma	77.0	96.7	77.0	96.7
Femoral hernia	72.7	97.8	80.0	96.8
Epigastric hernia	100.0	100.0	100.0	100.0
Abscess	66.6	100.0	100.0	96.9
Metastasis	85.7	98.0	85.7	98.9
Total hernias	85.0	93.8	98.5	91.0

Neg., negative; Pos., positive.

and a specificity of 97.8%, especially due to confusion with lymphoma (Table 8.1).

Because of its sensitivity in detecting epigastric and inguinal hernias, sonography constitutes an ideal aid in the diagnosis of hernias and pathologic findings of the abdominal wall. In comparison with CT or herniography, the ultrasonographic examination is time- as well as cost-saving and not burdened with risks such as contrast medium allergy.

Therefore, sonography can be used repeatedly by every examiner at any time. In the classification of small hernias or obese patients with palpable findings, sonography is an essential contribution to the differential diagnosis.

COMPUTED TOMOGRAPHY OF THE ABDOMINAL WALL

CT is an excellent method for evaluating the abdominal wall and its relations to the abdominal viscera. Lesions can be easily identified, owing to their different density. CT becomes the modality of choice in obese patients, after surgery, or if the hernia is located in an uncommon site (17). The examination allows cross-sectional visualization of the herniated bowel, abdominal wall defect, and the severity of the hernia. It can be useful in demonstrating the condition of bowel loops (Figs. 8.27 and 8.28) (4).

There are several reports in the literature concerning the primary diagnosis of spigelian hernia by CT (18,20). Hojer et al. examined 24 patients with suspected hernia of the abdominal wall by CT (7). They found a sensitivity of 0.83 and a specificity of 0.83. To achieve the highest diagnostic accuracy, they recommended using Valsalva's maneuver and oral radiopaque material.

CT examination allows exact evaluation of the volume and content of giant hernias. This information is often necessary when deciding on the operative procedure. CT is also used to differentiate postoperative findings such as hematoma, abscess, or recurrence of hernia after laparoscopic repair of ventral hernia (10).

One of the main advantages of CT is its ability to depict pathologic findings other than hernia that may be responsible for the patient's symptoms.

MAGNETIC RESONANCE IMAGING

Compared to CT, MRI offers the advantage of direct multiplane imaging without ionizing radiation and the use of contrast agents. A relative merit of MRI is the excellent demonstration of abdominal wall layers (Figs. 8.29–8.31) (1,8,15).

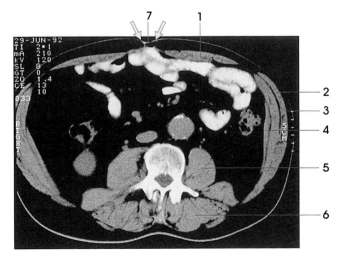

FIGURE 8.27. Transverse computed tomography section showing the anatomy of the abdominal wall with a midline hernia. *1,* rectus abdominal muscle; *2,* external oblique muscle; *3,* internal oblique muscle; *4,* transverse abdominal muscle; *5,* psoas major muscle; *6,* erector spinae muscle; *7,* midline hernia.

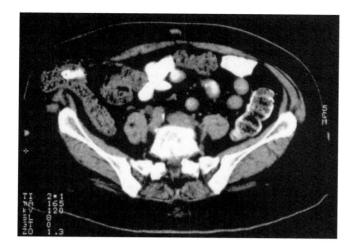

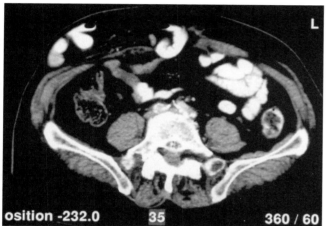

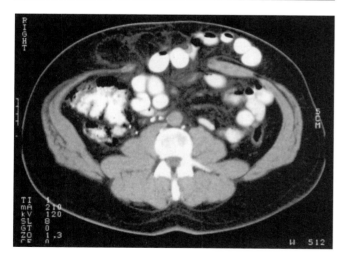

FIGURE 8.28. Computed tomography scan of an incisional hernia with protruding bowel.

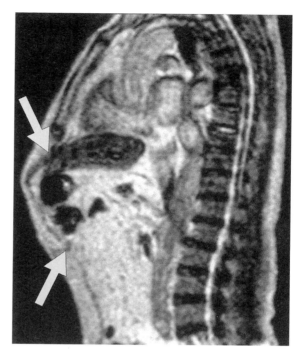

FIGURE 8.29. Magnetic resonance imaging scan of an incisional hernia indicated by the *arrows*.

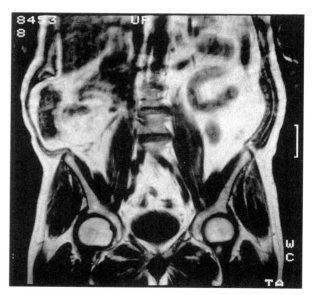

FIGURE 8.30. Magnetic resonance imaging scan of abdominal relaxation.

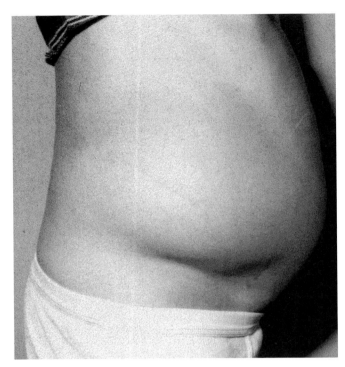

FIGURE 8.31. Patient with abdominal wall relaxation.

In conclusion, CT and MRI are not the first methods of choice in the diagnosis of abdominal wall hernia. However, these methods are useful in distinguishing hernias from benign, malignant, or inflammatory lesions of the abdominal wall and their correlation to the intraabdominal cavity, if clinical examination and sonography fail. In cases of abdominal wall relaxation, MRI allows direct comparison of the affected and the unaffected sides. The disadvantages include higher cost, limited availability, and potential allergic reactions to contrast medium.

HERNIOGRAPHY

According to the literature, herniography is used primarily in patients with unexplained groin pain, or to find nonpalpable, symptomatic cases of hernia recurrence (6,11,16,19). The technique of examination is described by Gullmo (5). A 20- to 22-gauge Veres needle is used to puncture the midline below the umbilicus. The catheter is guided into the lesser pelvis and 50 to 80 mL of contrast medium is injected. As the patient turns from side to side in the prone position, the contrast medium pools in the inguinal region.

Potential complications are caused by direct puncture of the abdominal cavity, the injection of contrast medium, and irradiation of the pelvic region. With the techniques now available, we believe that there is no indication for herniography, even if the complication rate is low. The order of our recommendations for the evaluation of abdominal wall is as follows:

1. Clinical history
2. Clinical examination
3. Sonography
4. CT/MRI

REFERENCES

1. Bennett HF, Balfe DM. MR imaging of the peritoneum and abdominal wall. *Magn Reson Imaging Clin N Am* 1995;3:99–120.
2. Deitch EA, Engel JM. Spigelian hernia, an ultrasonic diagnosis. *Arch Surg* 1980;115:93.
3. Deitch EA, Engel JM. Ultrasonic diagnosis of surgical diseases of the anterior abdominal wall. *Surg Gynecol Obstet* 1980;151:484–486
4. Goodman P, Raval B. CT of the abdominal wall. *AJR Am J Roentgenol* 1990;154:1207–1211.
5. Gullmo A. Herniography. The diagnosis of hernia in the groin and incompetence of the pouch of Douglas and pelvic floor. *Acta Radiol* 1980;361:1–76.
6. Harrison LA, Keesling CA, Martin NL, et al. Abdominal wall hernias: review of herniography and correlation with cross–sectional imaging. *Radiographics* 1995;15:315–332.
7. Hojer AM, Rygaard H, Jess P. CT in the diagnosis of abdominal wall hernias: a preliminary study. *Eur Radiol* 1997;7:1416–1418.
8. Johnson D, Dixon AK, Abrahams PH. The abdominal subcutaneous tissue: computed tomographic, magnetic resonance, and anatomical observations. *Clin Anat* 1996;9:19–24.
9. Lee GM, Cohen J. CT Imaging of abdominal hernias. *AJR Am J Roentgenol* 1993;161:1209–1213.
10. Lin BHJ, Vargish T, Dachman AH. CT findings after laparoscopic repair of ventral hernia. *AJR Am J Roentgenol* 1999;172: 389–392.
11. Makela JT, Kiviniemi H, Palm J, et al. The value of herniography in the diagnosis of unexplained groin pain. *Ann Chir Gynaecol* 1996;85:300–304.
12. Muller M, Truong SN, Schumpelick V. Sonographic diagnosis of abdominal wall relaxation. *J Clin Ultrasound* 1999;27:183–186.
13. Mufid MM, Abu-Yousef MM, Kakish ME, et al. Spigelian hernia: diagnosis by high-resolution real-time sonography. *J Ultrasound Med* 1997;16:183–187.
14. Ponka JL, Brush BE. Problem of femoral hernia. *Arch Surg* 1971; 102:417–423.
15. Rahmouni A, Chosidow O, Mathieu D, et al. MR imaging in acute infectious cellulitis. *Radiology* 1994;192:493–496.
16. Read RC. The development of inguinal herniography. *Surg Clin North Am* 1984;64:185–196.
17. Rose M, Eliakim R, Bar-Ziv Y, et al. Abdominal wall hernias. The value of computed tomography diagnosis in the obese patient. *J Clin Gastroenterol* 1994;19:94–96.
18. Shenouda NF, Hyams BB, Rosenbloom MB. Evaluation of Spigelian hernia by CT. *J Comput Assist Tomogr* 1990;14:777–778.
19. Smedberg SGG, Broome AEA, Elmer O, et al. Herniography in primary inguinal and femoral hernia: an analysis of 283 operated cases. *Contemp Surg* 1990;36:48–52.
20. Spangen L. Spigelian hernia. *World J Surg* 1989;13:573–580.
21. Truong SN, Pfingsten F, Dreuw B, et al. Value of ultrasound in the diagnosis of undetermined findings in the abdominal wall in inguinal region. In: Schumpelick V, Wantz GE, eds. *Inguinal hernia repair, expert meeting on hernia surgery.* St. Moritz–Basel: Karger, 1995:29–43.

9

ULTRASOUND EXAMINATION IN LAPAROSCOPIC/ENDOSCOPIC HERNIA SURGERY

REINHARD BITTNER
BARBARA KRAFT
BERND KUCKUK
BERNHARD LEIBL
KLAUS KRAFT

Next to a thorough physical examination, sonography is the method of first choice for the diagnosis of an unclear swelling in the inguinal region, as well as for exclusion of a hernia in case of inguinal pain and uncertain inguinal palpation findings.

If a hernia can be clinically diagnosed without any doubt, ultrasound becomes unnecessary. Sonography can be helpful, however, to differentiate a lipoma of the spermatic cord, which can simulate a protruding hernia sac during palpation.

Particularly for those who pursue a sophisticated tactical concept in surgery, the question arises as to whether ultrasound can provide the diagnosis of a certain hernia type and determine the size of the hernial defect.

While ultrasound examinations play a rather minor role postoperatively in conventional surgery, they are indispensable after endoscopic/laparoscopic hernia repairs. The objectives of ultrasound examinations are:

- Verifying the correct position of the mesh
- Diagnosing liquid collections between peritoneum and mesh, between mesh and inguinal region, within the inguinal canal, and in the region of the former hernia sac
- Diagnosing conditions of swelling along the spermatic cord, differentiating conditions of swelling in the testicle and its tunics
- Assessing the homogeneity of the testicular parenchyma as a parameter for its perfusion and determining the testicular volume
- Measuring the arterial blood flow to the testicle

R. Bittner: Department of Surgery, ULM University; Department of Surgery (General/Visceral), Marien Hospital Stuttgart, Stuttgart, Germany.

B. Kraft, B. Kuckuk, B. Liebl, and **K. Kraft:** Department of Surgery (General/Visceral), Marien Hospital Stuttgart, Stuttgart, Germany.

In conclusion, ultrasound examinations following laparoscopic/endoscopic hernia repair ensure a clarification of swellings in the inguinal region, the spermatic cord, and the testicle, and can thus give prognostic evidence of the surgical success.

TECHNIQUE OF EXAMINATION

Frequency and Penetration Depth

The frequency has a direct influence on the penetration depth. Penetration depth is defined as the maximum distance between a probe and the deepest structures within the tissue that can still be represented in the image without noise interference. Because of the frequency-dependent attenuation of the sound propagation within the tissue, the penetration depth is not only tissue dependent but, first and foremost, frequency dependent. Therefore, certain frequencies have proven advantageous for certain examinations. High frequencies are well suited for displaying superficial structures and low frequencies for deep imaging regions. Penetration depth is inversely proportional to frequency (Fig. 9.1).

Frequency Ranges of Sound

The term "audible sound" applies to the auditory range of human beings: 16 Hz to 20 kHz. Sound waves with frequencies below 16 MHz are classified as "subaudible" or "infrasound." Infrasound waves derive from the vibrations of earth, water, and air (earthquakes or vibrations of the ground caused by heavy machinery, waves, and winds). The ultrasonic frequency range starts above 20 kHz. The auditory range of a dog can reach up to 40 kHz and that of bats

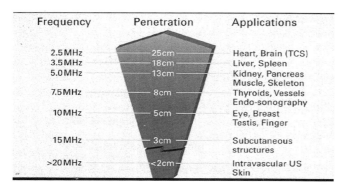

FIGURE 9.1. The influence of frequency on penetration depth. *TCS,* transcranial sonography; *endosonography,* vaginal and prostate sonography. (Courtesy of Siemens AG, 1999.)

up to 150 kHz. Bats are able to orient themselves in space by means of ultrasonic signals. Their auditory receptors can even deal with Doppler frequency shifts to control their flight velocity.

Diagnostic ultrasound uses frequencies between 2 and 30 MHz. Today's most frequent applications use a frequency range between 2 and 15 MHz, thus obtaining the necessary penetration depth and a high spatial resolution. Also, Doppler signals from blood flow happen to be within the kHz range and can therefore be made audible. Special applications such as intravascular ultrasound require frequencies up to 30 MHz and higher. The frequency range above 1 GHz is also called "hypersound" (Fig. 9.2).

Ultrasound examinations at our clinic are done with the high-end ultrasound system, Sonoline Elegra with optional SieScape (Siemens AG). The Sonoline Elegra ultrasound is equipped with the following broadband transducers:

- 5 MHz linear transducer with the option to extend the frequency range upward and downward; frequencies between 3.5 and 7.2 MHz can be chosen.
- 3.5 MHz transducer with the option to extend the frequency range upward and downward;
- frequencies between 2.8 and 5.1 MHz can be chosen.

A-, B-, and M-Mode Techniques

A-mode (A = amplitude) is the oldest image acquisition technique in ultrasound. In A-mode, the echo signals reflected by the body are demodulated, i.e., rectified, and appear as a function of depth.

In B-mode (B = brightness), the signal amplitude of the echo is transformed into the brightness of a picture element. These "pixels" are made visible in lines according to their tissue depth.

In Time Motion (TM- or M-mode), using a stationary transducer, the ultrasound lines formed by a series of transmitted pulses are recorded chronologically in B-mode.

This technique is used to recognize and evaluate fast organ movements (for example, cardiac walls and valves in echocardiography). The location of the echo signal is displayed on a time axis and allows an exact measurement of the motion velocities and wall thickness (Fig. 9.3).

Principal Scan Techniques

There are three principal scan techniques: parallel, sector, and convex.

A *parallel scan* is performed with a *linear array* (array of transducer elements): an active group of array elements is progressed step-by-step, and a rectangular image is created from parallel ultrasound lines. Since the image format is wide close to the probe, the linear array is the preferred choice for imaging superficial organs and structures.

In a *sector scan,* the ultrasound line swivels around a pivot point on or above the contact area, and a sector image is generated. Today, this is done primarily by utilizing *phased (linear) array* transducers that perform this rotation electronically. There are also mechanical sector scanners with one or more single transducer elements, which rotate or oscillate around an axis. Since these transducers have a small footprint, the sector scan is the preferred method when performing examinations under limited anatomic conditions (echocardiography, transcranial sonography).

A *convex scan* using a *convex array* combines the advantages of a sector scan in deeper body regions (large scanning

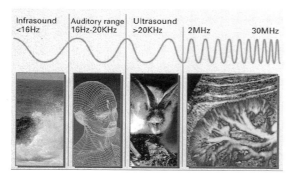

FIGURE 9.2. Frequency ranges of sound. (Courtesy of Siemens AG, 1999.)

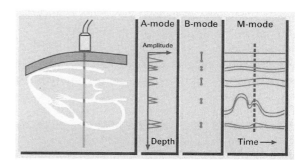

FIGURE 9.3. A-, B-, and M-mode techniques. (Courtesy of Siemens AG, 1999.)

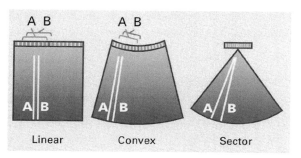

FIGURE 9.4. Principal scan techniques: linear, convex, and sector. (Courtesy of Siemens AG, 1999.)

width) with those of a linear array (large scanning width in superficial regions). Convex arrays are the preferred transducers for transabdominal examinations. The convex array is, in fact, a curved linear array with a point of origin at a distance above the contact area, depending on the radius of curvature (Fig. 9.4).

Variable Format with Linear Array

In addition to the principal scan formats obtained from linear, sector, and convex arrays, linear arrays can also be designed in such a way that they produce rectangular as well as sector image formats, combining the advantages of linear and convex arrays in a single transducer with variable image formats.

Technical requirements: the same high element density as in a phased array transducer (element spacing approximately 0.5 λ) but over the length of a standard linear array. Linear phased array transducers with up to 256 single elements fulfill these requirements. The ultrasound system used requires a corresponding number of channels for phase steering during the reception and transmission of signals (Fig. 9.5).

SieScape Panoramic Imaging

With the incorporation of high-speed image processors into ultrasound systems, new and more complex imaging procedures have become possible. SieScape has overcome the limited image formats of traditional ultrasound sonography by producing large-format images that provide a complete overview of the area under examination. The transducer is swept freehand in one plane over the body surface. The single images obtained in real time are formed into one large image without any loss of information. Any standard transducer and any scan format (parallel, sector, convex, trapezoidal) can be used, without any additional equipment to determine the transducer's position.

SieScape provides images up to a length of 60 cm. In addition to providing more distinct evaluation and measurement of large processes, this method serves as a valuable communication tool for physicians and their patients (Fig. 9.6).

Instrument Setting for Sonography of the Inguinal Region and the Testicle

1. *Inguinal region*: B-picture view with the 3.5-Mhz convex transducer. The transducer is set on a frequency of 5.1 MHz to offer the best resolution for close-ups (standard setting: 8 cm penetration depth). The focus is in a range between 2.5 and 5.5 cm.
2. *Inguinal region*: Quick shift to the 5-Mhz linear transducer, here operating with a standard virtual trapezoidal format. The 5-Mhz transducer is set on a 7.2-MHz frequency. The advantages of high frequency for an optimal detail and contrast resolution are thus combined with the virtual trapezoidal format for a better overall view.
3. *Testicle*: B-picture view with the same setting as in 2., high frequency for optimal resolution and virtual format for a better overall view. Thus, the determination of the testicular volume can be achieved in a quick and simple way.
4. *Duplex sonography of the testicles*: Ever since color Doppler ultrasonography was developed in 1982, sensitivity as well

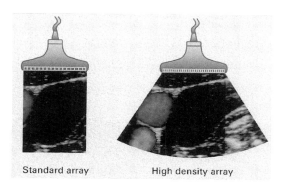

FIGURE 9.5. Variable format with linear array: standard and high density. See Color Plate 6. (Courtesy of Siemens AG, 1999.)

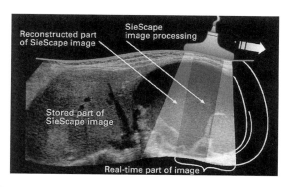

FIGURE 9.6. SieScape panoramic imaging. See Color Plate 7. (Courtesy of Siemens AG, 1999.)

as depth and time resolution of the direction-coded blood flow presentation in real time has been constantly improved. It is considered standard procedure for the ultrasound examination of the testicular blood supply pre- and postoperatively. The duplex examination of the testicles is done with a relatively low pulse rate so that even small and slow running blood vessels can be captured.

5. *Postoperative examination, as well as for extensive inguinal or scrotal findings*: Here the panoramic procedure SieScape is being used. In contrast to computer- and nuclear-resonance scanning, the conventional ultrasound technique can offer only small imaging details, which have a comparatively high resolution but are missing simple reference points. This disadvantage is compensated by the panoramic imaging SieScape (Siemens). During this procedure, the transducer is moved across the inguinal region along the planes of interest all the way to the scrotum. In contrast to other tomographic procedures, we can thus image body regions of up to 60 cm in length in any sectional plane. Extensive pathologic findings, as well as necessary landmarks for understanding and interpretation, can thus for the first time be imaged and measured.

PRACTICAL PROCEDURE

1. *Inguinal region*: The examination takes place with the patient in the supine position and the transducer set on the inguinal region. The assessment is always done in a longitudinal as well as in a transverse section. Also recommended is the assessment of the inguinal region under dynamic conditions, applying Valsalva's maneuver. The presentation of so-called landmarks or guiding structures facilitates orientation. First, a longitudinal section in the inguinal fold along the femoral blood vessels. Inspection of the same and compression of the femoral vein. Next, transverse section: presentation of the oval fossa and exclusion of a femoral hernia during Valsalva's maneuver. The given guiding structures here are, laterally, the femoral blood vessels, medially, the pubic tubercle, dorsally, the iliopsoas muscle (lateral) and the pectineus muscle (medial), and ventrally, resp. transducer close, the inguinal ligament. Then moving the transducer (transversal) above the pubic tubercle and the external inguinal ring: Valsalva's maneuver. Now we turn the transducer longitudinal and parallel to the course of the inguinal canal; guiding structures here are the edge of the internus muscle and the aponeurosis of the externus muscle. A simultaneous 2-finger palpation can ease the identification of the external inguinal ring for the beginner. During Valsalva's maneuver, we can now document the protrusion of a hernia in real-time mode and we can measure the size of the internal hernia opening (internal inguinal ring).

2. *Testicle*: Following palpation of the testicle, the patient now holds his penis across the lower abdomen. A folded towel is placed under the scrotum and the size of the testicles, the testicular parenchyma, possible foci, and the perfusion are measured and assessed.

DESCRIPTION OF FINDINGS

A hernia can be proved by ultrasound if a gap in the fascia with a hernia sac and movable contents can be identified. During Valsalva's maneuver, the inguinal hernia glides beyond the external inguinal ring; by analogy, the femoral hernia beyond the oval fossa (transverse section).

1. *Lateral (indirect) hernia*: At the inner inguinal ring, the hernia moves under the aponeurosis of the external muscle and appears at the external inguinal ring (longitudinal section) (Fig. 9.7).
2. *Medial hernia*: In this case, the hernia extends from dorsal to ventral, straight toward the transducer; combined hernias are difficult to judge (Fig. 9.8).

Portions of the omentum as hernia contents are rather echo dense, movable, or fixed. Intestines are characterized by peristaltic waves, as well as volume and air. Jejunum can be recognized by its typical Kerckring's folds (Fig. 9.9).

Lipomas of the spermatic cord protrude beyond the external inguinal ring during Valsalva's maneuver, but they do not disappear intraperitoneally at the inner inguinal ring (Fig. 9.10).

Lymph nodes are in no way connected to the hernia sac; they can be found subcutaneously or in the vicinity of the femoral blood vessels (Figs. 9.11 and 9.12).

Findings lateral to the femoral blood vessels never represent a hernia (possible differential diagnoses are hemorrhage, abscess in the iliopsoas muscle, and hip ganglion). Funiculoceles and hydroceles are echo-free structures with a dorsal sonar enhancement along the spermatic cord structures or situated in the scrotum (Fig. 9.13).

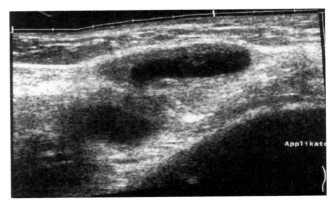

FIGURE 9.7. Irreducible lateral (indirect) hernia.

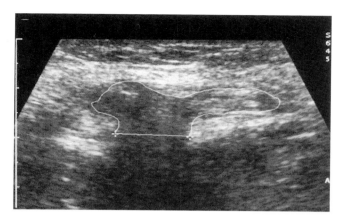

FIGURE 9.8. Medial (direct) hernia.

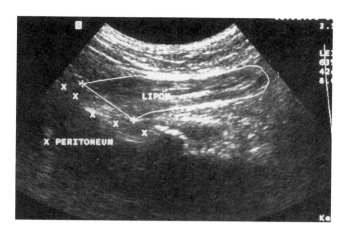

FIGURE 9.10. Lipomas of the spermatic cord protrude beyond the external inguinal ring during Valsalva's maneuver, but they do not disappear intraperitoneally at the inner inguinal ring.

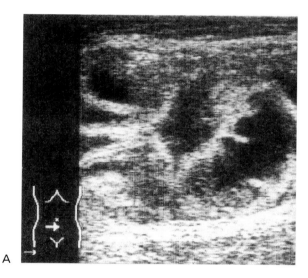

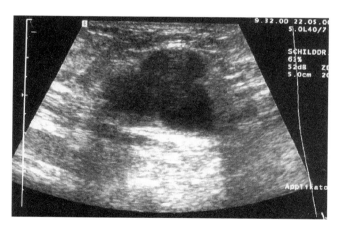

FIGURE 9.11. Multinodal resistance medial to the inner inguinal ring. Histology: highly differentiated leiomyosarcoma.

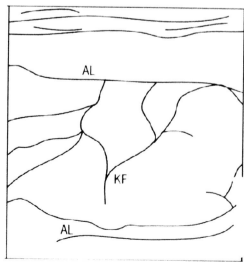

FIGURE 9.9. A: Incarcerated hernia with small intestine in the hernia sac. **B:** *AL,* external inguinal ring; *KF,* Kerckring's folds.

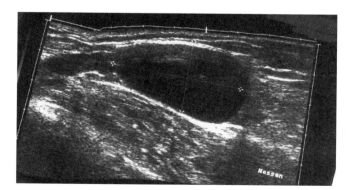

FIGURE 9.12. Varicose excavation of the vena saphena magna close to its inosculation.

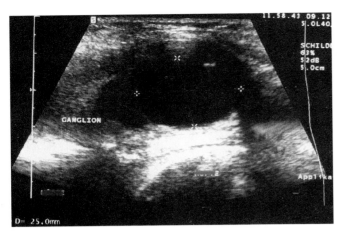

FIGURE 9.13. Hip ganglion.

REGULAR SONOGRAPHIC FINDINGS

Shadowing by Strong Reflector

One of the most common artifacts is the shadowing by a strong reflector distal to the transducer. Strong reflectors are, for example, bone, stones, calcifications, and air, i.e., substances whose acoustic impedances differ significantly from soft tissue. These reflectors return the greater part of the propagated ultrasound energy as echo signals.

If the reflector is hit vertically, it returns a strong, bright echo signal. The distal shadowing helps the user to identify the strong reflector as such and to define it (Fig. 9.14).

Echo Enhancement

If ultrasonic pulses travel through a laterally delimited region of lower attenuation (in comparison to that of the surrounding tissue), the echo signals emanating from the shadow behind this region appear enhanced. This artifact is due to the fact that the user has set the depth-dependent gain control of the ultrasound system for attenuation in normal tissue. Since this gain is too high for the weaker attenuating body region, the echo signals originating from

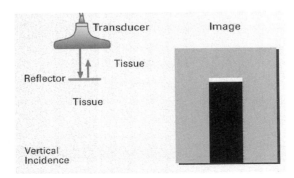

FIGURE 9.14. Shadowing by strong reflector.

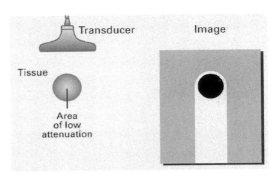

FIGURE 9.15. Echo enhancement.

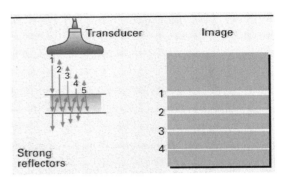

FIGURE 9.16. Reverberations.

behind that region are also presented at too high a gain and therefore appear brighter. It is understood that this "sound enhancement" is not a real enhancement of the ultrasound signal but, at best, a less strong attenuation than assumed.

These artifacts are used in the diagnostic differentiation of cystic and solid masses, for example (Fig. 9.15).

Reverberations

When a sonic pulse hits the borders between two media with different acoustic properties, one portion is always reflected while other portions traverse the borders. This may lead to internal reflections and, therefore, to multiple echoes from the same structure (Fig. 9.16).

NORMAL POSTOPERATIVE FINDINGS

Following laparoscopic hernia repair with mesh implantation: presentation of the mesh in two planes. The inserted mesh can be seen as an echo-dense, slightly waved reflex, sometimes even the lattice-shaped structures can be recognized (especially with accompanying hematoseromas). Dorsal to the mesh, there is a broad echo reduction across the whole depth of the picture (Fig. 9.17).

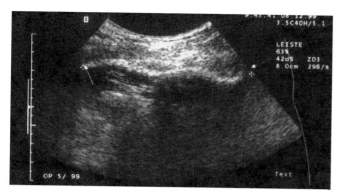

FIGURE 9.17. Normal postoperative finding of inserted mesh.

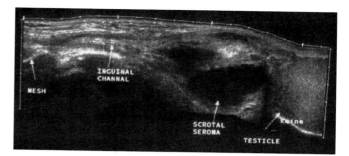

FIGURE 9.19. Large seroma in the scrotal compartment.

SONOGRAPHICALLY VERIFIABLE COMPLICATIONS FOLLOWING LAPAROSCOPIC HERNIA REPAIR

Hematoma resp. seroma can be found in the site of the former hernia sac and in the scrotum ventral to the mesh. Hematoseromas between mesh and peritoneum also present as echo weak, but they can be recognized by the ensuing dorsal echo enhancement. Infected hematomas can be recognized by the increase of echogenicity in the sonar structure, possibly even by air inclusions. Large hematoseromas show reticular fibrinous formations that are often mistaken for a septation of the findings. Large hematoseromas dorsal to the mesh can frequently force the urinary bladder in a dorsal direction within Retzius' space. Such findings cannot be recognized by palpation but only by ultrasound (Fig. 9.18).

Spermatic Cord Structures and Testicles

Swelling of the testicles, the testicular tunics, or the spermatic cord structures can be differentiated only by ultrasound (Figs. 9.19 and 9.20).

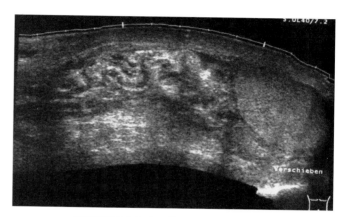

FIGURE 9.20. Swollen spermatic cord.

Congested blood vessels along the spermatic cord structures can be shown by color duplex sonography. Circulatory problems of the testicle are characterized by an inhomogeneity of the parenchyma. The affected testicle often shows a fan-shaped change in its echogenicity (Fig. 9.21).

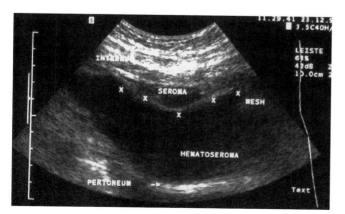

FIGURE 9.18. Mesh position correct; approximately 200 mL hematoseroma posterior to the mesh.

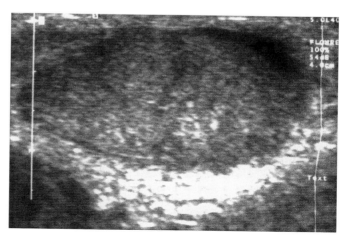

FIGURE 9.21. Affected testicle with inhomogeneity of the parenchyma.

RESULTS OF A PROSPECTIVE CLINICAL STUDY ON THE VALUE OF ULTRASOUND EXAMINATIONS IN THE DIAGNOSIS AND CLASSIFICATION OF INGUINAL HERNIAS

A total of 220 patients with 289 hernias were included in this study. All patients consecutively received a laparoscopic hernia repair and were compared for diagnosis leading to admission, preoperative clinical findings in the hospital, preoperative ultrasound results, and intraoperative laparoscopic findings.

The sonographic examination with the objective to detect an inguinal hernia showed a sensitivity of 0.97, a specificity of 0.87, and a total hit score of 0.94. In eight false-negative ultrasound findings, a very narrow hernia sac or a femoral hernia was found intraoperatively. In 19 false-positive ultrasound findings, no hernia was found but instead a spermatic cord lipoma. In those cases with a sonographic diagnosis of a spermatic cord lipoma, there was a 64% agreement with the intraoperative findings. The size of the hernia opening could be correctly determined in only 53% of all cases. The assessment of the type of hernia showed an agreement of 62% between ultrasound and intraoperative findings.

CONCLUSION

Ultrasound examination of the inguinal region and the testicle has become indispensable for the preoperative diagnosis of pathologic findings of the inguinal region, as well as for the postoperative control examinations after laparoscopic hernioplasty. Ultrasound has a high predictive value in the preoperative diagnosis of an inguinal hernia. While sensitivity is clearly higher in comparison to thorough clinical examination, specificity is correspondingly lower. The reason for the lower specificity can be found in the misinterpretation of spermatic cord lipoma as hernia pathology. Concerning the classification of inguinal hernias, only trend-setting statements are possible. A reliable classification can be achieved only by laparoscopy. In regard to the size of the hernia opening and the presence of lipomas, clinical and sonographic examinations have merely a small predictive value.

EDITORS' COMMENTS

Ultrasound has an important place in the evaluation of patients with groin problems, a fact that commonly escapes American physicians. This was underscored recently to me when a radiologist refused to perform an examination on a patient with questionable recurrent hernia because he had never heard of using it for this indication. Not only is sonography useful in cases of questionable recurrence, but it can also be helpful preoperatively in the differential diagnosis and as part of the management of postoperative pain problems. This chapter is especially valuable as a surgeon–author provides a unique perspective because of the appreciation of subtle surgical nuances. Dr. Bittner and his German colleagues are skilled in ultrasonography because it is mandated in their training programs. American surgeons need to come to grips with the fact that we should be similarly trained.

R.J.F., Jr.

Nyhus and Condon's Hernia, Fifth Edition, edited by Robert J. Fitzgibbons, Jr. and A. Gerson Greenburg. Lippincott Williams & Wilkins, Philadelphia © 2002.

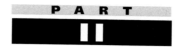

P A R T

II

CONVENTIONAL GROIN HERNIA REPAIRS

10

THE BASSINI REPAIR
AND ITS VARIANTS

ALENE J. WRIGHT
GLENN C. GARDNER
ROBERT J. FITZGIBBONS, JR.

It is widely agreed that the operation developed by Bassini in the late 1880s ushered in the modern era of hernia surgery. Before his contribution, a truss was the preferred treatment for an inguinal hernia, as operation was not routinely recommended because of the miserable results. The repair's foundation in basic anatomic principles changed these results dramatically, revolutionizing the field of herniology. The operation is used less frequently now because of the acceptance of the tension-free concept by many surgeons, especially in the United States. The original operation and its variations, which are described below, are of more than just historic interest, however, because there are situations when the use of a prosthesis is not appropriate. For example, in the presence of sepsis, in patients who are allergic, or in patients who refuse the use of any type of foreign material, these operations are an excellent option. In addition, many surgeons outside of the United States have not been so keen to accept the routine use of a prosthesis, fearing infection, rejection, erosion into surrounding structures, and even carcinogenesis (5). In this chapter, a detailed description of the original Bassini operation will be presented, as well as the most important modifications that have gained popularity from time to time since Bassini.

The description of the operations presented represents the authors' best consensus. This is because many of the techniques described were developed by surgeons who were not prolific writers, and some of the material must be quoted from secondary references. For example, Bassini himself only published a few illustrations in some rather obscure Italian journals. The drawings are difficult to interpret and are lacking detail. Textbooks vary significantly on the description of the procedures. Research in this area is further complicated by different illustrations by the surgeons themselves because of evolution in technique. The authors of this chapter welcome comments and corrections from readers, especially if specific reference material is available. Information can be sent to Robert J. Fitzgibbons, Jr., M.D., Department of Surgery, Creighton University School of Medicine, 601 North 30th Street, Suite 3740, Omaha, Nebraska 68131.

HISTORY

Edoardo Bassini (1844–1924) was born in Pavia, Italy, and received his doctorate in medicine from the University of Pavia at the age of 22. He joined the liberation forces of Garibaldi in the crusade for unification of Italy, and in combat suffered a bayonet wound to the groin that was complicated by a fecal fistula. After he recovered, he joined the staff at the University of Pavia and resumed his study of anatomy and surgical pathology, studying with Billroth, Langenbeck, Nussbaum, and Lister. At the age of 38, he became a professor of surgical pathology at the University of Padua and later advanced to the chair of clinical surgery to become the greatest Italian surgeon of his generation (1,2,7,9,10). Bassini's radical cure of a groin hernia resulted from his studies dealing with the anatomic and functional restoration of the inguinal canal, which he had pursued for more than a decade. His new technique was quite a departure from the accepted methods of repair that essentially involved closing the hernia sac at the subcutaneous ring. He had incorporated the principles of deep chloroform anesthesia and proper antiseptic techniques taught to him by Lister. His scientific approach to the problem led to the development of several distinct steps that he felt were essential for the procedure. These included:

A.J. Wright, G.C. Gardner, and **R.J. Fitzgibbons, Jr.:** Department of Surgery, Creighton University, School of Medicine, Omaha, Nebraska.

1. Splitting of the external oblique aponeurosis.
2. Division of the cremaster muscle lengthwise followed by resection so that an indirect hernia could not be missed, while exposing simultaneously the floor of the inguinal canal to more accurately assess for a direct inguinal hernia.
3. Splitting the floor or posterior wall of the canal for its full length. This step ensures examination of the femoral ring from above, but more importantly, it exposes the very tissue layers that will serve the purpose of a more solid reconstruction. In particular, it precludes the use of the "transversalis fascia," which is the poorest layer of the posterior wall. This step was largely ignored when the operation was imported to North America.
4. Resection of the indirect sac flush with the internal ring or even deeper. (We know today this is not necessary as simple reduction of the sac into the preperitoneal space is just as effective.)
5. Reconstruction of the posterior wall by suturing the transversalis fascia, the transversus abdominis muscle, the internal oblique muscle, and also the lateral border of the rectus abdominis (as emphasized by Bassini himself) medially to the inguinal ligament laterally (and possibly the iliopubic tract; this step is suggested in the drawings but not clarified in the original text of Bassini or Catterina) (14).

His series included 262 cases with only seven recurrences and greater than 90% follow-up at $4^1/_2$ years. These results were five times better than what was being reported at the time. Hospitalization decreased to 13 to 14 days, and a truss was not required (9). So many modifications of Bassini's original operation followed in the ensuing years that Attilio Catterina, one of his most celebrated students, felt compelled to publish an article in 1932 entitled "The Operation of Bassini." Catterina decided to do this because the classic operation was being performed incorrectly and was poorly described in surgical texts. This was causing inferior results, leading to criticism that he did not think was justified. What follows is paraphrased directly from Catterina's description of the original Bassini operation with the addition of accepted variations, e.g., reduction of an indirect inguinal hernia sac instead of high ligation.

TECHNIQUE

Cutaneous Incision

The important landmarks to be identified prior to incising the skin are the anterosuperior iliac spine, the symphysis pubis, and the pubic tubercle. In obese individuals, palpating through the base of the scrotum with a finger best identifies the latter two. A 7- to 10-cm incision is made along the line between the symphysis pubis and anterosuperior iliac spine. Alternatively, a more transverse incision can be used.

Incision of the External Oblique Aponeurosis

The skin incision is extended through Scarpa and Camper's fascia, and the external oblique aponeurosis is identified. The superficial ring of the inguinal canal is located, and the external oblique aponeurosis is incised at the upper margin of the superficial ring so that the reapproximated suture line does not overlap the deep sutures that are placed to repair the floor on the inguinal canal.

Isolating the Cord Structures

The upper flap of the external oblique aponeurosis is separated from the internal oblique muscle using blunt finger dissection or the handle of the scalpel. The iliohypogastric nerve is identified at this time and gently freed from the surrounding tissue. Care must be taken to avoid crushing the nerve with an instrument. A hemostat is used to keep it out of the field of surgery by passing the hemostat under the nerve and grasping the upper flap of the external oblique aponeurosis. This avoids injury to the nerve during surgery. The cord structures are then lifted en masse with the fingers of one hand exactly at the pubic tubercle so that the index finger can be passed gently underneath to meet the fingers of the other hand. Once this is done, a finger is slid all the way to the deep inguinal ring, completely isolating the cord structures. A Penrose drain or rubber loop is used to hold them out of the way.

Separation of the Cremaster Muscle and Other Coverings from the Sac

The cord structures are lifted with the help of the Penrose drain, and the cremaster muscle and spermatic cord with its vessels are gently separated from the hernia sac. Once the sac is identified, it is grasped with a pair of mosquito clamps and the cord structures are separated from it using DeBakey forceps. Extreme care must be taken to avoid injury to the vas deferens and the vessels. The cremaster muscle is separated beginning as close to the deep inguinal ring as possible. This simplifies the isolation of the spermatic cord. The cremaster muscle and other coverings are pulled aside from the spermatic cord and sac, clamped, divided, and ligated. Lipomas of the cord are removed at this stage.

Isolation of the Spermatic Cord from the Sac

Separation of the spermatic cord from the sac should begin adjacent to the internal ring. Again, care must be taken not to damage the vas deferens. Once the sac is free from the cord structures and the vas has been identified, the sac should be divided and the proximal end ligated. It is imperative to make sure that there are no peritoneal contents in the sac. If necessary, the sac can be opened and the contents reduced back into the abdominal cavity before ligating it. The distal sac may be left alone or may be slit in its entirety, exposing the inner surface so that the edges can be inverted around the cord and sutured behind it as in the treatment for a hydrocele. Many surgeons now prefer to simply reduce the sac back into the preperitoneal space, feeling that either opening or excising the sac is unnecessary. Bassini probably would have considered this hearsay, but experience has shown it to be as effective as excision. Proponents point out that simple reduction eliminates any possibility of damage to an incarcerated structure. Perhaps more importantly, some authorities feel that there is substantial decrease in pain when the richly innervated peritoneum is not incised.

Exposure and Incision of the Transversalis Fascia

Drawing the cord downward exposes the transversalis fascia. At the same time, the assistant draws the sac outward

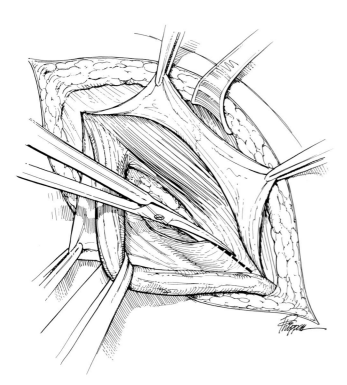

FIGURE 10.1. Bassini's repair. The inguinal floor has been exposed, and the transversalis fascia is being incised. The preperitoneal fat is visible beneath the fascia.

from the body. This stretches the transversalis fascia that covers the deep epigastric vessels near the neck of the sac. The fascia is then cut from the deep ring down to the pubis, creating a free edge of the transversalis fascia, transversus abdominis muscle, and internal oblique muscle. (Fig. 10.1) By sliding a finger between the fascia and the preperitoneal fat, the surgeon separates the two layers for 2 to 3 cm. This method of opening the inguinal floor by incising the transversalis fascia completes the creation of Bassini's famous "triple layer," which includes the edges of the transversalis fascia, transversus abdominis muscle, and the internal oblique muscle. Catterina was particularly disturbed by the common modification of not opening the transversalis in favor of using "good stuff" grasped blindly with an Allis clamp underneath the internal oblique muscle.

Suturing the Deep Layer and Closure of the Incision

The first stitch includes the transversalis fascia, transversus abdominis muscle, and internal oblique muscle (threefold layer), along with the external edge of the rectus abdominis muscle, with or without their aponeuroses. The stitch is passed through these tissues, about 2 cm from the edge, protecting the underlying structures at all times. The needle is then passed through the periosteum of the pubic tubercle and the rectus tendon and sheath very close to the medial side of the pubic tubercle. Early descriptions of the repair include mention of Colles' ligament or fascia as well as Henle's ligament. We prefer not to use these terms because their presence varies from patient to patient and their anatomic descriptions vary from text to text. A second suture is placed about 1 cm laterally and incorporates all the structure mentioned above. The third stitch includes the threefold layer and the reflected inguinal ligament (Poupart's ligament). Six to eight stitches are then placed through the threefold layer and Poupart's ligament so that the last suture is 1 cm below where the cord arises. The needle is passed through the triple layer approximately 2 cm from the edge, going in and out twice. This "purse-string"–like stitch is described in Catterina's translation; however, his illustrations by Orazio Gaigher seem to imply that the stitch went in and out only once. In addition, Bassini's original four drawings failed to show this step clearly at all (Fig. 10.2). Catterina emphasizes that Bassini's illustrations make no distinction between the iliopubic tract and Poupart's ligament. The cord is then repositioned, and the two flaps of the external oblique aponeurosis are sutured with a running stitch reconstructing the external ring. Interrupted sutures are used in the subcutaneous tissue, and the skin is closed (14).

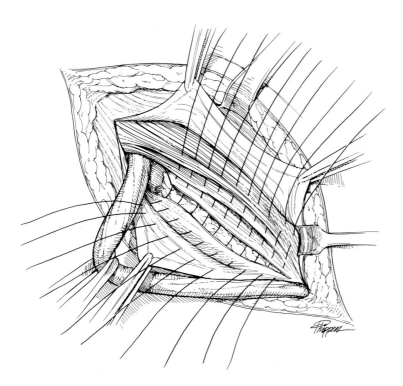

FIGURE 10.2. Bassini's repair. The "triple layer" (transversalis fascia, transversus abdominis muscle, and internal oblique muscle) is sutured to the inguinal ligament.

THE BASSINI VARIANTS

Following the introduction of Bassini's repair for inguinal hernias, there were a number of modifications to try to improve the procedure as an understanding of the anatomy became clearer. Most changes have been minor, but some were significant enough that they took on their own name. Many would consider these variants of historic interest only, but actually there are times that they can be used even in modern practice.

The Shouldice Repair

This pure tissue repair is based on the same principles as Bassini's repair but differs in certain details. Because of the outstanding results reported by the Shouldice clinic surgeons and others, the technique has become popular with many surgeons, especially in institutions where prosthetics are not routinely available. The operation is so important that it will be discussed in more detail in its own separate chapter. However, since it is a Bassini variant, it will be touched upon here briefly.

The initial approach is similar to Bassini's repair, with particular importance placed on freeing the cord from its surrounding adhesions, resection of the cremaster muscle, high dissection of the hernia sac, and division of the transversalis fascia. Continuous nonabsorbable suture is used to repair the floor. Traditionally, this has been monofilament steel wire. The Shouldice surgeons feel a continuous suture

distributes tension evenly and prevents defects that could potentially occur between interrupted sutures, resulting in a recurrence. However, this advantage has never been conclusively proven. The repair is started at the pubic tubercle by approximating the iliopubic tract laterally to the medial flap, which is made up of the rectus, internal oblique and transverse abdominis muscles, and the transversalis fascia. The running suture is continued to the internal ring, where the lateral stump of the cremaster muscle is picked up. The suture is then brought over to the other side to incorporate the transversalis fascia, transversus abdominis muscle, and internal oblique muscle, in that order, forming a new internal ring. The direction of the suture is then reversed back toward the pubic tubercle, approximating the medial edge of the internal oblique and transversus abdominis muscles to Poupart's ligament, and the ends of the wire are tied. Thus, there are two suture lines formed by the first suture. The second wire suture is started near the internal ring and approximates the internal oblique and transversus muscles to a band of external oblique aponeurosis superficial and parallel to Poupart's ligament. This forms the third suture line, which ends at the pubic crest. The suture is then reversed and a fourth suture line is constructed in a similar manner (3,13,14).

The Marcy Repair

The Marcy repair includes high ligation of the hernia sac plus narrowing the internal ring by approximating the surrounding muscular and aponeurotic layers on the medial side.

Removal of the Cremaster Muscle

This technique is used in men with well-developed cremaster muscles. The cremaster and internal oblique muscles are invested and bound together by a common thin fascia that can be displayed by grasping the cremaster at the level of the external ring and pulling it away from the internal oblique muscle. When the fascia is excised, a clean separation of the cremaster from the internal oblique is obtained. Upon elevating the cremaster, a thin sheet of fascia is seen anchoring it to the iliopubic tract. Incising this fascia along the iliopubic tract completely mobilizes the cremaster muscle and cord.

The cremaster muscle is incised longitudinally and dissected from the cord in upper and lower flaps. The lower flap is removed by an incision separating the fascial origin of the cremaster muscle from the iliopubic tract. The cremasteric vessels are ligated during this step. The upper flap is excised from the internal oblique, permitting optimal retraction of the arcuate edge of the confluence of the internal oblique and transversus abdominis for exposure of the ring superiorly.

Finding the Internal Ring

The sac and cord structures are handled as a unit that emerges from the internal ring and lies within the internal spermatic fascia. The sheath is incised longitudinally to permit dissection of the sac. Tracing the sheath proximally leads directly to the transversalis fascia and the internal ring. The transversalis fascia must be separated from the peritoneum above the neck of the sac and secured with clamps before the neck of the sac is ligated. During this dissection, the vas deferens and internal spermatic vessels are separated from the peritoneum and transversalis fascia. It is important to find strong fascia for the repair, and if the sac is large, further dissection and retraction may be needed.

High Ligation

This means ligating the sac above the internal ring so that the transversalis fascial edges may be sutured distal to the stump of the proximal portion of the sac. Before the sac is suture ligated, it is opened and explored to reduce any contents and to rule out a femoral or direct inguinal hernia.

Closure of the Ring

This involves displacing the cord structures laterally and placing sutures through the muscular and fascial layers, which narrows the internal ring. (Fig. 10.3) The reconstructed ring should admit only the tip of the hemostat. When the retractors are removed, the internal oblique muscles and transversus abdominis regain their normal positions and buttress the internal ring. The external oblique, subcutaneous tissue, and skin are then closed (4,11).

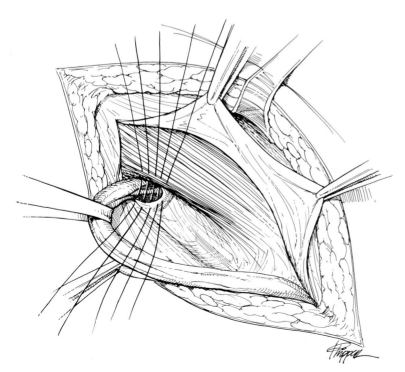

FIGURE 10.3. The Marcy repair. The internal ring is narrowed medial to the internal ring. (Some texts reflect this tightening with transversalis fascia only.)

Halsted Operation with Subcutaneous Transplantation of the Cord (Halsted I)

A long oblique incision parallel to the inguinal ligament is made to obtain adequate exposure, and the aponeurosis of the external oblique is identified and incised, preserving the iliohypogastric nerve. The external oblique aponeurosis is then separated from the underlying structures, and the flaps are dissected back laterally to the shelving edge of Poupart's ligament and medially as close to the midline as possible.

The sac is identified and separated from the surrounding tissues. The cord is carefully dissected from the sac, avoiding injury to the vas deferens and the internal spermatic vessels. The sac is then ligated as high as possible, closing the peritoneum.

Suturing the conjoint tendon to Poupart's ligament with interrupted nonabsorbable sutures completes the repair of the posterior wall. If the sac is very large and tissues are weak, a vertical paramedian relaxing incision in the rectus sheath is made. Placing sutures through the rectus muscle and the lateral edge of the rectus sheath and suturing them to Poupart's ligament completes the repair of the posterior wall. The cord structures are displaced superficially during this part of the procedure. Finally, the two edges of the external oblique are sutured together under the cord structures, thus placing the cord in a subcutaneous bed and creating a quadruple layer. This original technique would later be modified because of an unacceptable incidence of testicular atrophy, hydrocele, and infarction, as well as high recurrence rate through the new inguinal ring (8,12).

The Ferguson Operation

This modification was developed after witnessing some of the complications of the Halsted I. Ferguson said, "Leave the cord alone for it is the sacred highway along which travel vital elements indispensable to the perpetuity of our race"(10,12). An incision is made over Poupart's ligament 4 cm below the anterosuperior iliac spine, and the external oblique aponeurosis is identified. The external ring is located, and the aponeurosis is incised over the inguinal canal. The principal modification is that the spermatic cord is not transplanted. The sac of the hernia is identified and opened to reduce any contents. Ligature or suture is then used to close the peritoneum.

The transversalis fascia forms the internal ring, and the fibers are usually stretched when a hernia is present. As a result, the internal ring is abnormally large, and the fascia bulges. To reduce the slack in the fascia and make an accurately fitting internal ring, interrupted or continuous sutures are used. Care must be taken to avoid injuring the deep epigastric or iliac vessels.

The internal oblique and transversalis muscles are then sutured to the internal aspect of Poupart's ligament. If the conjoint tendon is deficient, the sheath of the rectus muscle is opened down to the pubic bone, and the rectus muscle is sutured to Poupart's ligament.

The external oblique aponeurosis edges are brought together in lateral folds or are overlapped, restoring the external ring, completing the repair.

The Andrews Operation

This operation differs in that the buttress overlying the weak part of the abdominal wall is made up of muscle and the aponeurosis of the external oblique. The incision is started at the external ring and extended for 7 to 9 cm upward and outward. The aponeurosis of the external oblique is identified and incised in the direction of its fibers through the external ring, preserving the iliohypogastric nerve. The lower flap is retracted and the cord lifted. Poupart's ligament is exposed up to the tubercle of the pubis. Following this, the cremasteric muscle and fascia are incised and the hernia sac identified and isolated after reducing its contents. High ligation of the sac is of utmost importance.

The posterior wall of the inguinal canal is buttressed by suturing the external oblique aponeurosis, internal oblique, and transversalis muscles or conjoint tendon to the shelving edge of Poupart's ligament (Fig. 10.4). This leaves the cord lying above the aponeurosis. The lower flap of the external oblique aponeurosis is then sutured to the anterior surface of the upper part of the aponeurosis to cover the cord. The subcutaneous tissue and skin can be closed in a routine manner (10,12,14).

Halsted II (Ferguson–Andrews Operation)

This was developed in the 1890s by Halsted after experience with the Halsted I and its complications of skeletonization and transplanting the cord. He incorporated Ferguson's procedure, which left the floor of the canal or transversalis fascia alone except lateral to the inguinal ring, and Andrews' concept of imbricating the flaps of the external oblique aponeurosis in front of the cord in performing the closure. The imbricated external oblique aponeurosis in front of the cord formed the anterior wall of the reconstructed oblique canal. The cremaster fibers are also preserved in this technique. This is often referred to as the Halsted II operation (10,12,14).

Nylon Darn Inguinal Hernia Repair

This procedure had a period of popularity in the United Kingdom and other parts of Europe and the Far East. It was introduced by Handley in 1918 as a darn–lattice procedure. Moloney first reported the double-layer darn technique in 1948. The Kinmonth modification involving a locked half stitch surfaced in the early 1970s and was investigated in at least one major trial in the United States (13). The usual principles of inguinal hernia surgery are adhered to, including high ligation of the sac and skeletonization of the cord.

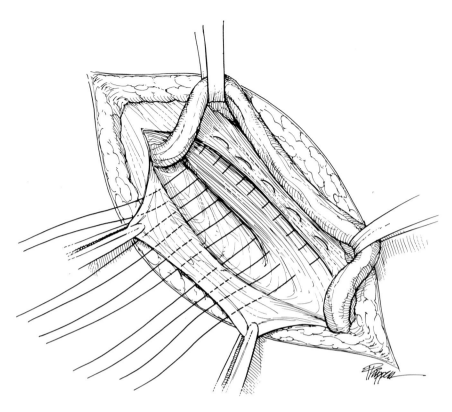

FIGURE 10.4. Andrews operation. The transversus abdominis muscle, internal oblique muscle, and external oblique aponeurosis are sutured to the inguinal ligament. (Some texts illustrate individual sutures through each layer.)

The procedure gets its name from the way the long nylon suture is repeatedly passed between the tissues to create a weave that one might consider similar to mesh. The initial layer consists of continuous nylon suture to oppose the conjoint tendon and rectus muscle to Poupart's ligament, and to reconstruct the fascia around the neck of the cord and internal ring. This first suture is continued into the muscle around the cord, weaving in and out to form reinforcement around the cord. On the lateral side of the cord, it is sutured to the inguinal ligament and tied (Fig. 10.5).

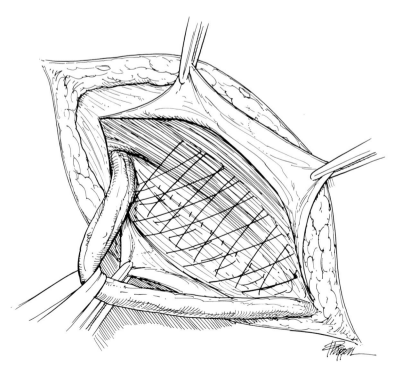

FIGURE 10.5. Maloney darn. Latticework-like weave opposing the conjoint tendon to Poupart's ligament and the rectus sheath medial to the pubic tubercle continued to the medial side of the internal ring. The deeper first layer can be seen beneath the weave.

The darn is a second layer on top of the first approximating layer. The sutures may be parallel or in a crisscross fashion, plicating well into the inguinal ligament below. The darn must be carried well over the medial edge of the inguinal canal. Once the darn is complete, the external oblique is closed over the cord structures. The rationale of the darn procedure is to form a meshwork of nonabsorbable suture that is well tolerated by the tissues and fills the interstices with fibrous connective tissue, producing a buttress across the weakened area of the inguinal canal (6).

The Relaxing Incision

In 1892, Wolfler described the relaxing incision. It later gained popularity for the repair of difficult inguinal hernias to relieve excessive tension on the sutures line(s). It is commonly used as an adjuvant to Bassini's repair or any of the variants described in this chapter. The relaxing incision is made through the anterior rectus sheath to the belly of the rectus muscle, extending from the pubic tubercle superiorly for a variable distance determined by the tension. Some surgeons prefer to hockey stick the incision laterally at the superior extent. The posterior rectus sheath is strong enough to prevent future incisional herniation. This relaxing incision works because when the anterior rectus sheath separates, the elements of the abdominal wall that one might be using for the various repairs can be displaced laterally and inferiorly with greater ease, resulting in less tension (14).

CONCLUSION

Surgeons should be familiar with the nonprosthetic repairs not only because of historic interest, but also because there are situations where prosthesis is not appropriate. In this chapter, Bassini's repair and its major variants have been described. There have been numerous modifications of the original Bassini procedure since the late 1800s, many with eponyms commonly more descriptive of the name of a surgeon who developed the change rather than the modification. It is not practical to include all of these procedures in a chapter such as this. The operations chosen for illustration were felt to be representative of classes of techniques. It is hoped that the reader who may have a particular interest in a named herniorrhaphy that has not been specifically included will be able to place it into perspective.

REFERENCES

1. Castrini G, Pappalardo G, Trentino P, et al. The original Bassini technique in the surgical treatment of inguinal hernia. *Int Surg* 1986;71:141–143.
2. Edoardo Bassini (1844–1924) [Editorial]. *JAMA* 1968;204: 329–330.
3. Glassow F. The Shouldice Hospital technique. *Int Surg* 1986;71: 148–153.
4. Griffith CA. The Marcy repair revisited. *Surg Clin North Am* 1984;64:215.
5. Klosterhalfen B, Klinge U, Hermanns B, et al. Pathology of traditional surgical nets for hernia repair after long-term implantation in humans. *Chirurg* 2000;71:43.
6. Lifschutz H. The inguinal darn. *Arch Surg* 1986;121:717–718.
7. Premuda L. The history of inguinal herniorrhaphy. *Int Surg* 1986;71:138–140.
8. Ravitch MM. The classic Halsted–Ferguson operation for inguinal hernia. In: *Repair of hernias.* Chicago: Year Book Medical Publishers, 1969:26–41.
9. Read RC. The centenary of Bassini's contribution to inguinal herniorrhaphy. *Am J Surg* 1987;153:324–326.
10. Read RC. The development of inguinal herniorrhaphy. *Surg Clin North Am* 1984;64:185–196.
11. Read RC. Marcy's priority in the development of inguinal herniorrhaphy. *Surgery* 1980;88:682–685.
12. Read RC. Inguinofemoral herniation: evolution of repair through the anterior approach to the groin. In: Zuidema G, ed. *Shackelford's surgery of the alimentary tract,* 4th ed. Philadelphia: WB Saunders, 1996:5:116.
13. Shearburn EW, Myers RN. Shouldice repair for inguinal hernia. *Surgery* 1969;66:450–559.
14. Wantz GE. The operation of Bassini as described by Attilio Catterina. *Surg Gynecol Obstet* 1989;168:67–80.

SPECIAL COMMENTS
Raymond C. Read

Today, inguinal herniation is routinely repaired around the world using mainly tension-free techniques. Plastic prostheses are inserted in the inguinal canal or the preperitoneal space, by open or laparoscopic methodology, with the patient awake or asleep. Why then, in this new millennium, do we bother with the details of an operation described by an obscure Italian academic surgeon over a century ago? He practiced in a small town (however, at a venerable university, attended by Fallopius, Harvey, Morgagni, Spigelius, Valsalva, Vesalius, and Scarpa), situated in the marshes west of Venice. Admittedly, on occasion, the use of a foreign body may be inadvisable. Nevertheless, the main reason this tissue repair, with its modifications, remains relevant today is that successful herniorrhaphy depends on much more than the simple introduction of an internal truss into the groin. This transition zone between trunk, limb, and genitalia is a surprisingly complex anatomic entity. Before the mesh can be placed, the protrusion has to be dealt with, defects defined, and surrounding musculofascial layers prepared to receive it. The plastic has to be attached in such a manner that it will stay put without damaging associated structures. Remarkably, the proper way to conduct this dissection remains that described by Bassini in the late 1880s. What Zimmerman and Heller stated in 1937, at the 50-year anniversary, remains true today: "The subject . . . is so completely and masterfully handled, that little of significance has since been added . . . . the fullness of the author's understanding of the problems involved is astounding . . . . contemporary herniographers could study this contribution with profit"(9).

This father of modern herniorrhaphy introduced a new era. He was the first to apply advances in anesthesia, antisepsis, and hemostasis, which allowed unroofing of the inguinal canal, reconstruction of its floor after high ligation of the sac(s), maintenance of obliquity, and closure of all defects. His outcomes not only were many times better than those achieved by his contemporaries with their "radical cures" (which, however, required the wearing of a truss postoperatively), but also rival many of ours today. None of the many modifications of his procedure have proved to be much better. In fact, the best results have been obtained with the Shouldice operation, which I (1985) and Wantz (1989) have labeled "the modern Bassini." Interestingly, this method was developed by Ryan, Obney, and Shouldice (1953), without their knowing the finer points of Bassini's operation—"a reinvention of the wheel," according to Wantz (8).

Bassini himself contributed to the inordinate delay before surgeons came to appreciate the finer points of his technique. His initial writings were in archaic Italian, nestled away in little-known publications. Only one article, a translation into German, became widely available. Unfortunately, the text and insufficient figures were short on details. Thus, excision of the cremasteric apparatus and division of the transversalis fascia were only implied, while no mention was made of nerves encountered during the dissection. Initially, his patients had large, neglected hernias with superimposed inguinal rings and a destroyed floor. Later, with earlier protrusions, he began to purposefully divide the transversalis fascia. As modifications blossomed, mainly in the United States, he remained silent even though he served as chairman of surgery at the University of Padua, publishing on a number of other procedures, for 30 more years.

A colleague, Catterina, in 1932 published, in Italian, an atlas describing Bassini's operation. This was later translated into English (London, 1934). However, it was not until 1989 that Wantz made the information widely available in this country (8). Nevertheless, the main reason Bassini's operation fell into disrepute was that a number of pernicious modifications associated with poor results bore his eponym. As Catterina stated, "If a surgeon doesn't follow the fundamental rules, he has no right to speak about a Bassini operation or attribute to the method recurrences resulting from the mistakes of the operator"(5). Perhaps the greatest accolade was bestowed by Halsted in 1922, just weeks before his death: "I have not seen a single paper since Bassini's which contributed anything new . . . . Prior to Bassini's publications, inguinal hernia had rarely been cured" (6).

What lessons can we learn from Bassini's epic achievement? The first is that advances in knowledge require dedication. Bassini, who introduced antisepsis into Italy, visited all the major surgical centers of Europe. He tried and gave up on the repairs of others: "A scar in the inguinal canal, weakened by the

passage of the spermatic cord within it, provides inadequate protection against recurrence" (3). He then spent 4 years perfecting his own technique, using extensive follow-up and autopsy studies before presenting a large series of cases in 1885 before the Italian Surgical Society. His focus on surgery of the groin was perhaps stimulated by being bayonetted in the groin while fighting for Italian independence. A prolonged fecal fistula ensued.

He insisted on strict adherence to surgical principles. After unroofing the inguinal canal and excising the cremaster apparatus, including its vascular and nerve supply, indirect, direct, femoral, and bilateral defects were differentiated, the latter being operated on at one setting. The true necks of the peritoneal sacs were dissected out 2 cm. proximal to the internal ring, "in the iliac fossa," by separating "subserous fat" 1 inch circumferentially from the incised transversalis fascia. All lipomata were removed. He thus followed Bogros (1823) (4) and Annandale (1876) (2), who, for iliac aneurysm or combined inguinofemoral herniation, entered the preperitoneal space anteriorly.

Hernial defects were repaired by reconstructing the floor of the inguinal canal rather than its roof or outlet. Bassini's triple layer included transversalis fascia. Its presence was important because it obviated strictly musculoligamentous healing (necessitated by the Ferguson and Halsted II operations), which was later shown experimentally to fail (7). These latter procedures, although eliminating skeletonization of the cord and failing to restore obliquity to the canal, unfortunately left the transversalis fascial floor undisturbed, making high ligation almost impossible. Bassini placed a finger intra- or extraperitoneally while stitching the triple layer, and protected the bladder and other viscera, besides making sure full thickness bites were obtained. Injury to the iliac vein encountered with the Halsted I procedure, which stimulated the latter and others to retreat from the preperitoneal space, was thus avoided. The fact that Bassini stitched, starting ³/₄ inch from the edges as a double purse-string or Lembert suture, both above and below enabled broad-based apposition as pointed out by Andrews, who later popularized imbrication (1). The former transplanted the cord 1 to 2 cm laterally at the internal ring by cutting the internal oblique muscle. This facilitated deep dissection of the cord and its contents (parietalization). Before closing the external oblique aponeurosis and skin, the repair was tested by lightening the anesthesia and having the patient retch. Drainage of the wound was rarely used, and then only in cases with giant protrusions. Cryptorchidism was managed. The same operation was carried out consistently in young and old. Ambulation was begun earlier than usual, with length of hospitalization being reduced by a third. Almost all of Bassini's patients were followed to document the results.

In conclusion, we are indebted to the authors from Creighton University for detailing Bassini's operation and its variants. I have attempted to point out whence they arose and why this pioneer resides in the surgeons' pantheon.

REFERENCES

1. Andrews EW. Imbrication or lap joint method: a plastik operation for hernia. *Chicago Med Rec* 1895;9:67–77.
2. Annandale T. Case in which a reducible oblique and direct inguinal and femoral hernia existed on the same side and were successfully treated by operation. *Edinburgh Med J* 1876;21: 1087.
3. Bassini E. Ueber de behandlung des listenbruches. *Arch Klin Chir* 1890;40:429–476.
4. Bogros JA. Essay on the surgical anatomy of the iliac region and description of a new procedure for the ligation of the epigastric and external iliac arteries. *Postgrad Gen Surg* 1995;6:4–14. Bendavid RA, translator.
5. Catterina A. *Bassini's operation for the radical cure of inguinal hernia.* London: Lewis, 1934.
6. Halsted WS. *Surgical papers,* vol 1. Baltimore: Johns Hopkins Press, 1924:308.
7. Seelig MG, Chouke KS. A fundamental factor in the recurrence of inguinal hernia. *Arch Surg* 1923;1:553.
8. Wantz GE. The operation of Bassini as described by Attilio Catterina. *Surg Gynecol Obstet* 1989;168:67–80.
9. Zimmerman LM, Heller RE. Landmarks in surgery: Edoardo Bassini—his role in the development of hernial surgery. *Surg Gynecol Obstet* 1937;64:971–973.

11

HERNIA SURGERY IN ITALY: HOW FAR HAVE WE COME SINCE BASSINI?

ENRICO NICOLÒ
ANTONIO GUARNIERI
FRANCESCO GUARNIERI

EDOARDO BASSINI

It may seem excessive to dare to write nowadays about the radical cure of inguinal hernia after all that has been already printed about it in the past, and with fervent activity in the present.

This is how Edoardo Bassini began his epoch-making monograph of 106 pages, "*Nuovo metodo operativo per la cura radicale dell'ernia inguinale*" (3). Bassini knew in his heart and mind that he had found the key to the problem of hernia, and he was fully aware of the greatness of his new idea, which was not simply a short step forward but a true revolution in the surgery of hernia. His results confirmed the accuracy of his intuition.

Edoardo Bassini became convinced that the current operations of Wood and Czerny (which consisted of introflexing the hernia sac and loosely closing the external inguinal ring, relying on a single layer of scar tissue, which was further weakened by the passage of the cord) were inadequate to resist intraabdominal pressure, and that the patients would show signs of recurrence as soon as they abandoned the use of the truss. All of this indicated to Bassini the need for another operative method to achieve and secure the radical cure of inguinal hernia, thus eliminating the necessity of wearing a truss.

Bassini recognized that in large external oblique hernias, the inguinal canal became shorter and straight, losing its obliquity, and both the internal and external inguinal rings became dilated. In this manner, the physiologic shutter mechanism was completely lost. Bassini emphasized the need to restore the obliquity and length of the inguinal canal. This consists of physiologically reconstructing of the inguinal canal, so that it once again possesses two openings,

abdominal and subcutaneous, and two walls, anterior and posterior, through which the spermatic cord passes. This is so simple an idea that it is hard to believe that in the "fervent activity" of research about hernia, no one had this insight before Bassini.

On Christmas Eve, 1884, Bassini operated for the first time on an inguinal hernia using his new method. The operation consisted of high ligation and excision of the hernia sac. Bassini separated, from the external oblique aponeurosis above and from the subjacent properitoneal fat, the rectus muscle and the "*triple layer*" corresponding to the internal oblique muscle, transversus muscle, and "*fascia verticalis Cooperi*" (transversalis fascia), and sutured the "*triple layer*" to the shelving edge of Poupart's ligament with interrupted, tension-free silk sutures. The two lowermost sutures included the outer margin of the rectus muscle, so that obliquity and the length of the canal were restored and plasty of the posterior wall would resist intraabdominal pressure. In 1889, Bassini published his monograph on inguinal hernia. His results were striking. An extensive follow-up of more than 90% of his patients for a period up to $4\frac{1}{2}$ years revealed in a series of 262 patients an infection rate of only 4%, no mortality, and seven recurrences (2.6%). His postoperative care orders included early ambulation, shortened hospitalization, and, most importantly, no truss—the so-called "radical cure."

In 1890, Bassini's comprehensive work was translated verbatim by his pupil, Attilio Catterina, and published in the leading surgical journal of the time, *Archiv für Klinische Chirurgie* (4). Eduardo Bassini's new method for the radical cure of inguinal hernia was instantaneously known, immediately accepted, and widely adopted by the surgical world.

A BRIEF BIOGRAPHY OF EDOARDO BASSINI

Edoardo Bassini (Figs. 11.1 and 11.2) was born April 14, 1844, in Pavia, Italy. At age 22, he received his doctorate in

E. Nicolò: Department of Surgery, University of Pittsburgh Medical Center, McKeesport, Pennsylvania.

A. Guarnieri and **F. Guarnieri:** Department of Surgery, Clinica Guarnieri, Rome, Italy.

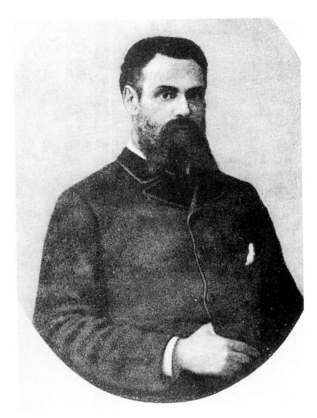

FIGURE 11.1. Edoardo Bassini (1884–1924).

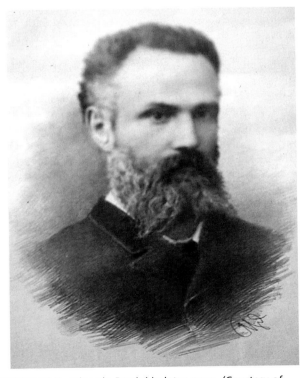

FIGURE 11.2. Edoardo Bassini in later years. (Courtesy of Francesco Battocchio, M.D.)

medicine. In 1866, Bassini participated in the movement of the liberation and unification of Italy.

Following the example of his uncle Angelo, colonel of the "Mille," Bassini enlisted in Garibaldi's army in Varese, at the rank of private, deliberately hiding his doctorate and participating in the campaign in Val Canonica on July 2, 1866, with courage and valor.

In September, after the famous "Obbedisco" by Garibaldi, armistice came first, then peace. Bassini returned to Pavia as a private citizen and volunteered at San Matteo Hospital, where he studied anatomy and pathology.

Rome was the only city left to be liberated. In 1867, Bassini joined a small army of 78 young intellectuals under the command of two brothers, Enrico and Giovanni Cairoli—his close friends—with the mission of going to Rome and helping the Roman people already in uprising, to finally liberate the city from the Pope, who was defended by the French troops.

"Bassini was in the first squadron of the III Section under the command of Giovanni Cairoli" (2). All of them were aware of the importance and gravity of the mission. The Supreme Commandant, Enrico Cairoli, just before leaving, instructed and encouraged them with such noble and great words that they responded with a frenetic "Hurrah!" On October 20, 1867, as night came, this handful of 78 courageous men began the march from Terni to the "Eternal City," Rome. When Enrico realized the disproportion to the number of the enemy, he ordered a bayonet attack in an impetus of heroism, and advanced crying, "Viva l'Italia, viva Garibaldi . . . ." ("Long live Italy, long live Garibaldi . . . ."). At once the Cairoli brothers, Bassini, and a few others climbed across the left side of the road. A series of duels followed, and Giovanni Cairoli was the first to fall, with a bullet wound to the head. As he fell, he saw Enrico surrounded by four or five enemy soldiers. A short time later, Enrico also fell, with bullet wounds to his head and lungs. Not far from them, Bassini and others also fell wounded. With Enrico lying dead in his arms, Giovanni Cairoli recalls, "I told my comrades, whom I could hear moaning around me, of the immense loss. Mantovani, Popassone, and Bassini answered with broken words of condolence. Bassini, expressing his deep sorrow after learning of the death of his commandant and friend, whispered these beautiful words to me: 'I am sorry that I'm not able to reach out and kiss him . . . .' How great a valor can be expressed in one moment!"

Later that night, Giovanni Cairoli, his head tangentially wounded, and Bassini, with a stab wound to the right lower quadrant of his abdomen, after many attempts were able to stand up and, arm by arm, help and hold each other, thereby reaching an old country house, where they found their companion, Moruzzi, wounded in the leg. Moruzzi begged them to help him, and Cairoli and Bassini did so as well as they could. Bassini lay down close to Moruzzi with just some sips of water that was brought to him by a peasant. The morning after the battle, Bassini was brought to the Villa Glori, where the body of Enrico was lying, and also found Mantovani and all the others who were wounded and who had been transported there from the battlefield after the enemy's retreat. Following the battle, they were left alone all that day without food or any help. Eight o'clock that evening, Bassini, Giovanni Cairoli, and Ferrari were transported to Santo Spirito Hospital in Rome; here, Bassini was visited by a banker, sent by his family to give him all the help he needed. Bassini had suffered a large stab wound, anteriorly and inferiorly to the anterosuperior iliac spine, penetrating the abdomen with a lesion to the cecum. After a few days in the hospital, Ferrari recalled, a military officer with a few soldiers came with an order to transfer Bassini, Cairoli, and Castagnini to jail. All attempts to explain to the officer that it was impossible to transfer Bassini were in vain, and he continued and insisted on carrying out the order. Finally, a doctor came and assessed the gravity of Bassini's wounds and took full responsibility for stopping the transfer. Indeed, Bassini's condition was critical for several days because of stercoraceous phlegmon and a localized septic peritonitis that externalized along the tract of the stab wound, resulting in a fecal fistula. Following a short stay at Castle Sant'Angelo, the three men were free to go back home. After several stops, Bassini arrived in his hometown of Pavia. There, he was followed very closely by Professor Luigi Porta, who immediately held him in great esteem. He continued to suffer from repeated episodes of partial bowel obstructions and reactivation of the inflammatory process. Finally, in 1868, the fistula closed, and the door of Bassini's surgical career was opening. We know enough now to enable us to understand the influences that molded his brilliant surgical career. His groin injury sparked an interest in the anatomy of this region, which ultimately determined the surgical destiny of Bassini. Following a few weeks of convalescence, Bassini began his surgical career. That same year, he became an assistant in the surgical clinic of Professor Luigi Porta. He visited Billroth in Vienna, Langenbeck in Berlin, and Lister in London. He then received teaching appointments in anatomy, pathology, and clinical surgery in Parma, La Spezia, and finally in Padova, where Bassini served as Chairman of the Department of Clinical Surgery for the next 35 years. It is worth mentioning that one morning when he learned that the victory was certain in the battle of Piave and Vittorio Veneto, Bassini was seen crying, and through his tears he said, "Now Italy is truly made, and I can die content and happy."

It is unknown what misunderstanding induced Bassini to remain in his teaching position for a few months after he reached 75 years of age, when "summa lex" (by law), he had to retire. One day, while he was walking back to his small locker room to change clothes after a long day in the operating room, Bassini found a telegram ordering him to leave his teaching position immediately and to give a full explanation of his delay in doing so. Bassini became pale for a

moment; then he took a deep breath and immediately ordered that his horse be prepared and brought outside the door of his clinic. So he left Padova, his clinic, and his works. This was November 1919.

In 1922, Bassini donated all of his assets to the Milan Institute of Hernia for the Poor (Istituto Milanese per gli erniosi poveri E. Bassini). Honored and admired by his students, colleagues, and the Italian government, Bassini died in 1924 at the age of 80 in Vigasio, Italy. We can conclude with the words of two of his pupils, Fasiani and Catterina. More than a century has passed, and ". . . the method of Bassini for the repair of inguinal hernia remains as the ultimate achievement that has withstood criticism, attempts on modification, and the daily appraisal and study repeated numerous times throughout the world" (6).

"Bassini unquestionably has the priority . . . . Prior to Bassini's publications, inguinal hernia had rarely been cured . . . . Indeed, I have not seen a single paper since Bassini's which contributed anything new . . . . The cure of inguinal hernia may be listed with the triumphs of surgery" (William Stuart Halsted) (13).

BASSINI'S DESCRIPTION OF HIS TECHNIQUE

In external (oblique) acquired inguinal hernias, I operate in the following manner: Understandably, I use the deep anesthesia, and strict antisepsis. I incise the skin over the inguinoscrotal hernia region; expose the aponeurosis of the external oblique over an area, which corresponds to the inguinal canal (aperture of the hernia), thus exposing the crura of the subcutaneous inguinal ring, and control bleeding. This is the first step in the operation.

In the second step, I divide the aponeurosis of the external oblique muscle from the external ring to the level of the internal inguinal ring, and mobilize the upper and lower flaps of the aponeurosis, isolate and elevate *in toto* the spermatic cord and the neck of the hernial sac. Keeping the index finger beneath these structures, I dissect the neck of the sac from the elements of the cord to the opening of the hernia. This dissection proceeds with little difficulty with the aid of blunt instruments, regardless of whether it is an acquired or congenital hernia. The isolation of the neck of the sac should extend to the iliac fossa, i.e., beyond the opening of the sac itself. Immediately afterward I dissect the body and fundus of the sac and draw it outwards, then open its fundus and inspect to see whether or not the viscera contained in the hernia show adhesions, and whether the omentum is thickened. If so, I separate the adhesions and remove the omentum as widely as is necessary. After reducing the contents I twist the sac (the neck), place a ligature proximal to it, and cut off the sac one half centimeter beyond it. If the hernia is very large, and the neck and mouth of the sac are broad, I use, in addition to the single ligature, two suture–ligatures placed distal to it, to assure

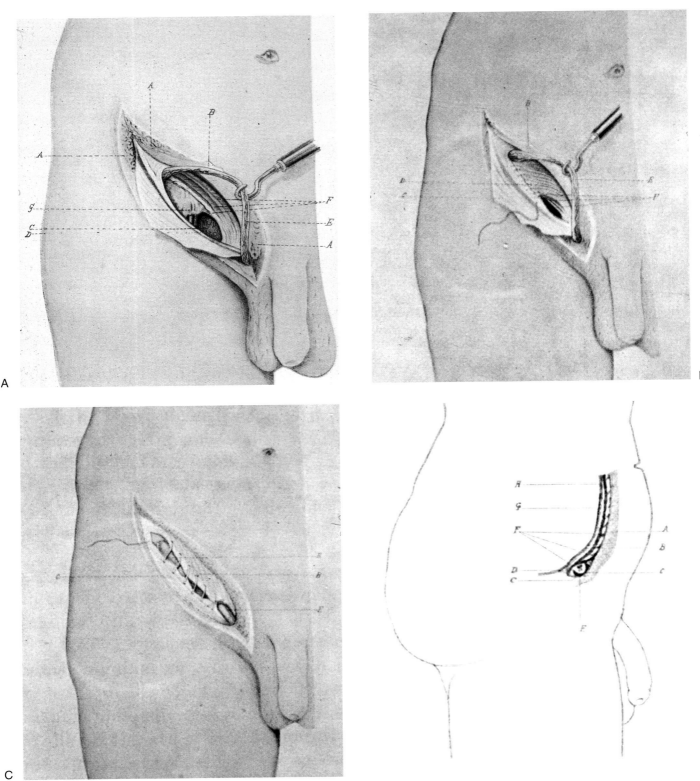

FIGURE 11.3. Bassini's operation. (From Bassini E. *Nuovo metodo operativo per la cura dell'ernia inguinale.* Padova: Prosperini, 1889, with permission.)

closure and prevent the slipping of the ligature. The peritoneum closed in this fashion becomes retracted into the iliac fossa. With the extirpation of the sac, and its ligation proximal to the opening, the second step of the operation is concluded.

In the third step, I elevate the cord onto the abdominal wall by gentle traction; and if necessary, do the same to the testicle, if it has been drawn out of the scrotum. With broad sharp retractors, I have an assistant pull the lower flap of the aponeurosis downward and the upper flap upwards, to expose the groove formed by the inguinal ligament and its posterior wall (shelf) to a level one centimeter above the point where the spermatic cord emerges from the iliac fossa. I then mobilize the outer edge of the rectus muscle and the triple layer, consisting of the internal oblique muscle, transversus abdominis muscle and the fascia verticalis of Cooper (transversalis fascia), from the external oblique aponeurosis and the peritoneal adipose tissue, until this united layer can be brought without difficulty to the shelf of Poupart's ligament. After this has been done, I sew these two parts together with interrupted sutures for a distance of 5 to 7 cm, from the pubic bone, laterally to the cord which has been pushed upwards approximately 1 cm toward the anterior superior iliac spine. This concludes the third step of the operation, and the interior or abdominal opening, and the posterior wall of the inguinal canal have been restored.

In connection with the above-mentioned suture, it is advisable to use interrupted silk and to grasp the triple layer 2 to 3 cm from its edge. The first two stitches placed on the pubis include also the lateral edge of the rectus muscle. If the patient is made to vomit after this phase of the operation has been concluded (I have tried this in the first 50 cases), one sees that the inguinal region is able to withstand the strongest intraabdominal pressure, and that the triple musculoaponeurotic layer which has been fixed to Poupart's ligament remains tightly stretched and immovable in its new position.

In the fourth step of the operation the spermatic cord is replaced and the testis also if necessary and the external oblique aponeurosis is reunited down to the pillars of the external ring. The skin is brought together, and finally a bandage is applied. I drain only in very voluminous old hernias in which the dissection and isolation of the sac is performed with difficulty (Fig. 11.3A–D). In this manner, the inguinal canal is reconstructed with an inner opening and a posterior wall, both formed by the union of the triple musculoaponeurotic layer to the shelving edge of Poupart's ligament, and with an anterior wall and narrowed external or subcutaneous opening formed by reuniting the flaps of the external oblique aponeurosis. In indirect hernias, especially when they have a considerable circumference, the inguinal canal loses its obliquity and becomes straight or almost straight. By the operation here described it regains its normal course; the spermatic cord, displaced slightly outwards passes obliquely through the abdominal wall where the

canal has been reconstituted. The deep suture lines are not superimposed on one another; the posterior remains below and the anterior above the spermatic cord.

AFTER BASSINI

Bassini's repair spread rapidly throughout Italy and, after its publication in German in 1890 (4), throughout the world. Many Italian and foreign authors, favorably impressed by the innovation, produced numerous variations, mostly detrimental, with a few exceptions. Some of the more interesting modifications were suggested by Italian authors who had, naturally, come into contact with the technique earlier than others.

Still in use and with a positive history behind it, it is opportune to recall the variation elaborated on by Postempski (17), an Italian surgeon at Rome's Santo Spirito Hospital, who in 1889 proposed reconstructing the posterior layer according to Bassini while suturing the external oblique aponeurosis behind the cord. As a result of this operation, the superficial inguinal ring is aligned with the deep ring. This variation seems to reduce the risk of recurrence involving the lower angle of the inguinal canal, one of the critical points in Bassini's repair.

Further variations, still applied, especially by pediatric surgeons, are the Mugnai (1891) and the Ferrari (1895) techniques. In both cases, the wall is repaired completely in front of the cord, which remains, therefore, in the preperitoneum, emerging at the pubic spine. Here, too, the superficial and deep rings are aligned below. The difference between Mugnai and Ferrari lies in the fact that the former sutured the wall on one layer only; the latter, on two: the posterior wall and external oblique aponeurosis.

It is to the Italian surgeon Margarucci that we owe the idea of superimposing the flaps of the external oblique aponeurosis (1901), who first reconstructed the back wall according to Bassini's technique. The lower external flap is sutured onto the internal oblique muscle. The upper internal flap is made to overlap it and the cord to pass between the two flaps.

It must be said that the most important variation on Bassini's repair was devised in Canada. This is the Shouldice (19) technique, developed in Toronto between 1945 and 1952, when a group of surgeons modified some steps of Bassini's technique: superimposing the flaps of the fascia transversalis, using six continuous sutures of steel thread, availing themselves of the proximal stump of the cremaster to strengthen the deep ring, and superimposing the flaps of the external oblique aponeurosis. This technique, which—when applied by experts—produces excellent results, obtained worldwide favor and is still generally used. Strangely enough, it spread to Italy only in the 1980s.

Among the Italian surgeons who, immediately after Bassini, made important contributions to the field, we must mention Ruggi, who in 1892 systematically sutured the inguinal ligament to Cooper's ligament through the inguinal approach. It should be pointed out, however, that this approach had already been used by Annandale in 1876 and by Zucherkandl in 1883, although in strangulated crural hernias only.

For years, Italian surgeons, most probably satisfied with Bassini's repair, did not feel the need to elaborate new ideas. Certainly up to the 1950s, Bassini's technique and its variations continued to dominate the Italian (perhaps even the worldwide) scene unrivaled. In the following years, however, techniques from other countries began to make their presence felt; among these, the first was that developed and divulged by the American McVay (15). This repair, used above all in crural hernias, became popular in Italy and is still applied today.

In the 1960s, despite considerable initial misgivings, techniques using biocompatible meshes were introduced and slowly but surely accepted. These techniques, though developed in the United States (14,23), were first introduced into Italy by the French (18).

During the second half of the 1980s and the 1990s, Italy witnessed an amazing spread of prosthetic methodologies devised by American (Lichtenstein, Gilbert, Robbins, and Rutkow) and French (Rives, Stoppa) surgeons, of laparoscopic techniques, and, above all, of the Italian surgeon Trabucco's mesh-plug technique.

Only over the past few years, after a long silence, have the Italian authors made a comeback on the international scene of hernial surgery. For example, Ermanno Trabucco has been a long-standing and well-known figure.

The Italian surgeon Trabucco, although he has practiced prevalently in the United States, is credited with pioneering, in January 1977, outpatient hernia surgery, a solution today considered routine but at the time of its introduction extremely daring. Outpatient surgery introduced the need for techniques that reduce surgical trauma to a minimum. Trabucco has devised an original autostatic retractor that permits the surgeon to operate without assistance, and he has also developed the "*mesh-plug*" technique (20–22), where the use of sutures is reduced to a minimum and is totally *tension free*. Furthermore, the simplicity of the methodology is such that even less expert surgeons may obtain good results. The Trabucco repair is described in detail in Chapter 15.

In December 1988, a time when prosthetic surgery was taking hold, the author (A.G.) proposed an inguinal hernia repair called *physiologic hernioplasty*, in contrast to the general trend. This technique, the chief aim of which was reducing prosthetic use to a minimum, is based on reconstructing the chief physiologic defense mechanisms of the inguinal region (sphincter and shutter mechanisms), which are usually compromised in hernia patients. Assuming a position decidedly remote from classic conceptions, we consider anatomic reconstruction negatively; in fact, we maintain that it is fundamental that the anatomic structure undergo modifications aimed at eliminating discrepancies *between anatomy and function* that cause hernias. We have also developed two interesting prosthetic techniques: the "*locked-plug*" technique for the repair of small defect hernias (femoral, umbilical, etc.) and the "*sandwich*" technique for large incisional hernias. The former is extremely simple to perform, while the latter prevents the prosthesis from coming into direct contact with the intestine and subcutaneous fatty tissue.

GUARNIERI'S PHYSIOLOGIC HERNIOPLASTY

Of the many surgical hernia repair methods, techniques aimed at reconstructing the "anatomy" and, more recently, tension-free repairs using biocompatible materials to replace tissue defects, have been established.

The physiologic hernioplasty technique came to light in 1988 thanks to the idea of *adapting the anatomic structure to functional necessity*, considering the inguinal region as a system subject to the physical laws of elastic containers (7–10).

Technique

The operation is normally carried out using local anesthesia. The approach is inguinal.

Preliminary Steps

The stages that precede isolation of the sac do not differ from those applied in other inguinal-approach methods. Two important steps are (a) opening the cribriform fascia to detect possible presence of crural hernias, and (b) ample separation of the external oblique aponeurosis from the rectus sheath.

In *indirect hernias,* the sac is completely isolated beyond the neck; it is not opened but simply abandoned in the preperitoneum without introflexion or suture.

In *direct hernias,* the anatomic layer that covers the hernial sac (fascia transversalis–transversus muscle aponeurosis) is excised. Then the fascia transversalis is incised up to the deep ring, so as to open the posterior wall of the inguinal canal completely. The hernial sac is abandoned in the preperitoneum.

Reconstruction of the Deep Layer

The reconstruction of the deep layer differs depending on whether the hernia is indirect with a medium-to-small defect, indirect with a large defect, or direct.

Indirect Medium-to-Small–Defect Hernias
The cord elements (testicular vessels and deferent duct) are isolated completely from the cremaster–internal spermatic

fascia proximal tract, which is not sectioned but retracted laterally.

The transversalis fascia–transversus muscle aponeurosis is held by two hemostatic curved forceps at the deep ring medial margin level, and isolated medially for a few centimeters from the preperitoneal fat below and the internal oblique muscle above.

The latter is then retracted medially. The more caudal of the hemostatic forceps is removed, passed below the cord elements, and then reinserted at the same point (Fig. 11.4A). Between the two forceps, a direct medial and cranial incision of about 2 cm is made on the transversalis fascia–transversus muscle aponeurosis, beginning with the deep ring.

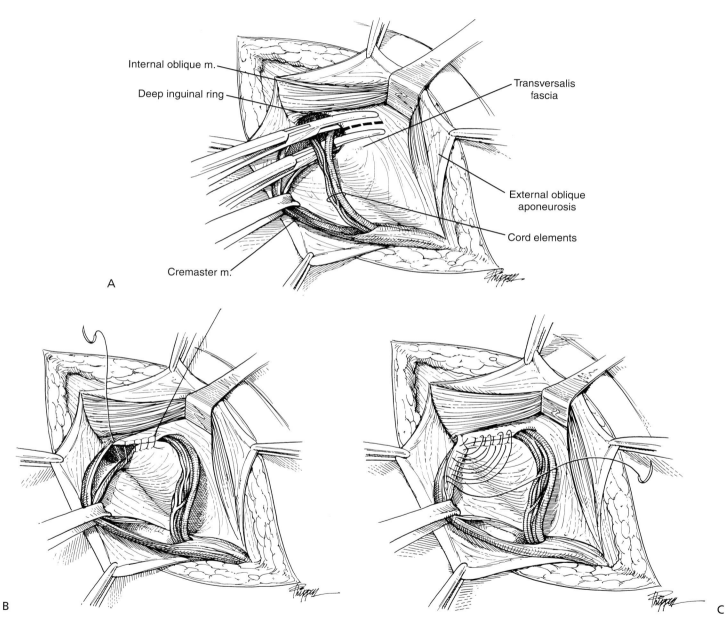

FIGURE 11.4. A: The right inguinal region (head above). The cord elements have been completely detached from the proximal tract of the cremaster, which is retracted laterally. The internal oblique muscle is retracted medially. At the deep ring, level two forceps, of which the lower passes beneath the cord elements, have been applied. On this plane, a medially directed incision of about 2 cm in width has been made. **B:** The cord elements have been moved to the medial corner of the incision. A continuous suture creates a calibrated neoring and closes the deep ring completely. **C:** The same suture "on the way back" takes in a short tract of the cremaster, which thus strengthens and protects the incision below.

The cord elements are positioned at the medial corner of the incision.

A continuous "forward-and-back" suture begins close to the cord elements, creating a new ring calibrated to fit around them, then, proceeding laterally, it reaches the deep ring, closing it completely (Fig. 11.4B). The same line of suture, on its "way back," takes in and joins to itself a brief tract of the cremaster (Fig. 11.4C).

Indirect Large-Defect or Direct Hernias.

Reconstruction of the inguinal canal's posterior wall is achieved by suturing the superimposed flaps of the transversalis fascia–transversus muscle aponeurosis layer *along the tract between the pubis and the inferior epigastric vessels only.* This transforms a large-defect hernia into a small-defect indirect one. The procedure, as described above, for indirect hernias is then performed.

Reconstruction of the Superficial Layers

Reconstruction of the superficial layers is the same in all types of hernia. While the cord is held aside, the inferolateral flap of the external oblique aponeurosis is freed completely of the fibrous tissues that restrain it on the outer side, and is sutured to the rectus sheath along the tract between the lower margin of the internal oblique muscle's intersection and the pubis (Fig. 11.5A).

Allowing a sufficiently large space for the exit of the cord, such as to create a new superficial ring, a second suture between the external oblique aponeurosis's inferolateral flap and the rectus sheath is performed (Fig. 11.5B).

Finally, the superomedial flap of the external oblique aponeurosis, previously detached from the rectus sheath, is overlapped and sutured onto the inferolateral flap both above and below the cord (Fig. 11.5C). This overlap is normally ample and practically tension free.

Use of Prostheses

If the tissues are very weak, a mesh containing an eyelet for the passage of the cord elements may be placed in the preperitoneum or, alternatively, in front of the transversus muscle aponeurosis. In the latter case, the long, narrow (2 × 6–cm) mesh is positioned along the posterior wall of the inguinal canal after the deep ring is closed but before the cremaster is superimposed. The superimposition of the cremaster will hold the mesh in place. During preparation of the mesh, a transverse incision is made in it at the deep ring level to allow for the passage of the cord elements.

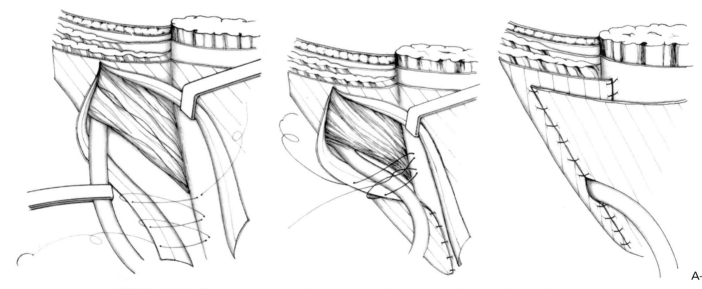

A–C

FIGURE 11.5. A: Note the lower margin of the internal oblique muscle's insertion "high" on the rectus sheath (one must not take into consideration the lower muscle fibers, which correspond more to the cremaster than to the internal oblique muscle and which are absolutely inefficient). The area devoid of muscular protection appears evident (inguinal triangle). A suture joins the inferolateral flap of the external oblique aponeurosis to the rectus sheath from the insertion of the internal oblique muscle's lower margin to the pubis. **B:** The new inguinal canal borders along the entire length of the edge of the internal oblique muscle. Having left sufficient space for the exit of the cord, a second suture between the inferolateral flap of the external oblique aponeurosis and the rectus sheath creates a superficial neoring and narrows the inguinal canal. **C:** The medial flap of the external oblique aponeurosis overlaps the lateral flap abundantly above and below the cord. Thus, a synergy between the two flaps is obtained.

The mesh serves a purely precautionary function; the reconstruction is carried out in the usual way.

During the first year, we used mesh in 49% of all cases. This was due to prudence because we were as yet uncertain of the validity of the technique, which was at the time absolutely new. As results demonstrated the trustworthiness of the surgical method, we began to reduce the use of meshes drastically. Since 1991, they have been applied, on average, in about 8% of all cases. The decision regarding whether to use mesh is made during the operation, after assessment of the condition of the tissues.

Patients and Results

Between December 1988 and June 1999, this technique was applied to 2,051 patients suffering from primary inguinal hernia. In 74% of the cases, the operation was performed using local anesthesia.

In December 1988, we began a follow-up program in which patients were scheduled for examination at 7 days, 1 month, and 1 year postoperatively, and then annually. The average percentage of patients thus controlled was 95% after 1 year, 86% after 2 years, and 55% after 10 years.

The postsurgical complications that occurred were subcutaneous seroma (6%), hematoma (0.4%), transitory testicular edema (1%), wound infection (0.4%), and testicular atrophy (0.1%). There were 14 cases of recurrence (0.6%). There were no recurrences in cases where mesh was used.

It is important to note that these results include patients who were operated on during improvement of the technique and patients of a relatively inexperienced surgeon who began applying this technique only 4 years ago, as of this writing.

Rationale

The operative stages that characterize this method are:

- *The elimination of the deep ring* and creation of a *neoorifice.*
- *The narrowing* and *shortening* of the inguinal canal to fit the internal oblique muscle.
- *The use of the external oblique aponeurosis* for autoplasty.
- *The preservation* of the cremaster.

The Elimination of the Deep Ring and Creation of a Neoorifice

In most hernia patients, the deep ring is surrounded by weak tissue unable to resist suture strain. Its reconstruction is almost always unreliable. For this reason, nearly all herniorrhaphy techniques seek to reinforce the deep ring, anchoring it to the inguinal ligament, thus immobilizing, stiffening, and defunctionalizing it. The weakness of the tissue, associated with defunctionalization and approximate

suture, is among the most frequent causes of recurrence. These considerations led to the idea of creating a new deep ring, easily calibrated around the cord elements and situated in a much stronger area. When the transversus muscle contracts, the neoring, *solely because collocated between the fibers of the aponeurotic arch,* is *tightened* by them *and drawn in a superolateral direction.* The medial collocation of the ring enhances the internal oblique muscle's protective action.

Even if the *sling effect* cannot occur, the *sphincter effect* is restored.

The Narrowing and Shortening of the Inguinal Canal

The shutter mechanism is obtained only if the inguinal canal is *narrow* and bordered on *along its entire length* by the internal oblique muscle. In hernia patients, the internal oblique muscle is nearly always hypotrophic and reaches the rectus sheath high relative to the pubic spine; the lower fibers actually belong to the cremaster and are totally inefficient. The lower area of the inguinal canal's posterior wall, known as the *inguinal triangle* (not to be confused with Hesselbach's triangle), remains *completely devoid of the protection of the muscle* both at rest and under exertion (Fig. 11.5A). The first suture of the external oblique aponeurosis onto the rectus sheath obtains the double effect of *reinforcing the depleted area and excluding it from the inguinal canal.* As a result, the inguinal canal grows *shorter* and narrower and thus more functional because it is *completely bordered by the oblique internal muscle.* The shutter mechanism is thus restored, also because the internal oblique muscle is not affected by stitching capable of limiting its movement.

The Use of the External Oblique Aponeurosis for Autoplasty

The external oblique aponeurosis is elastic along the fibers' transverse axis; additionally, the lateral aponeurotic flap easily reaches the rectus sheath, producing a moderate amount of tension. This flap enters into direct contact with the area devoid of muscular protection and soon forms an ample *scar layer* with it. The resulting overlap of the medial flap further distributes the already-moderate pull of the sutures and compensates for the poor resistance of this layer to transverse tension. Between these two layers, *a second scar layer* forms. The anatomic layers, joined by the two scar planes, become extraordinarily solid, as in prosthetic surgery.

The Preservation of the Cremaster

The cremaster–internal spermatic fascia's proximal portion, superimposed on the suture of the fascia transversalis between the deep ring and the neoorifice, in addition to strengthening the suture, guarantees the total closure of the deep ring and blockage of small lacerations, which might occur (even though never encountered by us) due to the passage of the suture along the underlying fascia transversalis. Below this point, the cremaster remains intact; therefore, besides maintaining its normal functions, the cremaster protects the testicular vessels from the risk of iatrogenic lesions in cases where recurrence makes further operations necessary, and guarantees a better collateral vascular bed, which is invaluable in cases of testicular vessel lesions.

Discussion

The chief criticisms drawn by this technique are:

1. Suture tension
2. Weakening of the posterior layer due to the incision carried out to medialize the deep ring
3. The technical difficulty

As far as the first item is concerned, we believe that the tension-free idea has been and continues to be overrated. One must, above all, note that the absence of suture tension *at rest* does not prevent the reestablishment of normal tension due to abdominal wall tone in the erect position or under exertion. Furthermore, *the ample noncontractile surfaces* left in the abdominal wall in the name of tension-free techniques, even if reinforced by mesh, *are considerably solicited by endoabdominal pressure.*

The contraction of the abdominal muscles, in fact, increases endoabdominal pressure while simultaneously reducing bend radius of the wall. The reduction of the bend radius lessens the strain on the wall, which is provoked by the increase of pressure. (According to *Laplace's Law*, the strain is proportional to the bend radius). On the contrary, the *noncontractile areas* subjected to abdominal pressure *are thrust outward* (with subsequent increase of the bend radius) *and do not reduce their surface.* Therefore, the strain, which is proportional to *the surface and to the bend radius, increases exponentially in relation to the increase in the surface.* It is no chance that in normal conditions the noncontractile areas of the abdominal wall are few and subtle (e.g., *linea alba*).

We believe that a *moderate tension* that does not produce ischemia and *reduces noncontractile areas* is the best possible choice. In fact, in this technique, the sutures undergo moderate tension; otherwise, they would cause laceration of the external oblique aponeurosis, which is very delicate along the fibers' transverse axis. Furthermore, the sutures take in small quantities of tissue and do not produce ischemia as they invest only the fasciae that are avascular. Besides, the suture lines are nonaligned and do not pass through the wall in all its depth, and therefore they do not favor the formation of new hernial defects.

As far as fear of *weakening of the posterior wall* is concerned, it must be pointed out that the strength of this part of the inguinal canal has been and continues to be over-

rated. The back wall is not strong. This can be plainly seen during operations. Its resistance to endoabdominal pressure in normal conditions is due to its *being narrow* and to the noteworthy support it receives from the anatomic layers above, in particular, the action of the internal oblique muscle. In our opinion, the posterior wall is meant fundamentally to "seal."

The incision we perform on the transversalis fascia–transversus muscle aponeurosis (an anatomic plane that is subtle and weak because of scarce pressure) is reinforced by the cremaster and covered by the internal oblique muscle: if anything, the area is made stronger. The weakest point remains the original site of the deep ring. It is in this area, in fact, that we have come across recurrences in patients we have operated on a second time. On the other hand, the low incidence of recurrence among our patients demonstrates that this "weakening" represents more of a fear than a concrete reality.

As far as this repair's *procedural difficulty* is concerned, we believe that the operation is more difficult to grasp than to perform. We perform it, on average, in about half an hour. Certainly, this operation is not for mediocre surgeons (in whose hands any technique will lead to poor results) because it requires a sound knowledge of anatomy, at least; however, each phase of the procedure is extremely clear, thus reducing the possibility of errors caused by the snares of hernia surgery.

THE LOCKED-PLUG TECHNIQUE

This technique suits a variety of hernia types: femoral, umbilical, direct recurrent, epigastric, small incisional, etc. It is important that the defect be small, its diameter equal to or less than about 2 cm (10).

Technique

The preliminary phases contemplate the resection or abandonment of the hernial sac after it has been properly isolated beyond the neck. In femoral hernias, the approach is anterosubinguinal.

A small square of polypropylene mesh, measuring about 4 × 4 cm in the case of larger defects, is cut. If the defect is small, the square may be as little as 1.5 × 1.5 cm. A thread of monofilament polypropylene is knotted to the center of the square; a loose end of roughly 10 cm is left, and the thread is not cut (Fig. 11.6).

The square is then folded twice along its orthogonal lines (Fig. 11.6), so that the thread remains on the inside. A further diagonal fold produces a roughly conical shape.

Using a curved hemostatic forceps, the "cone" is placed inside the hernial defect. When the forceps is removed, the cone tends to expand spontaneously. The mesh is unfolded with the help of the same forceps introduced into the defect, while the thread is pulled slightly.

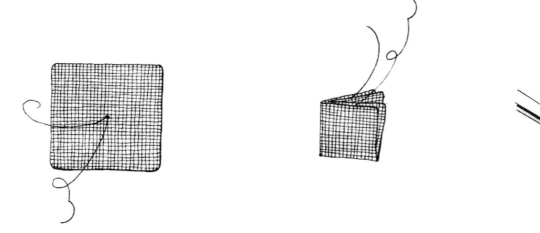

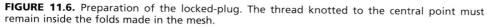

FIGURE 11.6. Preparation of the locked-plug. The thread knotted to the central point must remain inside the folds made in the mesh.

If the defect is very small, it is possible to use a mesh that exceeds the defect slightly and introduce it "unfolded" using the forceps, ensuring that the thread faces outward.

This thread is used to suture the edge of the hernial defect. Generally speaking, two stitches are sufficient (Fig. 11.7).

A traction on the thread attached to the needle, while the end beyond the knot is left slack, tightens the hernial defect and fixes the mesh onto it.

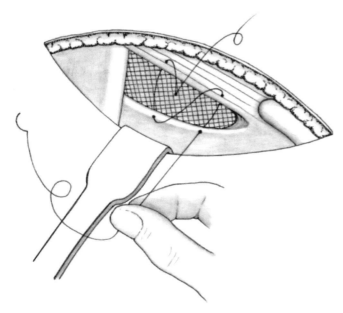

FIGURE 11.7. The locked-plug repair of a right femoral hernia using a subinguinal approach. Once the mesh has been inserted and unfolded within the hernial canal, the thread knotted to the mesh is passed twice between the inguinal ligament and the pectineal fascia. A traction on the needle end of the thread contemporaneously narrows the hernial defect and fixes the mesh onto it.

The two ends of the thread are then tied together.

As far as femoral hernias are concerned, it is not necessary to include Cooper's ligament and the iliopubic tract, which are difficult to reach through a small defect. It suffices to suture the inguinal ligament to the pectineal fascia; these two areas are easily brought together. It is not necessary that the suture approach the femoral vein.

Patients and Results

Between October 1989 and August 1999, we used this technique in 218 cases: 99 femoral, 50 recurrent direct, 30 umbilical, 22 incisional, seven spigelian, and 10 epigastric hernias. About 78% of the patients were examined 2 years after the operation. There was only one recurrence (0.4%) in the case of an umbilical hernia with considerable diastasis of the rectus muscles.

Discussion

It is not true that small-defect hernias never recur. Crural hernias recur frequently when treated using traditional herniorrhaphy (5). Umbilical hernias, too, have a certain tendency to recur because the defect is often surrounded by very subtle tissue that frays along the suture stitches, creating new defects.

This operation, in keeping with the *"moderate tension of sutures and narrowing of the noncontractile areas"* thesis, aims at creating synergy between two methodologies: direct suture and mesh. In fact, the hernial defect is simply narrowed (with very slight tension) but not necessarily "sealed" by the suture; the mesh acts as a "sealing" agent, even as far as the holes produced by the suture stitching are concerned.

The fact that the mesh is blocked along the suture and the defect is narrowed permits the use of a small mesh, without any risk of detachment or dislodgment.

THE SANDWICH TECHNIQUE IN INCISIONAL HERNIAS

This method, first published in 1988 (11,12), is particularly suited to cases of large incisional hernia and when defects have stiffened due to fibrosis of the wall. It may, however, be used in all incisional hernias by those who prefer to use mesh on principle.

Incisions

Cutaneous–subcutaneous excision by means of two incisions on scar-free tissue externally to the neck of the sac is generally preferable. This guarantees that the scar area that surrounds the sac is bypassed and that the fascial layer is reached. One then proceeds in the direction of the defect and sac.

Treatment of the Sac

In incisional hernias, the sac is a continuation of the aponeurotic muscle plane, from which it may not easily be separated. The sac must not be *transected*; on the contrary,

it must be isolated up to the neck and then divided longitudinally into two halves, along a plane perpendicular to the wall (Fig. 11.8). The contents of the sac are pushed back into the abdomen. It is indispensable to remove all adhesions from an ample tract of the parietal peritoneum surrounding the hernial defect.

The Sandwich Repair

The longitudinal division of the sac creates two flaps (Fig. 11.8). The free margin of the flap on the surgeon's side is brought within the hernial defect and sutured to the parietal peritoneum along the entire hemicircumference facing the insertion and at the greatest possible distance from the defect (Fig. 11.9A). Alternatively, the flap of the sac may be sutured onto the fascial–muscular layer if an incision is first made along the suture line on the parietal peritoneum. This suture of absorbable synthetic thread, because it follows the entire free margin of the sac, begins and ends at the edge of the hernial defect. The thread must not be cut because later it will be used again to suture the other flap of the sac on the outer side.

A polypropylene mesh is cut so that its shape resembles the outline of the defect, but its diameters should exceed it

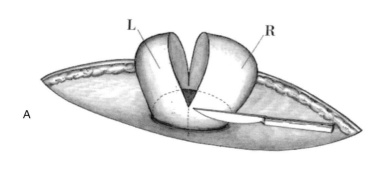

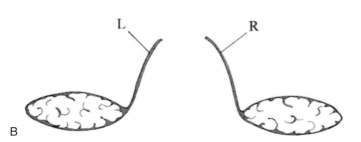

FIGURE 11.8. A: In the sandwich technique, the hernial sac, totally isolated, is divided into two halves (*L–R*) with an incision perpendicular to the abdominal wall. **B:** The scheme shows a cross section of the rectus muscles and the flaps of the hernial sac. The "*L*" flap is on the surgeon's side of the operating table.

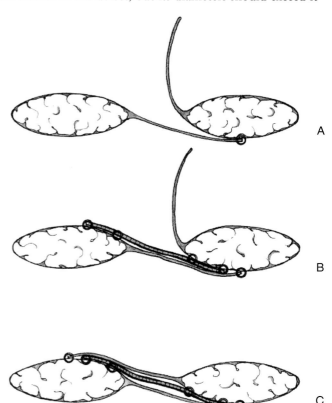

FIGURE 11.9. Views of the various phases of the sandwich repair. **A:** endoabdominal suture of the first flap of the sac. **B:** Positioning of the mesh and the fixing sutures. **C:** Suture of the other flap of the sac to the muscular fascia. The surgeon stands to the left side of the patient.

by 4 cm or more. The mesh must be positioned half within and half outside the defect. The hemicircumference of the mesh on the side opposite the surgeon is fixed to the parietal peritoneum using continuous nonabsorbable suture, concentric to the previous circle. The remaining hemicircumference is sutured to the premuscular fascial layer (and therefore external to the hernial defect) (Fig. 11.9B).

A further circle of continuous suture, using nonabsorbable thread, joins the mesh to the edge of the hernial defect (Fig. 11.9B).

The second flap of the hernial sac (on the side opposite the surgeon) is pulled over the mesh, covering it completely (Fig. 11.9C). Its edge is sutured to the fascial layer using the absorbable thread purposely left over after suturing the other flap.

Patients and Results

From December 1988 to August 1999, out of a total of the 118 incisional hernias treated by us, this technique was applied in 39 cases. The postsurgery complications that arose were 9 cases of seroma (23%), 1 hematoma (3%), and 1 wound infection (3%).

Follow-up examinations were carried out after a year (average of 93%), 2 years (average of 70%), and 10 years (average of 50%). There were four cases of recurrence (10%).

Discussion

In incisional hernias where prostheses are indispensable, depending on the level at which the mesh is collocated, the prosthesis may come into contact with the intestine or subcutaneous tissue, creating the risk of complications such as enteric fistulae and infection (1,16,24). The sandwich technique isolates the prosthesis from the intestine and subcutaneous tissue by using the flaps of the hernial sac as insulation.

The number of operations carried out using this technique is not particularly high because, as far as possible, in the presence of incisional hernias we usually prefer to shut the hernial defect completely, following the principle of the reduction of noncontractile surfaces, compatible with moderate suture tension.

As far as the rather high recurrence rate is concerned, one must take into account the fact that patients who undergo this type of procedure present, on average, a rather challenging condition due to obesity, large hernial defects, the particular weakness of their tissue, or fibrosis of the abdominal wall.

REFERENCES

1. Amid PK. Classification of biomaterials and their related complications in abdominal wall hernia surgery. *Hernia* 1997;1: 15–21.

2. Austoni A. *La vita e le opere di Edoardo Bassini*. Bologna: Cappelli Editore, 1922.

3. Bassini E. *Nuovo metodo operativo per la cura dell'ernia inguinale*. Padova: Stabilimento Prosperini, 1889.

4. Bassini E. Über de Behandlung des Leistenbruches. *Arch F Klin Chir* 1890;40:429–476.

5. Bendavid R. A femoral umbrella for femoral hernia repair. *Surg Gynecol Obstet* 1987;165:153–156.

6. Fasiani GM, Catterina A. *Scritti di chirurgia erniaria*. Padova: Tipografia del Seminario, 1937.

7. Guarnieri A, Moscatelli F, Guarnieri F, et al. A new technique for indirect inguinal hernia repair. *Am J Surg* 1992;164:70–73.

8. Guarnieri A, Guarnieri F, Moscatelli F. The functional repair of inguinal hernia. *Hernia* 1997;1:117–121.

9. Guarnieri A. Procédé original de plastie "fonctionnelle" des hernies inguinales primaires. *Chirurgie* 1997;122:534–538.

10. Guarnieri A. *La nuova chirurgia dell'ernia*. Milano: Masson, 1995.

11. Guarnieri A, Di Rosa P, Moscatelli F. Cura dei laparoceli con protesi: la nostra tecnica. *90º Congresso Soc It Chirurgia, 1988*. Comunicazioni vol 1: 199–202.

12. Guarnieri A, Guarnieri AE, Moscatelli F, et al. Una nuova tecnica chirurgica per la riparazione con mesh del laparocele. *Minerva Chir* 1994;49:967–970.

13. Halsted WS. An additional note on the operation of inguinal hernia. *Surgical papers by William Stewart Halsted*, vol 1. Baltimore: The Johns Hopkins Press, 1924:306–308.

14. Mahorner H, Goss GM. Herniation following destruction of Poupart's and Cooper's ligaments: a method of repair. *Ann Surg* 1962;155:741–747.

15. McVay CB. Inguinal and femoral hernioplasty: anatomic repair. *Arch Surg* 1948;57:524–530.

16. Molloy RG, Moran KT, Waldron RP, et al. Massive incisional hernia: abdominal wall replacement with Marlex mesh. *Br J Surg* 1991;78:242–244.

17. Postempski P. *Modificazioni alla cura radicale Bassini*. Rome: Bollettino Società Lancisiana, 1889.

18. Rives J, Nicaise H, Lardennois B. A propos du traitement chirurgical des hernies de l'aine. Orientation nouvelle et perspectives thérapeutiques. *Ann Med Reims* 1965;2:193–200.

19. Shouldice EE. The treatment of hernia. *Ontario Med Rev* 1953;20:670–684.

20. Trabucco E. The office hernioplasty and the Trabucco repair. *Ann It Chir* 1993;64:127–149.

21. Trabucco E, Trabucco A, Rollino R, et al. L'ernioplastica inguinale tension-free con rete presagomata senza suture secondo Trabucco. *Chirurgia* 1998;11:1–7.

22. Trabucco EE, Trabucco AF. Flat plug and mesh hernioplasty in the "inguinal box": description of the surgical technique. *Hernia* 1998;2:133–138.

23. Usher FC, Hill JR, Ochsner JL. Hernia repair with Marlex mesh. A comparison of techniques. *Surgery* 1959;46:718–724.

24. Wantz GE. Prosthetics: their complication and management. In: Bendavid R, ed. *Prostheses and abdominal wall hernias*. Austin: RG Landes Co, 1994:326–329.

EDITOR'S COMMENT

One might argue that Dr. Guarnieri's technique is merely a modification or perhaps a combination of some of the other classic operations. It is for this reason that the editors felt that the description should be incorporated into a larger work. What better than to ask these authors to provide a perspec-

tive on the contribution of Italian surgeons to the science of herniology? They have certainly delivered the goods with their detailed description of Bassini and others. This chapter contains many nuances of the lives of these important Italian surgeons that were heretofore unknown to me. Obviously, *there are other countries that have produced surgeons who have made tremendous contributions to the field. However, since Bassini and his protégés were so important in introducing the modern inguinal herniorrhaphy, we felt that this chapter was justified.*

R.J.F., Jr.
A.G.G.

12

THE SHOULDICE REPAIR

ROBERT BENDAVID

The study of hernias never ceases to present a myriad of challenges. Knowledge of the anatomy (no mean task) must be succinct. The mechanics of the muscles, ligaments, and sling (the shutter of Keith) require a logical aptitude. The formation and evolution of hernias, which imply the presence of aberrant tissue physiology, must impose a preemptive attitude in the choice of treatment. Eminent authors of the past have considered it a worthy intellectual and academic endeavor to devote their lives to understanding the many facets that hernias present. Some of these authors have left an indelible mark: Astley Cooper (1768–1841), Henry Marcy (1837–1924), Edoardo Bassini (1844–1924), Chester B. McVay (1911–87). Edward Earle Shouldice (1890–1965) belongs in this pantheon. His unique fascination with the treatment of abdominal wall hernias in the 1930s culminated in 1945 in the establishment of a hospital where more than 300,000 operations have been performed to date, providing a wealth of anatomic, clinical, and statistical observations.

HISTORIC SYNOPSIS

An interesting parallel often has been pointed out between the Shouldice and Bassini repairs. Wantz refers to the procedure as the Bassini–Shouldice repair. In 1887, Bassini presented a personal series of 42 patients at the Fourth Assembly of Italian Surgeons in Genoa. His textbook was published in 1889 and remained essentially unknown. It was Bassini's pupil, Attilio Catterina, who authored a superb monograph that appeared in Berlin (1933), Paris (1934), London (1934), and Madrid (1935). For some reason, publication in North America never took place. In the late 1930s, E.E. Shouldice's interest in hernias resulted in the presentation of 272 cases at the annual meeting of the Ontario Medical Association (September 1944). Modifications to his original repair were introduced by his colleague E.A. Ryan and, by 1952, the operation had taken on the

final character that we know today. Although similarities exist between the two procedures, so do differences, and these are appreciated best by gleaning from the improved results of many authors.

Certain steps in the operation, which are considered crucial, have been associated with eminent contributors to the field of hernia surgery. These steps are (a) resection of the cremaster (Bassini, Shouldice); (b) ligation of the indirect hernial sac (Lucas-Championniere, Marcy, Bassini, Shouldice); (c) incision of the entire posterior wall of the inguinal canal (Marcy, Bassini, Shouldice); (d) reconstruction of the inguinal floor (Marcy, Bassini, Halsted, Shouldice, Condon); and (e) incorporation of the iliopubic tract of Thomson in the reconstruction of the posterior inguinal floor (Bassini, Condon, Shouldice).

GENERAL PRINCIPLES

The Shouldice operation involves the use of local anesthesia, as well as a 48- to 72-hour period of convalescence in the hospital, which is described more accurately as a period of active rehabilitation during which patients ambulate early and perform exercises as a group. Because 7,500 operations are carried out yearly at the Shouldice Hospital by full-time surgeons, extensive experience has been acquired that translates into well-founded principles and practices. These have been corroborated and confirmed by others, and merit discussion here.

Weight Control

Controversy surrounding the ideal weight of a patient has polarized surgeons. Whereas obesity is agreed on as a major factor in the recurrence of incisional hernias, the same cannot be said of groin hernias. If anything, the overweight patient seems to have a protective mechanism, as can be seen in the follow-up studies of Abrahamson, Abramson, Thomas and Barnes, DeWilt, and Wantz. Disagreement has been expressed by Pietri, Sitzman, Stoppa, Weinstein, and Zimmerman. There is no doubt, however, that surgery on a

R. Bendavid: Elisha Hospital, Mount Carmel, Haifa, Israel.

thin patient is easier, a lesser volume of local anesthesia is required, a smaller incision is needed, and ambulation takes place sooner.

Local Anesthesia

In 1900, the use of local anesthesia already had been reported by Cushing, Halsted, and Bloodgood during 200 operations, 49 of which were herniorrhaphies. The reasons, now as then, include safety in elderly patients and those whose cardiac, pulmonary, and renal function is compromised. By its nature, local anesthesia also implies a benign procedure to patients who fear general anesthesia. An added advantage is that the patient retains the ability to cooperate during surgery and can strain on request to reveal secondary hernias and allow the surgeon to assess the quality of the tissues and the repair. Table 12.1 presents the age distribution of patients undergoing the Shouldice operation.

Early Ambulation

Early resumption of normal activities is not associated with an increased incidence of hernia recurrence. This was noted initially by Herzfeld in 1938 and subsequently confirmed by Blodgett, Ryan, Iles, Palumbo, and Kingsworth. The most comforting aspect of early ambulation was the disappearance of deep-vein thrombophlebitis and pulmonary complications in the postoperative period.

Ligation of the Hernial Sac

Ligation of the hernial sac has been well established for indirect sacs, but not for direct ones. Resection of an indirect sac is not an absolute necessity, as demonstrated by Glassow, Lichtenstein, and Welsh. It is essential, however, that the indirect sac be freed from the cord and the surrounding tissue layers deep to the internal ring (transversus aponeurosis, transversalis fascia, and posterior lamina) so that it disappears into the preperitoneal space of Bogros.

Incision of the Transversalis Fascia

Incision of the transversalis fascia is of paramount importance and was emphasized by Marcy, Bassini, and Shouldice. It allows exploration and detection of femoral,

interstitial, prevesical, and smaller direct inguinal hernias. This maneuver also exposes the myoaponeurotic layers needed for an adequate repair. Incision of the transversalis fascia is not as crucial in women. In a review of 27,870 external abdominal wall hernias, Glassow reported the use of this incision in 0.2% of cases. Still, the lateral third of the floor should be incised to allow examination of the femoral ring and assessment of the integrity of the posterior wall.

Reconstruction of the Internal Ring

Reconstruction of the internal ring was the mainstay of the Marcy repair and, combined with reconstruction of the entire posterior wall, it formed the basis of the Bassini, Condon, and Shouldice repairs. Marcy used only the transversalis fascia, but this tissue is relatively weak. Therefore, the transversus myoaponeurotic arch subsequently was included for reconstruction of the posterior inguinal wall.

Sliding Hernias

The various operations described for the treatment of sliding inguinal hernias have become historical footnotes. In a series of more than 3,000 cases, Ryan and Welsh provided conclusive evidence that simply freeing a sac and reducing it in the preperitoneal space is adequate. They recorded 11 recurrences, only one of which was a true recurrence of the previous repair, the others being femoral and direct inguinal hernias.

Relaxing Incisions

The relaxing incision, first described in 1892 by Wölfler, is an important adjunct to all repairs. This was emphasized by Tanner in 1942 and endorsed by Read and McLeod, Rutledge, Postlethwait, and Griffith. I believe fervently in using relaxing incisions if they are necessary. I have never seen a recurrence take place through what may have been identified as a relaxing incision.

Resection of the Cremaster

The longitudinal incision of the cremaster between the internal ring and the pubic crest is a crucial maneuver that ensures the detection of an indirect inguinal hernia. Overlooking such a defect is a significant technical error that has been reported by Obney and Chan to account for 37% of the recurrences identified in patients referred to the Shouldice Hospital.

Subsequent resection of the medial and lateral leaves of the cremaster exposes the posterior inguinal wall and allows accurate assessment of a direct inguinal hernia if one is present. A peritoneal protrusion on the medial aspect of the spermatic cord always should be identified, freed, and reduced into the preperitoneal space. This practice rules out

TABLE 12.1. PATIENT POPULATION OLDER THAN 50 YEARS (OF 7,159 OPERATIONS IN 1990)

Age Group (yr)	No. of Patients	No. of Operations	%
50–59	1,116	1,369	19.1
60–69	1,330	1,533	21.4
70–79	603	689	9.6
80–89	124	144	2.0

the presence of an indirect sac and removes any possibility of this protrusion becoming a lead point for a recurrence.

The Cribriform Fascia

At the upper medial end of the thigh, the fascia lata extends as a thin cribriform fascia. This fascia is incised routinely from the level of the femoral vein to the pubic crest for two reasons: (a) to allow examination of the femoral opening below the inguinal ligament, and (b) to free the lowermost fibers of the external oblique aponeurosis medially so that they may cover the medial aspect of the floor of the canal (a site that is known for its tendency to break down) during the inguinal repair. This practice results in a 2-cm lateral displacement of the superficial inguinal ring.

Stainless Steel Wire

Stainless steel wire has been a tradition, if not a trademark, of the Shouldice repair. Since it first was introduced in 1941 by Jones, it has been endorsed by both Abel and Goligher. It is an ideal material, elicits no inflammatory response, may remain *in situ* in case of infection, does not cause granulomas, and has a modest price. It is not a difficult suture to handle but does require some practice.

Continuous Suture

The use of continuous rather than interrupted sutures needs no further support from the surgical literature. Wantz was able to obtain better results after converting to the use of continuous sutures. Poole demonstrated a decided improvement in bursting pressure as well as a better distribution of tension. Bartlett reported that excessively tight sutures may contribute to the development of pressure necrosis and wound dehiscence, and recommended that tissue layers be approximated gently. Jenkins estimated that the length of a suture used should be four times the length of the incision to allow for adequate give. In the Shouldice Hospital experience, the continuous suture also has sealed fascial edges better, preventing a lead point for herniation, which may occur between interrupted sutures.

Search for Multiple Hernias

The search for secondary hernias must be sedulous. Our statistics reveal that 13.5% of patients have more than one hernia. Hernias that are overlooked are a source of both early recurrence and embarrassment.

TECHNICAL ASPECTS
Sedation

All patients are given diazepam, 10 to 20 mg orally, 90 minutes before surgery and pethidine hydrochloride (Demerol,

Sanofi Pharmaceuticals, Inc., New York, NY, U.S.A.), 25 to 100 mg 45 minutes before surgery.

Local Anesthesia

A solution of 1% procaine hydrochloride is used, to a maximum dose of 200 mL. Infiltration of the skin is carried out along a line joining the anterosuperior iliac spine and the pubic spine. This step requires 30 to 40 mL of procaine. When the skin incision has been made, another 15 to 30 mL is infiltrated deep to the external oblique aponeurosis. After the latter is incised, the ilioinguinal, iliohypogastric, and genitofemoral nerves are identified, and each is infiltrated again with 1 mL of procaine. Some sympathetic pain fibers are present along the transversus arch deep to the transversalis fascia, and 5 mL of procaine is injected at this site. The deep inguinal ring also is given 3 to 5 mL of procaine, and the loose areolar tissue of the spermatic cord near the internal ring receives another 2 to 5 mL. If an indirect inguinal sac is present, a few milliliters of procaine are injected around the base of the sac, as well as within it.

Dissection

The skin incision is made along a line joining the anterosuperior iliac spine and the pubic crest, and should extend to the pubic crest to expose eventually the medial aspect of the posterior inguinal floor. The external oblique aponeurosis is incised along the direction of its fibers from the superficial inguinal ring to a point 2 to 3 cm lateral to the deep inguinal ring. The medial flap of the external oblique aponeurosis is freed from its underlying loose areolar adhesions as far as the rectus sheath. Laterally, the fibers of the cremaster are freed from the underlying inguinal sulcus. The cremaster is incised along the direction of the muscular fibers from the level of the deep inguinal ring to the pubis and is separated from the contained spermatic cord. This results in medial and lateral muscular flaps. The lateral flap, which contains the external spermatic vessels and the genital branch of the genitofemoral nerve, is divided between two clamps, creating two stumps, a medial one near the pubis and a lateral one at the level of the internal ring. Each stump is doubly ligated with an absorbable tie. The medial flap of the cremaster near the transversus arch usually is less substantial and also is resected. If an indirect sac is present, it will become evident now and should be dissected free from the cord at the internal ring and deeper.

At this point, some surgeons resect the sac. It is essential to ascertain that the peritoneal sac is freed thoroughly of all attachments at the internal ring, so that the stump retracts deep to the plane of the deep inguinal ring.

The next step consists of incising the transversalis fascia. To accomplish this without injuring the deep inferior epigastric vessels, the transversalis fascia is picked up with a hemostat on the superomedial aspect of the internal ring. A gentle snip of the scissors will reveal a yellowish, diaphanous layer; this posterior lamina is incised and reveals the glistening, yellow preperitoneal fat situated in Bogros' space. The incision is extended inferomedially to the level of the pubis. Medial to the longitudinal incision, the preperitoneal fat is separated from the posterior aspect of the myoaponeurotic transversus arch. Laterally, the preperitoneal fat also is separated from the posterior aspect of the transversalis fascia. More laterally, the transversalis fascia can be seen to thicken and dip posteriorly as the iliopubic tract or bandelette of Thomson.

At this stage, the cribriform fascia of the thigh is incised below the inguinal ligament, from the level of the femoral vein to the pubis. It then is possible to examine the femoral ring from above the inguinal ligament and the femoral orifice from below. A fat pad lying in the femoral fossa should not be disturbed because this may set the stage for a femoral hernia. Deep to the iliopubic tract, the iliopubic vein, which sometimes is paired, is identified and avoided carefully because it may be the source of bleeding and hematoma.

The dissection is terminated and the internal oblique, transversus abdominis, and transversalis fascia can be identified medially, with the lateral border of the rectus in a deeper and more medial plane. Laterally, the iliopubic tract can be seen as a free border, leading to the cremasteric stump laterally.

Reconstruction of the Inguinal Region

The floor of the inguinal canal is reconstructed using stainless steel wire (gauge 32 or 34). Two strands of wire are required, each of which will provide two lines. The first strand approaches the lateral aspect of the iliopubic tract near the pubis without ever including the periosteum of the pubis, and crosses over to the full-thickness abdominal wall (Fig. 12.1). This wall consists of the transversalis fascia, the lateral edge of the rectus, the transversus abdominis, and the internal oblique. A knot is tied, and the longer wire becomes the continuous suture that will form the first line. This suture line is continued toward the deep ring, picking up alternately the iliopubic tract laterally and the full-thick-

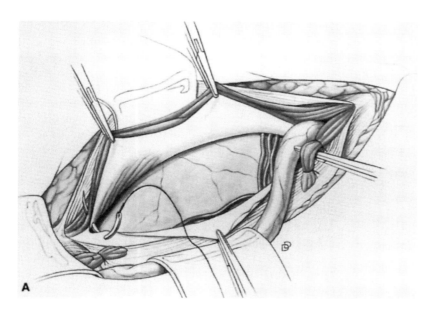

A

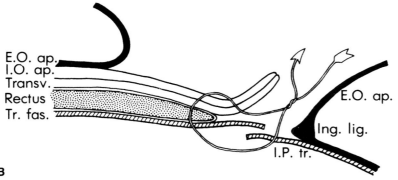

B

FIGURE 12.1. A: Dissection completed. Note the cremasteric stump and iliopubic tract laterally. Medially, the first suture incorporates the transversalis fascia, lateral border of the rectus, transversus abdominis, and internal oblique. **B:** Cross section at the site of the first suture. Laterally, the iliopubic tract (*I.P. tr.*) being incorporated. Medially, the transversalis fascia (*Tr. Fas.*), the lateral edge of the rectus, transversus abdominis (*Transv.*), and internal oblique are incorporated. *E.O. ap.,* external oblique aponeurosis; *Ing. Lig.,* inguinal ligament; *I.O. ap.,* internal oblique aponeurosis.

ness transversus arch medially, leaving a free edge to this arch. Halfway between the pubis and the deep inguinal ring, the edge of the rectus becomes too distant and is abandoned. Near the internal ring, this first suture line incorporates the cremaster stump and carries it across to form a new deep inguinal ring (Fig. 12.2). The suture now reverses itself, as the second line, and advances toward the pubic crest. To do this, it picks up the free edge of the transversus arch, approximating it to the inguinal ligament all the way to the pubic crest. Near the latter, the two ends of the wire are tied (Fig. 12.3).

The next strand of wire will become the third and fourth lines. The third line begins near the internal ring, goes through the internal oblique and transversus abdominis medially, then crosses to the inner aspect of the external oblique aponeurosis, creating an artificial inguinal ligament adjacent to the true one (Fig. 12.4). This line continues to the pubic crest before reversing itself as the fourth line toward the internal ring (Fig. 12.5). Near the pubic crest,

the medial 2 cm of the external flap of the external oblique aponeurosis is used to cover the medial end of the floor of the canal before proceeding along yet another artificial inguinal ligament superficial to the previous one. At the internal ring, the two ends of the wires are tied. Each suture line, as it is added on, serves the purpose of reducing tension on the previous one.

The spermatic cord is placed back in its usual anatomic bed, and the edges of the external oblique aponeurosis are approximated with an absorbable suture. The medial cremasteric stump is anchored near the pubis to prevent a low-lying testicle, which could become excessively pendulous with time.

The subcutaneous tissues are approximated with fine, absorbable sutures, and the skin edges are approximated with Michel clips. Half these clips are removed in 24 hours and the remainder in 48 hours. When surgery is terminated, the patient stands away from the table and walks to the recovery room.

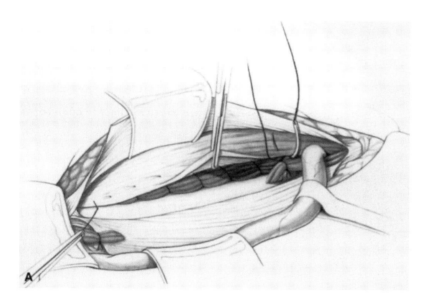

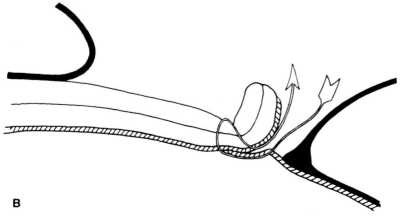

FIGURE 12.2. A: The first line of suture has approximated the iliopubic tract laterally to the full thickness transversus arch (i.e., the transversalis fascia, transversus abdominis, and internal oblique). The cremasteric stump laterally is also carried deep to the transversus arch before the first line of suture reverses to become the second line. **B:** Cross section at the level of the internal ring when the first line is being inserted. Note that the lateral edge of the rectus no longer is incorporated because it has become too medial and too distant.

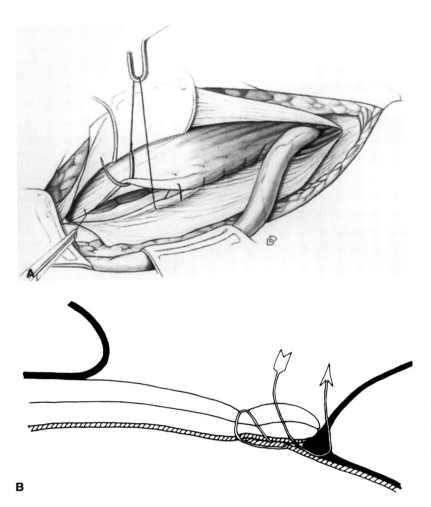

FIGURE 12.3. A: The second line of suture, approximating the free border of the transversus arch to the inguinal ligament. A knot is tied at the level of the pubic crest. **B:** Cross section showing the second line, which now incorporates the inguinal ligament and causes the free border of the transversus arch to abut against the inguinal ligament, thus filling the inguinal sulcus.

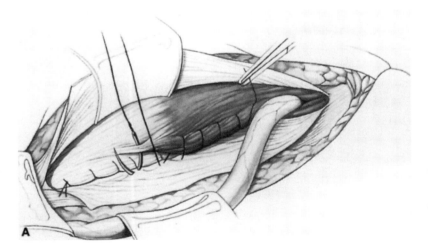

FIGURE 12.4. A: The third line of suture begins near the internal ring and advances toward the pubic crest, approximating the internal oblique and the deeper transversus to the external oblique aponeurosis along a line parallel to the inguinal ligament. *(Continued)*

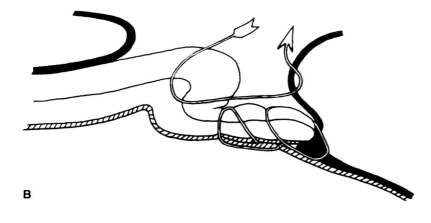

B

FIGURE 12.4. *(Continued)* **B:** Cross section of the third line. The suture approximates the transversus and internal oblique medially and the external oblique aponeurosis laterally. Gentle traction eliminates the dead space in between.

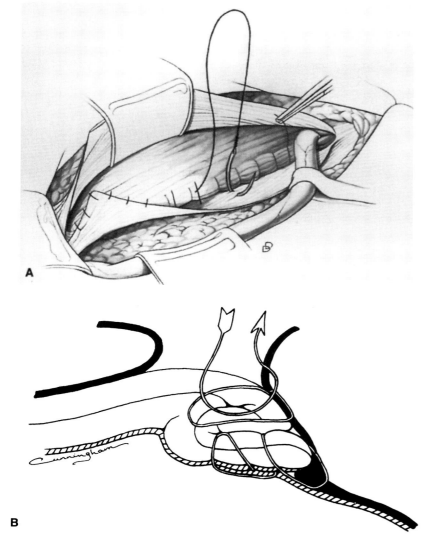

FIGURE 12.5. A: Fourth line showing apposition of the medial 2 cm of the external oblique aponeurosis on the medial portion of the inguinal floor and continuing laterally along a line parallel to the inguinal ligament. The two suture ends are tied at the level of the internal ring. **B:** Cross section with the fourth line in place showing the superimposition of two myoaponeurotic layers forming the new inguinal floor and sulcus.

POSTOPERATIVE PERIOD

Patients are allowed to remain in bed for 4 hours to allow the effect of preoperative drugs to dissipate. At that point, ambulation is encouraged. The first meal after surgery is brought to the patient's room, but all subsequent meals are taken in a cafeteria. Patients are brought together daily for a session of light physical exercises. Discharge from the hospital takes place 48 to 72 hours after surgery.

RESULTS

More than 300,000 Shouldice operations have been performed. The rate of recurrence depends on the accuracy and length of follow-up (Table 12.2). After a short follow-up period, recurrence may be less than 1%. In a group of patients from 1955 who were followed for 35 years, however, the rate of recurrence was 1.46% (Table 12.3). These results have been duplicated, supporting the efficacy of this operation (Table 12.4).

Many of the patients referred to the Shouldice Hospital have recurrent groin hernias. The number varies from 900 to 1,300 cases per year and amounts to 12% to 16% of the yearly total. For most patients, a standard Shouldice herniorrhaphy is adequate. Our statistics before 1983, however, reveal an average global recurrence rate of 2.3% for the first recurrent hernia and 11.4% for the third through the sixth recurrent hernias. These high recurrence rates are the result of extensive tissue destruction and the absence of an

TABLE 12.4. RECURRENCE RATE AFTER THE SHOULDICE OPERATION FOR PRIMARY INGUINAL HERNIAS, AS REPORTED BY VARIOUS AUTHORS

Author[a]	No. of Cases	% Follow-up	Follow-up (yr)	Recurrence (%)
Shearburn	550	100	13	0.2
Volpe	415	50	3	0.2
Wantz (a)	2,087	—	5	0.3
Bocchi	1,640	84	5	0.6
Myers	953	100	18	0.7
Devlin	350	—	6	0.8
Flament	134	—	6	0.9
Wantz (b)	3,454	—	1–20	1.0
Moran	121	—	6	2.0
Berlin	591	—	2–5	2.7

[a]Above sources are cited in Bendavid R. Expectations of brain surgery. In: Peterson-Brown S, Garden J, eds. *Principles and practice of surgical laparoscopy*. Philadelphia: W.B. Saunders, 1994:387.

intact inguinal ligament. Such cases now are treated by the insertion of prosthetic mesh, which produces better results and is associated with a recurrence rate of 2.2%.

COMPLICATIONS

The combination of local anesthesia, a short hospital stay, and a simple but effective herniorrhaphy through an anterior approach has created the belief that hernias are a minor surgical problem. This is true in most cases, and is supported further by the fact that complications are few and rarely life threatening (Table 12.5).

TABLE 12.2. RECURRENCES: THEIR TIMING

Yr	No. of Patients	%
0–4	27	65.8
5–8	7	17.1
9–13	7	17.1

TABLE 12.3. THIRTY-FIVE–YEAR FOLLOW-UP OF 2,748 REPAIRS ON 2,270 PATIENTS OPERATED ON IN 1955 (RECURRENCE RATE, 1.46%)

Year	No. of Recurrences Discovered	% Follow-up	Cumulative Total
1955	3	—	3
1956	4	95.6	7
1957	1	92.4	8
1958	3	88.9	11
1959	3	84.8	14
1960	2	81.0	16
1965	8	—	24
1975	7	—	31
1990	9	—	40

TABLE 12.5. SUMMARY OF POSTOPERATIVE COMPLICATIONS

Complication	Affected Patients
Infection	1.0%
Hematoma	0.3%
Hydrocele	0.7%
Dysejaculation	0.25%
Recurrence	1.46%
Phlebitis	Practically nonexistent as a result of early ambulation and exercise
Atelectasis	—
Pneumonitis	—
Pulmonary embolism	—
Cerebrovascular accident	5 patients
Coronary thrombosis	12 patients
Intestinal obstruction	4 patients
Acute mesenteric thrombosis	1 patient
Perforated duodenal ulcer	1 patient
Spontaneous rupture of gallbladder	1 patient
Pancreatitis	1 patient
Death	20 patients (0.009%)

Testicular Atrophy

Benign testicular and scrotal swelling is common after inguinal herniorrhaphy. Testicular atrophy can occur, however, and usually is characterized by a firm, woody, enlarged testicle 2 to 3 times its normal size, associated with severe pain and a low-grade fever. This complication arises within 24 to 48 hours. The pain resolves in 3 to 6 weeks, but the atrophy may take months. The manifestations of testicular atrophy vary; atrophy has been documented without associated pain or swelling. In some cases, what appears to be threatening testicular atrophy resolves with no adverse sequelae. Atrophy never should be predicted until a year has elapsed. The Shouldice Hospital reports the incidence of testicular atrophy to be about 0.5% after repair of a primary inguinal hernia and 1.5% after repair of recurrent inguinal hernias.

Hematomas

Hematomas are found in the preperitoneal or subcutaneous space. Preperitoneal hematomas are rare: only two have occurred in the last 15 years. Subcutaneous hematomas have been noted in 0.3% of 5,762 patients. They are a minor complication and should be treated with evacuation and a careful search for the source of bleeding.

Infections

The rate of wound infection after surgery at the Shouldice Hospital has always been low (less than 1%) because we avoid nosocomial contamination. Any patient known to harbor an infection (e.g., cutaneous, pulmonary, draining sinus) is not admitted to the hospital until the infection has cleared. This practice effectively limits the incidence of infection.

Dysejaculation

Dysejaculation is a syndrome characterized by severe burning and pain on ejaculation. Its incidence is probably 0.25%. Seventeen cases were reported in April 1992, and another six cases have been identified since then. Most patients improve without active treatment, although symptoms may persist for as long as 5 years.

Hydrocele

Hydrocele is seen occasionally after herniorrhaphy. Obney reported an incidence of 0.7% after 14,442 hernia operations. He also pointed out that lipomas around the spermatic cord should be dissected cleanly and resected, ligatures about the cord should be kept to a minimum, and both deep and superficial inguinal rings should not be too snug.

Mortality

Since 1945, 20 patients have died within 30 days of surgery. This represents a mortality rate of 0.009%. The diagnosis clinically or at autopsy was myocardial infarction in 15 patients (average age, 70 years: range, 56 to 85 years), cerebrovascular accident in one (age 66 years), and undetermined in four (ages 56, 66, 70, and 78 years).

CONCLUSION

No doubt exists in any surgeon's mind that a well-executed primary herniorrhaphy will yield excellent results. Good technique does not mean legerdemain, but a good understanding of the anatomy and the procedure. The Shouldice repair lends itself to easy execution with confirmed good results, but above all, to near perfection in terms of safety.

SELECTED READING LIST

Abel AL, Hunt AU. Stainless steel wire for closing abdominal incisions and for the repair of hernias. *Br Med J* 1948;2:379.

Bartlett LC. Pressure necrosis is the primary cause of wound dehiscence. *Can J Surg* 1985;28:27.

Bendavid R. The Shouldice method of inguinal herniorrhaphy. In: Nyhus LM, Baker RJ, eds. *Mastery of surgery,* 2nd ed. Boston: Little, Brown and Company, 1992:1584.

Bendavid R. Expectations of hernia surgery. In: Peterson-Brown S, Garden J, eds. *Principles and practice of surgical laparoscopy.* Philadelphia: W.B. Saunders, 1994:387.

Bendavid R, Andrews DF, Gilbert AI. Testicular atrophy: incidence and relationship to the type of hernia and to multiple recurrent hernia. *Probl Gen Surg* 1995;12[Part 2]:225–227.

Bendavid R. Dysejaculation. *Probl Gen Surg* 1995;12[Part 2]:238.

Blodgett JB, Beattie EJ. The effect of postoperative rising on the recurrence rate of hernia. *Surg Gynecol Obstet* 1947;84:716.

Bocchi P. Bassini, the man, the soldier, the surgeon. *Postgrad Gen Surg* 1992;4:175.

Cushing H. The employment of local anaesthesia in the radical cure of certain cases of hernia, with a note upon the nervous anatomy of the inguinal region. *Ann Surg* 1900;31:1.

Glassow F. Inguinal hernia in the female. *Surg Gynecol Obstet* 1963;116:701.

Glassow F. High ligation of the sac in indirect inguinal hernia. *Am J Surg* 1965;109:460.

Goligher JC, Irvin TT, Johnston D, et al. A controlled clinical trial of three methods of closure of laparotomy wounds. *Br Med J* 1975; 62:823.

Griffith CA. The Marcy repair of indirect inguinal hernia: 1870 to the present. In: Nyhus LM, Condon RE, eds. *Hernia,* 3rd ed. Philadelphia: JB Lippincott, 1989:106–118.

Herzfeld G. Hernia in infancy. *Am J Surg* 1938;39:422.

Iles JDH. Specialisation in elective herniorrhaphy. *Lancet* 1964;1:751.

Iles JDH. Convalescence after herniorrhaphy. *JAMA* 1972;219:385.

Jenkins TPN. Incisional hernia repair: a mechanical approach. *Br J Surg* 1980;67:335.

Jones TE, Newell ET, Brubaker RE. The use of alloy steel wire in the closure of abdominal wounds. *Surg Gynecol Obstet* 1941;72:1056.

Kingsworth AN, Britton BJ, Morris PJ. Recurrent inguinal hernia after local anaesthetic repair. *Br J Surg* 1981;68:273.

Lichtenstein IL. Herniorrhaphy. A personal experience with 6321 cases. *Am J Surg* 1987;153:553.

Marcy HO. *The anatomy and surgical treatment of hernia.* New York: D. Appleton & Co, 1892:100.

Obney N. Hydrocoeles of the testicle complicating inguinal hernias. *Can Med Assoc J* 1956;75:733.

Obney N, Chan CK. Repair of multiple time recurrent inguinal hernias with reference to common causes of recurrence. *Contemp Surg* 1984;25:25.

Palumbo LT, Sharpe WS. Primary inguinal hernioplasty in the adult. *Surg Clin North Am* 1971;51:1293.

Poole GV Jr, Meredith JW, Kon ND, et al. Suture techniques and wound bursting strength. *Am Surg* 1984;50:569.

Postlethwait RW. Recurrent inguinal hernia. *Ann Surg* 1985;202:777.

Read RC, McLeod PC. Influence of a relaxing incision on suture tension in Bassini's and McVay's repairs. *Arch Surg* 1981;116:440.

Rutledge RH. Cooper's ligament repair: a 25-year experience with a single technique for all groin hernias in adults. *Surgery* 1988;103:1.

Ryan EA. Recurrent hernias: an analysis of 369 consecutive cases of recurrent inguinal and femoral hernias. *Surg Gynecol Obstet* 1953;96:343.

Ryan EA. An analysis of 313 consecutive cases of indirect sliding inguinal hernias. *Surg Gynecol Obstet* 1956;102:45.

Shouldice EE. Surgical treatment of hernia. In: Program and abstracts of the Annual Meeting of the Ontario Medical Association; September 10, 1944; District Number 9; pp. 3–28.

Wantz G. The operation of Bassini as described by Attilio Catterina. *Surg Gynecol Obstet* 1989;168:67.

Welsh DRJ. Bilateral sliding inguinal hernias. *Postgrad Gen Surg* 1992;4:114.

EDITOR'S COMMENTS

Few can argue with the success achieved by the Shouldice group in refining and defining a cure for groin hernia. It is clear that their success is predicated on very sound surgical principles applied systematically and, to some degree, systemically in advancing a cure for inguinal herniation. However, it is clear from a review of the literature that not all centers achieve the same remarkable success as that reached in Toronto. There are clearly sporadic reports of failure rates quite in excess of those reported by the group at the Shouldice Clinic. It is not entirely clear that a uniform explanation for this difference exists. Surely, the sheer volume of repairs done far exceeds the capacity if not the ability of other centers to amass such numbers. While the author reports on failure of the original operation, there is little analysis to address the underlying factors for the failure of this otherwise useful operation.

I have employed a variation of the suture technique described for the past 18 years mostly in the repair of inguinal hernias with small direct defects and an indirect component.

This approach is used in younger individuals, usually less than 40 years of age, because of a desire to avoid the placement of prosthetic material in patients with significant longevity.

The determinants of applying the technique are the amount of weakness in the inguinal floor, defined at the time of open anterior surgical repair, and the degree of dilation of the internal ring. If weakness of the floor is perceived to exceed one third the length of the floor of the inguinal canal, a modification of the Shouldice repair is used to reinforce the floor. A tension distribution analysis of the angles of force in the floor would support this concept.

The modification in suturing is illustrated in the figure below. It essentially approximates the transversalis fascia by imbrication and then adds a more anterior layer of internal abdominal oblique fascia, sometimes the conjoint tendon, sewn to the shelving edge of the inguinal ligament. In essence, two layers of the abdominal wall are approximated with a single suture of 2-zero polypropylene. The suture is placed at the medial aspect of the floor, just below the pubic tubercle and then run in continuous fashion toward the internal ring, placed loosely so that the transversalis fascia or iliopubic band are always visible. When this layer of suture is completed, the loose suture is tightened, and invariably the floor of the inguinal canal is firm and noted to be reconstructed. The other arm of the double-armed 2-zero suture is then used to place the suture medially on the pubic tubercle, effectively closing this area—an area of frequent recurrence—minimizing the potential for a recurrent defect. Once this suture is placed, the fascia of the internal abdominal oblique is approximated to the shelving edge of the inguinal ligament, again loosely placed while tension is retained on the deeper layer approximation. Approaching the internal ring with this more ventrally placed suture, it is relatively easy to minimize the size of the ring without compromise to cord structures, while assuring closure of the area to prevent recurrence. The two ends of the single suture are then tied, creating the repair of the floor and reconstruction of the internal ring.

When this operation is performed under local anesthesia, immediate assessment of tension is possible, and relaxing incisions in the internal abdominal oblique fascia can be made. In my experience, this has been required less than 15% of the time. If there is any concern about the integrity of the repair or that the patient may place undo stress on the area through work or recreation (e.g., heavy-weight–class power weight lifting), on occasion I have added an anterior mesh reinforcement in the fashion of Lichtenstein. Recurrence rates for this variation, without the mesh, have been about 1%, all occurring after 5 or more years.

A.G.G.

Nyhus and Condon's Hernia, Fifth Edition, edited by Robert J. Fitzgibbons, Jr. and A. Gerson Greenburg. Lippincott Williams & Wilkins, Philadelphia © 2002.

13

THE COOPER'S LIGAMENT REPAIR

ROBB H. RUTLEDGE

A strong posterior inguinal wall is the best protection against a groin hernia in an adult. Normally, this is provided by the insertion of the transversus abdominis and the underlying transversalis fascia from the pubic tubercle to the medial margin of the femoral ring.

There is a weak area in this posterior wall that is protected only by transversalis fascia. Fruchaud named this the myopectineal orifice (6). It is bounded by the rectus muscle medially, the internal oblique and transversus abdominis superiorly, the iliopsoas muscle laterally, and Cooper's ligament and the pubis inferiorly. It is spanned and divided by the inguinal ligament, traversed by the spermatic cord and femoral vessels, and bridged on its inner surface by the transversalis fascia (Fig. 13.1) (24).

All groin hernias begin as a weak area in the myopectineal orifice. With a decrease in the area's aponeurotic fibers from defective collagen metabolism and a gradual attenuation from increased intraabdominal pressure, a hernia can result. The transversalis fascia deteriorates and allows a peritoneal protrusion through it. Depending on the length of the insertion of the transversus abdominis on Cooper's ligament, the presence of a patent processus vaginalis, and the width of the femoral ring, the hernia can be direct, indirect, or femoral, or any combination of the three (Fig. 13.2).

Groin hernias are treated by repairing all or part of the myopectineal orifice. Fruchaud favored a deep reconstruction of this entire groin area, not unlike a Cooper's ligament repair (23). Currently, hernia repairs can be divided into two main groups: (a) those that close all or part of the myopectineal orifice by suturing the tissues at its boundaries (Cooper's ligament, Shouldice, and Bassini), and (b) those that cover the unclosed orifice with prosthetic mesh (Lichtenstein, plug and patch, and laparoscopic). Low recurrence rates can be obtained with any of these repairs.

The Cooper's ligament method is the only anterior open repair that closes the complete myopectineal orifice. It is a more extensive operation and has a slower convalescence than any of the "tension-free" procedures, but it gives excellent results.

HISTORIC DEVELOPMENT

In 1784, at the age of 16 years, Sir Astley Cooper was apprenticed to Mr. Henry Cline, the leading surgeon at St. Thomas' Hospital in London. One night, when he was attending one of Mr. Cline's lectures on hernias he realized that he himself was the subject of that complaint. He ran home, dashed upstairs to his room, threw himself on the bed, elevated his legs on the bedpost, and waited for Mr. Cline to come home. When Mr. Cline arrived, he confirmed the diagnosis and fitted young Cooper with a truss that he wore faithfully for 5 years (2).

This episode stimulated Cooper's interest in hernias. In 1804, he published his classic hernia work and dedicated it to Mr. Cline (3). In this, he demonstrated the anatomic defects of groin hernias, described the transversalis fascia, and defined the superior pubic ligament that later bore his name. Anesthesia and asepsis were unknown then, and Cooper recommended surgery only for incarceration. He did not use his own ligament in his repairs, and he treated his own hernia with a truss. Cooper had no further trouble with his own hernia, and his autopsy findings showed only the fibrotic remains of a right indirect inguinal hernia (2).

In 1892, Giuseppe Ruggi was the first to use Cooper's ligament in any type of hernia surgery. He sutured the inguinal ligament down to Cooper's ligament in his femoral repairs (18).

In 1897, Georg Lotheissen was the first to suture the conjoined tendon to Cooper's ligament. He was operating in Innsbruck on a 45-year-old woman with a twice-recurrent inguinal hernia after previous Bassini's repairs. Lotheissen found that the patient's inguinal ligament had been destroyed, so he anchored the conjoined tendon to Cooper's

R. H. Rutledge: Department of Surgery, University of Texas Southwestern Medical Center Dallas, Texas; and Department of Surgery, John Peter Smith Hospital, Fort Worth, Texas.

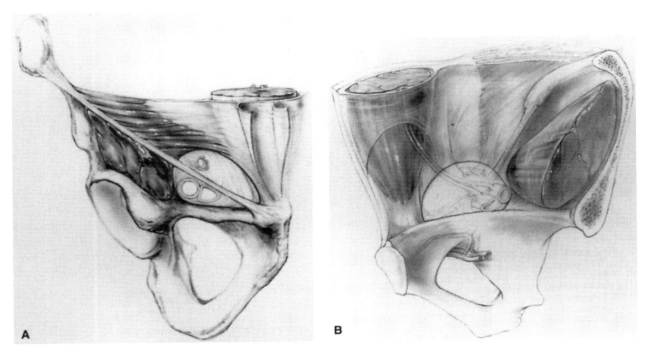

FIGURE 13.1. Anterior (**A**) and posterior (**B**) views of the myopectineal orifice. See text for boundaries. (From Wantz GE. Anatomy of hernias of the groin *Atlas of hernia surgery*. New York: Raven Press, 1991:1–10, with permission.)

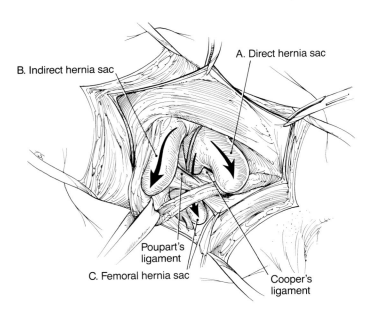

B. Indirect hernia sac

A. Direct hernia sac

Poupart's ligament

C. Femoral hernia sac

Cooper's ligament

FIGURE 13.2. Direct, indirect, and femoral hernias all present through the myopectineal orifice and can be repaired with one operation. (From Rutledge RH. Cooper's ligament repair: a 25-year experience with a single technique for all groin hernias in adults. *Surgery* 1988;103:1–10, with permission.)

ligament instead. He subsequently reported success with his Cooper's ligament technique for both inguinal and femoral hernias, but he did not use a relaxing incision (11).

In 1939, Chester McVay submitted his thesis on the anatomy of the inguinal and femoral areas for his doctorate at Northwestern University in Evanston, Illinois. He pointed out that the normal insertion of the transversus abdominis and the transversalis fascia was on Cooper's ligament, not the inguinal ligament. From these dissections, McVay developed his technique of a Cooper's ligament repair and reported this from Ann Arbor in 1942 while he was a surgical resident (12). He was unaware of Lotheissen's work then. McVay emphasized that Cooper's ligament was the anatomically correct anchor for a posterior wall reconstruction and recommended a Cooper's ligament repair for direct, large indirect, and femoral hernias. He used a relaxing incision to avoid tension. His work provided a sound anatomic basis for a Cooper's ligament repair and popularized its use in America (14).

A relaxing incision is an essential part of a Cooper's ligament repair. Although Anton Wolfler did not use the Cooper ligament in his hernia surgery, he is given credit for making the first relaxing incision. In 1892, in the Festschrift for Theodor Billroth, Wolfler described making an incision in the anterior rectus sheath whenever he noted tension approximating the conjoined tendon to the inguinal ligament. He did this to relieve tension and also to gain access to the rectus muscle to transplant it to reinforce his repair (Fig. 13.3) (25).

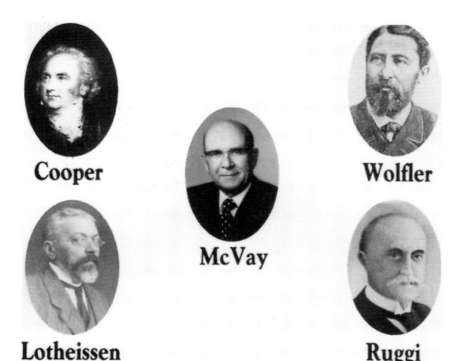

FIGURE 13.3. The developers of the Cooper's ligament repair. (From Rutledge RH. Cooper's ligament repair: a 25-year experience with a single technique for all groin hernias in adults. *Surgery* 1988;103:1–10, with permission.)

INDICATIONS FOR A COOPER'S LIGAMENT REPAIR

A Cooper's ligament repair should be considered whenever a posterior inguinal wall reconstruction is done. Many surgeons use a Cooper's ligament repair only for direct, large indirect, and femoral hernias. They do not use this repair for small or medium indirect hernias because they believe that a posterior wall reconstruction is unnecessary in these cases.

Using this selective approach, McVay and Chapp in 1958 reported a recurrence rate of 3.2% for abdominal ring repairs for small or medium indirect hernias, but only a 0.85% recurrence rate for Cooper's ligament repairs for the more difficult direct, large indirect, or femoral hernias (13). McVay's report is one of the few that has a higher recurrence rate for indirect hernias than for direct ones. A more complete repair on the small and medium indirect hernias should give better results.

Because of McVay's report, my preference was to do a Cooper's ligament repair on all groin hernias in adults. About 15% to 20% of patients have multiple ipsilateral defects at the original operation. Most recurrences are due to missed hernias, inadequate dissection, or subsequent further deterioration of the transversalis fascia. All the types of groin hernias present within inches of each other through the myopectineal orifice. Recurrences should be fewer if all possible defects are repaired and the myopectineal orifice completely closed at the original operation. Since 1959, I have done a Cooper's ligament repair on all groin hernias in

adults, primary or recurrent, regardless of the presenting type (20,21).

SURGICAL MANAGEMENT

Before operation, all patients are told of the possible use of Marlex mesh and the possible sacrifice of the ilioinguinal nerve. All male patients are told of the possible occurrence of ischemic orchitis and subsequent testicular atrophy regardless of careful technique.

General anesthesia has been used routinely, but local or regional anesthesia would be satisfactory. A short course of perioperative antibiotics is given, and the bladder is emptied immediately preoperatively. An identical repair is done whether the hernia is primary or recurrent, and direct, indirect, or femoral. More detailed remarks about recurrent hernias, bilaterality, relaxing incisions, the femoral vessels, and testicular problems follow under *Special Considerations*.

Operative Technique

A low, almost transverse incision is made. The external oblique is opened through the external ring. Small hemostatic clips mark the boundaries of the external ring as a guide for the new external ring diameter. The ilioinguinal nerve is usually preserved, but I clip and divide it laterally if I feel it has been injured during the surgery. The spermatic cord is mobilized in the canal but is not disturbed medial to the pubic tubercle in order to preserve testicular collateral circulation.

The posterior wall of the inguinal canal is incised completely, destroying the internal ring. The iliopubic veins are controlled, and Cooper's ligament is dissected free (Fig. 13.4A). The spermatic cord is retracted superiorly with a broad Deaver retractor, and the deeper portion of Cooper's ligament is cleared (Fig. 13.4B).

Then, starting lateral to the femoral vessels, the femoral sheath (anterior femoral fascia) is identified and dissected free. Working medially, the anterior surface of the femoral artery and vein are seen and cleared off as the femoral sheath is developed. The dissection continues medially, and the fat and lymph nodes are removed from the femoral canal. Any femoral sac is converted to an inguinal one. Finally, any vascular connections to the obturator circula-

tion are divided and ligated so they will not be torn during the repair.

After the inferior dissection is completed, the transversus abdominis arch is mobilized superiorly from the underlying preperitoneal tissues, and any attenuated transversalis fascia and internal oblique are excised. Then a relaxing incision is made at the point of fusion of the external oblique aponeurosis and the anterior rectus sheath. This starts at the pubic tubercle and extends superiorly about 4 to 5 inches (Fig. 13.4C).

The patient is placed in the Trendelenburg position to decrease the likelihood of intestinal injury. The spermatic cord is opened, and the cremaster fibers are divided at the internal ring (Fig. 13.4D). Any fat or lipoma is removed

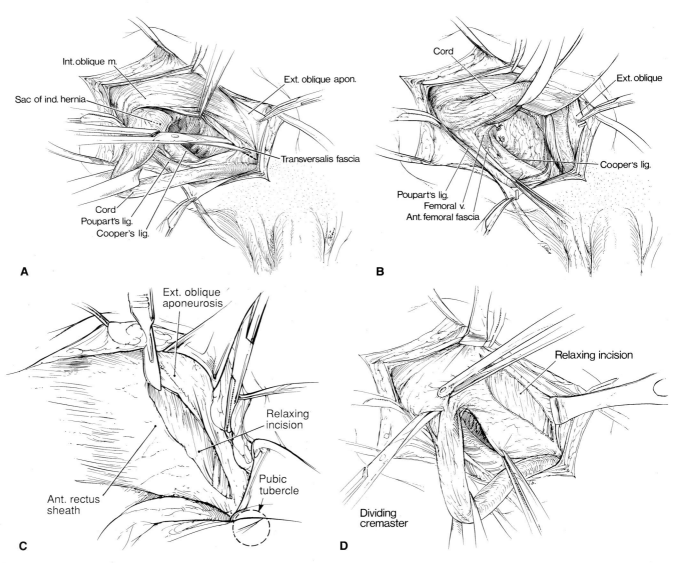

FIGURE 13.4. Basic steps in a Cooper's ligament repair. See text for current surgical technique. (From Rutledge RH. Cooper's ligament repair: a 25-year experience with a single technique for all groin hernias in adults. *Surgery* 1988;103:1–10, with permission.) *Continued on following pages*

from the cord. The external spermatic artery is divided as it comes off the inferior epigastric so the cord can be moved laterally during the repair (Fig. 13.4E).

Indirect sacs are opened and explored to evaluate any intraabdominal pathology and to ascertain that no intestine is adherent directly under the area of the repair. Small indirect sacs are removed and the peritoneum closed. Large indirect sacs are transected just distal to the internal ring. The proximal sac is freed from the cord by sharp dissection and closed. To decrease the chances of developing an ischemic orchitis, the distal sac is left in place and filleted on its anterior surface to prevent hydrocele formation. If no indirect sac is apparent, the anteromedial portion of the cord is dissected superiorly to identify and ligate the small peritoneal tab that is always present, to avoid overlooking an indirect sac.

Most direct sacs are inverted, but large ones are occasionally excised. Large combined direct and indirect sacs are joined by dividing the inferior epigastric vessels and closing the sacs as one defect.

Sliding hernias are reduced either by working through the sac or by freeing the sac from the cord by sharp dissection and then reducing the whole sac into the abdomen.

The repair is begun by inverting the preperitoneal tissues with a continuous 1-zero chromic catgut suture to reduce them away from the main repair (Fig. 13.4F). This must be done carefully to avoid injuring the underlying intestine. Then, beginning at the pubic tubercle, a layer of about ten interrupted sutures is placed between the transversus abdominis arch and Cooper's ligament, going as far laterally as the medial edge of the femoral vein (Fig. 13.4G). An Allis clamp is used to grasp the transversus abdominis arch to be

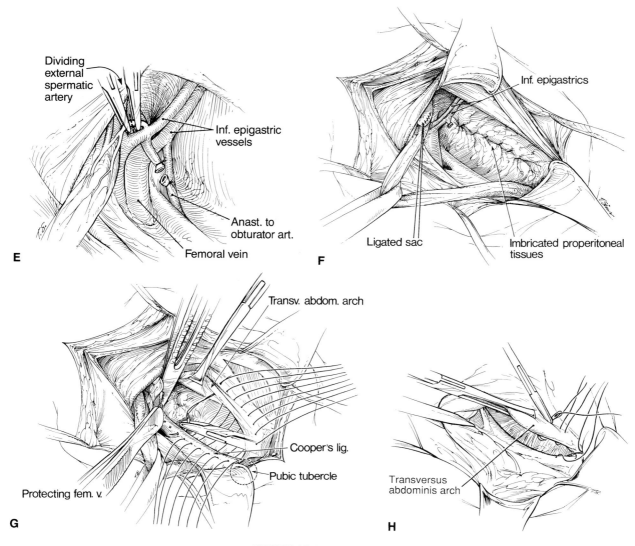

FIGURE 13.4. *Continued.*

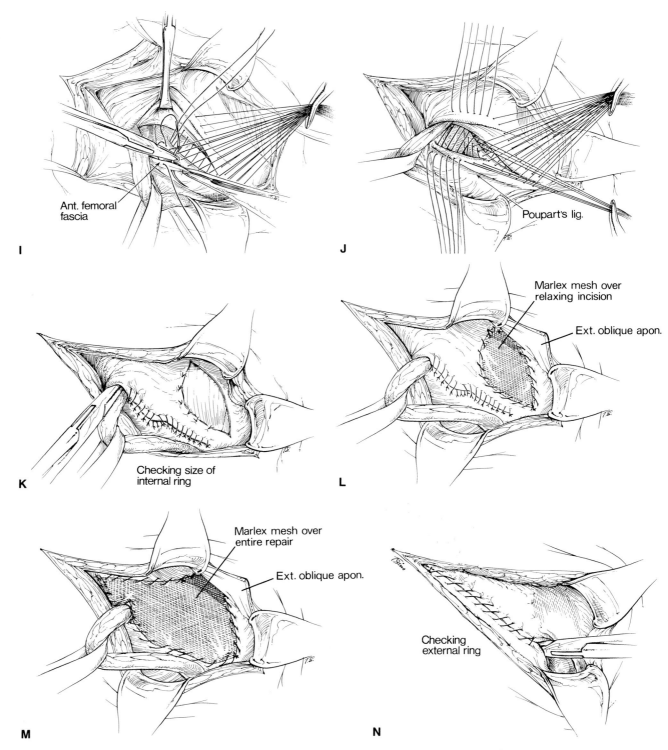

Ant. femoral
fascia

I

Poupart's lig.

J

Checking size of
internal ring

K

Marlex mesh over
relaxing incision

Ext. oblique apon.

L

Marlex mesh over
entire repair

Ext. oblique apon.

M

Checking
external ring

N

FIGURE 13.4. *Continued.*

certain that good bites are placed in it, not merely in the overlying internal oblique (Fig. 13.4H). A short thick tonsillectomy needle is used for the Cooper's ligament sutures. I prefer to place the sutures in Cooper's ligament right-handed on right-sided hernias and left-handed on left-sided hernias.

The femoral canal is closed by three transition sutures between Cooper's ligament and the femoral sheath (Fig. 13.4I). The lateral one is placed just lateral to the last suture previously placed in Cooper's ligament. The medial two are then placed medial to this between the Cooper's ligament sutures.

Using a larger needle, the repair is continued by placing sutures between the transversus abdominis arch and the femoral sheath, continuing laterally beyond any indirect sac so the spermatic cord comes out obliquely laterally at the new internal ring. No sutures are placed lateral to the cord in this layer (Fig 13.4J).

This entire layer is done with 1-zero silk sutures (siliconized, Davis & Geck, New Haven, CT, U.S.A.). They are tied from medial to lateral, and the patient is brought out of the Trendelenburg position. Many surgeons would prefer to use Prolene, but the silk is easier to tie and has given no problems.

The new internal ring is snug and admits only a Kelly clamp (Fig. 13.4K). Although the relaxing incision can be secured in position with a few interrupted sutures, I prefer to fill the defect with a Marlex mesh patch held in position by a continuous 1-zero Prolene suture (Figure 13.4L). Occasionally, a sheet of Marlex mesh is sutured on top of this whole basic layer as an onlay graft reinforcement if I am concerned about the repair (Fig. 13.4M). The cord is returned to its natural position, and the external oblique is closed over the cord with continuous 2-zero Vicryl (Fig. 13.4N). The new external ring is loose, easily admitting a finger. The soft tissues are closed, and the skin is closed with subcuticular 4-zero Dexon sutures and Steri-Strips.

Special Considerations

Recurrent Hernias

Currently, most surgeons repair recurrent hernias by a preperitoneal or laparoscopic approach because they can avoid the previous scarred operative field and are less likely to have problems with the spermatic cord and the sensory nerves. Ilzermans et al. reported a 23% 5-year recurrence rate using classic anterior methods for recurrent repairs and concluded that these techniques were not suitable (8).

In contradistinction to this, my experience has been that a Cooper's ligament repair can give excellent results repairing recurrent hernias. The old incision is opened, and dissection is begun laterally in clean tissues. Then, working medially, the previous repair is dismantled. The transversus

abdominis arch, Cooper's ligament, and anterior femoral sheath are dissected free. Frequently, they were not used in the previous operation. A long relaxing incision, rarely done at the first operation, is made, and the spermatic cord is carefully preserved. Nearly always, a good repair can be done.

Bilaterality

An underlying metabolic collagen defect is found in most adult hernia patients. Forty-six percent of my patients either had a bilateral repair or had a contralateral hernia that was repaired earlier or developed subsequently. This high percentage of eventual bilaterality emphasizes two points. First, all patients who have a unilateral repair must have the opposite side carefully checked before operation. Second, a complete repair should be done at the primary operation to avoid further problems with that side.

Most bilateral hernias are repaired at the same operation through two separate incisions, leaving a broad area between them to minimize scrotal swelling. If the first repair was prolonged or difficult, the second side is postponed until that repair is clinically indicated.

Relaxing Incisions

A generous relaxing incision is essential to prevent tension on the repair. This incision begins just above the pubis and extends 4 to 5 inches superiorly in the plane of fusion of the external oblique aponeurosis and the anterior rectus sheath. If there is tension while the posterior wall reconstruction sutures are being tied, the incision is lengthened superiorly. This nearly always gives enough relaxation. On the rare occasion that this is unsuccessful, I look for aberrant aponeurotic fibers lateral to the pyramidalis. Dividing these fibers provides adequate relaxation (15). Although a relaxing incision does not make the posterior wall reconstruction "tension-free," it reduces the tension enough to allow good healing.

Others have described patients in whom a Cooper's ligament repair could not be performed without tension despite all of the maneuvers just described. In such cases, a piece of Marlex mesh could be placed in the preperitoneal position as an inlay graft for a new posterior wall. It is attached to Cooper's ligament and the femoral sheath inferiorly, to the rectus medially, and to the transversus abdominis superiorly. This has not been necessary in my practice (Fig. 13.5).

A hernia through the relaxing incision is normally prevented by the medial extension of the transversalis fascia as the rectus fascia. Occasionally, a patient has a prominence of the rectus muscle through the relaxing incision. To prevent this, I routinely fill the relaxing incision defect with a Marlex mesh patch.

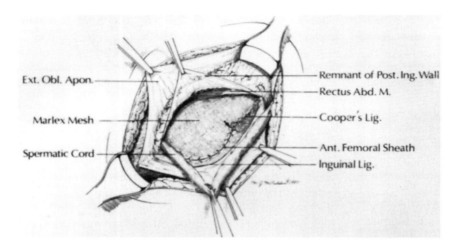

FIGURE 13.5. Marlex mesh inlay graft used when posterior wall is deficient for a primary Cooper's ligament repair. (From McVay CB. Abdominal wall. *Anson and McVay: surgical anatomy*, 6th ed. Philadelphia: WB Saunders, 1984:560, with permission.)

Femoral Vessels

Careful technique around the femoral vessels is required. Well-trained surgeons are familiar with basic vascular techniques and should have no trouble with this (22). I have found it easier to develop the femoral sheath lateral to the femoral vessels first. Then, working medially, the femoral sheath is developed, and the front surface of the femoral artery and vein are cleaned off; with the femoral vein clearly identified, the femoral canal is cleaned out. This gives excellent exposure to any tributaries to the obturator circulation. These are then divided and ligated so they will not be torn during the repair. Placement of sutures in Cooper's ligament is stopped at the medial edge of the femoral vein to prevent any venous constriction and decrease the likelihood of a thrombophlebitis (16).

Testicular Problems

To minimize risks to the testicle, several maneuvers are important. No dissection is done medial to the pubic tubercle. The external ring is left loose. An ipsilateral hydrocele is not removed unless an orchiectomy is done. Only sharp dissection is used around the cord. Large indirect sacs are transected at the internal ring and the distal portion left in place. Although the external spermatic artery is routinely divided and the internal ring made quite snug, no sutures are placed lateral to the cord so that it can move laterally without constriction. All these technical steps protect testicular circulation and decrease the chances of thrombophlebitis of the spermatic cord and ischemic orchitis.

Orchiectomy is rarely necessary in hernia surgery and is done only with prior consent. Examples include a patient with an undescended, painful, or atrophic testicle or an elderly patient with a large coexisting ipsilateral hydrocele. Patients with recurrent hernias only rarely require an orchiectomy. Nearly always, enough of the spermatic cord can be preserved to save a good testicle.

RESULTS OF A PERSONAL SERIES

My total experience from 1959 through 1994 is shown in Table 13.1. It includes 1,652 Cooper's ligament repairs. My last complete report was in 1988, on 1,142 Cooper's ligament repairs in 942 patients done between 1959 and 1984, with a 97% follow-up (20). The only operative death was in a 65-year-old man with a proven myocardial infarction on the fourth postoperative day. One hundred sixty-seven patients (202 hernia repairs) had died by the time of the follow-up. They were followed an average of 7.2 years before death, with one suspected recurrence. None of this group had an operation for a recurrence. The late death patients were not included in the statistics. Twenty-eight patients (34 hernia repairs) were lost to follow-up. The remaining 747 living patients (906 hernia repairs) were followed an average of 9 years. I personally examined 80% and talked to the remaining 20% on the telephone.

There were 18 recurrences, for a 2% overall recurrence rate. Seventeen of these were indirect along the cord in a subgroup of 147 repairs done with a subcutaneously transplanted cord. This method was discarded in 1972. There was one recurrence in 572 repairs with the cord in the natural position; there was no recurrence in 154 repairs in female patients; and there was no recurrence in 33 repairs

TABLE 13.1. COOPER'S LIGAMENT REPAIR 1959–1994 (1,682 REPAIRS)

	No. (%)	
	1,437 Primary	**245 Recurrent**
Direct	516 (36)	137 (56)
Indirect	868 (60)	100 (41)
Femoral	53 (4)	8 (3)
Total	1,437 (100)	245 (100)
	(85% of Total)	(15% of Total)

in male patients with an orchiectomy. Excluding the group with the subcutaneously transplanted cord, the recurrence rate is 0.13% for 759 repairs followed an average of 7.4 years.

The only three recurrences in the 127 recurrent repairs were indirect along the cord in the subcutaneously transplanted group. There has been no recurrence in a recurrent repair using the present technique that was begun in 1972.

Although a complete follow-up has not been done since my 1988 report, I followed my patients closely through 1994 and believe the recurrence rates are essentially unchanged (21).

ADVANTAGES OF A COOPER'S LIGAMENT REPAIR

The Cooper's ligament repair restores normal anatomic planes and provides the best anchor for a strong posterior wall reconstruction. It closes the femoral canal and displays the femoral vessels to protect them from injury. It is the only anterior repair that closes the complete myopectineal orifice. It repairs all the hernias that can occur in the groin.

DISADVANTAGES OF A COOPER'S LIGAMENT REPAIR

There are four disadvantages of a Cooper's ligament repair that are frequently cited. I agree with the first two of these but believe that the latter two can be prevented with careful technique.

1. *More extensive operation*: The Cooper's ligament repair has a longer operating time and requires more extensive dissection. A long relaxing incision is necessary to minimize tension to allow good healing.

2. *Slower convalescence*: Although most Cooper's ligament patients are cared for on an outpatient basis, they require more medicine for pain relief and have a slower early convalescence than do patients undergoing open tension-free or laparoscopic repairs. Although cultural and socioeconomic factors are the most important determinants of time off work, Cooper's ligament patients clearly have a longer recovery, especially if they undergo a bilateral repair. The fact that all of my patients who were self-employed physicians or lawyers were back at work in a week shows the importance of individual motivation.

After the initial 4 to 6 weeks, patients with Cooper's ligament repairs do not have any more pain than other hernia repair patients. Long-term results show no differences in comfort or function (4).

3. *Vascular injuries*: Careful technique around the femoral vessels is required. Since the artery and vein are displayed and protected, the chances of injury are minimal. In my series of 1,682 Cooper's ligament repairs, there has been no vascular injury.

4. *Thromboembolic complications*: If the most lateral suture in Cooper's ligament is placed just medial to the femoral vein, there should be no increased embolic risk. Two patients in my series had pulmonary emboli requiring anticoagulants, but phlebograms did not show the operative leg to be the source. One patient had a flare-up of her recurrent bilateral superficial thrombophlebitis treated by anticoagulants. A fourth patient had a venous constriction demonstrated by phlebogram. He was treated with elastic support and elevation but no anticoagulants. The swelling subsided, and he was asymptomatic for the remaining 6 years of his life. This last patient emphasizes the potential problem, but careful technique should prevent it.

DISCUSSION

Fifteen percent to 20% of hernia operations are done for recurrent hernias. It is cost-effective to keep recurrence rates as low as possible. Acceptably low rates can be achieved by several different types of hernia repairs. Consequently, the recurrence rate should be only one of the factors that are used to judge hernia repairs. Other factors include technical difficulty, complications, early and late postoperative pain and disability, medical costs, and societal costs (19).

Cost-effectiveness analysis is being used more and more to evaluate the relative value of different types of hernia operations, but comparing series of hernia repairs from different centers is difficult. Definitions of a recurrence differ, and methods of follow-up vary. Even the technique for a Cooper's ligament repair (equally well known as a McVay repair) is not standardized. Some reports mention that the posterior wall reconstruction is done with four or five absorbable sutures, and that a relaxing incision was made about 50% of the time (1,5). This is not the same Cooper's ligament repair that I have described. The results will not be the same. Physicians who are conducting these trials should realize that the operative technique is the main factor in preventing complications and obtaining good results (17).

Currently, the vast majority of groin hernia surgery in adults is done by one of the tension-free mesh repairs (9). The technical problems are fewer, the recovery is quicker, and the recurrence rate should be low. Whether or not these repairs will allow recurrences deep to the mesh, cause late deep infections, or result in increased inguinodynia (7) and fertility problems (10) is not clear. Some mesh plugs will migrate and may penetrate vascular or gastrointestinal structures.

Although most surgeons prefer a tension-free mesh repair most of the time, not all patients will be suitable candidates or require this. The surgeon should still be familiar with the anatomy of the groin so that he/she can do a good Cooper's ligament repair when indicated.

CONCLUSION

A Cooper's ligament repair provides the best anchor for a strong posterior wall reconstruction, closes the femoral canal, and repairs all of the hernia defects that can occur in the groin. It requires a generous relaxing incision and careful technique around the femoral vessels. It is a more extensive operation and is associated with a slower convalescence than most hernia repairs.

Because of the success of the easier tension-free mesh repairs, Cooper's ligament repairs are done less frequently than in the past. However, they will continue to give excellent results whenever a posterior inguinal wall reconstruction is done.

REFERENCES

1. Barbier J, Carretier M, Richer JP. Cooper ligament repair: an update. *World J Surg* 1989;13:499–505.
2. Brock RC. *The life and work of Astley Cooper.* London: E&S Livingstone Ltd, 1952:164.
3. Cooper A. *The anatomy and surgical treatment of inguinal and congenital hernia.* London: JT Cox, 1804.
4. Cunningham J, Temple WJ Mitchell P, et al. Cooperative hernia study. Pain in the postrepair patient. *Ann Surg* 1996;224:598–602.
5. Friis E, Lindahl F. The tension-free hernioplasty in a randomized trial. *Am J Surg* 1996;172:315–319.
6. Fruchaud H. *Anatomie chirurgicale des hernies de l'aine.* Paris: G. Doin, 1956.
7. Heise CP, Starling JR. Mesh inguinodynia: a new clinical syndrome after inguinal herniorrhaphy. *J Am Coll Surg* 1998;187:514–518.
8. Ilzermans JNM, de Will H, Hop WCJ, et al. Recurrent inguinal hernia treated by classical hernioplasty. *Arch Surg* 1991;126:1097–1100.
9. Kark AE, Kurzen MN, Belsham PA. Three thousand one hundred seventy-five primary inguinal hernia repairs: advantages of ambulatory open mesh repair using local anesthesia. *J Am Coll Surg* 1998;186:447–455.
10. Litwin D. Risks to fertility with laparoscopic mesh repair. In: Arregui ME, Nagan RF. *Inguinal hernia, advances or controversies.* New York: Radcliffe Medical Press, 1994:223–225.
11. Lotheissen G. Zur radikaloperation den schenkelhernien. *Centralbl Chir* 1898;25:548–550.
12. McVay CB, Anson BJ. A fundamental error in current methods of inguinal herniorrhaphy. *Surg Gynecol Obstet* 1942;74:746–750.
13. McVay CB, Chapp JD. Inguinal and femoral hernioplasty. *Ann Surg* 1958;148:499–512.
14. McVay CB. The anatomic basis for inguinal and femoral hernioplasty. *Surg Gynecol Obstet* 1974;139:931–945.
15. McVay CB. Abdominal wall. *Anson and McVay: surgical anatomy,* 6th ed. Philadelphia: WB Saunders, 1984:560.
16. Nissen HM. Constriction of the femoral vein following hernia repair. *Acta Chir Scand* 1975;141:279–281.
17. Pettigrew RA, Burns HUG, Carter DC. Evaluating surgical risk: the importance of technical factors in determining outcome. *Br J Surg* 1987;74:791–794.
18. Ruggi G. Metado operativo meovo per la cura radicale dell'ernia crurale. *Bull Sci Med Bologna* 1892;7:223–229.
19. Rutkow IM. The recurrence rate in surgery. *Arch Surg* 1995;130:575–577.
20. Rutledge RH. Cooper's ligament repair: a 25-year experience with a single technique for all groin hernias in adults. *Surgery* 1988;103:1–10.
21. Rutledge RH. The Cooper ligament repair. *Surg Clin North Am* 1993;73:451–485.
22. Shamberger RC, Ottinger LW, Malt RA. Arterial injuries during inguinal herniorrhaphy. *Ann Surg* 1984;200:83–85.
23. Stoppa R, Wantz GE. Henri Fruchaud (1894–1960): a man of bravery, an anatomist, a surgeon. *Hernia* 1998;2:45.
24. Wantz GE. Anatomy of hernias of the groin. *Atlas of hernia surgery.* New York: Raven Press, 1991:1–10.
25. Wolfler A. Zur radikaloperation des freien leistenbruches. In: Festschrift TB, ed. *Beitrage zur chirurgie.* Stuttgart: Verlag Von Ferdinand Enke, 1892:552–603.

EDITORS' COMMENTS

Dr. Rutledge has updated and improved his previous contribution to this text. This remains an operation of important historic interest, although less popular now because of the tension-free repairs. The main indication now is for the patient with destruction of the entire inguinal floor, in whom a prosthesis is contraindicated. Perhaps more important, though, is that this operation is the basis for what my residents like to call the "Fitztenstein" procedure. Instead of sewing the inferior border of a prosthesis to the shelving edge of the inguinal ligament as in a usual Lichtenstein hernioplasty, the inferior edge is sewn to Cooper's ligament with a transition to the shelving edge as Dr. Rutledge describes for his Cooper's ligament repair.

R.J.F., Jr. and A.G.G.

Nyhus and Condon's Hernia, Fifth Edition, edited by Robert J. Fitzgibbons, Jr. and A. Gerson Greenburg. Lippincott Williams & Wilkins, Philadelphia © 2002.

14

LICHTENSTEIN TENSION-FREE HERNIOPLASTY FOR THE REPAIR OF PRIMARY AND RECURRENT INGUINAL HERNIAS

PARVIZ K. AMID

Cooper, in the early 1900s, recognized that inguinal hernias were not simply caused by mechanical force of straining. Heredity, debility, and age also had adverse effects on the strength of the abdominal wall. Halsted emphasized the importance of the principle of avoiding tension in a successful hernia repair.

Harrison questioned the mechanical concept of herniation once again in 1922 by stating, "When we consider the dozens and hundreds of men who first showed hernias at 50–60, after their active life is over, the hypothesis becomes improbable to say the least."

Billroth speculated: "If only the proper material could be created to artificially produce tissue of density and toughness of fascia and tendon, the secret of the radical cure of hernia would be discovered."

This type of thinking inspired investigators to develop a host of prosthetic materials. Many were associated with disastrous complications related to rejection and infection. Usher is credited with popularizing the use of polypropylene mesh, which has been in use since the mid-1950s with a negligible complication rate. Although not tissue, this material would appear to otherwise meet the criteria suggested in Billroth's dream.

In 1984, Lichtenstein addressed the issue of tension by popularizing routine use of mesh, coining the term "tension-free" hernioplasty.

It was left to Nyhus to remove the fear of infection and rejection when he stated in 1989, "My concerns relative to the potentially increased incidence of infection or rejection of the polypropylene mesh have not been warranted to date" (21).

Today, understanding the role of protease–antiprotease imbalance in the pathogenesis of groin hernias has led to a new grasp of the pathology of groin hernias and the causes of their surgical failure (25). There is biochemical evidence that some adult male inguinal hernias are associated with impaired hydroxylation of proline, resulting in decreased levels of hydroxyproline. These changes lead to weakening of the fibroconnective tissue of the groin and development of inguinal hernias (25). To use this already defective tissue, especially under tension, is a violation of the most basic principles of surgery. Furthermore, approximation of the transverse tendon to structures such as the inguinal ligament or iliopubic tract results in widening of the femoral ring and development of iatrogenic femoral hernias.

In the tension-free hernioplasty, instead of suturing anatomic structures that are not normally in apposition, the entire inguinal floor is reinforced by insertion of a sheet of mesh. The prosthesis, which is placed between the inguinal floor and the external oblique aponeurosis, extends well beyond Hesselbach's triangle in order to provide sufficient mesh/tissue overlap. Upon increased intraabdominal pressure with straining, contraction of the external oblique applies counterpressure on the mesh, thus using the intraabdominal pressure in favor of the repair. The procedure is both therapeutic and prophylactic in that it protects the entire susceptible region of the groin to herniation from future mechanical and metabolic adverse effects.

Local anesthesia is preferred for all reducible adult inguinal hernias (1). It is safe, simple, effective, economical, and without the side effects of nausea, vomiting, and urinary retention. Furthermore, local anesthesia administered prior to making the incision produces a prolonged analgesic effect via inhibition of the build-up of local nociceptive molecules (1). Several safe and effective anesthetic agents are currently available. Our choice, however, is a 50:50 mixture of 1% lidocaine (Xylocaine, Astra Pharmaceuticals,

P. K. Amid: Department of Surgery, Harbor UCLA and Harbor UCLA Research and Education Institute, Torrance, California; Department of Surgery, Cedars–Sinai and Harbor UCLA Medical Centers; and Lichtenstein Hernia Institute, Los Angeles, California.

L.P., Wayne, PA, U.S.A.) and 0.5% bupivacaine (Marcaine, Abbott Laboratories, North Chicago, IL, U.S.A.), with 1/200,000 epinephrine.

TECHNIQUE OF ANESTHESIA

An average of 45 mL of this mixture is usually sufficient for a unilateral hernia repair and is administered in the fashion described below.

Subdermal Infiltration

About 5 mL of the mixture is infiltrated along the line of the incision, with a 5-cm long 25-gauge needle inserted into the subdermal tissue parallel with the surface of the skin. Infiltration continues as the needle is advanced. Movement of the needle reduces the likelihood of intravascular infusion of the drugs because even if the needle penetrates a blood vessel, the tip will not remain in the vessel long enough to deliver a substantial amount of the anesthetic agent intravenously. This step blocks the subdermal nerve endings and reduces the discomfort of the intradermal infiltration, which is the most uncomfortable stage of local anesthesia.

Intradermal Injection (Making of the Skin Wheal)

The needle in the subdermal plane is withdrawn slowly until the tip of the needle reaches the intradermic level. Without extracting the needle completely, the dermis is infiltrated by slow injection of about 3 mL of the mixture along the line of the incision.

Deep Subcutaneous Injection

A total of 10 mL of the mixture is injected deep into the subcutaneous adipose tissue through vertical insertions of the needle (perpendicular to the skin surface) 2 cm apart. Again, injections are continued as the needle is kept moving to reduce the risk of intravascular infusion.

Subaponeurotic Injection

About 10 mL of the anesthetic mixture is injected immediately underneath the aponeurosis of the external oblique muscle through a window created in the subcutaneous fat at the lateral corner of the incision. This injection floods the enclosed inguinal canal and anesthetizes all three major nerves in the region, while the remaining subcutaneous fat is incised.

It also separates the external oblique aponeurosis from the underlying ilioinguinal nerve, reducing the likelihood of injuring the nerve when the external oblique aponeurosis is incised.

Occasionally, it is necessary to infiltrate a few milliliters of the mixture at the level of the pubic tubercle, around the neck, and inside the indirect hernia sac to achieve complete local anesthesia.

The local anesthesia can be further prolonged by splashing 10 mL of the mixture into the inguinal canal before closure of the external oblique aponeurosis and in the subcutaneous space before skin closure (6).

Epidural anesthesia is preferred for repair of nonreducible inguinal hernias. Sedative drugs given by the surgeon, or preferably by an anesthetist as "conscious sedation" via infusion of rapid short-acting amnesic and anxiolytic agents such as propofol (Diprivan, manufactured by Zeneca Pharmaceuticals, Wilmington, DE, U.S.A.), reduce the patient's anxiety. This also reduces the amount of local anesthetic agents required, particularly for bilateral inguinal hernia repair.

TECHNIQUE OF THE OPERATION

A 5-cm skin incision, which starts from the pubic tubercle and extends laterally within Langer's lines, gives an excellent exposure of the pubic tubercle and the internal ring. After skin incision, the external oblique aponeurosis is opened and its lower leaf freed from the spermatic cord. The upper leaf of the external oblique is then freed from the underlying internal oblique muscle and aponeurosis for a distance of 3 cm above the inguinal floor.

The anatomic cleavage between these two layers is avascular, and the dissection can be done rapidly and nontraumatically. High separation of these layers has a dual benefit: (a) improved visualization of the iliohypogastric nerve and (b) creation of ample space for insertion of a sufficiently wide sheet of mesh that can overlap the internal oblique by at least 3 cm above the upper margin of the inguinal floor. The cord with its cremaster covering is separated from the floor of the inguinal canal and the pubic bone for a distance of about 2 cm beyond the pubic tubercle.

The anatomic plane between the cremasteric sheath and the aponeurotic tissue attached to the pubic bone is avascular, so there is no risk of damaging the testicular blood flow. When lifting the cord, care should be taken to include the ilioinguinal nerve, external spermatic vessels, and the genital nerve with the cord. This assures that the genital nerve, which is always in juxtaposition to the external spermatic vessels, is preserved (Fig. 14.1). I have found this method of preserving the genital nerve safer and easier than the originally described "lesser-cord" method (2) (a method in which the genital nerve and external spermatic vessels are separated from the cord in the form of a bundle referred to as "lesser cord" and passed through a gap along the suture line of the mesh with the inguinal ligament). The iliohypogastric nerves should also be preserved.

To explore the internal ring for indirect hernia sacs, the cremasteric sheath is incised longitudinally at the deep ring

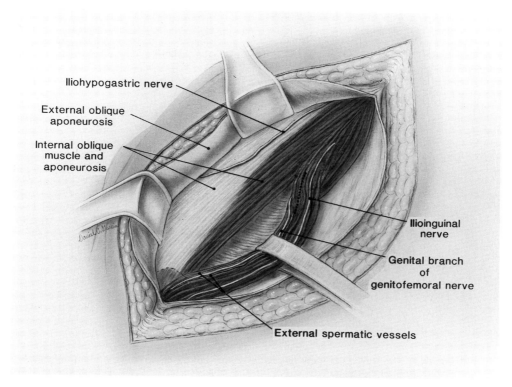

FIGURE 14.1. Spermatic cord together with its cremasteric covering, inguinal nerve, external spermatic vessels, and genital nerve is raised, and the cremasteric fibers are cut transversely or longitudinally at the level of the internal ring.

(Fig. 14.1). Complete stripping and excision of the cremasteric fibers is unnecessary, and can result in injury to the nerves, small blood vessels, and vas deferens. Furthermore, it can lead to the testicles hanging too low.

Indirect hernial sacs are freed from the cord to a point beyond the neck of the sac and inverted into the abdomen without ligation. Due to mechanical pressure and ischemic changes, it has been suggested that ligation of the highly enervated peritoneal sac is a major cause of postoperative pain (26). It has been shown that nonligation of the indirect hernia sac does not increase the chance of recurrence (26). To minimize the risk of postoperative ischemic orchitis, complete nonsliding scrotal hernia sacs are transected at the midpoint of the canal, leaving the distal section in place. However, the anterior wall of the distal sac is incised to prevent postoperative hydrocele formation.

In the event of direct hernias, if large, the sacs are inverted with an absorbable suture (Fig. 14.2). A thorough exploration of the groin is necessary to rule out the coexisting intraparietal (interstitial), low-lying spigelian or femoral hernias. The femoral ring is routinely evaluated via Bogros' space through a small opening in the canal floor. A sheet of 8 × 16 cm of mesh is used. We prefer monofilamented polypropylene meshes because their surface texture pro-

motes fibroplasia and their monofilamented structure does not perpetuate or harbor infection (3). The medial end of the mesh is cut to the shape of the medial corner of the inguinal canal. With the cord retracted upwards, the rounded corner is sutured, with a nonabsorbable monofilamented suture material, to the anterior rectus sheath above the pubic bone and overlapping the rectus sheath by 1 to 1.5 cm (Fig. 14.3). This is a crucial step in the repair because failure to cover this bone with the mesh can result in recurrence. The periosteum of the bone is avoided. This suture is continued (as a continuous suture with not more than 3 to 4 passes) to attach the lower edge of the mesh to the inguinal ligament up to a point just lateral to the internal ring. Suturing the mesh beyond this point is unnecessary and could injure the femoral nerve. If there is a concurrent femoral hernia, the mesh is also sutured to Cooper's ligament 1 to 2 cm below its suture line with the inguinal ligament to close the femoral ring (Fig. 14.3).

A slit is made at the lateral end of the mesh, creating two tails, a wide one (two thirds) above and a narrower (one third) below. The upper wide tail is grasped with a hemostat and passed toward the head of the patient from underneath the spermatic cord; this positions the cord between the two tails of the mesh (Fig. 14.4).

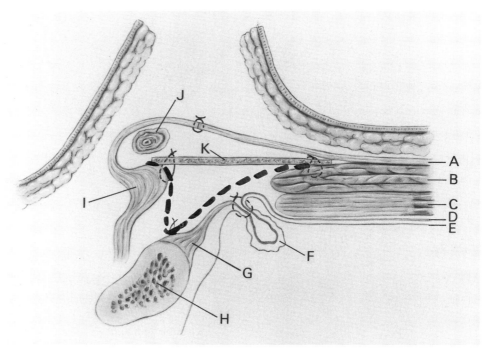

FIGURE 14.2. Fixation of the mesh to Cooper's ligament for closure of the femoral ring (*dotted line*). *A*, external oblique aponeurosis; *B*, internal oblique muscle; *C*, transversus aponeurosis; *D*, transversalis fascia; *E*, peritoneum; *F*, inverted direct sac; *G*, Cooper's ligament; *H*, pubis; *I*, inguinal ligament; *J*, spermatic cord; *K*, mesh patch bridging defect.

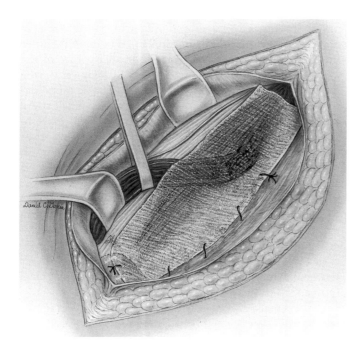

FIGURE 14.3. Medial corner of the patch overlaps the pubic bone by 1 to 1.5 cm.

The wider upper tail is crossed and placed over the narrower one and held with a hemostat (Fig. 14.5). With the cord retracted downward and the upper leaf of the external oblique aponeurosis retracted upward, the upper edge of the patch is sutured in place with two interrupted absorbable sutures, one to the rectus sheath and the other to the internal oblique aponeurosis just lateral to the internal ring. Occasionally, the iliohypogastric nerve has an abnormal course and stands against the upper edge of the mesh. In those instances, a slit in the mesh will accommodate the nerve. Upward retraction of the upper leaf of the external oblique during this phase of the repair is important because it results in the appropriate amount of laxity (in a dome-like configuration) for the patch when the retraction is released. This laxity assures a true tension-free repair and is taken up when the patient strains on command during the operation or resumes an upright position. More importantly, it compensates for the future shrinkage of the mesh, which, according to our clinical and laboratory studies, is approximately 20% (3).

Using a single nonabsorbable monofilamented suture, the lower edges of each of the two tails are fixed to the inguinal ligament just lateral to the completion knot of the lower running suture. This creates a new internal ring made of mesh (Fig. 14.6). The crossing of the two tails produces a configuration similar to that of the normal transversalis fascia sling, which is assumed to be largely responsible for

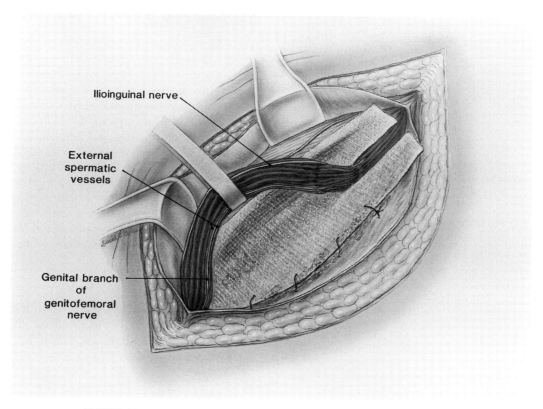

Ilioinguinal nerve

External
spermatic
vessels

Genital branch
of
genitofemoral
nerve

FIGURE 14.4. Spermatic cord is placed between the two tails of the mesh.

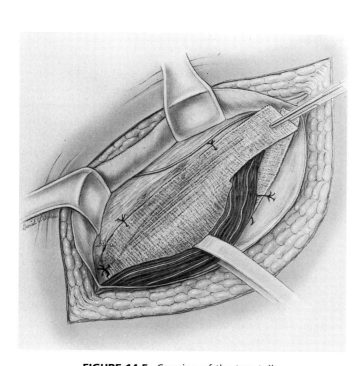

FIGURE 14.5. Crossing of the two tails.

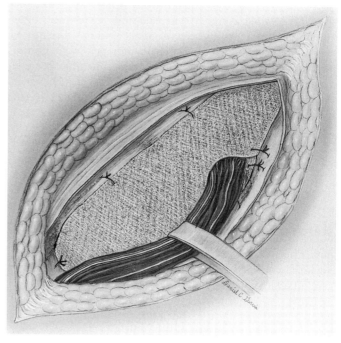

FIGURE 14.6. The lower edges of the two tails are sutured to the inguinal ligament for creation of a new internal ring made of mesh.

the normal integrity of the internal ring. In addition, it results in the creation of a dome-like sagittation (or tenting up) of the mesh in this area and assures a tension-free repair of the internal ring area.

The excess mesh on the lateral side is trimmed, leaving at least 5 cm beyond the internal ring. This is tucked underneath the external oblique aponeurosis (Fig. 14.6), which is then closed over the cord with an absorbable suture. Fixation of the tails of the mesh to the internal oblique muscle, lateral to the internal ring, is unnecessary and could result in entrapment of the ilioinguinal nerve with the fixation suture.

OUTCOME MEASURES

As reported by more than 100 authors from Europe and the United States, the results of open tension-free hernioplasty are outlined in sections titled "Postoperative Pain," "Return to Work," "Recurrence Rate," and "Complications," below.

Postoperative Pain

Regardless of the approach, laparoscopic or open, tension-free mesh repair of inguinal hernias results in minimal postoperative pain, requiring only moderate oral analgesic for a period of 1 to 4 days. Several prospective randomized studies, including those by Horeyseck (17) and Filipi et al. (13), show no statistical difference in postoperative pain following open tension-free hernia repair compared with the laparoscopic tension-free technique. In fact, a five-armed study by Kawji et al. (20), comparing Lichtenstein repair under local anesthesia, Lichtenstein repair under general anesthesia, laparoscopic repair, Shouldice repair, and open properitoneal repair, showed that postoperative pain and the postoperative analgesic requirement were lowest after Lichtenstein repair under local anesthesia, followed in order by Lichtenstein under general anesthesia, laparoscopic repair, Shouldice, and open properitoneal repair. This is not to say that one approach is less painful than the other; instead, it is only to conclude that tension-free repair (regardless of the approach) is associated with minimal discomfort, which results in a faster recovery and return to normal activities.

Return to Work

Returning to work after hernia operation is a complex socioeconomic issue that largely depends on preoperative patient education and patient motivation. In general, return to work after tension-free hernioplasty (regardless of the approach) is between 2 and 14 days, depending on the patient's occupation. As published in several major series, return to work after open tension-free repair for bilateral inguinal hernia is a maximum of 2 days longer than unilateral repair (5,19,27). This is equally comparable with return to work after laparoscopic repair of bilateral inguinal hernia.

Recurrence Rate

The reported recurrence rate for this procedure is less than 1%. Early in the development of tension-free hernioplasty, several patients at the Lichtenstein Hernia Institute developed recurrences as a result of technical errors. Three hernias recurred at the pubic tubercle because of a failure to overlap the bone with the mesh. One resulted from total disruption of the mesh from the inguinal ligament because the mesh was too narrow. Lessons learned from these recurrences led to overlapping the mesh with the pubic bone, increasing the width of the mesh to approximately 7.5 cm, and keeping the mesh slightly wrinkled. These refinements, adopted by this author in the late 1980s, served to further decrease the postoperative pain and compensate for the future shrinkage of the mesh in order to avoid recurrences (2,4).

Complications

Complications such as infection, hematoma, and seroma occur in approximately 1% of the cases. The most serious complications associated with the technique are chronic neuralgia and testicular atrophy, which occur in a fraction of 1%.

TECHNICAL CONSIDERATION

Using a wide piece of mesh to overlap tissues beyond the boundary of Hesselbach's triangle for 3 to 4 cm is important in order to reduce the chance of recurrence. After incorporation is complete, this overlap results in uniform distribution of intraabdominal pressure over the much wider surface of the overlapped area, rather than just the line where the mesh is joined to the tissue. More importantly, it compensates for future shrinkage of the mesh described previously (3). Placement of the mesh over the inguinal floor and behind the external oblique aponeurosis uses the intraabdominal pressure in favor of the repair. Contraction of the external oblique keeps the mesh tightly in place by acting as an external support when intraabdominal pressure rises with straining. Although a sound concept, placement of the mesh underneath the transversalis fascia, in the preperitoneal space, requires unnecessary dissection of this highly complex anatomic space and may lead to major bladder and neurovascular injuries. In fact, a recent prospective randomized study comparing Lichtenstein's repair with repair by placement of the mesh behind the transversalis fascia indicated no difference in the recurrence rate (7). In addition, the study concluded that Lichtenstein's repair was easier to perform, teach, and learn (7). Proper fixation of the margins of the mesh to the groin tissue is another important step in the prevention of recurrence. In mobile areas such as the groin, there is a tendency for the prosthesis to fold, wrinkle, or curl around the cord. Even the slightest movement of the mesh from the pubic tubercle, the inguinal ligament, or the area of the internal ring is a leading cause of failure of mesh repair of inguinal hernias. Adequate laxity of the mesh must be allowed during fixation to totally eliminate tension and compensate for increased intraabdominal pressure when the patient stands or strains, and for contraction of mesh which, according to our laboratory and clinical studies, is 20% after implantation of the mesh *in vivo* (3). A mesh that is completely flat with no ripple in a patient under sedation and in a recumbent position will be subject to tension when the patient strains or is in a standing position.

REPAIR OF RECURRENT INGUINAL HERNIAS

Our preferred method of repair for recurrent inguinal hernias was the mesh plug technique. The concept of the mesh plug technique was based on the assumption that recurrent inguinal hernias occur through a single defect in an otherwise intact inguinal floor, requiring minimal dissection limited to the area of the defect for the repair. This assumption was proved wrong by Greenburg's study, which demonstrated that 10% of recurrent inguinal hernias consisted of more than one defect (15). Furthermore, insertion of a plug behind the transversalis fascia and into the small Bogros' space places the plug in close proximity with the iliac vessels. In fact, erosion of the plug into these vessels has been reported (10). Mesh plug repair fails due to a variety of factors: (a) missing a second defect as a result of inadequate dissection; (b) failure of the repair due to shrinkage of the plug (4,14); depending on their looseness, mesh plugs [Lichtenstein's cigarette plug, Gilbert's umbrella plug, and Robin–Rutkow's Perfix plug (manufactured by Davol, Inc., Cranston, RI, U.S.A.)] lose up to 75% of their diameter; (c) infection of the plug requiring its explantation; and, more importantly, (d) serious complications such as 5.5% to 8.6% chronic postoperative pain, requiring explantation of the plug (23,24,28); migration of the shrunken plug to the scrotum (4,12); and erosion of the plug into the bladder (3), intestines (8,11,16), and femoral vessels (10). Therefore, in 1996, the mesh plug was completely abandoned by the Lichtenstein Group and all recurrent inguinal hernias were repaired by the patch technique, similar to the repair of primary inguinal hernias.

In 400 hernioplasties performed for the repair of recurrent inguinal hernias, there was only one recurrence in the parapubic region in a patient who had a previous open prostatectomy. The same recurrence rate has been reported by other authors (18).

CONCLUSION

Since the introduction of the open tension-free hernioplasty in 1984, the operation has been evaluated and compared to other types of hernia repairs in several studies with regard to postoperative pain, postoperative time off work, complications, costs, and recurrence rates. Comparison of papers from different institutions studying the same conventional herniorrhaphies are characterized by a considerable variation in results from institution to institution, whereas studies of the open tension-free hernioplasty report remarkably uniform results, a fact that increases the validity of the individual studies.

Published series, many from European universities, demonstrate that the open tension-free hernioplasty can safely be performed under local anesthesia and allows the patient's immediate mobilization, keeping hospital stay, cost, and patient discomfort to a minimum. Furthermore, published recurrence rates are uniformly low (1% or less) after tension-free operation performed as described above. Additionally, a metaanalysis of randomized controlled trials of laparoscopic versus conventional inguinal hernia repair demonstrated no difference when laparoscopic repair was compared with open tension-free repair (9).

More than 15 years after the beginning of the tension-free hernioplasty in 1984 and 12 years after the publication of the first series of open tension-free hernioplasty in 1989, the operation has been thoroughly evaluated in large series and has been gaining increasing acceptance with surgeons around the globe. In fact, a recent survey in England showed that 70% of British surgeons are now employing the Lichtenstein tension-free method of hernia repair (22).

Large series and randomized studies indicate that excellent results from the open tension-free operation are less dependent on the experience of the surgeon than results from conventional tissue repair and laparoscopic operation, an indication of the simplicity of the operation and short learning curve (17,27). The same technique can safely be applied to all inguinal hernias, indirect and direct, as well as recurrent hernias (4,18).

REFERENCES

1. Amid PK, Shulman AG, Lichtenstein IL. Local anesthesia for inguinal hernia repair step-by-step procedure. *Ann Surg* 1994; 220:735–737.
2. Amid PK, Shulman AG, Lichtenstein IL. Critical scrutiny of the open tension-free hernioplasty. *Am J Surg* 1993;165:369–371.
3. Amid PK. Classification of biomaterials and their related complications in abdominal wall hernia surgery. *Hernia* 1997;1:12–19.
4. Amid PK, Lichtenstein IL. Long-term result and current status of the Lichtenstein open tension-free hernioplasty. *Hernia* 1998;2: 89–94.
5. Amid PK, Shulman AG, Lichtenstein IL. Simultaneous repair of bilateral inguinal hernias under local anesthesia. *Ann Surg* 1996; 223:249–252.
6. Bays RA, Barry L, Vasilenko P. The use of bupivacaine in elective inguinal herniorrhaphy as a fast and safe technique for relief of postoperative pain. *Surg Gynecol Obstet* 1991;173:433–437.
7. Bonwich JP, Johnson DD, Read RC, et al. Randomized trial of superficial and preperitoneal prosthetic mesh placement in inguinal hernia repair. *Hernia*1998;1[Suppl]:S3.

8. Chuback JA, Singh RS, Sills C, et al. Small bowel obstruction resulting from mesh plug migration after open inguinal hernia repair. *Surgery* 2000;127:475–476.
9. Chung RS. Meta-analyses of randomized controlled trials of laparoscopic versus conventional inguinal hernia repair. *Surg Endosc* 1999;7:68–94.
10. Cristaldi M, Pisacreta M, Elli M, et al. Femoro-popliteal by-pass occlusion following mesh-plug for prevascular femoral hernia repair. *Hernia* 1997;1:197–199.
11. Danielli PG, Kurihara H, Montecamozzo G, et al. Le complicanze dei plugs: infezioni e recidive. *Hernia* 1997;1:55.
12. Dieter RA Jr. Mesh plug migration into scrotum: a new complication of hernia repair. *Int Surg* 1999;84:57–59.
13. Filipi CJ, Gaston-Johansson F, McBride PJ, et al. An assessment of pain and return to normal activity: laparoscopic herniorrhaphy vs open tension-free Lichtenstein repair. *Surg Endosc* 1996;10:983–986.
14. Gai H. Hernienoperation mach Lichtenstein. *Chir Praxis* 1998;54:183–195.
15. Greenburg AG. Revisiting the recurrent groin hernia. *Am J Surg* 1987;154:35–40.
16. Gilbert AI, Graham MF. The internal inguinal ring is nature's window into the preperitoneal space—why not use it? In: Chevrel JP, ed. *Hernias and surgery of the abdominal wall,* 2nd ed. New York: Springer–Verlag, 1998:210–214.
17. Horeyseck G, Roland F, Rolfes N. Die "spannungsfreie" reparation der leistenhernie: laparoskopisch (TAPP) versus offen (Lichtenstein) *Chirurg* 1996;67:1036–1040.
18. Horeyseck G, Pohl C. Lichtenstein-patch repair of recurrent inguinal hernia. *Hernia* 1998;2[Suppl]:S6.
19. Kark AE, Kurzer MN, Belsham PA. Three thousand one hundred seventy-five primary inguinal hernia repairs: advantages of ambulatory open mesh repair using local anesthesia. *J Am Coll Surg* 1998;186:447–456.
20. Kawji R, Feichter A, Fuchsjäger A, et al. Postoperative pain and return to activity after five different types of inguinal herniorrhaphy. *Hernia* 1999;3:31–35.
21. Nyhus LM. The preperitoneal approach and iliopubic tract repair of inguinal hernia. In: Nyhus LM, Condon RE, eds. *Hernia,* 3rd ed. Philadelphia: JB Lippincott Co, 1989:154–177.
22. O'Riordan DC, Morgan M, Kingsnorth AN, et al. The surgical management of inguinal hernias in England. *Hernia* 1998;2[Suppl]:S17.
23. Palot JP, Avisse C, Cailliez-Tomasi JP, et al. The mesh plug repair of groin hernias: a three year experience. *Hernia* 1998;2:31–34.
24. Pelissier EP, Blum D, Damas JM, et al. The plug method in inguinal hernia: a prospective evaluation. *Hernia* 1999;4:201–204.
25. Read RC. A review: the role of protease–antiprotease imbalance in the pathogenesis of herniation and abdominal aortic aneurism in certain smokers. *Postgrad Gen Surg* 1992;4:161–165.
26. Smedberg SGG, Broome AEA, Gullmo A. Ligation of the hernia sac? *Surg Clin N Am* 1984;64:299–306.
27. Wantz, GE. Experience with tension-free hernioplasty for primary inguinal hernias in men. *J Am Coll Surg* 1996;193:351–360.
28. Zdolsek JM, Kald A, Enebog J, et al. A prospective evaluation of mesh-plug hernioplasty in 385 consecutive inguinal hernias. Paper presented at: The International Hernia Conference: Hernia in the 21st Century; June 2000; Toronto, Ontario; p. 200.

SPECIAL COMMENTS

Muhammed Ashraf Memon

Lichtenstein first published his experience of "onlay sutured mesh tension-free hernioplasty" in 1986 (3). The experience involved 300 consecutive inguinal hernias with a 2-year follow-up. This experience was updated in 1989, when Lichtenstein and colleagues reported the use of this technique in 1,000 cases with minimal complications and a zero recurrence rate after a follow-up of between 1 and 5 years (4). However, they were ridiculed by the Anglo-American surgical community following this publication. Remarks such as ". . . results as presented are laughable" were allowed to appear in subsequent issues of the American Journal of Surgery (5). However these comments failed to deter Lichtenstein and colleagues, who continue to practice their craft to this day, with extremely impressive results (6).

One of the important changes in the modern inguinal hernia surgery is the advent of laparoscopic inguinal herniorrhaphy. Surgeons very early on realized that the only satisfactory way of repairing inguinal hernias laparoscopically was with the use of a large mesh. This provided the much needed boost for "anterior tension-free hernioplasty." This, combined with the ease of learning and mastering this technique, has resulted in widespread acceptance of anterior tension-free hernioplasty by surgeons on both sides of the Atlantic. The reproducibility of the superb results yielded by this technique outside of the Lichtenstein clinic was confirmed in two subsequent publications analyzing the incidence of wound infection, mesh rejection, and recurrence rate of nonexpert surgeons (7,8). These results no doubt testify to the simplicity and reliability of the Lichtenstein repair by surgeons with no special interest in hernia surgery.

I started using the Lichtenstein technique of tension-free hernioplasty in 1994 for both primary and recurrent inguinal hernias, with notably one difference, i.e., instead of using a monofilament nonabsorbable suture to secure the mesh to the floor of the inguinal canal, I started stapling it. I called this technique "anterior stapled mesh inguinal hernioplasty" (Figs. 14.7 and 14.8). I currently use the Multifire VersaTack (Autosuture, Ascot, U.K.) stapling gun, which comes with a reloading unit. This gun is especially designed for anterior her-

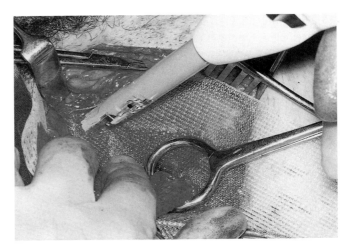

FIGURE 14.7. Stapling mesh with the Multifire VersaTack.

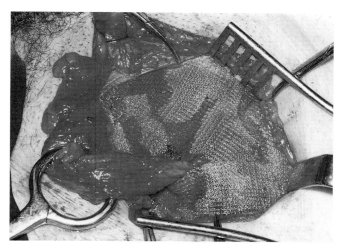

FIGURE 14.8. Mesh completely stapled to the inguinal floor.

nia repair and is very easy to use. Studies in the porcine model have unequivocally demonstrated that staples are safe, can be firmly attached to tissue, and are not dislodged by an increase in intraabdominal pressure (2). Carroll and Semel (1) have confirmed the security of stapled mesh in humans during Valsalva's maneuver and cough using fluoroscopy in the early postoperative period.

The potential benefits of stapling the mesh include:

1. Not inadvertently penetrating vessels such as the inferior epigastric artery with a needle, especially when anchoring the inferior border of the mesh to the inguinal ligament.
2. The avoidance of deep biting sutures reduces tissue manipulation and trauma, which may lead to reduced postoperative pain. Similar mechanisms may play a role in reducing postoperative pain in laparoscopic inguinal herniorrhaphy.
3. Because staples do not penetrate the various layers of the inguinal floor, the risk of spread of infection is virtually eliminated.
4. The use of interrupted small staples compared to continuous sutures has the potential advantage of avoiding nerve compression or entrapment. This, in turn, decreases the incidence of neuralgic pain both in the short and long term.
5. Preventing osteitis pubis. This has been reported with suturing of the mesh to the pubic tubercle. I think even with the greatest of care in the world, it is difficult to be certain if the needle has not traversed through the periosteum.

6. It is far easier, simpler, and faster to staple the mesh compared to suturing it. It takes me on average 20 minutes (results not published) to repair a primary unilateral inguinal hernia.
7. Titanium staples are more inert compared to any suture material used. This may decrease the incidence of foreign body granuloma or abscess.
8. The use of a stapling gun allows for a smaller skin incision to secure the mesh accurately and with ease over a much wider area compared to a sutured repair (at least in my experience) and thereby has some merit as far as the comesis is concerned.

The downside to this technique is the cost. On average, it costs £90 ($127.50 U.S.) to secure the mesh using the stapling gun, whereas the cost of suturing the mesh is £3.26 ($4.61), no doubt a big difference!

Of all the current repairs available for inguinal hernias, the Lichtenstein repair, whether sutured or stapled, is simple and reliable. However, I personally feel that the stapling method has certain potential advantages over the sutured repair. Only time will tell if staples will completely replace sutures for the Lichtenstein repair.

REFERENCES

1. Carroll BJ, Semel CJ. Stapled mesh herniorrhaphy. In: Arregui ME, Nagan RF, eds. *Inguinal hernia: advances or controversies?* New York: Radcliffe Medical Press, 1994:353–355.
2. Dion YM, Charara J, Guidoin R. Bursting strength evaluation of an experimental hernia repair using Prolene mesh attached to tissue with EMS stapler or with US surgical Endopath. Paper presented at: Annual Meeting of the Society of the American Gastrointestinal Endoscopic Surgeons; April 1993; Phoenix, Arizona.
3. Lichtenstein IL. *Hernia repair without disability*, 2nd ed. St. Louis: Ishiyaku EuroAmerica, 1986.
4. Lichtenstein IL, Shulman AG, Amid PK, et al. The tension-free hernioplasty. *Am J Surg* 1989;157:188–193.
5. Sarr MG. The tension-free hernioplasty [Letter]. *Am J Surg* 1990; 160:139.
6. Shulman AG, Amid PK, Lichtenstein IL. The Lichtenstein open "tension-free" mesh repair of inguinal hernias. *Surg Today* 1995; 25:619–625.
7. Shulman AG, Amid PK, Lichtenstein IL. The safety of mesh repair for primary inguinal hernias: results of 3,019 operations from five diverse surgical sources. *Am Surg* 1992;58:255–257.
8. Shulman AG, Amid PK, Lichtenstein IL. A survey of non-expert surgeons using the open tension-free mesh patch repair for primary inguinal hernias. *Int Surg* 1995;80:35–36.

15

TENSION-FREE, SUTURELESS, PRESHAPED MESH HERNIOPLASTY

ERMANNO E. TRABUCCO
ARNALDO F. TRABUCCO

Over the years, various surgical techniques, with or without prosthesis, have been utilized in inguinal hernia repairs. After Lichtenstein introduced the concept of a tension-free repair in 1986 (2), this became the procedure of choice. We began using a tension-free sutureless repair with a preshaped mesh in 1989.

From 1989 to 1997, all primary inguinal hernioplasties at the Trabucco Hernia Institute, of which there were 3,422, were performed using this technique (7). A preshaped mesh alone or in conjunction with a three-dimensional plug was used. The plug was formed by folding a circular mesh into the shape of a dart. This was then inserted into the deep ring of indirect inguinal hernias after the reduction of the sac.

From 1997 to 1999, 275 herniorrhaphies were performed. During this period, the use of the three-dimensional plug was abandoned. Flat sheaths of mesh, which were slit to accommodate cord structures, were implanted (8), or suture narrowing of the deep inguinal ring in small indirect hernias was used instead. A sutureless preshaped onlay mesh was implanted routinely in both groups of patients.

The principles of the sutureless preshaped hernioplasty are based on the following observations:

1. There is an anatomically closed space in the inguinal canal below the external oblique aponeurosis—a subaponeurotic space, which we have come to refer to as the "inguinal box" (Fig. 15.1) (8). It had been observed that the size and shape of this space has minimal variations from one individual to another.
2. It is possible to design and utilize a preshaped mesh in all primary inguinal repairs. In other words, a universal preshaped-size mesh that will virtually always fit into the subaponeurotic inguinal space of every individual (Fig. 15.2) (7,8).
3. In order for a sutureless preshaped mesh to be effective, it must be rigid in consistency and possess a controlled memory (remain flat without a tendency to wrinkle or curl) (6).

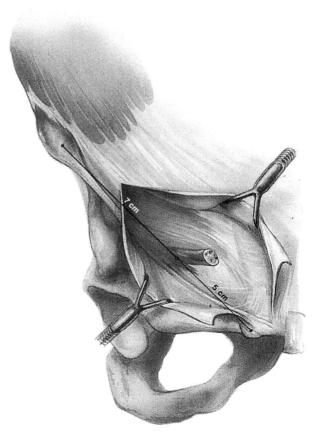

FIGURE 15.1. The open "inguinal box."

E. E. Trabucco: Department of Surgery, Trabucco Hernia Institute, Great Neck, New York.

A. F. Trabucco: Department of Surgery, Division of Urologic Surgery, Trabucco Institute, Rego Park, New York.

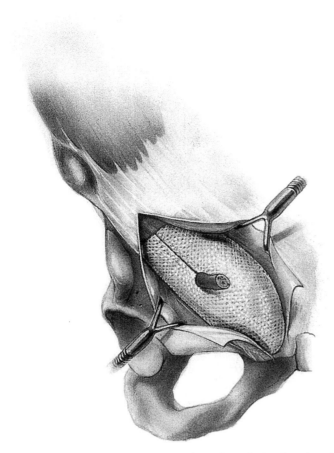

FIGURE 15.2. The sutureless preshaped mesh in the closed anatomic space of the inguinal box; cannot move.

SUBAPONEUROTIC INGUINAL SPACE

Its upper boundary is sealed by the insertion of the external oblique aponeurosis on the anterior rectus sheath. Its lower border ends in the concavity of the shelving edge of Poupart's ligament. The medial boundary is formed by the pubic tubercle and the lateral boundary by the blunt dissection of the subaponeurotic space, which usually ends 3.5 cm medial to the anterosuperior iliac spine. The bottom of this space is the floor of the inguinal canal, and the external oblique aponeurosis is the top of the space.

This anatomically closed space was measured during 800 hernioplasties (4–7). The average measurements were as follows: 12 cm from the anterosuperior iliac spine to the pubic tubercle, 7 cm from the anterosuperior iliac spine to the deep inguinal ring, 5 cm from the internal inguinal ring to the pubic tubercle, and 5 cm from the insertion of the external oblique muscle on the anterior sheath of the rectus muscle to the shelving edges of Poupart's ligament. The preshaped mesh was designed to fit a closed space with these measurements.

THE PRESHAPED MESH (USED AS AN ONLAY FOR THE INGUINAL CANAL)

This is made of monofilament polypropylene weaved into a mesh structure. The mesh is then treated with a combination of heat and traction in order to tighten the weave and flatten the mesh. This process allows the mesh to lose part of its memory (controlled memory) (6,7) and acquire a flat shape, thus losing its tendency to curl or wrinkle. The dimensions of the preshaped mesh are based on the average size and shape of the subaponeurotic inguinal space, which is 10 ± 4.5 cm. The mesh has a 1.2-cm in diameter circular opening for the exit of the spermatic cord. This opening is located 6 cm from the tip and 4 cm from the base of the mesh.

RIGIDITY OF THE MESH

Soft meshes placed on the floor of the inguinal canal without sutures will have a tendency to wrinkle or curl, thus increasing the potential for the formation of dead spaces and recurrences (6). Soft meshes such as Marlex (C.R. Bard, Inc., Murray Hill, NJ, U.S.A.) and Prolene (Ethicon, Inc., Somerville, NJ, U.S.A.) cannot be implanted without sutures. Curling from memory may also result from the manner in which the mesh is packaged. If the mesh is packaged folded, it will tend to fold and will not lie flat. All polypropylene prostheses have memory, even after sutures are applied.

In a sutureless technique, the mesh must lie flat when implanted and remain flat during the fibroblastic infiltration into its pores, a process that seals the mesh into place.

A rigid preshaped mesh with controlled memory does not need to be sutured when placed in a closed space. If implanted correctly, it will always lie flat and will not move or form dead space. Such a mesh is time saving and easy to implant. The postoperative discomfort is minimal and nerve injury rare. The prosthesis does not need to be shaped by hand at the time of surgery or fixed by sutures. Contamination due to handling or trimming a flat sheet of mesh is avoided, as well as tissue trauma produced by sutures. Most importantly, a sutureless prosthesis is always tension free and is not subject to tension along the suture line. Curling or wrinkling of a rigid mesh has never been observed.

SUTURELESS PROSTHESIS

A preshaped mesh of Marlex was first used in 1988. Later, this mesh was found to curl or wrinkle under the fascia, due to its soft consistency and presence of memory. The use of a double-layer preshaped mesh, a more rigid prosthesis, was proposed in 1990 (4). This preshaped mesh was made by placing two single sheets of Marlex (7), one on top of the other, and cutting them using an electric soldering tip. This double-layer mesh was found to have the desired rigidity and became very popular in Italy. The problem was that this preshaped mesh was not commercially available. Surgeons were forced to fabricate the meshes by themselves and to use illegal sterilization methods, which lack quality control. The U.S. Food and Drug Administration and C.E. (European Community) allow only approved industrial sterilization plants to sterilize medical devices. Both agencies have strict rules for quality control.

In the search for a single-layer mesh with the ideal rigidity and characteristics, 12 new single-layer polypropylene preshaped prostheses were fabricated and implanted in 36 patients undergoing inguinal hernioplasties in 1995 and 1996. Every type of mesh was implanted in three of these patients.

The prosthesis was made using monofilament polypropylene of 180 μm in diameter. A monofilament of 160 μm in diameter is used in soft meshes such as Marlex and Prolene. Each of the 12 meshes had a different knit structure. This accounted for differences in weight, thickness, and porosity. The traction and heat treatment the meshes were subjected to after weaving accounts for the "controlled memory."

The weight of each prosthesis was calculated in grams per square meter. Weights ranged from 90 to 240 g/m². The heavier the mesh, the greater the thickness and rigidity, and the lower the porosity. All meshes were observed during surgery for their ability to lie flat without wrinkling or curling. The ideal prosthesis was chosen on the basis of the following:

1. Weight—lower weights were preferred
2. Thickness—thinner meshes were preferred
3. Porosity—a greater porosity was preferred
4. Rigidity
5. Absence of memory
6. Tendency to remain flat after implant

Naturally, the final choice was a compromise. Nine of the meshes were discarded because of their tendency to curl when implanted without sutures. Their weights ranged from 90 to 168 g/m². The mesh of 240 g/m² was eliminated because it was too thick and its porosity too low. Two of the 12 meshes were eventually selected as being ideal for a sutureless technique. They were Hertra-R (rigid), of 223 g/m², and Hertra-S (semirigid), of 177 g/m². The Hertra preshaped prosthesis (7) always remained flat when implanted on the floor of the inguinal canal and was found not to shrink after implantation (3). It has been reported that other soft polypropylene meshes may shrink up to 20% (1). If a sutureless mesh shrinks, it may increase the risk of recurrence. The Hertra-S was used in individuals of normal weight and the Hertra-R in obese patients (Table 15.1).

CIRCULAR MESH FOR THE PREPERITONEAL SPACE

Primary inguinal hernias are flat defects of the thin transversalis fascia. They have no real depth. The use of a flat mesh should therefore be preferred to the use of a three-dimensional plug. Three-dimensional plug, such as the plug T2, is indicated only in repairs of tunnel-type defects such as a femoral or recurrent inguinal hernia (5). A flat mesh is a preperitoneal prosthesis that is placed around the spermatic cord. It is used in conjunction with a preshaped onlay mesh in the repair of medium-to-large indirect primary inguinal hernias (T4), or in large direct hernias with a loss of substance in the posterior wall (T5).

MESH T4 AND T5 (HERNIAMESH)

T4 is a 5-cm in diameter round preshaped mesh with a 1-cm eccentric hole. It is positioned around the spermatic cord in the preperitoneal space with the eccentric hole directed toward the iliac vessels, where the free space is limited. The enlarged deep ring is narrowed over the implanted T4. The mechanical containment of this mesh extends over the margins of the defect, unlike the containment of a

TABLE 15.1. CHARACTERISTICS OF PROSTHESES[a]

Mesh	Size of Monofilament	Weave	g/m2	Porosity	Thickness of Mesh
Hertra-R	180 μm	Two course Tuch mit Shuss	223	65.2%	0.68 mm
Hertra-S	180 μm	Two course Atlas Tuch	177	63.8%	0.53 mm
Hermesh 3	180 μm	Single course Atlas Tricot	127	69.7%	0.48 mm
Hermesh 4	180 μm	Single course Atlas	112	72.4%	0.45 mm
Hermesh 5	180 μm	Single course Atlas	107	68.3%	0.42 mm

[a]Herniamesh SRL, Via Cire 22/A, San Mauro Torinese, Torino, Italy 10099.

three-dimensional plug, which is limited to the inside of the defect. This mesh does not need suturing because it lies between the closed posterior wall above and the diverging elements of the spermatic cord below.

The mesh T5 is a preshaped mesh that is 5 cm in width and 10 cm in length. It has a 1-cm hole for the spermatic cord to pass through. It is used as a preperitoneal implant that is anchored to a preshaped Hertra mesh. The upper curved border of the mesh T5 reaches over the aponeurotic arch of the transversus muscle and its lower border follows Cooper's ligament. The distance between the hole for the exit of the spermatic cord and its medial aspect is 8 cm.

SUTURELESS PRIMARY INGUINAL HERNIOPLASTY

For the sake of simplicity, indirect hernias are classified as small, medium, or large. The direct hernias are classified as involving part of the posterior wall or all of the wall, and with loss of the posterior wall substance.

Small indirect hernias were repaired by dissection and reduction of the sac into the deep ring, which was then narrowed with sutures. A sutureless Hertra mesh was implanted and the external oblique aponeurosis closed over the mesh and under the spermatic cord.

Medium and large indirect hernias were repaired by dissection and reduction of the sac, followed by implantation of the T4 around the spermatic cord in the preperitoneal space. The posterior wall was closed over the mesh T4. A preshaped Hertra mesh was then implanted on the posterior wall of the inguinal canal. A Foley catheter was sometimes used to facilitate the placement of the mesh T4. The catheter was inserted into the deep inguinal ring and inflated with approximately 30 cc of air. The preperitoneal segment of the spermatic cord was exposed, allowing for an easier placement of the T4. The Foley was deflated and removed (Fig. 15.3).

Direct hernias with partial or total wall involvement were repaired by reduction of the sac with a continuous running suture, which flattened the floor of the inguinal canal, thus allowing for a better apposition with a preshaped Hertra mesh.

Direct hernias with loss of substance of the posterior wall were repaired using two anchored prostheses, a T5 and a Hertra. The posterior wall was opened and the preperitoneal fat dissected and retracted.

A Reverdin's needle carrying a suture material was introduced into the soft tissue near the pubic tubercle, directed toward the dissected preperitoneal space near the lacunar ligament. A loop suture was placed through the mesh T5, 2 cm from its medial aspect with the help of the needle (Fig.15.4). Both ends of the suture were pulled above the tubercle area by the Reverdin's needle and then inserted into the medial tip of the preshaped Hertra mesh.

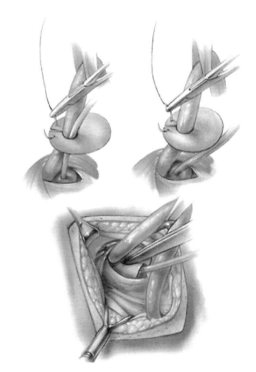

FIGURE 15.3. A Foley catheter facilitates the placement of a plug T4 around the spermatic cord in the preperitoneal space.

A Reverdin's suture needle, difficult to find in the United States but readily available in Europe, is an old valuable instrument for placing sutures in distant areas with good hand control. It is actually a combination of a needle holder and a needle. It comes in different sizes and curvatures and has a handle with a knob that controls the

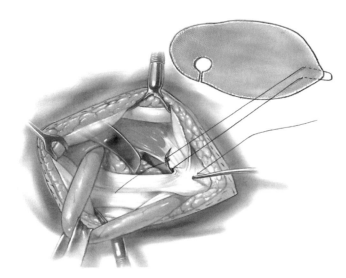

FIGURE 15.4. A Reverdin's needle facilitates the preperitoneal implant of a plug T0 by placing two loop sutures on the plug.

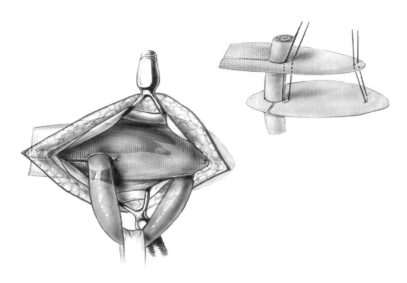

FIGURE 15.5. The posterior wall has been closed over the implanted plug T0. The two loop sutures are inserted in the preshaped mesh and are tied, controlling their tension.

opening and closure of the eye of the needle, similar to the eye of a sewing machine needle. Suture material placed in the needle's eye can easily and safely be pulled or pushed through tissues.

A loop suture was also placed near both openings for the exit of the spermatic cord in the T5 and the Hertra mesh. The posterior wall was closed without tension over the plug T5, and both sutures were tied over the preshaped Hertra mesh, controlling the tension between the two anchored prostheses (Fig. 15.5). Since the distance from the opening through which the cord passes to the medial tip is 6 cm in the Hertra and 8 cm in the T5, the medial aspect of the T5 is 2 cm longer and will reach Retzius' space.

After dealing with all kinds of direct or indirect hernial protrusions and the possible implants that could be used, the preshaped Hertra 1 or Herta 2 was selected. The mesh was implanted on the floor of the inguinal canal. The medial tip of the prosthesis was placed to overlap the pubic tubercle by at least 1 cm. The lateral aspect of the prosthesis ended about 3.5 cm lateral to the deep inguinal ring, and this is where the blunt dissection of the closed space ended. This preshaped mesh required adjustments in less than 1% of the cases (7). If the mesh was too long, trimming its proximal tip altered it. If the mesh was too short, its tip was pulled medially to overlap the pubic tubercle by 1 cm. In this case, the spermatic cord followed a short horizontal course on the floor of the inguinal canal before its exit trough the opening in the Hertra mesh. The external oblique aponeurosis was always closed over the mesh and below the spermatic cord (Fig. 15.6). The loss of obliquity of the inguinal canal, while important in pure suture repairs, plays no role in prosthetic repair. This closure allows the formation of a triple layer between the deep ring and the pubic tubercle, an area that is prone to recurrence. The

three layers are the transversalis fascia below, the aponeurosis of the external oblique above, and the preshaped mesh in the middle (Fig. 15.7).

RESULTS

A total of 3,422 hernioplasties were performed from 1989 to 1997, and 275 from 1997 to 1999.

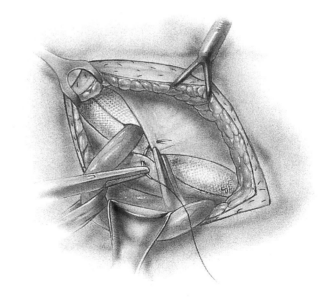

FIGURE 15.6. The external oblique aponeurosis is closed over the mesh, under the spermatic cord.

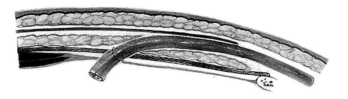

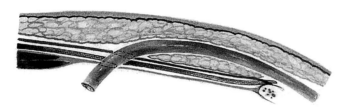

FIGURE 15.7. If the spermatic cord is in a subfascial position, the medial aspect of the floor of the inguinal canal is protected only by a mesh and transversalis fascia. If the spermatic cord is in a subcutaneous position, a triple layer is formed (transversalis fascia, mesh, and external oblique aponeurosis), a stronger protection against recurrences in an area where they occur more frequently.

In the first group, a Hertra mesh was used with or without a three-dimensional plug, which was placed in the deep ring of all indirect inguinal hernias.

In the second group, the T4 polypropylene prosthesis was used 130 times in medium and large indirect defects. A narrowing of the deep ring was performed 45 times in small indirect inguinal hernias. The T5 prosthesis was used six times in direct hernias with loss of substance of the posterior wall, instead of an unshaped preperitoneal mesh, which implanted in similar cases of the first group. The Herta mesh was implanted alone in all other direct hernias.

The results of the first group have been reported (7). The results of the second group were similar. The results of all 3,697 repairs are summarized as follows:

Ninety-seven percent of the patients were operated on under local anesthesia. The average stay of the patients at the surgical center was 150 minutes. All patients were instructed to walk 2 miles daily after surgery.

A total of 2,995 repairs (80%) were available for long-term follow-up and were actually examined by a surgeon. There were four recurrences, with a follow-up of 1 to 10 years. There were six persistent inguinal neuralgias, which were treated suc-

cessfully with neurectomies; all were in patients in whom a soft mesh was used. Two prostheses were removed due to persistent drainage, which resulted from wrinkled soft meshes. There were no mortalities, and other complications were minor. Minimal postoperative discomfort was observed, especially in those patients who ambulated immediately.

CONCLUSION

Three-dimensional plugs have been used with or without a mesh in the repair of primary inguinal hernias. This is the first time that a flat mesh has been used as a substitute for a three-dimensional plug in a totally sutureless repair. Sutures were used only six times for direct hernias with loss of substance in the posterior wall of the inguinal canal. The importance of rigidity in a preshaped sutureless mesh has been discussed.

The results demonstrate that this technique is simple and easy to learn. Compared to other tension-free repairs, there are fewer recurrences and complications, as well as less tissue trauma. The preshaped mesh technique saves surgical time. Its also prevents the possible contamination that results from handling a prosthesis that needs to be shaped by hand.

REFERENCES

1. Amid PK. Classification of biomaterials and their related complications in abdominal wall hernia surgery. *Hernia* 1987;1: 15–21.
2. Lichtenstein IL, Schulman AG, Amid PK, et al. The tension-free hernioplasty. *Am J Surg* 1989;157:188–193.
3. Petruzelli L, et al. Utilization of a rigid pre-shaped mesh according to the Trabucco technique: an experimental study. In: National Congress of SICADS. *Ambulatory Surgery in Italy, April 15–18, 1999*, Rome: Atti of Congress, 1999: p. 47.
4. Trabucco EE. The office hernioplasty and the Trabucco repair. *Ann It Chir* 1993;44:127–149.
5. Trabucco EE. Femoral and pre-peritoneal plugs. In: Bendavid R, ed. *Prostheses and abdominal wall hernias*. Austin: Landes, 1994: 411–412, 446–449.
6. Trabucco E, Campanelli GP, et al. Nuove protesi erniarie in polipropilene. *Min Chir* 1998;53:337–341.
7. Trabucco EE, Trabucco AF, Rollino R, et al. *Ernioplastica inguinale tension-free con rete presagomata senza suture secondo Trabucco*, vol II. Torino: Chirurgia Minerva Medica, 1998.
8. Trabucco EE, Trabucco AF. Flat plugs and mesh hernioplasty in the inguinal box: description of the surgical technique. *Hernia* 1998;2:133–138.

16

PLUG REPAIR OF INGUINAL HERNIA: INDICATIONS, TECHNIQUES, AND RESULTS

ULRIKE MUSCHAWECK

As early as from the beginning of advanced hernia surgery, the phenomenon of recurrence has repeatedly resulted in new approaches in terms of methodology and in modifications of existing techniques. It is anything but astonishing that the idea of bridging a hernia gap with synthetic material is more than 150 years old. In 1831, Belams had already made experiments with air bladders to correct an inguinal hernia. He tested this method on 30 dogs and finally also on three human patients—always with success. In 1900, Witzel (42) described the use of silver wire meshes on abdominal hernia, and in 1931, Fieschi used rubber sponges. Soon after World War II, synthetic polymer materials were developed for medical applications, which were used for various suture and mesh materials. In 1958, a woven polypropylene product (Marlex, C.R. Bard, Inc., Murray Hill, NJ, U.S.A.) was introduced. This material cleared the way for all future prostheses in hernia surgery. After positive experience had been gained with the application of mesh prostheses for incisional hernia, indications were extended to recurrent inguinal hernias: the value of tension-free patching of large defects in the fascia transversalis was superior to closing such defects with suture, which was destined to fail because of the tension created.

DEVELOPMENT OF THE MESH PLUG

Since the mid-1980s, the surgical techniques for repair of inguinal hernia have undergone a fundamental change. Aspects such as safety, recurrence rates, costs, and not least the comfort for the patients have been the repeated subjects of scientific studies (11,18,26,29,40). Within a few years, the application of mesh prostheses for hernia repair has become widespread. In 1997, a mesh prosthesis was used in more than 60% of all cases of inguinal hernioplasty. What is certainly decisive in this ever-increasing acceptance is the

availability of well-tolerated synthetic materials and the development of tension-free methods.

The idea of a tension-free hernia repair is mainly linked up with the words by Lichtenstein (18–21), Stoppa (37), Gilbert (11,12), and Amid (1–3). In distinction from the repair according to Bassini or Shouldice, the principle behind the "tension-free reconstruction" is the bridging of the defect with an alloplastic material, without closure of muscular or fascicle material above the hernia defect. The mesh prosthesis is not used as reinforcement of a hernioplasty with a primary suture, but rather represents the repair itself. The tension-free principle is applied by Lichtenstein and Stoppa, each in a different way: Lichtenstein places the prosthesis in the premuscular position, using a mesh at the extreme from the anterior iliac space to the rectus sheath; Stoppa, by contrast, applies the largest prosthesis size possible in the preperitoneal space in a retromuscular position. Newer modifications, which are spreading like mushrooms, can be traced back to the methodology developed by Lichtenstein and Stoppa.

Because the Lichtenstein patch merely covers the inguinal canal and the hernial orifice, it is smaller than a preperitoneal prosthesis. The Lichtenstein repair constitutes a straightforward operation for a primary hernia. However, dissection in scar tissue, which is required for spreading a flat prosthesis, is unnecessary for recurrent hernias. There is often a stable scar with a relatively small defect. This should not be destroyed just so that a large flat needle can be applied. In many cases, the surgical preparation is required. For this reason, Lichtenstein and Shore were the first, in 1974, to develop a cylindrically coiled mesh plug for the repair of recurrent femoral and inguinal hernias (21). This method permitted the very early establishment of a highly efficient repair with very low recurrence rates (31,33,34).

Several surgeons have improved and combined the Lichtenstein patch and plug techniques, creating very fanciful shapes of prostheses, such as an umbrella, a parachute, a butterfly, a mushroom, a flower, a bud, etc. After Bendavid had reported a mesh umbrella for the repair of

U. Muschaweck: Department of Hernia Surgery, Arabella-Klinik, Munich, Germany.

femoral hernia for the first time in 1987 (4), Gilbert established the tension-free "mesh plug method" in the late 1980s, using a polypropylene plug with the configuration of an umbrella for occluding initially indirect hernias only (11). He embedded the folded prosthesis through the inner inguinal ring into the preperitoneal space, assuming that the prosthesis would unfold there and occlude the inner inguinal ring without tension. In 1993, Rutkow and Robbins were the first to describe the tension-free mesh umbrella technique as a standard method for repair of primary inguinal hernia and recurrent inguinal hernia (26).

INDICATION FOR MESH PLUG APPLICATION

From the technical literature, widely varying information can be derived about the indications and techniques for repair of an inguinal hernia or a recurrent inguinal hernia by means of a plug. Worldwide, there are surgeons who use these prostheses only for repair of recurrent hernias (32) and those who employ the mesh plugs for any primary indirect or direct inguinal hernia (27). Which technique among the appropriate methods is employed and which form of prosthesis is selected among the great variety of different commercially available shapes will certainly depend mainly on the individual experience and results obtained by the individual surgeon.

As has been described above, Lichtenstein developed a patch for the repair of primary inguinal hernia and a plug in the form of a coiled polypropylene cylinder for repair of recurrent inguinal hernias and femoral hernias. Gilbert (11), by contrast, uses the tension-free "mesh plug method," using a polypropylene plug of umbrella-like configuration for occluding indirect hernias only. Rutkow and Robbins, on the other hand, apply the tension-free mesh umbrella technique to any primary inguinal hernia and recurrent inguinal hernias. Many surgeons have adopted this approach.

We consider recurrent inguinal hernias as well as femoral hernias to be the primary indications for a mesh umbrella application. When there is only a localized defect with the rest of the wall intact and sufficiently stable, the mesh umbrella implant provides a successful tension-free occlusion of the defect, without the need to resect stable scar tissue.

In 1995, we substituted this form of implantation for the flat Marlex mesh because the latter required too much dissection of normal healthy tissue, resulting in enlargement of the defect.

Today, we implant a mesh umbrella on approximately 80% of all patients suffering from a recurrent inguinal hernia. In 20% of the patients, the implantation of a mesh umbrella can be dispensed with because an intact fascia transversalis is encountered during the operation, which is frequently weakened. Even though a surgical operation had been performed previously, the fascia transversalis is not scarred, which means that it had not been affected by the preceding operation. In these cases, it is therefore easily possible to perform a classic Shouldice repair.

We have carried out a χ^2 test to study the problem of whether the application of a mesh plug is dependent on the type of the recurrence. At the 0.01% level, it became apparent with a high significance that the mesh plug application is preferred in the case of lateral and suprapubic recurrence, whereas there is a trend to dispense with the mesh in the case of medial and mediolateral recurrence.

Like Bendavid (4) and Amid (3), we deem femoral hernias and recurrent femoral hernias to be indications for mesh umbrella application.

SURGICAL TECHNIQUES

The technique of repairing recurrent hernias as described by Lichtenstein in 1974 (21) is performed with local anesthesia and with the smallest incision possible above the hernial orifice. With the patient actively straining to demonstrate the hernia, the external aponeurosis is exposed and lanced only in the region of the location where the hernia can be seen. Moreover, the spermatic cord is dissected only to an extent that is necessary for detaching the hernial sac. The hernial sac is pushed back through the hernial orifice into the preperitoneal tissue. The plug is then prepared by coiling one or two polypropylene strips with a dimension of 20 × 2 cm. It must fit into the hernial orifice so tightly that the patient cannot push it out even before the suture is fixed. The cylinder is fixed in the hernial annulus by six Prolene sutures placed above. Due to its depth, the cylinder diverges the hernial sac and the preperitoneal fat out of their direction of impact. Above the cylinder, the external aponeurosis, the subcutaneous tissue, and the skin are closed in the conventional manner.

Gilbert, by contrast, applies a "sutureless technique" in cases of small- and medium-sized indirect inguinal hernia. To this end, a polypropylene patch measuring 6 × 6 cm is slit over its half from one edge. The patch is then coiled to form a circular cone around the incision, grasped with a clamp, and advanced through the inner inguinal ring into the preperitoneal cavity. When the patient coughs, the patch unfolds and gets wedged behind the internal inguinal ring. If the hernia does not come out during this coughing maneuver, the patch is correctly positioned in the preperitoneal cavity in a properly unfolded form. The inguinal canal is then additionally reinforced with a second layer of flat Marlex mesh in the sense of an "onlay patch." The onlay mesh part is not intended to constitute an integral element of the repair, but it should rather serve to prevent the formation of a hernia in the future. Replacement is performed without any suture, the spermatic cord structures are placed on the front face of the "onlay patch," and a continuous absorbable suture is applied on the external aponeurosis.

Rutkow implants a preshaped mesh umbrella, in distinction from Gilbert, not only in cases of indirect hernia, but also in cases of direct hernia. With indirect hernias, including scrotal hernias, the hernial sac is first approached by longitudinally lancing into the fibers of the cremaster muscle along the spermatic cord. The high preparation of the hernial sac, which is characterized by the exposure of the preperitoneal fatty layers at the base of the indirect hernial sac, must be considered to constitute the most important step. It is this step that creates a pocket for plug positioning. The closed hernial sac, which is thus exposed, is then simply pushed back through the internal hernial ring into the abdominal cavity. The preshaped mesh umbrella is inserted through the internal inguinal ring, with the tapering end leading, and positioned just below the shanks of the inguinal ring. In the case of small indirect hernias, the plug is fixed by means of one or two isolated end-to-end sutures (Vicryl 3-zero, polyglactin 910, Ethicon, Inc., Somerville, NJ, U.S.A.) through the mesh and the inguinal shanks. In the case of large indirect hernias and scrotal hernias, the plug should always be fixed with several isolated end-to-end sutures at the edges of the inguinal ring. This fixation prevents the plug from possibly migrating. In cases of direct hernia, the thinned fascia transversalis is lifted with a clamp, and the hernial sac is circularly excised for exposure of the preperitoneal fat. This dissection must not be carried too far down into the intact fascia transversalis. The freed hernial sac and the overlapping thinned fascia transversalis are inverted to the inside. In a way similar to the repair of the indirect hernia, a plug is introduced into the defect, with the narrow end leading, and fixed by several isolated interrupted sutures at the surrounding intact tissue.

The mesh umbrella is fixed in accordance with the inguinal hernia type (following Rutkow's classification). In cases of type 1 inguinal hernia, i.e., indirect inguinal hernias with a narrow inguinal ring, the mesh plug is placed entirely without any suture because it remains in the proper position by itself. In all other cases of indirect and direct hernias, the mesh plug is fixed with interrupted sutures. Additionally, all primary hernioplasties and some of the recurrent hernioplasties are reinforced with a second layer of a flat Marlex mesh in a fashion similar to the "onlay patch" of Lichtenstein.

As has been mentioned previously, we prefer the Shouldice technique whenever possible for our patients suffering from primary, direct, or indirect hernias at our Munich Hernia Center. In cases with particularly large defects, we occasionally place a Marlex mesh under the fascia transversalis and incorporate this mesh into the first suture.

In cases of recurrent hernia we proceed as follows:

Under local anesthesia, the previous skin incision is opened and scar tissue excised. The external aponeurosis is longitudinally opened. Next, neurolysis of the nervus iliohypogastricus and the nervus ilioinguinals from the cicatricial tissue is carried out, and neurectomy is performed when needed. The ductus deferens, together with the plexus pampiniformis, is then carefully freed from its adhesions and encircled by means of an elastic cord. The floor of the inguinal canal is exposed, and the hernial sac is identified and exposed down to its base (Fig. 16.1). It is then reduced without opening it (Fig. 16.2).

The hernial orifice in the fascia transversalis is grasped with sharp small clamps. This allows the fascia to be lifted so that the mesh umbrella can be inserted into the defect (Fig. 16.3) and anchored with a circular continuous suture

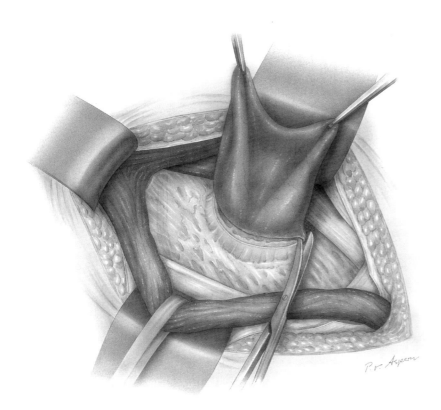

FIGURE 16.1. After exposure of the hernial sac, the base is circularly peritomized.

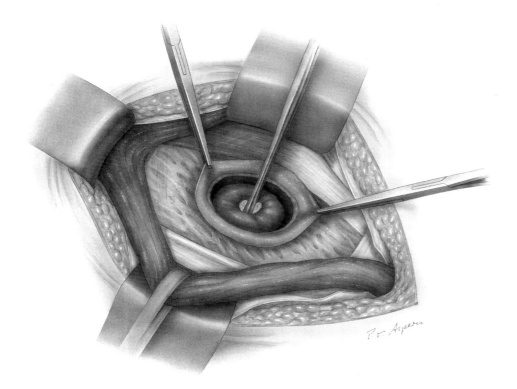

FIGURE 16.2. The hernial orifice is seized with sharp small clamps, and the hernial sac is repositioned in a closed form.

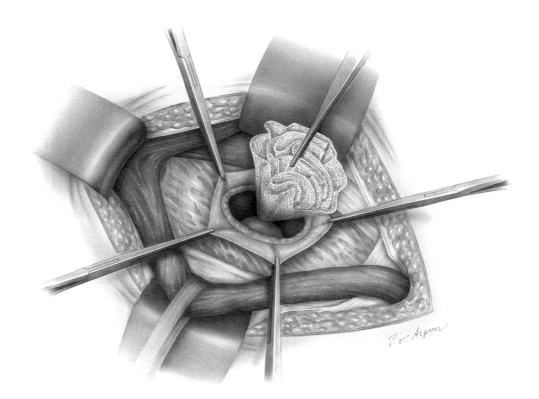

FIGURE 16.3. The fascia transversalis, which is located in the depth of the circumference of the hernial orifice, is seized with sharp small clamps. Insertion of the mesh umbrella in the defect at the level of the fascia transversalis.

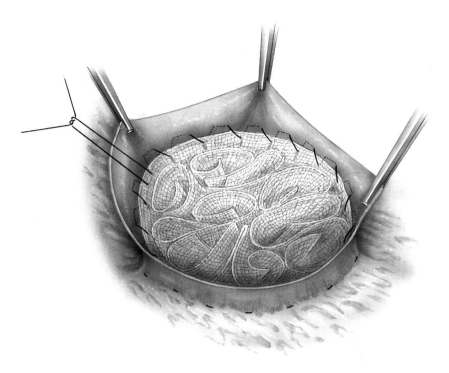

FIGURE 16.4. The mesh umbrella is anchored by means of a continuous circular suture. This is done in a way that a free flap of the fascia transversalis is retained.

(Fig. 16.4). This is done in a way that a free flap is retained on the transversalis, which can then be occluded above the mesh umbrella in a second suture line (Fig. 16.5). Next, the internal oblique muscle is fixed to the inguinal ligament, using continuous suture.

The cord structures are repositioned, and the external aponeurosis is closed with a double suture line. Polypropylene 2-zero is used as suture material. The wound is closed with a combination of subcutaneous sutures and subdermal interrupted end-to-end sutures.

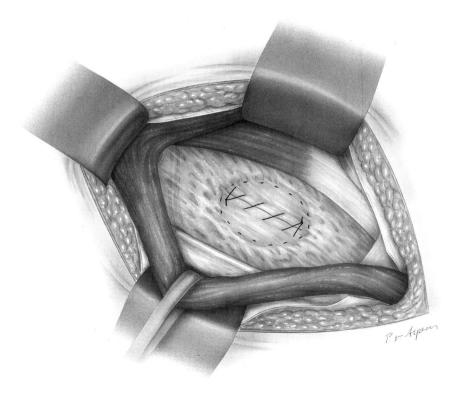

FIGURE 16.5. The retained free flap of the fascia transversalis is closed over the mesh umbrella by continuous suture and can be additionally fixed in a second line on the inguinal ligament.

In the majority of surgical techniques for repair of recurrent inguinal hernia that do not use an umbrella, healthy aspects of the inguinal floor must be incised again. This is true even with implantation of flat meshes because the defect must be unintentionally enlarged. With the application of a mesh umbrella, the repair can be restricted to the defect insert.

RESULTS AND DISCUSSION

Since December 1993, we have devoted our practice exclusively to hernia repair in our Hernia Center in Arabella-Klinik in Munich. Recurrent hernia accounts for approximately 15% of our workload. Out of this, 81.7% of the patients have suffered a first recurrence, 13.9% a second recurrence, and 4.4% a third or higher recurrence.

With a total number of hernia operations of more than 6,000, our own recurrence rate is lower than 0.5% and hence within the lower range of the frequencies quoted in literature to occur after an operation with the original Shouldice technique, which vary between 0.2% and 2.7% (5,39,41).

The recurrence rates after repair of a primary hernia with mesh application in the sense of a "tension-free repair" are comparable to these results, ranging from 0% to 1.65% (18,25,38).

In view of our low recurrence rates with the Shouldice repair, we are convinced that the general application of mesh implants for repair of all hernia types is not necessary, and we assess the problems occurring after mesh implantation to be critical.

As meshes made of monofilar polypropylene have been employed for hernia surgery since 1962, and with polypropylene having been used as suture material in surgery since approximately 1970, extensive documentation of their biocompatibility is available. In particular, the manufacturer has developed tests for cytotoxicity and chronic toxicity, and above all for genotoxicity, and passed all of these tests. The producer also warrants that not a single case of carcinogenic or neoplastic response has been reported. The team working under Schumpelick in Aachen recently published electron-microscopic, immunohistochemical, and histologic data on persisting inflammatory foreign body reactions, based on 121 flat meshes, including polypropylene meshes, that had to be removed (16,17). Following these results, a chronic inflammatory tissue response with the growth of connective tissue and macrophages manifested even several years later.

Isolated reports are available (8,10) in relation to plug migration into neighboring areas such as the scrotum or the small intestine. We did not observe a single case of migration because we anchor the plug by means of a continuous nonabsorbable suture in the *fascia transversalis* and cover the plug additionally in a second row of sutures through one flap of the *fascia transversalis* completely. With such an approach, we can operate without a mesh patch.

The problem of whether the transitions and edges created by preshaping the material into the form of a "plug" may trigger physical erosion on the tissue is another question. In this respect, not any hint may be found in the technical literature. Rutkow and Robbins (28) did not find any indication of plug-induced tissue erosion in the retrospective analysis of 407 cases. We noted a single case of peritonitis occurring 5 days after the operation among our own patients; in that case, plug-induced intestinal erosion cannot be precluded as the cause with ultimate certainty.

Numerous studies have dealt with the problem of mesh shrinkage. The inflammation that is induced by the mesh, which is mainly determined by the material and the size of the mesh, influences the extent of shrinkage. For instance, Amid (3) reported mesh shrinkage of 20% in length and 30% to 40% of total area. For prevention of recurrence, a sufficiently large mesh must therefore be implanted, which may create the sensation of a foreign body, particularly when the patient is leptosomatic. Recurrence induced by the strong shrinkage of the mesh can never be precluded. As a result of the occurrence of inflammation, the healing of the wound may be retarded.

Another disadvantage of mesh implants is the creation of stiffness of the abdominal wall by this mesh. This effect is a function of the mesh material employed, as has been demonstrated by three-dimensional stereographic studies (15).

Since the adoption of the mesh plug in 1995, and after more than 1,100 implantations, we have not observed a single case of recurrence in patients in whom this device has been implanted.

The technical literature reports a recurrence rate after mesh plug implantation between 0.5% and 1.6% (22,31). Similar results are described by authors employing other tension-free techniques, who report recurrence rates of 0% to 3.4 % in their patient populations (11,13,14,38).

The recurrence rates after application of traditional techniques have been reported in the literature. For instance, Cevese et al. (7) evaluated a recurrence rate of 13.4 % with Bassini's repair. The authors employing the Shouldice method in cases of recurrent hernia reported recurrence rates between 3.9 % and 6.4% (23,41).

Just as with primary repair, we have observed low rates of wound infection after mesh umbrella implantation. In our center, the rate of wound infection of less than 0.1% for both recurrent hernia and primary repair is extremely low compared with the figures reported in current literature, where rates between 0% and 2.4% are reported (9,30,35, 36). As has been described by several authors, one can establish that the mesh application and the rate of wound infection are independent of each other.

In roughly 8% of our patients undergoing mesh plug implantation, a *seroma* occurs, which is tapped under sterile conditions only in exceptional cases.

The application of meshes or mesh plugs does not result in an increased frequency of postoperative hematoma formation. Incidences between 0.4% and 18.7% are reported in literature (9,29,30,36). It is interesting to note that most of the studies report a similar hematoma incidence for hernioplasty with mesh and without mesh. The rates of complications seem rather to be correlated with the extent of dissection in repair with large prostheses and with the application of heparin.

It is extremely seldom that a transient ischemic orchitis occurs (less than 0.1%). Rates between 0% and 0.9% are reported in literature (9,30,36).

We have the further advantage that postoperative traumatic pain is distinctly lower after application of a mesh umbrella. This is due to reduced exposure, less strain on the tissue, and the conservation of intact cicatricial sections.

Several studies (6,24) have proved that patients undergoing repair with a mesh umbrella experience extremely light postoperative pain.

We did not observe chronic inguinal pain, which we have noted only in very rare cases (less than 0.2%) after hernioplasty, on a single patient after mesh umbrella implantation.

Mesh umbrella implantation by an experienced surgeon is a safe method. Particularly in cases of lateral recurrence, it is definitely required to ensure that the mesh umbrella will not cause injury on the vasa epigastrica. In cases of doubt, resection of the vasa epigastrica should be performed.

CONCLUSION

We consider the mesh umbrella implantation to be a substantial improvement for the repair of recurrent inguinal hernia.

In our hands, sufficient stability is achieved with the Shouldice technique in the majority of patients suffering from primary, direct, or indirect hernia. Because mesh application may give rise to potential disadvantages such as mesh shrinkage and changes in the mobility of the muscles of the anterior abdominal wall, we do not consider routine mesh implantation in any case of inguinal hernia to be justified.

Plug implantation in cases of recurrent hernia, by contrast, is a safe and reliable technique that offers many advantages. As the implantation of flat meshes requires the destruction of normal scarred areas, the defect is actually made worse. With the application of mesh umbrellas, it is possible to restrict the repair to the actual defect, which results in a tension-free occlusion of the defect.

Because of the light postoperative pain and the immediate physical exercise tolerance following tension-free closure of the wound, the patient can return to professional activities as early as 0 to 4 days postoperatively, can return to

physical exercise immediately, and can even resume sports activities without any restrictions.

REFERENCES

1. Amid PK, Shulman AG, Lichtenstein IL. Die Herniotomie nach Lichtenstein. *Chirurg* 1994;65:54–58.
2. Amid PK, Shulman AG, Lichtenstein IL, et al. The goals of modern hernia surgery. How to achieve them—open or laparoscopic repair? *Probl Gen Surg* 1995;12:165.
3. Amid P. Classification of biomaterials and their related complications in abdominal wall hernia surgery. *Hernia* 1997;1:5–8.
4. Bendavid R. A femoral "umbrella" for femoral hernia repair. *Surg Gynecol Obstet* 1987;165:153–156.
5. Berliner S, Burson L, Katz P, et al. An anterior transversalis fascia repair for adult inguinal hernias. *Am J Surg* 1978;135:633–636.
6. Brooks DC. A comparison of laparoscopic and tension-free open herniorrhaphy. *Arch Surg* 1994;129:361–366.
7. Cevese PG, Lise M, Spatari V. La chirurgia delléernia inguinale. Paper presented at: International Congress in Honour of E. Bassini; November 28–29, 1986; University of Padova, Padova, Italy.
8. Chuback JA, Singh RS, Dick LS. Small bowel obstruction resulting from mesh plug migration after open inguinal hernia repair. *Surgery* 2000;127:475–476.
9. Coda A, Ferri F, Fillipa C, et al. Open mesh-plug repair for primary inguinal hernia. *Hernia* 1999;3:57–63.
10. Dieter RA. Mesh plug migration into scrotum: a new complication of hernia repair. *Int Surg* 1999;84:57–59.
11. Gilbert A. Sutureless repair of inguinal hernia. *Am J Surg* 1992;163:331–335.
12. Gilbert A. Overnight hernia repair: updated consideration. *South Med J* 1987;80:191–195.
13. Gruwez JA. Lichtenstein repair with e-PTFE. Paper presented at: Xth Grensland Symposium; March 1992; Leuven, Belgium; p. 43.
14. Kaufman M, Weissberg D, Bider D. Repair of recurrent inguinal hernia with Marlex mesh. *Surg Gynecol Obstet* 1985;160:505–506.
15. Klinge U, Conze J, Klosterhalfen B, et al. Changes in abdominal wall mechanics after mesh implantation. Experimental changes in mesh stability. *Langenbecks Arch Chir* 1996;381:323–332.
16. Klinge U, Klosterhalfen B, Müller M, et al. Foreign body reaction to meshes used for repair of abdominal wall hernias. *Eur J Surg* 1999;165:665–673.
17. Klosterhalfen B, Klinge U, Hermanns B, et al. Pathology of traditional surgical nets for hernia repair after long-term implantations in humans. *Chirurg* 2000;71:43–51.
18. Lichtenstein IL, Shulman AG, Amid PK, et al. The tension-free hernioplasty. *Am J Surg* 1989;157:188–193.
19. Lichtenstein IL, Shulman AG. Ambulatory outpatient hernia surgery, including a new concept, introducing tension-free repair. *Int Surg* 1986;71:1–4.
20. Lichtenstein IL. Herniorrhaphy: a personal experience with 6,321 cases. *Am J Surg* 1987;153:553–559.
21. Lichtenstein IL, Shore JM. Simplified repair of femoral and recurrent inguinal hernia by a "plug" technique. *Am J Surg* 1974;128:439–444.
22. Lichtenstein IL, Shulman AG, Amid PK, et al. The tension-free hernioplasty. *Am J Surg* 1989;157:188–193.
23. Obney N, Chan CK. Repair of multiple time recurrent inguinal hernias with reference to common causes of recurrence. *Contemp Surg* 1984;25:25.
24. Pélissier EP, Blum D. The plug in inguinal hernia: prospective

evaluation of postoperative pain and disability. *Hernia* 1997;1: 185–189.

25. Peyton-Barnes J. Inguinal hernia repair with routine use of Marlex mesh. *Surg Gynecol Obstet* 1987;165:33–37.

26. Robbins AW, Rutkow IM. The mesh-plug hernioplasty. *Surg Clin North Am* 1993;73:501–512.

27. Rutkow IM, Robbins AW. Hernioplastik mit Netzplombe. *Chirurg* 1997;68:970–976.

28. Rutkow IM, Robbins AW. The mesh plug technique for recurrent groin herniorrhaphy: a nine-year experience of 407 patients. *Surgery* 1998;124:844–847.

29. Rutkow IM. Laparoscopic hernia repair: the socioeconomic tyranny of surgical technology. *Arch Surg* 1992;127:1271.

30. Schmitz R, Treckmann J, Shah S, et al. Die "tension-free-Technik" bei offener Leistenhernienoperation. *Chirurg* 1997;68:259–263.

31. Shulman AG, Amid PK, Lichtenstein IL. The "plug" repair of 1402 recurrent inguinal hernias: a 20-year experience. *Arch Surg* 1990;125:265–267.

32. Shulman AG, Amid PK, Lichtenstein IL. Patch or plug for groin hernia—which? *Am J Surg* 1994;167:331–336.

33. Shulman AG, Amid PK, Lichtenstein IL. Prosthetic mesh plug repair of femoral and recurrent inguinal hernias: the American experience. *Ann R Coll Surg Engl* 1992;74:97–99.

34. Shulman AG, Amid PK, Lichtenstein IL. Plug repair of recurrent inguinal hernias. *Contemp Surg* 1992;40:30–33.

35. Soler M, Stoppa R, Verhaeghe P. Polyester (Dacron) mesh. In: Bendavid R, ed. *Prostheses and abdominal wall hernias*. Austin: RG Landes Co, 1994:26.

36. Spier N, SD Berliner. The open tension-free mesh repair of inguinal hernia. Analysis of 1235 cases. *Hernia* 1998;2:81–83.

37. Stoppa RE. The treatment of complicated groin and incisional hernias. *World J Surg* 1989;13:545–554.

38. Trabucco E. ATTI updating course in general and GI surgery. March 20–22,1991; Milan, Italy; p. 45.

39. Volpe L, Galli T. The Shouldice repair—our experience. Paper presented at: Acts of the Congress on General and Gastrointestinal Surgery. March 20–22,1991; Hospital San Carlo Borremeo di Milan, Italy.

40. Wantz GE. Laparoscopic herniorrhaphy. *J Am Coll Surg* 1997; 184:521–522.

41. Wantz GE. The Canadian repair of inguinal hernia. In: Nyhus LM, Condon RE, eds. *Hernia*, 3rd ed. Philadelphia: JB Lippincott, 1989:236–248.

42. Witzel O. Über den Verschluß von Bauchwunden und Bruchpforten durch versenkte Silberdrahtnetze. *Zbl Chirurg* 1900;10: 257–260.

Nyhus and Condon's Hernia, Fifth Edition, edited by Robert J. Fitzgibbons, Jr. and A. Gerson Greenburg. Lippincott Williams & Wilkins, Philadelphia © 2002.

17

TENSION-FREE HERNIOPLASTY USING A BILAYER PROSTHESIS

ARTHUR I. GILBERT
MICHAEL F. GRAHAM

Abdominal wall and groin hernia repairs are no longer mundane operations, as surgeons are challenged to decide between many successful techniques that have evolved in the past 20 years. They ask, should I use mesh? If so, should I use it occasionally or routinely? If tension-free procedures are really the current gold standard for hernia repair, why does the Shouldice repair continue to have so many devoted proponents? If mesh prostheses are the answer to the age-old problem of recurrence, is mesh best used as a plug, a patch, or both? Should mesh be used anterior or posterior to the defect in the groin? Why not use it in both planes to doubly protect the repair? And when considering open tension-free techniques versus laparoscopic methods, which procedure is easiest to learn, can be performed by most general surgeons more safely and successfully, will least incapacitate patients, and can be done at less expense to each country's national health care budget?

The senior author (A.I.G.) first became seriously interested in the details of hernia surgery in 1976. Prior to then, from 1962, when he finished residency training, until 1976 he used the modified Bassini operation to repair all types of primary and recurrent inguinal hernias. Though he did not keep a record of results during that early phase of his surgical career, approximately 15% of his primary hernia repairs and at least 25% of his recurrent hernias repairs failed. Until 1976, most surgeons practicing in Miami did not perform hernia surgery using local anesthesia. General anesthesia was preferred; regional anesthesia was used occasionally.

In 1976, he received an invitation to visit the Shouldice clinic in Toronto, Canada, from Dr. Nicolas Obney, its surgical director at that time. That invitation followed a patient being referred there who needed to have a hernia repaired but whose general condition did not permit anything but a local anesthetic. Dr. Obney's invitation was accepted, and 3 days were spent observing the talented her-

nia surgeons of the Shouldice Clinic perform groin herniorrhaphies using local anesthesia. It became quickly evident that the success of their operation stemmed from a few factors. Those surgeons clearly understood the inguinal region as evidenced by their knowledgeable dissection of the various tissue planes of the inguinal anatomy. They operated using local anesthesia with the patient awake enough to cooperate in demonstrating the hernial defects and the completeness of the repair by testing it before the wound was closed. And the essential step of the Shouldice dissection is to open the posterior wall from the internal ring partway or completely to the pubic tubercle. Seeing them operate introduced those three components and allowed a better understanding of the anatomy of the groin, particularly Bogros' space.

When the senior author returned to Miami, he began to employ the Shouldice operation using a local anesthetic with intravenous sedation. He used the Shouldice repair for all primary and most recurrent inguinal hernias from 1976 to 1984. The only two specifics of the Shouldice technique that were altered were that 3-zero Prolene suture material was used rather than stainless steel wire, and that the skin was closed with staples rather than Michel clips. The first 25 patients were kept in the hospital for 3 nights following the Shouldice format. Because they did so well, the next group of 25 was kept for only 2 nights. That group did so well that the next group was kept for just 1 night. The results using the Shouldice technique were published in an article entitled "Overnight Hernia Repair: Updated Considerations" (3). Patients on whom Shouldice repair was employed were followed mostly by annual recalls and yearly examinations. Failure of repairs for primary hernias in this group was 2%; and for recurrent hernias, 8%. In the group of indirect hernias repaired, the peritoneal sac was ligated and divided unless a sliding component complicated them.

In 1984, at the first 3-day surgical meeting devoted exclusively to herniology, improved results were reported after switching from the modified Bassini repair to the Shouldice repair (8). Everett Shockett, a Miami surgeon, suggested that

A. I. Gilbert: Department of Surgery, University of Miami; and Hernia Institute of Florida, Miami, Florida.

M. F. Graham: Hernia Institute of Florida, Miami, Florida.

since the posterior wall of the canal was already being opened for a Shouldice repair, a swatch of polypropylene mesh could be used in the properitoneal space to reinforce the suture lines of the repair. Shockett's suggestion was adopted and polypropylene mesh became used routinely in essentially every primary hernia repair. For direct hernias, the posterior wall was still opened through the defect, separating the properitoneal fat from the under surface of the transversalis fascia and thereby actualizing the potential Bogros' space. A 1.5 × 3-inch swatch of polypropylene mesh was placed in the space between the underlying properitoneal fat and the overlying tissues, which was imbricated with four rows of continuous Prolene suture. Annual follow-up examinations were conducted, and over the next 5 years there was a reduction in failures to 0.3% for primary hernias and 3.0% for recurrent hernias.

Later in 1984, the senior author borrowed Lichtenstein's concept of a hand-rolled polypropylene plug and used it in the internal ring to repair indirect hernias. (Lichtenstein had used the plug to repair femoral and small direct hernias, but never in the internal ring for indirect hernias.) He no longer ligated the sac. Instead, it was invaginated through the internal ring. He next placed the hand-rolled plug in the internal ring and secured it in place to the surrounding tissues with a few sutures. That accomplished the immediate repair of the presenting hernia. He soon began to question the rationale of the traditional next step of the Bassini and Shouldice repairs of indirect hernias, that of opening the intact posterior wall of Hesselbach's triangle, and then having to repair or reinforce it. If it wasn't broken, why break it and then need to fix it?

In conjunction with the plug repair at the internal ring, he elected to stop opening the intact posterior wall of indirect hernias. To reinforce it against deformation with possible future direct herniation, he placed a swatch of polypropylene mesh as an onlay patch anterior to it. The plug worked well to repair primary and recurrent inguinal hernias; however, it was not completely free of problems. Occasionally, thin patients complained of feeling their plug. Responding to that complaint and a fortuitous event that occurred one day during repair of an indirect hernia under local anesthesia, he altered the procedure. After dissecting the peritoneal sac free and reducing it through the internal ring, he unintentionally inserted the rolled plug a bit too deep, getting it completely through the internal ring into Bogros' space. Feeling that this error needed immediate correction, he instructed the patient to cough and strain to push the plug out. The patient was unable to push either the plug or the peritoneal sac out. The possibility of using the internal inguinal ring as an access route to the properitoneal Bogros' space was immediately recognized. From that time on, and for the various modifications of that original technique, he has used the internal ring as the avenue to place mesh behind the abdominal wall, thereby doing a posterior mesh repair through an open anterior approach. The plug in the properitoneal space acted as a barrier. No sutures were required for effectiveness. Added to

the posterior plug, he continued to protect the intact posterior wall of Hesselbach's triangle with a polypropylene onlay mesh patch. Like the rolled plug in the properitoneal space, he believed the onlay mesh patch did not require suture fixation. The spermatic cord and the sutured external oblique aponeurosis held the onlay patch securely in place.

After a few months of success with the rolled plug, there was some concern reagarding the possibility of damage to the urinary bladder or the bowel by the wadded mesh of the plug. This promoted the next modification of the technique. With some help from engineers at the University of Miami, the unrolled plug was converted to an umbrella plug for the posterior component of the repair. Actually, "umbrella plug" was a misnomer for the patch developed and used for the posterior repair. It would better have been named an "umbrella patch" because it was designed to open into a flat mesh once it was passed through the internal ring.

This technique was described as the *sutureless repair of inguinal hernia* in an article published in 1991 (4). For many years, it was displayed at scientific exhibit sections of the annual meetings of the American College of Surgeons. Surgeons who viewed it remarked that they believed it worked, but they were reluctant to try it because of concern that the unsutured underlay patch would migrate.

Until 1998, for indirect hernias, the senior author used the Prolene umbrella plug and onlay patch repair for all indirect hernias. For direct hernias, he continued to use the Shouldice repair, protecting it with a Prolene underlay patch. Our repair for indirect hernias was completely tension free and sutureless. Our repair for direct hernias was not tension free until 1998, when he began using the latest generation of the repair, the Prolene Hernia System, a bilayer one-piece mesh device. Incorporated in the new one-piece device are all of the components of previous generations of our technique, while it most notably eliminates surgeons' concerns about migration of the underlay patch. The preliminary dissection is styled after that performed at the Shouldice Hospital and is part of the best pure-tissue repair currently being done.

In 1987, 1990, and 1993, he proposed to Ethicon, Inc. (Somerville, NJ, U.S.A.) that it consider manufacturing the design of the mesh umbrella plug and patch into a single device. It wasn't until 1997, some years after other manufacturers had introduced products designed around the principles of his internal ring mesh repair, that Ethicon decided to become involved. This led to his becoming the clinical surgeon–consultant to Ethicon, Inc. in its development of the Prolene Hernia System device. He designed its shape and the dimensions of its patches and connector for the three sizes that are currently available. He continues to be a consultant to Ethicon for its mesh products, without proprietary interest in any of its products. Since 1986, when he gave up doing general surgery, his surgical interest has been devoted exclusively to hernial problems of the abdominal wall. Together with two associates, who also restrict their work to hernial surgery, he annually operates on more than a thousand patients who need groin and other abdominal wall hernia repairs.

DEFINITIONS

Certain terms have become part of the parlance of modern-day hernia surgery. A *prosthesis* is an artificial replacement for a body part. A *graft* is derived from natural tissue. A *plug* is a hand-rolled or prefabricated mesh device that is shaped like a cylinder or a shuttlecock. A *patch* is a flat swatch of mesh. An *onlay patch* is a swatch of mesh placed anterior to the inguinal canal's posterior wall. An *underlay patch* is a swatch of mesh placed in the properitoneal space posterior to the inguinal canal's posterior wall. The *myopectineal orifice* is the natural aperture in the pelvic–groin area through which the spermatic cord and femoral vessels pass. It is bounded medially by the rectus muscle and fascia, inferiorly by Cooper's ligament, laterally by the iliopsoas muscle, and superiorly by the internal oblique and transversus abdominus muscles. The *lateral triangle* is the area bounded by the middle third of the inguinal ligament, the deep epigastric vessels, and a reach from the junction of the upper and middle thirds of the inguinal ligament to where the deep epigastric vessels pass behind the rectus muscle. To *actualize* a space is to open a potential space that exists in a normal tissue plane, such as Bogros' space. *Plasticity* is the ability of tissues to resume their natural state and shape after they have been stretched. *Deformation* is the progressive process of tissue degeneration that can eventually result in a clinical hernia.

It is important that surgeons appreciate the concepts and consequences of plasticity and deformation when considering their functional significance to tissues affected by any repair. Appreciation of these natural physical qualities in tissues is even more critical as pertains to mesh repairs. Prosthetic mesh plugs placed in the internal ring of an indirect hernia, or in the defect of a direct hernia, will barricade the space in which the plug is set. The problem created by a plug is that the unprotected tissue surrounding it, especially in the lateral triangle, must shoulder considerable intraabdominal force around the fixed point of the plug without losing its plasticity and progressing to form a recurrent hernia. Mesh applied to protect the entirety of the lateral and medial triangles can accomplish this. In patients who returned with a recurrence following our own repairs, we found that most failures developed lateral to the internal ring. These recurrences do not represent breakdown of the sutured plug or rupture in the medial mesh patch. They developed because there were areas of imbalance of resistance of the posterior wall between the double bellies of the transversus abdominus and internal oblique muscles that originate from the lateral one third of the inguinal ligament and the mesh protection we had placed in the medial triangle. The tissues within the lateral triangle, protected only by the thinner fibers of the internal oblique muscle, progres-

sively weakened until clinical herniation developed. This could have been avoided, and can be prevented by using anterior and posterior patches that reach far enough lateral and medial to protect the entire myopectineal orifice.

GILBERT REPAIRS OF INGUINAL HERNIA

The internal ring is nature's window into the properitoneal space (5). The basic principle of this repair, and subsequent generations of the repair, is applicable to every type of indirect inguinal hernia. The herniated peritoneum and its contents must be reduced to within the abdominal cavity. Then, to prevent either from reherniating through the musculoaponeurotic plane of the anterior abdominal wall, the internal ring is buttressed with a properitoneal mesh patch. To avoid insult to the testicle or distal spermatic cord in cases of a larger or longer peritoneal sac, the sac's proximal or middle portion is divided and the distal sac left untouched. The proximal sac is fully dissected, ligated, and reduced. Regardless of how the distal portion of the sac is treated, a meticulously high dissection to the level of the true neck of the sac is required to free it from its attachments at the musculofascial threshold of the deep ring (Fig. 17.1). The level of ligation of the sac need not be too high, similar to a peritoneal

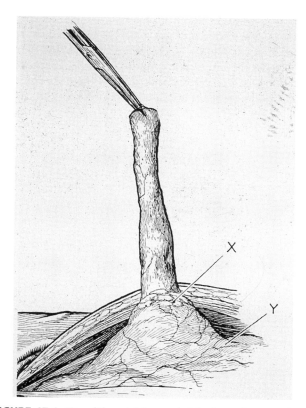

FIGURE 17.1. True (*Y*) and false neck (*X*) of sac. (Henry's drawing from *Lancet* 1936, Fig. 5:533.)

sac with a sliding component. In all cases, the peritoneal sac should be closed to prevent contact between the mesh and any viscus.

Prior to insertion of the mesh, it is necessary to actualize the properitoneal Bogros' space. The sac is separated from the elements of the spermatic cord and from the transversalis fascia deep to the internal ring. Conceptually, it is similar to Stoppa's "parietalization" of the spermatic cord from the peritoneum in his "giant prosthetic reinforcement of the visceral sac" (GPRVS) procedure (2). Dissecting the "shoulders" of the peritoneal sac through the internal ring actualizes the properitoneal space (Fig. 17.2). This step is essential to allow easy insertion of the prosthetic patch. Once placed in that space, the patch will seat itself against the abdominal wall to protect the myopectineal orifice, including the incompetent internal ring. Completion of the repair requires absolute assurance that no portion of the intraabdominal peritoneal sac or any properitoneal fat protrudes through the deep inguinal ring.

Of the various modifications we have made to our basic technique over the past 15 years, each supports the fundamental theory that the model repair is accomplished by interposing a mesh prosthesis between the peritoneum and the defect in the abdominal wall (Fig. 17.3). To accomplish that, a swatch of polypropylene mesh is used. Like a rubber stopper held in place by the pressure of water within a tub, the properitoneal mesh in the pelvis is held in place against the abdominal pelvic wall by hydrostatic pressure (Pascal's law). When supine, the mean intraabdominal pressure in a human subject is 8 cm of water. Severe coughing or straining pushes it as high as 80 cm of water (1). When the subject stands, the intrapelvic pressure is further increased by the added load of the abdominal viscera and its contents. This amount of intraabdominal outward force is more than

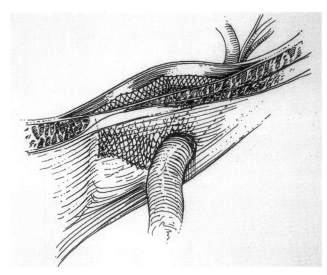

FIGURE 17.3. Gilbert's drawing of mesh between peritoneum and defect.

sufficient to flatten a pliable mesh, unless it has been manufactured to remain as a fixed plug (Fig. 17.4). Fibroplasia through the interstices of the mesh permanently binds it in place within the abdominal wall.

Each generation of the Gilbert technique has incorporated the same three features: (a) the deep inguinal ring is an available and convenient passageway to the properitoneal retromuscular space; (b) polypropylene mesh patch is a permanent barrier to protect the deep inguinal ring; and (c) the body's intraabdominal pressure is sufficient to permanently fix the mesh patch in its properitoneal position. Since its original description in 1985, and modifications in its later generations, the principle of using the internal ring as an avenue to the properitoneal space has been used to

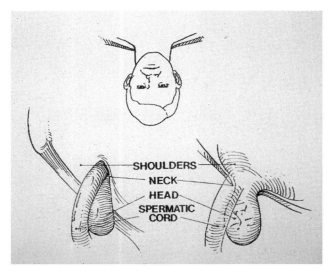

FIGURE 17.2. Head, neck, and shoulders of the sac.

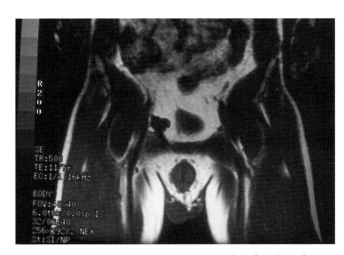

FIGURE 17.4. Magnetic resonance imaging showing plug.

successfully repair all types of primary and recurrent indirect inguinal hernias (6).

GENERATIONS OF THE GILBERT REPAIR

The first version, a polypropylene rolled plug, was put into the deep inguinal ring and fixed there with two Prolene sutures (5). The transversus arch was approximated to the shelving edge of the inguinal ligament. The posterior wall was reinforced with an onlay patch. The tissue reinforcement of Hesselbach's triangle was abandoned because it was unnecessary. The second version of the technique employed

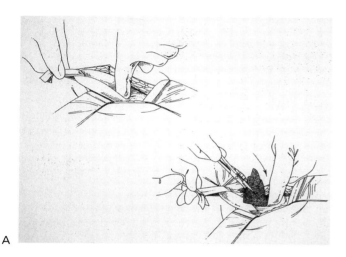

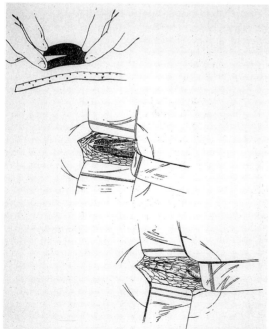

FIGURE 17.5. A: Insertion of umbrella patch. **B:** Application of onlay patch.

the umbrella patch in Bogros' space and the onlay patch to reinforce the posterior wall medially, as described previously. The third and fourth versions of the Gilbert technique differed by one suture. In the third version, to repair type 1 and type 2 inguinal hernias, a flat polypropylene mesh measuring 2 and one half × 4 and one half inches was divided into two pieces (5). One piece was cut to twice the size of the other. The larger piece was shaped into an unopened umbrella and inserted through the deep inguinal ring into the properitoneal space, where it was designed to open and block the deep ring (Fig. 17.5A,B). The remaining one third of the mesh was placed flat as an onlay patch. This technique did not require suture fixation of either the umbrella patch or the onlay patch. Accordingly, it was described as "Gilbert's sutureless repair." The fourth version, designed to repair all indirect hernias, including Gilbert type 3 hernias, simply added a single Marcy suture at the deep inguinal ring to reduce the breadth of the defect. This technique and its modifications worked well from 1985 until 1998 to successfully repair 6,351 indirect inguinal hernias at the Hernia Institute of Florida with a 99% success rate. For direct hernias, we continued to use the Shouldice method reinforced with a polypropylene underlay patch.

A BILAYER PROSTHETIC DEVICE

The bilayer polypropylene device known as the Prolene Hernia System, released in April 1998 by Ethicon, Inc., is constructed as a three-in-one model (Fig. 17.6). Its underlay component is designed to protect the canal's posterior wall, just as a laparoscopic repair attempts to do. Its diameter exceeds the dimensions of the myopectineal orifice. Inferiorly, it will reach beyond Cooper's ligament to protect the femoral triangle; superiorly, it will reach well above the transversus arch; medially, it reaches behind the pubic

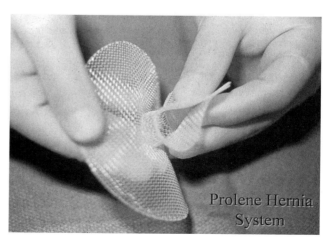

FIGURE 17.6. Photograph of the Prolene Hernia System.

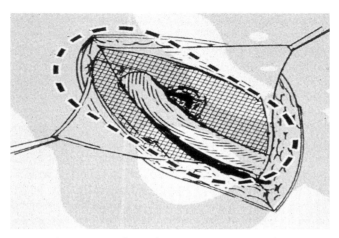

FIGURE 17.7. The Prolene Hernia System in place.

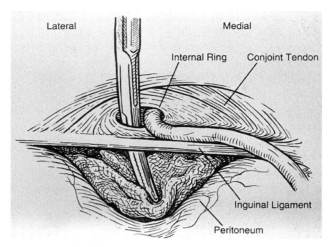

FIGURE 17.8. Slide of anterior space.

ramus; and laterally, it reaches to well beyond the internal ring. It is flat and pliable, and in Bogros' space it will cover and protect the entire myopectineal orifice. It should be placed deep to the deep epigastric vessels. Its 2-cm diameter connector will sit within the defect or the internal ring. The onlay component of the device covers and protects the entire posterior wall. Laterally, it is positioned between the internal and external oblique muscles, and medially, it extends over the transversus arch and the pubic bone. It extends along the shelving edge of the inguinal ligament, protecting the entirety of Hesselbach's (medial) triangle and the tissues of the lateral triangle. The design of the onlay patch makes it wide enough and long enough to cover the full width and breadth of the vulnerable posterior wall (Fig. 17.7).

Technique

Usually with local, occasionally with regional, and rarely with general anesthesia, a low 2-inch transverse incision is made in the groin. The external oblique aponeurosis is opened. Dissecting beneath the medial and lateral flaps of the external oblique aponeurosis creates the *anterior* space. This dissection should extend from over the pubic tubercle medially up to the upper one third of the inguinal ligament, then down the shelving edge of the inguinal ligament clearing the cord and cremasteric components, including the genital branch of the genitofemoral nerve (Fig. 17.8). The cremasteric branch of the ilioinguinal nerve is retracted alone or left on the lateral flap of the cremasteric fascia. The medial flap of the cremasteric fascia is excised. The anterior space will eventually house the onlay patch of the device. Sharp dissection is used to separate the indirect sac from the cord, and from the investing fibers of the transversalis fascia at its neck. Dissection high in the spermatic cord and at the neck of a sac or lipoma is essential, but invariably and unavoidably it damages the protective sling mechanism of the internal ring and the tissues lateral to it. The double

patches of the device were designed considering that the area lateral to the internal ring needs to be protected.

To actualize the posterior space, the peritoneum is freed from its attachments to the posterior wall (the shoulders of the sac) by inserting a 4 × 4-inch gauze sponge through the internal ring (Fig. 17.9). For direct hernias, Gilbert types 4 and 5, the hernia protruding through Hesselbach's triangle is opened, and the contents are dissected from it with a 4 × 4-inch sponge to actualize the space. The latter approach can also be used for indirect hernias but must include ligation of the peritoneal sac. Cooper's ligament can be visualized after completion of dissection through the posterior wall. The deep epigastric vessels are usually not disturbed unless the hernia is a pantaloon presentation, in which case they are divided and the two defects are converted to one. Attempts to actualize the posterior space using the prosthetic device or by using only the gloved finger usually frustrate the surgeon and are often inadequate. In all types of indirect and direct hernias the posterior space is best created using an opened sponge. The sponge provides sufficient traction to displace the properitoneal fat, and has proven most effective. It is a key element to the ease and success of the operation. The properitoneal space need not be developed to the full 10-cm diameter of the underlay patch; there will be sufficient space for the underlay component to deploy if a 4 × 4-inch sponge can be inserted.

Using the insertion maneuver, with the finger in the defect of a direct hernia, or the deep inguinal ring of an indirect hernia, pulsations of the iliac artery can be felt laterally (7). The device is slid down the medial side of the forefinger into the properitoneal space (Fig. 17.10). In the case of a direct hernia, the device is pointed directly into the defect. When inserting the device through the internal ring for an indirect hernia, it is helpful for the surgeon to lift up the abdominal wall with the finger that is through the ring. The sponge stick carrying the device should be angled

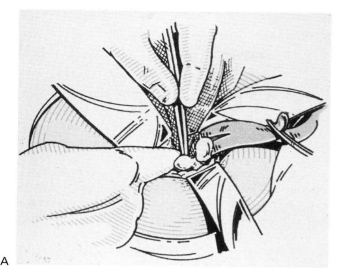

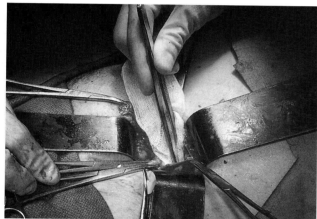

FIGURE 17.9. Illustration **(A)** and photograph **(B)** depicting sponge dissection.

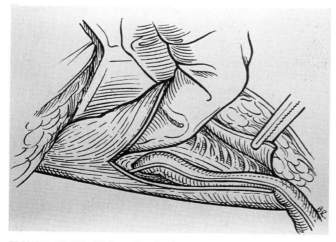

FIGURE 17.10. Sliding the Prolene Hernia System down the finger.

toward the umbilicus to facilitate its passage, after which the surgeon removes his/her finger from the properitoneal space. The two leaves of the onlay patch are extracted while holding a finger in its connector to keep the underlay patch in place. After both leaves of the onlay patch have been extracted, they are held like a bridle while any visible part of the edge of the underlay patch is deployed. It is unrealistic to expect that the underlay patch will lie exactly flat. It is not being fastened against a wall as in the laparoscopic approach, but rather into an irregular space containing fat. It is unnecessary to remove every fat globule from between the mesh patch and the abdominal wall. The technical goal of deployment is to spread the edge of the underlay patch circumferentially at maximum distraction from the connector. The connector remains in the internal ring of an indirect hernia or in the defect of a direct hernia.

Next, the lateral leaf of the onlay patch is stored in the anterior space beneath the external oblique aponeurosis. An army–navy retractor is most helpful for this step. This flattens it and greatly facilitates the remainder of the procedure. The medial part of the onlay patch is flattened against the transversus arch, and the end of its medial leaf is positioned approximately 2 cm over the pubic bone. The underlay patch will be seated against the interior muscular wall by the patient's intra-abdominal pressure. Effectiveness of the underlay patch alone can be evaluated before suturing the onlay component. By having the patient cough and perform Valsalva's maneuver, it will be obvious that the defect has been repaired. To ensure permanence of the repair, we suggest the onlay patch be sutured over the pubic tubercle, at the middle of the transversus arch, and at the middle of the inguinal ligament. To accommodate the spermatic cord through the onlay patch for indirect and direct hernias, we usually use a centrally placed slit. Occasionally, a lateral slit is used (Fig. 17.11A,B). At minimum, we use three sutures for indirect hernias and four for direct hernias. Additional sutures can be placed in the onlay patch, depending on need. Any excess of the onlay patch is trimmed before closing the external oblique aponeurosis. Fixation of the onlay patch ensures immobility of the entire three-piece device. After final testing of the repair, the spermatic cord and nerves are laid on the onlay patch, and the leaves of the external oblique aponeurosis are approximated. The subcutaneous tissues are opposed, and the skin is closed with absorbable subcuticular suture and a topical adhesive.

Results

We began using this prosthesis in April 1998. From that time through February of 1999, 759 bilayer devices were used to repair inguinal hernias: 405 for indirect hernias, of which 32 (8%) were recurrent; and 354 were for direct hernias, of which 45 (12.7%) were recurrent. Bilateral primary hernias were repaired simultaneously in 17 patients using separate devices through separate incisions. Sixteen other

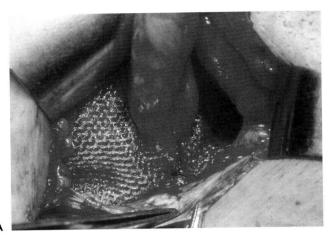

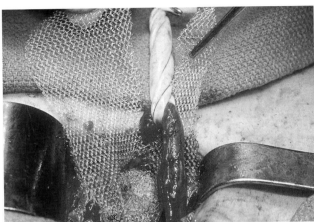

FIGURE 17.11. A: Central slit in onlay patch. **B:** Lateral slit in onlay patch.

patients had bilateral hernias that were repaired on separate days, from 2 to 6 weeks apart; of these, eight were bilateral primary and four were bilateral recurrent hernias. Four patients had unilateral primary and unilateral recurrent hernias when they came for consultation. Local anesthesia was used for 512 repairs, regional for 244 repairs, and general anesthesia for three repairs. Follow-up by the operating surgeon was done at 1 week and 1 month postoperatively for patients who were geographically close. Telephone inquiry and progress reports were used with others. There were no recurrences reported. Seromas developed in 32 repairs, all of which subsided without event. Hematomas occurred in six repairs and wound infections in six repairs. In all cases of infection or hematoma the wounds were opened and irrigated, and in all patients the prostheses were left in place. All wounds healed without further event. No case of severe or sustained postoperative pain was reported. The average level of postoperative discomfort was controlled with small doses of acetaminophen or propoxyphene. A few patients experienced temporary testidynia that gradually subsided in

3 to 8 weeks. None developed testicular atrophy. There has not been a recurrence in this group to date.

DISCUSSION

Lasting hernia repair, especially with newer mesh tension-free techniques, requires that surgeons have a better appreciation for the concept of plasticity of the entire vulnerable area of the groin. Surgical trauma created by dissection around and lateral to the internal ring is unavoidably necessary for the detection of an indirect hernia and to remove lipomas that penetrate the internal oblique muscle. Such created weaknesses must be reinforced to protect against lateral recurrences. Only by complete protection of the entire myopectineal orifice can disparity of resistance and deformation of the remainder of the posterior wall be avoided. A new bilayer hernia repair device that protects the inguinal and femoral areas has been used for 3 years with impressive results. It is easy to apply using local anesthesia in ambulatory patients. Postoperative activities, including strenuous efforts, are not limited. Discomfort following surgery is minimal. Considering the strategy incorporated in the device and the early encouraging results of its clinical trials, it seems that failures should be rare. The device, different than others currently available, has a double protective mechanism built into its design. Like the double support of wearing a belt and braces, or wearing two parachutes when sky diving, the Prolene Hernia System gives double protection. It is competitively priced with other hernia repair devices. Its recurrence rate is so impressively low that it essentially eliminates the lost time and expense related to even a 1% failure rate. Attention to the advice of this operative technique will minimize the learning time for surgeons who use it.

REFERENCES

1. Caix M. Functional anatomy of the muscles of the anterolateral abdominal wall electromyography and histoenzymology. In: Chevrel JP, ed. *Surgery of the abdominal wall.* New York: Springer–Verlag, 1985:27–40.
2. Drye JC. The intraperitoneal pressure in the human. *Surg Gynecol Obstet* 1948;87:472–475.
3. Gilbert AI. Overnight hernia repair: updated considerations. *South Med J* 1987;80:191–195.
4. Gilbert AI. Inguinal hernia repair: biomaterials and sutureless repair. *Perspect Gen Surg* 1991;2:113–129.
5. Gilbert AI. Sutureless repair of inguinal hernia. *Am J Surg* 1992; 163:331–335.
6. Gilbert AI. An anatomic and functional classification of inguinal hernia. *Am J Surg* 1989;157:331–333.
7. Gilbert AI. Improved sutureless technique—advice to experts. *Probl Gen Surg* 1995;12:117–119.
8. Gilbert AI. Shouldice repair in preference to other tissue repairs. Presented at *Advances and Improvements in Hernia Surgery,* February 1984, Miami.

18

PREPERITONEAL HERNIA REPAIR

KONSTANTINO PAPADAKIS
A. GERSON GREENBURG

A BRIEF HISTORIC NOTE

In the years 1800 to 1500 before the Common Era, Hindu "surgeons" approached the surgical treatment of groin hernia by celiotomy. The success rate and complications, if the patients survived, were not reported. A few centuries later, Greek physicians and surgeons modified this approach, employing anterior inguinal incisions without entering the abdominal cavity. This duality between the inguinal and transabdominal routes for the repair of groin hernias remains a central issue in the current debate regarding the best surgical approach to this common clinical entity. As technologic advances associated with laparoendoscopic surgery broaden, increasing its applicability in many aspects of general surgery, its role in the repair of groin hernia continues to evolve. Whether employing a transabdominal (see Chapter 23) or preperitoneal approach (see Chapter 22), the argument over *the best surgical repair* using laparoendoscopic methods is the modern expression of the age-old duality.

The pioneering efforts of many surgeons involved in the development and refinement of the preperitoneal approach over the past 100 years or so clearly laid an essential foundation for transabdominal preperitoneal prosthetic (TAPP) repair, totally extraperitoneal prosthetic (TEPP) repair, and other nonanatomic posterior approach repairs currently in vogue. Absent these early and often well-documented efforts, the anatomic basis for these "modern" repairs—with or without the use of mesh—would be unknown. The very basis of the technologically oriented approach to groin hernia repairs is rooted in basic surgical principles applicable independent of technique:

an understanding of the "normal" anatomy and an appreciation of the defect in that anatomy so that appropriate repair options can be considered and applied. For many technologically or mesh-based repairs, the concept of "one operation fits all" is implied. The authors consider this subject open to debate, preferring to argue that the repair should be tailored to the anatomic findings and the individual patient.

Identification of the transversalis fascia layer and the iliopubic tract are essential elements of a successful "anatomic hernia repair." The term "anatomic" is used here to differentiate the sutured, tissue-to-tissue approximation techniques from the plug with or without patch or patch-reinforcing bolstering mesh repairs that do not involve closure of the identified and defined fascial defect.

The term "preperitoneal" is preferred to its synonyms (properitoneal, extraperitoneal, and posterior approach) for describing this procedure.

In 1886, Annandale of Edinburgh introduced the concept of a preperitoneal approach for groin hernia repair using a transverse incision. He did not invoke a fascial repair, using the approach simply to reduce incarcerated bowel and ligate the peritoneal sac. A fascinating commentary on his role in the early development of this approach for groin hernia repair has been published by Read (14). Tait of Birmingham in 1883 and again in 1891 touted the advantages of hernia cure by "median abdominal section," adding the requirement that the defect in the tendinous aperture had to be closed to effect a cure—a sound observation. In that fledgling era of rapidly developing surgical skills and techniques, synthetic patches and useful and usable mesh were not in the surgeon's armamentarium. Nonetheless, his concept of the operation remains valid today. Others in that era wrote in praise or condemnation of the posterior approach, arguments that continue to this day. In historic context, this was a most interesting time in the evolution of surgical thinking, especially related to the treatment of groin hernia. Proponents of a posterior approach for the repair of groin her-

K. Papadakis: Department of Surgery, University of Tennessee; Department of Surgery, East Tennessee Children's Hospital, Knoxville, Tennessee.

A. G. Greenburg: Department of Surgery, Brown Medical School; Department of Surgery, The Miriam Hospital, Providence, Rhode Island.

TABLE 18.1. METHODS OF ANATOMIC REPAIR OF A DEFECT WITH A PREPERITONEAL APPROACH TO HEMIOPLASTY

Author	Type of Hernia	Method of Repair
Annandale (1876)	Indirect	Ligation of hernial sac
	Direct	Ligation of hernial sac
	Femoral	Obscure
Tait (1883)	Groin	Obscure
Maunsell (1887)	Femoral	Suture of pectineus fascia and pectineal line to Poupart's ligament
Tait (1891)	Indirect	Suture of fascial defect, "external column of ring to inner column"
	Femoral	Obscure
Bates (1913)	Indirect	Suture of transversalis fascia of internal ring
Cheatle (1920)	Indirect	Occlusion of internal ring by suture
	Femoral	Flap periosteum of pubis to Poupart's ligament
Cheatle (1921)	Indirect	High ligation of sac only
	Femoral	Flap periosteum of pubis to Poupart's ligament
Henry (1936)	Indirect	Plastic to internal ring—transversalis fascia to fascia deep surface internal oblique muscle
	Femoral	Flap of pectineus fascia to Poupart's ligament
Jennings et al. (1942)	Indirect	Plastic closure of internal ring—suture of transversalis fascial sling lateral to the cord
Musgrove and McCready (1949)	Femoral	Suture of Poupart's ligament to Cooper's ligament
McEvedy PG (1950)	Femoral	Suture of conjoined tendon to Cooper's ligament
Riba and Menn[a] (1952)	Indirect	Plastic closure of internal ring—suture of transversalis fascial sling
	Direct	Suture of transversalis fascia to Cooper's ligament
Hull and Ganey (1953)	Femoral	Suture of Poupart's ligament to Cooper's ligament or pectineus fascia flap technique of Henry
Mikkelsen and Berne (1954)	Femoral	Suture of transversalis fascia and transversus aponeurosis to Cooper's ligament
	Small, indirect	Plastic repair of internal ring—transversalis fascia
	Large, indirect	Similar to femoral closure
Mouzas and Diggory (1956)	Femoral	Suture of conjoined tendon to Cooper's ligament
McEvedy BV (1958)	Femoral	As described by his father in 1950
	Indirect	Suture of inguinal ligament to transversalis fascia and reinforced by conjoined tendon to Cooper's ligament
	Direct	Suture of conjoined tendon to Cooper's ligament
Nyhus et al. (1959)	Indirect	Suture of transversalis fascial sling medial to the cord
	Direct	Suture of transversalis fascia or conjoined tendon or both to Cooper's ligament
	Femoral	Suture of transversalis fascia to Cooper's ligament
Nyhus et al. (1960)	Indirect	Suture of transversalis fascial sling medial or lateral to the cord or both
	Direct	Suture of transversalis fascia, arch of transversus abdominis aponeurosis, or both to iliopubic tract
	Femoral	Suture of iliopubic tract to Cooper's ligament
Sheehan (1961)	Femoral	Suture of transversalis fascia and conjoined tendon to Cooper's ligament
Smith (1962)	Medial, recurrent	Suture of transversalis fascia to Poupart's ligament
	Lateral, recurrent	Same
Estrin et al. (1963)	Femoral	Suture of transversalis fascia to Cooper's ligament
	Indirect	Suture of transversalis fascia to inguinal ligament
	Direct	Suture of transversalis fascia to Cooper's ligament
Stoppa et al. (1972)	Indirect, direct	Preperitoneal insertion of large Dacron prosthesis without fascial repair
Stoppa et al. (1984)	Femoral, recurrent	Same
Ger (1990)	Indirect	Laparoscopic closure neck of sac
Greenburg (1995) (Current)	All types plus recurrent	Similar to Nyhus (below)
Nyhus (1995) (Current)	Small, indirect (type II)	Suture of transversalis fascial sling medial to the cord
	Large, indirect (type IIIB)	Suture of transversalis fascia and transversus abdominis aponeurosis to iliopubic tract medial to cord. Occasionally, 1 or 2 sutures placed between transversalis fascial sling and iliopubic tract lateral to cord to ensure adequate closure of internal ring. Cord at level of femoral vessels. If massive, use components of direct repair as well. Buttress with Marlex mesh.
	Direct (type IIIA)	Suture of transversalis fascia and transversus abdominis aponeurosis to iliopubic tract.
	Femoral (type IIIC)	Suture of iliopubic tract to Cooper's ligament
	Recurrent (type IV)	Repair defect, and buttress with Marlex mesh

[a]Performed in conjunction with retropubic prostatectomy.
For complete references, see Nyhus LM. The peritoneal approach and iliopubic tract repair of inguinal hernias. In: Nyhus LM, Condon RE, eds. *Hernia*, Fourth edition. Philadelphia: J.B. Lippincott Company, 1995:153–174.

nia found themselves in direct conflict with the recently reported and rapidly adopted Bassini's repair. The latter, an anatomically based anterior groin repair, would come to dominate this area of surgery for many decades to follow (see Chapters 10 and 11).

Table 18.1 provides a rather complete chronology, including the major contributors to the development of the preperitoneal repair of groin hernia. Many of these contributions have stood the test of time, remaining relevant, useful, and applicable in surgery to this day. Significant events in the evolution of the preperitoneal concept and operative variations are noted. This table is included to provide a more detailed historic perspective of this important surgical technique.

Cheatle in 1920 first described the definitive preperitoneal procedure. Initially, using a lateral rectus-splitting incision with the patient in the Trendelenburg position, Cheatle retracted the rectus muscle laterally and developed the extraperitoneal Retzius' space to observe the posterior wall of the inguinal region. The operation was originally designed for the elective radical cure of unilateral or bilateral femoral hernia, and shortly thereafter extended to include inguinal herniation. The following year, he reported his technique using the transverse bilateral Pfannenstiel's incision, adding a concomitant appendectomy if the appendix was in the hernia sac; at this time, he proposed the operation for the relief of strangulated hernias. Cheatle had remarkable insight into the pathophysiology of groin herniation and was prescient regarding the relationship of the anatomy, the pathology, and the needs of the surgeon to effect a quality outcome. In 1936, Henry described and expanded on Cheatle's approach. He placed an emphasis on high closure of peritoneal sacs and transversalis or pectineal fascial repairs of bilateral femoral herniation. Henry's reflections on his contributions, taken in historic context, are noted in a special comment found in the 4th edition of *Hernia* (pages 184–186).

With global conflicts on the horizon and developments in surgery taking a more physiologic scientific-based approach in research, there was little interest in refining the preperitoneal hernia repair, or any hernia repair for that matter. Bassini's repair, with variations, had taken a firm hold in the surgical management of groin hernia. Just after World War II, interest in the preperitoneal approach was once again ignited. The objective now was to minimize recurrence following groin hernia repair, an end point and outcome measure still the subject of great debate.

The most important postwar contribution to preperitoneal herniorrhaphy was that of P.G. McEvedy in 1950. He described an operation for femoral hernia through an oblique incision in the rectus sheath with medial, rather than lateral, retraction and displacement of the rectus

muscle. McEvedy took advantage of an anatomic fact: below the linea semicircularis, there is no posterior rectus sheath; only a weak layer of preperitoneal fat and some very poorly defined preperitoneal fascia covers the peritoneum once the rectus muscle is retracted medially. For all intents and purposes, the base of the incision is the peritoneum. Closure of the femoral ring was accomplished by suturing the conjoined tendon to Cooper's ligament. Whether this was really the "conjoined tendon" or the iliopubic tract tracing anteriorly is not clear. Anatomically, the conjoined tendon, a fusion of the aponeuroses of the internal abdominal oblique and transversalis muscles, is too anterior and possibly too superior from this vantage point to be used. Moreover, it is an inconstant structure at best, making its use somewhat speculative. The variations in this structure were well cataloged by Anson and Maddock (2). Indeed, in a superbly written and elegantly illustrated description of groin anatomy, Condon illustrates this point very well (Fig. 18.1) (6). If, indeed, the conjoined tendon was sutured to Cooper's ligament, the almost certain resulting tension would contribute to a high rate of recurrence, a not-uncommon observation at that time.

Mouzas and Diggory modified the skin incision from vertical to oblique, repairing all types of groin hernias from this surgical vantage point. In 1956, Reay-Young changed the skin incision to "half a Pfannenstiel incision," the rectus sheath being incised transversely rather than vertically or obliquely. Today, the skin incision is made more cephalad than described by these authors to accommodate the variable location of the internal ring, an essential landmark for the use of this approach.

In 1960, Nyhus and colleagues reported a series of groin hernia repairs using a modification of the McEvedy approach: a transverse incision 3 cm above the inguinal ligament extended across the midline for bilateral defects. The internal inguinal ring was closed with sutures placed laterally, essentially reconstructing the internal ring. In this series, the iliopubic tract (transversalis fascia) repair was introduced; relaxing incisions were not used because excessive tension was not observed. Further, they recommended the preperitoneal approach be used for all recurrent hernias, thus avoiding the previously scarred anterior groin, a position that we hold as well. Nyhus indicated he had adopted the transverse "lateral to rectus" incision because it was less liable to postoperative herniation than the median suprapubic incision. Indeed, this is the case: the authors have not seen an incisional hernia in this area in the total experience with this approach in over 4,000 cases. Nyhus, his colleagues, and his disciples—including the senior author of this chapter—deserve credit for popularizing the preperitoneal herniorrhaphy as a safe, secure, and reliable technique of groin hernia repair.

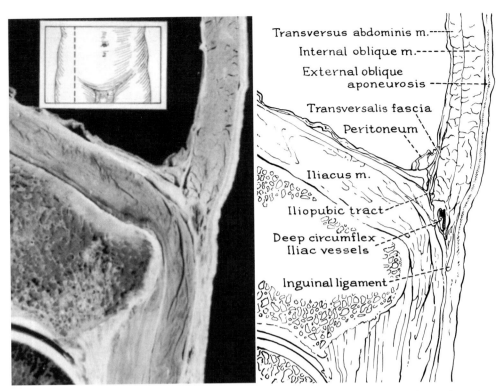

FIGURE 18.1. A parasagittal section of the right groin through the iliacus muscle just lateral to the femoral sheath, viewed from its lateral aspect. An embalmed cadaver was frozen, and then a parasagittal slice of tissue was cut, laid flat on its medial surface, and photographed under water. The relations of the layers of the anterior abdominal wall in the lateral portion of the groin are well shown. Note particularly the relative positions of the inguinal ligament (superficial musculoaponeurotic lamina) and the iliopubic tract (deep musculoaponeurotic lamina).

DEFINITIONS AND REVIEW OF THE CRITICAL ANATOMY

A hernia is an abnormal protrusion of a peritoneal-lined sac through the musculoaponeurotic covering of the abdomen.

The modern era of hernia surgery has been characterized by a better understanding of the abdominal wall anatomy, especially by defining the relationship of the muscular, aponeurotic, and fascial layers of the lower abdominal wall, the area that constitutes the commonly called groin (see Chapters 5 and 6). It is now generally agreed that the most important tissue layer in the groin, *relative to hernia repair*, is the transversus abdominis muscle and its aponeurosis and fascial coverings. The more superficial layers of the anterior abdominal wall appear to play no role in the support of the inguinal floor. The objective of any groin hernia repair should be the return the transversus abdominis layer to a normal anatomic and functional role. As an aside, while the anatomy of the groin continues to be a subject of study with refinement of detail, the physiology of the abdominal wall in both normal and pathologic states is a sadly underinvestigated area. There are little reliable data to use in the design of function–structure solutions to anatomic problems in this area.

Transversus Abdominis Muscle

The integrity of the transversus abdominis muscle prevents the formation of most groin hernias. The transversus abdominis muscle in the inguinal area arises from the iliopsoas fascia and not from the inguinal ligament. The transversus abdominis fascia is a useful anatomic entity for the repair of inguinal hernias. The arch is formed by the free aponeurotic and muscular lower margin of the muscle. Medially, the arch is aponeurotic, whereas toward the internal ring, it is both muscular and aponeurotic. In the vicinity of the internal ring, the internal oblique is muscular and the transversus abdominis is aponeurotic. The transversus abdominis muscle inserts on Cooper's ligament. Further, medially in the inguinal area, all the aponeurotic layers of the three flat muscles pass anterior to the rectus muscle and form the anterior lamina of the sheath.

The aponeurosis of this muscle is bilaminar; both laminae (anterior and posterior) fuse together. If this fails to occur in normal development, attenuation of the posterior layer results, creating the potential for weakness to develop.

Transversalis Fascia

A direct inguinal hernia results from a disruption and/or relaxation of the transversalis fascia. This is a fundamental concept in understanding the anatomy and, by logical extension, the repair of all groin hernias generally. Independent of the repair technique employed, fascia to fascia, mesh overlay, plug and/or patch, or a combination of all of these, restoration of the anatomic integrity of the transversalis fascia is the surgical objective. Failure to appreciate this principle is but one of a host of factors contributing to the recurrence rates observed following inguinal herniorrhaphy.

The anatomic structures used for repair must, therefore, all lie within the transversalis laminae of the inguinal region—in the posterior inguinal wall. This layer forms the essential guide to repair because it defines the lamina upon which the repair is based. This concept applies to all types of groin hernias. Often used in hernioplasty are a group of ligamentous and aponeurotic structures closely associated with the transversalis fascia. They should be of sufficient integrity to retain sutures, and generally provide the strength and support required for reapproximation and restoration of continuity of the transversalis fascia.

The list of "*good stuff*" for groin hernia repair is noted in Table 18.2. While not all of the structures and materials noted in the table are accessible from the preperitoneal vantage point, the essential components for a secure and lasting repair are on the list. For the most part, an awareness of these structures is useful and applicable to the management of the more complex multiply recurrent groin hernia. In this situation, the surgeon's experience and, to a degree, creativity will play a major role in restoring the anatomy without a fascial defect and with reduced recurrences.

While it is preferable and even desirable to repair complex groin hernias using the preperitoneal approach, there are occasions when a more "*creative*" solution is required. In those instances, knowledge of tissues potentially useful in repair, with our without mesh, is necessary.

Internal Inguinal Ring

The internal ring has an elliptic shape by the presence on its anterior and posterior aspects of a double fold of transversalis fascia that cradles and supports the spermatic cord in this region. Transversalis fascia can be delineated on all sides of the internal inguinal ring. The posterior crus consists of fibers that parallel the iliopubic tract and finally fuse with it. The anterior crus is a dense band that has an extensive origin in the transversalis fascia above the internal ring. The two crura are, of course, continuous with each other on the medial aspect of the internal ring near the vas deferens testicular vessels. Because they are more prominent at this level, a sling effect is perceived, giving rise to the term "transversalis fascial sling of the internal ring." Lateral movement of this sling when straining, any increased intraabdominal pressure, or Valsalva's maneuver closes the fascial ring around the elements of the spermatic cord. In theory, this action prevents descent of a peritoneal sac through the ring. This natural protective mechanism should be enhanced during hernioplasty by placement of sutures only into the posterior lamina of the transversus muscle and fascia, avoiding cross-laminar sutures between the anterior crus and the inguinal ligament.

Iliopubic Tract

The iliopubic tract is an aponeurotic band that extends from the iliopectineal arch to the superior ramus of the pubis. It forms the inferior margin of the deep musculoaponeurotic layer made up of the transversus abdominis muscle and aponeurosis and the transversalis fascia. Perhaps the best description of this structure and its role in the repair of groin hernias is that of Condon in Chapter 2 of the 4th edition of this text. Quoting from Nyhus (*Hernia*, 4th edition, Chapter 8): "The iliopubic tract is a strong fascial band that begins laterally along the crest of the ilium and at the anterior superior iliac spine. In this area, it gives origin to the iliacus muscle and the lowermost fibers of the transversus abduminus muscle. The iliopubic tract arches over the psoas muscle and the femoral vessels; at the arch, it forms an integral part of the anterior femoral sheath. In its midportion, the iliopubic tract lies immediately subjacent to the inguinal ligament. It is, however, completely separated from the inguinal ligament, and the relation is one of proximity only. Continuing medially, the iliopubic tract inserts fanwise into the superior ramus of the pubis and into the Cooper ligament. The most inferior fibers of the iliopubic tract—those that insert most laterally into the Cooper ligament—are sharply recurved in the normal groin. It is this recurved portion of the iliopubic tract that defines the medial bor-

TABLE 18.2. THE "GOOD STUFF" FOR GROIN HERNIA REPAIR

Inguinal ligament
Lacunar ligament (Gimbernat's)
Pectineal ligament (Cooper's)
Transversalis fascia and transversus aponeurosis
Ileopubic tract
Anterior femoral sheath
Transversalis fascia
Conjoined fascial "area"
Arch of the internal oblique and transversus abdominis
   aponeurosis
"Prosthesis"

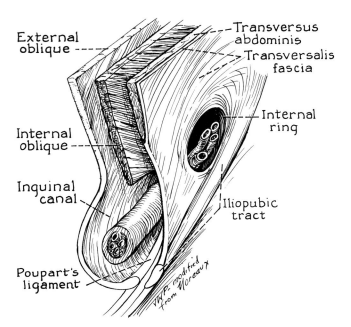

FIGURE 18.2. Parasagittal section through the right midinguinal region illustrating the separation of the musculoaponeurotic lamina into the anterior and posterior inguinal walls. All figures in this chapter are drawn on the right side.

der of the femoral canal, not the lacunar (Gimbernat) ligament of classic description.

"The fundamental importance of the iliopubic tract in understanding the anatomy of groin hernias is appreciated when one realizes that the iliopubic tract forms one of the margins of the hernial defect in each of the common groin hernias. Direct and indirect inguinal hernia defects are limited on their posterior aspects by fibers of the iliopubic tract; femoral hernial defects are similarly limited on their medial and anterior aspects" (Figs. 18.2 and 18.3).

Hesselbach's Triangle

Hesselbach's triangle is defined today as having the inferior (deep) epigastric vessels as its superior or lateral border, the rectus sheath as its medial border, and the inguinal ligament as its lateroinferior border. This is a more refined definition than that originally described, no doubt the result of decades of interest in this anatomic area relative to hernia repair.

Two layers of fascia cover Hesselbach's triangle: the transversalis fascia and fibers of the transversus abdominis aponeurosis. These tissues are almost always adhered to one another, forming the heavy, curved arch of the transversus abdominis aponeurosis. These structures are not easily isolated and are usually sutured as one layer in the repair of the defect.

This historically identified anatomic area is very well visualized from the posterior approach, and continues to serve as a reference for defining and classifying groin hernias.

Inguinal Herniation

An indirect hernia is congenital in origin; it requires a preformed or potential hernial sac, namely, the processus vaginalis. The processus vaginalis is the tubular anlage along

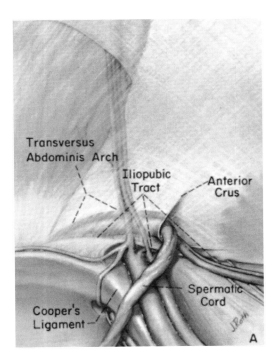

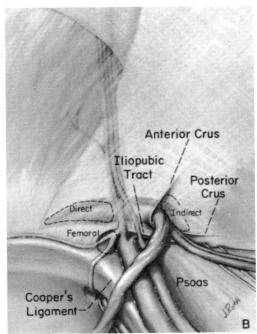

FIGURE 18.3. A: The important anatomic structures of the posterior inguinal wall as seen from the preperitoneal approach. **B:** The same view demonstrating sites of common groin hernias.

which the fetal testis descends into the scrotum from the retroperitoneum. In female fetuses, this may be the descent of the round ligament. Normally, the processus vaginalis obliterates to form a fibrous cord, the ligamentum vaginale, which extends from the parietal peritoneum deep to the internal ring through the inguinal canal to the testis. Depending on the length of the patent processus vaginalis, an indirect inguinal hernia may extend into the inguinal canal through the external ring or protrude into the scrotum. Anomalies of descent of the testes are frequently related to the presence of an indirect groin hernia (see Chapter 38).

Direct inguinal hernias are usually not considered "congenital" in origin. Rather, current thought considers them to be acquired, although the exact mechanisms are neither well understood nor well defined (see Chapters 1 and 2). Acquired, possibly genetically programmed, metabolic tissue deficiencies or other physiologic metabolic responses to external or internal perturbations may predispose fascia generally, and the groin specifically, to weakening. The result is often direct herniation.

Two anatomic mechanisms act to preserve the structural integrity of the inguinal canal, and to prevent herniation of abdominal contents through the transversalis fascia of Hesselbach's triangle and the internal abdominal ring. Movement of the transversus aponeurotic arch produces the shutter mechanism of the internal ring. This arch, which is normally convex at rest, straightens and flattens when the transversus and obliquus internus abdominis muscles are tensed. This tensing action moves the arch toward or in apposition to the iliopubic tract, thereby reinforcing the floor of the inguinal canal.

The internal abdominal ring is attached to the transversus abdominis muscle by the transversalis fascia sling. In the sphincter mechanism, when the transversus abdominis contracts, the transversalis fascia sling is pulled superiorly and laterally to close the internal ring around the cord structures. For the coordinated actions of the sphincter and shutter to occur, the transversalis fascia and related structures must be free to move in their respective laminar planes. Therefore, any operative repair that secures by sutures the posterior lamina to a superficial fixed structure such as the inguinal ligament disrupts the shutter and sphincter mechanisms.

While these descriptions may be helpful in gaining an appreciation of the function and physiology of the abdominal wall, the functional anatomy of the groin is neither well documented nor well understood. This is especially true in the context of relating clinical outcomes to specific surgical interventions. These comments should be recognized as speculative, for they assume relationships between anatomy and function that have not been scientifically validated. While the hypotheses may be valid, there is scant data to support the actual function as described. How various patches, plugs, and other "nonanatomic repairs" interact with these presumed mechanisms is, at the moment, unknown.

Classification of Groin Hernias

Nyhus classified groin hernias based on observations from the posterior vantage point. In our opinion, it is very clearly the best way to define the groin anatomy and classify defects. The preperitoneal approach affords direct observation of the entire groin area, making all defects readily identifiable. The practical classification Nyhus derived is detailed elsewhere (see Chapter 7).

The purpose of a classification schema needs iteration. For a defined set of criteria, a more precise stratification of the anatomic defect is possible. When the specific defect is related to a specific repair, and the data then adjusted for various patient risk factors, a more accurate assessment of that is possible. A classification schema provides a basis for comparison of techniques stratified as they are applied to specific anatomic defects. Two schools of thought compete in the world of hernia repair: one repair for all defects versus tailored repairs for specific defects. For a variety of reasons, the authors prefer the latter as it seems more logical, rational, and cost-effective.

Indications

The indications for the preperitoneal approach to repair of groin hernia are recurrence, incarceration, strangulation with obstruction, femoral herniation, and a "high-risk" patient. The technique of most anterior approach hernia repairs, especially those that dominated this area of surgery for over a century, usually avoided violation of the posterior wall, the floor, of the inguinal canal. Thus, a transversalis arch to iliopubic tract repair, with or without mesh reinforcement, is feasible in almost every instance when approaching the hernia from the preperitoneal vantage point.

The iliopubic tract repair from the preperitoneal approach *is ideal* for Nyhus hernia types III and IV, with or without prosthetic buttress, as well as femoral hernia. Because the preperitoneal approach provides exposure of the entire groin area, visualization of all areas of inguinal herniation, as well as other confounding structures including elements of sliding hernias, is possible. Repair is readily effected while minimizing the potential for injury to bowel and bladder, anatomic structures that are often elements of the peritoneal hernia sac. When meticulous knowledge of the anatomy is applied, the preperitoneal approach is perfectly acceptable and safe for primary repair of simple or complex inguinal hernias. Indeed, in the experience of the senior author, no injury to bowel or bladder has been observed in over 30 years of experience with this approach in the repair of primary or recurrent groin hernia. It should be noted that injury to these organs has been reported for both TAPP and TEPP repairs.

Anesthesia

General endotracheal anesthesia is preferred for the preperitoneal hernia repair. It is a safe technique, with well-controlled patient physiology, providing effective analgesia and anesthesia for even the most physiologically deranged patient. This anesthetic technique is acceptable for both ambulatory surgery—the majority of cases—and short-stay hospitalization. Modern general anesthetic techniques use agents that afford smooth induction and emergence with minimal retching and less confusion. Continuous epidural anesthesia is an excellent alternative technique for this procedure. However, it does demand and require additional skill and careful monitoring, especially in the older patient. This form of regional anesthesia is not recommended for patients with significant heart disease or cardiovascular instability requiring multidrug therapy. These patients do better with well-controlled general anesthesia techniques. Local anesthesia is not an acceptable alternative for the preperitoneal repair because there is direct traction on the peritoneum during the procedure. Since the peritoneum is sensitive and responsive to both touch and stretch, it is difficult to anesthetize it effectively with local anesthesia alone. The instillation of topical anesthetic agents into the preperitoneal space before closure is generally not effective, although there are sporadic reports of benefit. The authors do not use it.

Technique

A transverse incision is placed sufficiently cephalad to be above the internal ring. However, precise localization of the internal ring on physical examination is not always possible. Indeed, the anatomic localization of the internal ring varies greatly, primarily as a function of the pelvic anatomy and in some cases because of previous surgery. In some patients the internal ring is located more laterally, while in others it is more inferior. The location is defined by the angle of the pelvis and the length of the posterior inguinal floor, two variables not easily defined preoperatively. Generally, the internal ring is located below a perpendicular line running from the anterior iliac crest to the midline, about halfway below this line and the pubis, in a line with the femoral vessels. As the pelvis narrows and deepens or broadens and flattens, the location of the internal ring varies vertically and horizontally. In essence, the length of the inguinal canal changes, and the angle between the external and internal rings of the groin also varies.

Considerable attention has been paid to this area by many surgeons and anatomists in the past. The musculopectineal opening so nicely described by Fruchaud (9) was noted to vary significantly. Associated with this variation, and clearly related to both the depth and width of the pelvis, is variability in the location and size of the internal ring. Stoppa (see Chapter 19) indicates that these efforts formed, in part, the basis for his approach to the repair of complex recurrent hernias.

The incision must be superior to the internal ring to permit inspection and identification of the cord, ring, and contents. The skin incision is started in the midrectus muscle

and carried 10 to 15 cm laterally, essentially centering the lateral aspect of the rectus muscle in the middle of the incision. This incision is made approximately 5 to 7 cm above the pubic tubercle, adjusted for individual patient anatomy and pelvic configuration. The authors choose not to invoke the "three fingerbreadths above the tubercles" rule for placement of the incision because surgeons with different hand sizes span different distances with three fingers.

The skin incision is made with a scalpel and carried down to the fascia of the external abdominal oblique. Hemostasis is obtained with electrocautery, while the wound edges are elevated with rake retractors. Once the fascia of the external abdominal oblique is reached, it is cleared of adjacent tissue, fat, and fibrous scar. No attempt is made to identify the external ring; it is not a critical part of the repair. The anterior rectus sheath is opened transversely.

Starting at about the midrectus muscle, the fascial incision is carried laterally across the lateral margin of the rectus. If necessary for exposure, the rectus fascial incision can be extended medially to effect better medial retraction of the rectus muscle. This is most often necessary in the larger patient. The two layers of the anterior rectus sheath, external and internal abdominal oblique, are incised over the rectus muscle. These layers of fascia and the transversalis muscle are then opened laterally along the natural cleavage planes to expose the peritoneum (Fig. 18.4). A curved retractor is placed in the corner to maximize exposure. Large Kocher clamps are used to grasp the fascia, three on the inferior edge of the incised rectus sheath, one medially, one at the lateral margin of the rectus and the transversalis, and a final one lateral to the internal ring. The third Kocher clamp grasps all layers of the abdominal wall lateral to the internal ring, including the transversalis fascia as part of the inferior leaf of the fascial incision. The fourth clamp is placed on the superior edge of the rectus incision at its lateral border.

At this stage of the procedure the anatomy is visualized as follows: rectus muscle is medial, preperitoneal fat and/or peritoneum is lateral to it, and the fascia of the abdominal wall is lifted superiorly with the Kocher clamps.

The rectus muscle is now retracted medially with a curved retractor to maximize exposure. The lateral and inferior margin of the rectus muscle may require sharp dissection to mobilize the adjacent peritoneum or scar tissue to gain access to the medial portion of the preperitoneal space. Caution is advised here, particularly in recurrent hernia repair, because the bladder may be adherent to the peritoneum. This may be the area of previous surgical intervention if, indeed, the posterior wall was fully dissected during the previous procedure.

With the rectus muscle retracted medially and the inferior leaf of the abdominal wall elevated, a sweeping motion with dissectors and/or sponge sticks with sharp dissection, as needed, will free the peritoneum from the posterior aspect of the abdominal wall. The periosteum of the ilium

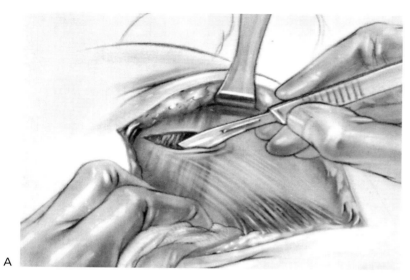

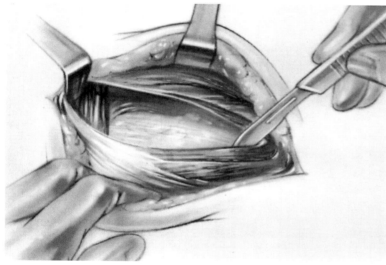

FIGURE 18.4. Transverse fascial incision. **A:** The incision begins at the midrectus muscle of the affected side. **B:** The surgeon enlarges the incision by separating and cutting fascia and muscle fibers of the external oblique, internal oblique, and transversus abdominal muscles. The transversalis fascia is seen in the depth of the wound. When the transversalis fascia is cut, the preperitoneal space is entered and the proper plane of dissection is achieved.

is an excellent landmark, and it should be visualized as the first step in the dissection and exploration. Visualization of this key and, fortunately, remarkably constant anatomic landmark is essential to the operation's success. Should Cooper's ligament not be visible while examining the posterior wall, a direct inguinal hernia is most likely present. This is confirmed with dissection of a peritoneal sac from its entrance into the defect in the abdominal wall. The sac is dissected free, primarily using blunt dissection techniques, with cephalad retraction on the peritoneum (Fig. 18.5A–C). If the distal sac does not free easily, amputation of the sac, leaving the cut margin of the distal end open, is a reasonable option. While there is a slightly increased incidence of seroma formation associated with this option, it is generally not a persistent problem.

In some cases, the peritoneal sac is incarcerated, not readily dissected free of the fascial hernia defect. The following sequence of procedures facilitates sac removal. First,

an incision is made to enlarge the transversalis fascia defect. A right-angle clamp is slipped under an identified edge of the defect and the fascia incised, away from the sac, for a distance sufficient to free the peritoneal sac, usually 1 or 2 cm in length. The defect can be enlarged medially and laterally, or extended to the medial aspect of the internal ring if needed.

A second approach to dealing with the incarceration involves opening the peritoneum and reducing the sac contents from within. This maneuver may also require the use of a fascial incision to free the incarcerated bowel, omentum, or sliding element of the sac. Reducing the contents of the sac facilitates visual identification of an edge of the defect. The incision to enlarge the defect can be made from the intraperitoneal vantage point safely if needed.

The peritoneum is closed after the sac, without contents, is removed from the hernia defect. The sac can be amputated and the distal end left open. The open distal end will not

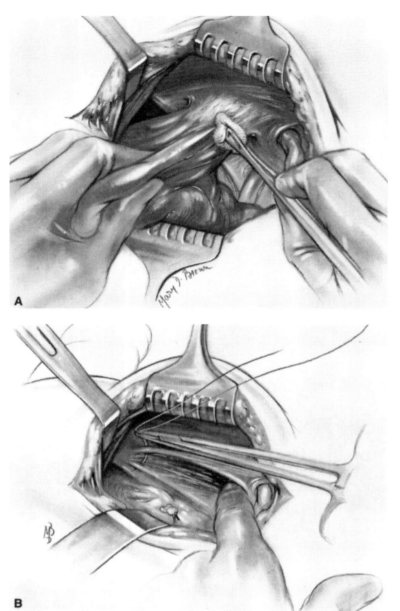

A

B

FIGURE 18.5. A: Direct hernia. The peritoneal sac is removed from the direct defect by traction and blunt dissection. The junction between the peritoneum and the weakened transversalis fascia is usually seen as a definite fold or white line. The peritoneum in a direct hernia usually has a broad base and does not need to be excised. The redundant peritoneum may be inverted into a purse-string suture if desired. **B:** The superior edge of this direct defect is the fused transversalis fascia–transversalis abdominis aponeurosis layer. A suture is being placed into this upper edge and into the iliopubic tract below. One may delineate these structures by placing a finger into the direct defect and placing lateral traction on the tissues.

likely cause any problem. However, there is frequently (2% to 5% incidence) an accumulation of fluid, a seroma, in this retained open-ended sac that may be confused with an early postoperative recurrence. The approach to management is expectant, waiting at least 6 weeks and then reexamining the patient. In most instances, the seroma will have resorbed and will no longer be detectable. Early imaging with ultrasound or computed tomography (CT) scan is not advised, and percutaneous drainage by needle aspiration is not recommended. This mass may indeed be a recurrent hernia.

Proximal preperitoneal ligation closure of the sac, ligature or suture ligature, prevents the abdominal contents from obscuring the view while the repair to the posterior wall is effected.

Access to the peritoneal cavity and its contents is excellent with this approach, affording relative ease to observe or resect bowel with vascular compromise frequently noted in an acutely incarcerated or strangulated hernia. Should evidence of vascular compromise to the bowel or any other structure be observed, the peritoneal incision is extended. Through this extended peritoneal incision, access to the small bowel, colon, omentum, or bladder is excellent. The intraabdominal organs are readily examined. If intestinal infarction is noted, resection is readily accomplished without the use of counterincisions in the style of LaRoque or a separate incision for access to the peritoneal cavity. Bowel with "apparent" vascular compromise can be observed to "pink up" or regain peristalsis through the peritoneal incision.

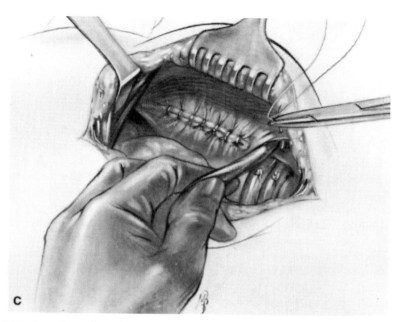

FIGURE 18.5. *(continued)* C: The direct defect has been closed. The transversalis fascial sling of the internal abdominal ring is tightened as a prophylactic measure.

Following the periosteum of the ilium laterally from the pubic tubercle, the iliopubic band is noted just above Cooper's ligament. Near the femoral vein—technically, the distal iliac vein—the iliopubic band begins to bifurcate, passing both under and over the femoral vein. The iliopubic tract runs essentially parallel, and for all practical anatomic purposes is part of the periosteum of the ilium. At the bifurcation, the superior element curves anteriorly, crossing over the femoral vessels to become part of the femoral fascia. The space between this diversion and the medial wall of the femoral vein is normally small and without named contents. This is, however, the site of femoral herniation (Fig. 18.6).

A peritoneal hernia sac can descend into this canal, rarely as a congenital defect, most commonly as an acquired defect. Once a peritoneal sac enters this space, the hydraulic forces of increased intraabdominal pressure—for whatever reasons—work, over time, enlarging the opening. When this action is combined with other hernia-related etiologic factors (e.g., metabolic defects, malnutrition, smoking, trauma) (see Chapters 1 and 2), a femoral hernia eventuates. Strictly speaking, this is not a fascial defect in the sense of the definition previously offered. However, if the iliopubic tract is considered part of the transversus abdominus complex of muscle, fascia, tendons, and aponeurosis, then this defect at the bifurcation of the iliopubic band must be considered a true hernia. The defect is medial to the femoral vein, more technically, the distal iliac vein proximal to the inguinal ligament, the structure that defines the two veins.

As the hernia sac descends into the femoral canal, extending below the inguinal ligament as it enlarges and lengthens, the *true* femoral vein is compromised along its medial aspect.

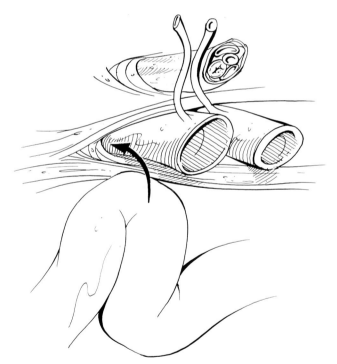

FIGURE 18.6. Following the periosteum of the ilium laterally from the pubic tubercle, the iliopubic band is noted just above Cooper's ligament. Near the femoral vein—technically, the distal iliac vein—the iliopubic band begins to bifurcate, passing both under and over the femoral vein. The iliopubic tract runs essentially parallel to and, for all practical anatomic purposes, is part of the periosteum of the ilium. At the bifurcation, the superior element curves anteriorly, crossing over the femoral vessels to become part of the femoral fascia. The space between this diversion and the medial wall of the femoral vein is normally small and without named contents. This is, however, the site of femoral herniation.

As an aside, the use of ultrasound imaging in the area of the femoral vessels with the patient performing Valsalva's maneuver can often demonstrate this lateral displacement of the femoral vein with the descent of the sac and its contents into the canal. This diagnostic approach is useful in differentiating infrainguinal mass lesions of the groin, allowing the planning of appropriate surgical intervention. It must be noted that a large percentage of femoral hernia patients present as urgent or emergent cases, most often elderly women with incarceration or strangulation of bowel. The opportunity for preoperative imaging in these cases is limited and is usually not required. Imaging of the patient with a symptomatic mass in the groin is not unreasonable.

Approaching the femoral hernia sac from the preperitoneal vantage point requires careful dissection and a delicate teasing of the sac from the femoral canal, as the lateral border of the sac is in intimate proximity to the medial wall of both the iliac and femoral veins. Dissection begins on the ventral and medial aspect of the femoral vein, the distal external iliac vein, retracting the hernia sac medially and slightly cephalad as illustrated in Fig. 18.7.

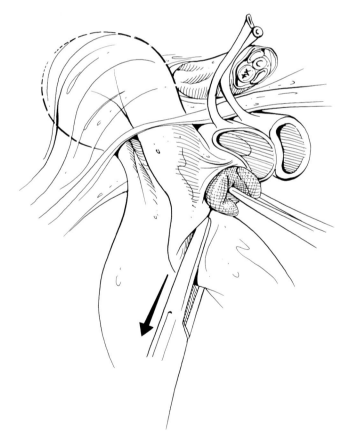

FIGURE 18.7. Approaching the femoral hernia sac from the preperitoneal perspective requires careful dissection and a delicate teasing of the sac from the femoral canal, as the lateral border of the sac is in intimate proximity to the medial wall of both the iliac and femoral veins. Dissection begins on the ventral and medial aspect of the femoral vein, distal external iliac vein, retracting the hernia sac medially and slightly cephalad as illustrated by the *arrow.*

With the sac removed from the femoral canal—or the canal found free of hernia—identification of the internal ring is the next step. Good superior retraction on the inferior leaf of the abdominal wall is required to expose the internal ring. Recall, the position of the internal ring is highly variable, a function of the shape of the pelvis and the angle between the internal and external inguinal rings, as well as the length of the canal itself. The location of the transverse abdominal wall skin incision must be selected to be cephalad the critical anatomic site of the internal ring to facilitate identification of indirect defects, as well as to effect a complete repair of all defects encountered.

If there is an indirect defect—an enlarged ring with a peritoneal sac entering it—the peritoneal sac is usually identified laterally and slightly ventral to the femoral vessels. The sac is removed from the internal ring with cephalad traction again coupled with blunt and sharp dissection as necessary to remove the sac from the internal ring. As with an incarcerated direct sac, an incision to enlarge the internal ring may be necessary. Removal of the sac is desirable to minimize the seroma and hematoma formation, but is not essential. Once the sac is removed from the internal ring, and thus out of the inguinal canal, the cord structures (vas, arteries, and venous pampiniform plexus) are readily separated. The sac is then ligated, avoiding easily any sliding components, and redundant sac removed. This ligation is "very high" relative to the location of the internal ring, usually 5 to 6 cm away from the internal ring of the anterior abdominal wall. Cord structures, without muscle or investing fascia, are readily identified and preserved in the course of the procedure. It is not possible to skeletonize the cord structures, for they have no investing fascia or muscles when approached from the posterior aspect (see Chapters 5 and 6).

REPAIR OF DEFECTS

Direct Hernias

Direct hernial defects are repaired based on the specific findings. Some defects of the direct wall, most frequently encountered in the repair of recurrent hernias, are well above the iliopubic tract and periosteum of the ilium, truly in the floor of the inguinal canal.

If the floor appears otherwise solid and the margins of the defect are clearly identifiable, simple interrupted suture closure using a vertical or horizontal suture line—dictated by the appearance and topology of the defect—is acceptable, especially for defects of 3 to 4 cm in length and 1 to 2 cm in width (Fig. 18.8). Over 77% of direct recurrent hernias in the senior author's initial experience with 413 recurrent groin hernias repaired preperitoneally were noted to be 4.0 cm or less in maximum diameter (10). In that series, 58% of the recurrent hernias were purely direct. Of those, 41.9% were observed at the pubic tubercle, 28.6% in the midfloor, and 15.2% adjacent to the internal ring. Of particular note, disruption of the entire posterior wall of the

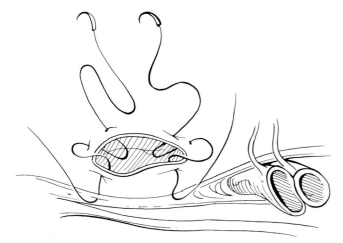

FIGURE 18.8. If the floor appears otherwise solid and the margins of the defect are clearly identifiable, simple interrupted suture closure using a vertical or horizontal suture line—dictated by the appearance and topology of the defect—is acceptable, especially for defects of 3 to 4 cm in length and 1 to 2 cm in width.

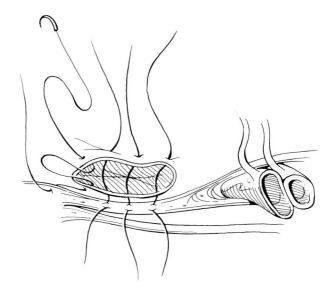

FIGURE 18.9. A running or interrupted suture technique is used, securing the transversus arch to the iliopubic tract. It is desirable to place the corner suture past the edge of the defect in either direction. The "corners" of the defect are rolled in with a "crown stitch." This stitch wraps the ends of the defect by rolling a lip of tissue in and is then secured to the iliopubic tract of periosteum, especially when the defect is medial.

inguinal canal was noted in only 11.4%, and multiple defects were seen in 2.8% of cases. In a later analysis of the series, expanded to over 750 recurrent groin hernia repairs using the preperitoneal approach, these numbers essentially remained the same. The anatomy of primary hernia repair direct defects, as observed from the posterior vantage point, is remarkably similar in the 500 or so cases cataloged during the past 20 years.

Nonabsorbable, running or interrupted suture material is preferred, typically a suture with tensile strength at least equal to that of the tissue being approximated, for example, at least that of 2-zero polypropylene.

For recurrent or primary repair of medial defects of the direct wall, those at or near the pubic tubercle (42% of all recurrent hernias repaired), the transversus arch and/or the edge of the defect is approximated to the iliopubic tract or periosteum of the ilium. A running or interrupted suture technique is used, securing the transversus arch to the iliopubic tract. It is desirable to place the corner suture past the edge of the defect in either direction. The "corners" of the defect are rolled in with a "crown stitch." This stitch wraps the ends of the defect by rolling a lip of tissue in and is then secured to the iliopubic tract of periosteum, especially when the defect is medial (Fig. 18.9).

For larger defects in the direct wall, the transversus arch is secured to the iliopubic tract and/or periosteum of the ilium with interrupted or running nonabsorbable sutures, again employing the corner stitches medially and laterally to reinforce the repair.

It is considered critical to approximate the edges of the defect if the inferior margin is not the iliopubic tract or periosteum. Repair of direct groin hernias that are more lateral, perhaps involving the medial aspect of the internal ring, uses a similar suturing technique. The superior and

inferior aspects of the defect are fixed to the iliopubic tract as it begins to cross over the femoral vein (Fig. 18.10). The use of mesh to buttress the suture repair is discussed in Mesh Placement, below.

Femoral Hernia

Closure of a femoral hernial defect is readily achieved using the following approach. After definition of the anatomy, especially the medial wall of the femoral vein, and the diversion or apparent bifurcation of the iliopubic tract anteriorly and posteriorly, sutures to close the defect, the femoral canal space, are readily placed. The iliopubic tract, medial to the femoral vein and femoral canal space, as it begins its ventral ascent towards and ventral to the femoral vein, is sutured to the periosteum of Cooper's ligament as the latter courses laterally and inferiorly to the femoral vessels. Interrupted nonabsorbable sutures are preferred (Fig. 18.11).

Those familiar with the true McVay repair, an innovation almost of pure historic interest, (see Chapter 13) will recognize the most lateral suture of this repair as the crucial "transitional stitch," one of the important elements of that repair. This suture in particular approximates the transversus arch to Cooper's ligament adjacent to the femoral vein, effectively obliterating the canal. Usually only two or three sutures are required to close this defect. The femoral canal is closed in a fashion to avoid compression of the femoral vein, minimizing the potential for thrombotic complications. Because of the heavy-gauge needle used to secure the suture to the periosteum and the large (2-zero or zero) suture material used to secure the repair, caution is exercised in the extreme

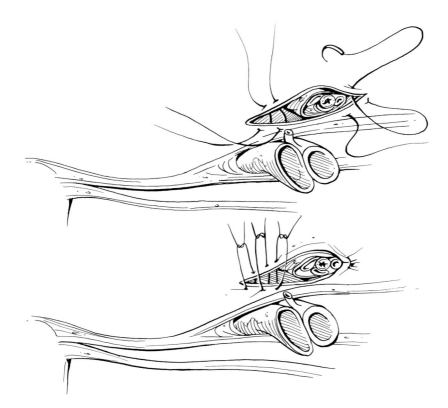

FIGURE 18.10. It is considered critical to approximate the edges of the defect if the inferior margin is not the iliopubic tract or periosteum. Repair of direct groin hernias that are more lateral, perhaps involving the medial aspect of the internal ring, uses a similar suturing technique. The superior and inferior aspects of the defect are fixed to the iliopubic tract as it begins to cross over the femoral vein.

to prevent accidental puncture or laceration of the femoral vein, which is radically exposed and vulnerable in this operation. In the senior author's personal series of thousands of hernia operations done with the preperitoneal approach, there has not been a laceration of this vessel.

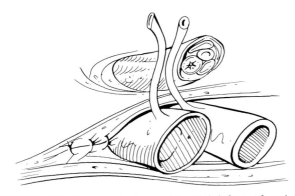

FIGURE 18.11. Closure of a femoral hernial defect. After definition of the anatomy, especially the medial wall of the femoral vein and the diversion or apparent bifurcation of the iliopubic tract anteriorly and posteriorly, sutures to close the defect, the femoral canal space, are readily placed. The iliopubic tract, medial to the femoral vein and femoral canal space, as it begins its ventral ascent toward and ventral to the femoral vein, is sutured to the periosteum of Cooper's ligament as the latter courses laterally and inferior to the femoral vessels. Interrupted nonabsorbable sutures are preferred.

Indirect Hernia

From the preperitoneal approach, the anatomy of the internal ring and its relationship to the cord structures is very clear. Not obscured by the cremaster muscle, the "bare" cord structures are seen as they pass through the internal ring. Some internal rings are quite narrow and small, while others are relatively large and wide, often dilated by a peritoneal sac with intestinal contents. Similar to the approach for direct defects, "individualization" of the repair, based on sound anatomic principles, is desirable. Defining the extent of the defect is an essential element of any repair; for an indirect defect especially, identifying the lateral limits is necessary. Placement of a crown stitch at the lateral extent of the internal ring to prevent possible extension is strongly recommended.

The cord structures are retracted laterally and the medial aspect of the internal ring defect is then closed. The upper edge (internal ring and transversalis arch) is secured to the anterior or most ventral element of the iliopubic tract that here is part of the femoral fascia. The thought behind closing the medial aspect of the internal ring is the preservation or maintenance of an adequate length of floor of the inguinal canal to avoid any crimping or kinking of the vas deferens or other cord structures. While not frequently observed as a cause of postoperative discomfort or patient dissatisfaction, injury or alteration of these structures has been noted (Fig. 18.10).

Mesh Placement

In a prospective sequential study of the preperitoneal repair of recurrent groin hernias, only 6% of the repairs were deemed to require mesh support (10). Primary suture repair for first-time groin hernia recurrence was effective in most cases (98.4%) *without* the addition of mesh to reinforce the tissue to tissue apposition. If the suture approximation of a primary or recurrent hernia is considered suspect by the experienced surgeon, a buttress of mesh (polypropylene) can be readily positioned against the deepest layer of the abdominal wall, the transversalis fascia, in the fashion of Wantz and Stoppa. Usually, a smaller size of mesh is used.

Mesh placement for support of a direct defect is shown in Fig. 18.12. Anchored inferiorly to the periosteum, Cooper's ligament, or iliopubic tract with continuous or interrupted suture, the mesh will be incorporated into the posterior abdominal wall. In this position, it not only covers the closed defect, but it also serves to generally reinforce this area of the abdominal wall.

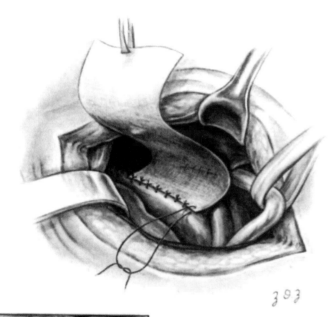

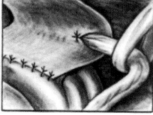

FIGURE 18.12. A polypropylene mesh buttress is attached posteriorly to Cooper's ligament (after repair of the recurrent defect in the wall) with 1-0 polypropylene suture material. If there is concern about closure of the internal abdominal ring (in direct recurrences), the mesh may be folded around the spermatic cord **(inset)**.

The extent of the superior or cephalad extension of the mesh remains an area of interest and discussion. In general, we have elected to use mesh patches smaller than those recommended for TAPP, TEPP, or Kugel repairs (see Chapters 21 to 24). Indeed, in perusing the literature of those repairs, it would appear that the size of the mesh placed does correlate to the incidence of recurrence. This has not been our experience.

In the open preperitoneal repair, mesh is used to *reinforce* a tissue approximation repair; it is not used to span the defect as the repair *per se*. The techniques advocated by Stoppa (see Chapter 19), involving the use of large mesh reinforcement, are not always appropriate for straightforward primary or first-time recurrent groin hernia and should, in our opinion, be reserved for the more complex situations of multiply recurrent hernia. Dr. Stoppa's contributions to this approach and those of George Wantz are fully recognized as significant to the overall evolution of this operation. It must be noted that the recurrence rates quoted in the more recent literature for these repairs in general fall into the same 1% to 2% range reported for first-time recurrent hernia repair using this technique.

Obturator hernias are well managed by the preperitoneal approach. After the defect is identified, its contents are removed most frequently by opening the peritoneum and reducing the contents of the sac from within. Placement of the mesh onto Cooper's ligament with a 4- to 5-cm inferior excess covers this area of the pelvis, adequately reinforcing it. It must be noted that direct suture repair of the obturator defect is difficult, if not impossible. There are reports of obturator hernia repair employing laparoendoscopic techniques that are interesting. This is a rare hernia of the groin, and few surgeons have encountered it in any large volume.

In this instance, the use of the mesh to span the "defect" is effective for the following reasons (Fig. 18.13). By covering the defect with an excess area of mesh while securing it to Cooper's ligament ventrally, the mesh is effectively held in place between the peritoneum and the rather solid pelvis, minimizing potential mesh migration. It must be noted that variations on the placement of mesh into this area have been reported, and the question of securing the mesh at all—even in those repairs that are technologically defined—remains unanswered (see Chapters 22 and 23).

As for the superior or cranial extent of mesh, once sutured to the iliopubic tract or Cooper's ligament, cephalad location becomes the surgeon's judgment. Securing the mesh to the anterior abdominal wall, with continuous or tacking sutures into the transversalis fascia, 4 to 5 cm above the arch, is reasonable in most cases. At times, as in the primary closure of a large whole floor direct defect, complete blowout of the floor, large internal ring, and enlarged defect to free an incarceration, there is a shortening of the inferior flap of the abdominal wall. This effectively produces a gap in the rectus sheath fascial incisions used to enter the preperitoneal space. At times, this can be from 2 to 6 cm or more in size. In that

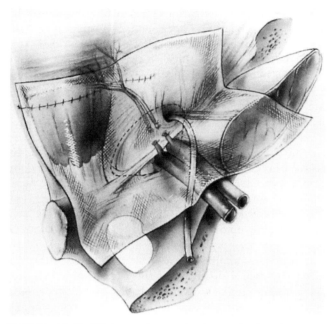

FIGURE 18.13. With patch prosthetic repair, hernias recur through the unrepaired portion of the myopectineal orifice and at the borders of the prosthetic suture attachment. With giant prosthetic reinforcement of the visceral sac, recurrent herniation is difficult to conceive. (From Wantz GE. Prosthetic repair groin hernias. *Atlas of hernia surgery*. New York: Raven Press, 1991: 94–151, with permission.)

instance, the mesh is secured to the rectus sheath inferiorly and superiorly as part of the closure. In all cases of mesh placement, a hole for the cord structures is made.

Complex and Combined Primary and Recurrent Groin Hernias

This group of hernias represents for the surgeon a challenge of major magnitude. The preperitoneal approach is ideal for these cases. The preperitoneal approach permits a complete dissection of the abdominal wall, providing identification of any structural weakness in the three critical areas: indirect, direct, and femoral. Repairing defects individually is thus possible. At times, a large defect from the pubic tubercle to the lateral aspect of the internal ring must be repaired. Here, closure is accomplished with running or interrupted sutures and the defect buttressed with mesh that is secured to the iliopubic tract or ilium inferiorly.

Complex groin hernias, or those with multiple defects, make up approximately 10% of our experience. Over half (56.4%) were combinations of direct and indirect defects. The combination of direct and femoral hernia made up 18% and indirect and femoral another 18%. The remaining 7% were truly complex, often involving all three areas and elements of tissue loss as well. It is not clear how these would be classified, given the various schema available today.

PERSONAL PREFERENCES

Suture Material

The authors prefer repair with nonabsorbable, minimally reactive suture material. Certain small heavy needles (Mayo No. 7) facilitate repair in this limited space. Minimally reactive sutures appear to be associated with a very low incidence of suture granuloma and infection. While the incidence of wound complications related to infection is low, when there is an infection, the patient's course is not easy. In the authors' series, significant wound infections were rarely observed (fewer than five total). This incidence is lower than values reported for infection in many of the anterior mesh repairs and TAPP and TEP series as well. This low incidence of infection may be related to the deep placement of sutures, the suture type, and, when mesh is used, the proximity to the peritoneum, a known biologically active membrane surface.

Closure of the Fascial Incision/Skin

A simple running suture of zero or No. 1 polypropylene is used to close the anterior fascia (rectus sheath and external abdominal oblique). At the lateral margin of the rectus, all layers are closed to avoid creating an iatrogenic spigelian hernia. The transversalis and external abdominal oblique are closed lateral to the rectus as one layer. If a "relaxing incision" is needed, it can be accomplished by sewing both internal and external anterior rectus sheaths superiorly to only the external rectus sheath inferiorly. The mesh placement will reinforce this area if it is assessed prior to cutting off the excess mesh cephalad so that a sufficient length is present to cover this area. Suture knots are buried to keep the firm ends of the cut polypropylene from irritating the patient. The skin is closed with subcuticular polyglycolic acid suture (4-zero), and skin tapes are applied. Antibiotics are not used unless mesh is placed; in that case, systemic parenteral antibiotics are given and the wound is irrigated with an antibiotic solution prior to closure. Patients can usually be discharged the same day, making the operation feasible as an outpatient procedure. They can resume normal activities and return to work by week 6, including heavy lifting, and often earlier if the work does not involve significant physical labor.

Personal Experience

The senior author has used the open preperitoneal hernia operation, as described and taught to him by Professor Nyhus, to repair more than 750 recurrent groin hernias and in over 3,000 primary repairs of inguinal hernias. Over a course of nearly 30 years of experience with this operation, the technique has been acquired and passed on to younger generations of surgeons. It has been used almost exclusively as an element of surgical resident education and occasionally to educate practicing surgeons. In the series of recurrent hernia repairs (over 750 cases), the observed failure rate (recurrence rate) *for first-time repair of a recurrent hernia* is 1.6%. This figure is comparable to, and perhaps slightly better than, results reported from other centers using the entire gamut of surgical options in the repair of groin hernia.

A few, albeit small, randomized prospective studies of groin hernia repair have included an "open preperitoneal repair" arm (1,4,11,12). In these studies, the "open preperitoneal repair" was compared to a variety of anterior or laparoscopic repairs, usually, but not always, constant within a study. The use of mesh was another variable in the analysis. In other reports, the "open preperitoneal repair" was the operation advocated by Stoppa or Wantz. While recurrence was not the primary end point of many of these studies, the reported failure rates of some anterior repairs were at variance with numbers reported from single-experience, longitudinal reports from various centers. It must be noted that the number of trials that included the preperitoneal surgical approach described here are actually few (3,5,7,8,15).

A computer-generated literature search, searching for the terms "groin hernia," "randomized trial," "complications," and "outcome," conducted in early January 2001 had a yield of nearly 400 entries for the years 1995–2000. While many of the cited and retrieved articles were not relevant to the specific question of comparing the open preperitoneal repair to other repairs, a few actually did include this procedure in the study. One important observation is the generally small number of patients or hernia repairs completed in each of these studies. Without questioning the skills of the surgeons involved, it is clear that the surgeons' experience with any specific procedure refines the eventual outcome. For the preperitoneal repair described here, the individual series report of Patino (13) clearly supports this approach as valid in the contemporary surgical armamentarium.

With respect to the randomized trials, in general they involved few patients, often 50 or less, and frequently had a follow-up of less than 3 years. From an experimental design vantage point, these studies usually lack the power, due to insufficient numbers of patients, to identify real differences in recurrence rates, assuming there really are clinically significant differences (see Chapter 49).

Ten reports in which an open preperitoneal repair was done were reviewed. Recurrence rates ranged from 0% to as high as 21.6%. The incidence of recurrence appears to be a function of length of follow-up. In some reports, the patients were randomized as they entered the study; in others, the type of hernia defined clinically or at surgery determined randomization. Still others compared the repair of specifically classified groin hernias, the classification defined preoperatively.

It is interesting to note that not one study, randomized or prospective single series, reported an experience similar to that of the senior author, who has repaired over 750 recurrent groin hernias with the preperitoneal approach. It is also not clear that this experience can be transported to another site, for the learning curve has not been well established.

The recurrence rate for complex, multiply recurrent hernias in this series is 3% to 5%, a valid reference value by any comparison since recurrence rates of 5% to 10% or more are being reported for many of the more modern hernia repairs. Significant morbidity, femoral nerve injury, ischemic orchitis, and chronic pain have been rare complications, with two femoral nerve injuries and one testicular infarct in the entire series (orchiectomy accompanied the repair on two occasions).

There have been two rather extensive literature reviews of hernia surgery in recent years. They have attempted to answer some of the vexing questions surrounding recurrence, complications, and other aspects of morbidity and mortality associated with surgical repair of groin hernia.

In the article comparing methods of repair, the variable rate of recurrence with many operations is obvious. The article that addresses the use of mesh finds data to support the role of mesh use in decreasing the incidence or recurrence, independent of the technique used for the repair. A point obvious in both reviews is the rather short follow-up period in the studies analyzed. In our experience, and that of some others, patients who have a recurrent hernia frequently do not return for additional surgery for 13 to 15 years for most asymptomatic hernias. There is an incidence of groin hernia recurrence, found on routine follow-up, that represents technical failure but may be without clinical implications.

In reviewing this massive body of literature, the anonymous adage, "When two people do the same thing, it is not the same thing after all" begins to ring true.

As with any new operation, and perhaps more so for the technologically sophisticated mesh-only repairs, there is a significant learning curve associated with this procedure. Given the variation in human groin anatomy, a reasonable, but for the moment undefined, volume of experience is necessary to gain familiarity and comfort with this approach to treating groin hernia. Once a level of comfort based on experience is attained, the open preperitoneal approach should be *the preferred option* for repair of any recurrent groin hernia and any femoral or incarcerated/strangulated hernia because it is based on anatomic principles combined with sound surgical concepts.

REFERENCES

1. Aitola P, Airo I, Matikainen M. Laparoscopic versus open preperitoneal inguinal hernia repair: a prospective randomised trial. *Ann Chir Gynaecol* 1998;87:22–25.
2. Anson B, McVeigh C, eds. In: *Callander's surgical anatomy.* Philadelphia: WB Saunders, 1958:353–414.
3. Beets GL, Dirksen CD, Go PM, et al. Open or laparoscopic preperitoneal mesh repair for recurrent inguinal hernia? A randomized controlled trial. *Surg Endosc* 1999;13:323–327.

4. Bostanci BE, Tetik C, Ozer S, et al. Posterior approaches in groin hernia repair with prosthesis: open or closed. *Acta Chir Belg* 1998;98:241–244.

5. Champault GG, Rizk N, Catheline JM, et al. Inguinal hernia repair: totally preperitoneal laparoscopic approach versus Stoppa operation; randomized trial of 100 cases. *Surg Laparosc Endosc* 1997;7:445–450.

6. Condon RE. The anatomy of the inguinal region and its relationship to groin hernia. In: Nyhus LM, Harkins HN, eds. *Hernia*. Philadelphia: JB Lippincott Co, 1964:14–72.

7. European Union Hernia Trialists Collaboration. Laparoscopic compared with open methods of groin hernia repair: systematic review of randomized controlled trials. *Br J Surg* 2000;87:860–867.

8. EU Hernia Trialists Collaboration. Mesh compared with non-mesh methods of open groin hernia repair: systematic review of randomized controlled trials. *Br J Surg* 2000;87:854–859.

9. Fruchaud H. *Anatomie chirugicale des hernies de l'aine*. Paris: Doin, 1956.

10. Greenburg AG. Revisiting the recurrent groin hernia. *Am J Surg* 1987;154:34–40.

11. Janu PG, Sellers KD, Mangiante EC. Recurrent inguinal hernia repair: preferred operative approach. *Int Surg* 1999;84:57–59.

12. Johansson B, Hallerback B, Glise H, et al. Laparoscopic mesh versus open preperitoneal mesh versus conventional technique for inguinal hernia repair. *Ann Surg* 1999;230:225–231.

13. Patino JF, Garcia-Herreros LG, Zundel N. Inguinal hernia repair. The Nyhus posterior preperitoneal operation. *Surg Clin North Am* 1998;78:1063–1074.

14. Read RC. Annandale's role in the development of preperitoneal groin herniorrhaphy. *Hernia* 1997;1:111–115.

15. Velasco JM, Gelman C, Villina VL. Preperitoneal bilateral inguinal herniorrhaphy: evolution of a technique from conventional to laparoscopic. *Surg Endosc* 1996;10:122–127.

19

THE MIDLINE PREPERITONEAL APPROACH AND PROSTHETIC REPAIR OF GROIN HERNIAS

RENÉ E. STOPPA

Around the year 1965, hernia recurrences continued to plague the patients and humiliate surgeons, hence I became convinced of a possible revolution for repairing even the worst cases. This led me to propose a method mixing some important concepts, the advent of which I had been a direct witness to: (a) My mentor, Henri Fruchaud (1956), had described his myopectineal hole, which expressed an evident structural weakness of the groin, due to the absence of voluntary striated muscle fibers in this area. (b) Convenient synthetic meshes had been used in France by Don Acquaviva since 1949 (1) and by one of my mentors, René Bourgeon (1955) (4), and then, in the United States, by Usher (1959) (21) and Koontz (1960) (6) for direct repair of hernia defects. My friend Jean Rives enthusiastically introduced the use of polyester (Dacron, Ethicon Ethnor) mesh in France (14). (c) I personally observed that the used pieces of mesh were of insufficient dimensions: whether by small patches of the same dimensions as those of the defect, or by larger pieces covering the myopectineal hole. (d) Moreover, synthetic fabrics, though well answering biologic tolerance criteria, could not thoroughly replace the anatomic living structures, nor assume their tonic and motor functions. By elimination of the possibility of restoring the wall, I realized that a supple mesh could preferably be used only as an artificial fascia able to widely enwrap the visceral sac, as does the natural endoabdominal fascia. An interesting tactical advantage was provided when proceeding this way: instead of making the difficult attempts required to repair the defective wall, the surgeon could now render the peritoneal sac inextensible so that herniation could no longer appear. The conflict between the intraabdominal pressure and a more or less defective wall was abolished by the interposition of a mesh barrier. Such have been the circumstances that led to the introduction of an almost absolute weapon

against recurrence of herniation in the groin region at first, and then in other locations in the abdominal wall (ventral and incisional hernias).

In this chapter, I present my original method, introduced 30 years ago, combining a midline preperitoneal approach and the entrapment of the inferior part of the visceral sac into a very large bilateral piece of polyester (Dacron) mesh.

I do not propose this operation as a panacea but rather as a worthwhile method for the treatment of difficult cases. In the name of efficacy, there is no doubt that the reinforcement or replacement of the transversalis fascia by a synthetic mesh arrived in the nick of time for rendering possible the repair of irremediably damaged inguinal walls.

ANATOMIC PURPOSES

Good anatomic knowledge is a basic principle for improving operations for hernia. Fruchaud (5a) proposed a possible unification of groin hernias: whatever their superficial emergence (inguinal or femoral), they pass through the inguinal wall across the musculopectineal opening (Fig. 19.1). The size of this hole varies according to the structure of the inguinal muscular triangle, shown in the work of Condon and Nyhus, and Gaston, and the variations of the "inguinal angles" of Radojevic and Barbin, or the "pubic height" of Ami (Fig. 19.2).

Within the weak area of the musculopectineal opening, deprived of voluntary striated muscle fibers, the transversalis fascia (the inguinal portion of the endoabdominal fascia) and its analogs represent the only (and often poorly) resistant layer—the intraabdominal, pressure-tight layer—of the wall. This is the best depth for inguinal repairs, in which the wall must be sutured without tension or reinforced. I believe that perfect and permanent tightness of the deep inguinal layer, in this weak area, can easily be ensured by a piece of synthetic mesh.

R. E. Stoppa: Department of Surgery, University de Picardie Jules Verne; Department of Surgery, Centre Hospitalier Universitaire, Amiens, France.

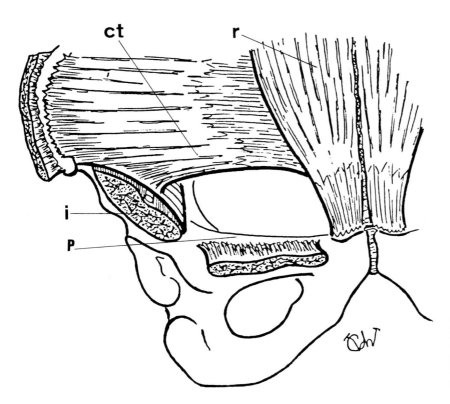

FIGURE 19.1. Schematic constitution of Fruchaud myopectineal hole, limited by a regional solid frame: the rectus muscle (*r*), its medial pillar; the iliopsoas muscle (*i*), its lateral pillar; the conjoined tendon arch (*ct*), its superior limit; and the pectineal crest (*p*), its inferior bony margin.

Behind the transversalis fascia is a wide cleavable cellular space that spreads to the two sides of the infraumbilical midline—the retrofascial preperitoneal and prevesical spaces—which widely overspread the Retzius' and Bogros' spaces. With Odimba (10), we have made precise measure-

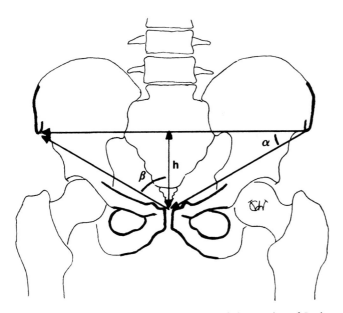

FIGURE 19.2. Schematic representation of the angles of Radojevic (α) and Barbin (β) and the pubic height of Ami (*h*), which are related to the dimensions of the musculopectineal opening described by Fruchaud.

ments of its shape, dimensions, and variations by dissection and radioanatomic study. Thus, we have been able to show the practicing surgeon the shape and size of the retrofascial space, a natural site for large prostheses replacing or reinforcing the transversalis fascia (Fig. 19.3), and at the same time a fine route for placing them.

An interesting anatomic detail related to a key gesture in our prosthetic repair is the retroparietal anatomic disposition of the elements that constitute the spermatic cord. Every surgeon operating through a posterior route has observed that, of the two pedicles that pass through the musculopectineal opening, the iliofemoral vascular pedicle is a parietal element, whereas the spermatic pedicle, surrounded by its cellular sheath, traverses the inguinal retroparietal space when the preperitoneal cleavage has been performed. The elements of the cord can be separated from the peritoneum and parietalized when a preperitoneal prosthesis is placed. There are three advantages to this technique: (a) The zigzag course of the cord is transversely enlarged, and consequently its deeper angle is transferred several centimeters more laterally. (b) Consequently, the inguinal passage is better protected against a dangerous sudden increase in intraabdominal pressure (3). The need to cut the mesh for passage of the spermatic cord is eliminated; the prosthesis can be easily placed in a retroparietal and retrofunicular location (Fig. 19.4).

On the whole, one must remember the anatomic conditions naturally favorable to the logical use of prostheses: (a) the frequent propensity to weakness of the inguinal structures that sustain the tight layer of the wall, the transversalis

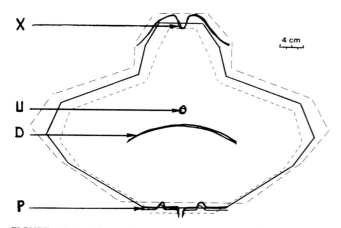

FIGURE 19.3. Schematic plane projection on the abdominal wall of the preperitoneal prevesical retrofascial space after anatomic and roentgenographic measurements. The *continuous line* represents the median size and shape of this cleavable space. The *outer dashed line* represents the maximal dimensions, and the *inner dashed line* represents the minimal size. *D*, Douglas linea arcuata; *P*, pubis; *U*, umbilicus; *X*, xiphoid appendix.

fascia itself being of variable strength, and (b) the existence of a retroparietal, easily cleavable wide space, a natural site for insertion of large prostheses underlying the wall.

PATHOLOGIC PURPOSES

In the field of prosthetic repairs by the preperitoneal approach, we restrict ourselves to discussing the respective efficiency of the two main methods of treatment of groin hernias—herniorrhaphy and prosthesis insertion. If herniorrhaphies, elective by nature, call for a precise study of hernial orifices, prosthetic repair accommodates itself to Fruchaud's singular concept: that all groin hernias, inguinal or femoral, pass through the musculopectineal opening. From this point of view, there are two types of groin hernias: *congenital* hernias, caused by persistence of the peritoneovaginal channel, and *weakness* hernias, always resulting from the failure of the musculofascial layer (Fig. 19.5). In addition to congenital abnormalities of the transversalis fas-

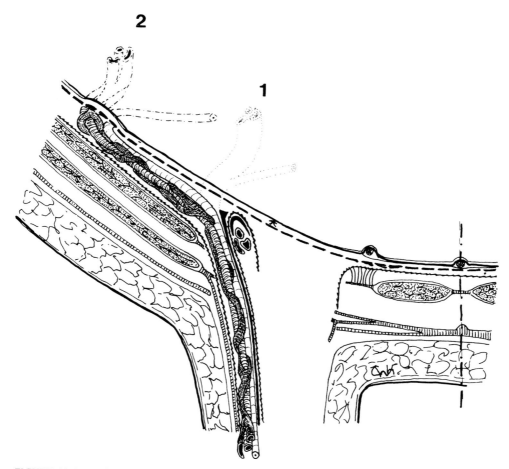

FIGURE 19.4. Horizontal cross section of the inguinal region and of the relative disposition of the cord after "parietalization" of its constitutive elements. Note the more lateral position of the deep cord angle, so that its zigzag course is enlarged transversely: before *1* and after *2* parietalization.

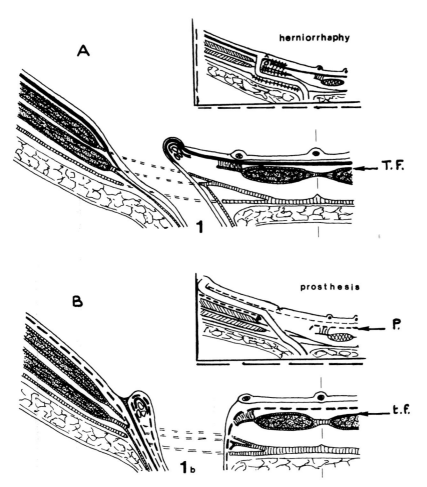

FIGURE 19.5. Schematic horizontal cross sections of the inguinal region, showing a congenital indirect inguinal hernia **(A)** and one caused by direct weakness **(B)**. The **insets** show the proposed methods of treatment: herniorrhaphy **(A)** and prosthetic repair **(B)**. *1, 1b,* hernial sacs; *T.F.,* strong transversalis fascia; *t.f.,* weakened transversalis fascia; *P.,* prosthesis.

cia and the internal oblique muscle arch, one hears more and more of a probable biologic insufficiency of the groin, a sort of "fascial diathesis" predisposing mostly to direct hernias, a weakening by aging of the aponeurotic structures, or diverse progressive deficiencies of scars.

Hernial lesions are diverse and call for diverse methods of repair. Herniorrhaphy is nearly always appropriate for congenital hernias. Prosthetic repair of the transversalis fascia is logical for weakness hernias caused by deterioration of the inguinal musculofascial layer. The best reason for the use of prostheses is their radical efficacy. They solve instantly and definitively the mechanical problem created by the deficiency of the impervious layer of the abdominal wall in hernias caused by weakness because they reinforce the endoabdominal fascia or replace it. They are also a definitive solution against scar aging.

PURPOSE OF THE PREPERITONEAL APPROACH

Among the abdominal or posterior approaches, the preperitoneal approach offers the richest well-known resources nicely exposed by Nyhus. Since 1965, Rives, in France, has emphasized the approach. Since 1967, I have used the preperitoneal subumbilical approach (16,17). The advantages of the approach are facility of separation of the retrofascial cellular space, direct access to the posterior inguinal structures, clear understanding of hernial lesions, and good exposure of the musculopectineal opening. The movements in placing a prosthesis are easily carried out. This is most noticeable when one repairs multirecurrent hernias, which proceed from normal anatomy (of the midline) toward abnormal anatomy (of the hernial lesions)—there is no additional deterioration of the already-weakened inguinal structures and no risk of injury to the cord or the superficial nerves. Familiarity with this approach and with prostheses encourages us to distinguish no longer between the different types of groin hernias (inguinal or femoral). The main interest in this approach is the ability to place a large piece of synthetic mesh behind the weak groin area for tightening the wall, whatever the damage to its structural layers, at the same time widely wrapping the visceral sac—rendering it inextensible—so that herniation can no longer occur. The preperitoneal approach is perfectly convenient for even the most difficult hernial repairs, such as those of multirecurrent, prevascular, sliding, enormous, and bilateral hernias.

In the preperitoneal approach one avoids the nerves and cord dissection; thus, the number of testicular atrophies and painful sequelae is decreased (11,12). In the same way, this technique preserves the mechanisms that protect the inguinal region from the effects of intraabdominal pressure (Keith's inguinal shutter, Lytle's Hesselbach ligament sling, Ogilvie's cord lifting).

The median preperitoneal approach may induce the risk of incisional hernia, and I respond to this risk by using large bilateral pieces of prosthetic material, which tighten the weak inguinal areas of both sides and at the same time protect the subumbilical midline closure. I have had limited experience with Nyhus's suprainguinal incision (7) because I prefer to use the retroparietal large bilateral prosthesis, which cannot be placed by this approach. Nyhus's approach has the advantage of not damaging the median raphe, but in my experience, it does not secure the repair from the risk of eventration after wound suppuration. I, followed by Rignault and coworkers, have used a Pfannenstiel's incision, but opening and closing the wall are time-consuming, the risk of damaging superficial nerves is present, and I believe that there is only a cosmetic advantage to this transverse incision.

One must distinguish between the here-described preperitoneal approach and preperitoneal placement of mesh through inguinal incision, which is used in France (12–14). As in all inguinal approaches, this procedure requires identification of the nerves and dissection of the spermatic cord, inguinal layers, and hernial sac; this dissection may be difficult in recurrent hernias. The square prosthesis used is small (6 to 10 cm) and must be carefully sewn laterally to the iliac fascia, with care taken to avoid the crural nerve; to Cooper's ligament and the femoral vessel sheath, with care to avoid the femoral vein; and to the medial and superior edges of the musculopectineal hole. The prosthetic mesh is cut to let the cord through, which creates a risk of recurrence through the gap in the patch. This technique is more difficult than insertion of the large bilateral prosthesis by the preperitoneal approach and must be used only by experienced surgeons. I do know that Rives and associates have been successful, and I have some personal experience with the technique (18), with less consistent results than with the use of our large bilateral prosthesis.

In conclusion, I use the preperitoneal approach—well known in the United States for elective repair of hernial orifices—for the placement of large pieces of mesh that reinforce or replace the damaged transversalis fascia. Prosthetic repair by this method is easier than by the inguinal approach. I prefer the median approach over others because it allows the surgeon to approach both sides at once, quickly and with good exposure, and to insert large bilateral pieces of Dacron mesh. Wantz proposed the unilateral giant prosthetic repair, which is the same as our bilateral procedure, but cut in half; the preperitoneal space is reached by a transverse incision extending from the midline laterally for 8 to 9 cm, made 2 to 3 cm below the level of the anterosuperior iliac spines.

HOW TO USE PROSTHESES

Choosing a Good Prosthesis

Good prostheses replace or reinforce the tight inguinal layer (the transversalis fascia) and are a fundamental modern therapeutic option. Classic research and clinical experience have produced well-known data, which are not reproduced here. A good prosthetic material must provoke a moderate inflammatory reaction and have strong fibroblastic activity. Macroporous mesh must be preferred because of its fast invasion by the connective tissue and its good biologic tolerance of septic conditions.

I routinely have used Dacron mesh, advocated in France by Rives and associates, for 30 years. Our experiments with Petit (11) and Soler showed the good biologic tolerance of Dacron mesh. Arnaud and colleagues (2) stressed the quality of the fibroblastic-to-inflammatory cell ratio. Marlex (C.R. Bard, Inc. Murray Hill, NJ, U.S.A.) or Prolene (Ethicon Ethnor) mesh and Rhodergon 8000 (Rhone Poulenc, France) can be used, but they are less supple than Dacron and less convenient for groin hernia repair by giant prostheses as assessed by Wantz (22). Other materials, such as Vicryl (Ethicon Ethnor) mesh (low absorbency), offer only a temporary buttress, and silicone sheets (impervious), and Rhodergon velours (joining a sheet of Silastic and synthetic velvet) should never be used because they are badly tolerated by the body. I do not recommend microporous expanded polytetrafluoroethylene (ePTFE) mesh, which is not penetrated by fibrocytes, but simply encapsulated, and thus does not fix, and is responsible for frequent seromas.

Important Principles of Prosthesis Use

I conceive the prosthetic repair of groin hernias, like that of eventrations, as the placement of synthetic nonabsorbable mesh between the deeper inguinal layer and the visceral sac in the retroparietal cleavable space described earlier. In so doing, I do not place a simple patch, but make a large interposition of prosthetic mesh able to hold face to face with the neighboring layers and to support instantly and permanently the inguinal wall. For this purpose, the prosthesis must extend broadly beyond the weak inguinal area in all directions (Fig. 19.6) so that when the peritoneal sac is replaced, the prosthesis is pressed by intraabdominal pressure against the inner face of the abdominal wall and quickly attached by the development of the connective tissue through the mesh. By this method, the surgeon uses the force that has created the hernia—the intraabdominal pressure—to obtain a radical cure.

I and my colleagues have demonstrated that in accordance with Pascal's hydrostatic principle, abdominal pressure procures a stability that exempts the surgeon from fixation of the prosthesis, provided it is large. Gosset wrote that the prosthesis was like "a gaiter between the inner tube and the tire," and Van Damme compared the

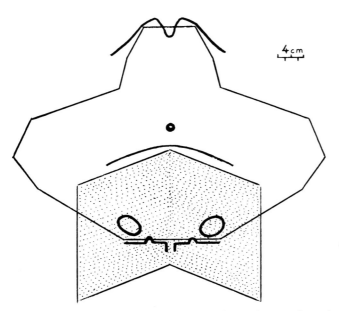

FIGURE 19.6. Schematic superposition of our chevron-shaped prosthesis over the plane projection of the retrofascial–preperitoneal cleavable space. The chevron-shaped pattern of the prosthesis provides better centering and broader overlapping of the two musculopectineal openings. (See also Fig. 19.11.)

tactic with "plugging a leak in a bathtub." The central principle of our method is this: the larger the prosthesis, the more efficient the repair. In our conception, there are two possible types of operations that use Dacron mesh as a piece of artificial endoabdominal fascia placed by the preperitoneal approach: the unilateral patch, which needs to be fixed carefully because of its rather small size, and the large bilateral prosthesis, widely wrapping the visceral sac, which needs no suture because it holds instantly and definitively with the intraperitoneal pressure.

TECHNICAL ASPECTS OF PROSTHETIC REPAIR

Preoperative Preparation

Operations for extremely large hernias necessitate respiratory preparations and, exceptionally, the use of the progressive pneumoperitoneum, as suggested by Goñi-Moreno. General anesthesia is usually used, as is spinal or peridural anesthesia in patients at respiratory risk. Some useful surgical instruments are: mounted swabs for the retroparietal cleavage, two straight retractors (6 and 10 cm long) for the abdominal wall, Ombrédanne's forceps or tape for handling the cord, a sterilized scale and scissors for measuring and cutting the prosthesis, and long curved Rochester's forceps for no-touch handling and easy positioning of the prosthesis.

The Operation

Medial Preperitoneal Approach

The patient is placed supine in a light Trendelenburg position. The surgeon is on the opposite side of the hernia. An adhesive field is applied as the usual protection against skin contamination. A median subumbilical incision is made, and the umbilicoprevesical fascia is cut with Mayo scissors (Fig. 19.7). The preperitoneal cleavage starts from the lower portion on the median line in the retropubic Retzius' space. It continues laterally, posteriorly to the rectus abdominis muscle on the far side of the operator, and proceeds behind the epigastric vessels. The dissection advances downward in front of the bladder, up to the prostatic compartment, and then outward behind the iliopubic ramus in Bogros' space. Thus is the hernial pedicle isolated (Fig. 19.8), and the spermatic cord is either united to or distinct from the hernial sac, depending on the type of hernia. This dissection does not necessitate a difficult search even in recurrent her-

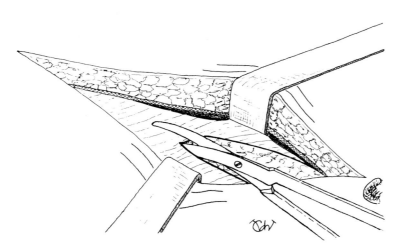

FIGURE 19.7. The section downward of the umbilicoprevesical fascia, with Mayo scissors.

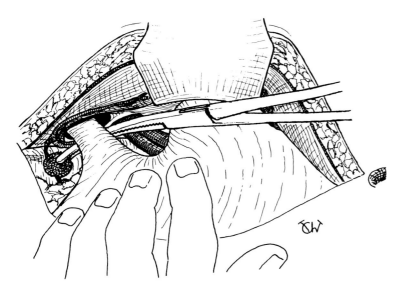

FIGURE 19.8. The right indirect hernial pedicle lifted on a forceps with a small swab.

nias, which is pleasing for all operators regardless of their experience. The iliac vessels and crural nerve in their sheath do not incur any injury.

Direct hernial sacs (inguinal, femoral or rarely obturator) are inverted with a purse-string suture. An interesting detail of surgical anatomy of direct hernias is to be dealt with at this stage of the operation: after the management of the peritoneal sac, another fascial sac is visible, like a superficial lining of the reduced hernial sac; turning inside out this fascial sac and fixing it to the inner surface of the abdominal wall eliminates the dead space and prevents serosanguinous collection, which may give the appearance of an early pseudorecurrence. *Indirect sacs* are opened for introducing a finger in order to simplify their dissection. Small sacs are managed by resection or invagination. After reduction of their contents, larger sacs should be preferably transected and closed at their proximal level, and their distal part left undisturbed in the scrotum, being careful not to dissect the sac below the level of the pubis, which carries the risk of ischemic orchitis due to the trauma of the distal spermatic vascularization. The anterior aspect of the distal sac should be opened as widely as possible to promote drainage into the surrounding tissues, and a suction drain is placed within it at the end of that step of the procedure. The preperitoneal approach opens a large exposure of the whole region and uncovers other clinically nonapparent hernias (e.g., obturator hernias). The peritoneum is closed after eventual resection of the hernial sac, and the preperitoneal dissection continues rapidly and without difficulty under the external iliac vessels and laterally to the ureter. It is not necessary to pursue the dissection above the Douglas linea arcuata, where the peritoneum is adherent or may tear. When an iliac appendectomy scar is present, dissection may become somewhat difficult but is easily overcome with scissors. On the whole, the surgeon can perform the dissection of the

Bogros' and Retzius' spaces quickly and easily without bleeding, using a single straight retractor under the inner wall while depressing the peritoneal sac with the left hand.

Joining the constituting elements of the spermatic cord with the pelvic wall simplifies placement of the large prosthesis and eliminates the need to cut it for passage of the spermatic cord. The cord is seized in its retroparietal course with an Ombrédanne's forceps or a tape, with moderate traction applied, so that the scissors and a blunt swab may dissociate the different elements of the cord, contained into their carefully preserved sheath, from the peritoneal sac. At the end of the dissection, one finds a triangular cellular spread (Fig. 19.9) with a posterosuperior base, the sides of which contain the deferent canal, on its medial side, and the spermatic vascular pedicle on its lateral side. When they are released, as when the Ombrédanne's forceps are opened, the elements of the spermatic cord join by gravity with the lateral wall so that no element now crosses the preperitoneal prevesical space and the spermatic sheath covers the external iliac vessels. During this operative time, preperitoneal and cordal lipomas should be suppressed in the aim to avoid the deceiving cough impulsion of a false recurrence. To perform the retroparietal dissection on the other side, the operator and assistant change sides and proceed in the same manner as for the first side.

Placement of the Prosthesis

Unilateral Patch. Rives, who routinely uses the inguinal approach for prosthetic repairs, scarcely uses the preperitoneal approach for the placement of a unilateral piece of mesh. In this case, he places two to three stitches to close the musculopectineal orifice, joining the arch to Cooper's ligament. Then, a 10-cm^2 piece of Dacron mesh is cut up and inserted in the angle formed by the abdominal wall and

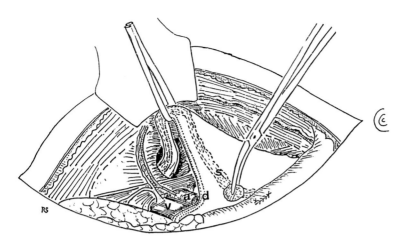

FIGURE 19.9. Intraoperative aspect of the right cord, within its spermatic triangular sheath, elevated by a tape, during its separation from the peritoneum. *s,* spermatic vessels; *d,* ductus deferens; *a,* femoral artery; *v,* femoral vein.

the fascia iliaca (Fig. 19.10). Differently than I do, Rives does not parietalize the cord; the prosthesis is usually split to let the cord through, then attached to the wall of the inguinal region by a few carefully executed sutures. If a hernia exists on the opposite side, the operator changes sides and proceeds in the same manner as for the first side; in this situation, two symmetric pieces are placed.

Wantz, whose technique is presented later, places a 12-cm piece of Dacron mesh unilaterally, without splitting it (for the passage of the cord), owing to the parietalization of the cord elements (the same maneuver as mentioned earlier).

Large Bilateral Prosthesis. This technique, which I have used for 30 years, does not require any attempt at repair of the hernial orifice. The size of the prosthesis is measured on the patient. The correct transverse dimension is equal to the distance between both anterosuperior iliac spines minus 2 cm, the height of the prosthesis being equal to the distance between the umbilicus and the pubis. The mean values are 24 cm transversally and 16 cm vertically; the extreme values

are 20 to 30 cm and 14 to 19 cm. The prosthesis is cut with straight scissors, using a no-touch technique, taking into account the main dimensions, which are chevron shaped, so that its lateroinferior angles will later be placed far down behind the two pelvic obturator frames (Fig. 19.11) and its superior convex border will fit to the concavity of the line of Douglas.

The patch is then seized by all angles and by the middle of the lateral borders with eight long Rochester's forceps that facilitate placement (Fig. 19.12). The patch is first placed on the opposite side of the operator. The assistant retracts the parietal wall up as the operator depresses the peritoneal sac with his or her left hand, pulling it upward; this opens the parietoperitoneal cleavage space. The prosthesis is then pushed into this space with the Rochester's forceps. The inferior median forceps is first placed between the pubis and bladder, followed by the inferior angle forceps, median lateral forceps, and superior angle forceps, while pushing them as far back as possible. This maneuver

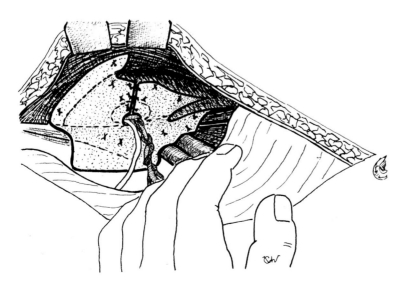

FIGURE 19.10. Schematic anteromediolateral view of a unilateral prosthesis placed by the medial prepertioneal approach. The operator's left hand depresses the peritoneal sac. The prosthesis, split to let the cord pass through, is sewn to the parietal wall, Cooper's ligament, the femoral sheath, and the fascia iliaca.

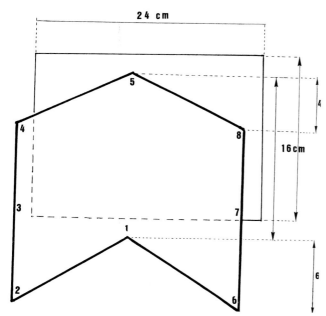

FIGURE 19.11. The chevron-shaped prosthesis is cut with regard to the mean dimensions (in centimeters) of the rectangle measured on the patient. The numbered points (*1 to 8*) will be seized by eight long Rochester's clamps for easy placement of the mesh prosthesis. The numbers also indicate the order of using the clamps for positioning the prosthesis.

unfolds the prosthesis on all points of the parietoperitoneal cleavage space, surrounding the part of the visceral sac opposite the operator (Fig. 19.13). Every time one of the forceps is pushed into its correct place, the assistant immobilizes it until the operator releases the visceral sac with his or her left hand, which enables it to take its place. The valve is removed from under the parietal wall. The forceps used to place the prosthesis are then delicately removed at the same angle in which they were placed, while passing along the inner facet of the parietal wall.

The operator and the assistant again change sides and perform the same maneuvers on the opposite side (Fig. 19.14). The Dacron mesh prosthesis is fully unfolded and inserted to surround the visceral sac, generously overlapping the hernial orifices and protecting the median subumbilical incision (Fig. 19.15). Then, the middle of the superior border of the prosthesis is fixed with a synthetic absorbable suture to the inferior border of the Richet's umbilical fascia. No other stitch is used for fixation of the prosthesis, simplifying the technique. No antibiotic agents are used in the surgical wound.

Closure and Drainage

The parietal suture is made with a continuous slowly absorbing synthetic suture, the subcutaneous fat is padded with small sutures, and the skin is sewn with fine nylon. When suction drainage tubes are necessary, they are placed in front of the prosthesis.

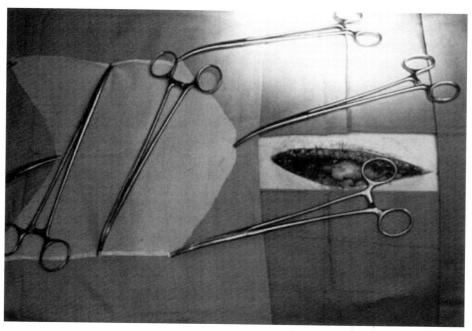

FIGURE 19.12. The large chevron-shaped Dacron mesh prosthesis, cut to the correct dimensions, has been seized by eight long Rochester's forceps for no-touch handling. The subumbilical midline incision is to the right.

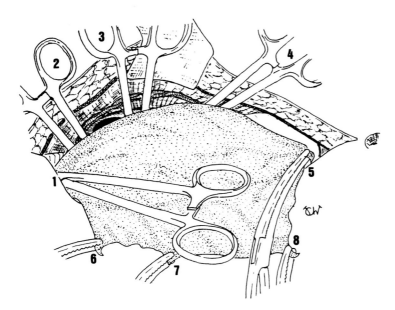

FIGURE 19.13. The right part of the giant bilateral mesh prosthesis has just been pushed, with no. 8 Rochester's forceps, into the right part of the parietoperitoneal cleavage space. The numbers (*1* to *8*) show the order in which the forceps have been used (right side, *1* to *5*) or will be used (left side, *6* to *8*).

Postoperative Care

The patient is encouraged not to restrict activity. Recovery of activity is usually not a problem because postoperative discomfort is minimal. Nevertheless, slow-acting heparin is used for a few days. Prophylactic antibiotic therapy is never used. Eventual suction drainage and dressings are discontinued on the second postoperative day. Hospital discharge occurs between the third and fifth days.

Miscellaneous Remarks

A huge inguinoscrotal sac may be freed by an associated direct high scrotal approach, leaving the lower portion of the sac adherent to the scrotal fundus, with the possible risk

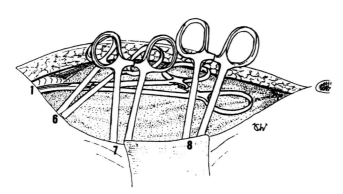

FIGURE 19.14. The mesh prosthesis has been pushed into the two sides of the parietoperitoneal cleavage space. Forceps *6* to *8* have just pushed the left side of the prosthesis and still have not been removed. Forceps *1* is the medioinferior (prevesical) one still in place. A single stitch is visible at the upper part of the incision to the right, fixing the medial point of the superior border of the mesh prosthesis to the Richet's umbilical fascia.

of hematoma formation not regularly avoided despite careful suction drainage.

In unilateral hernias, one must carefully observe the clinically uninvolved side. A tip of hernia is frequently discovered, usually when the hernia being operated on is direct or large or when preperitoneal lipomas exist. One may be tempted to use a unilateral patch, but for patients older than 50 years, we routinely insert a large bilateral prosthesis because of the frequent later appearance of a contralateral hernia.

The Trendelenburg position is helpful in obese patients. It is impossible not to recognize other hernias when the preperitoneal approach is used.

Hernias in unusual locations are identified precisely from the inner hernial orifice and easily treated, no matter what the location—laterofemoral, prevascular, mediofemoral, or obturator. The same is true for low eventration.

Most problems related to sliding hernias are solved by the preperitoneal approach. One obtains the correct diagnosis by opening the sac at the appropriate level. Reduction of the contents and eventual limited resection of the sac are performed without difficulty. The prosthetic repair abolishes the hazards resulting from the large hernial orifice.

Although hernias in elderly patients have a low recurrence rate in our experience, when the hernias are bilateral, elderly patients profit from a large prosthetic repair, which can be done quickly.

We have developed a prosthetic repair by the preperitoneal approach for multirecurrent hernias. This technique is irreplaceable when previous attempts by the inguinal approach have destroyed Poupart's and Cooper's ligaments. The preperitoneal approach also avoids the difficult dissection by the inguinal approach of modified groin structures and saves time.

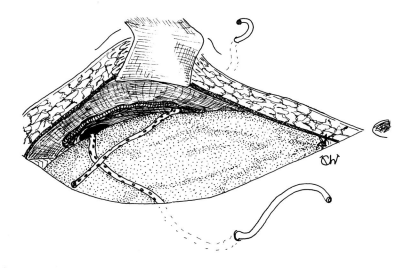

FIGURE 19.15. The large prosthesis, bilaterally overlapping the hernial orifices, protecting the subumbilical midline incision. Note the suction drains.

In technique, associated pelvic abdominal intraperitoneal or extraperitoneal lesions can be treated if no potentially septic maneuver is required.

One may summarize our method in the following way: The *giant bilateral prosthesis* repair is the placement of a wide piece of Dacron mesh in the large bilateral interparietoperitoneal cleavable space. The prosthesis has large dimensions; thus, its stability is excellent without any fixation, and there is no need for a direct repair of the wall. The surgeon's only concerns are to separate the retroparietal cellular spaces, to cut a prosthesis of the needed size, and to surround the visceral sac while at the same time reinforcing the endoabdominal fascia by placing the mesh barrier across the different hernial orifices and the midline laparotomy wound, so that there is no possibility of recurring hernia or eventration (Figs. 19.16 and 19.17). The operative time is short (30 to 40 minutes), which is important for elderly patients and those at risk.

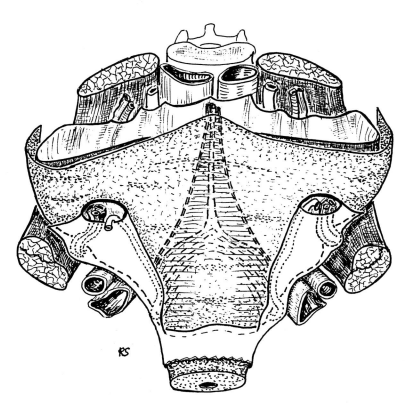

FIGURE 19.16. Schematic anteroposterior view of the giant bilateral Dacron mesh prosthesis surrounding the inferior part of the visceral sac as an artificial endoabdominal fascia, logically and radically forbidding reherniation. Note the correct position of the prosthesis behind the spermatic bundles (within their spermatic sheaths) and in front of the umbilicoprevesical fascia.

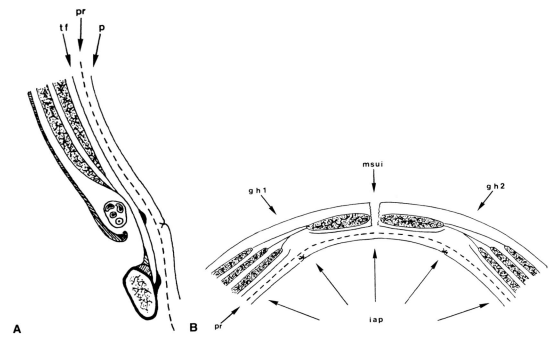

FIGURE 19.17. Schematic representations of the giant bilateral prosthesis at the end of the operation. **A:** Sagittal paramedian cross section of the inguinal wall showing the deep position (underlay) of the mesh (*pr*) between peritoneum (*p*) and transversalis fascia (*tf*). **B:** Horizontal cross section of the abdominal wall, at the level of the inguinal regions, showing how intraabdominal pressure (*iap*), acting in all directions (*arrows*) and following Pascal's hydrostatic principle, fixes the prosthesis (*pr*), which involves the peritoneal sac, rendering it inextensible, and at the same time reinforces the endoabdominal fascia. *msui,* midline subumbilical incision; *gh1* and *gh2* arrows indicate the locations of two groin hernias. (Adapted from Stoppa R. In: Nyhus LM, Baker RJ, eds. *Mastery of surgery,* 2nd ed, vol 2. Boston: Little, Brown and Company, 1992, with permission.)

DO PREPERITONEAL PROSTHESES CARRY SPECIAL RISKS?

We have not found prosthetic repair by the preperitoneal approach to be a risky or complex procedure. The most elaborate herniorrhaphies (e.g., the Shouldice technique) require thorough dissection, which is useless in our method. Moreover, certain complicated hernias, such as huge, sliding, bilateral, or recurrent hernias, are more easily treated by a preperitoneal prosthetic repair than by a standard herniorrhaphy. They are also treated more quickly and more reliably. In addition, the preperitoneal prosthetic repair avoids some rather frequent and medicolegal complications of inguinal herniorrhaphies—femoral vein thrombosis, testicular atrophy, and persistent pains. Like any technique, however, this hernial repair must be well studied and well understood before it is well executed.

Septic complications are more disagreeable when they occur after prosthetic repair than after nonprosthetic approaches. The suppurations observed do not represent rejection, but are the consequences of bacterial contamination. Thus, rigorous vigilance before, during, and after operation is imperative. Before operation, the patient's skin must be carefully and extensively disinfected. No attempt at Dacron repair should be made in the presence of an obstinate dermatosis. During operation, the no-touch technique and the frequent use of antiseptic agents should be followed. During the postoperative course, no dressing should be applied to the wound, to allow better observation. A superficial inflammation requires an early and generous opening of the skin incision. In the case of a deep infection related to the prosthesis, fortunately a rare occurrence, the wound must be opened widely. On the other hand, one must not remove the prosthesis immediately; when the drainage is done precociously and correctly, the prosthesis can be penetrated and covered by the connective tissue, and healing can take place.

The inclusion of the prosthesis between wall and peritoneum does not impede subsequent operations on the abdomen, which can be performed with the usual blade and sutured normally, as in a primary laparotomy, and normal healing should occur. In our experience, several patients have had to undergo subsequent operations for prostatectomy or intraabdominal diseases, mostly colonic cancers, without any disadvantage. Three patients have withstood transprosthetic peritoneal dialysis for later renal insufficiency.

RESULTS

Personal Experience

In my contribution to the third edition of this text, my staff and I reviewed a series of 1,522 patients with 2,108 groin hernias operated on from 1970 to 1984. We compared, using a computerized study of 140 items, the results of four techniques in our hands—Bassini's operation (BO), Cooper's ligament repair (CLR), inguinal patch (IP), and our preperitoneal prosthetic repair (PPR). Patients were 16 to 103 years of age, the median ages being 55.8 years for men and 61.5 years for women. The sex ratio was 5.32 men to 1 woman. The anatomic and clinical breakdown of types of hernia was 40.1% indirect hernias, 30% direct hernias, 6.6% groin eventrations, 6.3% femoral hernias, and 17% diverse hernias; 12.6% of the hernias were recurrent; 9.7% of the operations were for acute complications. The breakdown by techniques was 99 BOs, 549 CLRs, 213 IPs, and 604 PPRs; 42 modified Shouldice operations were also performed.

Postoperative Course

Uncomplicated courses were followed in 91 BOs (92%), 525 CLRs (95.6%), 191 IPs (89.6%), and 572 PPRs (94.7%); that is, each of the techniques had a similarly favorable success rate. (Note that BO was used for some complicated hernias and PPR for the most unfavorable instances.)

Hematoma rates were 2.2% after BO, 2.8% after CLR, 4% after IP, and 3.2% after PPR; there was no important difference between the techniques.

Sepsis rates were 5.6% after BO, 2.2% after CLR, 6.1% after IP, and 2.1% after PPR (BO was used in complicated hernias).

Other complications reported were 16 chest infections (eight after herniorrhaphies, seven after PPR, one after IP), four instances of phlebitis (three after CLR, one after PPR), and two pulmonary embolisms (one after CLR, one after PPR).

Twenty deaths occurred during the first postoperative month (1.3%), related to 14 herniorrhaphies (2%) and six PPRs (0.7%) in elderly patients and complicated operations (18).

Use of Dacron does not much lengthen the median hospital stay, especially when taking into account the use of PPR in the most unfavorable situations. Since 1985, 97.3% of operated patients have been discharged between the second and fifth postoperative days in my department.

Comparison of off-work periods for diverse operations in my department has shown that prostheses are not responsible for the longer off-work periods.

Follow-up Data

Of 1,522 patients reviewed in 1984, 1,330 (87.4%) had their repairs intact 1 to 10 years after the operation. One hundred thirteen (8.5%) had recurrences: 22.5% after BO, 15.3% after CLR, 10.7% after IP, and 1.4% after PPR. The recurrences after PPR were caused by prostheses that were too small or that had split. Of the recurrences after 1 year, 27.8% were after BO and 31.4% after CLR, whereas there was no worsening of results after Dacron herniorrhaphy. The sequelae observed were four testicular atrophies and two hydroceles, all occurring after an inguinal approach. The late migration into the bladder of a preperitoneal prosthesis placed during a prostatectomy emphasizes that septic gestures and prosthetic herniorrhaphy should not be associated with each other. The study of our 1984 series demonstrates the favorable results of the preperitoneal prosthetic repair of groin hernias when compared with other techniques. These are emphasized by my 1989 control of another 529 PPR personal series, which has found the following recurrence rates: 1.1% for recurred hernias and 0.56% for primary repairs.

Results Reported in the Literature

Tables 19.1 and 19.2 report results obtained by other surgeons using diverse prosthetic repair techniques. The results found in these studies do not contradict our own good results with prosthetic repair. Most interestingly, Nyhus's report demonstrated "a dramatic difference in recurrence rates when prosthetic material is used and particularly if the operative approach is preperitoneal or posterior (9a)."

PATIENT SELECTION FOR PREPERITONEAL PROSTHETIC REPAIR

It is often said that the treatment of hernias must be as simple as possible, restoring the wall with the support of a perfect knowledge of regional anatomy and technical details, with the aim of opposing the mechanisms of herniation and avoiding recurrence. The preperitoneal prosthetic repair fits these principles, but one should keep in mind the potential of septic accidents. Thus, a logical attitude includes selective indications for repairs with prostheses and careful attention to the prevention of septic complications. If the surgeon makes efforts to avoid septic risk, he or she cannot do much more than use Dacron to improve the strength of a weakened transversalis fascia. Reasonably, the respective indications for repairs using prostheses must be founded on the evaluation of the recurrence risk, restricting prosthetic repairs to hernias with high risks of recurrence. As are many others (8), we are still trying to finalize recurrence risk by a classification of groin hernias through their morphologic characteristics; but rational arguments have to be assessed by consistent results.

Contraindications to prosthetic repair occur when septic risk cannot be controlled and when general or spinal anesthesia cannot be used. We do not consider a previous median laparotomy a contraindication, nor do we consider

TABLE 19.1. RECURRENCE RATES AFTER INGUINAL PATCH

Author	Technique	No. of Hernias Operated on	Control Rate (%)	Follow-up Duration (yr)	Recurrence Rate (%)
Bapat[a]	Steel	95	84.2	0.5–5.5	1.0
Barthes (1971)[b]	Nylon	273		3	9.9
Cerise[a]	Dacron	100	100.0	1–4.5	1.0
Courtot[a]	Rhodergon	31		1	7.0
Martin[a]	Marlex	365		1–10	0.0
Nahas[a]	Nylon	51			2.0
Notaras[a]	Dacron	246		1–8	0.4
Piper[a]	Skin	246	67.7		12.2
Rives et al. (1978)[b]	Dacron	65			0.0
Rives et al. (1982)[b]	Dacron	183	66.1	1–9	1.6
Saliba[a]	Dacron	204			0.0
Snidjers[a]	Teflon	150	93.0	1–8	2.7
Warlaumont (1982)[b]	Dacron	208	87.3	1–10	10.9
Usher[a]	Marlex	541	44.4	1	10.2
Zagdoun (1959)[b]	Nylon	185	80.0	1–7	7.0

[a]Cited in Stoppa R, Houard C. *Le traitement chirurgical des hernies de l'aine.* Paris: Masson, 1984.
[b]Cited in Stoppa RE. The preperitoneal approach and prosthetic repair of groin hernias. In: Nyhus LM, Condon RE, eds. *Hernia,* Fourth edition. Philadelphia: J.B. Lippincott Company, 1995:188–206.

the sequelae of an iliocaval thrombosis (the supply shunts do not embarrass the midline) contraindications. However, one must be extremely selective in using prostheses in emergency operations or when treating strangulated hernias.

The practical indications for the preperitoneal prosthetic repair include the following:

1. The patient is preferably a man who is not younger than 40 years of age.

2. The hernia is intricate, as are some types of groin hernia, bilateral hernia, and hernia associated with single or multiple lower eventrations.
3. The hernia is complicated by nature, as in sliding hernias, enormous inguinoscrotal hernias, and recurrent or multirecurrent hernias; when a recurred hernia is associated with a destroyed Poupart's or Cooper's ligament, it is the last resort.
4. The hernia is femoral prevascular.

TABLE 19.2. RECURRENCE RATES AFTER PREPERITONEAL PROSTHETIC REPAIR

Author	Technique	No. of Hernias Operated on	Control Rate (%)	Follow-up Duration (yr)	Recurrence Rate (%)
Blondiaux et al. (1979)[a]	Teflon, mid. ap.	91	52.7	0.5–3.5	0.0
Brismoutier[b]	Silicone, mid. ap.	101		4	6.0
Calne (1967)[a]	Dacron, Pfannenstiel	30		1–7.5	13.3
Champault (1996) (4a)	Polypropylene, mid. ap.	49	93	3	2.0
Detrie[b]	Nylon, mid. ap.	50	100	0.5–4	0.0
Fagot[b]	Dacron, mid. ap.	29	100	0.5–3	1–3
Gosset (1972)[a]	Rhodergon, mid. ap.	7	100	2	0.0
Mathonnet (1997) (6a)	Dacron, mid. ap.	198		2–6	1.6
Read (1975)[a]	Marlex, mid. ap.	83		4	7
Rignault et al. (1983)[a]	Dacron, Pfannenstiel	658	86.3	4	4.6
Saint Julien[c]	Dacron, mid. ap.	309	63.0	0.5–6	2.9
Stoppa et al. (1973)[a]	Dacron, mid. ap.	168	88.1	1–7	3.3
Stoppa (1990) (18a)	Dacron, mid. ap.	529		1–12	1.1
Warlaumont (1982)[a]	Dacron, mid. ap.	285	91.3	1–10	1.2

mid. ap., midline approach.
[a]Cited in Stoppa RE. The preperitoneal approach and prosthetic repair of groin hernias. In: Nyhus LM, Condon RE, eds. *Hernia,* Fourth edition. Philadelphia: J.B. Lippincott Company, 1995:188–206.
[b]Cited in Stoppa R, Houdard. Le traitement chirurgical des hernies de l'aine. Paris: Masson, 1984.
[c]Cited in Salinier L. Etude comparative du traitement des hernies inguanales par prosthese: a propos de 309 observations. *Thèse Med* 1983;II(233).

5. The hernia has recurred after repair by an inguinal patch.
6. The conditions are such that the surgeon must aim for a guaranteed result. Obesity, advanced age, and cirrhotic disorders are such conditions.
7. The operation must be performed quickly, as in bilateral hernias or in elderly or high-risk patients.
8. Ehlers–Danlos or Marfan's syndrome with multirecurrent hernia is present (22).

RECURRENCE

The six recurrences in my series occurred because the prostheses used were too small. Thus, the recurrent sac made its way through the insufficient fascia under the lower edge. Because of these recurrences, we now cut the piece of mesh into a chevron shape, which results in a larger downward interposition. A reoperation by the inguinal approach has allowed us to suture the displaced lower edge of the prosthesis to Cooper's ligament. Satisfactory results have been obtained in all patients. Failure of the inguinal patch can easily be eliminated by a large prosthesis inserted by the preperitoneal approach.

CONCLUSION

Prosthetic repairs are an important development in herniology because of their excellent results. When I hear "prosthetic repair," I think of reinforcement or replacement of the transversalis fascia; this means the interposition of a synthetic mesh underlay between muscles and peritoneum for the restoration of the tightness of the abdominal wall against intraabdominal pressure. Not all synthetic materials are equally efficient; Dacron mesh is the best fitting one for giant prosthesis repair. The midline preperitoneal approach allows the surgeon to reach the deep hernial orifice quickly and easily and with a wide exposure while also managing a deep cleaved site for the placement of a large bilateral prosthesis. Large prostheses are kept in place by intraabdominal pressure; following Pascal's hydrostatic principle, they need not be fixed or associated with a repair of the hernial orifice. It is an easy operation that allows repair of badly damaged inguinal walls in multirecurrent hernias.

Because of the disagreeable septic accidents that can occur after prosthetic repair (neither to be neglected nor exaggerated), the indications for the procedure must be selective. The operation may be used logically and reservedly in instances in which other techniques may fail, usually recurrences and rerecurrences, multiple and complex hernias.

In regard to the future of preperitoneal prosthetic repairs, we do not believe that randomized studies comparing the diverse techniques will lead us to an exclusive choice because hernias are polymorphous lesions. Evidence based data are deservedly appreciated in the field of medicine nowadays. It

may go differently in surgical fields, particularly in hernia surgery. Randomized studies are inconsistent with the principle of personalization of hernia cure. In addition, they pose a quasimetaphysical problem to the surgeon, who, as a craftsman, is prone to practice his best "savoir faire" and reluctant to proceed at random. Thus, I have not reported comparative studies (although they exist) including our method of hernia repair. Nevertheless, considering its logically based conception, its proper application of a physical rule (Pascal's principle)—a valuable scientific base—its easy correct performance, and its reproducible satisfactory results, the above described and discussed method can be trusted as an irreplaceable one in the mentioned elective indications—a reason to continue teaching it among other classic procedures of the current arsenal of hernia repairs.

ACKNOWLEDGMENTS

I would like to express my sincere thanks to Dr. Christian Warlaumont, hernia surgeon and friend, for having thoroughly studied one of my series in his excellent medical thesis, and provided his talent in some illustrations of this chapter.

REFERENCES

1. Acquaviva DE, Bourret P, Corti F. Considérations sur l'emploi des plaques de nylon dites crinoplaques comme matériel de plastie pariétale. *52e Congrès Fr. de Chirurgie.* Paris: Masson, 1949:453–457.
2. Arnaud JP, Eloy R, Weill-Bousson M, et al. Résistance et tolérance biologique de 6 prothèses "inertes" utilisées dans la réparation de la paroi abdominale. *J Chir* 1977;113:85–100.
3. Bendavid R. *Prostheses and abdominal wall hernias.* Austin: RG Landes Co, 1994.
4. Bourgeon R, Pantin JP, Guntz M, et al. Notre expérience de la thérapeutique des vastes hernies inguinales par plaque de nylon. *Afr Chir Fr* 1955;4:423–429.
4a. Champault G. Revue de 16,177 cures laparoscopiques de hernies de l'aine réalisées chez 13,132 patients. In: Estour E, ed. *J Coelic Chir* 1999;30:70–76.
5. Chevrel JP. *Hernias and surgery of the abdominal wall,* 2nd ed. Paris: Springer, 1997.
5a. Fruchaud H. *Anatomie chirurgicale des hernies de l'aine.* Paris: Doin, 1956.
6. Koontz AR, Kimberley RC. Tantalum and Marlex mesh (with a note on Marlex thread): an experimental and clinical comparison. Preliminary report. *Ann Surg* 1960;151:796–804.
6a. Mathonet M, Antarieu S, Gainant A, et al. Prothèse intra-ou extrapéritonéale? *Chirurgie* 1998;123:154–161.
7. Nyhus LM, Condon RE, Harkins HN. Clinical experiences with preperitoneal hernia repair for all types of hernia of the groin. *Am J Surg* 1960;100:234.
8. Nyhus LM, Klein MS, Rogers FB. Inguinal hernia. *Curr Probl Surg* 1991;29:403–450.
9. Nyhus LM, Condon RE. *Hernia,* 4th ed. Philadelphia: JB Lippincott Co, 1995.
9a. Nyhus LM. The recurrent groin hernia: therapeutic solutions. *World J Surg* 1989;13:541.
10. Odimba BFK, Stoppa R, Laude M, et al. Les espaces clivables sous-pariétaux de l'abdomen. *J Chir* 1980;117:621–627.

11. Petit J, Stoppa R. Evaluation expérimentale des réactions tissulaires autour des prothèses de la paroi abdominale en mesh de Dacron. *J Chir* 1974;107:667–676.

12. Rives J. Surgical treatment of the inguinal hernia with Dacron patch: principles, indications, technic and results. *Int Surg* 1967;47:360–361.

13. Rives J, Stoppa R, Fortesa L, et al. Les pièces en Dacron et leur place dans la chirurgie des hernies de l'aine. *Ann Chir* 1968;22:159–171.

14. Rives J, Fortesa L, Drouard F, et al. La voie d'abord abdominale sous-péritonéale dans le traitement des hernies de l'aine. *Ann Chir* 1978;32:245–255.

15. Soler M, Verhaeghe P, Essomba A, et al. Le traitement des éventrations post-opératoires par prothèse composée (polyester-polyglactine 910). Etude clinique et expérimentale. *Ann Chir* 1993;47:598–608.

16. Stoppa R, Quintyn M. Les déficiences de la paroi abdominale chez le sujet âgé: colloque avec le praticien. *Semain Hop Paris* 1969;45:2182–2185.

17. Stoppa R, Petit J, Abourachid H. Procédé original de plastie des hernies de l'aine: l'interposition sans fixation d'une prothèse en tulle de Dacron par voie médiane sous-péritonéale. *Chirurgie* 1973;99:119–123.

18. Stoppa RE, Warlaumont CR. The midline preperitoneal approach to and the prosthetic repair of groin hernias. In: Nyhus LM, Baker RJ, eds. *Mastery of surgery*, 2nd ed. Boston: Little, Brown and Company, 1992:1859–1869.

18a. Stoppa R. Technical and scientific objections to laparoscopic herniorrhaphy. In: Gilbert AI, Graham MF, eds. *Prob Gen Surg* 1995: 12:209–214.

19. Stoppa R, Diarra B, Mertl P. The retroparietal spermatic sheath. An anatomical structure of surgical interest. Hernia 1997;1:55–59.

20. Stoppa R, Diarra B, Verhaeghe P, et al. Some problems encountered at reoperation following repair of groin hernias with preperitoneal prostheses. Hernia 1998;2:35–38.

21. Usher FC. A new plastic prosthesis for repairing tissue defects of the chest and abdominal wall. Am J Surg 1959;97:629–633.

22. Wantz GE. Giant reinforcement of the visceral sac. Surg Gynecol Obstet 1989;169:408–417.

23. Wantz GR. Prosthetic repair groin hernioplasties. In: Atlas of hernia surgery. New York: Raven Press, 1991:94–151.

SPECIAL COMMENT: PERSONAL EXPERIENCE WITH THE STOPPA TECHNIQUE

George Wantz

René E. Stoppa's operation—the operation he calls giant prosthetic reinforcement of the visceral sac (GPRVS)—is the solution to the difficult problem of recurrent and rerecurrent inguinal herniations and selected other hernias of the groin at high risk for recurrence. Conceptually, it is correct. Recurrences are inconceivable. Personal experiences with it are gratifying (3).

I gave up the Shouldice repair of rerecurrent inguinal hernias when an analysis of my personal experience revealed an unacceptably high recurrence rate, averaging 13.25%, and instead adopted the posterior approach to this truly difficult problem (6).

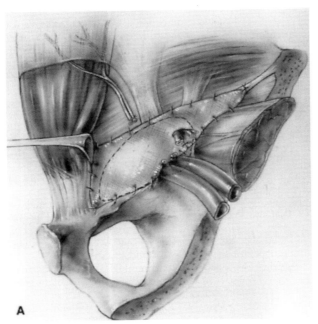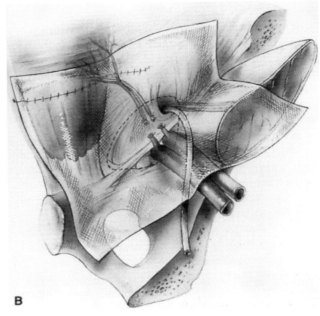

FIGURE 19.18. Patch preperitoneal hernioplasty **(A)** is contrasted with unilateral giant prosthetic reinforcement of the visceral sac (GPRVS) **(B)**. With patch prosthetic repair, hernias recur through the unrepaired portion of the myopectineal orifice and at the borders of the prosthetic suture attachment. With GPRVS, recurrently herniation is difficult to conceive. (Wantz GE. Prosthetic repair groin hernias. *Atlas of hernia surgery.* New York: Raven Press, 1991:94–151, with permission.)

The preperitoneal access of Nyhus and colleagues (1) was chosen, and the repair was reinforced with a triangular piece of polypropylene mesh sutured in place as described by Read (2) (Fig. 19.18A). This approach has important advantages. It reduces the chances of testicular atrophy by avoiding redissection of the spermatic cord; it provides an unparalleled view of the posterior inguinal canal; it is the ideal site for the prosthesis; and the repair can still be done with local anesthesia.

Sixty-eight operations for rerecurrent inguinal herniations were performed. There were five recurrences, for a rate of 7.4%. Although this rate is the same as that reported by Read in his patients with mesh, it was again discouragingly high when it became evident. The recurrences were at the sutured edge of the mesh and were of the following types: two indirect, one femoral, and two through the oblique muscles lateral and superior to the mesh. They would not have occurred had the mesh been larger (5).

At about the time the disappointing results became known, I became aware of Dr. Stoppa's operation, and a patient coincidentally sought my help who was a perfect candidate for it. The patient, with multiple recurrences, had Ehlers–Danlos syndrome and was cured by the operation. No other operation would have worked in this patient in whom sutures would not hold. I became an immediate enthusiast for the Stoppa operation.

Early in my experience with GPRVS, I used knitted polypropylene mesh and even Gore-Tex (W.L Gore & Associates, Newark, DE, U.S.A.), which are synthetic prosthetic soft tissue materials favored by American surgeons. I had no experience with Mersilene (Ethicon Ethnor) and failed to appreciate the importance this mesh plays in the success of GPRVS (5).

Mersilene is the preferred prosthesis for GPRVS. It is a knitted, lace-like, supple mesh composed of loosely braided fine fibers of pure uncoated Dacron (polyester). It has a texture that grips the tissue and prevents slippage. Fibroblastic infiltration is fast and does not cause the mesh to crinkle or curl at the edges. Buckling when bent in two directions at once is minimal. Consequently, the Mersilene is able to conform readily without distortion to the complex curvatures of the pelvis. Contrary to the fears of many surgeons, Mersilene is tolerant of infection. Surgeons distrustful of Dacron forget the enormous success of Dacron aortic prostheses.

To date, 121 of Stoppa's bilateral GPRVS procedures have been successfully performed. Unfortunately, most of these patients require 1 or 2 days of hospitalization, and this fact has restricted its routine use. Its chief indication is for patients with bilateral recurrent inguinal hernias.

A reliable ambulatory surgical procedure for recurrent hernias and other hernias at high risk of recurrence was needed. The procedure developed was unilateral preperitoneal hernioplasty with a large piece of Mersilene. It evolved from my experience with Read's preperitoneal patch repair and Stoppa's preperitoneal GPRVS. By combining the operations, unilateral GPRVS was born (Fig. 19.18) (5,6).

TECHNIQUE OF UNILATERAL GIANT PROSTHETIC REINFORCEMENT OF THE VISCERAL SAC

The preperitoneal space is accessed by a lower-quadrant transverse incision similar to that of Nyhus. The preperitoneal space is widely cleaved in all directions, and the elements of the spermatic cord are parietalized as described by Stoppa (Fig. 19.18B). The inferior epigastric vessels are usually preserved. Parietal defects are not closed. When necessary, the dead space of a direct hernia sac can be minimized by withdrawing the transversalis fascia, which envelops the peritoneal sac in the abdominal wall. Surplus preperitoneal fat should be cleared away from the abdominal wall. Closed-suction drainage is needed if hemostasis is incomplete or dead space from a large retained indirect sac remains.

The prosthesis is arranged so that the material stretches transversely. The prosthesis is shaped somewhat like a diamond (Fig. 19.19). The width of the superior edge of the prothesis equals the distance from the midline to the anterosuperior iliac spine minus 1cm. The vertical distance is about 14 cm. Distances of the inferolateral corner increase the measured dimensions by 2 to 4 cm. The exaggerated elongated lateral inferior corner ensures a solid prosthetic grip on the lateral visceral sac. The shape of the mesh is different from that described in the original publication.

The prosthesis is secured to the abdominal wall 2 to 3 cm above the incision by three absorbable synthetic sutures appropriately placed along the upper border of the mesh (Fig. 19.20). The inferior portion of the mesh is implanted with the aid of three long clamps, which grasp the two corners of the middle

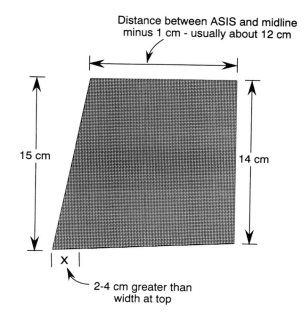

FIGURE 19.19. Diagram illustrating the size and shape of the permanent prosthesis.

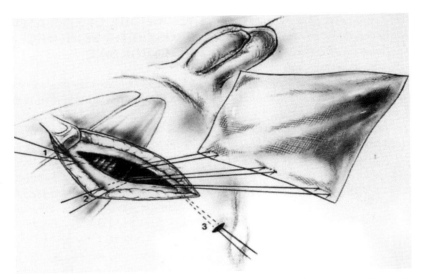

FIGURE 19.20. The mesh is drawn into the superior retromuscular space by three absorbable sutures. One suture attaches the mesh to the linea alba 2 to 3 cm above the incision and another at the semilunar line 2 to 3 cm above the incision; a third is placed in the oblique muscles 2 to 3 cm lateral and above the incision. (Adapted from Wantz GE. Prosthetic repair groin hernias. Atlas of hernia surgery. New York: Raven Press, 1991:94–151.)

lower edge. Retracting the abdominal wall opens the preperitoneal space, enabling the clamps to unfold the mesh and slide it into place: medially, deep into Retzius' space and in front of the bladder; inferiorly, over the peritoneum facing the deep ring (Fig. 19.21). Wrinkling of the mesh occurs with clamp removal

if the preperitoneal space is insufficiently cleaved or the prosthesis incorrectly positioned. After inspecting the position of the prosthesis and the closed suction drain, if used, the incision is closed without tension.

RESULTS OF EXPERIENCE

A total of 340 patients with 358 hernias of the groin at high risk of recurrence after classic repair were treated by unilateral GPRVS. There were 16 recurrences. Mostly, the recurrences were the result of technical errors and were corrected with experience with this new procedure: two resulted (presumably) from hematomas displacing the mesh, one was an overlooked interstitial hernia near the anterosuperior iliac spine, one resulted from mesh displacement due to premature disruption of a large parietal defect closed with excess tension, three were pseudorecurrences and consisted of fat only, and eight were due to errors in the shape and size of the mesh.

PREVENTION OF RECURRENCE

Because most of the recurrences were technical, it is important that the procedure be carried out correctly to avoid pitfalls. The preperitoneal space must be cleaved sufficiently to center smoothly the prosthesis over the myopectineal orifice of Fruchaud. Previous preperitoneal dissection, and especially suprapubic prostate surgery, inhibits a wide cleavage. Previous preperitoneal prostate or bladder surgery may be a contraindi-

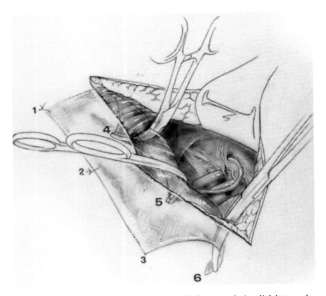

FIGURE 19.21. The distal portion of the mesh is slid into place with three long clamps. (Wantz GE. Prosthetic repair groin hernias. Atlas of hernia surgery. New York: Raven Press, 1991: 94–151, with permission.)

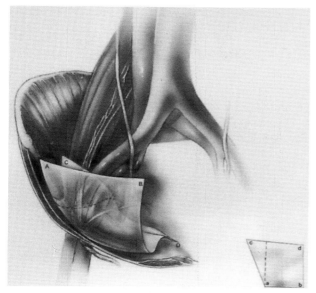

FIGURE 19.22. The illustration demonstrates the complex curves to which a prosthesis must conform. It also shows that the diamond-shaped prosthesis adequately covers the myopectineal orifice, whereas a rectangular prosthesis might not.

cation for unilateral GPRVS. Dissection of Retzius' space may be difficult or impossible, and there is a good chance of unintentionally opening the bladder.

Large parietal defects should not be closed. Invariably, there is tension that becomes excessive when the lower-quadrant access incision is closed. Also, there is surplus preperitoneal fat from passing in and out of small aponeurotic defects or the deep ring and mimicking a peritoneal protrusion.

Finally, the original suggested rectangular shape of the mesh may prove inadequate and is no longer recommended. Repair of the recurrence and review of pelvic anatomy revealed why this was so. The pelvic contours make the distal mesh twist and deflect medially, thereby exposing the lateral border of the myopectineal orifice and inadequately retaining the peritoneum in this region. This flaw in the original procedure was

corrected by elongating the inferolateral corner of the mesh, which allows it to be implanted up into iliac fossa, cover adequately the myopectineal orifice, and retain the visceral sac (Fig. 19.22). No recurrences have occurred since the prosthesis was enlarged and reshaped.

REFERENCES

1. Nyhus LM, Condon RE, Harkins HN. Clinical experiences with preperitoneal hernial repair for all types of hernia of the groin. *Am J Surg* 1960;10:234.
2. Read RC. Bilaterality and the prosthetic repair of large recurrent inguinal hernias. *Am J Surg* 1979;138:788–793.
3. Wantz GE. Personal experience with the Stoppa technique. In: Nyhus LM, Condon RE, eds. *Hernia,* 3rd ed. Philadelphia: JB Lippincott Co, 1989:221–225.
4. Wantz GE. The Canadian repair of inguinal hernia. In: Nyhus LM, Condon RE, eds. *Hernia,* 3rd ed. Philadelphia: JB Lippincott Co, 1989:236–248.
5. Wantz GE. Giant prosthetic reinforcement of the visceral sac for the management of hernias of the groin at high risk for recurrence. *Surg Gynecol Obstet* 1989;169:408–417.
6. Wantz GE. Prosthetic repair groin hernias. *Atlas of hernia surgery.* New York: Raven Press, 1991:94–151.

EDITOR'S COMMENT

Professor Stoppa's contribution to the field of inguinal herniorrhaphy has long been significant. It seems even timelier now because of the advent of the newer repairs that take advantage of the preperitoneal space, which Dr. Stoppa popularized. Indeed the laparoscopic repairs, the bilayer polypropylene prosthesis repair, and the Kugel procedure are at least in part based on Dr. Stoppa's teachings.

The other reason why Dr. Stoppa's work is so timely is because his principles were so completely embraced by the late Dr. George E. Wantz. Given Dr. Wantz's recent death, the editors feel it is entirely appropriate to reprint his outstanding critique and description of his own experience with the Stoppa technique, which he published in the last edition of this book.

R.J.F., Jr.

UNILATERAL GIANT PROSTHETIC REINFORCEMENT OF THE VISCERAL SAC

GEORGE E. WANTZ
EVA FISCHER

René Stoppa's operation—giant prosthetic reinforcement of the visceral sac (GPRVS: La *g*rande *p*rothese de *r*enforcement du *v*isceral *s*ac)—is the solution to the difficult problems of recurrent and rerecurrent inguinal herniation and selected other hernias of the groin at high risk of recurrence. Conceptually, it is correct. Recurrences are inconceivable. Personal experiences with it are gratifying.

Unilateral GPRVS is the Stoppa procedure applied to a single groin (Fig. 20.1). The properitoneal mesh in unilateral GPRVS may be implanted through a lower quadrant transverse abdominal incision or through an anterior groin incision either transinguinally or subinguinally (1,2,4–6).

Recently, Franz Ugahary described the technique for unilateral GPRVS performed through a short gridiron abdominal incision (3). Originally, unilateral GPRVS was developed for the treatment of complex hernias of the groin (e.g., recurrent hernias) in an ambulatory setting, with local anesthesia and a minimal chance of the complications of testicular atrophy and chronic neuralgia. Currently, the chief indication for unilateral GPRVS is when the Stoppa operation is unnecessary or inapplicable, when an unanticipated complex hernia is encountered during hernioplasty with an anterior groin incision, or for repair of the groin after removal of a previously implanted prosthesis. Unilateral GPRVS via an abdominal incision or via Ugahary's gridiron incision is the hernioplasty we use for primary and recurrent groin hernias whenever regional or general anesthesia is used in adult male patients.

PERMANENT PROSTHESIS FOR UNILATERAL GPRVS

The permanent prosthesis for unilateral GPRVS must conform to the complex curves of the pelvis and therefore should be soft, elastic, supple, and conforming. Also, it must become integrated rapidly, be tolerant of infection, have a

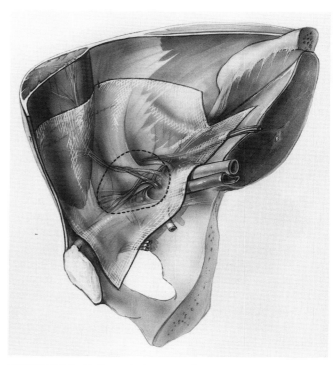

FIGURE 20.1. Unilateral giant prosthetic reinforcement of the visceral sac is the Stoppa procedure cut in half. (From Munshi IA, Wantz GE. Management of recurrent and perivascular femoral hernias by giant prosthetic reinforcement of the visceral sac. *J Am Coll Surg* 1996;182:417–422, with permission.)

G. E. Wantz and **E. Fischer:** Department of Surgery, Joan and Sanford Weill Medical College of Cornell University; Department of Surgery, New York Presbyterian Hospital, New York, New York.

surface texture that will grip the tissues, and be available in large pieces. To date, the only prosthetic mesh meeting these criteria is Mersilene (Ethicon, Inc. Somerville, NJ, U.S.A.), which is composed of polyfilamented fibers of the polyester Dacron (2). Meshes of other materials are not suitable substitutes. Polypropylene meshes currently available are semirigid and nonconforming. Moreover, intraabdominal pressure may be insufficient to prevent unfixed polypropylene mesh inside the properitoneal space from deforming from the contracture of the investing scar tissue. Gore-Tex (W.L. Gore & Associates, Flagstaff, AZ, U.S.A.) is conforming but intolerant of early infection and, rather than being rapidly integrated, is only slowly encapsulated in the tissues. Therefore, it is not a suitable prosthesis for GPRVS.

TECHNIQUES OF UNILATERAL GPRVS

Transverse abdominal incision. The properitoneal space is reached by a transverse incision extending from the midline laterally for 8 to 9 cm. It is made 2 to 3 cm below the level of the anterosuperior iliac spine and should be well above the deep ring and any hernias that might present (Fig. 20.2). The rectus sheath and oblique abdominal muscles are incised for the length of the skin incision. The rectus muscle is bluntly dissected from the rectus sheath and the lower abdominal wall retracted (Fig. 20.3). The transversalis fascia will be seen adjacent to the lateral border of the rectus muscle. It is thin, covers the inferior epigastric vessels and the yellow properitoneal fat, and passes deep to the rectus muscle. Incising the transversalis fascia along the border of the rectus muscle frees the muscle, permits entrance into the properitoneal space, and exposes the inferior epigastric vessels, which do not necessarily require division.

The properitoneal space is cleaved in all directions, medially and superiorly, behind the rectus muscle and the oblique muscle of the abdominal wall, and inferiorly and deeply, into the pelvis, exposing Retzius' space, the superior ramus of the pubis, the obturator foramen, the iliac vessels, and the iliopsoas muscle.

Hernia sacs are dealt with in conventional ways. The sacs of direct, femoral, or other rare hernias, such as obturator, are easily identified and teased from adjacent tissues. If the sacs are large, they are amputated or inverted beneath a purse-string suture in order to smooth the external surface of the visceral sac. The pedicle of simple indirect inguinal hernias is divided and the proximal peritoneum oversewn. The distal peritoneal sac is left in place, undissected, and attached to the cord. Of course, all sliding indirect hernia sacs will require dissection from the cord. An incision in the anterior inguinal canal may be required to release voluminous incarcerated hernias.

The vas deferens and the testicular vessels are freed from the peritoneum from the level of the deep ring proximally

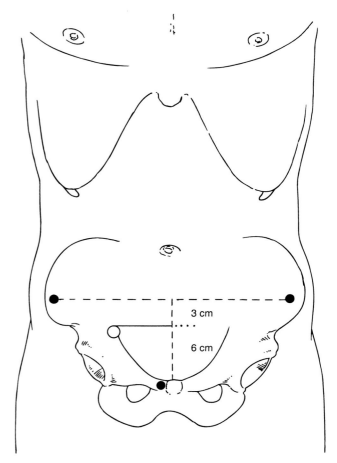

FIGURE 20.2. The location of the abdominal incision for properitoneal unilateral giant prosthetic reinforcement of the visceral sac. (From Wantz GE. Preperitoneal hernioplasty with Mersilene—unilateral giant prosthetic reinforcement of the visceral sac. In: Schumpelick V, Wantz GE, eds. *Inguinal hernia repair.* Basel: S. Karger, 1995:222–232, with permission.)

at least 10 cm. This technique, first described by Stoppa, is called parietalization of the elements of the spermatic cord (Fig. 20.4).

The defects in the abdominal walls are not closed. If necessary, the dead space created by the hernia sac can be eliminated by inverting the transversalis fascia, which envelops the peritoneal sac in the abdominal wall, and suturing it to the abdominal wall. In this process, the spermatic cord should not be withdrawn. Surplus properitoneal fat should be cleared away from the abdominal wall.

The Mersilene is arranged so that the material stretches transversely. In the developmental stages of the operation, the mesh was shaped as a square or rectangle and was considerably smaller than what is used nowadays. Experience (recurrence) showed that the mesh was incorrectly shaped and too small. Currently, the prosthesis is shaped like a diamond (Fig. 20.5). It is important that the bottom edge is wider than the top and that the lateral side is longer

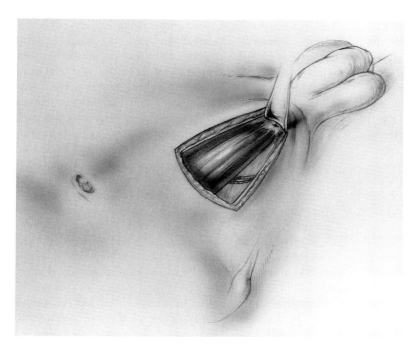

FIGURE 20.3. The rectus sheath has been dissected from the rectus muscle and the abdominal wall lifted, revealing the rectus muscle and lateral to it the thin transversalis fascia covering the inferior epigastric vessels and properitoneal fat. (From Wantz GE. Preperitoneal hernioplasty with Mersilene—unilateral giant prosthetic reinforcement of the visceral sac. In: Schumpelick V, Wantz GE, eds. *Inguinal hernia repair*. Basel: S. Karger, 1995:222–232, with permission.)

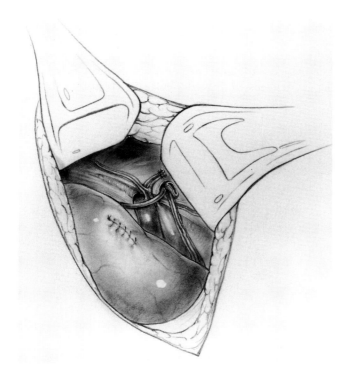

FIGURE 20.4. The complete dissection of the properitoneal space showing parietalization of the vas deferens and testicular vessels. (From Wantz GE. *Atlas of hernia surgery*. New York: Raven Press, 1991, with permission.)

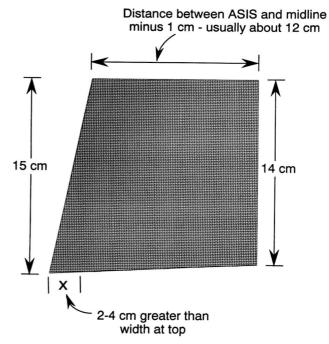

Distance between ASIS and midline minus 1 cm - usually about 12 cm

15 cm

14 cm

X

2-4 cm greater than width at top

FIGURE 20.5. The dimensions of the Mersilene mesh for transabdominal unilateral giant prosthetic reinforcement of the visceral sac. (From Wantz GE. Preperitoneal hernioplasty with Mersilene—unilateral giant prosthetic reinforcement of the visceral sac. In: Schumpelick V, Wantz GE, eds. *Inguinal hernia repair*. Basel: S. Karger, 1995:222–232, with permission.)

than the medial side. The width of the superior edge of the prosthesis equals the distance from the midline to the anterosuperior iliac spine minus 1 cm. The vertical distance medially is approximately 14 cm. The inferolateral corner is extended 2 to 4 cm. This elongates the lateroinferior corner of the mesh and ensures a solid prosthetic grip on the lateral visceral sac.

In lieu of the diamond-shaped mesh, a square of Mersilene 15 × 15 cm may be used. In this case, the lateral absorbable suture attaching the mesh to the anterior abdominal wall should be omitted and the mesh should instead be implanted with a long clamp because the width of the mesh will exceed the distance from the midline to the anterosuperior iliac spine.

The prosthesis is drawn into place under the rectus muscle and the superior abdominal wall by three successively placed absorbable sutures appropriately placed along the upper border of the mesh. The sutures secure the mesh to the abdominal wall 3 to 4 cm or more above the incision. The medial corner suture is near the linea alba, the middle suture is in the semilunar Spieghel's line, and the lateral corner suture passes through the oblique abdominal muscles near the anterosuperior iliac spine. A Reverdin's suture needle facilitates the placement of the sutures. Lacking this instrument, very large curved needles can be used.

The inferior portion of the mesh is implanted with the aid of three long clamps, which grasp the two corners and the middle lower edge (Fig. 20.6). Retracting the abdom-

inal wall opens the properitoneal space, enabling the clamps to unfold the mesh and slide it into place. The clamp grasping the medial corner is placed into Retzius' space and unfolds the mesh behind the rectus and in front of the bladder. It is steadied by an assistant. Next, the clamp that grasps the middle of the inferior edge is pushed deeply into the wound to unfold the mesh over the peritoneum facing the superior ramus of the pubis, the obturator foramen, and the iliac vessels. It is also steadied by an assistant. Finally, the clamp grasping the lateral corner of the mesh slides the prosthesis up into the iliac fossa and over the peritoneum facing the deep ring, the parietalized spermatic cord, and the iliopsoas muscle. This is steadied by the surgeon. The retractors are removed, and the clamps are released and carefully withdrawn. Wrinkling and folding of the mesh will occur with removal of the clamps if the properitoneal space is insufficiently cleaved. Closed suction drainage is used when hemostasis is incomplete or there remains a large distal indirect hernia sac. The access incision is loosely closed with continuous absorbable suture.

The important feature of GPRVS via a transverse abdominal incision is that dissection or redissection of the inguinal canal and its contents is avoided, thereby eliminating trauma to the spermatic cord and sensory inguinal nerves. Another advantage is that, in many cases, the procedure can be done with local anesthesia when necessary. Anesthetizing the peritoneum adjacent to the pelvic wall, the vas deferens, and the testicular vessels may be difficult

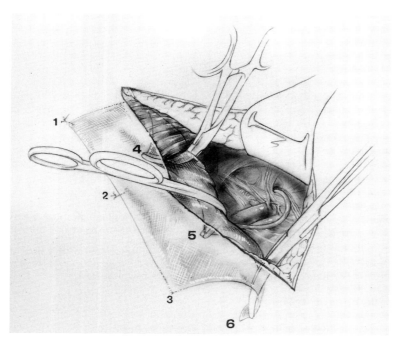

FIGURE 20.6. The distal mesh is implanted with three long clamps (*4–6*). The mesh envelops the visceral sac. (From Wantz GE. *Atlas of hernia surgery*. New York: Raven Press, 1991, with permission.)

and incomplete. Supplementation of the local anesthesia by an anesthesiologist is advisable. Drugs that may cause abdominal breathing, such as fentanyl, can severely restrict exposure and should not be administered.

TRANSINGUINAL GPRVS

Transinguinal GPRVS is similar to the Rives hernioplasty but differs from it in that the mesh is not sutured circumferentially and the vas deferens and testicular vessels are parietalized. The main indication is for unexpected complex hernias of the groin. Also, it is the procedure of choice to repair the groin after painful polypropylene patches and devices previously implanted from the anterior have been removed.

The properitoneal space is reached by division of the posterior wall of the inguinal canal in exactly the same way as in the classic hernioplasties and repairs. Division of the cremaster muscle, cremaster vessels, and genital nerve assists exposure but is not essential. Wide cleavage of the properitoneal space is easily accomplished bluntly with the index finger or sponge stick in all directions. Division of the inferior epigastric vessels facilitates this dissection and the implantation of the prosthesis, but is not always necessary.

Parietalization eliminates the need for a slit in the mesh to accommodate the spermatic cord and is done exactly as described above. If parietalization is not done, the operation can be completed as described by Rives. A

lateral slit is made in the mesh to accommodate the cord. The lateral bisected tails of the mesh are sutured around the cord and circumferentially to Cooper's ligament and the abdominal wall.

The Mersilene prosthesis should be as large as possible and not less than 10 × 10 cm. It should be arranged so that it stretches transversely. The prosthesis is drawn into the properitoneal space underneath the superior abdominal wall by three to five sutures of permanent or slowly absorbable synthetic suture (Fig. 20.7). The sutures that suspend the prosthesis are placed medially, superiorly, and laterally far beyond the borders of the myopectineal orifice (MPO) of Fruchaud. The sutures not only expedite the correct placement of the prosthesis superiorly, but also ensure its position during the manipulation required to insert the inferior portion of the prosthesis. The inferior border of the prosthesis is implanted with long curved clamps (Wiley or Rochester Pean) that grasp the prosthesis on the corners and in the middle of the distal edge (Fig. 20.8). The long curved clamps push the prosthesis medially deep into Retzius' space and laterally far up into the iliac fossa. The clamp in the middle edge aids implantation of the prosthesis over the peritoneum facing the obturator canal. The clamps are then carefully removed and the position of the prosthesis checked to make sure that it has not been dislodged (Fig. 20.9). The posterior wall of the inguinal canal is closed without tension, with a permanent monofilament synthetic suture. A formal hernioplasty is not essential. The hernioplasty is finished in a conventional way.

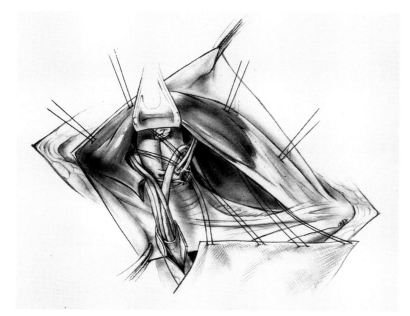

FIGURE 20.7. Unilateral giant prosthetic reinforcement of the visceral sac can be done through an anterior groin incision. In this case, the floor of the inguinal canal is completely incised, the properitoneal space is bluntly dissected, and the cord is parietalized. The mesh is fixed to the anterior abdominal wall with three or five sutures. (From Wantz GE. The technique of giant prosthetic reinforcement of the visceral sac performed through an anterior groin incision. *Surg Gynecol Obstet* 1993;176:497–500, with permission.)

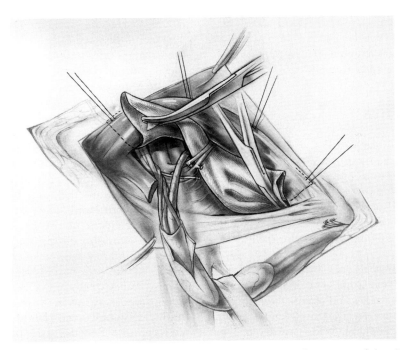

FIGURE 20.8. The distal mesh in transinguinal giant prosthetic reinforcement of the visceral sac is implanted with long clamps to envelop the visceral sac. (From Wantz GE. The technique of giant prosthetic reinforcement of the visceral sac performed through an anterior groin incision. *Surg Gynecol Obstet* 1993;176:497–500, with permission.)

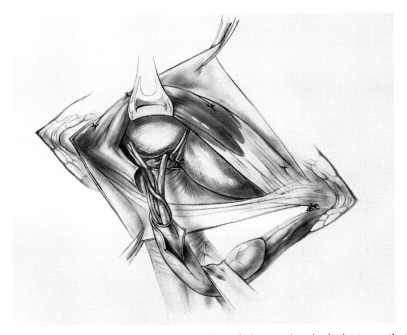

FIGURE 20.9. The appearance of the implanted mesh in transinguinal giant prosthetic reinforcement of the visceral sac. The transversalis fascia and aponeurosis are loosely approximated to complete the procedure. (From Wantz GE. The technique of giant prosthetic reinforcement of the visceral sac performed through an anterior groin incision. *Surg Gynecol Obstet* 1993;176: 497–500, with permission.)

SUBINGUINAL GPRVS

Subinguinal GPRVS is used when unanticipated perivascular femoral hernias are encountered in frail elderly women during femoral hernioplasty, and in patients with perivascular femoral hernias following successful prosthetic inguinal hernioplasty. It is easily done with unassisted local anesthesia. The need for subinguinal GPRVS is rare, yet knowing the technique is important.

The technique of subinguinal GPRVS resembles the other methods of unilateral GPRVS. The femoral region is reached through an anterior groin incision. The femoral hernia sac is dissected from adjacent tissues and from the edge of the parietal defect. The sac may be ligated and amputated or merely inverted if empty. The properitoneal space is entered through the parietal defect and cleaved by gentle blunt-finger dissection in all directions. The dissection, however, is limited on the anterior surface of the iliac vessels by the origin of the inferior epigastric vessels. A square of Mersilene mesh approximately 6 to 8 cm square is arranged so that the stretch is transverse. A larger piece of mesh is not needed because the parietal defect is relatively small compared to the size of the mesh. It is placed in the properitoneal space and secured to the anterior abdominal wall 3.0 cm above the inguinal ligament with 3 sutures (Fig. 20.10). A demitasse spoon is a useful instrument to retain and protect the peritoneum during suturing. Reverdin's needle facilitate placement of the sutures. These sutures, which need not be permanent, are very useful because they ensure the position of the superior portion of the mesh during implantation of the distal border. The distal mesh is implanted with two long clamps, which grasp the far edge of the mesh at the corners. The clamps push the mesh into place, medially deep in Retzius' space and laterally up into the iliac fossa (Fig. 20.11). The inferior epigastric vessels prevent deep implantation of the midportion of the mesh. Injury of the inferior epigastric vessels does not occur because the Mersilene is elastic and pliant and can bunch up around them. Closure of the parietal defect is not necessary (Fig. 20.12).

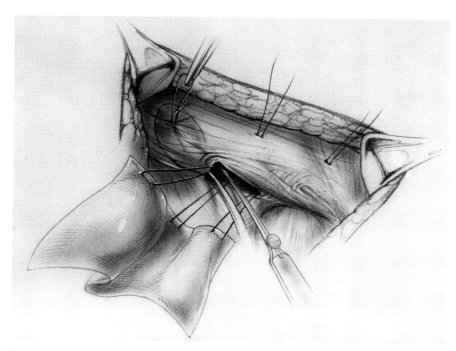

FIGURE 20.10. Subinguinal giant prosthetic reinforcement of the visceral sac to repair the parietal defect of femoral hernias. The mesh is fixed to the anterior abdominal wall with three sutures. (From Munshi IA, Wantz GE. Management of recurrent and perivascular femoral hernias by giant prosthetic reinforcement of the visceral sac. *J Am Coll Surg* 1996;182:417–422, with permission.)

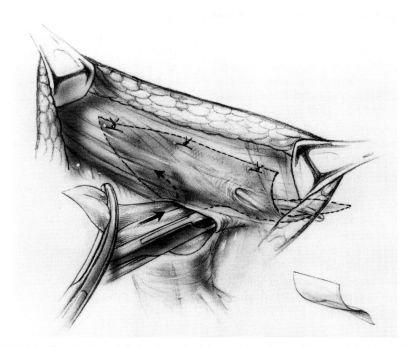

FIGURE 20.11. The distal mesh is implanted with two long clamps. The medial clamp places the mesh in Retzius' space, and the lateral clamp puts the mesh deep into the iliac fossa. (From Munshi IA, Wantz GE. Management of recurrent and perivascular femoral hernias by giant prosthetic reinforcement of the visceral sac. *J Am Coll Surg* 1996;182:417–422, with permission.)

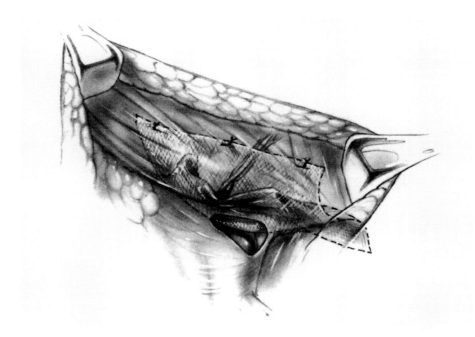

FIGURE 20.12. The soft pliable Mersilene mesh bunches up around the inferior epigastric vessels. (From Munshi IA, Wantz GE. Management of recurrent and perivascular femoral hernias by giant prosthetic reinforcement of the visceral sac. *J Am Coll Surg* 1996;182:417–422, with permission.)

RESULTS OF TRANSABDOMINAL UNILATERAL GPRVS

Unilateral GPRVS via a transverse abdominal incision was used to manage 455 complex and recurrent hernias of the groin with an overall recurrence rate of 1.8% in the period 1986–97. It was not recognized until six recurrences became apparent among the first 127 repairs that the rectangular-shaped mesh did not ensure against recurrence. Draping the mesh in the properitoneal Bogros' space in a cadaver revealed that inadequate coverage of the MPO occurred due to twisting of the mesh as it accommodated the curves of the pelvis. When the mesh was elongated at the inferolateral corner to correct this fault, no recurrences occurred in the subsequent 328 repairs.

Experience with the other methods of performing GPRVS is not large, but there have been no recurrences. Surgeons need to know these techniques because they never know when they will be called upon to use them.

RECURRENCE AFTER UNILATERAL GPRVS

Recurrent herniations after GPRVS are caused by technical errors. For success, the pitfalls of the procedure must be avoided. These are inadequate cleavage of the properitoneal space; closure of the defect in the abdominal wall; and incorrect sizing, shaping, and placement of the mesh. Buckling of the mesh indicates inadequate cleavage or poor placement of the mesh. When implanting the mesh, the surgeon should picture the mesh enveloping and retaining the peritoneum rather than being applied to the defective abdominal wall. Too small a piece of mesh is probably the most common cause of recurrence. Hematomas and seromas prevent rapid integration, may displace the mesh, and provide a rich medium for bacterial growth. They can be prevented by closed suction drainage when hemostasis is incomplete.

REFERENCES

1. Munshi IA, Wantz GE. Management of recurrent and perivascular femoral hernias by giant prosthetic reinforcement of the visceral sac. *J Am Coll Surg* 1996;182:417–422.
2. Stoppa RE, Rives JL, Warlaumont CR, et al. The use of Dacron in the repair of hernias of the groin. *Surg Clin North Am* 1984;64:269–285.
3. Ugahary F, Simmermacher RKJ. Groin hernia repair via a grid-iron incision: an alternative technique for preperitoneal mesh insertion. *Hernia* 1998;2:123–125.
4. Wantz GE. *Atlas of hernia surgery.* New York: Raven Press, 1991.
5. Wantz GE. Giant prosthetic reinforcement of the visceral sac. *Surg Gynecol Obstet* 1989;169:408–417.
6. Wantz GE. The technique of giant prosthetic reinforcement of the visceral sac performed through an anterior groin incision. *Surg Gynecol Obstet* 1993;176:497–500.

21

THE KUGEL APPROACH TO GROIN HERNIAS

ROBERT D. KUGEL

Over the years, numerous "innovations" have been advocated as answers to the problems associated with groin hernia surgery. Each of these innovations has had its proponents as it has claimed some great advantage in the application of a new modification. If anything has been the result of these advances, it should be the realization that there is no perfect repair and no repair equally applicable in every case. Certain principles, however, have risen to the top.

BACKGROUND

In every technique for hernia repair, the purpose is the same. The hernial defect must be eliminated by closing, bridging, plugging, and/or patching. This is the difference between surgical *repair* and nonoperative *management,* as with a truss. For many years, the primary, and essentially only, alternative to repair was to surgically close the defect. This has been done in a variety of ways, but collectively these techniques have been referred to as the "traditional" repairs. The primary concern with traditional repairs has been the risk of recurrence (12,14). Tension on the repair was recognized as a potential problem and modifications were introduced in an attempt to reduce tension (9,11).

Despite the earlier contributions by surgeons such as Usher and Gannon (16), Rives (13), and Stoppa et al. (15), it was the pioneering efforts and persistent message of Irving Lichtenstein and colleagues (6) that resulted in the eventual acceptance of the concept of "tension-free" hernia surgery in the United States and elsewhere. Essentially, all of the newer repairs for hernia are considered "tension free" and utilize a prosthetic piece of mesh to bridge, plug, and/or patch the hernia defect.

The prevention and treatment of femoral hernias has attracted attention in recent years (3). As laparoscopic and other preperitoneal approaches have confirmed the presence of both occult femoral hernias and wide femoral canals

without hernia, the femoral hernia may prove to have greater significance than previously thought. The exact association between occult femoral hernias and groin pain without obvious physical findings has yet to be demonstrated, but the possible connection adds to the importance of reconstructing the entire groin, including the femoral canal, at the time of herniorrhaphy.

Long before the advent of the laparoscopic hernia repair, many surgeons had advocated the advantage of the preperitoneal approach, both with and without mesh (2,5,10). The professed advantages have included ease of access in recurrent hernias, sliding hernias, large incarcerated hernias, and femoral hernias. The preperitoneal approach sometimes allows for a more complete evaluation of the groin and identification of all of the defects and potential defects. In addition, the preperitoneal approach can use intraabdominal pressure to its advantage, rather than as an impediment.

One other emerging concept or principle in hernia repair is the idea of "minimal invasion." This has generally been used in conjunction with endoscopic surgery. It should suggest that the least amount of "damage" be done during the course of the procedure. It should also include the concept of minimal risk. The term should be used not simply because the procedure is endoscopic, but because the surgery involves the least dissection and disruption of normal tissues. It should, therefore, be applicable to the procedure that is indeed least invasive, regardless of the technique or instrumentation used.

In 1992, Arthur Gilbert described what he called a sutureless repair (4). This idea had been suggested earlier, but only in conjunction with a relatively major operation (13,15). A "sutureless" repair means that rigid suture closure of a hernia defect or rigid fixation of prosthesis is not needed. The advantage to the surgeon not only includes simplified placement, but also allows the prosthesis to take advantage of intraabdominal pressure and hydrostatic tissue forces without interference from rigid fixation of the prosthesis as in sutured repairs. This should, at least in theory, decrease postoperative pain and disability and allow the prosthesis to more perfectly conform to the patient's anatomy.

R. D. Kugel: Hernia Treatment Center Northwest, Olympia, Washington.

METHOD AND MATERIALS

Patients

Between January 1, 1994, and July 1, 1999, 902 inguinal hernia repairs were performed in 775 patients using the Kugel approach. Of these repairs, 804 were performed for primary hernias (89%) and 98 for recurrent hernias (11%). An extensive discussion about the procedure was held with patients and informed consent obtained. Prophylactic antibiotics were not used routinely.

Most procedures were performed under epidural anesthesia and occasionally under spinal or local anesthesia. General anesthesia was rarely used. Most patients were released home within 1 to 2 hours after the procedure, depending on the type of anesthesia. In general, no specific restrictions were placed on these patients after surgery. They were informed that their only limitation was relative to their discomfort.

Patients were seen in follow-up 1 to 2 weeks following surgery and repeatedly thereafter if there was a questionable finding at the first postoperative visit. Regular attempts to follow these patients have been made at 3 months, 1 year, and 3 years.

The Patch

The Kugel Patch (Davol, Inc., Cranston, RI, U.S.A.) was developed over a period of 2 years. It has been used in its present form with limited change since January 1994. The patch evolved to facilitate performance of a "minimally invasive," "tension-free," "sutureless," preperitoneal approach to repair of groin hernias. The patch was then utilized for "tension-free" repair of ventral hernias. This resulted in a uniform approach to repair of all abdominal wall hernias.

The patch is composed of two layers of a knitted, monofilament polypropylene mesh material (Fig. 21.1). The two overlapping layers are bonded together near their outer circumference with a narrow weld. There is a free "apron" of mesh outside of this weld into which are cut several radial slits. This allows the outer edge of the patch to fold over irregular structures and surfaces (i.e., iliac vessels).

An important part of the patch is a monofilament spring contained between the outer weld and a second inner weld. This stiffens the patch similar to a trampoline, with greatest rigidity concentrated near the outer edge. This monofilament fiber helps keep the patch in its intended configuration while still allowing it to conform to the patient's groin.

Multiple small holes extend through both layers of the patch to allow greater tissue apposition through the patch. In addition, there are small V-shaped cuts in the top layer of the patch at these apposition holes to increase friction and resistance to movement. The monofilament spring, outer apron, tissue apposition holes, and V-shaped cuts are all designed to keep the patch in place and allow a "sutureless" repair.

There is a single cut placed transversely in the top layer of the patch to allow insertion of a single digit or instrument between the layers of the patch as an aid to placement of the patch into the patient.

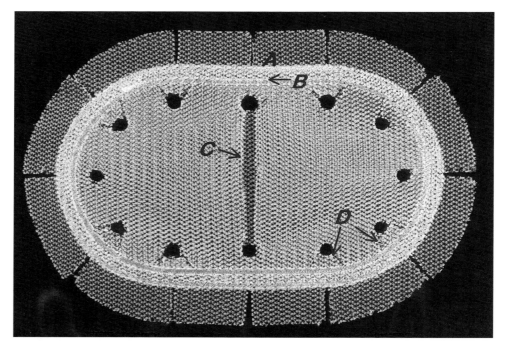

FIGURE 21.1. Mesh patch: *A*, outer "apron"; *B*, monofilament spring; *C*, transverse slit; *D*, tissue apposition holes and "V-shaped" cuts.

OPERATIVE TECHNIQUE

Incision

The pubic tubercle and anterior superior iliac spine are identified by palpation and marked. A third mark is made at a point about halfway between these two points. An oblique skin incision is made about one third lateral and two thirds medial to this third mark (Fig. 21.2). In an average-sized adult, the procedure can usually be done through a 3- to 4-cm incision. A larger incision may be necessary in obese patients and while learning the procedure. Because the goal is to approach the transversalis fascia at a point just superior to the internal ring, it is wise to err on the side of making the incision a little too high rather than too low.

Scarpa's fascia and subcutaneous tissues are divided using electrocautery. The fascia of external oblique is opened a short distance parallel with its fibers but not through the external ring. The underlying internal oblique muscle is bluntly separated, as would be done with a "muscle-splitting" approach for an appendectomy, just lateral to the edge of the rectus sheath. There is usually very little, if any, transversus abdominus muscle at this level and it can easily be separated or divided. This allows exposure of the transversalis fascia, which is opened vertically, but not through the internal ring.

Dissection

The preperitoneal space can then be entered using blunt dissection. Gentle traction is placed on the peritoneum while bluntly pulling away the preperitoneal fat and trans-

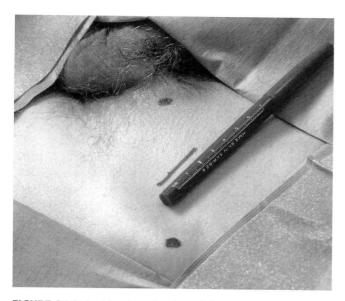

FIGURE 21.2. Incision location for a left inguinal hernia showing the pubic tubercle, incision, and anterior superior iliac spine. © Steve Vento. Reproduced with permission.

versalis fascia, which is then retracted anteriorly. A plane of dissection is created between the peritoneum and overlying preperitoneal fat and transversalis fascia, taking special care to retract the inferior epigastric vessels anterior and medial with the transversalis fascia. With difficult dissections, particularly in obese patients, placing the patient in the Trendelenburg position will improve exposure.

This dissection is started anteriorly and laterally. The cord structures will be visible on the lateral and posterior aspect of the peritoneum and should be gently teased away from the peritoneum for a distance of about 3 cm posterior to the internal ring. The peritoneum is dissected from the preperitoneal tissues in a lateral and superior direction, and then continued anteriorly and medially. Cooper's ligament is then followed, over to the symphysis, while sweeping the loose connective tissue off the ligament, anteriorly and posteriorly, using a single digit (Fig. 21.3). The completed preperitoneal pocket should be only slightly larger than the size of the patch.

Indirect Hernias

With indirect hernias, the hernia sac will come into view as traction is placed on the peritoneum (in a superior direction) while dissecting it free from the preperitoneal fat. The sac will usually pull through the internal ring and out of the inguinal canal with ease. If the hernia sac will not reduce easily, it is divided at the level of the internal ring and the resulting peritoneal defect is closed with a running stitch using absorbable suture. With easily reduced but large and redundant sacs, the sac is excised.

The cord structures will need to be completely separated from the hernia sac as it is pulled out of the inguinal canal (Fig. 21.4). Any large "lipoma" of the cord should be excised to prevent it from being confused with a recurrent hernia at a later date. The internal ring is sometimes difficult to palpate from the preperitoneal space, but it can be entered by sliding an index finger along the lateral aspect of the dissected pocket over the top of the cord structures.

Direct Hernias

Direct hernias are identified by finding a defect medial to the inferior epigastric vessels. With direct hernias, there is usually a "pseudosac" formed from the attenuated transversalis fascia. This will frequently evert as traction is placed on the peritoneum. The preperitoneal fat and peritoneum are completely separated from this pseudosac. The dissection and exposure may be improved by placing a dry gauze sponge into the partially completed preperitoneal pocket and retracting the peritoneum out of the way with a narrow malleable retractor.

To be sure that the pseudosac is completely separated from the preperitoneum, Cooper's ligament must be visualized. This is a useful exercise while doing the medial por-

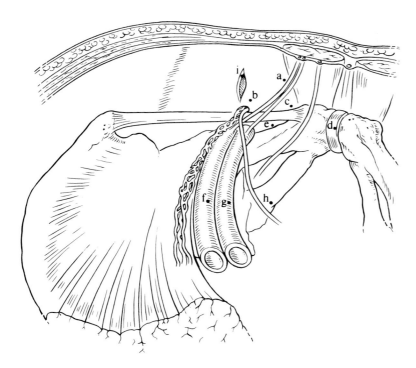

FIGURE 21.3. Preperitoneal view of the left groin showing *a,* inferior epigastric vessels; *b,* internal ring; *c,* direct space; *d,* symphysis pubis; *e,* femoral canal; *f,* iliac artery; *g,* iliac vein; *h,* vas; and *i,* transversalis incision. (Reproduced from Kugel RD. Minimally invasive, non-laparoscopic, preperitoneal, and sutureless, inguinal herniorrhaphy. *Am J Surg* 1999;178:298–302, with permission from Davol, Inc.)

tion of the dissection even when there is no direct hernia. The loose connective tissue attached to the posterior edge of Cooper's ligament should be carefully stripped off. This can usually be done bluntly using an index finger, but occasionally some sharp dissection, under direct visualization, may be required. Care is taken to avoid injury to the aberrant obturator vessels that occur here about 25% of the time.

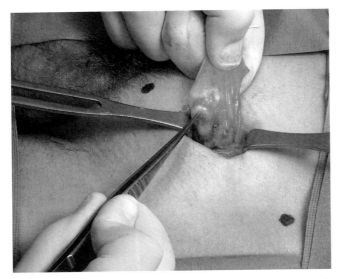

FIGURE 21.4. Indirect hernia sac with cord structures, thumb forceps pointing to vas. © Steve Vento. Reproduced with permission.

Femoral Hernias

Although an infrainguinal approach might be preferred for an isolated femoral hernia identified on physical examination, sometimes these are not easily diagnosed preoperatively or they may be encountered as an incidental finding at the time of inguinal hernia repair. The hernia patch will not lie correctly in the preperitoneal space unless the femoral canal medial to the femoral vein is cleared of any herniated material. This can usually be done with careful blunt dissection using finger dissection and thumb forceps. Care is taken to avoid any possible injury to the iliac vein. Pressure over the femoral canal below the inguinal ligament will help reduce an incarcerated hernia, but in rare cases a counterincision below the inguinal ligament may be necessary.

Patch Placement

The dissected preperitoneal pocket lies between the peritoneum, which is superior and posterior, and the internal ring, cord structures, femoral canal and Hesselbach's triangle, which are inferior and anterior. The oval-shaped pocket extends from just superior and lateral to the transversalis incision made to enter this space over to the symphysis pubis medially (Fig. 21.5).

An 8 × 12-cm mesh patch is used in most cases. With unusual or very large hernia defects (particularly direct hernias), an 11 × 14-cm patch can be used, but it is rarely necessary.

A dry gauze sponge is placed over the peritoneum and a narrow malleable retractor is used to retract the peri-

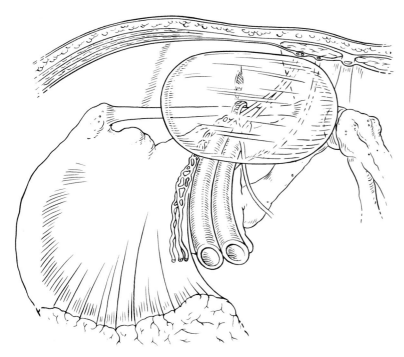

FIGURE 21.5. Area of dissection in the preperitoneal space. (Reproduced from Kugel RD. Minimally invasive, nonlaparoscopic, preperitoneal, and sutureless, inguinal herniorrhaphy. *Am J Surg* 1999;178:298–302, with permission from Davol, Inc.)

toneum out of the way (Fig. 21.6). A single index finger (right-sided hernias use the left finger and left-sided hernias use the right finger) is passed through the slit in the anterior layer of the patch. The end of the patch is then folded over the tip of the finger (Fig. 21.7). The patch is inserted into the preperitoneal pocket, sliding on top of the malleable retractor and along Cooper's ligament

(which can be felt through the patch with the palmar surface of the index finger) toward the pubic bone (Fig. 21.8). The finger is removed (as is the sponge) and replaced with the narrow malleable retractor, which is used to complete insertion of the patch (Fig. 21.9).

The superior edge of the patch is pushed up under the transversalis fascia into the superior portion of the preperi-

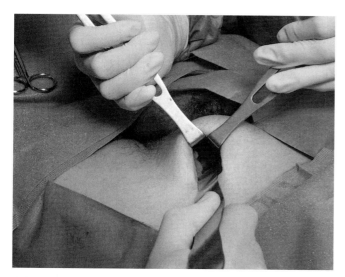

FIGURE 21.6. A narrow malleable retractor is used to retract the peritoneum out of the way. © Steve Vento. Reproduced with permission.

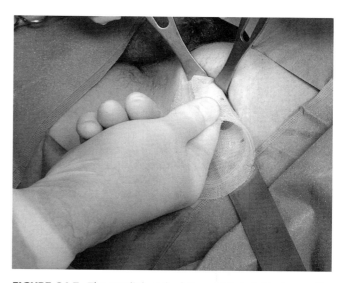

FIGURE 21.7. The medial end of the patch is folded over the fingertip. © Steve Vento. Reproduced with permission.

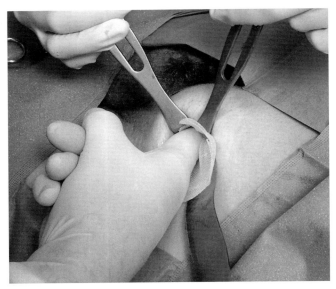

FIGURE 21.8. The patch is inserted by sliding it over the malleable retractor. © Steve Vento. Reproduced with permission.

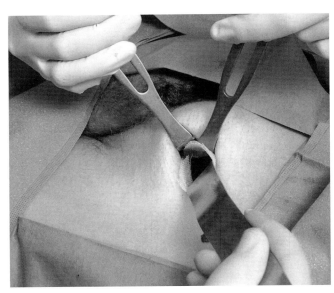

FIGURE 21.9. The malleable retractor is used to complete insertion of the patch. © Steve Vento. Reproduced with permission.

toneal pocket. The patch should lie completely "open" with no kinks in the outer ring. If the patch will not completely open, it is because the pocket is incomplete. This can usually be corrected by following the periphery of the patch with a single finger and breaking any fibers that are restraining it, while manipulating the patch into position. Occasionally, the patch will have to be removed to complete the pocket.

When properly placed, the medial edge of the patch will lie behind (superior to) the pubic bone and against Cooper's ligament. The posterior edge of the patch folds under the peritoneum, onto the iliac vessels. The mesh sits between the peritoneum and the cord structures (round ligament) and does not encircle them (Fig. 21.10).

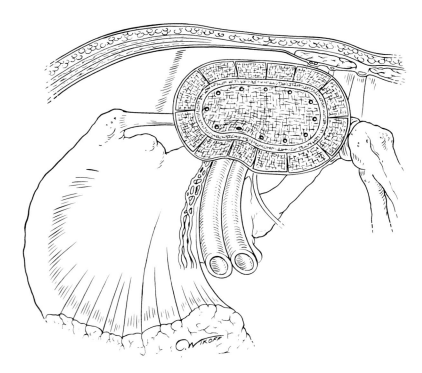

FIGURE 21.10. The 8 × 12-cm mesh patch positioned in the preperitoneal space. (Reproduced from Kugel RD. Minimally invasive, nonlaparoscopic, preperitoneal, and sutureless, inguinal herniorrhaphy. *Am J Surg* 1999;178:298–302, with permission from Davol, Inc.)

Closure

The transversalis fascia is closed with a single interrupted stitch using an absorbable material. The anterior layer of the patch, near the mediosuperior edge, is caught in this stitch to discourage the patch from floating anteriorly. With a very large direct hernia, it is occasionally of benefit to place an anchor stitch between Cooper's ligament and the patch *instead* of transversalis fascia. Stitches placed in two or more separate locations will create two-point fixation and interfere with hydrostatic tissue forces that help keep the patch in position. A long-acting local anesthetic is sprayed into the preperitoneal space.

The fascia of external oblique is closed using a simple running stitch with an absorbable material, taking care to avoid catching an underlying nerve. Additional local anesthetic is infiltrated into the subfascial, subcutaneous, and deep dermal tissues. Scarpa's fascia is approximated with a single interrupted stitch, as is the deep dermis. The skin edges are reapproximated using a running, buried subcuticular stitch with absorbable suture.

At this stage, the patient is encouraged to cough while testing the repair. A pressure dressing is applied over the wound site to minimize ecchymosis and hematoma formation.

RESULTS

No recurrences have been identified in any patient undergoing this technique in the last 3 years. Previously, there were five total recurrences (overall recurrence rate of 0.55%). All of these were in primary hernias (none in recurrent hernias). There were three in right inguinal hernias and two in left inguinal hernias.

Two patients developed wound infections that required drainage of purulent material, but in no case did the patch have to be removed.

DISCUSSION

As with every hernia repair, the likelihood of success is linked to the surgeon's understanding of the anatomy involved. The anatomy is key to this repair. When properly understood, this procedure is simple to perform, but if the patch is improperly placed, the risk of recurrence increases significantly.

This repair represents an open, tension-free, and essentially sutureless preperitoneal groin hernia repair. It is minimally invasive, requiring less dissection and a smaller pocket than that ordinarily created for a totally extraperitoneal prosthetic (TEPP) repair (8), and it does not enter the abdominal cavity as with a transabdominal preperitoneal prosthetic (TAPP) repair (1). It does not require general anesthesia, which, in fact, is discouraged. Compared with other open repairs, this approach protects the entire groin, including the internal ring, Hesselbach's triangle, and the femoral canal. There is less manipulation of the cord structures, which are not encircled.

When evaluating a hernia repair, the recurrence risk must not be the only consideration (7). Safety, ease of performance, disability period, and cost are also important considerations. Although the experience with this repair is still relatively early, it appears to provide an ideal balance of these factors.

REFERENCES

1. Arregui ME, Davis CJ, Yucel O, et al. Laparoscopic mesh repair of inguinal hernia using a preperitoneal approach: a preliminary report. *Surg Laparosc Endosc* 1992;2:53–58.
2. Cheatle GI. An operation for the radical cure of inguinal and femoral hernia. *Br Med J* 1920;2:68.
3. Crawford DL, Hiatt JR, Phillips EH. Laparoscopy identifies unexpected groin hernias. *Am Surg* 1998;64:976–978.
4. Gilbert AI. Sutureless repair of inguinal hernia. *Am J Surg* 1992; 163:331–335.
5. Henry AK. Operation for femoral hernia by a midline extraperitoneal approach. *Lancet* 1936;1:531.
6. Lichtenstein IL, Shulman AG, Amid PK, et al. The tension-free hernioplasty. *Am J Surg* 1989;157:188–193.
7. Memon MA, Fitzgibbons RJ Jr. Assessing risks, costs, and benefits of laparoscopic hernia repair. *Ann Rev Med* 1998;49:95–109.
8. McKernan JB, Laws HL. Laparoscopic repair of inguinal hernias using a totally extraperitoneal prosthetic approach. *Surg Endosc* 1993;7:26–28.
9. McVay CB, Chapp JD. Inguinal and femoral hernioplasty. *Ann Surg* 1958;148:499.
10. Nyhus LM, Condon RE, Harkins HN. Clinical experiences with preperitoneal hernial repair for all types of hernia of the groin. *Am J Surg* 1960;100:234.
11. Ponka JL. The relaxing incision in hernia repair. *Am J Surg* 1968;115:552–557.
12. RAND Corp. *Conceptualization and measurement of physiologic health of adults.* Santa Monica, CA: RAND Corp Publications, 1983:15.
13. Rives J. Surgical treatment of the inguinal hernia with Dacron patch: principles, indications, technic and results. *Int Surg* 1967;47:360–361.
14. Rulli F, Percudani M, Muzi M, et al. From Bassini to tension-free mesh hernia repair. Review of 1409 consecutive cases. *G Chir* 1998;19:285–289.
15. Stoppa R, Petit J, Abourachid H, et al. [Original procedure of groin hernia repair: interposition without fixation of Dacron tulle prosthesis by subperitoneal median approach.] *Chirurgie* 1973;99:119–123.
16. Usher FC, Gannon JP. Marlex mesh: a new plastic mesh for replacing tissue defects. *Arch Surg* 1959;78:131.

EDITOR'S COMMENT

The Kugel approach is another in the ever-evolving development of open prosthetic groin hernia repairs. Here, the variation is placement of a specifically designed prosthetic mesh patch into the preperitoneal space to buttress the posterior inguinal wall and block the femoral canal. This patch has the added feature of a reinforcing ring that helps keep it flat, allowing it to contour to the wall after placement. Performing this repair requires a detailed understanding and appreciation of the anatomy of the groin from the posterior aspect, including knowledge of significant variations. Moreover, an understanding of the pitfalls associated with hernia surgery from the posterior approach is essential.

While Dr. Kugel has had excellent results with his repair, sporadic reports of complications, similar to those reported for most of the purely open prosthetic repairs, are beginning to appear as broader use of the technique takes hold. Confirmation of the initial reports as well as an assessment of the durability of the repair over time will be paramount in determining the place of this approach in the surgical armamentarium of the future.

Another open posterior approach using a mesh buttress is that reported by Ugahary (1). The variation here is the use of a small lateral abdominal wall "gridiron" incision to gain access to the preperitoneal space for exposure of the posterior wall of the inguinal canal. As in the Kugel approach, there appears to be a significant amount of blunt digital dissection in the process. Indeed, it is perceived that application in the obese patient may be limited using either of these approaches. Once access is attained, a rather large piece of mesh, 10 × 15 cm, is placed into the area, reinforcing the wall. This is "standard mesh," polypropylene, and is neither specifically designed for nor unique to this operation. Clearly, the surgeon using this approach has options as to material, porosity, weave, and firmness. In many ways, this approach is similar to the totally extraperitoneal prosthetic (TEPP) concept. However, it lacks the direct visualization achieved with instrumentation—a potential economic benefit—substituting the aforementioned digital dissection with attendant risks. There are few reports by others describing experience with this repair, which is not surprising, considering its relatively recent appearance on the surgical scene. This repair needs broader application and the combined experience of other surgeons to place it contextually in the evolution of groin hernia surgery.

Given my personal experience with the open posterior approach in this area, I have reservations about the techniques used to gain access in both of these procedures. Having observed numerous anatomic variations that could turn a straightforward operation into an exercise in trauma management if a blunt dissection is attempted, I would advise extreme caution and a detailed review of the anatomy before undertaking either of these operations for the first time.

A.G.G.

REFERENCE

1. Ugahary F, Simmermacher RKJ. Groin hernia repair via a gridiron incision: an alternative technique for preperitoneal mesh insertion. *Hernia* 1998;2:123–125.

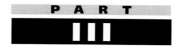

P A R T

III

LAPAROSCOPIC AND ENDOSCOPIC GROIN HERNIA REPAIRS

22

LAPAROSCOPIC TOTALLY EXTRAPERITONEAL HERNIORRHAPHY

DAVID L. CRAWFORD
EDWARD H. PHILLIPS

HISTORIC OVERVIEW

Extraperitoneal herniorrhaphy began in 1920, when Cheatle (8) introduced his extraperitoneal technique of inguinal hernia repair to deal with the multiply recurrent hernia. The magnitude of the operation and the technical difficulty of the approach limited its application to complex cases. In the 1980s, Stoppa (45) and Nyhus et al. (36) used the extraperitoneal approach but bridged the hernia defects with prosthetic mesh. The prosthetic mesh covers the entire inguinal floor and does not place the patient's weakened tissues under any additional tension. Published recurrence rates are low (1.4% to 2.2%), even in patients with prior recurrences.

The first report of a laparoscopic hernia repair was in 1982, when Ger et al. (18a,19) used a Michel staple applied with a Kocher clamp to close the peritoneal opening of a hernia sac under laparoscopic guidance. In this early report, the authors envisioned several potential advantages of laparoscopic herniorrhaphy, including the ability to repair bilateral hernias concurrently, the ability to perform diagnostic laparoscopy, earlier return to activity, and reduced postoperative pain. In 1989, Bogojavlensky (5) reported filling an indirect hernia defect with a plug of polypropylene mesh followed by laparoscopic suture closure of the internal ring. In 1990, Popp (40) reported closing an indirect hernia with extracorporeally tied sutures, then reinforcing the closure by placing a 4 × 5-cm dural patch over the area. Schultz (43) conducted the first large series of laparoscopic herniorrhaphy. Prior to the introduction of the hernia staplers, he incised the peritoneum adjacent to the indi-

rect hernia defect, filled the inguinal canal with a mesh plug, and closed the sac with suture. Because of mesh migration and unacceptable recurrence rates (25%), he began fixing the mesh anatomically. Also in the early 1990s, Phillips et al. (39) and McKernan and Laws (35) independently developed totally extraperitoneal prosthetic (TEPP) techniques, with and without peritoneoscopy, respectively. In 1991, Arregui (2) was the first to publish the transabdominal preperitoneal prosthetic (TAPP) approach, with full exposure of the inguinal floor and placement of a large preperitoneal mesh prosthesis. In 1992, Fitzgibbons (17) performed a series of intraperitoneal onlay mesh (IPOM) repairs, in which polypropylene mesh was secured to the abdominal wall with staples. Franklin (18) still performs an IPOM technique and has published good results.

The application of minimally invasive technology to the repair of inguinal hernias is a natural extension of the surgical skills acquired during the development of laparoscopic cholecystectomy. These operative techniques are based on the results achieved by the "open" extraperitoneal techniques of Cheatle, Stoppa, and Nyhus. Though the laparoscopic approach is not "minimally invasive," it has several advantages over its "open" counterparts. First, and often the most important from the patient's standpoint, is the reduced postoperative incisional pain and resultant disability. Second, the entire myopectineal orifice can be inspected bilaterally, allowing for repair of any unexpected contralateral hernias (reported to occur in 25% to 40% of patients) (10). Third, for patients with a previous anterior herniorrhaphy, laparoscopic herniorrhaphy avoids the previous operative site in patients with recurrent hernias, decreasing the chance of vascular and nerve injury or testicular ischemia. The disadvantages of laparoscopic herniorrhaphy include the need for general anesthesia, the need for prosthetic mesh, the violation of the peritoneal cavity (TAPP repair), the cost of the procedure, and the time and skill required to learn the technique in order to perform it in a safe and efficient manner.

D. L. Crawford: Department of Surgery, University of Illinois at Chicago, College of Medicine at Peoria, Peoria, Illinois.

E. H. Phillips: Department of Surgery, University of Southern California School of Medicine; Department of Surgery, Cedars–Sinai Medical Center, Los Angeles, California.

TOTALLY EXTRAPERITONEAL PROSTHETIC TECHNIQUE

Phillips Technique (TEPP with Peritoneoscopy)

Peritoneoscopy provides a diagnostic laparoscopy and a complete view of the hernia repair without added risk. In a small number of TEPP repairs, the peritoneum is inadvertently torn. There have been reports of bowel obstructions from herniated small bowel. Inspection of the peritoneum at the conclusion of the case allows for identification and closure of any breaches in the peritoneum. It also identifies the rare case of hernia reduction "en masse."

Patient and Team Position

Patients receive a single prophylactic dose of intravenous antibiotics to cover *Staphylococcus*. They are asked to void immediately preoperatively, so urinary catheters are rarely used. The patient is secured to the operating table in the supine position with both arms tucked. The monitor is located at the foot of the bed. The surgeon stands on the side opposite the hernia to be repaired. The first assistant stands opposite the surgeon with the scrub nurse toward the patient's legs on either side. The abdomen is shaved from 3 cm above the umbilicus to 5 cm below, and then it is prepared in the usual fashion.

Surgical Technique

After induction of general anesthesia, pneumoperitoneum is established using a Veress needle technique through an infraumbilical incision. A 10/11-mm laparoscopic trocar is then inserted into the peritoneal cavity while being directed toward the pelvis. Through this trocar, a 30-degree laparoscope is introduced and a general inspection of the abdomen and pelvic floor is made. A 10-mm scope is sturdier when used to bluntly develop the preperitoneal space, and it provides better illumination during the procedure.

Under laparoscopic direction, sites directly lateral to the rectus muscle and in line with the infraumbilical trocar site are chosen for the two working ports (see Fig. 22.1). Preemptive local anesthesia (0.5% bupivacaine) is injected into the abdominal wall and preperitoneal space, creating a preperitoneal "blister" at the planned trocar site. A 10-mm skin incision is made at both locations, and a curved hemostat is used to dissect through the abdominal wall until the transversalis fascia is reached. At this point, to decrease the likelihood of peritoneal perforation, a large Kelly clamp is exchanged for the hemostat. Dissection is continued until the tip of the clamp or "metal sign" is seen through the peritoneum (see Fig. 22.2). The larger clamp is turned with its curve pointing up toward the underside of the abdominal wall. It is opened with two hands and withdrawn while still open to create a muscle-splitting pathway through the abdominal wall (see Fig. 22.3). A blunt probe is then placed through a 10/11-mm cannula and slowly guided into the preperitoneal space under laparoscopic guidance while being rocked back and forth in a rowing motion parallel to the abdominal wall (see Fig. 22.4). With the blunt probe still in place, the 10/11 trocar is rotated 360 degrees around it and advanced into the preperitoneal space. The valve on the trocar must be

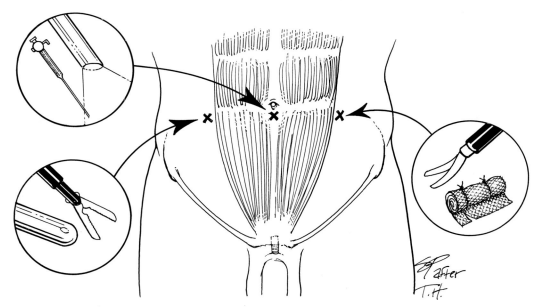

FIGURE 22.1. Trocar positions and instrumentation (Phillips technique). (From Friedman R, Phillips E. Laparoscopically guided total extraperitoneal inguinal hernioplasty. In: Maddern G, Hiatt J, Phillips E, eds. *Hernia repair: open vs laparoscopic approaches.* Philadelphia: WB Saunders, 1997, with permission.)

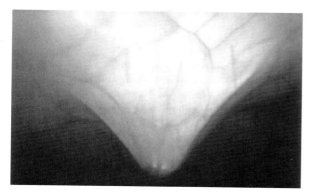

FIGURE 22.2. Tip of clamp "metal sign" visible in preperitoneal space.

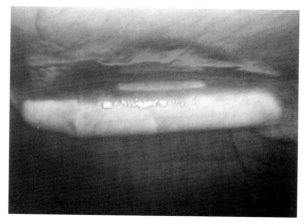

FIGURE 22.4. Blunt probe being advanced into preperitoneal space.

opened before probe removal to prevent a suction tear of the peritoneum.

A 10/5-mm reducer cap is placed on the cannula and a blunt grasper is carefully advanced into the preperitoneal space under direct visualization. The grasper is carefully advanced between the peritoneum and the epigastric vessels toward the pubic symphysis while staying cephalad to the direct and indirect hernia spaces (see Fig. 22.5). This procedure is repeated on the opposite side. If difficulty is encountered during grasper placement, a small amount to CO_2 can be instilled through the trocar in question, dissecting out the potential space nicely and facilitating grasper placement. Prior lower abdominal incisions frequently present challenging peritoneal scars that necessitate sharp dissection in the preperitoneal space with CO_2 and laparoscopic scissors while viewed and guided by the intraabdominal laparoscope.

The preperitoneal space is then insufflated to 15 mm Hg through the lateral cannulas in sequence while the intraperitoneal carbon dioxide is allowed to escape and the laparoscope is backed into the infraumbilical (transparent) can-

nula. This cannula and the laparoscope are then drawn back until the peritoneum slips past the trocar tip and its overlying preperitoneal fat is seen. The laparoscope is oriented with the 30-degree angle facing down, then advanced blindly but gently into the preperitoneal space, hugging the anterior abdominal wall until it touches the pubic symphysis. The cannula is then advanced over the laparoscope, the scope withdrawn approximately 2 cm, then rocked gently side to side, further developing the preperitoneal space. The laparoscope is then withdrawn, cleaned, and reinserted.

Orientation in the preperitoneal space is established by identifying the pubic symphysis in the midline and one or more of the graspers. If neither is seen, the operator must decide whether the laparoscope is above or below the muscle and/or fascia. When the 30-degree laparoscope is facing upward the rectus muscle should be seen, and when facing downward one should see preperitoneal fat. If the laparoscope is improperly placed in a position anterior to the fascia, fat is seen anteriorly and fascia is seen below. If the

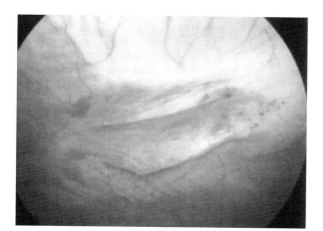

FIGURE 22.3. Clamp opening prior to forceful removal from the preperitoneal space.

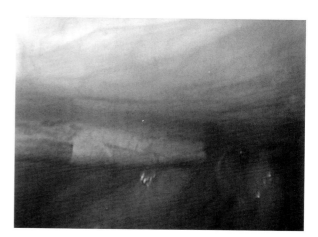

FIGURE 22.5. Grasper in preperitoneal space.

proper plane cannot be entered after several attempts, a small incision should be made 2 cm below the umbilical port, and a 10-mm Hasson cannula can be placed into the preperitoneal space under direct visualization and secured to the fascia. A blunt rod can then be used through the Hasson cannula to develop the preperitoneal space. Balloon dissection can also be used with this technique.

Once the graspers are seen extraperitoneally, the space is further developed by sliding the laparoscope up the anterior surface of each grasper while applying gentle posterior pressure on each instrument. This motion in combination with CO_2 insufflation quickly creates a large work area. The pubic symphysis is identified in the midline, followed by Cooper's ligaments, which are followed laterally until the femoral canal is identified. The inferior epigastric vessels are encountered anteriorly on the underside of the abdominal wall. Identification of the epigastric vessels prevents over-dissection into the femoral vessels. If the anatomy becomes confusing during the procedure, the surgeon need only return to the midline where the pubic symphysis and Cooper's ligaments serve as the central reference point (see Fig. 22.6).

When present, an indirect hernia sac is identified medial and anterior to the cord structures (lateral to the epigastric vessels) and is dissected free of the cord structures using the same blunt teasing dissection technique used in "open" surgery. Large indirect sacs may be proximally ligated with an endoscopic loop ligature and amputated, leaving the distal sac open. Cord "pseudolipomas" are located inferior and lateral to the cord structures, and are reduced in a fashion similar to indirect hernia sacks. These "pseudolipomas" do not need to be excised. The contents of and preperitoneal fat within direct hernias are reduced until the edges of the fascial defect are clearly seen and all hernial defects are identified. At this time, 10 cc of 0.5% bupivacaine local anesthetic is instilled into the tissues directly above Cooper's ligament and the posterior aspect of the abdominal wall bilaterally.

Polypropylene mesh is then cut in a square of 13 × 13 cm with a slit cut for the cord structures. In our earlier experience, we slit the mesh to allow placement beneath and around the cord and approximated the slit with staples to provide better fixation. Concern over the possibility that encircling of the cord might increase pain and morbidity from scar formation, patients with mesh repairs using encircled and nonencircled techniques were examined prospectively. We found that closing the slit around the spermatic cord was not essential for prevention of early recurrence. Chronic pain (greater than 2 weeks) and fluid collections tended to be more frequent when the mesh was closed around the cord (27). The mesh is fashioned as shown in Fig. 22.7. The mesh is partially rolled up, and two chromic sutures are used to hold it in position. The mesh is then held with a locking grasper on its medial end and pushed through the lateral trocar toward the pubis into the preperitoneal space. Having the mesh rolled up makes it easier to pass through the trocar, and easier to position in the preperitoneal space. The mesh is positioned with the lateral slit and its corresponding suture directly over the cord structures at the base of the epigastric vessels. The lateral flap is then grasped at its medial tip with the ipsilateral grasper and slid beneath the cord structures as they are gently retracted medially. Care is taken that no medial or lateral tension is placed on the cord by the mesh. The lower medial

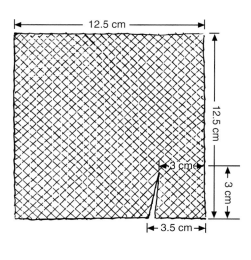

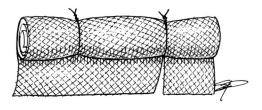

FIGURE 22.7. Mesh dimensions for Phillips technique. (From Crawford D, Phillips E. Laparoscopic extraperitoneal hernia. In: Zucker K, ed. *Surgical laparoscopy*, 3rd ed. Philadelphia: Lippincott Williams & Wilkins, 2000:571–584, with permission.)

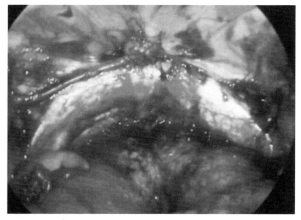

FIGURE 22.6. Preperitoneal view during dissection shows central location of pubic symphysis.

mesh flap is then secured to Cooper's ligament with staples before it is unrolled (see Fig. 22.8). In bilateral hernia repairs, both pieces of mesh are secured to Cooper's ligaments before unrolling. After the mesh is secured to Cooper's ligaments on both sides, the chromic sutures are cut and the mesh prostheses are unrolled and stapled to one another in the midline and sparingly to the underside of the abdominal wall (see Fig. 22.9). No staples are placed lateral to the epigastric vessels; this avoids potential injury of the ilioinguinal and lateral femoral cutaneous nerves. In this configuration, the femoral, direct, and indirect spaces are well covered with mesh.

The laparoscope and infraumbilical trocar are then withdrawn from the preperitoneal space and reinserted into the peritoneal cavity. The preperitoneal space is decompressed via the lateral cannulas as the peritoneal cavity is refilled with CO_2. The repair is then inspected from the intraperitoneal position to ensure no reduction en masse of the hernia has occurred and that the mesh is in good position (see Fig. 22.10). At the same time, the peritoneum is inspected for inadvertent lacerations. If present, the laparoscope is reinserted into the preperitoneal space and the defects are closed with loop ligatures, sta-

ples, or sutures. Occasionally, it is necessary to push the lateral cannulas through the peritoneum and close the defects in the peritoneum from an intraperitoneal position with either sutures or staples.

The lateral cannula site fascial defects are closed at two levels. First, a 2 × 2-cm mesh square is cut with a chromic suture anchored to it at its center, leaving a 10 cm tail. The knot is held with a grasper, and the plug is pushed down through the lateral trocar into the preperitoneal space. The cannula is removed and the suture is used to position the plug beneath and within the fascial defect under direct laparoscopic visualization (see Fig. 22.11). An attempt to close the external oblique can be made with zero polyglycolic acid suture, but this is not always possible in the obese patient. The infraumbilical site is closed under direct vision with zero polyglycolic acid suture because the peritoneum is open at that site. Skin incisions are closed with absorbable suture in a subcuticular fashion.

McKernan Technique

This approach, first described in 1993 by McKernan and Laws (35), totally avoids the peritoneal cavity.

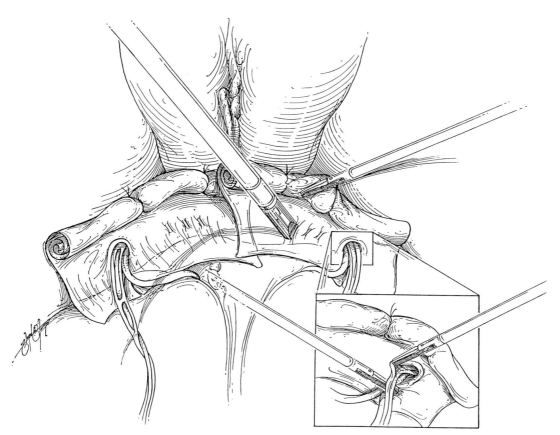

FIGURE 22.8. Stapling mesh to Cooper's ligament. Tucking mesh beneath cord structures **(inset)**. (From Crawford D, Phillips E. Laparoscopic extraperitoneal hernia. In: Zucker K, ed. *Surgical laparoscopy*, 3rd ed. Philadelphia: Lippincott Williams & Wilkins, 2000:571–584, with permission.)

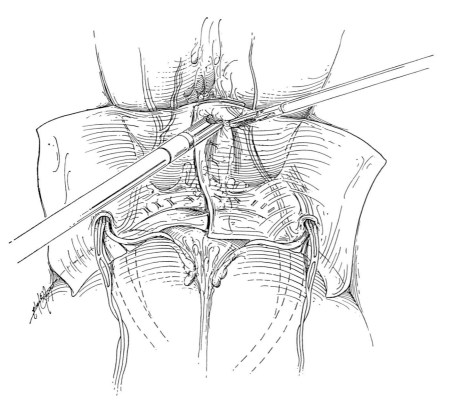

FIGURE 22.9. Fixing mesh prostheses to one another in midline. (From Crawford D, Phillips E. Laparoscopic extraperitoneal hernia. In: Zucker K, ed. *Surgical laparoscopy*, 3rd. ed. Philadelphia: Lippincott Williams & Wilkins, 2000:571–584, with permission.)

Positioning of Patient and Team

Patients receive prophylactic antibiotics and urinary catheters preoperatively. They are secured to the table in the supine and Trendelenburg positions. The arms can be either tucked at the side or at 90 degrees from the table. The surgeon stands opposite the side to be repaired, with the assistant (camera operator) opposite the surgeon.

Surgical Technique

A 2-cm infraumbilical skin incision is made, and the fascia is exposed. The fascia is elevated and incised vertically, exposing the rectus muscles, which are separated bluntly. The fascia is secured with stay sutures of zero polyglycolic acid. Retractors are placed beneath the rectus muscles, and a tunnel is bluntly developed between the rectus muscle and

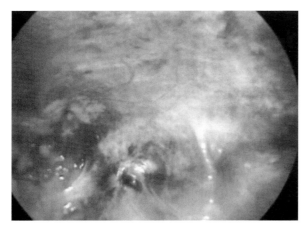

FIGURE 22.10. Intraperitoneal view confirms accurate mesh placement and lack of peritoneal tears (right inguinal hernia).

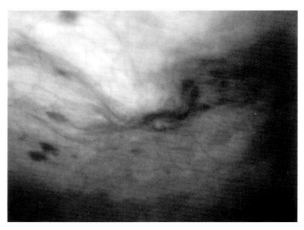

FIGURE 22.11. Intraperitoneal view of mesh plug in lateral trocar site.

the underlying preperitoneal fat. A transparent disposable 10/11-mm Hasson cannula is inserted into this tunnel and secured with the stay sutures. A 10/11-mm operating laparoscope is placed into the preperitoneal space with a 5-mm blunt probe, extending 2 cm beyond the optics, being used to dissect down to the pubic symphysis and then laterally to expose both of Cooper's ligaments. Insufflation is begun with a pressure setting of 8 to 10 mm Hg and should be kept below 12 mm Hg to avoid excessive subcutaneous emphysema.

The simpler and more commonly used alternative to the above technique of dissection is the use of a balloon dissection device. The same incision is made; the balloon is inserted beneath the rectus muscle to the pubic symphysis and inflated, thus performing most of the preperitoneal dissection. Most balloons have a guide rod for initial placement, and some allow laparoscopic visualization during inflation with either air or saline. A fairly large, bloodless workspace is quickly obtained using these devices.

Whether the balloon or manual dissection technique is used, the result is that the peritoneum has been dissected off the posterior aspect of the rectus muscle and the pubic symphysis is exposed. Next, two working ports are placed into the preperitoneal space. First, a 5-mm port is placed approximately one fingerbreadth above the pubis and a second 10/11-mm trocar is placed halfway between the pubis and the upper trocar (see Fig. 22.12). This third trocar must be carefully inserted, as it is associated with the greatest risk

of invading the peritoneal cavity. After the skin incision is made, a hemostat is used to bluntly dissect through the subcutaneous fat down to the fascia. The shielded trocar is placed through the fascia, and the shield is engaged then advanced bluntly through the rectus. This method lessens the likelihood of injuring the peritoneum.

The operative telescope is exchanged for a zero-degree 10-mm laparoscope. Bimanual dissection is carried along Cooper's ligament to the femoral canal. Dissection continues until Cooper's ligament, the femoral canal, the direct floor, and the epigastric vessels are exposed. At this point, a 10-mm 45-degree viewing laparoscope is substituted for the zero-degree scope. Using a sweeping motion, the peritoneum is further dissected away from the abdominal wall cephalad, exposing the internal ring and indirect sac, if present. Dissection is continued preperitoneally in a cephalad direction to the level of the iliac crest. The cord structures are inspected and an indirect sac, if present, is reduced. If the sac is large, it is entered anteromedially, separated from the cord structures, severed, and ligated proximally, leaving the distal sac in place. The distal sac is not ligated. If a cord lipoma is found, it is reduced through the internal ring.

To cover the hernial defect, a 7.5 × 12.5-cm piece of polypropylene mesh is fashioned by cutting a 4.5-cm slit vertically in the mesh 5 cm from the cephalad portion in the mesh. A 12-mm hole is made for the cord structures (see Fig. 22.13A). The cord structures are carefully dissected free from the lateral pelvic wall, enabling the mesh to be placed easily behind them. The mesh is folded and a suture is placed to facilitate mesh placement (Fig. 22.13B). The mesh is brought into the preperitoneal space in proper orientation for easy positioning. The mesh is brought behind the cord structures and is positioned so that the structures pass through the precut hole (Fig. 22.13C). The stay sutures are cut and the mesh is elevated into position. The first staple is placed to close the keyhole, then the mesh is secured to Cooper's ligament (see Fig. 22.14).

In the case of a bilateral hernia, two mirror image pieces of polypropylene mesh are prepared. The two are stapled to one another in the midline. In the case of a very large defect, an additional piece of mesh (5 × 15 cm) can be placed cephalad to the pubis, connecting the two pieces in the midline. This prevents protrusion of mesh through a large direct defect. The mesh is stapled around the opening of the fascial defect in addition to the previously described placement of staples.

After inspecting all trocar sites and areas of dissection for hemostasis, 30 mL of 0.25% bupivacaine is instilled into the preperitoneal space, and the pneumopreperitoneum is released. The periumbilical fascia and the fascia at the middle trocar are closed with zero polyglycolic acid sutures. The skin is then closed with 4-zero subcuticular sutures.

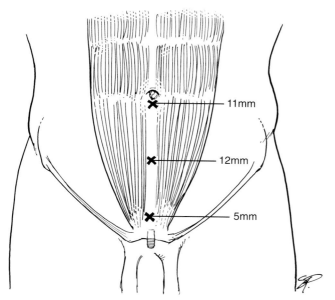

FIGURE 22.12. Trocar positions (McKernan technique). (From Friedman R, Phillips E. Laparoscopically guided total extraperitoneal inguinal hernioplasty. In: Maddern G, Hiatt J, Phillips E, eds. *Hernia repair: open vs laparoscopic approaches.* Philadelphia: WB Saunders, 1997, with permission.)

11mm
12mm
5mm

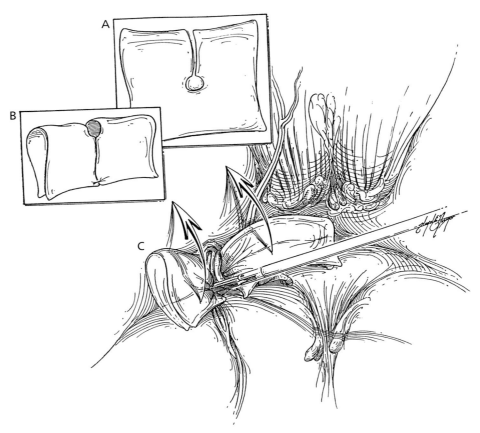

FIGURE 22.13. Mesh shape **(A)**, preparation **(B)**, and positioning **(C)** (McKernan technique). *Arrows* indicate elevation of mesh anteriorly against abdominal wall. (From Crawford D, Phillips E. Laparoscopic extraperitoneal hernia. In: Zucker K, ed. *Surgical laparoscopy,* 3rd ed. Philadelphia: Lippincott Williams & Wilkins, 2000:571–584, with permission.)

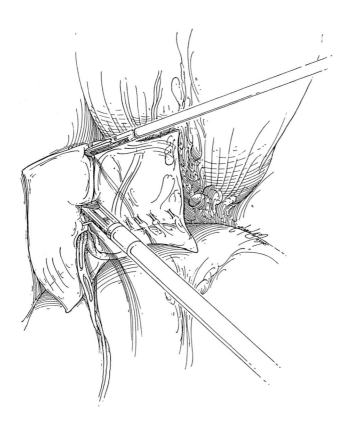

FIGURE 22.14. Slit in mesh is closed, then entire mesh is secured to Cooper's ligament. (From Crawford D, Phillips E. Laparoscopic extraperitoneal hernia. In: Zucker K, ed. *Surgical laparoscopy,* 3rd ed. Philadelphia: Lippincott Williams & Wilkins, 2000:571–584, with permission.)

Published Series

"Open" Versus Laparoscopic

Many randomized prospective studies have been published comparing open and laparoscopic techniques for the repair of inguinal hernias. These studies are listed in Tables 22.1 and 22.2.

In one prospective randomized study (21), both open and laparoscopic repairs were performed under general anesthesia and then compared in relation to operative time and costs, hospital stay, postoperative pain, return to work, and patient satisfaction. Differences that reached significance between the two repairs were as follows: laparoscopic repairs took longer, had higher operative costs, resulted in less postoperative pain and analgesic consumption, allowed patients to return to work earlier, and had fewer complications.

Kozol et al. (28) performed a prospective, randomized, blinded comparison of both repairs with regard to postoperative pain using two standardized pain scales and the cumulative dosages of analgesics during the first 48 hours. In these 62 patients, all of whom had general anesthesia, postoperative pain was significantly less in those undergoing laparoscopic repair. No difference was found in complications between the two groups.

In another study (33), 105 patients were prospectively randomized (48 open, 57 TEPP) to accurately determine ability to return to normal activity by measuring their muscular performance with exercise testing. These results were then compared to questionnaires assessing activities of daily living (ADL) and return to normal activity. The results of the exercise tests and ADL questionnaires after operation in patients who underwent laparoscopic herniorrhaphy were significantly better. Patients undergoing laparoscopic herniorrhaphy returned to normal activities sooner (6 versus 10 days; $p = 0.0003$). At 1 week postoperatively, the laparoscopic herniorrhaphy patients were able to perform more repetitions of sit-ups and straight leg raises ($p < 0.0001$), and their ADL scores were significantly better ($p = 0.0001$) than those of patients undergoing open repairs. The authors concluded that laparoscopic herniorrhaphy results in a quicker recovery.

The largest and best-executed prospective randomized trial was conducted by Liem et al. (32). In this large multicenter trial, 487 patients were treated by TEPP and 507 were treated by reduction of the hernia, ligation of the sac, if necessary, and reconstruction of the inguinal floor with nonabsorbable sutures or mesh if needed. All patients had unilateral inguinal hernias (primary or recurrent). Those with bilateral hernias were excluded. Complete follow-up in 97% of patients and a median follow-up of 607 days yielded the following results. Patients in the laparoscopic group had a more rapid recovery (median time to the resumption of normal daily activity, 6 versus 10 days; time to return to work, 14 versus 21 days; and time to the resumption of athletic activities, 24 versus 36 days; $p < 0.001$ for all comparisons). Patients in the laparoscopic group also had fewer recurrences than the open group: 17 (3%) in laparoscopic versus 31 (6%) in open. A breakdown of the complications experienced by the two groups is shown in Table 22.3. The authors concluded that patients

TABLE 22.1. OPEN VERSUS LAPAROSCOPIC HERNIORRHAPHY: PROSPECTIVE RANDOMIZED STUDIES 1994–1996

Reference	Year	Technique	No. of Patients (O/L)	Postoperative Pain	Return to Activity (d) (O/L)	Complications % (O/L)	Recurrence (O/L)	Follow-up (mo)
Stoker et al. (44)	1994	D/TAPP	75/75	< lap[a]	28/14[a]	21/8[a]	0/0	7[b]
Payne et al. (38)	1994	L/TAPP	52/48	NR	17/9[a]	18/12	0/0	10[c]
Champault et al. (6)	1994	S/TEP	89/92	< lap[a]	24/12[a]	NR	0/0	12[b]
Maddern et al. (34)	1994	D/TAPP	44/42	ND	30/17[a]	47/40	0/2	8[c]
Vogt et al. (48)	1995	B/V/IPOM	31/30	< lap	18/7	16/17	2/1	8[b]
Barkun et al. (3)	1995	SC/TAPP	49/43	ND	11/9	12/22	1/0	14[c]
Lawrence et al. (29)	1995	D/TAPP	66/58	< lap[a]	28/22	2/12[a]	0/1	1.5
Leibl et al. (30)	1995	S/TAPP	48/54	< lap[a]	38/21[a]	6/4	0/0	16[b]
Schrenk et al. (42)	1996	S/TAPP/TEP	34/28/24	< lap[a]	ND	6/8/6	0/1/0	3[b]
Bessell et al. (4)	1996	S/TEP/TAPP	72/29/3	< lap[a]	32/30	10/12	0/2	7[c]
Filipi et al. (16)	1996	L/TAPP	29/24	ND	ND	10/8	2/0	11[b]
Tschudi et al. (47)	1996	S/TAPP	43/44	< lap[a]	48/25[a]	26/16	2/1	7[c]
Wright et al. (51)	1996	SC/TAPP	64/67	< lap[a]	NR	71/22	NR	NR
Hauters et al. (20)	1996	S/TAPP	35/35	< lap	10/6	NR	9/3	30

lap, laparoscopic; O, open; TAPP, transabdominal preperitoneal repair; TEP, totally extraperitoneal; IPOM, intraperitoneal onlay mesh; S, Shouldice; D, darn; L, Lichtenstein; B, Bassini; V, McVay; SC, surgeon's choice of repair; ND, no difference; NR, not reported.
[a]$p < 0.05$ open vs. laparoscopic.
[b]Values are means.
[c]Values are medians.

TABLE 22.2. OPEN VERSUS LAPAROSCOPIC HERNIORRHAPHY: PROSPECTIVE RANDOMIZED TRIALS 1997–1999

Reference	Year	Technique	No. of Patients (O/L)	Postoperative Pain	Return of Activity (d) (O/L)	Complications % (O/L)	Recurrence (O/L)	Follow-up (mo)
Kozol et al. (28)	1997	SC/TAPP	32/30	< lap[a]	NR	22/20	NR	1.5[b]
Liem et al. (32)	1997	SC/TEP	507/487	< lap[a]	10/6[a]	20/15	31/17[a]	20[c]
Heikkinen et al. (21)	1997	L/TAPP	18/20	< lap[a]	19/14[a]	83/20[a]	NR	2
Liem et al. (33)	1997	SC/TEP	48/57	NR	10/6[a]	NR	NR	1.5
Kald et al. (24)	1997	S/TAPP	100/100	NR	23/14[a]	ND	3/0[a]	12
Champault et al. (7)	1997	SC/TEP	49/51	< lap[a]	35/17[a]	30/4[a]	1/3	36[b]
Tanphiphat et al. (46)	1998	B/TAPP	60/60	< lap[a]	14/8[a]	ND	0/1	32[b]
Zieren et al. (52)	1998	S/P/TAPP	80/80/80	< lap and P[a]	26/18/16[a]	ND	0/0/0	25[b]
Wellwood et al. (49)	1998	L/TAPP	200/200	< lap[a]	21/17[a]	< lap[a]	0/0	3[b]
Heikkinen et al. (22)	1998	L/TAPP	20/20	ND	21/14[a]	40/25[a]	0/0	17[c]
Paganini et al. (37)	1998	L/TAPP	56/52	ND	ND	ND	0/2	28[c]
Aitola et al. (1)	1998	PPO/TAPP	25/24	< lap[a]	5/7	8/21	2/3	18[c]
Dirksen et al. (12)	1998	B/TAPP	87/88	< lap[a]	27/17[a]	ND	22/7[a]	24[b]
Khoury (26)	1998	P/TEP	142/150	< lap[a]	15/8[a]	23/13[a]	4/3	17[c]
Juul and Christensen (23)	1999	S/TAPP	130/138	< lap[a]	18/13[a]	ND	3/4	12[c]
Total Tables 2 and 3			2,365/2,233				83/49	

lap, laparoscopic; O, open; TAPP, transabdominal preperitoneal repair; TEP, totally extraperitoneal; S, Shouldice; L, Lichtenstein; B, Bassini; SC, surgeon's choice of repair; P, plug and patch; PPO, preperitoneal open; ND, no difference; NR, not reported.
[a]$p < 0.05$ open vs. laparoscopic.
[b]Values are means.
[c]Values are medians.

with inguinal hernias undergoing laparoscopic repair recover more rapidly and have fewer recurrences than those undergoing open anterior repair.

A recent study by Zieren et al. (52) compared TAPP, Shouldice, and plug-and-patch (Rutkow–Robbins) repairs in a prospective randomized fashion. A total of 240 patients were evenly divided between the three techniques. The laparoscopic approach had significantly longer operation times and material costs were higher ($p < 0.01$ for both comparisons). Postoperative pain, analgesia requirements, limitation of daily activities, and return to work did not differ between TAPP and plug-and-patch repairs but were sig-

nificantly lower in both groups compared with Shouldice's repair ($p < 0.05$). Postoperative complications did not differ significantly between the groups. The authors concluded that the plug-and-patch repair is a promising technique in adults because it offers the same excellent patient comfort as laparoscopic repair but is less expensive and can be performed under local anesthesia.

Another study by Khoury (26) compared plug-and-patch (n = 142) to TEPP (n = 150) with an 89% follow-up at 17 months (median) postoperatively. Initially, laparoscopic repair was slower than open but became 10 minutes faster during the last 75 repairs. Patients undergoing TEPP

TABLE 22.3. COMPLICATIONS: ANTERIOR AND LAPAROSCOPIC HERNIORRHAPHY

Complication	Anterior		Laparoscopic		*p* value
	No.	%	No.	%	
Seroma (6 wk)	0	0	7	1	0.007
Wound infections	8	1.5	0	0	0.03
Chronic pain	70	14	10	2	< 0.001
Hematoma (6 wk)	14	3	24	5	0.07
Urinary retention	2	<1	5	1	0.28
Bleeding	1	<1	1	<1	1.0

From Liem MSL, Van Der Graaf Y, Van Steensel CJ, et al. Comparison of conventional anterior surgery and laparoscopic surgery for inguinal hernia repair. *N Engl J Med* 1997;336:1541–1547, with permission.

repair consumed less narcotic analgesic and returned to their normal activities 1 week earlier than their open counterparts ($p < 0.01$). Hospital stay did not differ between the two groups. Postoperative complications occurred in 23% of open patients and 13% of TEPP patients ($p < 0.01$). Recurrence rates at follow-up were 3% for plug-and-patch and 2.5% for TEPP. The author concluded that patients with inguinal hernias who undergo extraperitoneal laparoscopic repair have the same hospital stay and recurrence rates but recover faster, use less pain medication, and have fewer minor complications than those who undergo plug-and-patch repair.

Wellwood et al. (49) reported a large study in which 400 patients were prospectively randomized to undergo either TAPP or Lichtenstein repairs. Patients with both unilateral and bilateral hernias were included. Follow-up in 86% of patients at 3 months revealed the following data. More patients in the open group (96%) than in the laparoscopic group (89%) were discharged on the same day as the operation ($p = 0.01$). Although pain scores were lower in the open group while the local anesthetic effect persisted, scores after open repair were significantly higher for each day of the first week, on day 7, and during the second week ($p < 0.01$). At 1 month, there was a greater improvement in mean SF-36 scores (measurement of well-being) over baseline in the laparoscopic group compared with the open group on seven of eight parameters, reaching significance on five ($p = 0.01$). For every activity considered, the median time until return to normal was significantly shorter for the laparoscopic group. Patients randomized to the laparoscopic repair were more satisfied with surgery at 1 and 3 months postoperatively. An elaborate cost comparison of the two techniques showed that laparoscopic repair was £335 ($502) more expensive than open repair. The authors concluded that laparoscopic hernia repair has considerable short-term clinical advantages after discharge compared to open mesh herniorrhaphy, even though it was more expensive.

Other randomized studies support those above in showing reduced postoperative pain (1,4,6,7,12,20,23,29,30,44, 46–48,51,52), reduced analgesic requirements (4,12,26, 46–48,52), earlier return to work (7,12,22–24,26,30,38, 44,46–49,52), and fewer complications (7,22,26,30,34,38, 44,47,49) when compared to standard open approaches. These very same studies in many cases have shown laparoscopic herniorrhaphy to be more costly (3,29,31,37,38,46, 49), have more complications (1,3,4,29,42,48), and demonstrate no significant difference in convalescence (1,3,4,16, 20,29,37,42,48) or postoperative pain (3,22,34,37,47). As the number and size of the prospective randomized studies regarding laparoscopic herniorrhaphy grow, evidence in favor of the laparoscopic approach is rapidly accumulating. Recurrence, perhaps the most important standard for comparison of techniques, is only beginning to be looked at with adequate follow-up, but initial laparoscopic herniorrhaphy results are encouraging (35).

TAPP versus TEPP

The TAPP technique is easier to learn and therefore more frequently performed in most surgical communities. However, there is a significant body of literature developing that shows TEPP to have several advantages over TAPP. Several nonrandomized studies compare the TAPP and TEPP techniques (Table 22.4).

One such study by Felix and Michas (14) compared 733 TAPP with 382 TEPP procedures. The TEPP procedure had no complications and one recurrence, while TAPP had nine complications (one small-bowel obstruction, two small-bowel injuries, six trocar hernias), and two recurrences. Five TEPP patients had their procedures converted

TABLE 22.4. TAPP VERSUS TEPP COLLECTED SERIES

Author (year)	Repair Type	No. of Hernias	Recurrence (%)	Complications (%)
Felix and Michas (1995)	TAPP	733	0.2	1.2
	TEPP	382	0.2	0
Ramshaw et al. (1996)	TAPP	300	2	4.3
	TEPP	600	0.3	0.8
Dellemagne et al. (1996)	TAPP	254	1.5	NR
	TEPP	371	0	NR
Fielding (1996)	TAPP	386	1	0.5
	TEPP	218	0.9	0
Kald et al. (1997) (25)	TAPP	339	2	11
	TEPP	87	0	8
Cocks (1998)	TAPP	148	2	27
	TEPP	313	0.3	12
Felix et al. (1999)	TAPP	472	NR	5.6
	TEPP	678	NR	1.0

NR, not reported; TAPP, transabdominal preperitoneal prosthetic repair; TEP, totally extraperitoneal prosthetic.

to TAPP due to technical difficulties. The median time to return to work for both groups was similar.

Ramshaw et al. (41) compared 300 TAPP with 600 TEPP procedures. Recurrence rates were 2% for TAPP and 0.3% for TEPP. Complication rates also favored the TEPP approach, with only 0.8% of patients being affected versus 4.3% in the TAPP group. When patients with a history of prior lower abdominal surgery were examined separately, they were found to have increased rates of recurrence (2.2%) and complications (8.7%) when undergoing a TEPP procedure. The authors concluded that TEPP is the procedure of choice, except in cases with history of prior lower abdominal surgery.

In another study (15), 386 TAPP and 218 TEPP procedures were compared. There were two recurrences in the TEPP group and four in the TAPP group. TAPP procedures were complicated by two small-bowel obstructions. Operative times for both groups were similar.

In a similar large study by Dellemagne et al. (11), 254 TAPP and 371 TEPP repairs were compared. There were no recurrences in the TEPP group and four in the TAPP group. The TAPP repair was associated with a higher incidence of complications, including small bowel obstruction.

Kald et al. (25) compared 339 TAPP to 87 TEPP procedures. Recurrence was more common in TAPP than TEPP (2% versus 0%) with follow-ups of 23 versus 7 months. Fifteen major complications, including one postoperative death, two bowel obstructions, one severe neuralgia, three trocar hernias, one epigastric artery bleeding episode, and seven recurrences, were recorded; all except one (epigastric artery bleed) were in the TAPP group. The authors concluded that TEPP "may be the method of choice in laparoscopic hernia repair."

Cocks (9) sequentially compared 129 patients undergoing TAPP procedures to 254 having the TEPP procedure. The patients were examined at 1 day, 1 week, 5 weeks, and 1 year postoperatively. No significant differences were found in length of hospital stay, postoperative analgesia, or the rate of early or late operative complications. The operating time was shorter, and the return to normal activities was quicker for the TEPP patients. The author now favors the TEPP technique over the TAPP.

Felix et al. (13) again recently reviewed their experience with laparoscopic herniorrhaphy and compared TAPP (n = 395) and TEPP (n = 692) with regard to complications; recurrence was not discussed in detail. The incidence of complications varied significantly with the year in which the operation was performed. The overall incidence of complications was 2.7% over the 6 years of the study: 5.6% during the first 3 years and 0.5% during years 4 to 6. Complications also varied with technique (TAPP, 5.6%; TEPP, 1%). The authors admit, however, that their selection was biased with those difficult hernias (incarcerated, giant scrotal) being repaired with TAPP. They also state that the first TEPP repairs were not performed until a large (n = 333)

experience with TAPP had been completed. Thus, the experience gained with TAPP definitely decreased the learning curve for the TEPP repair. The authors concluded that the incidence of complications following laparoscopic herniorrhaphy could be substantially reduced by experience to less than 1%. They also stated that the risk of complications following TEPP may be less than after TAPP but that a randomized prospective study would be needed to accurately answer this question.

Complications

Complications unique to laparoscopic herniorrhaphy are those associated with the use of general anesthesia and the presence of a peritoneal incision (TAPP). Most complications from general anesthesia are cardiopulmonary in nature. When examining TAPP series, especially those that include the authors' learning phase, a noticeable incidence of small-bowel obstruction is present. Although small-bowel obstruction is more common in TAPP, there is otherwise no difference in the types of complications occurring in TAPP and TEPP repairs. Comparison of open and laparoscopic techniques by Liem et al. (32) (Table 22.3) and our own experience shows that anterior repairs have a higher incidence of wound infections and chronic pain while laparoscopic repairs have more seromas. Comparison of our own complication data to those of other TEPP series shows that the results are similar (Table 22.5).

Cost

Cost is an issue that must be considered when deciding between techniques of hernia repair. The direct operating room cost of laparoscopic herniorrhaphy has generally been shown to be $500 to $1200 higher than that of traditional open repair (3,21,22,29,37,38,44,46,49,52). This is primarily due to longer operating room times, anesthesia charges, the price of laparoscopic instrumentation, and consumables. The reduced postoperative disability associated with laparoscopic herniorrhaphy has the potential to reduce the societal cost of hernia repair by returning patients to work earlier. This potential is especially high in those patients with physically demanding jobs (38).

This complicated question of societal cost has been best evaluated by studies taking place in countries with socialized medical practices, where charges and costs are nationally standardized. Kald (24) and Heikkinen (22) et al. analyzed direct hospital cost and then included indirect cost analysis associated with return to work in the postoperative period. Both groups found that in employed patients, the earlier return to work experienced by the laparoscopically treated patients actually saved money when the cost of paid sick leave was considered. Kald et al. found that these savings in indirect cost exceeded the higher direct cost of laparoscopy at 3 days off work, and Heikkinen et al. calcu-

TABLE 22.5. COMPLICATIONS OF LAPAROSCOPIC EXTRAPERITONEAL HERNIORRHAPHY: COLLECTED SERIES

	Author (Year)/No. of Patients					
	Felix and Michas (1995) 382	Massaad (1996) 316	Heithold (1997) 346	Cocks (1998) 254	Phillips[a] (1998) 278	McKernan[b] (1998) 638
Recurrence	1 (0.3)	5 (1.6)	2 (0.6)	1 (0.4)	1 (0.4)	4 (0.6)
Complications						
Seromas/hematomas	38 (9.9)	4 (1.3)	0	19 (7.5)	22 (7.9)	45 (7.1)
Urinary retention	0	8 (2.5)	7 (2.0)	1 (0.4)	11 (4.0)	21 (3.3)
Neuralgia (transient)	0	1 (0.3)	0	2 (0.8)	3 (1.1)	4 (0.6)
Bleeding	0	0	3 (0.9)	0	0	4 (0.6)
Wound infection	0	1 (0.3)	0	2 (0.8)	0	1 (0.2)
Testicular swelling /pain	0	2 (0.6)	0	0	2 (0.7)	19 (3.0)
Postoperative pain	0	0	0	14 (5.5)	12 (4.3)	0
Hydrocele	2 (0.5)	0	0	0	4 (1.4)	0
Enterotomy	0	0	2 (0.6)	0	0	0
Cystotomy	0	1 (0.3)	2 (0.6)	1 (0.4)	1 (0.4)	0

[a]Personal review of hernia patient database by the authors.
[b]Personal review of Dr. B. McKernan's hernia patient database by the authors.
Number in parentheses is percentage.

lated the same to occur at 7 days. It should be noted, however, that no cost savings were realized in the retired population, and neither author recommended laparoscopic herniorrhaphy for this group of patients.

Liem et al. (31) performed an elaborate prospective randomized cost-effectiveness analysis of 273 patients using the number of averted recurrences and quality of life as the main outcome measures. The authors analyzed every imaginable direct and indirect, cost including costs for time off work, cost of follow-up visits, cost of medications, and the cost of treating a recurrence. The quality of life for the laparoscopic group was significantly better at both 1 and 6 weeks after surgery. Recurrence after laparoscopic repair was 2.6% lower than after conventional repair. This then implies that one recurrence is averted for every 38 patients undergoing laparoscopic repair instead of conventional repair, resulting in a cost-effectiveness ratio of Dfl 9557.58 per averted recurrence, seen from a societal point of view. In summary, the authors found laparoscopic hernia repair to be more expensive than conventional repair from a hospital perspective, but from a societal point of view 75% of these extra costs were offset, leaving the laparoscopic repair only Dfl 251.50 more expensive. They felt that the better quality of life in the postoperative period and the possibility of replacing parts of the disposable kit with reusable instruments may result in the laparoscopic repair becoming dominantly better, that is, less expensive and more effective from a societal standpoint.

In the United States, the ability to realize these cost savings will largely depend on patient, physician, and employer education about laparoscopic herniorrhaphy. However, it has been suggested (50) that time off work is frequently more dependent on the type of insurance plan a patient has and how much time off is approved by his or her employer than by how much physical disability the patient is experi-

encing. With better education of both patient and employer, ideally this disparity will narrow.

CONCLUSION

Prospective randomized trials have proven that laparoscopic herniorrhaphy can be performed with a low incidence of recurrence and complications. Postoperative pain and disability is less than after anterior repairs, but these small differences come at a price—increased direct costs, longer operating times (for a unilateral hernia), and increased demands on the laparoscopic skill of the surgeon. Of the two most frequently used techniques, the TEPP technique has the advantage of not violating the peritoneal cavity and a lower recurrence rate but the disadvantage that it is more difficult to learn.

With graduating surgical residents knowledgeable about the various laparoscopic techniques and existing laparoscopic skills in the surgical community increasing, many primary care physicians and surgeons are faced with the question of when to recommend laparoscopic herniorrhaphy to their patients. Accepting the caveat that a surgeon's best hernia repair is the one with which they have the greatest experience and thus lowest recurrence and complication rates, when should that surgeon refer a patient to a different surgeon who has the skill and experience to perform a laparoscopic repair? Certainly, the patient with multiple recurrent hernias, in whom a preperitoneal repair is appropriate, is best served with a laparoscopic repair. On the other end of the spectrum, a young patient with a small indirect hernia should not be referred for a laparoscopic repair. Many times, laparoscopic herniorrhaphy is too much surgery for a patient with a unilateral hernia. In such a case, repair is best performed under local anesthesia. Also, young patients in whom it is advantageous to avoid mesh should not undergo laparoscopic herniorrhaphy. A giant scrotal hernia, an incarcerated hernia, or the presence of cardiopulmonary disease is a contraindication to the laparoscopic technique, whereas the healthy, working patient with bilateral hernias or unilateral hernia with a suspected contralateral hernia can be repaired by either technique but will have less pain and disability with laparoscopy.

REFERENCES

1. Aitola P, Airo I, Matikainen M. Laparoscopic versus open preperitoneal inguinal hernia repair: A prospective randomised trial. *Ann Chir Gynaecol* 1998;87:22.
2. Arregui ME. Laparoscopic preperitoneal herniorrhaphy. Paper presented at: Annual Meeting of the Society of American Endoscopic Surgeons; April 18–20, 1991; Monterey, CA.
3. Barkun JS, Wexler MJ, Hinchley EJ, et al. Laparoscopic versus open inguinal herniorrhaphy: preliminary results of a randomized controlled trial. *Surgery* 1995;118:703.
4. Bessell JR, Baxter P, Riddell P, et al. A randomized controlled trial of laparoscopic extraperitoneal hernia repair as a day surgical procedure. *Surg Endosc* 1996;10:495.
5. Bogojavlensky S. Laparoscopic treatment of inguinal and femoral hernias. Video presented at: 18th Annual Meeting of the American Association of Gynecological Laparoscopists; 1989; Washington, DC.
6. Champault G, Benoit J, Lauroy J, et al. Hernies de l'aine de l'adulte. Chirurgie laparoscopique vs opération de Shouldice. Étude randomisée contrôlée: 181 patients. Résultats préliminaires. *Ann Chir* 1994;48:1003.
7. Champault GG, Rizk N, Catheline JM, et al. Totally preperitoneal laparoscopic approach versus Stoppa operation: randomized trial of 100 cases. *Surg Laparosc Endosc* 1997;7:445.
8. Cheatle GL. An operation for the radical cure of inguinal and femoral hernia. *Br Med J* 1920;2:68.
9. Cocks JR. Laparoscopic inguinal hernioplasty: a comparison between transperitoneal and extraperitoneal techniques. *Aust N Z J Surg* 1998;68:506.
10. Crawford DL, Hiatt JR, Phillips EH. Laparoscopy identifies unexpected groin hernias. *Am Surg* 1998;64:976.
11. Dellemagne B, Markiewicz S, Iehaes C, et al. Extraperitoneal laparoscopic inguinal hernia repair: technique and results. *Surg Endosc* 1996;10:228.
12. Dirksen CD, Beets GL, Go PMNYH, et al. Bassini repair compared with laparoscopic repair for primary inguinal hernia: a randomised controlled trial. *Eur J Surg* 1998;164:439.
13. Felix EL, Harbertson N, Vartanian S. Laparoscopic hernioplasty. *Surg Endosc* 1999;13:328.
14. Felix EL, Michas CA. Laparoscopic hernioplasty: totally extra-peritoneal or transabdominal preperitoneal? *Surg Endosc* 1995;9:984.
15. Fielding GA. Laparoscopic hernia repair—600 cases with a median 30 month follow-up. *Surg Endosc* 1996;10:231.
16. Filipi CJ, Gaston-Johnson F, McBride PJ, et al. An assessment of pain and return to normal activity. Laparoscopic herniorrhaphy vs open tension-free repair. *Surg Endosc* 1996;10:983.
17. Fitzgibbons RJ. Laparoscopic inguinal herniorrhaphy. Postgraduate course: Society of American Gastrointestinal and Endoscopic Surgeons, April 1992; Washington, DC.
18. Franklin M. Laboratory rationale for intraperitoneal placement of mesh in inguinal repair. Paper presented at: Hernia 93: advances or controversies; 1993; Indianapolis, IN.
18a. Ger R. The management of certain abdominal herniae by intra-abdominal closure of the neck of the sac. *Ann R Coll Surg Eng* 1982;64:342.
19. Ger R, Monroe K, Duvivier R, et al. Management of indirect inguinal hernias by laparoscopic closure of the neck of the sac. *Am J Surg* 1990;159:370.
20. Hauters P, Meunier D, Urgayan S, et al. Prospective controlled study comparing laparoscopy and the Shouldice technique in the treatment of unilateral inguinal hernia. *Ann Chir* 1996;50:776.
21. Heikkinen T, Haukipuro K, Leppälä J, et al. Total costs of laparoscopic and Lichtenstein inguinal hernia repairs: a randomized prospective study. *Surg Laparosc Endosc* 1997;7:1.
22. Heikkinen TJ, Haukipuro K, Hulkko A. A cost and outcome comparison between laparoscopic and Lichtenstein hernia operations in a day-case unit. *Surg Endosc* 1998;12:1199.
22a. Heithold D, Ramshaw B, Mason E, et al. 500 total extraperitoneal approach laparoscopic herniorrhaphies: a single-institution review. *Am Surg* 1997;63:299.
23. Juul P, Christensen K. Randomized clinical trial of laparoscopic versus open inguinal hernia repair. *Br J Surg* 1999;86:316.
24. Kald A, Anderberg B, Carlsson P, et al. Surgical outcome and cost-minimization-analyses of laparoscopic and open hernia repair: a randomized prospective trial with one year follow up. *Eur J Surg* 1997;163:505.
25. Kald A, Anderberg B, Smedh K, et al. Transperitoneal or totally extraperitoneal approach in laparoscopic hernia repair: results of 491 consecutive herniorrhaphies. *Surg Laparosc Endosc* 1997;7:86.
26. Khoury N. A randomized prospective controlled trial of laparoscopic extraperitoneal hernia repair and mesh-plug hernioplasty: a study of 315 cases. *J Laparoendosc Adv Surg Tech* 1998;8:367.
27. Korman JE, Hiatt JR, Feldmar D, et al. Mesh configurations in laparoscopic extraperitoneal herniorrhaphy: a comparison of techniques. *Surg Endosc* 1997;11:1102.
28. Kozol R, Lange PM, Kosir M, et al. A prospective, randomized study of open vs laparoscopic inguinal hernia repair: an assessment of postoperative pain. *Arch Surg* 1997;132:292.
29. Lawrence K, McWhinnie D, Goodwin A, et al. Randomised controlled trial of laparoscopic versus open repair of inguinal hernia: early results. *BMJ* 1995;311:981.
30. Leibl B, Däubler P, Schwarz J, et al. Standardisierte laparoskopische Hernioplastik vs. Shouldice-Reparation. *Chirurg* 1995;66:895.
31. Liem MSL, Halsema JAM, Van Der Graf Y, et al. Cost-effectiveness of extraperitoneal laparoscopic inguinal hernia repair: a randomized comparison with conventional herniorrhaphy. *Ann Surg* 1997;226:668.
32. Liem MSL, Van Der Graaf Y, Van Steensel CJ, et al. Comparison of conventional anterior surgery and laparoscopic surgery for inguinal hernia repair. *N Engl J Med* 1997;336:1541.
33. Liem MSL, Van Der Graaf Y, Zwart RC, et al. A randomized comparison of physical performance following laparoscopic and open inguinal hernia repair. *Br J Surg* 1997;84:64.
34. Maddern GJ, Rudkin G, Bessell JR, et al. A comparison of laparoscopic and open hernia repair as a day surgical procedure. *Surg Endosc* 1994;8:1404.
34a. Massad A, Fiorillo M, Hallak A, et al. Endoscopic extraperitoneal herniorrhaphy in 316 patients. *J Laparoendosc Surg* 1996;6:13.
35. McKernan JB, Laws HL. Laparoscopic repair of inguinal hernias using a totally extraperitoneal prosthetic approach. *Surg Endosc* 1993;7:26.
36. Nyhus LM, Stevenson JK, Listerud MB, et al. Preperitoneal

herniorrhaphy: a preliminary report in 50 patients. *West J Surg Obstet Gynecol* 1959;67:48.

37. Paganini AM, Lezoche E, Carle F, et al. A randomized, controlled, clinical study of laparoscopic versus open tension-free inguinal hernia repair. *Surg Endosc* 1998;12:979.

38. Payne JH Jr, Grininger LM, Izawa MT, et al. Laparoscopic or open inguinal herniorrhaphy? A randomized prospective trial. *Arch Surg* 1994;129:979.

39. Phillips EH, Carroll BJ, Fallas MJ. Laparoscopic preperitoneal inguinal hernia repair without peritoneal incision. *Surg Endosc* 1993;7:159.

40. Popp LW. Endoscopic patch repair of inguinal hernia in a female patient. *Surg Endosc* 1990;4:10.

41. Ramshaw BJ, Tucker JG, Duncan TD, et al. Laparoscopic herniorrhaphy: a review of 900 cases. *Surg Endosc* 1996;10:255.

42. Schrenk P, Woisetschläger R, Rieger R, et al. Prospective randomized trial comparing postoperative pain and return to physical activity after transabdominal preperitoneal, total preperitoneal or Shouldice technique for inguinal hernia repair. *Br J Surg* 1996;83:1563.

43. Schultz LS. Laser laparoscopic herniorrhaphy. *J Laparoendosc Surg* 1990;1:41.

44. Stoker DL, Spiegelhalter DJ, Singh R, et al. Laparoscopic versus open inguinal hernia repair: randomised prospective trial. *Lancet* 1994;343:1243.

45. Stoppa RE. The preperitoneal approach and prosthetic repair of groin hernias. In: Nyhus LM, Condon RE, eds. *Hernia,* 4th ed. Philadelphia: JB Lippincott Co, 1995:118.

46. Tanphiphat C, Tanprayoon T, Sansubhan C, et al. Laparoscopic versus open inguinal hernia repair: a randomized, controlled trial. *Surg Endosc* 1998;12:846.

47. Tschudi J, Wagner M, Klaiber C, et al. Controlled multicenter trial of laparoscopic transabdominal preperitoneal hernioplasty vs Shouldice herniorrhaphy. Early results. *Surg Endosc* 1996;10:845.

48. Vogt DM, Curet MJ, Pitcher DE, et al. Preliminary results of a prospective randomized trial of laparoscopic onlay versus conventional inguinal herniorrhaphy. *Am J Surg* 1995;169:84.

49. Wellwood J, Sculpher MJ, Stoker D, et al. Randomized controlled trial of laparoscopic versus open mesh repair for inguinal hernia: outcome and cost. *BMJ* 1998;317:103.

50. Wexner SD. Laparoscopic hernia repair: a plea for statistics. *Surg Endosc* 1993;7:150.

51. Wright DM, Kennedy A, Baxter JN, et al. Early outcome after open versus extraperitoneal endoscopic tension-free hernioplasty: a randomized clinical trial. *Surgery* 1996;119:552.

52. Zieren J, Zieren HU, Jacobi CA, et al. Prospective randomized study comparing laparoscopic and open tension-free inguinal hernia repair with Shouldice's operation. *Am J Surg* 1998; 175:330.

23

THE TRANSABDOMINAL PREPERITONEAL LAPAROSCOPIC HERNIORRHAPHY

ROBERT J. FITZGIBBONS, JR.
CHARLES J. FILIPI

The preperitoneal space is ideally suited for the repair of an inguinal hernia. It can be widely dissected so that the entire myopectineal orifice of Fruchaud, including the direct, indirect, and femoral hernia spaces, can be exposed. This results in the ability to perform a variety of herniorrhaphies ranging from simple tissue approximation to prosthetic repairs that use such a large implant that fixation is not necessary. The most important argument for using the preperitoneal space is that mechanical advantage is gained by performing the repair on the abdominal side of the defect in the inguinal floor, lessening the deleterious influence of abdominal pressure. This is especially true for the prosthetic preperitoneal repairs because intraabdominal pressure is exerted equally against the entire prosthesis, helping to fix the material at the normal tissue interfaces with the implant after wide overlap of the defect. A variety of conventional (open) completely extraperitoneal preperitoneal herniorrhaphies have been described. The most notable are the operations popularized by Nyhus (22), Malangoni (17), Stoppa et al. (25), and, more recently, Kugel (15) and Ugahary et al. (26), which are discussed in Chapters 18 and 21.

Soon after the introduction of laparoscopic cholecystectomy, because of its unprecedented rapid acceptance, surgeons began to envision ways to adapt many commonly performed general surgical procedures for use with laparoscopic methods. Inguinal herniorrhaphy was no exception. An intraabdominal herniorrhaphy, as is implied by the use of the term "laparoscopy," is not a new concept. Surgeons have been repairing inguinal hernias found incidentally during laparotomy for other conditions for years (1). Marcy (18) and LaRoque (16) advocated the intraabdominal

approach as a primary method for herniorrhaphy. However, most surgeons think that the morbidity associated with a laparotomy is far too great for repair of a primary inguinal hernia. Laparoscopy changed this because, despite the fact that the procedure is intraabdominal, little perioperative discomfort is the rule due to the minimally invasive nature of this type of surgery. The preperitoneal space is the logical target for the laparoscopic surgeon because it can be entered so neatly using laparoscopic instrumentation.

Two laparoscopic preperitoneal herniorrhaphies have emerged as the most popular. They are called the transabdominal preperitoneal (TAPP) and the totally extraperitoneal (TEP) laparoscopic inguinal herniorrhaphies. Both are modeled after the conventional preperitoneal operations described elsewhere in this book. They begin with a radical dissection of the preperitoneal space, followed by the placement of a large prosthesis widely overlapping the entire inguinal floor. The purpose of this chapter is to describe the TAPP procedure. Pertinent anatomy, patient selection, operating room set up, operative technique, and complications will be presented. The chapter concludes with a brief discussion of the advantages and disadvantages compared to the TEP procedure and conventional herniorrhaphy. The TEP procedure is outlined in detail in Chapter 22.

PERTINENT ANATOMY

A successful laparoscopic inguinal herniorrhaphy (LIHR) is not possible without a thorough understanding of the groin anatomy as seen laparoscopically. In fact, many of the early complications seen with laparoscopic herniorrhaphy were a direct result of a lack of appreciation of the locations of the lateral cutaneous nerve of the thigh and the genitofemoral nerve (Fig. 23.1). The important anatomic features will be discussed in reverse manner to how one usually learns the

R. J. Fitzgibbons, Jr. and C. J. Filip: Department of Surgery, Creighton University School of Medicine, Omaha, Nebraska.

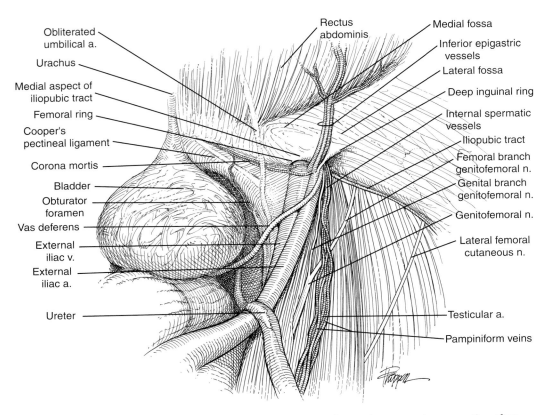

FIGURE 23.1. Anatomy of the preperitoneal space as seen from a laparoscopic perspective after the peritoneum has been removed.

anatomy of the groin, because this is the vantage point of the laparoscopic surgeon.

The deep surface of the abdominal wall above the iliopubic tract is covered by peritoneum that forms five folds (Fig. 23.2). The median umbilical ligament, which is the obliterated remnant of the urachus, lies in the midline extending from the bladder fundus to the umbilicus. The medial umbilical ligament consists of a fold of peritoneum that covers the obliterated umbilical artery. The lateral umbilical ligament makes up a fold of peritoneum around the inferior epigastric vessels. On each side of the midline, the medial and lateral umbilical ligaments delineate two laparoscopically significant fossae. The medial fossa is the space between the lateral and medial umbilical ligament and is the site of development of direct inguinal hernias. The lateral fossa lies lateral to the inferior epigastric vessels (lateral umbilical fold) and is the site where indirect hernias pass through the internal inguinal ring.

Once the peritoneum has been stripped away, one can appreciate the critical anatomic structures that should be identified in any laparoscopic herniorrhaphy. These include the inferior epigastric vessels, Cooper's pectineal ligament, and the rectus sheath that represents the original anatomic borders of the weak area where direct inguinal hernias occur, Hesselbach's triangle. When described from the anterior aspect, the inguinal ligament is usually called the base

of Hesselbach's triangle, but this structure is not readily appreciated from the laparoscopic vantage point. Therefore, we prefer the original description.

The key to preperitoneal space for the laparoscopic surgeon is the inferior epigastric vessels because this landmark is so useful in reorientation should confusion arise. The inferior epigastric vessels arise from the external iliac vessels just before they pass under the inguinal ligament to become the femoral vessels. The inferior epigastric vessels run superomedially along the medial margin of the internal ring toward the rectus sheath and give rise to two branches in the inguinal region, the external spermatic (cremasteric) artery and the pubic branch, which anastomose with the obturator artery, forming what is known as the "corona mortis." The corona mortis or death's crown is important because of the significant bleeding that can occur if it is damaged when stapling or suturing around Cooper's ligament.

The iliopubic tract is another important landmark for the surgeon intent on performing a laparoscopic herniorrhaphy because most surgeons feel that if staples are not placed below it, neuralgia can be prevented (23). Although this concept has recently been challenged, we continue to feel it is a useful guide (11). The iliopubic tract is the thickened band of transversalis fascia formed at the zone of transition between the deep surfaces of the iliac and transversus abdominis muscles. Its course is parallel to the more super-

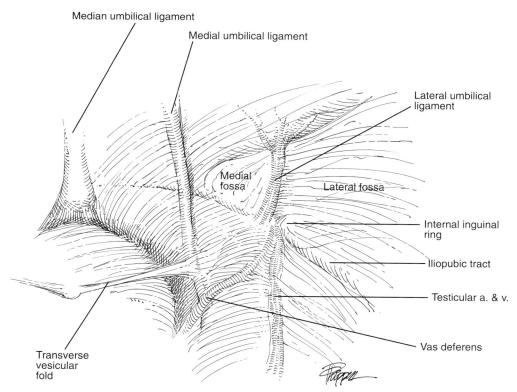

FIGURE 23.2. The appearance of the inguinal floor from a laparoscopic perspective before the peritoneum has been opened. Five peritoneal folds delineate the borders of the medial and lateral fossae on either side of the midline.

ficially located inguinal ligament. It is attached to the iliac crest laterally, and inserts on the pubic tubercle medially. At its insertion on the pubic tubercle, it curves backward slightly to blend with Cooper's pectineal ligament. Cooper's ligament, or the pectineal ligament, is actually a condensation of periosteum.

Important anatomic landmarks below the iliopubic tract include the internal spermatic vessels and the vas deferens, which join at the inferomedial corner of the internal ring and/or indirect inguinal hernia defect. The genitofemoral nerve, arising from lumbar plexus (L1-3 nerves) pursues a course obliquely and downward through the body of the psoas muscle. It then emerges on the anteromedial surface of this muscle covered by peritoneum. It divides into the femoral and the genital branches at a variable distance proximal to the internal inguinal ring. The femoral branch enters the femoral sheath and innervates the skin of the proximal anterior thigh. The genital branch passes through the internal inguinal ring at its lateral border and supplies sensory innervation to the scrotum and medial aspect of the thigh. The lateral cutaneous nerve of the thigh also arises from the lumbar plexus. It courses toward the groin along the iliacus muscle and enters the thigh in close proximity to the midportion of the iliopubic tract and innervates the skin of the lateral side of the thigh. The femoral nerve is deeper compared to the above-mentioned nerves, and supplies the skin and the muscles of the anterior thigh.

Patient Selection for Laparoscopic Herniorrhaphy

All adult patients fit for general anesthesia can be considered candidates for LIHR. Although there may be a role for laparoscopy in the pediatric patient, primarily as a tool for evaluation of the opposite side, this has yet to become accepted. It is not clear that there are sufficient advantages for patients with uncomplicated inguinal hernias to outweigh the major disadvantages of the procedure, which include (a) a laparoscopic accident, (b) bowel obstruction secondary to adhesions or an internal or ventral hernia, and (c) the increased cost. Currently, we do not recommend laparoscopy for every hernia, i.e., unilateral and nonrecurrent. However, certain types, such as those that are recurrent, bilateral, or otherwise complicated, are particularly suited to the laparoscopic approach.

Absolute contraindications include any signs of intraabdominal infection and peritonitis. Relative contraindications include intraabdominal adhesions from previous surgery, ascites, obesity, coagulopathy, and previous "Retzius' space" surgery due to the increased risk of bladder injury. Severe underlying medical illness is also a relative contraindication because of the added risk of general anesthesia. These patients are better suited to a conventional operation under local anesthesia. An incarcerated sliding scrotal hernia is a relative contraindication, especially when it involves the sigmoid colon due to the high risk of perforation during the dissection.

OPERATING ROOM SET-UP

Figure 23.3 depicts the operating room set-up most commonly employed for the TAPP procedure. The surgeon usually stands on the opposite side of the table from the hernia. This position provides an appropriate angle for dissection and staple placement. After induction of general anesthesia,

a Foley catheter is placed to ensure continuous decompression of the bladder. This can be omitted if the patient voids immediately before being transferred to the operating room. The cannula placement is depicted in Fig. 23.3. The initial cannula is placed at the umbilicus. It can be either 5 or 10 mm. After generalized exploration of the abdomen, the patient is placed in the Trendelenburg position to allow the abdominal contents to fall away from the inguinal region. Two additional 5-mm cannulas are placed lateral to the rectus sheath on either side at the level of the umbilicus.

Operative Technique

Adhesions are taken down as necessary. Both inguinal regions are inspected, and the median umbilical ligament (remnant of the urachus), medial umbilical ligament (remnant of the umbilical artery), and lateral umbilical fold (peritoneal reflection over the inferior epigastric artery) are

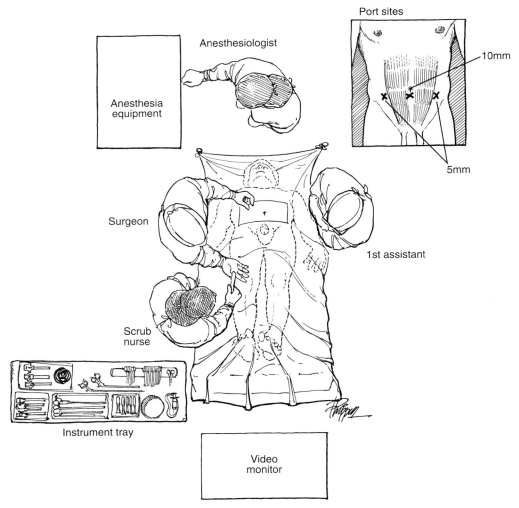

FIGURE 23.3. Operating room set-up and cannula placement for the transabdominal preperitoneal prosthetic repair.

identified (Fig. 23.2). The internal inguinal ring and cord structures are immediately evident. Commonly, the inferior epigastric vessels and the vas deferens can be seen through the intact peritoneum.

The peritoneum is incised using scissors approximately 2 cm above the superior edge of the hernia defect (Fig. 23.4A). Occasionally, the median umbilical ligament is divided if it appears to compromise exposure. The peritoneal flap incision extends from the median umbilical ligament to a point just medial to the anterosuperior iliac spine, where it is sometimes best to "hockey stick" it downward. The flap is mobilized inferiorly using blunt and sharp dissection. The inferior epigastric vessels are exposed. Next, the pubic symphysis and lower portion of the rectus abdominis muscle need to be identified. Cooper's ligament is then dissected to its junction with the femoral vein. The iliopubic tract is identified and dissection continued inferiorly with care taken to avoid injuring the femoral branch of the genitofemoral and lateral femoral cutaneous nerves, which enter the lower extremity just below the iliopubic tract. Finally, skeletonizing the cord structures from the peritoneum completes the dissection. For a direct hernia, the sac and preperitoneal fat are reduced from the hernia orifice by gentle traction, separating the peritoneal sac from the thinned out transversalis fascia, which lines the abdominal wall portion of the hernia defect. This characteristic layer is sometimes referred to as the "pseudosac" (Fig. 23.4B). It is important that this layer be teased away from the hernia sac and allowed to retract back into the defect, as needless bleeding will be the result of an attempt to resect it. Some surgeons feel that the pseudosac should be tacked or stapled to Cooper's ligament to decrease the incidence of seroma with large direct hernias. For indirect hernias, there are two options. A small sac is easily mobilized from the cord structures and reduced back into the peritoneal cavity. A large sac may be difficult to mobilize because of dense adhesions between the sac and the cord structures due to chronicity of the hernia, resulting in undue trauma to the cord if an attempt is made to remove the sac in its entirety. In this situation, the sac can be divided just distal to the internal ring, leaving the distal sac *in situ,* with dissection of the proximal sac away from the cord structures. The division of the sac is most easily accomplished by opening the sac on the side opposite the cord structures. The division of the sac can then be performed from the inside.

Upon completion of the dissection, a large piece of mesh, at least 15×7.5 cm, is placed over the myopectineal orifice so that it completely covers the direct, indirect, and femoral spaces. Either the mesh can simply be laid over the cord structures, or a slit can be made in the mesh to wrap around the cord structures. Most surgeons now avoid the slit in the prosthesis because recurrences have been noted through these slits even when they have been repaired around the cord. The use of a large prosthesis allows the intraabdominal pressure to act uniformly over a large area, thus preventing its herniation through one point, i.e., the hernial defect.

Fixation of the prosthesis represents a matter of ongoing controversy. Some experts argue that it is completely unnecessary if the prosthesis is large enough to provide extensive overlap (7). The major advantages of avoiding fixation are the elimination of the complications such as neurologic or vascular injury associated with fastening and the decreased cost because a disposable item does not need to be used. Many surgeons remain unconvinced. Prosthetic migration or roll-up as well as prolapse into a large direct defect are cited as potential problems. Regardless, all agree that the surgeon should use as few fastening devices as possible.

When a fastening system is preferred, the medial edge is stapled or tacked to the contralateral pubic tubercle and the symphysis pubis. The medial, inferior border is secured to Cooper's ligament. Next, the mesh is fastened along its superior border to the posterior rectus sheath and transversalis fascia at least 2 cm above the hernia defect. If staples are used, they are placed horizontally for the superior border of the prosthesis to correspond to the direction of the ilioinguinal and iliohypogastric nerves to decrease the incidence of neuralgia. They are placed vertically when stapling laterally as this is the direction of the lateral cutaneous nerve of the thigh and the femoral branch of the genitofemoral nerve. It is again emphasized that staples or tacks should not be placed below the iliopubic tract when lateral to the internal spermatic vessels to avoid neuralgias involving the lateral cutaneous nerve of the thigh or the femoral branch of the genitofemoral nerve. A useful maneuver is to palpate the head of the instrument through the abdominal wall with the nondominant hand. This ensures that fasteners are placed above the iliopubic tract. A point just lateral to the anterosuperior iliac spine is the preferred location for the lateral edge of the prosthesis, completing coverage of the myopectineal orifice with a wide overlap. Following the completion of the fixation, redundant mesh on the inferior border can be trimmed *in situ* to tailor it to the preperitoneal space (Fig. 23.5). The purpose of trimming the mesh is to prevent roll-up of the inferior border when closing the peritoneum.

Finally, the peritoneal flap is pulled over the mesh and stapled or sutured in order to isolate the prosthesis from intraabdominal viscera (Fig. 23.6). We do not feel that linear approximation of the peritoneum is necessary for all patients, especially if the result is tenting of the peritoneum, because of the excessive tension required to approximate the two edges. The tenting effect may leave a space between the peritoneal flap and the prosthesis. The concern is that bowel might migrate into this space, resulting in a bowel obstruction. Occasionally, it is necessary to simply cover the prosthesis with the inferior flap, leaving exposed transversalis fascia. Excessive gaps between the staples should also be avoided because (a) bowel can herniate between these gaps and/or (b) bowel can adhere to the exposed mesh. In either situation, small-bowel obstruction may result. Decreasing the pneumoperitoneum before closing the peritoneal flap is felt by some authorities to aid the closure.

(text continues on page 263)

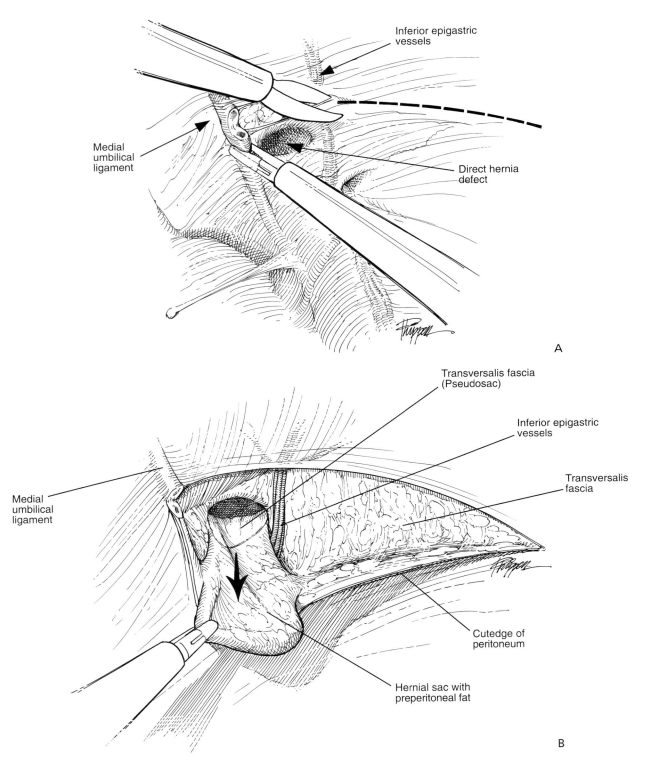

Inferior epigastric vessels

Direct hernia defect

Medial umbilical ligament

A

Transversalis fascia (Pseudosac)

Inferior epigastric vessels

Transversalis fascia

Medial umbilical ligament

Cutedge of peritoneum

Hernial sac with preperitoneal fat

B

FIGURE 23.4. A and **B:** Dissection of the preperitoneal space for repair of a right direct inguinal hernia. Note the so-called "pseudosac."

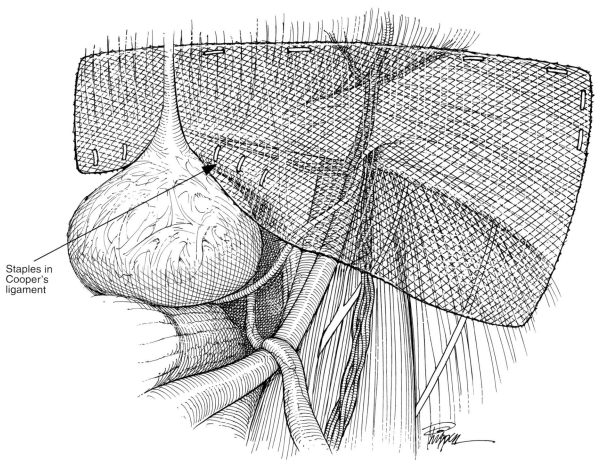

FIGURE 23.5. The appearance of the prosthesis after it has been secured in the preperitoneal space.

Staples in Cooper's ligament

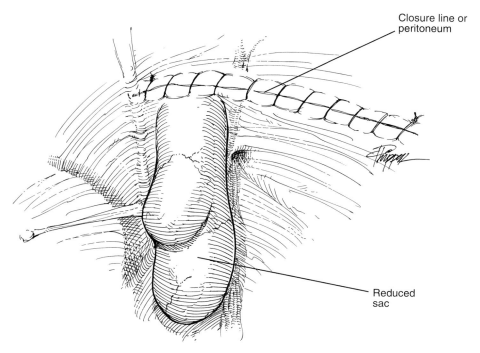

Closure line or peritoneum

Reduced sac

FIGURE 23.6. Completed transabdominal preperitoneal prosthetic repair after peritoneal closure.

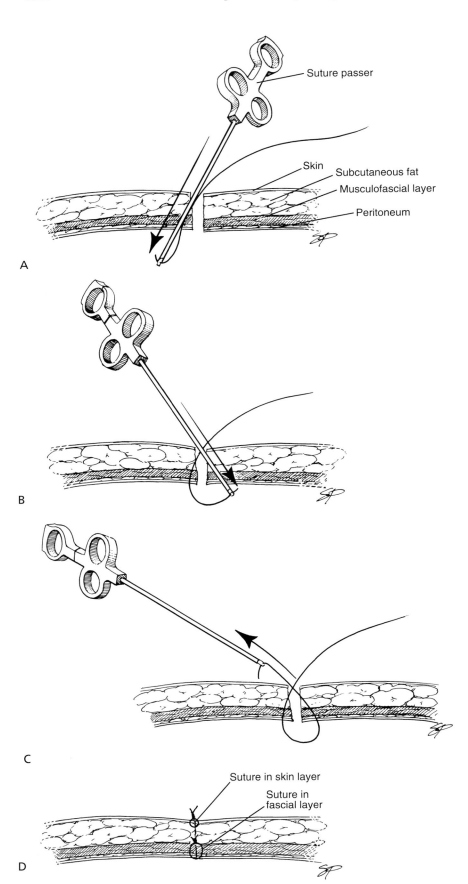

Suture passer

Skin
Subcutaneous fat
Musculofascial layer
Peritoneum

A

B

C

Suture in skin layer
Suture in fascial layer

D

FIGURE 23.7. A simple device for closing the fascial layer of trocar sites greater than 5 mm. Not shown is a cone shaped device that is placed through the defect to prevent gas loss while placing the suture. The suture passer is introduced through strategically placed holes 180 degrees apart from each other. To prevent injury to an intraabdominal organ, the procedure is performed under direct vision with the laparoscope in another cannula. **A:** The sharp-pointed grasping tips of the suture passer with a suture held are pushed through the full thickness of the abdominal wall except the skin on one side of the trocar site defect. **B:** The suture is released and the suture passer is passed through the abdominal wall on the opposite side of the trocar defect. The previously placed suture is regrasped. This step is facilitated with a grasping instrument brought from an accessory cannula to actually place the suture in the jaws of the suture passer. **C:** The suture is pulled out of the abdomen. **D:** The suture is tied, closing the fascia in a full-thickness manner. The skin is closed over the fascia suture. (Adapted from Fig. 52.30 in Greenfield, with permission.)

(text continued from page 259)

A long-acting local anesthetic is injected into the preperitoneal space before completing the closure of the peritoneum prior to deflating the abdomen to reduce postoperative discomfort. Similarly, local anesthetic is used in all trocar sites. Cannula sites greater than 5 mm should be closed at the fascial level. Otherwise, an excessive rate of trocar site herniation will be observed. Direct suture is difficult, especially in obese patients, but there are a variety of reusable or disposable devices available to facilitate fascial closure (Fig. 23.7). Finally, the pneumoperitoneum is released and the skin of all trocar sites closed with absorbable, intracuticular sutures.

Bilateral hernias can be repaired using one long transverse peritoneal incision extending from one anterosuperior iliac spine to another on the opposite side. We prefer to use the same peritoneal incision and preperitoneal dissection used for a unilateral hernia on either side, preserving the peritoneum between the medial umbilical ligaments. The symphysis pubis is completely dissected so that both preperitoneal dissections communicate with each other. This allows the placement of one large prosthesis (usually 30×8 cm or larger) essentially covering the entire lower pelvis, similar to Dr. Stoppa's procedure performed conventionally. By not incising the peritoneum between the two medial umbilical ligaments, one avoids the theoretic complication of dividing a patent urachus. Some surgeons prefer two separate pieces of mesh to avoid placing the mesh in front of the bladder. Also, it is easier to manipulate two pieces separately and tailor them more accurately to fit the preperitoneal space on either side.

Complications

In addition to the usual complications of inguinal herniorrhaphy, the laparoscopic approach implies a set of unique complications that are related to the laparoscopy itself. Such complications are exceedingly rare but, when they do occur, can be life threatening. This fact is the basis for one of the most serious challenges to the whole concept of laparoscopic herniorrhaphy.

Vascular injuries are considered first. The most serious injuries occur to vessels that reside in the retroperitoneum (3,6). Mintz quotes a risk of injury to these vessels requiring operative intervention at 0.05% (20). The vessels most at risk are the distal aorta, the common iliac arteries and veins, and the inferior vena cava. Injuries to the renal vessels have also been reported. These vessels are fixed and may be penetrated even if the safety mechanisms of the needle or trocar are working properly. The mesenteric and omental vessels are also at risk, especially in the presence of adhesions.

Visceral injuries are uncommon, occurring in 0.05% to 0.4% of all laparoscopic procedures. A mortality rate of 5% mandates that the surgeon take every precaution to avoid them. We believe that it is this complication that most

severely retards the growth of laparoscopic herniorrhaphy because it is virtually unheard of with the conventional operation. Visceral injury should be extremely rare with laparoscopic herniorrhaphy because of an algorithm that steers the surgeon toward the conventional operation in a high-risk patient. Unfortunately, there probably is an irreducible number of these accidents associated with laparoscopy even in a patient without injury risk factors.

Bladder injury with closed peritoneal access is rare but possible. It usually is the result of failure to decompress the bladder. Less commonly, it is associated with a congenital bladder abnormality. The most common offender is the Veress needle, followed by the initial trocar. Bladder injury has not been reported with the open access technique. The bladder is at significant risk for injury if there has been previous dissection in the preperitoneal space or Retzius' space, such as for a previous laparoscopic herniorrhaphy or a prostatectomy. As noted above, these both are considered relative indications because of this risk.

Trocar site wound problems are the most common abdominal wall complications. Infection and hematoma are occasionally seen. Most abdominal wall vascular complications such as epigastric vessel injury occur with careless secondary cannula placement and can be avoided with placement under direct vision.

Bowel obstruction is almost unheard of with a conventional groin herniorrhaphy, and its association with the laparoscopic approach is another argument made by detractors against the laparoscopic procedure. Indeed, the major advantage of the TEP procedure is the theoretic avoidance of this problem. The complication was frequent in the developmental stages of the laparoscopic procedure because of the lack of appreciation of the need to close trocar sites greater than 5 mm at the fascial level, resulting in trocar site hernias (24). Inadequate peritoneal closure over the prosthesis allowed bowel to migrate into the preperitoneal space, which also resulted in intestinal obstruction on occasion. These problems were soon resolved by better technique and are now rare. The incidence of delayed bowel obstruction related to adhesions because of the intraabdominal nature of the procedure has yet to be determined but would appear to be extremely low as very few reports have appeared.

Diaphragmatic dysfunction has been reported with other laparoscopic procedures as well as herniorrhaphy (21). It manifests as phrenic nerve palsy and is usually transient but has been known to require a short period of mechanical ventilation. Stretching because of the pneumoperitoneum probably causes it. Hypercapnia is the result of inadequate compensatory ventilation, given the fact that the vast majority of laparoscopies are performed using carbon dioxide as the insufflating agent.

The general anesthetic necessary to perform a TAPP procedure introduces a group of complications that are more common than the incidence for a conventional procedure performed under local anesthesia. Urinary retention is not rare and has important socioeconomic implications because it commonly results in unscheduled admissions. Age and a history of urinary symptoms are predisposing factors. Overhydration with intravenous fluid and opiates may also contribute to this problem (14). Ileus can be seen with any laparoscopic procedure. The occurrence of this complication is unpredictable, just as its etiology is unclear and largely a matter of speculation. Nausea and vomiting occur in a fixed percentage of patients undergoing laparoscopy for any reason. Aspiration pneumonia and cardiorespiratory complications occur at about the same rate as for any other operative procedure performed under general anesthesia. Prevention by careful preoperative assessment looking for underlying medical illness is the best approach.

The recurrence rates for the laparoscopic repairs, when performed by experienced surgeons are low (see Table 23.1). These rates are nearly identical to those reported from specialty centers using a conventional method. Clearly, the operation is effective when performed properly.

Various neuralgias may develop, usually from incorporation of a nerve during the application of staples or tacks. The nerves that are usually involved are the ilioinguinal nerve, iliohypogastric, both the genital and femoral branches of the genitofemoral nerve, and the lateral cutaneous nerve of the thigh (5). The former two are especially prone to injury if a vigorous bimanual technique is used for stapling, while the latter are most likely damaged by stapling below the iliopubic tract when lateral to the internal spermatic vessels. A femoral nerve injury is extremely rare and is almost always the result of a gross technical misadventure. This is fortunate because of the motor component of this structure. Pain and/or paraesthesia in their distribution characterize patient's symptoms for the more common nerves. There is significant overlap of these nerves, and therefore it is commonly difficult to sort out exactly which nerve is damaged, a fact that makes these neuralgias particularly difficult to treat. Reassurance and con-

TABLE 23.1. NONCOMPARTATIVE TRIALS OF LAPAROSCOPIC INGUINAL HERNIORRAPHY (SERIES WITH >100 REPAIRS)

Authors	Technique	Source	Recurrent Hernias at Enrollment %	Hernias No.	Recurrence Rate %	Follow-up Mo
Arregui et al.	TAPP/EXTRA	*Surg Clin North Am* 1993;73:513–527	14	147	1.3	[a]
Corbitt	TAPP	*Surg Clin Endosc* 1993;7:550–555	12	100	0	18
Felix et al.	TAPP	*Surg Endosc* 1994;8:100–103	13	205	0	21
Felix	TAPP	*Surg Endosc* 1995;9:984–989	14	733	0.3	24
Geis et al.	TAPP	*Surgery* 1993;114:765–772	11	450	0.6	30
Hawasli	TAPP + plug and patch	*J Laparoendosc Surg* 1992;2:137–143	10	143	1.4	7
Himpens	TAPP	*Surg Endosc* 1993;7:315–318	17	100	2	[a]
Kald et al.	TAPP	*Br J Surg* 1995;82:618–620	17	200	3.5	24
Kavic	TAPP	*Surg Endosc* 1995;9:12–15	10	244	1	34
Newman et al.	TAPP	*J Laparoendosc Surg* 1993;3:121–128	14	102	[a]	1
Paget	TAPP	*Med J Aust* 1994;161:249–253	15	222	1.8	18
Panton	TAPP	*Am J Surg* 1994;167:535–537	18	106	0	12
Quilici et al.	TAPP	*Am Surg* 1993;59:824–830	5	173	0	[a]
Ramshaw et al.	TAPP	*Am Surg* 1995;61:279–283	14	290	2.1	[a]
Wheeler	TAPP Mesh + plug	*J Laparoendosc Surg* 1993;3:345–350	5	135	0	18
Ramshaw et al.	TEP	*Am Surg* 1995;61:279–283	16	118	0.5	[a]
Begin	EXTRA	*Endosc Surg Allied Technol* 1993;1:204–206	53	200	0.5	18
Ferzli et al.	EXTRA/balloon CO_2/blunt	*Surg Endosc* 1998;12:1311–1313	11	326	1.6	22
Voeller et al.	EXTRA/balloon CO_2	*Surg Rounds* 1995;18:107–112	12	365	0	15
Rubio	IPOM	*Int Surg* 1994;79:293–295	[a]	120	48	0
Fitzgibbons et al.	TAPP/EXTRA IPOM	*Ann Surg* 1995;221:3–13	14.5	867	4.5	34
Philips et al.	TAPP/EXTRA IPOM Plug and patch Simple closure	*Surg Endosc* 1995;9:16–21	1.6	3,229	1.6	22

CO_2, carbon dioxide; EXTRA, extraperitoneal; IPOM, intraperitoneal onlay mesh; TAPP, transabdominal preperitoneal repair; TEP, totally extraperitoneal.
[a]Information not available.

servative treatment with antiinflammatory medications and local nerve blocks is preferred initially, as commonly these will resolve spontaneously. The only exception might be the patient who complains of severe pain immediately, i.e., in the recovery room, after the procedure. This patient may be best treated by immediate reexploration before scar tissue develops. Otherwise, we scrupulously avoid reexploration before 1 year to allow the possibility of spontaneous resolution. When groin exploration is required, neurectomy and neuroma excision is performed. The results are often less than satisfying.

The blood supply of the testicle, if interfered with, can lead to ischemic orchitis and testicular atrophy (4). The vas deferens is occasionally transected or obstructed. Reanastomosis should be attempted immediately if this occurs (5). The dysejaculation syndrome develops following handling of the vas with forceps, producing a fibrosis of varying severity throughout the muscular wall of the vas (4). This syndrome consists of a searing, burning, painful sensation throughout the groin around the time of ejaculation. The incidence is about 0.04%.

Wound infection is a surprisingly rare complication of groin herniorrhaphy. The reason for this "protected status" of the groin is unknown and would not be predicted given the proximity to the perineum and rectum. Nevertheless, in almost all reported series of groin hernia repairs, wound infection rates are very low even when prosthesis is used. Seromas are particularly common with the use of synthetic mesh in laparoscopic hernia repairs. This is possibly related to the size of the mesh that is used. Initially, these seromas were treated very actively with repeated aspirations, but it has been found that this is not necessary and the fluid eventually resorbs spontaneously. Fluid collections in the scrotum are also common, especially when a large inguinoscrotal sac is completely mobilized. These, too, will usually resolve spontaneously. Aspiration is performed for symptomatic relief only. Hydroceles requiring formal surgical correction are occasionally the result, but the etiology is unclear. Therefore, preventive measures or a preemptive treatment strategy is impossible.

Bleeding can occur producing a wound or scrotal hematoma. This is usually the result of delayed bleeding from the cremasteric, internal spermatic, or branches of the inferior epigastric vessels (5). Although this complication can be quite disabling, conservative treatment with reassurance is the best course of action. Evacuation is rarely required. Injuries to the deep circumflex artery, the corona mortis or the external iliac vessels may result in a large retroperitoneal hematoma. Again, conservative treatment is the best course of action, but the patient must be cautioned about the development of distressing bruising, and a paralytic ileus may be the result.

Osteitis pubis seems to have disappeared as a complication following the elimination of sutures through the periosteum. The staples or tacks used to attach the mesh to Cooper's ligament may sometimes produce discomfort.

Chronic postoperative groin pain occurs in a small subset of patients undergoing groin herniorrhaphy regardless of the type of repair performed. These patients are notoriously difficult to treat but a recent report suggests that some might be improved by prosthesis removal (12).

TAPP VERSUS TEP

One of the major criticisms of the laparoscopic TAPP procedure is the need to enter the peritoneal cavity. The result is the possibility of a laparoscopic accident resulting in injury to an intraabdominal organ or intestinal obstruction secondary to adhesive complications or ventral herniation. The TEP operation was developed to address this concern. Technically, it is not a laparoscopic operation because the peritoneal cavity is never entered. However, since laparoscopic instrumentation is used, it is classified as a "laparoscopic" herniorrhaphy. Instead of entering the preperitoneal space from the abdominal cavity, as is done with the TAPP operation, dissection is confined to the space deep to the rectus muscle but above the posterior rectus sheath without intentionally entering the abdomen. Once the surgeon is below the arcuate ligament, the preperitoneal space is entered. The procedure is more demanding than the TAPP because of the limited working space. Most authorities believe that the laparoscopic surgeon should be comfortable with the TAPP herniorrhaphy before attempting a TEP. Inadvertent breaches of the peritoneum are common, especially in patients with thin peritoneum or those who have scar tissue associated with previous lower abdominal surgery. The peritoneal lacerations can be difficult to recognize because they are not in the visual field of the limited working space. The consequences of these unrecognized peritoneal holes are as yet unclear. Intestinal obstruction secondary to bowel finding its way into the preperitoneal space has now been reported. Thus, it is yet to be proven that the TEP procedure will actually substantially decrease the incidence of the complications it was designed to prevent. Further patient follow-up is needed before the question can be completely settled. The authors tend to recommend the TEP procedure for smaller, simpler hernias, while patients with large hernias and those with previous lower abdominal incisions or any other complicating situation usually undergo a TAPP herniorrhaphy.

TAPP VERSUS CONVENTIONAL HERNIORRHAPHY

The proponents of LIHR cite the following potential advantages: less postoperative discomfort/pain; reduced recovery time, allowing earlier return to full activity; easier repair of a recurrent hernia because the repair is performed in tissue that has not been previously dissected; the ability to treat bilateral hernias concurrently; the performance of a simultaneous diagnostic laparoscopy; the highest possible ligation of the hernia sac; and improved cosmesis (8,9,13). In addition, it is felt that LIHR might have a lower recurrence rate than conventional inguinal herniorrhaphy (CIHR) because of the mechanical advantage gained by placing the prosthesis in the preperitoneal space and the "tension-free" nature of the repair (2,10,19).

These potential advantages of laparoscopic herniorrhaphy must be interpreted in light of the disadvantages of a laparoscopic approach, which have already been pointed out in this chapter. These include complications related to the laparoscopy, such as bowel perforation or major vascular injury; potential adhesive complications at sites where the peritoneum has been breached or prosthetic material

has been placed; the apparent need, at least at the present time, for a general anesthetic; and increased cost because of the expensive equipment needs. On the other hand, the conventional operation can be performed under local anesthesia on an outpatient basis with minimal risk of intraabdominal injury, and the cost is less.

The question is, "Can one ever justify a laparoscopic TAPP herniorrhaphy?" Several commonly cited prospective trials comparing the laparoscopic TAPP procedure to conventional hernia repairs have been summarized in Table 23.2 (conventional tension free) and Table 23.3 (conventional nonmesh). Most demonstrate a statistically significant advantage for LIHR patients over both tension and

TABLE 23.2. TAPP VERSUS MESH CONVENTIONAL HERNIORRHAPHY COMPARATIVE TRIALS

Author (Year)	No. Analyzed	Source	Important Features (Laparoscopic/Conventional)
Payne (1994)	100 p	*Arch Surg* 1994;129:973–979	↑ return to work (9 vs. 17 d) ↑ straight-leg raising at 1 wk ↑ cost
Brooks (1994)	100 p/116 h	*Arch Surg* 1994;129:361–366	Nonrandomized ↑ time ↑ cost No difference in pain medication Earlier return to work
Wilson (1995)	242 p	*Br J Surg* 1995;82:274–277	Nonrandomized Earlier return to activity (7 vs. 14 d) Earlier return to work (10 vs. 21 d) No difference in analgesic requirements or pain scale
Filipi (1996)	53 h	*Surg Endosc* 1996;10:983–986	↓ pain score[a] ↑ HRQoL score
Johansson (1999)	613 p	*Ann Surg* 1999;230:225–231	Earlier full recovery, return to work ↓ restriction in physical activities ↑ complications ↑ cost
Sarli (1997)	108 p	*Acta Biomed Ateneo Parmense* 1997;68:5–10	Same patients as Paganini? Opposite-sided occult hernias detected Nd in pain or period of disability
Aitola (1998)	49 h	*Ann Chir Gynaecol* 1998;87:22–25	↑ complications ↑ recurrences (13% vs. 8%) ↑ cost ↓ pain Nd in period of disability
Beets (1998)	79 p/108 h	*Surg Endosc* 1999;13:323–327	TAPP vs. GPRVS ↑ time Earlier return to physical activities, work ↑ recurrence rate (12% vs. 1%) Costs same
Paganini (1998)	108 p	*Surg Endosc* 1998;12:979–986	↓ pain score ↑ cost
Wellwood (1998)	400 p	*Br Med J* 1998;317:103–110	↓ pain score for first 2 wk ↑ SF-36 scores ↑ return to normal activity ↑ patient satisfaction ↑ cost

HRQoL, health-related quality of life; Nd, no difference; GPRVS, giant prosthetic reinforcement of the visceral sac; p, patients; h, hernias; ↑, increased; ↓, decreased; SF-36, Medical Outcome Survey Short Form 36; TAPP, transabdominal preperitoneal repair.
[a]Not statistically significant.

TABLE 23.3. TAPP VERSUS NONMESH CONVENTIONAL HERNIORRHAPHY COMPARATIVE TRIALS

Author (Year)	No. Analyzed	Source	Important Features (Laparoscopic/Conventional)
Maddern (1994)	86 p	*Surg Endosc* 1994;8:1404–1408	↑ discharge time Pain scores, activity levels, analgesia requirement, and time to return to work were not significantly different
Stoker (1994)	150 p	*Lancet* 1994;343:1243–1245	Maloney darn ↓ pain score, medication use Earlier return to activities (3 vs. 7 d) Earlier return to work (14 vs. 28 d)
Millikan (1994)	126 h/106 p	*Surg Laparosc Endosc* 1994;4:247–253	Nonrandomized ↓ time off work ↓ pain medication ↓ complications Hospital days better ↑ cost
Lawrence (1995)	125 p	*Br Med J* 1995;311:981–985	Maloney darn SF-36, pain analog scores better early No difference in return to activity ↑ complication rate ↑ cost
Kald (1997)	200 p	*Eur J Surg* 1997;163:505–510	Better quality of life ↑ time Earlier return to work (10 vs. 23 d) ↓ overall cost ↑ direct cost
Kozol (1997)	62 p	*Arch Surg* 1997;132:292–295	↓ pain at 24 and 48 h using McGill Pain and Visual Analog Pain Scale score ↓ pain medication
Dirksen (1998)	170 p/217 h	*Eur J Surg* 1998;164:439–447	↑ time Maloney darn Earlier return to physical activities, work ↓ recurrence rate (6% vs. 21%) ↑ cost

↑, increased; ↓, decreased; h, hernias; p, patients; SF-36, Medical Outcome Survey Short Form 36.

tension-free CIHR in one or more of the parameters studied, i.e., decreased analgesia requirement in the immediate postoperative period, and/or earlier return to normal activity, and/or improvement in the overall quality of life as measured by validated instruments. This is the justification. Despite these findings, many surgeons continue to feel that the potential risks of a laparoscopic disaster are greater than the benefits. The question will not likely be settled until the results of additional randomized prospective trials are reported. Several such trials have been funded and are currently accruing participants. The results of these trials should provide a better understanding of the precise indications for this procedure.

REFERENCES

1. Andrews E. A method of herniotomy utilizing only white fascia. *Ann Surg* 1924;80:255.
2. Arregui ME, Navarrete J, Davis CJ, et al. Laparoscopic inguinal herniorrhaphy. Techniques and controversies. *Surg Clin North Am* 1993;73:513–527.
3. Baadsgaard SE, Bille S, Egeblad K. Major vascular injury during gynecologic laparoscopy. *Acta Obstet Gynecol Scand* 1989;68:283–285.
4. Bendavid R. Complications of groin hernia surgery. *Surg Clin North Am* 1998;78:1089–1103.
5. Condon RE, Nyhus LM. Complications of groin hernia. In: *Hernia,* 4th ed. Philadelphia: JB Lippincott Co, 1995:269–282.
6. Crist DW, Gadacz TR. Complications of laparoscopic surgery. *Surg Clin North Am* 1993;73:265–289.
7. Ferzli GS, Frezza EE, Pecoraro AM Jr, et al. Prospective randomized study of stapled versus unstapled mesh in a laparoscopic preperitoneal inguinal hernia repair. *J Am Coll Surg* 1999;188:461–465.
8. Filipi CJ, Fitzgibbons RJ Jr, Salerno GM, et al. Laparoscopic herniorrhaphy. *Surg Clin North Am* 1992;72:1109–1124.
9. Fitzgibbons RJ Jr, Salerno GM, Filipi CJ, et al. A laparoscopic intraperitoneal onlay mesh technique for the repair of an indirect inguinal hernia [comments]. *Ann Surg* 1994; 219:144–156.
10. Ger R, Mishrick A, Hurwitz J, et al. Management of groin hernias by laparoscopy. *World J Surg* 1993;17:46–50.
11. Gilroy A, Marks SC Jr, Quinfang L, et al. Anatomical characteristics of the iliopubic tract: implications for repair of inguinal hernias. *Clin Anat* 1992;5:255–263.
12. Heise CP, Starling JR. Mesh inguinodynia: a new clinical syndrome after inguinal herniorrhaphy? *J Am Coll Surg* 1998;187:514–518.
13. Johnson A. Laparoscopic surgery. *Lancet* 1997;349:631–635.

14. Kozol RA, Mason K, McGee K. Post-herniorrhaphy urinary retention: a randomized prospective study. *J Surg Res* 1992;52:111–112.

15. Kugel RD. Minimally invasive, nonlaparoscopic, preperitoneal, and sutureless, inguinal herniorrhaphy. *Am J Surg* 1999;178:298–302.

16. LaRoque GP. The intra-abdominal method of removing inguinal and femoral hernia. *Arch Surg* 1932;24:189–203.

17. Malangoni MA, Condon RE. Preperitoneal repair of acute incarcerated and strangulated hernias of the groin. *Surg Gynecol Obstet* 1986;162:65–67.

18. Marcy HO. The cure of hernia. *JAMA* 1887;8:589–592.

19. McKernan JB, Laws HL. Laparoscopic repair of inguinal hernias using a totally extraperitoneal prosthetic approach. *Surg Endosc* 1993;7:26–28.

20. Mintz M. Risks and prophylaxis in laparoscopy: a survey of 100,000 cases. *J Reprod Med* 1977;18:269–272.

21. Mouton WG, Bessell JR, Otten KT, et al. Pain after laparoscopy. *Surg Endosc* 1999;13:445–448.

22. Nyhus LM. Iliopubic tract repair of inguinal and femoral hernia. The posterior (preperitoneal) approach. *Surg Clin North Am* 1993;73:487–499.

23. Page DW, Gilroy A, Marks SC Jr. The iliopubic tract: an essential guide in teaching and performing groin hernia repairs. *Contemp Surg* 1996;49:219–222.

24. Patterson M, Walters D, Browder W. Postoperative bowel obstruction following laparoscopic surgery. *Am Surg* 1993;59:656–657.

25. Stoppa RE, Rives JL, Warlaumont CR, et al. The use of Dacron in the repair of hernias of the groin. *Surg Clin North Am* 1984;64:269–285.

26. Ugahary F, Simmermacher RKJ. Groin hernia repair via a grid-iron incision: an alternative technique for preperitoneal mesh insertion. *Hernia* 1998;2:123–125.

24

THE INTRAPERITONEAL ONLAY MESH PROCEDURE FOR GROIN HERNIAS

MORRIS E. FRANKLIN, JR.
JOSÉ A. DÍAZ-ELIZONDO

HISTORY

For the past century, following the lead of Henry O. Marcy (1837–1924) and Edoardo Bassini (1844–1924), surgeons have repaired groin hernias by positioning a musculoaponeurotic, fascial curtain over the defective posterior aspect of the inguinal canal and anchoring it to fascial or aponeurotic structures, close to the superior pubic ramus.

Acceptable results have been reported using Bassini, McVay, Shouldice, or any one of the many variations based on these techniques, provided the exact nature of the hernia is recognized and the "repair" is done without tension, using healthy tissues. Hernias occurring in men, whether direct or indirect, have a tendency to recur compared to those of women and children. This is for a variety of reasons, the most important being underestimation of tension present at the repair line.

Notwithstanding the excellent results reported by some individual series, the rate of recurrence for hernias in adult males repaired by the techniques mentioned above range from 5% to 10%, with some series worldwide in the 15% range. Repairs following a recurrence tend to break down at a much higher rate (20% to 25%) (6).

The introduction of synthetic mesh in 1900 by Geopel in Germany (silver wire prosthesis) for tension-free hernia repair started a new era in hernia surgery. The use of synthetic mesh for the repair of recurrent hernias, and then for the primary repair of hernias, has gradually gained acceptance among surgeons after the results advocated by Lichtenstein in 1989 (8).

The surgical concept that the common pathway leading to groin hernias is a defect in the fascia transversalis is widely accepted today (22). Replacing a deficient transversalis fascia with a sheet of resistant nonbiodegradable layer of synthetic mesh tailored to fit and cover the hernia defect without tension appears to be anatomically and biologically the proce-

dure of choice for repairing inguinal hernias in adults (particularly men) by a growing number of surgeons (1,3–5).

Various techniques using synthetic mesh for hernia repairs are described in the literature (8,10,18,19). The technique most frequently used consists of suturing without tension an adequate piece of mesh to the "conjoined" muscle and tendon superiorly and to the inguinal ligament inferiorly. A medially placed slit in the mesh allows for the egress of the cord, which then lies deep to the aponeurosis of the external oblique. This repair championed by Lichtenstein is attended by excellent results (18).

The history and rationale of the properitoneal repair of groin hernias has been described in detail by Millelsen (11), Musgrove (13), and Nyhus et al. (15), and Read (16). The absence in the properitoneal area of adequate fascial or aponeurotic structures that could be approximated to bridge the hernia defect led to the abandonment of this particular technique. Stoppa in Amiens, and Rives in Reims revived interest in the properitoneal area to repair the hernia defect by placing a large sheath of mesh in this area (22). This technique has gained wide acceptance in France for the treatment of many inguinal hernias. In the United States, its use had been generally limited to recurrent groin hernias (12).

Placing a prosthetic veil in the properitoneal area for repair of a recurrent hernia alleviates the need to reenter previously divided planes and dissect the cicatrized cord. This avoids the ever-present incidence of ischemic testicular and nerve injuries occurring after such dissections (9,24). The mesh placed properitoneally, if large enough, not only will cover the area of recurrence, but also will cover other potential groin herniation sites, including the femoral canal (Fig. 24.1) (23). The properitoneal placement of mesh for "first-time" and recurrent hernias has been well described in numerous publications (17,19,22).

With the development of laparoscopic surgery and continuous refinements in techniques occurring in that field, the authors tried to establish whether the principles of properitoneal placement of synthetic mesh could be used expeditiously and safely laparoscopically (5).

In the laboratory, a piece of polypropylene mesh was placed intraperitoneally over the internal right lower quadrant of 20 pigs. The mesh was secured to the peritoneum using

M. E. Franklin, Jr.: Texas Endosurgery Institute; Department of Surgery, University of Texas at San Antonio, Texas.

J. A. Díaz-Elizondo: Department of General Surgery, Instituto Tecnológico y de Estudios Superiores de Monterrey; Department of General Surgery, Hospital San José–Tec de Monterrey, Monterrey, Mexico.

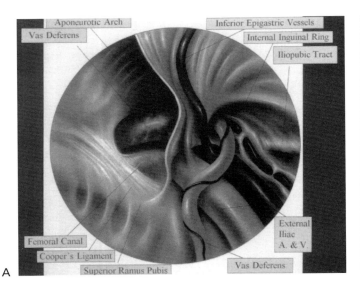

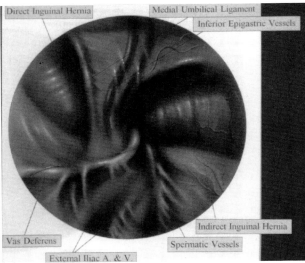

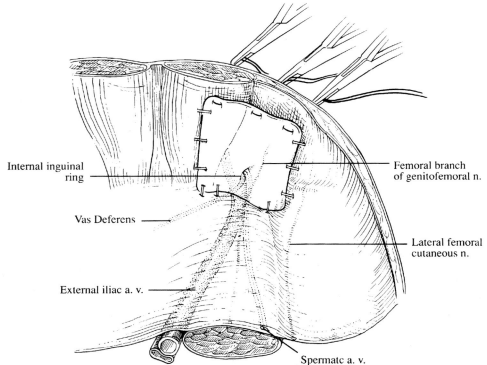

FIGURE 24.1. A: Anatomy of inguinal region. **B:** Inguinal hernia sites. **C:** Mesh placement.

stitches and metal staples. Of major interest to the authors was the fate of the mesh with the parietal peritoneal surface over which it was placed and the extent of adhesions the mesh would potentially contract with neighboring loops of bowel.

The pigs were sacrificed 1 to 2 months later, after laparoscopic examination at 1 and 2 weeks post–mesh placement. Good ingrowth of peritoneum over the mesh was noted, and few if any adhesions between loops of bowel and the mesh were found. These findings parallel those of Salerno (21) and Laymen et al. (7), who found that the use of intraperitoneal

material in swine models resulted in minimal adhesion formation. There was also no alteration of testicular growth or function and good incorporation of prosthetic material.

Interestingly, in a group of animals who had the mesh placed properitoneally with adequate peritoneal coverage of the mesh, 70% developed significant adhesions with the omentum and bowel to the peritoneal closure site. Durstein-Decker et al. (4a) noted adhesions to mesh that was placed properitoneally and the peritoneum closed, but a scarcity of adhesions to exposed mesh. The conclusion from our work, as well as others, was that in pigs, at least, intraperitoneal polypropylene mesh did not stimulate adhesion formation to a significant degree.

When we began studying a procedure for laparoscopic mesh placement in humans in early 1990, attempts at placing the large portion of mesh (12 × 15 cm) properitoneally required a large amount of dissection. The postoperative scrotal discomfort experienced by some patients undergoing this technique led us to try the much simpler intraperitoneal placement of the mesh (14). Arbitrarily, we decided not to operate on patients under 18 years of age or patients with large inguinoscrotal hernias. Later, we dropped the latter exclusion.

TECHNIQUE

With the patient under general anesthesia, a catheter is placed in the bladder and a nasogastric tube is placed in the stomach; both are removed at the end of the procedure. The surgeon places himself or herself on the contralateral side of the hernia. After inflating the peritoneal cavity using a Veress needle, a laparoscope with an attached video camera is placed through a 10/12-mm trocar at the umbilicus. A 5-mm trocar is placed approximately at McBurney's point on the opposite side of the hernia, and on the ipsilateral side, lateral to the umbilicus. For bilateral repairs, the same configuration applies.

After inspecting the peritoneal cavity, the hernia site and the contralateral inguinal area are carefully evaluated. For proper orientation, the surgeon should recognize the median, medial, and lateral umbilical ligaments. Just below the posterior parietal peritoneum, the external iliac vein and artery, the gonadal vessels, and, in men, the vas deferens should be identified. The hidden course of the genitofemoral nerve and the approximate course of the lateral femorocutaneous nerve should be recalled and mapped and care taken to avoid cross or rough dissection in this area. The exact location of the ureter bilaterally should also be noted.

We now routinely remove direct and indirect hernia sacs since in our experience leaving the sac may perpetuate a bulge in the groin, a bulge that patients and inexperienced surgeons interpret as an operative failure despite repeated assurances that no bowel can enter the sac or space. Division of the sac also gives access to the properitoneal area, where a "lipoma" of the cord, if present, can be excised. When operating for left-sided hernias, we often find it necessary to divide the embryonic adhesions that the sigmoid colon contracts with the parietal peritoneum next to the hernia defect. We excise the sac using laparoscopic scissors connected to an electrosurgical unit.

First, the sac is progressively inverted into the peritoneal cavity using gentle traction. Once the inversion is complete, the sac is incised starting 1 or 2 cm from its base at the 12-o'clock position and proceeding clockwise to about the 4-o'clock position. The incision is then restarted at the "top" and carried in a counterclockwise fashion until approxi-

mately the 8-o'clock position. The inversion of an indirect inguinal hernia sac drags within it the fatty areolar tissue in which the gonadal vessels and the vas may be embedded. This tissue must be bluntly and carefully swept away from the sac anteriorly. Once fully separated from the elements of the cord, the sac can now be safely circumferentially excised and removed through a 10/12-mm port.

Small or capillary vessel bleeding during this phase of the operation is easily controlled by pinpoint electrocoagulation. Large inguinoscrotal sacs and sacs in multiple recurrent hernias are ringed at the neck (incising the peritoneum circumferentially) and are left in place as bleeding and extensive edema may ensue if these sacs are aggressively pursued.

Once the sac is removed, a piece of polypropylene mesh is prepared. The size of the mesh should be such that it covers the hernia defect and extends 3 cm beyond its rim at a minimum. We have found that a 12 × 15-cms portion of mesh covers most defects adequately. The folded mesh is introduced into the abdominal cavity; if the mesh is folded rather than rolled, once opened it will not have a tendency to curl and will be much easier to manipulate and hold in place. Once the mesh is unfolded, it is placed over the defect and held there with grasping forceps.

The superior border of the mesh in its midportion is then tightly held against the anterior abdominal wall. A Keith needle attached to a 2-zero strand of polypropylene suture is pushed through the abdominal wall and through the mesh (Fig. 24.2) (20).

The spot where the incision is to be made and where the needle is to pierce the abdominal wall can be established by gently depressing the abdominal wall and visualizing the indentation laparoscopically. Through the same incision, a 13-gauge needle is then placed through the abdominal wall and the mesh, parallel to the Keith needle. Once the Keith needle is passed through the abdomen and mesh, it is grasped, turned around, and pushed back through the lumen of the 13-gauge needle exiting through the small skin incision. A clamp is applied to the polypropylene suture at skin level, holding the mesh tightly against the abdominal wall. The same procedure is repeated at both upper corners of the mesh.

Once placed, these three sutures hold the mesh securely in place, spreading it evenly and allowing for the rest of the mesh to be precisely and easily stapled in place. The staples are placed first on vertical sides of the mesh approximately 1 to 1.5 cm apart, then along its lower edge. Care should be taken to place the staples vertically along the inferior edge of the mesh to minimize the chances of entrapping the femoral branch of the genitofemoral nerve or the laterofemoral cutaneous nerve. Along the lower margin of the mesh, staples should be placed lightly and further apart (2 cm) to avoid damage to the iliac vessels and the vas deferens. A few staples are also used to fix the superior and central portion of the mesh to the anterior abdominal wall. Medially, every effort should be made to secure the mesh to Cooper's ligament. The anteriorly placed inferior epigastric vessels immediately

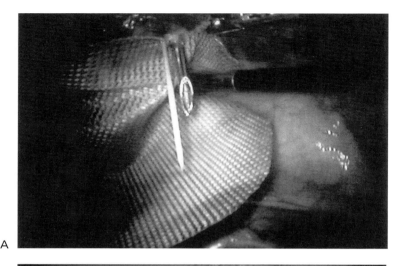

A

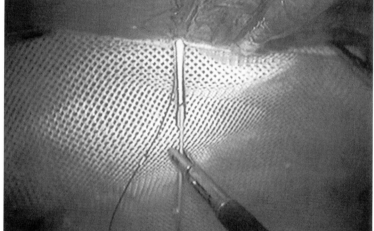

B

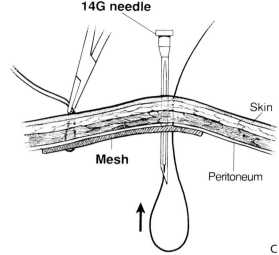

C

FIGURE 24.2. A: Keith needle passing through mesh and abdominal wall adjacent to 13-gauge spinal needle. **B:** Keith needle (with suture) exiting through 13-gauge needle. **C:** Diagrammatic representation.

beneath the peritoneum should be avoided in the stapling process. Staples should not be used near the inferior and inferolateral aspect of the internal ring for fear of injuring the structures passing through it (Fig. 24.3).

The area is irrigated with saline solution and inspected for hemostasis. The subcutaneous fat below the skin incisions through which the polypropylene strands were placed is spread with a fine tip hemostat, allowing the sutures to be tied over the external oblique aponeurosis. Firm anchoring of the mesh by transabdominal stitches and staples in Cooper's ligament prevents, in our opinion, displacement of the mesh when the abdomen is deflated and when the patient assumes the erect position (Fig. 24.3). We firmly believe that it is early migration of the mesh away from its intended position that causes recurrences; therefore, we do not rely solely on staples, grasping only mesh and peritoneum, to hold the mesh in place.

To repair a contralateral hernia, the same procedure is carried out on the opposite side. We do not combine this type of surgery with operations on the bowel or the biliary tree.

As the trocars are sequentially removed, the video camera examines the trocar sites to ensure that no bleeding is present.

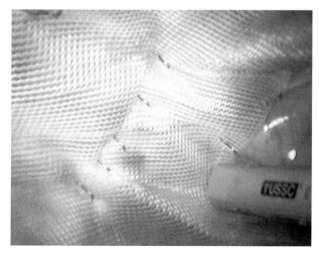

FIGURE 24.3. Staples should not be used near the inferior and inferolateral aspect of the internal ring for fear of injuring the structures passing through it. Mesh being stapled to Cooper's ligament.

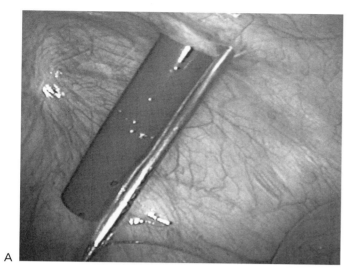

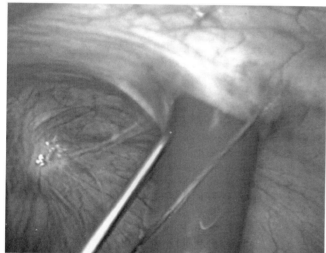

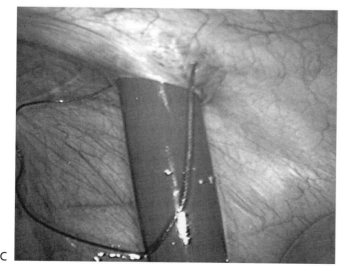

FIGURE 24.4. All ports 10 mm or larger are closed to prevent hernias at trocar sites.

Finally, the umbilical insertion site is observed by slowly withdrawing together the camera and its cannula. To prevent potential herniation, all 10-mm trocar sites are closed by repairing the underlying fascia or aponeurosis with zero Vicryl (Ethicon, Inc., Somerville, NJ, U.S.A.) or Polysorb (U.S. Surgical, Norwalk, CT, U.S.A.) sutures (Fig. 24.4). The skin edges are approximated using adhesive tape. The patients are generally discharged the evening of surgery or the following morning.

PATIENTS AND METHODS

Our experience with laparoscopic mesh hernioplasty consists of 520 hernia repairs performed on 413 patients from January 1990 through October 1998 (Table 24.1).

Our follow-up extends for up to 84 months with a median of 68 months. There were 81 women and 332 men.

The female group had, for the most part, unilateral hernias, as well as 12 femoral hernias; one of the femoral hernias was recurrent and four were incarcerated. Seven women had bilateral hernias.

In the male group, there were 394 hernias not previously repaired. Twenty-five patients had recurrent hernias and 107 had bilateral hernias, of which 10 were bilaterally recurrent.

Excluded from the study were patients under 18 years of age and, for the first 12 months, large or incarcerated

TABLE 24.1. LAPAROSCOPIC INTRAPERITONEAL ONLAY MESH HERNIA REPAIR (JANUARY 1990 TO JUNE 1999)

Total repairs	520
Total No. patients	413
Male	332
Female	81
Weight (94–340 lb)	
Avg. ≥ 180.31 lb (81.96 kg)	

Type hernia	Patients	No.
Unilateral	306	306
Recurrent	(25)	
Bilateral	107	214
Recurrent	(10)	
Total	413	520

Site	Type	No. of Patients	No. of Repairs
Right		169	(32.5%)
	Direct		23
	Indirect		134
	Pantaloon		4
	Femoral		8
Left		137	(26.35%)
	Direct		15
	Indirect		118
	Pantaloon		0
	Femoral		4
Bilateral		107	(20.5%)

inguinal scrotal hernias that had been treated with standard open McVay repairs. Two patients refused laparoscopic repair and were offered McVay-type repairs.

Hospitalization at our institution for most advanced laparoscopic procedures (i.e., those that are more extensive than tubal ligation or diagnostic laparoscopy) is a minimum of overnight, and 388 of 413 (94.0%) of our patients were discharged less than 23 hours after surgery. Most of these patients were kept overnight at the surgeon's request and could have been discharged sooner. Twenty-five (6.0%) patients required longer hospitalization for reasons shown in Table 24.2.

We have had, to date, five (0.96%) recurrences after a unilateral laparoscopic mesh hernioplasty. One was performed on a nonpreviously operated hernia, and at reoperation the obvious technical mistake that caused the recurrence was the use of an inadequate-sized patch applied only partially over the hernia defect.

The second case was that of a 67-year-old man with three recurrent right inguinal hernias prior to a laparoscopic repair (Bassini, McVay, Lichtenstein). A large direct hernia was repaired with a 14 × 18-cm portion of mesh without difficulty. Six weeks postoperatively, the patient had a recurrence at the same site, and upon laparoscopic/open repair the entire abdominal wall had given way. The entire right side of the abdominal wall was reinforced with a gigantic mesh extending from just below the rib margin to 6 cm to the left of the midline and well onto the pelvic and posterior abdominal wall. He has had no recurrences since the massive abdominal wall reinforcement; however, he has developed a hernia in a previously well-healed trocar site on the left side. It is felt by several observers that this patient has a mesothelial tissue problem, resulting in congenital weakness of the entire abdominal wall. He has had no recurrence on the right side at his 12-month postoperative follow-up visit.

It is noteworthy that surgeons reporting their experiences with the properitoneal placement of mesh claim that their recurrences occur early in the postoperative period, generally within the first 3 months of surgery. Few, if any, occur later (6,24).

This recurrence pattern is certainly at odds with the recurrence pattern associated with standard repairs (6). It can be explained by the fact that once the mesh is well fixed in place by local tissue ingrowth the hernia defect is somewhat permanently sealed.

Tension at the suture line, tissue "fatigue," and contiguously created weaknesses are all causes of recurrence after standard hernia repair; these causes are not present when properitoneal or intraperitoneal mesh is used. Recurrences seen after using properitoneal mesh are due to either too small a piece of mesh, poor placement, or inadequate fixation of the mesh. Recurrences in these cases will universally appear shortly after surgery.

Other complications associated with this series included three large scrotal and four large abdominal wall hematomas. One of the very large abdominal wall hematomas occurred in a patient who was taking aspirin daily but failed to disclose that information prior to surgery; the patient required 2 units of blood. The other three large hematomas and eight other minor ones required no intervention.

Three neuropraxias involving the femoral branch of the genitofemoral nerve subsided, one each at 3 months, 3 weeks, and 5 days, with one patient requiring steroid injections for pain control. The pain began more than 1 year postrepair after a severe strain. Our patients in this series did not experience clinical pulmonary, cardiovascular, venous, or testicular complications, impotence, or lack of virility.

There were no conversions from laparoscopic to open methods other than the last recurrence.

RETURN TO FULL FUNCTION

Evaluation of return to work is very difficult and subjective at best. Because of a great discrepancy in activities in our patients from college and professional athletes to retired gardeners, we evaluated this aspect based on the patients' concept of their ability to return to full activity. The results are tabulated in Table 24.3.

TABLE 24.2. REASONS PATIENTS REQUIRE ADDITIONAL HOSPITALIZATION AFTER LAPAROSCOPIC MESH HERNIOPLASTY

Hospital Stay	No. (%)	
<23 h	388 (94)	
≥23 h	25 (6)	
Reason for prolonged hospital stay	**No.**	**Median**
Cardiopulmonary	8	3 d
Urinary retention	7	2 d
Bleeding abdominal wall	3	2.5 d
Ileus	7	3 d
Total	25	

TABLE 24.3. RETURN TO FULL ACTIVITY AFTER MESH HERNIOPLASTY

	Average Return	Range
Patient profile: Age <60 yr (N = 111 ≥ 27%)		
Type of activity: Lifting		
Limited (<10 lb)	2.5 d	1–6 d
Normal (10–30 lb)	3.5 d	1–15 d
Full (>30 lb)	6.8 d	1–45 d
Patient profile: Age ≥60 yr (N = 402 ≥ 73%)		
Type of activity: lifting		
Limited (<10 lb)	2.8 d	1–8 d
Normal (10–30 lb)	3.6 d	1–12 d
Full (>30 lb)	7.2 d	1–40 d

TABLE 24.4. COMPLICATIONS OF LAPAROSCOPIC MESH HERNIOPLASTY

Recurrent hernia	5/520	(0.96%)
Neuropraxia	12/520	(2.31%)
Seroma	15/520	(2.88%)
Testicular pain	3/520	(0.58%)
		(2 with properitoneal)
Infection	0	
Trocar site hernia	0	
Abdominal wall hematoma	4/520	(0.77%)
Total complication rate: 7.5%		
Neuropraxia[a]	12/520	(2.31%)
Genitofemoral	3	
Lateral femorocutaneous	9	
Pain in distribution of nerve	3	

[a]All resolved in 3 wk except two: resolved with cortisone injection and one was chronic.

FOLLOW-UP TECHNIQUES

Our follow-up extended for up to 84 months with a median of 68 months. Attempts were made to see all patients in the follow-up period and we were very successful in this endeavor. All patients were seen at 1 week, 1 month, 3 months, 6 months, 9 months, and yearly after surgery. Each patient was initially interviewed and examined by the surgeon and examined at the above intervals. The patients were questioned in person with regard to pain, hypersensitivity, bulge, resumption of activity, and satisfaction with results.

Patients not returning for appointments were called, and most subsequently were seen (80%) or at least interviewed (13%). Twenty-nine patients (7%) were lost to follow-up and could not be found after 2 years (eight of these had died of cardiac and/or pulmonary disease not related to the hernia repair, and one had died of cancer of the lung). One patient has been seen and operated upon by another surgeon; he complained of recurrent hernia and was found to have a residual sac but no defect to the abdominal cavity. The remaining 25 patients have moved out of town or could not be located by telephone or direct visit inquiry.

Some of the complications have already been described; the total of the complications are summarized in Table 24.4.

DISCUSSION AND CONCLUSION

On the basis of our present experience, we feel that the described laparoscopic approach to groin hernias in adults stands on solid anatomic and physiologic grounds. On the negative side, this operation requires a general anesthetic, costs marginally more to perform than standard repairs, has the potential problems inherent to laparoscopy, and requires experience in laparoscopic surgery. The ultimate fate of the intraperitoneal mesh (even though proven harmless to date in the laboratory and in clinical practice) has yet to be established.

The lack of a major scar, avoiding dissection of the cord structures, the practically pain-free postoperative course, and the prompt return to unrestricted work/activities more than make up for the negative aspects mentioned above.

Despite laboratory findings of minimal adhesions to or surrounding the mesh, great concern has been raised on the part of the surgeons involved regarding adhesion formation in the human after intraperitoneal placement of the polypropylene mesh. Review of the literature reveals little in the way of complications (migration, carcinomatous transformation, intestinal obstruction, or erosion of the mesh into vessels) in mesh placed without other complicating factors.

Interestingly, we have been able to reexamine laparoscopically 21 different operative sites (Fig. 24.5): before repairing an ipsilateral recurrence (three), while looking

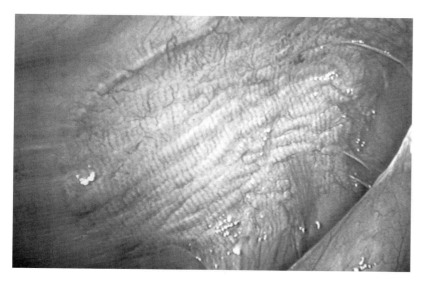

FIGURE 24.5. In all patients the mesh was completely incorporated into the peritoneum, and in three patients it was hardly visible.

TABLE 24.5. PROBLEMS OF ADHESIONS

Second-look procedures (N = 21)
- 10 Patients—clean
- 6 Patients—flimsy omental adhesions to edge of mesh
- 1 Patient—severe adhesions, nondissectable bowel and omentum (Gore-Tex)
- 4 Patients—moderately dense adhesions, all with prior surgery where adhesions were taken down to obtain exposure

for a suspected recurrence (four), during the performance of a subsequent cholecystectomy (five), during a subsequent diagnostic laparoscopy (four), and in the process of a subsequent colon resection (five). A solitary patient repaired with polytetrafluoroethylene [we attempted Gore-Tex (W.L. Gore & Associates, Flagstaff, AZ, U.S.A.) repair in two patients early in the experience] had severe adhesions to the bowel and omentum. Five patients had a small portion of omentum stuck to a corner of the mesh that had not been stapled flush with the anterior parietal peritoneum. Seven patients had no adhesions whatsoever. Four in whom adhesions had to be taken down for exposure at the first procedure had recurrence of their adhesions. In all patients, the mesh was completely incorporated into the peritoneum, and in seven patients it was hardly visible (Table 24.5).

REFERENCES

1. Annibali R, Camps J, Nagan R, et al. Anatomical considerations for laparoscopic inguinal herniorrhaphy. In: *Principles of laparoscopic surgery: basic and advanced techniques.* New York: Springer–Verlag, 1995.
2. Arreguie M, McKernan B, et al. *Inguinal hernia—advances or controversy?* Oxford, England: Radcliffe Medical Press Ltd, 1994.
3. Camps J, Nguyen N, Annibali R, et al. Laparoscopic inguinal herniorrhaphy: current techniques. In: *Principles of laparoscopic surgery: basic and advanced techniques.* New York: Springer–Verlag, 1995.
4. Condon RE, Carilli S. The biology and anatomy of inguinofemoral hernia. *Semin Laparosc Surg* 1994;1:75–85.
4a. Durstein-Decker C, Brick WG, Gadacz TR, et al. Comparison of adhesion formation in transperitoneal laparoscopic herniorrhaphy techniques. *Am Surg* 1994;60:157–159.
5. Gadacz T, Chase J, Duke S. Technology of prosthetic material. *Semin Laparosc Surg* 1994;1:123–127.
6. Ijzermand JNM. Recurrent inguinal hernia treated by classical hernioplasty. *Arch Surg* 1991;126:1097–2000.
7. Laymen ST, Burns RP, Chandler KE, et al. Laparoscopic inguinal herniorrhaphy in a swine model. Paper presented at: Southeastern Surgical Congress; June 2, 1992; Atlanta, GA.
8. Lichtenstein IL, Shulman AG, Amid PK, et al. The tension free hernioplasty. *Am J Surg* 1989;157:188–193.
9. MacFayden B Jr, Mathis C. Inguinal herniorrhaphy: complications and recurrences. *Semin Laparosc Surg* 1994;1:128–140.
10. Martin R, Shureih S. The use of Marlex mesh in primary hernia repair. *Surg Rounds* 1983;6:52–62.
11. Millelsen WP, McCready FJ. Femoral hernioplasty. *Surgery* 1954;35:743–748.
12. Mozingo DW, Walters MJ, Otchy DP, et al. Properitoneal synthetic mesh repair of recurrent inguinal hernias. *Surg Gynecol Obstet* 1992;174:33–35.
13. Musgrove JE, McCready FJ. The Henry approach to femoral hernia. *Surgery* 1949;26:601–611.
14. Nguyen N, Camps J, Fitzgibbons R. Laparoscopic intraperitoneal onlay mesh inguinal hernia repair. *Semin Laparosc Surg* 1994;1.
15. Nyhus LM, Condon RE, Harkins HN. Preperitoneal hernia repair for all types of hernia of the groin. *Am J Surg* 1960;100:234–244.
16. Read RC. Preperitoneal exposure of inguinal herniations. *Am J Surg* 1968;116:653–658.
17. Rignault DP. Properitoneal prosthetic inguinal hernioplasty through a Pfannenstiel approach. *Surg Gynecol Obstet* 1986;163:465–468.
18. Rives J. Surgical treatment of the inguinal hernia with the Dacron patch. *Int Surg* 1967;47:360–361.
19. Rosenthal D, Watlers M. Properitoneal synthetic placement for recurrent hernias of the groin. *Surg Gynecol Obstet* 1986;163:285–286.
20. Rosenthal D, Franklin ME Jr. Use of percutaneous stitches in laparoscopic mesh hernioplasty. *Surg Gynecol Obstet* 1993;176:491–492.
21. Salerno GM, Fitzgibbons RJ, Filipi CJ. Laparoscopic inguinal hernia repair. In: Zucker KA, Bailey RW, Reddick EJ, eds. *Surgical laparoscopy.* St. Louis: Quality Medical Publishing, 1991:290–291.
22. Stoppa RE, Rives JL, Warlaumont CR, et al. The use of Dacron in the repair of hernias of the groin. *Surg Clin North Am* 1984;64:269–285.
23. Toy FK, Smoot RT, Carey SD. Intraperitoneal inguinal hernioplasty. In: MacFadyen BV Jr, Ponksy JL, eds. *Operative laparoscopy and thoracoscopy.* Philadelphia: Lippincott–Raven Publishers, 1996:759–775.
24. Wantz GE. Testicular atrophy as a risk of inguinal hernioplasty. *Surg Gynecol Obstet* 1982;154:570–572.

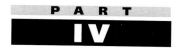
COMPLICATIONS OF GROIN HERNIA

25

WOUND INFECTION IN HERNIA REPAIR

DONALD E. FRY

Repair of hernias of the abdominal wall is one of the most common procedures performed by general surgeons. It is likely that millions of groin and ventral hernias are repaired annually around the world. Hernia repairs are performed in large tertiary care hospitals, and they are performed in the smallest of hospitals. They may be repaired laparoscopically, or they may require extensive open incisions. Hernia repair may require only a couple of interrupted sutures for adequate repair or may require extensive dissection and suturing. In recent years, synthetic meshes have been used with increasing frequency in both inguinal hernia (23,33) and ventral hernia repairs (4,34). The diversity in the size of hernias, the variability of techniques employed, and the different environments where hernia repair is undertaken all speak to the dramatic differences in complications and recurrence rates that are reported in the literature.

Infection is one of the most common complications following hernia repair. Infection as a complication may be recognized as only a minimal discharge of pus from around a single cutaneous suture, or it may be an extensive and invasive process requiring lengthy hospitalization, intravenous antibiotics, and repeated operations. While most surveillance programs and epidemiologists would define infection after hernia repair as any discharge of pus from the surgical site, it is clear that there are dramatic differences in the severity of wound infection. Unfortunately, this dramatic difference in the severity of infection makes interpretation of infection rates very difficult. Clinically significant infections after hernia repair are those in which antibiotics are required, hospitalization is necessary, or reoperation for debridement/drainage is needed. It is the prevention and timely treatment of significant wound infections at the site of hernia repair that should be understood by all who perform these procedures.

PATHOGENESIS OF WOUND INFECTION

Infection following hernia repair is nearly always secondary to bacteria that contaminate the wound during the operative procedure. Contaminants gain access to the wound from the patient's skin, from surgical instruments or the surgeon's gloves, or from environmental contamination via the air within the operating room. While considerable concern has existed regarding secondary contamination of the wound from hematogenous or lymphatic channels after wound closure, little evidence supports this as a significant route. Primary contamination from the events during the procedure is of paramount significance.

Culturable bacteria are present in the wound at the conclusion of every clean procedure (19) and are certainly present in every hernia repair. Fortunately, in most procedures, these bacterial contaminants do not result in clinical wound infection. The mobilization of the elements of the human inflammatory response within the surgical wound results in phagocytic cells, which eradicate the casual contaminants within the wound during the course of the routine procedure. It is only when this inflammatory response is exceeded in its capacity to eradicate the contaminants, or that the response is defective for either intrinsic or acquired reasons, that clinical infection is the result.

The probability of clinical infection of the hernia wound is the biologic summation of four variables: (a) the number of bacterial contaminants within the wound, (b) the virulence of the bacterial contamination, (c) the microenvironment within the wound that favors infection as an outcome, and (d) the integrity of the host. The intricate interaction of these variables underscores why prediction of wound infection in a given procedure is very difficult.

Bacterial Inoculum

It is intuitively obvious that the more bacteria that contaminate a given surgical wound, the greater will be the likelihood of a wound infection. Quantitative biopsies of open surgical wounds at the completion of procedures have demonstrated that the larger the number of bacteria per

D. E. Fry: Department of Surgery, University of New Mexico School of Medicine, Albuquerque, New Mexico.

gram of tissue, the higher the probability of infection. Over the years, the concept has developed that a critical threshold of bacterial contamination exists beyond which infection will occur. This threshold of bacteria has been 10^5 bacteria per gram of tissue (30).

Contamination of the magnitude of 10^5 bacteria per gram of tissue is an enormous inoculum following an appropriately prepped surgical site where the operation is being performed in an operative suite with conventional practices of surgical infection control. While biopsies of the surgical wound from clean surgical procedures will demonstrate higher bacterial infection rates in those that ultimately are clinically infected, quantitative bacteriology seldom demonstrates concentrations of bacteria at 10^5 bacteria per gram of tissue. This level of contamination would require the most extreme degree of departure from infection control practices in the repair of an elective groin hernia. Other clinical variables must amplify the bacterial effects other than numbers of contaminants.

Bacterial Virulence

All bacterial species do not have the same potential to cause clinical infections. Specific strains require very high concentrations of bacteria since their intrinsic virulence factors are of minimal consequence to the host. Other strains require only minimal numbers to cause invasive infection, particularly when the environmental conditions in the wound are especially suited to the pathogen.

Staphylococcus aureus is unquestionably the most common pathogen to be encountered as a pathogen in elective groin or ventral hernia repair. Staphylococci are ubiquitously found on the skin of patients and as nonpatient contamination from the operating room team or environment. Most clinically relevant, *S. aureus* produces coagulase as a virulence factor. Coagulase activates the human coagulation cascade and results in the precipitation of fibrin as the end-product of the coagulation process. This precipitation of fibrin creates a perimeter of protection about the pathogen and thus interferes with opsonic proteins and phagocytic cells gaining access to the contaminant. Given this protection from host inflammation and phagocytic function, microbial replication is able to continue. Replication begets the production of more coagulase, which precipitates more fibrin, but also creates an inflammatory milieu that attracts more leukocytes and more nonspecific vasodilatory responses of the host. The result is the thick, turbid environment of a staphylococcal wound abscess. The process tends to be localized within the wound, often associated with adjacent skin and soft tissue necrosis, a mild-to-moderate perimeter of induration and erythema, and seldom with a systemic bacteremic event.

Staphylococcus epidermidis is a less commonly seen pathogen in hernia infection, even though it is a more commonly cultured bacterium from the skin of patients under-

going these procedures. These staphylococcal species do not have the capacity to produce coagulase. Selected *S. epidermidis* strains can produce a glycocalyx "slime" that may increase their frequency of being a pathogen in patients with prosthetic materials (8,9). This glycocalyx about the microorganism that is seeded on a foreign body surface retards phagocytosis.

Group A streptococcal infection can infrequently be the cause of a postoperative wound infection following hernia repair. However, the virulence factors present in this microbe can make infection rapid and catastrophic. Streptococci have M proteins on their surface, which accounts for their virulence (14). Digestion of the M protein from the surface of the bacterium eliminates its virulence. These M proteins are different between different species of streptococci and have differing virulence potential. M proteins primarily retard phagocytosis by host neutrophils. Other important virulence factors among streptococci include hemolysins and other potent exotoxins. While quite uncommon, the rapid progression of these infections results in early fever, pain out of proportion to what should be experienced by the postoperative hernia patient, rapidly developing toxemia, and commonly systemic bacteremia.

Escherichia coli and other gram-negative colonists of the human intestinal tract can be pathogens. The gram-negative enterobacteriaceae have endotoxin as their primary virulence factor. This lipopolysaccharide is located in the outer membrane of the gram-negative organism and has a lipid A moiety of varying virulence (5). The proximity of the groin hernia procedure makes the gram-negative an identified pathogen. Ventral hernia repairs where enterotomy occurs will have much greater rates of *E. coli* infection and may also have obligate anaerobic bacteria present (e.g., *Bacteroides fragilis*). The gram-negative colonic bacteria with the obligate anaerobe creates a very pyogenic combination due to the capsular polysaccharide that is contributed for the infection by *B. fragilis* (22).

Thus, bacterial virulence becomes a very important consideration in elective hernia repair. More virulent organisms require a smaller inoculum to result in clinical infection. Common skin colonists with minimal virulence factors (e.g., *Corynebacterium acne*) are rarely if ever identified as pathogens in these infections.

The Microenvironment of the Wound

In this author's opinion, the most critical host factors that lead to infection in the hernia incision are microenvironmental factors created by the surgeon in the conduct of the procedure. Adjuvant factors, which are for the most part avoidable, create a local milieu that permits otherwise insignificant inocula of bacteria to achieve pathogenic potential in the wound.

Hemoglobin is probably the most potent adjuvant factor that promotes infection in the hernia wound. Hemoglobin is rich in protein and ferric iron, which creates an ideal pablum for microbial proliferation in the hernia wound (28). The availability of iron to some bacteria is a rate-limiting factor to bacterial growth. Wound hematoma from shoddy hemostasis requires an otherwise inconsequential number of bacteria to lead to wound abscess. In addition to the influence of iron in promoting proliferation, one report identifies a toxic end-product of microbial metabolism of hemoglobin, which is toxic to the host phagocytic cells (29).

Dead space in the hernia wound can be a particularly difficult problem in the ventral hernia patient (2). Dead space results in the accumulation of serum (and likely red blood cells as well), which becomes a liquid medium that is not well penetrated by phagocytic cells. Accumulated serum is commonly opsonin free. Infection rates increase for real biologic reasons with unattended dead space in the wound.

Foreign bodies in the wound clearly increase hernia wound infection rates. Suture material commonly becomes the nidus about which wound infections occur. Braided suture material such as silk will clearly reduce the number of bacteria necessary to create infection, as demonstrated in experimental models (13). Monofilament materials are generally perceived to have less of an adjuvant effect, but an overabundant number of knots in monofilament material can create a "braiding" effect. The adjuvant effects of nonabsorbable suture material appear to be secondary to poor phagocytic efficiency of human neutrophils for microbes on synthetic surfaces. Parsimony in the use of suture material in the hernia wound is generally advised.

The foreign material of greatest concern to the hernia surgeon is synthetic mesh. There is certainly the concern that infection rates in hernia repairs with mesh are higher than those without mesh, and repairs using mesh commonly have more risk factors for infection. Infections appear to be greater when the mesh material has a fine weave (e.g., polytetrafluoroethylene) as opposed to coarsely woven mesh (e.g., polypropylene). Infections in coarsely woven mesh seem to occur more commonly around the perimeter of the mesh. These infections may relate to braiding effects from the suture, which are used to secure the mesh in place, and may also relate to "crinkling" of redundant mesh, which creates pockets of dead space at the site of placement.

Necrotic tissue within the wound increases infection rates. Devitalized areas of subcutaneous tissue from extensive dissections of the abdominal wall become havens for microbial proliferation. Overenthusiastic utilization of the electrocautery also creates foci of dead tissue, which increases infection (10). Dead tissue does not develop edema, which then does not provide the aqueous conduits necessary for phagocytic cells to access microbial contaminants within the necrotic focus.

The Host

The integrity of host defenses in the surgical patient remains the most elusive variable to quantitate in the equation of infection in the hernia patient. It is clear that there are both intrinsic and acquired differences between patients. Acquired variables are well known to increase infection rates, although the mechanisms for this effect remain less well defined. Obesity increases infection rates in hernia patients, most likely because of the relatively avascular character of the large subcutaneous reservoir that is presented to potential bacterial contaminants. Preexisting diseases such as diabetes, renal failure, alcoholism, and malnutrition are additional variables that may affect the timing of operation or the risks of pursuing hernia repair at all.

Intrinsic host differences between patients are likely to exist but remain very difficult to define. Clinical studies of human monocytes identify highly variable and constant variability among different volunteers in their responsiveness to standardized proinflammatory stimuli (26). Others have suggested that selected elements of intrinsic responsiveness may potentially vary on a cyclical basis, which suggests that which day that is selected for operation in a given patient could be significant in terms of the probability of infection (3). The era of molecular genetics may permit a better characterization of the differences in individual host responsiveness and may provide evidence to define host variables in hernia wound infection rates.

Thus, the "equation of infection" in the hernia patient is certainly more than just a quantitative paradigm of bacteria in the wound at the time of operation. The interaction of these four sets of variables with each other in this complex surgical wound means that precise dissection of the responsible variable or variables in a given patient may be very difficult, if not impossible. The complexity of understanding the biology of wound infection in the hernia patient should suggest exercise of considerable caution when interpreting infection rates in a given report without fully characterizing the risk factors of the population and the techniques used during the operative procedure.

INCIDENCE AND EPIDEMIOLOGY

The incidence of wound infection after hernia repair is clearly inconsistently reported and is influenced by population-specific variables that may affect observations. Dramatically different infection rates are reported by different investigators. Trivial discharge of pus from the wound is often of limited significance to the patient and may not be identified at all by the surgeon or by even the most aggressive infection surveillance team. The small discharge of seroma fluid always is a debatable issue with regard to whether this constitutes a wound infection. Purists say that it is an infection. Pragmatists say that it is not. Others suggest that it does not matter. It would seem reasonable that the definition of wound infection in the hernia patient needs to have some relevance to outcome if it is to be of concern.

Postoperative infection rates following inguinal hernia repair are reported to be from 0.5% to 9%, depending upon the clinical variables of the population, such as whether mesh was used and whether preventive antibiotics were employed. Several reports from the United Kingdom identify relatively higher rates of infection following inguinal hernia repair. Holmes and Readman (17) reported a 4% rate with 1-month postoperative surveillance among an unstratified group of patients. Karran et al. (21) noted an 8% rate of infection and identified that it was four times greater than when they had previously studied infection rates by retrospective audit. Bailey et al. (7) noted a 9% infection rate when community-based surveillance was implemented, but only a 3% rate when standard inpatient surveillance was used. While the case for surveillance process to accurately reflect infection rates is understandable, it is not clear from these studies whether more accurate reporting really identified infections that resulted in either adverse outcome or increased utilization of medical resources.

Special conditions for patient management of hernia repair may affect wound infection rates. A French study noted a 4% wound infection rate when patients were hospitalized, compared to a 1% rate for outpatients (6). Obviously, hospitalized patients in the contemporary medical environment were likely to have other compounding variables. Deysine et al. (11) noted a 90% reduction of wound infections rates from 5.9% to 0.5% when a dedicated hernia service was organized with a dedicated senior hernia surgeon performing all procedures. The rate of 5.9% was seen among a group of general surgeons who were engaged in a broadly based general surgery practice. A large population study among a large group of providers in Belgium and Netherlands noted 1.2% and 0.4% hernia infection rates, respectively (25). No explanation could define the differences. Either regional practices in different countries are different, or the definition of infection may be different.

Other variables may affect wound infection rates. The use of drains in the wound has been reported to offer no benefit to the patient and may actually increase infection rates (31). The use of mesh is thought by most surgeons to increase wound infection rates, but has largely been supported only by testimony. Both Gilbert and Felton (15), and Janu et al. (20) found no increase in wound infection with mesh compared to those procedures where mesh was not used. Overall wound infection rates for hernia repair were 1% in both of these studies. Whether mesh-associated infections are more severe is still an unanswered question in need of objective clinical studies. The use of preventive antibiotics may or may not influence infection rates and become another variable when evaluating infection rates. This will be discussed further subsequently. While most surgeons believe that children have lower rates of infection after hernia repair in large part because of lesser subcutaneous fat, Tiryaki et al. (32) reported a 1.9% rate, which does not appear to be dramatically different than many adult studies.

Ventral hernia repair can be expected to have higher infection rates than inguinal hernia operations. Virtually all represent reoperations and will have scar tissue and more extensive dissection. Dead space within the wound is usually greater. Repair of these hernias usually requires longer surgical times. The expectation of contamination may be greater, particularly if repair is part of a procedure where intestinal resection is performed.

Houck et al. (18) noted that infections following ventral hernia repair were 16%, while rates of infection for inguinal hernia procedures were only 0.8%. They noted that patients who had prior wound infections were at increased risk of having the subsequent ventral hernia repair infected. Simchen et al. (31) reported no difference in wound infection rates among either inguinal hernia or ventral hernia (about 5%) repairs. They noted that advanced patient age, recurrent or incarcerated hernia, coexistent infections, and the use of drains were the four variables associated with infections. Medina et al. (24) from Spain reported an 8% infection rate among 497 patients and noted that the length of the procedure and the surgeon performing the procedure were the major variables associated with infection. White et al. (35) reported a rate of 34% for all wound complications, which included both seroma and clinical infection together. They noted that complications increased with the use of mesh and with hernias that were greater than 10 cm in diameter. They also noted that variables such as chronic obstructive lung disease, obesity, steroid therapy, and prior wound infection did not increase infection rates, and they noted no observable benefit from preventive antibiotics. Abramov et al. (1) noted a 44% rate of wound infection when preventive antibiotics were not used, and that the rate declined to 6% with a single dose of preventive systemic antibiotics preoperatively. From all of these studies, one can only conclude that infection (and seroma) rates are reported at dramatically different rates, and that the clinical variables present in individual patients require better definition.

DIAGNOSIS

The diagnosis of infection in the hernia wound is usually easily achieved. The classic signs of inflammation will usually be present. Induration and erythema are usually present. Pain that is persistent and more intense than customary is a common feature. The discharge of pus from the wound is the standard physical finding that indicates that infection is present. The diagnosis can be more difficult in the very obese patient. Deep-seated wound abscess may have very little erythema at the surface of the incision. Palpation of induration may be the only real clue of infection, and even induration may not be readily evident in the very obese patient. Attempts at direct aspiration of the indurated area may yield pus, but evolving deep-seated infection requires watchful waiting until the infection declares itself.

Fever and leukocytosis are variable features that may or may not be identified in the patient with surgical site infection following hernia repair, and generally lack the specificity to have any value for the diagnosis in these patients.

When mesh has been used for the hernia repair, the diagnosis is still made in the majority of cases by clinical findings of purulent discharge. Occasionally, a seroma may spontaneously drain from dead space in a large ventral hernia repair that is not infection. An immediate Gram's stain can be useful in the identification of bacteria within neutrophils. The absence of neutrophils means that infection is likely not present and a more conservative posture toward management can be undertaken.

As is true of foreign body infections in other locations of the body, infections from surgical mesh may not become evident for months to years following placement. These delayed infections may declare themselves with the eruption of a draining sinus that drains purulent material (Fig. 25.1). A large abscess with fluctuation may become palpable with or without systemic signs of fever and leukocytosis. Infections presenting as either draining sinuses or wound abscess will usually be identified about the perimeter of the mesh rather than from the body of the material. In inguinal hernia infections, it is commonly not possible to identify the infection as arising from any specific area of the mesh.

The utility of cultures in the diagnosis and subsequent therapy of these patients remains a source of contention between traditionalists in the management of infection and those who are somewhat more pragmatic. Cultures of small stitch abscesses are of no value. Small loculated collections of pus that are readily drained and have neither evidence of cellulitis nor wound necrosis will not be more successfully

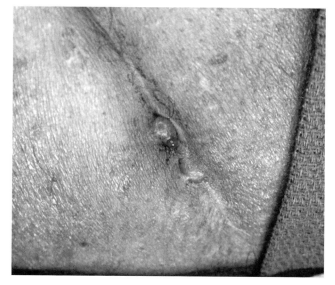

FIGURE 25.1. Healed inguinal hernia wound following a mesh repair that has a chronically draining sinus. These sinuses commonly have granulation tissue around the cutaneous opening.

treated because of culture information. If the patient appears to have an infection that is sufficiently severe to require antibiotic therapy, then cultures are prudent. Antibiotics will usually be employed when significant cellulitis is present around the wound or when wound necrosis requires debridement of tissue. Cultures should certainly be performed when evidence of fascial necrosis is present at the time of wound drainage.

PREVENTION

Prevention of infection in the surgical wound following hernia repair is of obvious value. The strategies to be used in prevention include both preoperative and intraoperative considerations. An important component of prevention is to have a fully informed patient who is knowledgeable about the risks of wound infection so that patient participation in the preventive strategy can be utilized.

Preoperative strategies should begin before the patient arrives for the operation. Most hernia procedures are performed as ambulatory operations. The patients should be instructed to take a preoperative shower with antiseptic soap the evening before or the morning of the operation. Scrubbing of the proposed surgical site is desirable. The site of the operation should not be shaved the night before the procedure, and should only have hair removed immediately prior to the operation. Patients with active remote infections and patients who have recently taken a course of antibiotics should have the operation deferred to a later date if possible. Even a seemingly insignificant paronychia of a finger may translate into higher infection rates at the surgical site. Prior antibiotic therapy will change the colonization of the patient to more resistant organisms and may pose a special problem if infection occurs. Preoperative hospitalization has been shown to increase clean wound infection rates (10), so incidental performance of hernia repair should not be undertaken because of the convenience of having the patient in the health care facility. While no data are available to guide the interval of delay after hospitalization or an antecedent course of antibiotic therapy, an interval of several weeks before elective repair seems prudent.

In the operating room, the surgical site is prepared with a standard antiseptic preparation. The site is scrubbed and an antiseptic is then applied over the proposed surgical site. Povidone iodine, chlorhexidine, or even isopropyl alcohol is used. Isopropyl alcohol is discouraged if the electrocautery is to be used.

Intraoperative strategies need to focus upon the reduction of bacteria being introduced into the wound and upon the elimination of adjuvant factors. Adherence to conventional infection control practices is always important. Minimizing pedestrian traffic in the operating room will minimize the risk of airborne contamination in the wound. A recent study reports reduced surgical wound infection rates with the use of higher concentrations of oxygen during and following the surgical procedure (16).

Reduction of adjuvant factors will have the greatest effect upon reducing infection rates. Hemostasis is obviously important but also requires an appropriate balance between controlling any bleeding into the wound without creating other problems. For example, the generous use of the electrocautery may achieve appropriate control of bleeding but only at the expense of creating a wound with significant superficial necrosis. Similarly, the liberal use of ligatures may reduce bleeding but potentially increase infection because of the foreign body effect. Nevertheless, large veins encountered in the wound should be tied, preferably with absorbable monofilament suture material. This has become more important in the era of ambulatory surgery since cauterized veins may bleed when immediate postoperative ambulation is expected of the patient. Parsimony in the use of sutures within the hernia wound should generally be observed, with subcutaneous sutures not being a requirement.

Dead space is a particular problem in the patient with a large ventral hernia. With or without mesh, bilateral abdominal wall flaps of subcutaneous tissue are commonly mobilized to achieve a cutaneous cover of the repair. The residual dead space will accumulate serum, and either a seroma or wound infection will commonly occur. This is usually best combated by the use of a closed suction draining system. The drain is introduced through a stab wound separate from the surgical incision, and is attached to continuous suction. Patients can be provided appropriate instruction for managing the suction catheter after discharge with a minimum of morbidity. The lack of a standard draining system and a standard method for placement of the drain means that additional prospective studies in the use of wound drains, particularly in patients with large ventral hernias requiring mesh, are necessary. Open Penrose drains become efficient conduits to introduce bacteria into the wound and should not be used.

An important but poorly studied area of infection involves the technical factors that lead to infection in the hernia repair with mesh. Three technical considerations are thought to be important by this author. First, place a minimum number of knots in the monofilament suture material that is being used to suture the mesh in place. The placement of eight to ten knots per placed suture is excessive in that it adds nothing to the repair. Multiknot sutures seem to be present in large numbers of mesh infections. Second, avoid redundancy in placing the mesh material. The completed mesh repair should be smooth, but also without tension. Redundant and folded mesh causes biologic dead space for the sequestration of serum and bacteria for infection. Finally, crinkled and bunched mesh around the perimeter of the repair increases infection rates. With inguinal hernia, do not have redundant and crinkled mesh along the shelving portion of the inguinal ligament or along Cooper's ligament. With ventral hernias, it is desirable to lay the mesh as flat as possible. Crinkled mesh at the edge

of the repair and at the site of the native fascia is asking for infection and failure of the repair.

Perhaps the most controversial area in the prevention of wound infection in hernia surgery is the use of systemic preventive antibiotics. The most notable study of this issue was performed by Platt et al. (27), in a multiinstitutional, prospective, randomized trial. They compared patients receiving a single preoperative dose of cefonicid versus placebo. The data are illustrated in Table 25.1. An apparently small, statistically insignificant reduction in wound infection rates was identified in those patients receiving the preoperative dose of the antibiotic. Infections at other anatomic sites appeared to be less in the group of patients receiving antibiotics as well. While the authors concluded that overall infection rates were reduced in the hernia patients, the differences even including the urinary tract and pneumonia infections were not statistically significant between the two groups.

The results of this largest randomized trial of inguinal hernia patients studied for the benefits of preventive antibiotics deserve several comments. First, even though the study was very large in terms of the number of patients, it remained insufficient to be a truly adequate sample for answering the question. If wound infection rates for elective inguinal hernia are at the 2% level that is usually identified for elective clean surgical procedures, the numbers of randomized cases that would be necessary to statistically prove the point would be very large.

Second, the severity of infections identified in the study patients was not stratified. Draining suture sinus infections versus catastrophic deep infections of the groin were not differentiated. To advocate the generalized use of preventive antibiotics for every elective hernia procedure would require a much more thorough analysis of the potential cost-effectiveness of the strategy than simply counting superficial wound infections.

Third, it is not appropriate to be evaluating infections that are not surgical site infections as part of the analysis of systemic preventive antibiotics. Postoperative urinary tract infections and pneumonia events after inguinal hernia proce-

TABLE 25.1.

Complication	Placebo Group (N = 311)	Antibiotic Group (N = 301)
Wound infection	6 (1.9%)	4 (1.3%)
Urinary tract infection	2 (0.6%)	1 (0.3%)
Pulmonary infection	1 (0.3%)	0
All infections	13 (4.2%)	7 (2.3%)

From Platt R, Zaleznik DF, Hopkins CC, et al. Perioperative antibiotic prophylaxis for herniorrhaphy and breast surgery. *N Engl J Med* 1990;322:153–160, with permission. These data have become the main justification for surgeons to use preventive systemic antibiotics in patients undergoing inguinal hernia repair. The differences in wound infection and the differences in total infections are not statistically significant.

dures are highly unusual in the absence of coexistent prostatic disease or obstructive lung disease. The literature on preventive systemic antibiotics has generally discredited their use for the prevention of urinary tract and pulmonary infection.

What is the appropriate strategy for preventive antibiotics in elective inguinal hernia repair? It is recommended that an individualized strategy be used. Elective inguinal hernia in younger patients who are of modest body habitus should not have preventive antibiotics. The risks of antibiotic-associated complications may actually exceed the rate of a superficial wound infection. Patients who have been operated on for a previously failed hernia repair, diabetic patients, obese patients, and those with major coexistent diseases may benefit from a single dose of a systemic antibiotic that has activity against *S. aureus* and the common gram-negative bacteria (e.g., *E. coli*). Cefazolin 1g in the immediate preoperative period remains the drug of choice. Systemic antibiotics must not be continued into the postoperative period.

Should systemic preventive antibiotics be used if mesh is to be used in the procedure? Most surgeons are of the opinion that mesh increases infection rates after hernia repair. Several studies have failed to validate that infection rates are higher with mesh repair (15,20). Because of the concern about placement of the foreign body in the wound, most surgeons would use preventive antibiotics in this situation, even though prospective randomized trials have not demonstrated their efficacy.

With ventral hernia repair, a separate consideration makes the use of preventive antibiotics more attractive than for patients undergoing inguinal hernia repair. Large ventral hernias with intestines within the hernia sac, or those that are the consequence of multiple previous abdominal operations, will be complicated by the potential risk of the inadvertent enterotomy. Major enteric contamination of the wound cannot be predicted and is a complication that can happen to the very best of technical surgeons. Preoperative systemic antibiotics should reduce infection from the enterotomy. In very-high-risk patients with multiply operated abdomens, some would even advocate a mechanical bowel preparation and the use of oral poorly absorbed intestinal antibiotics in the preoperative period to reduce the consequences of colotomy, and to add to the safety of primary repair of the injury. Even with this rationale in favor of using preventive antibiotics, the literature on this subject is very limited and conflicting. Randomized and well-stratified studies of ventral hernia repair with and without mesh would seem to be necessary to answer this question.

TREATMENT OF INFECTION

Infection in the surgical wound following hernia repair can span a broad continuum, from that of a very simple process requiring a minimal amount of treatment to a very complex infection requiring lengthy hospitalization and repeated

operation. A simple localized wound infection is characterized by the discharge of purulent material from a specific area of the wound. This small discharge of purulence is commonly from an area around a single suture, or may be from a localized area of tissue injury from the electrocautery. These simple infections are not associated with a generalized induration of the wound and are not associated with extensive cellulitis. Some may be associated with prolonged presence of cutaneous sutures or staples in the skin and resolve with removal of the foreign body and local drainage of the small focus of pus. Complete opening of the wound is not necessary. Systemic antibiotic therapy is not necessary. Gram's stain of the drainage will show polymorphonuclear phagocytic cells and small numbers of gram-positive cocci. Cultures are not necessary.

A simple generalized wound infection is one where the extent of the infection involves the majority if not the entire length of the hernia incision. Palpable induration along the length of the wound is usually present, and varying degrees of erythema can be seen depending upon the virulence of the pathogen and the duration of the infection process. These infections are more likely to cause fever and moderate leukocytosis than the localized simple infection discussed above. When discharge of pus is identified, probing the area of discharge with either a surgical instrument or a cotton-tipped probe results in the discharge of very large amounts of pus. The extent of the erythema and induration, and usually the pain and discomfort experienced by the patient from the infection, are clear signs that the entire skin and subcutaneous tissue must be opened to effect adequate drainage of the infection. In most of these infections, *S. aureus* will be the pathogen, although the occasional inguinal hernia wound will be infected by *E. coli*, and the ventral hernia wound subjected to enteric contamination will have a polymicrobial infection. The simple generalized wound infection will commonly have thick, shaggy, fibrinous debris that is adherent to the subcutaneous interface of the opened wound, particularly if *S. aureus* (coagulase-positive) organisms are the cause of the infection. Debridement of this shaggy exudate is important to expedite resolution of the inflammatory process and promotion of wound healing. Any evident suture material within the wound should be removed. Gram's stains are done. Cultures are performed only if it is anticipated that antibiotic therapy is necessary.

The determination to use antibiotics requires clinical judgment. Evidence of extensive cellulitis around the wound or evidence of soft tissue necrosis is an indication for antibiotic therapy. Gram-positive cocci identified by Gram's stain within a thick, purulent discharge usually confirms *S. aureus* as the pathogen. Antibiotic therapy with oral nafcillin or cephalexin is commonly prescribed for these infections. Many can be managed by drainage alone, and antibiotics for minimal cellulitis are used to make both the patient and the physician feel better but probably do not hasten resolution of the process when effective drainage has been implemented. *S. epidermidis* is an unusual pathogen for the simple generalized wound infection in the absence of synthetic mesh. Methicillin-resistant *S. aureus* (MRSA) is quite unusual as a wound infection pathogen after hernia surgery, since the MRSA have undergone a chromosomal mutation that not only confirms methicillin resistance, but also attenuates microbial virulence. MRSA are identified only in the very immunosuppressed hernia patient, usually in the patient who has had a recent hospitalization.

E. coli can be seen as a pathogen, and the clinical infection may share many of the features seen with staphylococcal wound infection. Oral quinolone therapy is useful because of the activity of this group of antibiotics against *E. coli* and because of the efficient absorption of these antibiotics from the gastrointestinal tract. If the infection is severe enough to require hospitalization, then intravenous antibiotic therapy may be useful. A large array of cephalosporins, advanced-spectrum penicillins, and other antibiotics that are active against *E. coli* can be chosen. Cultures are certainly warranted for the hospitalized patient to validate the antibiotic selection.

Anaerobes should not be participants in the simple infection of the hernia incision unless enteric contamination was present. Ventral hernia repair at the time of a simultaneous bowel resection and inadvertent enterotomy during elective ventral hernia repair would be situations where enteric anaerobes could be pathogens. Ventral hernia repair at the time of colostomy takedown, or repair in the presence of an existing colostomy would make enteric anaerobes a real possibility. Anaerobic participation in these infections is characterized by an especially putrid infection, often with some evidence of soft tissue or fascial necrosis, and almost always involves an aerobic partner in the synergistic infection. Gram's stains of the wound exudate will show polymicrobial pathogens. Oral quinolones plus metronidazole is the therapy of choice after drainage of all pus and mechanical debridement of all dead tissue and fibrinous debris. Metronidazole is chosen over clindamycin because of comparable anaerobic activity but at dramatically lower cost. These polymicrobial infections are commonly so severe from associated soft tissue necrosis that hospitalization and intravenous antibiotics are required.

Necrotizing Fasciitis

Necrotizing fasciitis can rarely be seen following elective inguinal hernia repair, but appears to be a more common event to complicate wound infection of ventral hernias. The greater frequency of necrotizing infection following ventral hernia repair is due to the greater probability of polymicrobial infections as well as poorer blood supply to the abdominal wall caused by multiple previous abdominal operations commonly seen in these patients.

Necrotizing fasciitis is suspected when drainage of a clinical wound infection from the hernia repair results in the identification of necrotic fascia, or the recognition that the infection has extended into the perifascial space. The investing fascia of the abdominal wall musculature has only a loose areolar connective tissue that attaches the subcutaneous fat to its anterior surface. Under normal circumstances, the surgeon can easily tease the subcutaneous tissue off the anterior surface of the rectus fascia with a gentle dissecting finger. This potential space between the subcutaneous fat and the anterior surface of the fascia is termed the perifascial space, and presents a plane for rapid advancement of infection. When the infection remains anterior to the fascia, then the underlying fascia may actually maintain its viability. Infection above and beneath the fascia concurrently results in necrosis of the fascia and potentially of the muscle as well. Infection can extend along the fascial plane with little visible evidence of the extent of the advancing process by just surface examination of the wound alone.

Necrotizing fasciitis is suspected in the infected hernia wound when palpable tenderness extends well beyond the visible evidence of cellulitis or induration that is present on examination of the hernia wound. Fasciitis will have a greater probability of systemic signs of fever and leukocytosis. However, this complication tends to occur more often in diabetic patients, and systemic signs may be absent in this group of patients until the infection is far advanced. The diagnosis is confirmed by exploration of the wound and identification of infection extending along the perifascial space, with or without evidence of actual necrotic fascia itself.

The treatment of necrotizing fasciitis is surgical debridement of all dead tissue. This means a return to the operating room under adequate anesthesia and complete excision of dead tissue until only viable, bleeding tissue remains. Debridement cannot be abbreviated in the expectation of subsequent reconstruction, since inadequate debridement means further extension of the process and more tissue destruction. The underlying muscle may or may not require debridement, and the degree of muscle excision must be individualized for each patient.

Hernia infection can rarely be caused by Group A streptococci with a rapid and fulminant necrotizing infection. Similarly, a rare case of clostridial gas gangrene may be seen when ventral hernia repair is subjected to contamination from either the biliary or the intestinal tract. These rapidly advancing necrotizing infections are characterized by early postoperative fever, extensive wound pain and tenderness, and rapidly evolving systemic toxicity. Objective evidence of severe wound infection can be subtle with only a brawny edema present, and a frothy but nonpurulent discharge from the wound. The most important factor in the diagnosis is a keen sense of awareness of this complication, and immediate reexploration of the wound. Extensive debridement of the groin or abdominal wall is usually required if recovery is to be achieved.

Polymicrobial necrotizing infections tend to be more indolent, but are serious infections usually in the ventral hernia patient. Debridement of fascia and muscle usually results in inadequate abdominal wall for primary closure. Temporary placement of synthetic mesh should be avoided during the early debridement of these infections since the suturing of synthetic material into a marginally viable or actively infected fascia may promote advancement of the necrotizing process. Temporary wound management can be achieved by several methods. Xeroform gauze over the surface of the omentum and/or bowel, followed by saline gauze dressings and a plastic, adhesive cover is one preferred method. Reoperation is then pursued on a daily basis until no evidence of advancing infection is seen. At this point, the placement of a permanent synthetic mesh for reconstruction can be entertained.

Systemic antibiotics for necrotizing fasciitis should cover the offending organism. Antibiotics are of no value in the absence of effective and comprehensive debridement of the wound. Topical antibiotics and topical antiseptics are not of proven value. The open wounds are simply managed with saline dressings. Wound desiccation must be avoided, or additional debridement will be necessary.

Toxic Shock Syndrome

The toxic shock syndrome was initially identified as a complication of staphylococcal infection associated with the use of vaginal tampons during the menses. Specific strains of *S. aureus* have the genetic capacity to produce a potent toxic shock toxin that causes a fulminant systemic inflammatory response syndrome. Profound hypotension and multiple organ failure are the consequences.

Increasing numbers of cases of toxic shock syndrome are now being reported among surgical patients, with gauze packing of open wounds being the clinical scenario. Staphylococcal infection within the gauze foreign body results in the liberation of the toxin, and all the subsequent sequela. While not a common event, the patient with a wound infection following hernia surgery secondary to *S. aureus* who then has gauze packing placed into the wound during management is at risk for this complication. Infrequent changes of the gauze packing in the self-managed outpatient is the scenario in which this syndrome can occur. Wound dressing changes on a twice-daily basis should eliminate this infrequent complication.

Toxic shock is suspected with the rapid onset of fever, chills, prostration, and rapidly advancing systemic inflammatory response syndrome. *S. aureus* is the pathogen, unchanged gauze packing in the wound is the setting, as stated previously. Blood cultures are rarely positive since the toxin, not the microbe, is released systemically. Treatment is removal of the packing, systemic antistaphylococcal antibiotic therapy, and aggressive systemic supportive care. Volume administration must be very aggressive, and inotropic support is commonly necessary.

A toxic shock–like syndrome is also seen with Group A streptococcal infection. The syndrome is similar in presentation, but a foreign body in the wound is not required. Treatment requires wound debridement, systemic clin-

damycin and penicillin therapy, and aggressive systemic supportive care. Unlike the staphylococcal toxic shock syndrome, the streptococcal variant is usually associated with bacteremia. However, positive blood culture information is available too late in the process to be of any clinical value.

INFECTED MESH

One of the most vexing problems in hernia surgery is infection of synthetic surgical mesh (12). While mesh has been useful in allowing tension-free repairs of inguinal and ventral hernias, and doubtlessly has reduced recurrence rates, the infected mesh poses a series of special management problems.

Infected Mesh in the Inguinal Hernia Wound

Infection of the wound that has had mesh used for repair requires an initial assessment as to whether the mesh itself is involved in the infection (Fig. 25.2). Simple localized

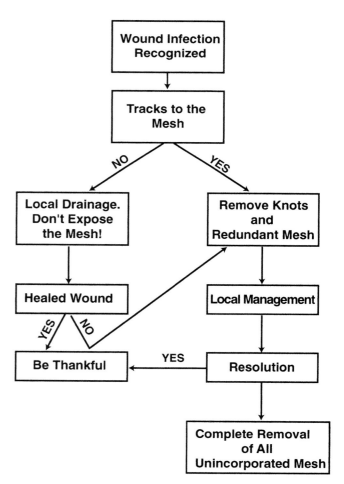

FIGURE 25.2. General algorithm for the management of wound infections following mesh placement in hernia surgery.

infection of the subcutaneous tissue can occur, and simple local drainage suffices without any long-term problems. However, the more common scenario is for the infection to track down to the mesh itself.

Mesh infection in the inguinal hernia wound often leads to removal of the entire mesh. Some inguinal hernia repairs require only 25 cm² of synthetic mesh. Open drainage of the infected wound with mesh leads to potential healing of much of the wound, but inevitably results in a clinically draining sinus or larger draining defect in the wound. Partial removal of the mesh seldom, if ever, leads to eradication of the infection, but partial removal always results in recurrence of the hernia. The infection will usually be found to track down to sutures used to secure the mesh, or to areas of redundant or crinkled mesh around the perimeter of the repair. Systemic antibiotics are used to treat the cellulitis of the infection, but are essentially of no value in the management of the open draining wound.

These patients will require a return to the operating room for removal of the mesh. This reoperation may be delayed until such time as the majority of the wound induration and other evidence of inflammation have resolved. The complete mesh is removed, including the sutures used to secure it. The mesh is seldom incorporated into the tissue, but rather can be bluntly freed because of the sustained infection. Anatomic landmarks are quite obscured, and care must be taken to avoid permanent damage to the cord structures or inadvertent entry into the femoral vein.

A healed wound can usually be achieved only by removal of the infected foreign body. Systemic antibiotics will not achieve wound closure if infected portions of the mesh or infected sutures remain. Lengthy courses of antibiotics have been used in the hope that elimination of the microbe will occur. This does not happen. Antibiotics may have some utility in getting the patient through the acute wound infection at the time of diagnosis. Antibiotics may be useful in a more rapid resolution of acute cellulitis around the wound. Antibiotic therapy may result in a short period of apparent epithelization over a draining sinus, but the area will inevitably break down and chronically drain.

On occasion, a small stitch sinus may erupt through the healed wound months to years after apparently successful repair of a groin hernia. Local exploration of the wound may suffice in these circumstances with removal of the festering stitch that is responsible for the infection (Fig. 25.3). Any unincorporated mesh should be debrided. Local exploration of the sinus tract with a crochet hook may allow return of the offending stitch, but commonly hooks onto the mesh itself. If the infected sinus tract leads deeply to the inferior aspects of the repair toward either Cooper's ligament or the shelving portion of the inguinal ligament, then removal should be undertaken in the operating room and not with local probing. These deeper sinuses commonly result in removal of the mesh and recurrence of the hernia.

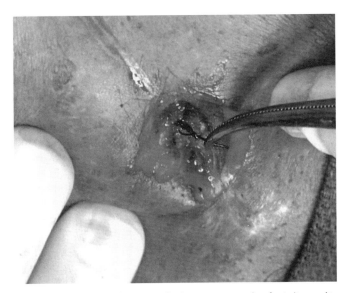

FIGURE 25.3. This photograph demonstrates the fortuitous situation in which local exploration identifies a single stitch at the superior margin of the mesh after inguinal hernia repair. Removal of the stitch will result in healing of the wound if there are not other infected stitches remaining in the area, and there is not redundant mesh.

Infected Ventral Hernia Mesh

Therapy must be individualized for these infections. Early infection within the first few weeks following placement requires that the surgical wound be opened and the entire infected space around the mesh be drained. The open wound is allowed to granulate and may be subsequently closed with full thickness coverage after successful granulation of the mesh surface. A key point for this strategy to be successful is not to have redundant, folded, or crinkled mesh around the perimeter of the repair. Mesh redundancy is a key to persistent drainage and failure. Similarly, six or more knots in suture used to secure the mesh will commonly resist incorporation into the granulation tissue and will result in persistent draining sinuses in the future.

Infections may declare themselves months to years after ventral hernia repair and assume highly variable degrees of severity. Local draining sinuses may erupt and persistently drain. These ordinarily will track to the edge of the repair to "bunched" mesh or to a suture. Local exploration with a hooked probe or with a small incision under local anesthesia may allow removal of the infected stitch. Local excision and debridement of redundant and unincorporated mesh may be necessary. Rarely do these sinus tracks arise from the midportion of flatly positioned mesh. Abscesses of the mesh can also be seen remote from the time of mesh placement. These may require incision and drainage. Failure to manage the stitch or redundant mesh that is the provocateur of these late infections will lead to a chronically draining sinus. Neglected management of the ventral hernia infection may result in mesh extruding through the wound (Fig. 25.4).

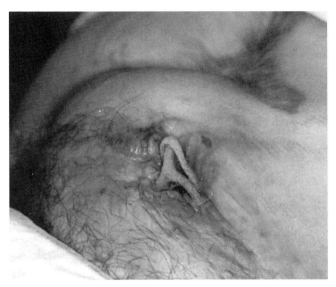

FIGURE 25.4. Extruding mesh from a ventral hernia. This situation requires general anesthesia and complete removal of the mesh.

These kinds of infections arise when very redundant or multiple layers of mesh or mesh plugs have been used in the repair. Local excision of the extruding mesh does not result in wound closure as the festering infection results in continued drainage and progressive exposure of infected edges of the mesh. Treatment of these catastrophic infections requires general anesthesia and complete removal of the mesh. Recurrent hernia is inevitable but a definitive attempt at repair must be delayed until complete healing of the infected wound has occurred.

Antibiotic therapy is of limited value in these ventral hernia mesh infections. Draining sinuses may transiently respond, but breakdown and recurrent drainage almost always occur following cessation of the drug therapy. Cellulitis may respond to antibiotics in the acute postoperative mesh infection, but those infections that occur months after mesh placement are chronic processes, and antibiotics are not of value.

Fistula Through Mesh

The ultimate disaster in the use of mesh for repair of a ventral hernia is an enteric fistula through the mesh. Fistula occurs when partial thickness injury to the intestinal wall occurs during dissection at hernia repair. Abrasion of the partial thickness injury by the mesh surface may be the responsible mechanism for this complication. Resection of bowel or inadvertent enterotomy that results in an acute suture line in the bowel wall cannot be in immediate proximity to the mesh surface without a risk of this complication. If available, placement of omentum between the mesh and the intestinal suture line is very desirable to avoid fistula.

When fistula occurs, treatment requires removal of all mesh around the site of fistulization, and control of the drainage from the intestine to avoid extensive digestion of soft tissue around the opening of the fistula. After removal of a margin of mesh around the fistula opening, a stomal bag or cannulation of the fistula with continued suction may be necessary. Some situations may permit use of an aluminum-based paste to protect intact skin around the fistula opening from enteric digestion. Most fistulas in association with mesh usually have a short track, and often have everted mucosa, which means that spontaneous closure from local management will not occur. Surgical repair of the fistula 5 to 6 months after the last operation is the best strategy. Patience is required in any attempted repair, since premature surgical approaches before the inflammatory process has completely resolved from the prior operation will result in additional risks of intestinal injury and failed attempts at fistula repair.

Nutritional support for the patient with fistula through mesh must be considered. Total parenteral nutrition may be needed when the fistula is in the midportion of the small intestine. Proximal fistulas may allow cannulation of the fistula tract itself and distal enteral feeding of the gut. Distal small bowel fistulas may benefit from proximal feedings with elemental feeding formulations. No standard strategy can be applied to all patients, and each circumstance requires an individualized approach to allow the 5- to 6-month interval before repair is attempted.

REFERENCES

1. Abramov D, Jeroukhimov I, Yinnon AM, et al. Antibiotic prophylaxis in umbilical and incisional hernia repair: a prospective randomized study. *Eur J Surg* 1996;162:945–948.
2. Alexander JW, Korelitz J, Alexander NS. Prevention of wound infection: a case for closed suction drainage to remove wound fluids deficient in opsonic proteins. *Am J Surg* 1976;132:59–63.
3. Alexander JW, Dionigi R, Meakins JL. Periodic variation in the antibacterial function of human neutrophils and its relationship to sepsis. *Ann Surg* 1971;173:206–213.
4. Amid PK, Shulman AG, Lichtenstein IL. A critical evaluation of the Lichtenstein tension-free hernioplasty. *Int Surg* 1994;79:76–79.
5. Apte RN, Galanos C, Pluznik DH. Lipid A, the active part of bacterial endotoxins including serum colony stimulating activity and proliferation of splenic granulocyte/macrophage progenitor cells. *J Cell Physiol* 1976;87:71–78.
6. Audry G, Johanet S, Achrafi H, et al. The risk of wound infection after inguinal incision in pediatric outpatient surgery. *Eur J Ped Surg* 1994;4:87–89.
7. Bailey IS, Karren SE, Toyn K, et al. Community surveillance of complications after hernia surgery. *Br Med J* 1992;304:469–471.
8. Christensen GD, Simpson WA, Bisno AL, et al. Experimental foreign body infections in mice challenged with slime-producing *Staphylococcus epidermidis*. *Infect Immunol* 1983;40:407–410.
9. Christensen GD, Baddour LM, Simpson WA. Phenotypic variation of *Staphylococcus epidermidis* slime production *in vitro* and *in vivo*. *Infect Immunol* 1987;55:2870–2877.
10. Cruse PJ, Foord R. A five-year prospective study of 23,649 surgical wounds. *Arch Surg* 1973;107:206–210.
11. Deysine M, Grimson RC, Soroff HS. Inguinal herniorrhaphy:

reduced morbidity by service standardization. *Arch Surg* 1991; 126:628–630.

12. Deysine M. Pathophysiology, prevention, and management of prosthetic infections in hernia surgery. *Surg Clin North Am* 1998;78:1105–1115.

13. Elek SD, Conen PE. The virulence of *Staphylococcus pyogenes* for man: a study of the problem of the wound. *Br J Exp Pathol* 1957; 38:573.

14. Fox EN. M proteins of Group A streptococci. *Bacteriol Rev* 1974;38:57–86.

15. Gilbert AI, Felton LL. Infection in inguinal hernia repair considering biomaterial and antibiotics. *Surg Gynecol Obstet* 1993;177: 126–130.

16. Greif R, Akca O, Horn E-P, et al. Supplemental perioperative oxygen to reduce the incidence of surgical wound infection. *N Engl J Med* 2000;342:161–167.

17. Holmes J, Readman R. A study of wound infection following inguinal hernia repair. *J Hosp Infect* 1994;28:153–156.

18. Houck JP, Rypins EB, Sarfeh IJ, et al. Repair of incisional hernia. *Surg Gynecol Obstet* 1989;169:397–399.

19. Howe CW. Bacterial flora of clean wounds and its subsequent sepsis. *Am J Surg* 1964;696–700.

20. Janu PG, Sellers KD, Mangiante EC. Mesh inguinal herniorrhaphy: a ten-year review. *Am Surg* 1997;63:1065–1069.

21. Karran SJ, Karran SE, Toyn K, et al. Antibiotic prophylaxis in clean surgical cases and the role of community surveillance. *Eur J Surg* 1992;567[Suppl]:31–32.

22. Kasper DL, Hayes ME, Reinap BG, et al. Isolation and identification of encapsulated strains of *Bacteroides fragilis. J Infect Dis* 1977;136:75–81.

23. Liakakos T, Karanikas I, Panagiotidis H, et al. Use of Marlex mesh in the repair of recurrent incisional hernia. *Br J Surg* 1994; 81:248–249.

24. Medina M, Sillero M, Martinez-Gallego G, et al. Risk factors of surgical wound infection in patients undergoing herniorrhaphy. *Eur J Surg* 1997;163:191–198.

25. Mertens R, Van den Berg JM, Veerman-Brenzikofer ML, et al. International comparison of results of infection surveillance: the Netherlands versus Belgium. *Infect Control Hosp Epidemiol* 1994; 15:574–578.

26. Molvig J, Baek L, Christensen P, et al. Endotoxin-stimulated human monocyte secretion of interleukin 1, tumor necrosis factor alpha, and prostaglandin E2 shows stable interindividual differences. *Scand J Immunol* 1988;27:705–716.

27. Platt R, Zaleznik DF, Hopkins CC, et al. Perioperative antibiotic prophylaxis for herniorrhaphy and breast surgery. *N Engl J Med* 1990;322:153–160.

28. Polk HC Jr, Miles AA. Enhancement of bacterial infection by ferric iron: kinetics, mechanisms, and surgical significance. *Surgery* 1971;70:71–77.

29. Pruett TL, Rotstein OD, Fiegel VD, et al. Mechanisms of the adjuvant effect of hemoglobin in experimental peritonitis: VII. A leukotoxin is produced by *Escherichia coli* metabolism in hemoglobin. *Surgery* 1984;96:375–383.

30. Robson MC, Krizek TJ, Heggers JP. Biology of surgical infection. *Curr Probl Surg* 1973:1–62.

31. Simchen E, Rozin R, Wax Y. The Israeli study of surgical infection of drains and the risk of wound infection for hernias. *Surg Gynecol Obstet* 1990;170:331–337.

32. Tiryaki T, Baskin D, Bulut M. Operative complications of hernia repair in children. *Ped Surg Int* 1998;13:160–161.

33. Usher FC. New technique for repairing incisional hernia with Marlex mesh. *Am J Surg* 1979;138:740–741.

34. Usher FC. Technique for repairing inguinal hernias with Marlex mesh. *Am J Surg* 1982;143:382–384.

35. White TJ, Santos MC, Thompson JS. Factors affecting wound complications in repair of ventral hernias. *Am Surg* 1998;64: 276–280.

26

CORD AND TESTICULAR COMPLICATIONS OF GROIN HERNIORRHAPHY

ALAN T. RICHARDS

"The heart is the beginning of life, but the testicles of a better life; for it is farre more noble to live well, than simply and absolutely to live." Ambroise Paré (Surgeon) (1582)

In the United States of America, where approximately 700,000 hernia repairs are performed each year, the incidence of complications varies between 1% and 26%. A review of various reports has indicated that approximately 10% of hernia repairs develop complications (9). This translates to 70,000 patients per year. The prevalence is very low in specialized hernia centers. Because the majority of groin hernias occur in male patients, complications involving the spermatic cord and the testis form an important subset.

ANATOMY

The spermatic cord emerges from the deep inguinal ring just above the midpoint of the inguinal ligament and runs through the inguinal canal down to the scrotum, where it joins the testis. The layers of the abdominal wall continue down to form the coverings of the cord. Within the cord are the vas deferens, the testicular (internal spermatic) artery, the pampiniform plexus of veins, and lymphatics. The ilioinguinal nerve runs on the anterior surface of the cord and the genital branch of the genitofemoral nerve on its posterior surface. One or more of these structures may be injured during hernia repair in the groin (13,17).

The blood supply of the testis is particularly vulnerable during surgical procedures on hernias in the groin. The major blood supply to the testis is the testicular artery

(internal spermatic artery), which has its origin from the aorta, a little below the renal arteries. Each testicular artery passes obliquely down laterally in the retroperitoneal area, on the psoas major muscle. On each side, the artery passes in front of the genitofemoral nerve, the ureter, and the lower part of the external iliac artery to reach the deep inguinal ring, where it enters the spermatic cord. With the other constituents of the cord, it traverses the inguinal canal and enters the scrotum. At the upper end of the posterior aspect of the testis, it divides into two branches that pass onto the medial and the lateral surfaces, pierce the tunica albuginea, and end in the tunica vasculosa. From here, terminal branches pass into the substance of the testis at various points over the free surface (13,17).

A rich collateral supply exists, communicating with the testicular artery (Fig. 26.1) (6,8). The external spermatic artery from the inferior epigastric artery supplies the cremaster muscle and is found at the deep ring, or at the iliopubic tract, and runs close to the vas deferens. The artery to the vas from the superior vesical artery communicates freely with the other arteries. A rich collateral network is found above the testis between the vesical and prostatic branches and the testicular and deferential vessels. In addition, scrotal vessels from the internal and external pudendal arteries freely communicate with the vessels in the spermatic cord just external to the superficial inguinal ring (13,17).

The testicular veins emerge from the back of the testis and unite to form a convoluted mass, the pampiniform plexus, which ascends in the spermatic cord in front of the ductus deferens. Below the superficial inguinal ring, the veins of the plexus are drained by three or four veins, which coalesce to two veins at the deep ring. These run upward on either side of the testicular artery. These veins become a single vein before they enter the inferior vena cava on the right side and the left renal vein on the left side (13,17).

A. T. Richards: Department of Surgery, Creighton University School of Medicine; Department of Surgery, Saint Joseph Hospital, Omaha, Nebraska.

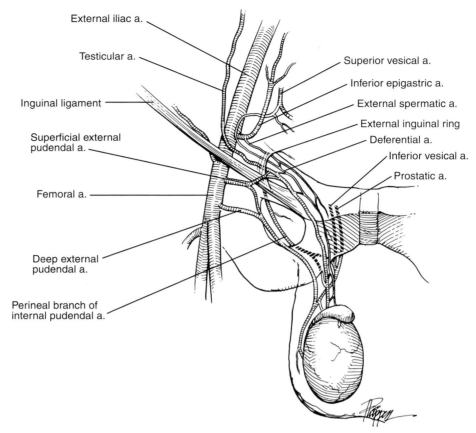

FIGURE 26.1. The primary and the collateral arterial supply to the testis. (Adapted from Koontz AR. Atrophy of the testicle as a surgical risk. *Surg Gynecol Obstet* 1965;120:511–513.)

HYDROCELE

If a patent processus vaginalis is present, then the potential exists for hydrocele formation after repair of an indirect inguinal hernia. This occurs especially if the distal sac is ligated; conversely, if the distal sac is left unclosed, the incidence decreases. A hydrocele can be diagnosed quite easily clinically by demonstrating that it transilluminates brilliantly. Once this has been done, a needle can be inserted and straw-colored fluid will be aspirated. Should a hydrocele develop in a pediatric patient after previous hernia repair, simple aspiration is all the treatment that is required.

HEMATOCELE

This is a collection of blood in the distal sac in a patient with a patent processus. It presents early postoperatively, usually within the first 12 to 24 hours. There is swelling of

the cord and scrotum with associated pain. Bruising becomes evident involving the scrotum as well. The source of the bleeding in these patients is either from the cut edges of the distal sac, from the testicular artery, from the pampiniform plexus of veins, or sometimes from veins injured in Bogros' space (Fig. 26.2) (3). Treatment may be expectant unless it becomes very tense. If this should be the case, surgical evacuation may be required. This is done by opening up the wound and expressing the clot from the processus. The source of the bleeding is then sought and controlled, usually by electrocautery.

COMPLICATIONS INVOLVING THE VAS DEFERENS

The Dysejaculation Syndrome

The dysejaculation syndrome results from trauma to the vas during surgery, which results in scarring and narrow-

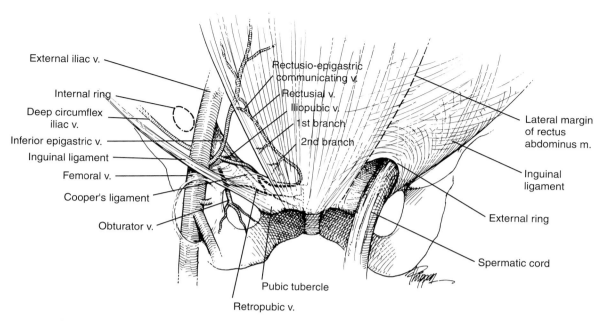

FIGURE 26.2. The deep inguinal vasculature in Bogros' space. *V,* vein. (Adapted from Bendavid R. The space of Bogros and the deep inguinal circulation. *Surg Gynecol Obstet* 1992;174:355–358.)

ing of the lumen of the vas. Clinically, the patient experiences a searing pain at the time of ejaculation. This will be dealt with in more detail in Chapter 30.

Transsection of the Vas

Transsection of the vas (12) can occur during hernia surgery when the sac is being mobilized from within the cord. If it is detected, it is imperative that the two ends of the severed vas are freshened by cutting them across and an end-to-end anastomosis performed over a small stent, such as a length of nylon suture, which can be brought out of the vas further along and through the skin of the groin as a pullout. The anastomosis is done using magnifying loupes or an operating microscope to obtain exact apposition. Should one vas be damaged, it is unlikely that the patient will develop infertility because the opposite vas will be intact.

NERVE INJURIES

The genitofemoral nerve and the *ilioinguinal nerve* are not infrequently injured during hernia surgery, particularly with the repairs done under tension. Injuries involving

these will be dealt with in more detail in Chapters 2 and 29.

DAMAGE TO THE BLOOD SUPPLY OF THE TESTICLE

Testis Appears Gangrenous at the Time of the Surgery

Gangrenous-appearing testes are usually seen in patients undergoing emergency surgery for torsion of a testis or for a strangulated inguinal hernia in infancy (10,11,13). In children, the incidence of incarceration and strangulation is higher. In a series of 2,764 pediatric patients, Rowe and Clatworthy found a 12% incidence, two thirds occurring in the first year of life (13). The greatest risk was in the neonatal period, where 28% of infants under 3 months of age had strangulation (13). In 89 premature babies with hernias, strangulation occurred in 13% (9). The testis appears dusky and probably nonviable. Because no large series of such patients exists, it is not possible to use clinical data to back up recommendations. However, most clinicians would replace this nonviable-appearing testis within the scrotum. A certain proportion of these will atrophy as time goes, but some will return to normal size. Atrophy of the testis in infants and children occurred in 1% of all hernia repairs in Fahlstrom's series (5).

Ischemic Orchitis and Testicular Atrophy

Incidence

In a series of 4,114 groin hernioplasties, Wantz reported ischemic orchitis occurring in 25 patients (0.61%) and testicular atrophy in 14 (0.34%) (14). In a review of a series of 59,752 hernia repairs at the Shouldice Hospital, Bendavid et al. found 52 patients with testicular atrophy (0.08%) (2). They found that the type of hernia (direct, indirect, or combined type) was not a significant factor for the development of a testicular atrophy. Testicular atrophy was 12.7 times more common following repair of recurrent hernias compared to primary hernia repairs. With reoperations for recurrence, it was found that the incidence of testicular atrophy increases by a factor of 3 to 4 with each successive recurrence.

Clinical Features

This develops insidiously, only becoming obvious between 2 and 5 days postoperatively. The patient complains of pain and swelling, and on examination a hard tender cord, epididymis, and testis are found. The testis is also retracted upward in the scrotum (15). The pain and tenderness lasts for several weeks. The swelling lasts even longer and may not resolve even after several months (16).

The ischemic orchitis may subside completely without any residual damage to the testicle, but in some patients testicular atrophy occurs. Should the testicle return to normal size after the initial pain and swelling, this does not mean that the patient will not develop atrophy. It is important that he be reassessed periodically for at least 12 months because atrophy may become apparent during that time (16). Atrophy may develop even after mild ischemic orchitis. The atrophic testis itself is pain free and nontender.

Pathophysiology

The process begins with an intense venous congestion of the testicle with thrombosis of the veins in the spermatic cord, resulting in infarction of the testis.

It was initially thought that the cause of this venous congestion was too tight reconstruction of the inguinal rings, and at the time it was recommended that the patient be taken to the operating room and the rings made wider by releasing the sutures. Wantz suggests it is more likely that extensive dissection within the cord and the cremaster for removal of the sac of the hernia that damages the venous plexus and the venous blood flow (16). He has demonstrated that division of the sac without removal of the distal sac decreases the incidence of ischemic orchitis and subsequent testicular atrophy. Also, patients with varicocele who have the pampiniform plexus of the veins ligated as treatment of their condition do not develop atrophy of the testis. The ligation is done at one level, so the cord is not extensively dissected.

Histologic examination of atrophic testes following ischemic orchitis has revealed that the Leydig's cells and Sertoli's cells are present and appear normal (4). The seminiferous tubules, however, are absent.

Management

Past reports have emphasized the necessity of decompressing the cord by opening the external and internal inguinal rings widely and by incising the capsule of the testicle, but these are no longer utilized. Prevention of this problem is the best option (16). Because of the extensive collateral blood supply of the testicle and the cord, as long as the testicle and cord are not mobilized too extensively and the testicle remains within the scrotum during the hernia repair, the arterial supply should be intact. Removal of the testis from the scrotum or dissection of the spermatic cord distal to the external ring may jeopardize the collateral supply. Under these circumstances, if the testicular artery is ligated, atrophy of the testis could result. In order to completely close the inguinal canal in difficult hernioplasties, Heifetz undertook division of the spermatic cord in 112 patients over a 20-year period (7). He reported swelling and tenderness of the testicles in two thirds of these patients. In 39 patients, testicular atrophy developed. Although the blood supply to these 39 testicles was jeopardized, in the remaining 73 the testicles returned to normal, indicating that the collateral blood supply was quite adequate. The other important preventive measure is not to attempt to remove the distal hernial sac unless it is very small. If it is a large sac, particularly extending into the scrotum, ligation of the neck and division of the sac are adequate (16). The distal sac can be left open and does not usually produce any problems.

For a patient with established ischemic orchitis, there is controversy about certain aspects of its management. All are in agreement that the testicle should not be removed and that surgical intervention does not appear to change the course of events (1,4,10,11,15,16). A Doppler study of the blood flow would be in order to ascertain whether the arterial flow is reaching the testicle. Opening the deep inguinal ring is not a factor to consider because the ring is not a fibrous circular band. Its lateral border is soft, elastic, and muscular, and so indistinct it cannot be palpated, and it would therefore be impossible for it to constrict the cord. The superficial inguinal ring is reconstructed to its original size at the end of the procedure, so it could not really be incriminated as a factor in causing the venous obstruction.

Antibiotics and antiinflammatory drugs have been used, but there is no case on record where actual suppuration of the testicle was found. Steroids have also been given, but it is not certain whether they have a beneficial effect.

CONCLUSIONS

Although these complications involving the testicle are not life threatening, they are frequently the reason for litigation by the patient. It is obvious that they can be avoided in a great majority of patients. This depends on meticulous surgical technique and avoidance of excessive mobilization of the cord and testicle in order to preserve the blood supply. Cord structures must be clearly seen and great care taken not to damage them.

REFERENCES

1. Bendavid R. Complications of groin hernia surgery. *Surg Clin North Am* 1998;78:1089–1101.
2. Bendavid R, Andrews DF, Gilbert AI. Testicular atrophy: incidence and relationship to the type of hernia and to multiple recurrent hernias. *Probl Gen Surg* 1995;12:225–227.
3. Bendavid R. The space of Bogros and the deep inguinal venous circulation. *Surg Gynecol Obstet* 1992;174:355–358.
4. Bohde YG. Condition of testicle after division of cord in treatment of hernia. *Br Med J* 1959;1:1507–1510.
5. Fahlstrom C, Holmberg L, Johansson H. Atrophy of the testis following operations upon the inguinal region in infants and children. *Acta Chir Scand* 1963;126:221–224.
6. Fong Y, Wantz GE. Prevention of ischemic orchitis during inguinal hernioplasty. *Surg Gynecol Obstet* 1992;174:399–402.
7. Heifetz CJ. Resection of the spermatic cord in selected hernias: 20 years' experience. *Arch Surg* 1971;102:36–39.
8. Koontz AR. Atrophy of the testicle as a surgical risk. *Surg Gynecol Obstet* 1965;120:511–513.
9. McFadyen BV, Mathis CR. Inguinal herniorrhaphy: complications and recurrences. *Semin Laparosc Surg* 1994;1:128–140.
10. Misra D, Hewitt G, Potts SR, et al. Inguinal herniotomy in young infants, with emphasis on premature neonates. *J Ped Surg* 1994;29:1496–1498.
11. Murdoch RWG. Testicular strangulation from incarcerated inguinal hernia in infants. *J R Col Surg Edinb* 1979;24:95.
12. Pollak R, Nyhus LM. Complications of groin hernia repair. *Surg Clin North Am* 1983;63:1363–1371.
13. Rowe M, Clatworthy HW. Incarcerated and strangulated hernias in children. *Arch Surg* 1970;101:136.
14. Wantz GE. The Canadian repair of inguinal hernia. In: Nyhus LM, Condon RE, eds. *Hernia,* 3rd ed. Philadelphia: JB Lippincott Co, 1989:236–252.
15. Wantz GE. Testicular atrophy and chronic residual neuralgia as risks of inguinal hernioplasty. *Surg Clin North Am* 1993;73:571–581.
16. Wantz GE. Testicular complications of inguinal hernioplasty. *Probl Gen Surg* 1995;12:219–224.
17. Williams PL, Warwick R. *Gray's anatomy,* 36th ed. London, U.K.: Churchill Livingstone, 1980:718.

SPECIAL COMMENT

Maurice E. Arregui

Although testicular and cord complications are infrequent, they do occur with both open and laparoscopic hernia repairs. This chapter by Dr. Richards very nicely details the more tradition-

ally discussed complications and their explanations. There are other complications that may occur but are less common or more difficult to study. These include transient postoperative testicular pain, infertility, and constriction of the cord at the internal ring. Although infrequent and often clinically not apparent, it is important that we understand how they may occur to avoid these potential injuries.

ENERVATION OF THE TESTIS AND VAS

In most discussions of anatomy and complications of hernia repair, the somatic enervation of the inguinal area is described. What is usually left out is the enervation of the testis and vas deferens via the spermatic plexus. The nerves of the spermatic plexus transmit nociceptive impulses via predominantly sympathetic postganglionic afferent fibers. The spermatic plexus is contributed to from three nerve groups. The superiormost group is from the aortic and renal plexus, the intermediate group is from the superior hypogastric plexus, and the inferiormost group is from the inferior hypogastric plexus, including the vesical plexus supplying mostly parasympathetic fibers to the distal portion of the vas deferens, epididymis, and seminal vesicles. These lower nerves travel along the vas deferens to enter the inguinal canal. The higher spermatic nerves are intimately wrapped around the spermatic artery (2,3).

TESTICULAR PAIN

While usually not a long-term or debilitating problem, testicular pain can be present in up to 2% of patients who have had a laparoscopic extraperitoneal or transperitoneal repair (6,7). The pain most likely is due to the dissection required to separate the peritoneum off the vas deferens and the spermatic artery and vein. Fortunately, the testicular pain is transient, lasting from 1 to 3 weeks. Chronic orchalgia, which is a known complication of vasectomy and other urologic procedures in the scrotum and inguinal area, has not been reported in the hernia literature. One of the listed causes of orchalgia is presence of an inguinal hernia (1). It is uncertain whether this complication does not exist, is underreported, or is mistaken to be genitofemoral, ilioinguinal, or iliohypogastric neuralgia.

FERTILITY PROBLEMS

Although infertility is not usually reported as a complication of hernia repair, a few reports from fertility clinics have shown an association of infertility with previous hernia repair (5,8). Animal studies have shown that overmanipulation or grasping the vas deferens with a clamp can lead to occlusion and infertility. Even unilateral injury to the vas deferens can affect fertility due to the development of antisperm antibodies (4). In laparoscopic and open preperitoneal approaches for placement of a large mesh, and for that matter, open anterior repairs with mesh, the resulting fibrosis of the mesh placed on or in proximity to the vas may have an unknown effect on the function of the vas. Because of the potential injury, it is important that surgeons cautiously handle the vas deferens and spermatic cord contents to avoid potential fertility problems in young men.

CONSTRICTION OF THE CORD STRUCTURES

Although this chapter suggests that constriction of the cord is not a problem with traditional hernia repairs because of the soft muscular outer border that serves to cushion the internal ring, with the increased use of mesh in both open and laparoscopic approaches the resulting fibrosis and contraction of incorporated mesh may lead to a tight internal ring. This may create testicular problems. Although it may not result in ischemia, swelling from venous congestion and testicular pain can occur as it did in one of my patients who underwent a laparoscopic repair with a slit made in the mesh to go around the cord structures. Because of persistent testicular pain and swelling, he underwent laparoscopic exploration. The mesh around the cord at the site of the internal ring had formed a tight band. Following release of the constricting mesh, postoperatively the edema and testicular pain resolved. For this reason, I no longer place slits in preperitoneally placed mesh. I do perform the Lichtenstein repair, which uses a slit to recreate a new internal ring. The new internal ring is so constructed to form an oblique tunnel rather than a ring or slit. This perhaps prevents a constricting band from devel-

oping. As of yet, I have not seen this complication with the Lichtenstein repair.

CONCLUSION

Although seemingly an innocuous operation and commonly performed, inguinal hernia repair done carelessly can result in significant complications. We should constantly remind ourselves of the complexity of the area and the ease with which the inguinal structures can be injured.

REFERENCES

1. Cadeddu JA, Bishoff JT, Chan DY, et al. Laparoscopic testicular denervation for chronic orchalgia. *J Urol* 1999;162:733–735.
2. Choa RG, Swami KS. Testicular denervation. A new surgical procedure for intractable testicular pain. *Brit J Urol* 1992;70:417–419.
3. Gee WF, Ansell JS, Bonica JJ. Pelvic and perineal pain of urologic origin. In: Bonica JJ, ed. *The management of pain.* Philadelphia: Lea & Febiger, 1990:1368–1373.
4. Litwin D. Risks to fertility with laparoscopic mesh repair. In: Arregui ME, Nagan RF, eds. *Inguinal hernia: advances or controversies?* Oxford, England: Radcliffe Medical Press, 1994:191–194.
5. Matsuda T, Horii Y, Yoshida O. Unilateral obstruction of the vas deferens caused by childhood inguinal herniorrhaphy in male infertility patients. *Fertil Steril* 1992;58:609–613.
6. Schurz JV, Tetik C, Arregui ME, et al. Complications and recurrences associated with laparoscopic inguinal hernia repair. *Probl Gen Surg* 1995;12:191–196.
7. Tetik C, Arregui ME, Castro D, et al. Complications and recurrences associated with laparoscopic repair of groin hernias. A multi-institutional retrospective analysis. *Surg Endosc* 1994;8: 1316–1322.
8. Yavetz H, Harash B, Yoger L, et al. Fertility of men following inguinal hernia repair. *Andrologia* 1991;23:443–446.

Nyhus and Condon's Hernia, Fifth Edition, edited by Robert J. Fitzgibbons, Jr. and A. Gerson Greenburg. Lippincott Williams & Wilkins, Philadelphia © 2002.

27

THE PHYSIOLOGY AND ANATOMY OF CHRONIC PAIN AFTER INGUINAL HERNIORRHAPHY

JOHANN CUNNINGHAM

This chapter on chronic pain will give the reader a basic understanding of the issues at hand in the patient with chronic pain after an inguinal hernia repair. First, the physiology of chronic pain and how it relates to the groin is discussed. Second, the nervous anatomy is reviewed, showing the areas where damage to structures may result in chronic pain. Finally, specific causes of chronic pain that do not fall into the previous groups are outlined.

It is estimated that in 1996 approximately 696,000 inguinal hernia repairs were done in the United States. The occurrence of chronic pain has been estimated at 5% to 15% (7,16,18). This means that 34,800 people per year develop chronic pain. This is a huge number for such a benign procedure. Not all are incapacitated by it. Some just notice it on occasion, reminding them that they have had a repair. Others limit their activity, either out of fear that they may get a recurrence because they feel pain, or because the pain is of such severity that the anticipation of it is enough to alter their lifestyle. In some patients, the pain is so constant and severe that their "tasks of daily living" are affected. They need a cane, can no longer drive, and often are very litigious. Nothing seems to work when trying to alleviate them of their pain. They end up in chronic pain clinics, using copious amounts of narcotics, and weigh upon their surgeon. In all probability, the surgeon did an excellent operation in which nothing went wrong. However, all too often the hernia repair is squeezed in at the end of a long list. Residents go "solo" for the first time with a hernia repair. The surgeon must understand that hernia repair is not a simple procedure but one requiring precise skill and judgment to give the patient a repair that is not only durable but also enjoyable. Even then, there will be those who develop chronic pain despite the best possible management. Those who have chronic pain are more likely to be depressed or have anxiety. They are more likely to have psychological illness (9). This is a huge social and economic cost to society as a result of an operation that was only meant to correct a small defect in the lower abdomen.

Pain, and in particular chronic pain, following inguinal herniorrhaphy is one of the least appreciated and yet most common complications of inguinal herniorrhaphy (7). Most research has focused on the prevention of recurrences. This is an easy end point for studies as this is an easily measured outcome. Yet pain is more common and can be more debilitating, affecting the quality of life more dramatically than a simple recurrence. Surgeons have long recognized chronic pain as a complication of inguinal hernia repair (13,18) and, as with all surgical procedures, advances have been made to reduce the amount of postoperative pain, both acute and chronic. Attempts to alleviate chronic pain have been primarily preventive in nature. There are, however, no good prospective controlled studies on the prevention or management of chronic pain (3,15). Emphasis has rightly been on preventing damage to the surrounding tissues (such as placing stitches in the symphysis pubis or around the ilioinguinal nerve, or not making the internal ring too tight), for once the pain is established it is difficult to manage (1,19). An understanding of the anatomy and physiology of chronic pain in the inguinal region helps to provide the best management plan for this potentially disabling complication (11). There is extensive literature on the incidence of pain in the immediate and early postoperative period. There are also a large number of studies looking at the different techniques of managing pain in the immediate postoperative period. A lot of the outcome studies comparing different operative techniques look at the early postoperative pain as a measure of how good the techniques are relative to each other (3). None, however, considers the incidence or severity of

J. Cunningham: Department of Surgery, University of British Columbia; Trauma Services, Vancouver General Hospital, Vancouver, British Columbia.

chronic postoperative pain as an outcome measure. Few studies differentiate as to the etiology of the pain, preferring to group all sources of pain together as a single entity. Chronic pain in general has been poorly studied by surgeons and is seldom reported in the surgical literature. Those who do report it do not differentiate between neuropathic and nociceptive pain, though they are quite different in their presentation and findings. Neuropathic pain can best be described as a brief, sharp, jabbing or electrical pain. It is of nervous etiology. There is an abnormality in conduction. Nociceptive pain is a dull, burning, tugging type of pain. It is akin to ligamentous or tendon injury. It can be somatic or visceral in origin. The nervous conducting system is intact. Classic causes of chronic pain, such as osteitis pubis and ilioinguinal nerve entrapment, are reported, not for their incidence as a complication of the multitude of new repairs, but rather from a management perspective (5,11). The majority of chronic pain has been attributed to ilioinguinal nerve entrapment. This ignores the large number of patients who have only intermittent episodes of pain that is not disabling on a day-to-day basis, yet can be severe enough that it has resulted in a lifestyle change for the patient. A lot of these patients have nociceptive pain from sutures or staples in ligamentous structures. It is well recognized that severe pain in the groin, genitalia, or upper thigh can lead to sexual dysfunction and loss of libido, and so loss of well-being. Injury to the vas deferens can lead to just such a situation (2). No surgeon would think of including the inability to continue playing sports because of chronic pain as a complication of their hernia repair, yet there are patients who, when taking a golf swing, get a sharp shooting pain in the groin. This affects their swing, so that they can no longer play to their previous caliber. A thorough understanding of the anatomy of inguinal region and its innervation is necessary to correctly diagnose the etiology of a patient's chronic pain.

PHYSIOLOGY

Pain is defined as "an unpleasant sensory and emotional experience associated with actual or potential tissue damage, or described in terms of such damage" by the International Association for the Study of Pain (14). This means that several components must be in place. First, there must be an intact neural path from the nociceptor to the brain (Fig. 27.1). This means that there is an event that causes a nerve

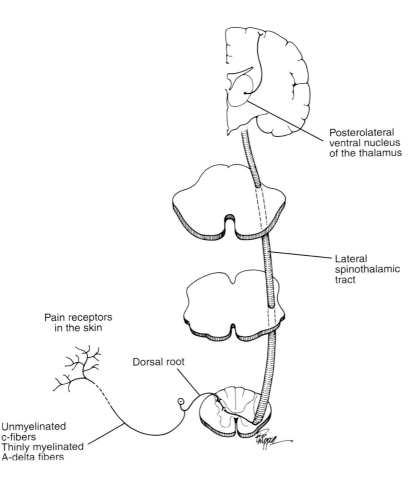

FIGURE 27.1. A diagram of an intact neural pathway. The stimulus originates in the nociceptor. It is then transmitted along the primary afferents. They synapse in the dorsal horn. The secondary afferent then decussates and travels along the lateral spinothalamic tract to the thalamus. From there, the message is transmitted to the cortical level.

receptor (nociceptor) to convert the event (heat, stretch, position, etc.) into an electrochemical message that travels along the spinothalamic tract to the thalamus and on to the cortex. Next, the stimulus must then be perceived as painful. If there is no perception with the associated emotional response, we do not have pain. Finally, the perception and expression of the pain in a patient is affected by the person's emotional state and environment. The same stimulus in a calm, reassuring environment may be perceived as less painful than the identical stimulus when the patient is alone, worried, and overwhelmed. Pain itself can be divided into two types: nociceptive and neuropathic (Table 27.1). Nociceptive pain can be subdivided into two groups: somatic and visceral. Four processes are required for somatic pain perception: transduction, transmission, modulation, and perception. There are specific nociceptors in the cardiovascular, respiratory, gastrointestinal, and genitourinary systems. Neuropathic pain is a result of injury to a neural structure. This injury results in the spontaneous and atopic firing of the nerves. Neuropathic pain is subdivided into three subgroups: peripherally generated, centrally generated, and sympathetically maintained. This is characterized by autonomic dysregulation. A classic example is reflex sympathetic dystrophy, where one sees vasomotor changes, edema, sweating, and eventual atrophy. It is important that the various types of pain be differentiated as their management can be quite different. Groin pain as a result of a high lumbar disc protrusion will not respond to a neurectomy of the ilioinguinal nerve, even though the pain felt is very similar.

Pain itself can be acute or chronic: in acute pain there is a stimulation of a nociceptor. This can be a pain receptor in the skin or a stretch receptor in the bowel wall. This results in an appropriate physiologic response of pain perception as well as the associated autonomic hyperactivity: hypertension, tachycardia, sweating, vasoconstriction, etc. It implies an intact neurologic system. The acute pain is a response to actual or impending tissue damage and ceases when the threat is removed or the damage ceases. Its purpose is to protect the organism from harm.

Chronic pain is the perception of pain when there is little or no threat to the tissue, yet the patient perceives the pain as if the area were being damaged. There is no associated autonomic response. This is both a psychological as well as a physiologic alteration in response. The actual function of the nervous system is reorganized (neuroplasticity). This is not just a peripheral event secondary to tissue damage, but a central sensitization where target cells modify their gene expression, resulting in enhanced response to future stimuli (6). There are physiologic, biochemical, cellular, and molecular changes that occur in the central nervous system, resulting in a "reprogramming" of the perception of pain rather than just a continuance of noxious stimuli. Furthermore, as there are cortical changes, factors such as stress, secondary gain, or financial compensation may all affect change here. There is lowering of the threshold for excitation of neurons and nociceptors. Therefore, one can get excitation of neurons without stimulation of the nociceptor (atopic firing), or one can have a lowering of the excitation threshold so that nerves and nociceptors fire at lower levels of stimuli. All this results in a reduction of the pain threshold (allodynia). There is also an exaggerated or increased response to noxious stimuli (hyperalgesia). The pain is deemed to be chronic if it persists more than 3 to 6 months after the injury. The irony of the situation is that the initial injury may have long since healed. Chronic pain is an inappropriate response to an innocuous stimulus. Though there is no reason to suppose that the nerves of the groin are in any way privileged, Kennedy et al. (10) showed that some patients who had chronic inguinal pain for at least 3 years did well after ilioinguinal and genitofemoral neurectomy. If these patients had central neuroplasticity, one would not expect to see improvement. It may be that there is a variable degree of neuroplasticity, as 40% of patients did not show complete resolution of their symptoms. One must remember that even if a patient has longstanding pain, it may not be chronic pain. For example, patients who have a hernia recurrence, abscess, foreign body granuloma, impaired flow to the testis from too tight an internal ring, or a stitch through the periosteum of the symphysis pubis (osteitis pubis) may have ongoing pain of a chronic nature but not necessarily chronic pain. These patients have recurring painful events or continuous pain because there is ongoing tissue damage with every movement. Once the underlying cause is identified and fixed,

TABLE 27.1. CLASSIFICATION OF CHRONIC PAIN

Classification	Symptoms	Example
Nociceptive		
Somatic	Aching, gnawing, throbbing, cramping	Incisional pain
Visceral dysejaculation	Colicky, squeezing	Early appendicitis
Neuropathic	Sharp, electrical, burning	
Centrally generated		Spinal cord injury
Peripherally generated		Postherpetic pain
		Ilioinguinal neuralgia
Sympathetically maintained		Reflex sympathetic dystrophy

their pain should resolve. It is therefore of vital importance to be able to identify those patients who have ongoing pain from a correctable cause from those who have chronic pain with neuroplasticity. Unfortunately, many in the former group, simply because of the duration of the pain, may develop chronic pain. This entity is a lot more difficult to treat and in many cases does not resolve despite the best medical and surgical interventions. Some of these patients stay on lifelong medication for the pain (7,18).

The surgeon who wants to be able to identify and manage chronic pain in the postoperative patient must do a careful history and physical to delineate the nature and the source of the pain. This includes associated signs and symptoms, such as the nature and duration of the pain, as well as localization and reproducibility of the areas of hyperalgesia, hyperesthesia, hypoesthesia, and anesthesia. Local areas of anesthesia and hyperesthesia are not uncommon in patients with chronic pain after hernia repair. Dysesthesia and allodynia are less common. Patients who have postoperative anesthetic areas are also more likely to have chronic pain. Careful examination may reveal which of the nerves, if any, are involved. However, up to 20% of patients with inguinal incisions have associated numbness up to 2 years postoperatively. Most of these have no associated concurrent nerve or tendon injury, but rather have an area of anesthesia caused by the division of the small nerve fibers that innervate the skin just inferomedial to the incision. This area is

about 2 to 5 cm wide and runs the length of the incision along its inferior border (Fig. 27.2). At 1 year post–hernia repair, 25% of patients have the anesthetic area. At 2 years, there is a small decrease to 20%. Interestingly enough, most patients are unaware that they have this anesthetic area, and they do not complain about it.

Nociceptive Pain

Nociceptive somatic pain is akin to ligamentous or tendon injury. As in other parts of the body, the pain is a tugging, burning, dull type of pain, which is brought on by lifting or stretching. The patient may have a dull background ache not associated with activity. The flares of pain could last for several hours and could be aggravated by abdominal muscle use or stretch. Most patients prevent or reduce the severity of pain on standing up by pressing over the tender area. This also works for other activities involving abdominal muscle contraction or stretching. On a visual analog pain scale, patients have an average of "2," with the worst pain being "7" ("0" being no pain and "10" being the worst pain possible). These patients on physical examination have an area of tenderness over the medial insertion of the inguinal ligament. Carnett's maneuver may worsen the patient's pain (4). Here, the examiner palpates the affected part of the anterior abdominal wall with the patient tensing the abdomen by raising his head off the bed or doing a partial sit-up. Carnett's sign (relief of ten-

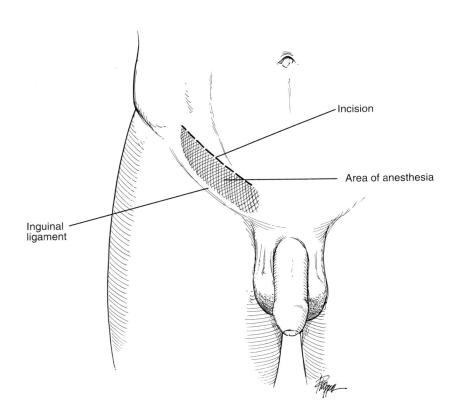

FIGURE 27.2. Normal area of postoperative anesthesia after inguinal hernia repair.

derness or pain) is indicative of intraabdominal pathology. Worsening of the pain with tension (muscle contraction) is consistent with nociceptive abdominal wall pathology. These patients have poor results with ilioinguinal or iliohypogastric nerve blocks or neurectomy. Heat, antiinflammatories, and local injection help these patients somewhat (18). The etiology is not clearly understood. It may be a strain of the pectineal muscle. Others suggest that the suture material is at fault (Silen W, personal communication, 1999). Either the suture is too unyielding and cuts into the tissue when tension (such as a sneeze or cough) is applied, or the sutures are spaced too far apart, resulting in a concentration of force over a relatively small area when increased strain is applied. Either way, these patients obtain relief of their pain with the removal of the suture.

Visceral neuropathic pain is rare in the groin. Bendavid (2) has described a syndrome of "dysejaculation," where the patient feels a searing, burning sensation just prior to, during, or after ejaculation. The incidence is about 0.04%. It is probably caused by a partial obstruction of the vas deferens from trauma or scar, though another etiology is that the somatic sacral or sympathetic nerves are damaged, resulting in dyssynergia of the ejaculatory effector muscles (7).

Neuropathic Pain

Neuropathic pain presents as jabbing, electrical, or brief, sharp pain. It may be provoked by movement, or it may

occur spontaneously. The jabs of pain may be single or may occur as multiple bursts of jabbing pain over a span of time. It is unpredictable and may have no associated trigger. In some patients, there may be a defined movement or position that triggers the pain. The pain is maximal almost instantaneously and then is gone 30 to 60 seconds later. There is rarely any residual pain, but frequently the patient's activity is interrupted. Furthermore, patients who have a specific trigger avoid the motion or position that causes the pain, altering their lifestyle and affecting the quality of life despite the brevity of the actual painful stimulus. These symptoms can occur concurrently with those of somatic ligamentous pain. It is important to identify these as two separate types of pain requiring individual management, for the management of one may not result in the relief of the other. Physical examination may show an area of anesthesia or hypoesthesia associated with the respective affected inguinal nerve (Fig. 27.3). This may include numbness on the medial thigh (which is innervated by the genitofemoral nerve). The area of anesthesia must be carefully delineated, as it must not be confused with the periincisional anesthetic area previously described. Chevrel and Gutt (5) have further divided the neuropathic pain into three groups by the anatomic defect (Table 27.2). The symptoms are different for each cause, even though there is a large amount of overlap between presentations. This allows one to better approach the patient with neuropathic pain. If the pain is that of a neuroma, local injection or a simple division of the

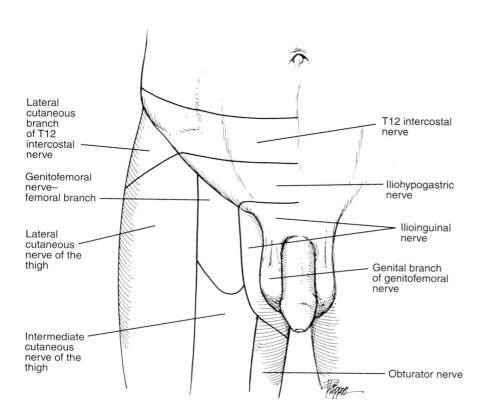

FIGURE 27.3. Sensory innervation of the groin and anterior thigh.

Lateral cutaneous branch of T12 intercostal nerve

Genitofemoral nerve–femoral branch

Lateral cutaneous nerve of the thigh

Intermediate cutaneous nerve of the thigh

T12 intercostal nerve

Iliohypogastric nerve

Ilioinguinal nerve

Genital branch of genitofemoral nerve

Obturator nerve

TABLE 27.2. ANATOMIC CLASSIFICATION OF NEUROPATHIC PAIN IN THE POSTHERNIORRHAPHY PATIENT

Neuroma pain	Most common Proliferation of nerve fibers outside the neurolemma after complete or partial division of the nerve	Hyperesthesia along corresponding dermatome Exquisite pain at neuroma Electrical in nature
Deafferentation pain	Partial or complete transection of nerve or entrapment in a suture or staple Chronic paroxysmal episodes	Burning pain Initial area of anesthesia with adjacent hypoesthesia Later hyperesthesia and contact dysesthesia in the innervated dermatome
Projected pain	Intact nerve entrapped in scar, staple, or suture	Pain elicited by light touch along course of the nerve

nerve just lateral to the neuroma should be adequate. If the pain is consistent with scarring of the nerve, with no well-defined point, local injection will have little effect and neurolysis has to be done more laterally to ensure that the nerve is free from scar. Patients with onlay mesh and tension-free repairs are not immune from chronic pain. Patients report neuropathic pain despite the fact there are few stitches or staples. The likely causes for this are either that the large amount of scar that a mesh provokes envelops the nerves, or as the divided nerve ends regenerate they come in contact with the mesh and become irritable (1). Finally, many patients, though not disabled by the repair, are quite aware that they have a mesh plug in place.

ANATOMY

The nervous anatomy of the region is quite variable, with 60% of patients showing variations of greater and lesser degree from the norm (15). However, an understanding of the normal anatomy and the areas in which the various nerves are at risk will prevent damage to them and prevent the potential for chronic pain. The inguinal region is innervated by the ilioinguinal, iliohypogastric, and genitofemoral nerves (Figs. 27.4 and 27.5). A fourth nerve, the femoral nerve, though not technically part of the inguinal region as it lies deep to the ligament, is at risk as well. It is these nerves that also are at greatest risk of injury during surgery or during the healing phase.

The lumbar plexus lies in the posterior part of the psoas major muscle. It consists of the ventral rami of L1-3 and most of L-4. It also has a branch from T-12. The gray rami communicantes join adjacent to the origin of the rami. The first lumbar ramus then divides in two, the upper branch forming the iliohypogastric and ilioinguinal nerves, the lower branch joining with the second lumbar ramus to form the genitofemoral nerve. The remainder of the second as well as the third and fourth rami fuse into ventral and dorsal trunks. The ventral trunk becomes the obturator

nerve and the dorsal trunk becomes the lateral femoral cutaneous nerve of the thigh. The lumbar plexus is well protected by muscle and retroperitoneal fat and so is out of harm's way during both open and laparoscopic herniorrhaphy. It is at risk of damage during epidural anesthesia. Disc herniation or foraminal impingement on the nerve roots as they exit the spinal canal may be a source of referred pain to the groin. L1-4 disc herniation or osteophyte impingement is uncommon, but certainly may be cause for chronic pain. This must be entertained in the patient with previous hernia repair and new onset of chronic pain in whom other modalities of treatment have failed.

The iliohypogastric nerve emerges as the upper branch of the first lumbar ramus. It emerges lateral to the psoas muscle and runs in front of the quadratus lumborum muscle. Above the iliac crest, it perforates the transversus abdominus to provide the musculature with its innervation. Here, it divides into two branches, the lateral branch passing through internal and external oblique just above the iliac crest to supply the posterolateral gluteal skin. The anterior cutaneus branch runs between the transversus abdominus muscle and internal oblique muscle until about 2 cm medial to the anterosuperior iliac spine, where it passes through the internal oblique muscle. It then proceeds medially and pierces the external oblique aponeurosis above the external ring. It innervates the suprapubic skin and has branches to the subcostal and ilioinguinal nerves. The nerve is at risk of damage in two areas. Laparoscopically, it can be damaged internally as staples are placed through the transversus abdominus, anchoring in the internal oblique muscle. This has been recognized as a cause of postoperative and chronic pain in laparoscopic hernia repair. It can be avoided by minimizing the number of staples placed laterally and ensuring that they do not penetrate too deeply. A low, laterally placed trocar may also damage this nerve. It is again at risk during open herniorrhaphy when dissecting above the inguinal canal after dividing the external oblique aponeurosis, especially if a high incision is used initially. Other incisions such as appendectomy incisions, C-section incisions, and previous hernia incisions may all alter the

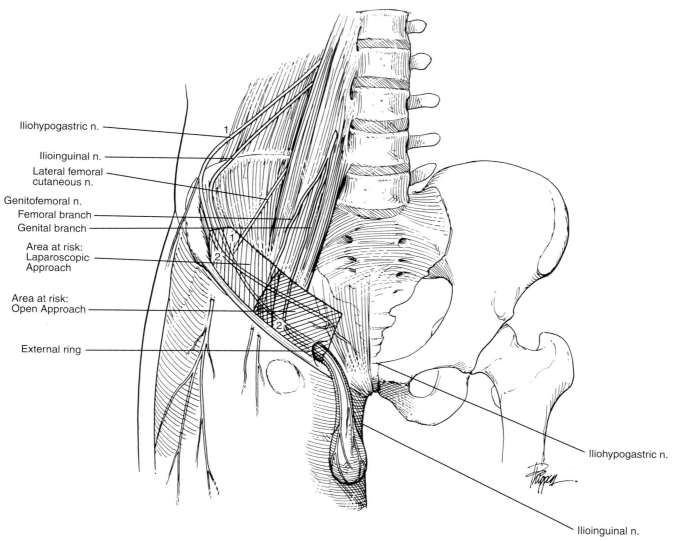

FIGURE 27.4. Iliohypogastric and ilioinguinal nerves showing the areas at risk in laparoscopic and open herniorrhaphy. *1*, point at which the nerve pierces the transversus abdominus muscle; *2*, point at which the nerve pierces the internal oblique muscle.

course of the nerve or even entrap the nerve, putting it at risk of damage and chronic pain.

The ilioinguinal nerve is the inferior branch of the L-1 ramus. It emerges from behind the psoas along with or just inferior to the iliohypogastric nerve. It passes obliquely across the quadratus lumborum muscle, perforates the transversus abdominus muscle near the anterior end of the iliac crest, and then pierces the internal oblique muscle to run along the inguinal canal until it leaves by the external ring. It may do so by exiting directly through the ring or by piercing the fascia just adjacent to the ring. It provides motor function to the internal oblique and sensory innervation to the medial thigh and scrotum or mons pubis and adjacent labia majora. It is this nerve that is classically described as the primary cause of chronic pain. Certainly, its course is straight through the center of the operative field. However,

in our study of chronic pain, we could not identify a specific cause for the nerve becoming involved (7). It did not matter if the surgeon had identified and protected the nerve, divided the nerve, or simply ignored the nerve; all had the same incidence of chronic pain. Intuitively, dividing the nerve should have the lowest incidence of chronic pain, as this is a means of treatment for ilioinguinal neuralgia. However this was not borne out in the results, indicating that nerve encasement by scar is probably a more common cause of chronic pain than direct injury to the nerve.

The genitofemoral nerve arises from the L-2 ramus. It passes obliquely through the psoas muscle, exiting on the medial border near the L-4 spinous process. It then travels caudally on the psoas, passing behind the ureter and dividing superior to the inguinal ligament. The genital branch follows the external iliac artery, passes through the internal

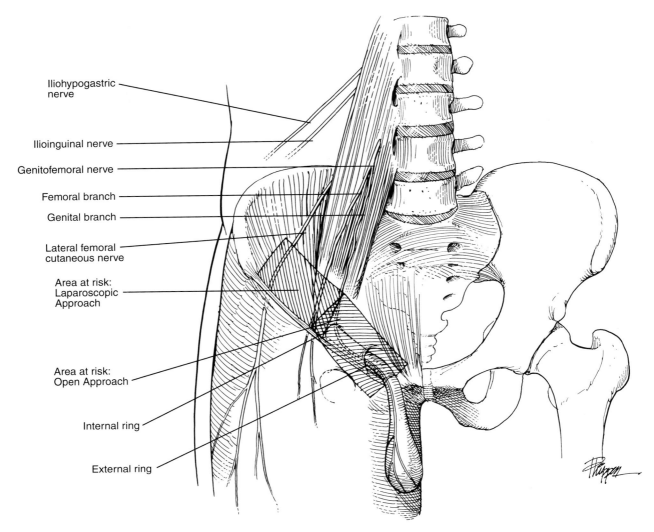

FIGURE 27.5. Genitofemoral nerve and lateral cutaneous nerve to the thigh showing the areas at risk in laparoscopic and open herniorrhaphy. *1*, internal ring; *2*, point at which the nerve pierces the deep fascia.

Iliohypogastric nerve

Ilioinguinal nerve

Genitofemoral nerve

Femoral branch

Genital branch

Lateral femoral cutaneous nerve

Area at risk: Laparoscopic Approach

Area at risk: Open Approach

Internal ring

External ring

ring into the inguinal canal and innervates the cremasteric muscle and scrotal skin or mons pubis and labia majora. There is a lot of cross innervation of the nerves, so that even when one nerve is divided proximally, there is seldom complete anesthesia, but rather hypoesthesia in the affected area. The femoral branch passes laterally to the iliac artery then behind the inguinal ligament, then traverses the femoral sheath anterior to the femoral artery and supplies the skin anterior to the femoral triangle. If the cord is skeletonized one can get anesthesia on the scrotum from division of the genital branch. This is routine in a Shouldice repair. It is sacrificed when doing hernia repairs in women; however, they may have decreased sensation in the labia majora.

The lateral femoral cutaneous nerve is formed from the dorsal branches of L-2 and L-3. It emerges at the lateral border of the psoas muscle. It traverses the iliacus muscle and

passes through or behind the inguinal ligament just medial to the anterosuperior iliac spine. It then divides with the anterior branch, supplying the anterior and lateral thigh to the knee, the posterior supplying the lateral thigh from greater trochanter to midthigh. It is at the extreme lateral edge of the surgical field in open herniorrhaphy, but can be at risk for damage and chronic pain if an incision is extended too far laterally, redo surgery is done, or the surgeon infiltrates laterally, injuring the nerve in the process. It has a distinctive distribution in that it innervates the leg below the inguinal ligament. It is at greater risk of damage in laparoscopic hernia repair, where a laterally placed staple may catch the nerve, causing chronic pain (neuralgia paresthetica) remote from the operative area.

The femoral nerve runs its course lateral to the iliac artery. It lies deep to the inguinal ligament. It provides motor function to the iliacus, pectineus, sartorius, and quadriceps muscles. Articular branches supply the hip and knee joints. Cutaneous sensory branches are the intermediate and medial cutaneous nerves and the saphenous nerve. They supply sensation to the anterior and medial aspect of the thigh distal to the genitofemoral nerve and medial to the lateral cutaneous nerve of the thigh. The saphenous nerve supplies sensation to the medial aspect of the knee and calf as far as the ankle. The femoral nerve is at risk during laparoscopic herniorrhaphy if the surgeon decides to place a staple low and lateral to the iliac vessels. It is also at risk with open herniorrhaphy if the surgeon decides to tighten the internal ring with a laterally placed stitch. If it is placed too deeply, one can catch the nerve, resulting in chronic pain.

OTHER CAUSES OF PAIN

Ligation of the hernia sac has been implicated in chronic pain from the constriction of the suture on the sac. Smedberg et al. (17) did a prospective randomized study of the complications of a high ligation of the hernia sac. They found a significant difference in the amount of postoperative pain at 6 weeks. They also showed that there was no difference in the early recurrence rate. Our study, in which all sacs were ligated, failed to show a difference in chronic pain between patients with a direct and indirect inguinal hernia. As it is no longer common practice to close the peritoneum on abdominal surgery, it behooves us to apply the same standard in an inguinal hernia repair and not ligate the sac. The added benefit is that it reduces the risk of bowel or bladder injury from an injudiciously placed stitch or tie.

Osteitis pubis has almost become of historic interest. As inguinal surgery has evolved, surgeons no longer place sutures through the periosteum at the symphysis pubis. This has resulted in a marked decrease of osteitis pubis. It still must be carefully differentiated from a pectineus insertion injury (12). The latter usually resolves spontaneously, whereas the former is a lot more persistent and may require surgery to remove the offending suture or staple. Patients, however, are at greater risk of recurrence at the medial end of the posterior wall repair as stitches are placed more laterally, leaving a small opening at the medial end. Furthermore, as more and more surgeons do tension-free repairs, less suture, especially suture under tension, is being placed in or near the periosteum. Laparoscopic surgery with the use of larger staples is again putting the periosteum within reach and the patient at risk for osteitis pubis. Staples should never be placed directly into bone.

CONCLUSION

Chronic pain has long been underestimated, in both its frequency and its severity. We looked at 883 hernia repairs, of which we were able to examine 315 at 1 and 2 years postoperatively. Our recurrence rate was less than 5%, yet at 1 year 63% and at 2 years 54% of patients still complained of mild, moderate, or severe pain. Mild pain was defined as an occasional pain or discomfort that did not limit activity, with a return to prehernia lifestyle. Moderate pain was defined as pain preventing return to normal preoperative activities (i.e., inability to continue with prehernia activities such as golf, tennis, or other sports, and inability to lift objects, without pain, that the patient had been lifting before the hernia occurrence). Severe pain was defined as pain that incapacitated the patient at frequent intervals or interfered with the activities of daily living (i.e., a pain constantly present or intermittently so severe as to impair normal activities such as walking). Greater than 10% of patients had pain 2 years postoperatively that caused them to alter their lifestyle. As our understanding of chronic pain improves, surgeons will start to include chronic pain as an outcome in their studies. It is a more significant problem than recurrence or immediate postoperative pain. There is a lot of literature on the management of acute pain in the post-herniorrhaphy patient. Lichtenstein et al. (12) and Geis (8) have proposed algorithms for the management of chronic pain. If a surgeon treats a herniorrhaphy with the same respect as a total thyroidectomy or an aortobifemoral bypass, then and only then will the patient have the best possible result. If a patient does develop chronic pain, then using the anatomy and physiology presented here, the surgeon should be able to diagnose the cause of the pain.

REFERENCES

1. Bendavid R. Complications of groin hernia surgery. *Surg Clin North Am* 1998;78:1091–1103.
2. Bendavid R. Dysejaculation. *Probl Gen Surg* 1995;12:237–238.
3. Callesen T, Kehlet H. Postherniorrhaphy pain. *Anesthesiology* 1997;87:1219–1230.
4. Carnett JB. Intercostal neuralgia as a cause of abdominal pain and tenderness. *Surg Gynecol Obstet* 1926;42:625–632.
5. Chevrel JP, Gutt MT. The treatment of neuralgias following inguinal herniorrhaphy: a report of 47 cases. *Postgrad Gen Surg* 1992;4:142–147.
6. Coderre TJ, Katz J, Vaccarino AL, et al. Contribution of central neuroplasticity to pathological pain: review of clinical and experimental evidence. *Pain* 1993;52:259–285.
7. Cunningham J, Temple WJ, Mitchell P, et al. Co-operative hernia study: pain in the postrepair patient. *Ann Surg* 1996;224:598–602.
8. Geis WP. Pain and neurological findings following inguinal herniorrhaphy: an algorithm for treatment. Paper presented at: Hernia Repair: Annual Meeting of the American Hernia Society: Las Vegas, February 1999.
9. Gureje O, Von Korff M, Simon GE, et al. Persistent pain and well being: a World Health Organization study in primary care. *JAMA* 1998;280:147–151.
10. Kennedy EM, Harms BA, Starling JR. Absence of maladaptive

neuronal plasticity after genitofemoral-ilioinguinal neurectomy. *Surgery* 1994;116:665–671.

11. Kraehenbuehl L, Striffeler H, Baer HU, et al. Retroperitoneal endoscopic neurectomy for nerve entrapment after hernia repair. *Br J Surg* 1997;84:216–219.

12. Lichtenstein IL, Shulman AG, Amid PK, et al. Cause and prevention of postherniorrhaphy neuralgia: a proposed protocol for treatment. *Am J Surg* 1988;155:786–790.

13. Magee RK. Genitofemoral causalgia (a new syndrome). *Can Med Assoc J* 1942;46:326—329.

14. Merskey H. Classification of chronic pain descriptions of chronic pain syndrome and definitions of pain terms. *Pain* 1986;[Suppl 3]:S217.

15. Moosman DA, Oelrich TM. Prevention of accidental trauma to the ilioinguinal nerve during inguinal herniorrhaphy. *Am J Surg* 1977;133:146–148.

16. Pollack R, Nights LM. Complications of groin hernia repair. *Surg Clin North Am* 1983;63:1363–1371.

17. Smedberg SGG, Broome AEA, Gullmo A. Ligation of the hernial sac? *Surg Clin North Am* 1984;64:299–306.

18. Wantz GE. Complications of inguinal hernial repair. *Surg Clin North Am* 1984;64:287–298.

28

AN ALGORITHM FOR THE TREATMENT OF CHRONIC GROIN PAIN AFTER INGUINAL HERNIORRHAPHY

W. PETER GEIS
KULDEEP SINGH
G. KEVIN GILLIAN

The occurrence of chronic pain in the inguinal area following inguinal hernia repair has been known for many years. In various literature reports over the past 60 years, the prevalence of chronic pain or neuralgia ranges from approximately 2% to 12% (2,3,5,9). The three nerves most commonly implicated in postoperative inguinodynia following open hernia repair are the ilioinguinal, iliohypogastric, and genitofemoral (9). In the absence of signs of infection, inguinodynia following open hernia repair prior to 1980 was usually limited to physical injury to one of the nearby nerves during the procedure, direct trauma to the pubic bone, or a hidden/incarcerated hernia either missed during the initial procedure or immediately recurrent following the procedure. Since 1980, a gradual increase in the routine use of mesh in the inguinal space during inguinal and/or femoral hernia repair has occurred. The additional fibroblastic stimulus caused by the polypropylene-type meshes added a fibrotic entrapment mechanism to the list of causes of postoperative inguinal pain. Finally, the addition of laparoscopy in approximately 1990 added the laparoscopic staple and other transfixing mechanisms as possible causes of nerve entrapment and subsequent pain. Further, the addition of the laparoscopic route added the risk of injury to the laterofemoral cutaneous nerve of the thigh, the femoral nerve, and the obturator nerve. Clearly, the mechanism of pain, the pattern of pain development, and the distribution of pain must be considered in the etiology and treatment of postherniorrhaphy inguinodynia.

MECHANISM OF PAINFUL SYNDROMES

Chronic pain after inguinal hernia repair may have its origin from many structures. Inguinodynia is the recommended generic term for chronic groin pain after hernia repair and should replace neuralgias or mesh inguinodynia for the sake of uniformity and avoidance of confusion in the literature.

The most common type of chronic pain is "somatic-type" pain (3). This is a dull, sharp, aching, pulling, etc., type of pain that is usually localized and pinpoint, and becomes aggravated by physical activity. It lasts more than a few hours and gradually subsides in 3 to 4 days (3). The commonly cited mechanisms are pulling or tension on osseoligamentous structures, and prevention of gliding mechanism of three layers of abdominal wall by transfixing sutures as in anterior repairs. Though Cunningham et al. have alluded to this problem and suggested preventive techniques (avoidance of periosteal tissue), there is no suggested method of treatment in the literature (3).

The second most common type of pain is neuralgic or neuropathic. It is described as burning, constant pain with no physical aggravating or relieving factors (3). This occurs due to injury, entrapment, stretching, or chronic irritation of the peripheral nerve or nerves. Since both ilioinguinal and iliohypogastric nerves are in harm's way in anterior repairs, they are the most common nerves involved in neuralgic pain syndromes. These injuries are often associated with a Tinel's sign on physical examination. In 1942, Magee described genitofemoral neuralgia, which is now being recognized more often as a cause of

W. P. Geis: St. Joseph Medical Center, Jordan Center, MISTI, Towson, Maryland; Department of Surgery, Saint Peters University Hospital, New Brunswick, New Jersey.

K. Singh: Department of Surgery, St. Agnes Healthcare, Baltimore, Maryland.

G. K. Gillian: Division of General Surgery, Southern Maryland Hospital Center, Clinton, Maryland.

chronic groin pain after hernia repairs (10). Despite different dermatome involvement, clinical differentiation of ilioinguinal–iliohypogastric neuralgia from genitofemoral neuralgia can be very difficult and confusing (15). The best way to distinguish these two entities is by selective nerve blocks (15).

The reported incidence of inguinodynia following open anterior repair is 2% to 12% (Table 28.1) (1–3, 5,9,12,13,17). Studies by Starling and Harms suggest involvement of both ilioinguinal–iliohypogastric and genitofemoral nerves in these syndromes (15). The introduction of laparoscopic hernia repair added another facet to this equation. Fitzgibbons et al. noted a rather dramatic decrease in postoperative neuralgias following laparoscopic hernia repair, from 12% to 4%, and attributed the decrease to better understanding of groin anatomy, associated with avoidance of nerves while stapling the mesh (5). Further, two other studies have demonstrated either similar or fewer groin pain syndromes following laparoscopic inguinal hernia repair (Table 28.1) compared to anterior approaches to herniorrhaphy.

Sporadic reports of femoral nerve entrapment or obturator nerve entrapment have been published following laparoscopic hernia repair, implicating laparoscopic staples as the causative agent for entrapment and neuralgia. Postoperative inguinodynia may also be caused by the technical and/or physiologic results of the surgical procedure that do not entrap specific nerves.

Suture or staple placement into the periosteal tissue of the pubic bone seems to be the most common cause of postherniorrhaphy inguinal pain (3). Further, a missed or hidden hernia may be the cause of persistent postoperative pain. Other traumatic events, including chronic inflammation of the appendix associated with a laparoscopic staple or suture that has transfixed the tip of the appendix, may cause pain in the inguinal area. We have observed two femoral hernias that were missed during inguinal hernia repairs, each of which caused a chronic and persistent inguinal pain. We have also identified two patients with chronic appendicitis secondary to a staple placed through the peritoneum during a preperitoneal laparoscopic hernia repair, causing chronic appendicitis and persistent pain in the inguinal area for many months (Table 28.2).

Over the past 20 years, synthetic mesh, usually polypropylene derivatives, has been used with increasing regularity in the performance of inguinal and femoral hernia repair. Rectangles of mesh have been placed during anterior hernia repair, as well as during laparoscopic hernia repair. "Keyholes" have been described as a mechanism to allow transmission of the cord structures through the mesh (4). In addition, double buttress of mesh has been placed in the preperitoneal space in order to cover and reinforce the potential weakness at the keyhole and the slit associated with the keyhole. Lastly, a variety of plug and/or patch techniques have been used to "plumbage" the inguinal hernia defects in the last few years, often resulting in a three-dimensional plug of mesh adjacent to neural structures in the inguinal region (14).

Finally, it should be mentioned that inguinal pain caused by other noninguinal mechanisms may be present in patients who simultaneously exhibit inguinal hernias. The most common example is the group of patients with lumbosacral back disease who have pain along an inguinal distribution and simultaneously have an inguinal hernia. Following inguinal hernia repair, the pain persists—and is

TABLE 28.1. INCIDENCE OF CHRONIC GROIN PAIN FOLLOWING INGUINAL HERNIA REPAIR

Author	Year	No. of Repairs	Type of Repair	Follow-up	Incidence of Pain (Chronic)
Lichtenstein et al.	1988	N/A	Lichtenstein repair	N/A	1% to 2%
Payne et al.	1994	100	Anterior (open) 52 Lap (TAPP) 42	7–18 mo Median 10 mo	Open—4 of 52 Laparoscopic—0 of 48
Panton and Panton	1994	106	Lap	1–12 mo	1%
Barkun et al.	1995	92	Anterior (open) 49 Lap (TAPP) 43	Mean 14 mo	Open—0 of 49 Laparoscopic—1 of 43
Fitzgibbons et al.	1995	869	Lap (TAPP, IPOM, EXTRA)	Minimum 15 mo	Overall—1.6% IPOM—12% TAPP—4.2% EXTRA—0%
Swanstrom	1996	158	Lap (not specified)	Mean 12 mo	Staple pain—5% Nerve injury—2% (GF)
Cunningham et al.	1996	315	Anterior (open)	12–24 mo	12% moderate-to-severe pain
Callesen et al.	1999	500	Anterior (open)	Mean 12 mo	6%—severe 19%—mild

EXTRA, totally extraperitoneal; GF, genitofemoral; IPOM, intraperitoneal onlay mesh; Lap, laparotomy; N/A, not available; TAPP, transabdominal preperitoneal.

TABLE 28.2. INGUINODYNIA FOLLOWING INGUINAL HERNIORRHAPHY[a]

Cause of Pain	Initial Type of Repair	Onset of Pain	Solution
Missed incarcerated femoral hernia	Anterior; plug and patch	No change from preoperatively	Laparoscopy and repair
Missed incarcerated femoral hernia	Anterior; plug and patch	No change from preoperatively	Laparoscopy and repair
Missed reduction—mass: inguinal hernia	Anterior; plug and patch	No change from preoperatively	Laparoscopy and repair
Chronic Appendicitis with hernia staple at tip	Preperitoneal, laparoscopic	Immediate, postoperatively	Laparoscopy and appendectomy
Mass ligature through inguinal floor	Transperitoneal, laparoscopic with suture	Immediate, postoperatively	Anterior suture removal[b]
Staple injury to urinary bladder; urinoma	Preperitoneal, laparoscopic	Immediate and progressive	Laparoscopy and transperitoneal repair
Chronic appendicitis at inguinal space	Lichtenstein with mesh	Delayed, postoperatively	Laparoscopy and appendectomy
Suture and mesh at pubic tubercle	Anterior; plug and patch	Delayed, postoperatively	Anterior suture and mesh removal[b]
Mesh—cicatrix to pubic tubercle	Anterior; plug and patch	Delayed, postoperatively	Anterior suture and mesh removal[b]

[a]Selected cases referred to authors due to postherniorrhaphy inguinodynia.
[b]Denotes Simultaneous performance of laparoscopy.

eventually demonstrated to be caused by lumbosacral orthopedic disease.

TEMPORAL PATTERNS OF PAIN AND TIMING OF ONSET

The timing of onset of pain following inguinal hernia repair, as well as the pattern of pain, seems to provide clues as to the etiology, and—often—possible solutions. Pain that persists for long intervals (3 to 6 months) following herniorrhaphy seems to follow one of three patterns: (a) new onset of pain immediately following the surgical procedure; (b) persistence of inguinal pain immediately following herniorrhaphy, which is similar to pain that was present prior to the inguinal hernia repair; and (c) pain that is delayed in onset for many weeks following herniorrhaphy—and gradually increases in intensity.

Immediate Onset of New Pain Following Herniorrhaphy

Abrupt onset of new pain immediately after inguinal hernia repair strongly suggests local trauma to the tissue involved—including nerve entrapment or direct nerve injury. Nonspecific pain in the inguinal region may be caused by ilioinguinal or iliohypogastric nerve trauma or entrapment, as well as by genitofemoral nerve trauma or entrapment. Pain in the area of the upper anterolateral or lateral thigh associated with numbness in this region suggests entrapment or injury to the laterofemoral cutaneous nerve of the thigh. This latter nerve is more likely to be injured in laparoscopic

hernia repairs or giant indirect hernia repairs that disrupt the integrity of the inguinal structures laterally toward the iliac spine. Abrupt onset of postoperative pain may also be caused by soft tissue or fascia injury due to tearing of a suture or staple abruptly away from tissue that has been transfixed with or without mesh. A mass ligature through the abdominal wall musculature has also been implicated in abrupt onset of pain postoperatively. The first circumstance is transfixation of mesh (usually laparoscopically) at the corners with a large U-stitch placed through the abdominal wall and tied anteriorly. A second circumstance includes the closure of a lateral laparoscopic port site in which a large U-stitch traverses all three layers of muscle and fascia in order to close the trocar defect. This suture transfixes three muscle layers that contract in three different directions.

Unexpected injuries to other structures in the inguinal region and lower abdomen have also been observed to cause onset of new pain following herniorrhaphy. Two key examples include a staple placed through the peritoneum during a preperitoneal hernia repair, which transfixed the apex of the appendix in two cases. In each of these circumstances, initial pain is presumed to be caused by acute peritoneal irritation followed by chronic inflammation irritating the structures in the inguinal region. Abrupt onset of pain following laparoscopic hernia repair or anterior hernia repair has also been associated with injury to the urinary bladder near the medial aspect of the inguinal floor, resulting in rapid onset of urinoma in the preperitoneal or intraperitoneal space shortly after completion of the procedure. Occasionally, a hidden large hematoma may occur in the preperitoneal space, causing abrupt onset of pain. However, in circumstances of enlarging hematomas following hernia repair, the hematoma most often distributes itself, at least partially, into the scrotum, resulting in an ecchymosis or intensely discolored and tender scrotum.

Inguinal Pain Immediately Following Hernia Repair that is Similar/Identical to the Preoperative Inguinal Pain

In circumstances in which patients exhibit inguinal pain prior to inguinal hernia repair, the surgeon and the patient both assume most often that the pain is associated with the hernia—and the hernia and the pain will be eliminated following the operative procedure. When pain persists following inguinal hernia repair, the nature of the pain needs careful reevaluation. The most common occurrence is in patients who have lumbosacral spine disease, pain along an inguinal distribution, and an inguinal hernia. In the absence of other localizing findings suggesting nerve root irritation, the pain may often be attributed to the inguinal hernia. Reassessment of disease of the lumbosacral spine is absolutely necessary when pain is not diminished. A variant on this theme occurs quite often when the spine surgeon cannot explain the inguinodynia based on spine disease, and consults with the general surgeon to evaluate the patient for an occult inguinal or femoral hernia. These patients occasionally are explored for the possibility of an inguinal hernia, which may or may not be present.

Other observations include a missed hernia during the initial operative procedure. Clearly, other causes of pain in the inguinal region should be investigated in these circumstances utilizing computed tomography (CT) scan, ultrasound, and other appropriate modalities as are indicated.

Delayed Onset of Pain, Increasing in Intensity, Following Inguinal Hernia Repair

Following hernia repair, all patients have minimal-to-moderate discomfort. Most often, the symptoms diminish over a period of days and do not impose on the progress of patients to their normal lifestyle. Following the initial postoperative interval, patients occasionally develop a gradual onset of inguinodynia, which often begins many weeks following the operative procedure. The pain increases in intensity with time. It is often associated with tenderness on physical examination. The occurrence of this pain pattern seems to have increased in its prevalence since the advent of the use of mesh for anterior repairs, laparoscopic hernia repairs, and the use of plug–patch techniques. Heise and Starling (7) and others have studied this pain pattern in many patients and have concluded that the increased fibroblastic response caused by the foreign body mesh results in eventual cicatrix, which entraps nerves in the inguinal region, resulting in neuralgia. Investigators have variously performed nerve blocks with local anes-

thetic, neurectomies, and/or removal of the majority of the mesh in order to resolve this pain.

The progressive intensity of this type of inguinodynia is often incapacitating to the patient, resulting in inability to perform normal and work activities. These patients often have point of maximum tenderness in the groin near the area of cicatrix. Rarely, the progressive onset of pain of this sort may be caused by an occult recurrent hernia.

In contrast, however, abrupt onset of pain many weeks or months after a hernia repair suggests an acute event. In these circumstances, the surgeon should increase the suspicion for a recurrent hernia and/or an abrupt separation of strong tissue layers from scar tissue or mesh. This possibility is less likely currently since the benefit of mesh seems to be associated with "tensionless" hernia repairs that diminish the risk of an abrupt rupture of tissue planes.

DIAGNOSTIC AND THERAPEUTIC STRATEGIES

The key to success in evaluating patients with inguinodynia following inguinal hernia repair is to first place the patient into a group based on the pattern and timing of development of pain, as described earlier. Secondly, physical examination will further aid in the assessment of the possible cause of pain.

The final goal of designing a strategy or algorithm for assessment and treatment of inguinal pain following hernia repair is to identify the cause of the pain as best as is possible, utilize diagnostic studies as is appropriate, decide whether surgical intervention is appropriate for diagnosis and/or therapy, and decide whether neurectomy is an appropriate adjunctive and/or primary treatment modality.

The *first pathway* is *abrupt onset* of *new pain* immediately *following hernia repair* (Fig. 28.1).

Physical examination should be performed, focusing on a variety of rationales. The first is to assess whether the pain is intense (almost intolerable), moderate (tolerable, but unable to perform daily activities with ease), or mild (able to perform many activities, pain may possibly be postoperative musculofascial discomfort). The intensity allows the surgeon to identify a time-frame perspective regarding diagnosis and treatment of the pain. Secondly, physical examination should include a detailed assessment of associated new neurologic findings. If motor-sensory findings are present, urgent reexploration should be considered to evaluate and remove sutures or staples that may have transfixed or entrapped specific nerves. Examples include an anterior McVay hernia repair in which the patient develops pain along with quadriceps muscle group motor weakness. In this circumstance, a search for a suture that transfixes the femoral nerve should be the highlight. Sensory loss along the anterolateral upper thigh following a laparoscopic hernia repair provides a second example. Reexploration laparo-

Post Operative Inguinodynia

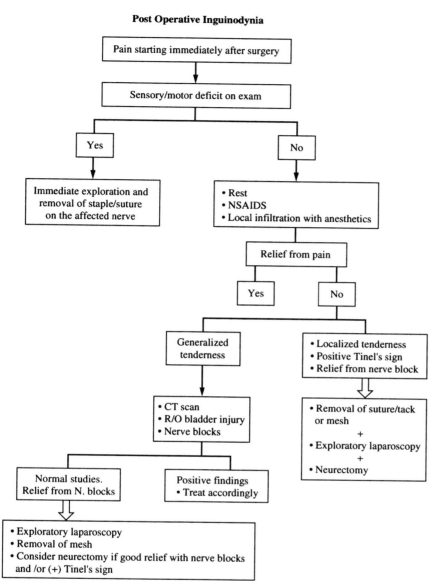

FIGURE 28.1. Algorithm I. Postoperative inguinodynia.

scopically should be considered urgently to find a staple that has transfixed the lateral cutaneous nerve of the thigh.

If no motor or sensory deficients are observed, then a regional nerve block of the ilioinguinal and iliohypogastric nerves should be considered. The local anesthetic is placed within the muscle layers of the anterior abdominal wall slightly medial and cephalad to the anterosuperior iliac spine. The technical details required to perform this nerve block are identified in many texts (11). Since these nerves are most frequently involved, the nerve block often provides a diagnostic clue as to injury of these nerves along with a therapeutic temporizing benefit by relieving pain. Further, if the regional nerve block relieves pain, then the ultimate possible therapeutic intervention might be neurectomy of these two nerves, although the pain may diminish dramatically over time, suggesting operative trauma to the nerve as the cause.

Prior to recommendation for neurectomy, other physical findings should be included in the equation. Point tenderness with a Tinel's sign suggests neuralgia and further indicates the use of a regional nerve block. However, point tenderness in the area of the operative procedure without a Tinel's sign suggests a localized musculofascial somatic cause of the pain. In this circumstance, the use of local infiltration anesthesia in the specific area of the tenderness is helpful therapeutically and reinforces the specific surgical cause of this pain—which may be a suture, a staple, or a direct traumatic insult to the bony pubic arch. Patient support with antiinflammatories and other pain medications may provide a time frame to observe a gradually diminishing pain intensity. The somatic pain may disappear altogether or may require a decision to reexplore the wound, focusing on the removal of a suture or staple. This decision may be made over weeks to months if the intensity of the pain is only moderate. If reexploration is performed, simultaneous exploration of the abdominal component of the inguinal–femoral space should be performed with a 5-mm laparoscope and 5-mm port. Unsuspected transfixation of an intraabdominal structure will be diagnosed and/or eliminated using this technique.

Alternately, if physical examination reveals generalized inguinodynia and diffuse, nonspecific tenderness, then other types of mishaps should be considered. These include a suture–laceration of the urinary bladder with a urinoma in the preperitoneal space, hematoma in the preperitoneal space, transfixation of an intraabdominal structure with a suture or staple—including the tip of the appendix, the wall of the small bowel, etc., or pain due to irritation of a mesh plug. Appropriate diagnostic studies include a urinalysis to assess for red blood cells, ultrasound to assess for a hematoma or urinoma, and a CT scan to evaluate intraabdominal/pelvic pathology; recommendation for surgical reexploration is determined based on results of these studies. Bloody urine, oliguria, and a preperitoneal fluid density suggest a urinary bladder injury; a retrograde cystogram followed by transperitoneal laparoscopic evaluation and/or anterior exploration should be performed to repair the bladder and remove the offending suture or staple. The presence of a preperitoneal hematoma may not require treatment other than analgesia, but might be benefited by the addition of a regional ilioinguinal and iliohypogastric nerve block. Resolution of the hematoma will be associated with resolution of pain. Continued pain of uncertain etiology should be treated with eventual reexploration of the wound anteriorly and/or laparoscopically. Transperitoneal laparoscopic assessment of the undersurface of the inguinal area has revealed such injuries as stapling of the tip of the appendix causing chronic appendicitis, and stapling of the wall of the small intestine. With no etiology observed during exploration in patients who have received a plug mesh hernia repair, detailed assessment of the location of the mesh and its surrounding tissues should be performed. If the mesh seems to have migrated or to be imposing on surrounding structures, then the mesh may be removed to bring relief from chronic pain.

The *second pathway* in the algorithm is the patient who has *continuation of the same pain* immediately after inguinal hernia repair that existed prior to the hernia repair. (Fig. 28.2) The first step is reexamination, focusing on the following possibilities:

The attempt to diagnose a "missed hernia"—which was not identified during the preoperative examination or during the operative procedure itself. Two key diagnoses include femoral hernia or a "reduction in mass" of an incarcerated hernia. If either of these are considered to be possibilities and are not observed on physical examination, then ultrasound of the inguinal area or herniogram might be diagnostic possibilities. Notably, however, the ultrasound studies are highly dependent on the individual ultrasonographer, and the herniogram is,

in many cases, a "lost art." If repeat physical examination does not suggest an inguinal–femoral etiology, then lumbosacral spine disease should be considered and evaluated by a spine surgeon. Final diagnostic possibilities include CT scan of the pelvis and inguinal spaces, and nuclear medicine bone studies.

If a "missed hernia" continues to be a diagnostic possibility, then a diagnostic laparoscopy should be seriously considered. A transperitoneal diagnostic laparoscopy will provide diagnosis and will allow definitive treatment. It should be noted that the preperitoneal space must be explored—especially if there is no evidence for a sack as viewed from the transperitoneal perspective.

The time frame for diagnosis and treatment of continued pain after an inguinal hernia repair will be dependent on the intensity of the patient's discomfort. However, diagnostic possibilities should be assessed within days to weeks to demonstrate a clear focus on the pain. Further, the patient should be supported with antiinflammatory agents and other pain medication.

Table 28.2 describes missed incarcerated femoral hernias in two patients who underwent anterior inguinal hernia repairs. In these circumstances, the diagnosis of the cause of the persistent and identical pain that occurred following anterior hernia repair was made using a laparoscopic exploration—both transperitoneally and preperitoneally. Following laparoscopic intervention, reduction of the incarcerated soft tissue, and repair of the femoral hernias, both patients became rapidly asymptomatic.

The *third pathway* addresses *pain* that *gradually develops after* a time delay of *weeks or months* following the hernia repair (Fig. 28.3).

In this pathway, the patient exhibits a pain-free interval following recovery from the hernia repair, only to exhibit new pain in the inguinal area that occurs many weeks or months after the hernia repair. This pain may be abrupt in onset and, and may even be associated with a specific physical activity—suggesting either musculoskeletal strain or injury, or possibly the occurrence of a recurrent hernia. Alternately, the pain of delayed onset may be gradual in its occurrence. Gradual onset of pain suggests an event associated with maturation of the healing process, including the contraction of scar tissue.

Abrupt onset of pain that occurs in delayed fashion should be occasioned by detailed physical reexamination of the patient. If there is evidence for recurrent hernia, then it is the likely cause of the pain. A "hidden" recurrent hernia is a possibility, even if physical examination does not reveal a recurrent hernia. If there is no evidence for a recurrent hernia, then expectant treatment including pain medication, rest, and antiinflammatory medication is appropriate. If the pain is due to muscle or fascial strain, then the discomfort will gradually abate. If the pain continues to increase in intensity, then a search for a significant injury is appropriate. If the pain becomes moderately severe or

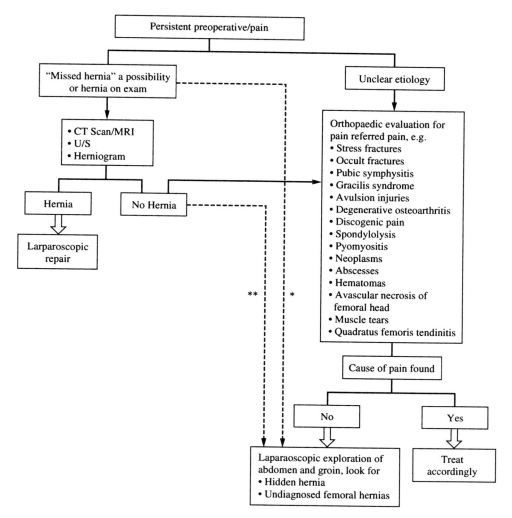

FIGURE 28.2. Algorithm II. Persistent preoperative pain. *, alternate pathway if expertise in computed tomography/magnetic resonance imaging/ultrasound, herniogram is not available and suspicion for missed hernia is high; **, alternate pathway if suspicion for missed hernia is high and/or no obvious orthopedic pathology is suspected.

severe, a diagnostic and therapeutic nerve block of the ilioinguinal and iliohypogastric nerves might be helpful. If the nerve block totally relieves the discomfort, then the pain should be considered to be either musculofascial and somatic in origin, or—more likely—due to irritation of the ilioinguinal and/or iliohypogastric nerves (neuralgia).

If the pain persists at elevated intensity for 4 to 6 weeks, a CT scan of the groin and pelvis may help to elucidate a hematoma or a dislodgment/migration of a mesh plug. If the CT scan delineates no abnormalities or somatic tissue reaction/hematoma, then expectant treatment with medications and rest should be continued. If, on the other hand, the CT scan shows migration of the mesh associated with pain and tenderness in the specific area, then consideration of reexploration either laparoscopically (transperitoneal) and/or anteriorly with removal and replacement of the mesh would seem to be the best approach.

Alternatively, if the patient develops delayed onset of pain in the inguinal region in a gradual fashion, then reexamination of the groin should focus on whether there is the presence of a bulging, tender, mesh patch or plug; whether there is a Tinel's sign; and whether there is evidence for a recurrent hernia. In the absence of evidence for recurrent hernia, pain of mild-to-moderate magnitude may be treated with antiinflammatory medications and rest. If the pain persists for many weeks and increases in intensity, then other diagnostic studies are appropriate.

In delayed onset of pain group, the combination of a Tinel's sign and pain that is totally eliminated by this regional nerve block is likely to be neuralgia secondary to cicatrix involving the ilioinguinal and/or iliohypogastric nerves. It should be noted that nerve entrapment by scar tissue may occur intimately associated with the foreign body mesh (especially if the mesh is of large plug geometry), or

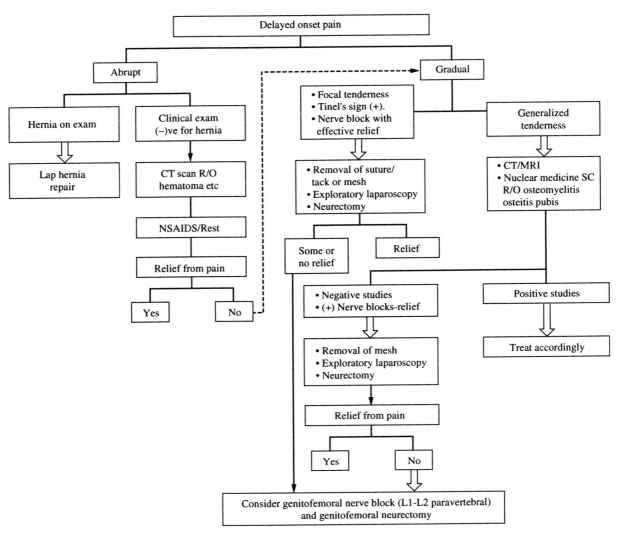

FIGURE 28.3. Algorithm III. Delayed pain onset.

the nerves may be entrapped by scar tissue not associated with mesh. Therefore, the association of a three-dimensional, tender mesh plug, Tinel's sign, and pain that is eliminated by regional nerve block (iliohypogastric and ilioinguinal) should be ultimately treated by removal of a large amount of the mesh and simultaneous ilioinguinal–iliohypogastric neurectomy. Even in the absence of a Tinel's sign, or absence of absolute resolution of pain during a regional nerve block, the combination of removal of the mesh and neurectomy of ilioinguinal and hypogastric nerves is the most likely approach to result in successful resolution of pain because the pain may be partially of somatic musculofascial origin and partially of neurogenic origin (neuralgia due to entrapment and/or irritation of nerves) (Table 28.3) (7,8,15). Further, we strongly recommend that the patient undergo a laparoscopic transperitoneal exploration with a single 5-mm port and 5-mm scope in order to evaluate the intraperitoneal floor of the inguinal and femoral space at

the time of neurectomy and mesh removal. The rationale is to ensure that an aberrant suture and/or staple has not caused one of the intraabdominal occult causes of inguinodynia as listed in Table 28.2.

Occasionally, gradual onset of pain following hernia repair will not be associated with a tender mass of synthetic mesh, will not exhibit a Tinel's sign, and will not be relieved by ilioinguinal and iliohypogastric nerve block. If this circumstance occurs, the important considerations should be either scar entrapment of the genital branch of the genitofemoral nerve, intraabdominal occult pathology as noted in Table 28.2, or an occult recurrent hernia. If the pain persists and is intense, diagnosis using a genitofemoral (L1-2 paravertebral) nerve block has diagnostic and therapeutic value (16). If the nerve block diminishes or eliminates the pain, then consideration of a combination of laparoscopic exploration of the abdomen and a retroperitoneal neurectomy of the genitofemoral nerve is the best combination to

TABLE 28.3. RESULTS OF TREATMENT OF INGUINODYNIA

Author	Year	No. of Procedures	Type of Preoperative Hernia Repair	Treatment Received	Results
Starling and Harms	1989	36	Hernia repairs (not pecified)—3 Blunt trauma—1 Nephrectomy—1 Appendectomy—1	ILN + IHG neurectomy—19 GF neurectomy—17	ILN + IHG neurectomy: good result—12 of 17 GF, ILN + IHG: good result— 17 of 19
Kennedy et al.	1994	23	Anterior inguinal herniorrhaphy	GF neurectomy	Good result—62.5%
Heise and Starling	1998	20	Anterior (open)—17 Laparoscopic—3	Neurectomy +/– mesh removal	Neurectomy + mesh removal: excellent 62% Mesh removal only: excellent 50%

+/–, with or without; GF, genitofemoral; IHG, iliohypogastric; ILN, ilioinguinal.

exact the best result (6). The details of genitofemoral neurectomy have been described (15).

Clearly, none of these syndromes involving inguinodynia are pure neuralgia versus pure somatic musculofascial etiology, or pure recurrent hidden hernia disorders, or pure occult disease in the abdominal component of the inguinal space. For this reason, combinations of diagnostic and therapeutic approaches, which have been extracted from reports in the literature by experienced surgeons and by deductive approaches, will accomplish the best ultimate goal with minimum morbidity. Clearly, it is presumed that nerve blocks, neurectomies of the nerves described, and exploration of the abdominal cavity using a 5-mm laparoscope and trocar should have minimum or nonexistent morbidity and/or disadvantages. The removal of a three-dimensional mass of tender mesh may, however, disrupt the structural integrity of the hernia repair and this possibility should be considered and discussed at the time of reexploration.

REFERENCES

1. Barkun JS, Wexler MJ, Hinchey EJ, et al. Laparoscopic versus open inguinal herniorrhaphy: preliminary results of a randomized controlled trial. *Surgery* 1995;118:703–710.
2. Callesen T, Bech K, Kehlet H. Prospective study of chronic pain after groin hernia repair. *Br J Surg* 1999;86:1528–1531.
3. Cunningham J, Temple WJ, Mitchell P, et al. Cooperative hernia study—pain in the post repair patient. *Ann Surg* 1996;224: 598–602.
4. Felix E, Scott S, Crafton B, et al. Causes of recurrence after laparoscopic hernioplasty. A multicenter study. *Surg Endosc* 1998; 12:226–231.
5. Fitzgibbons RJ Jr, Camps J, Cornet DA, et al. Laparoscopic inguinal herniorrhaphy—results of multicenter trial. *Ann Surg* 1995;221:3–13.
6. Harms BA, Haas DR Jr, Starling JR. Diagnosis and management of genitofemoral neuralgia. *Arch Surg* 1984;119:339–341.
7. Heise CP, Starling J. Mesh inguinodynia: a new clinical syndrome after inguinal herniorrhaphy. *J Am Coll Surg* 1998;187: 514–518.
8. Kennedy EM, Harms BA, Starling JR. Absence of maladaptive neuronal plasticity after genitofemoral-ilioinguinal neurectomy. *Surgery* 1994;116:665–671.
9. Lichtenstein IL, Shulman AG, Amid PK, et al. Cause and presentation of post herniorrhaphy neuralgia: a proposed protocol for treatment. *Am J Surg* 1988;155:786–790.
10. Magee RK. Genitofemoral causalgia (a new syndrome). *Can Med Assoc J* 1942;46:326–329.
11. Mulroy MF. *Peripheral nerve blockade: clinical anesthesia.* Philadelphia: Lippincott–Raven Publishers, 1996:669–697.
12. Panton ONM, Panton RJ. Laparoscopic hernia repair. *Am J Surg* 1994;167:535–537.
13. Payne JH, Grininger LM, Izawa MT, et al. Laparoscopic or open inguinal herniorrhaphy? A randomized prospective trial. *Arch Surg* 1994;129:973–981.
14. Robbins AW, Rutkow IM. The mesh-plug hernioplasty. *Surg Clin North Am* 1993;73:501–512.
15. Starling JR, Harms BA. Diagnosis and treatment of genitofemoral and ilioinguinal neuralgia. *World J Surg* 1989;13:586–591.
16. Starling JR, Harms BA, Schroeder ME, et al. Diagnosis and treatment of genitofemoral and ilioinguinal entrapment neuralgia. *Surgery* 1987;102:581–586.
17. Swanstrom LL. Laparoscopic herniorrhaphy. *Surg Clin North Am* 1996;76:483–491.

EDITOR'S COMMENT

Dr. Geis and his colleagues have done a wonderful job of trying to find a way to evaluate this most difficult group of patients in an orderly manner. These patients as a group are so heavily burdened by psychosocial factors that even the most empathetic physician has to be skeptical about the pain at times. The authors point out that legitimate pain can be caused by a variety of factors. It is important that the physician try to determine if it is related to foreign body reaction, such as is seen with suture or mesh material, or related to scar tissue, or perhaps some pathology involving a single or multiple nerves in the area of the groin. Finally, the authors also emphasize the importance of looking for either missed or alternative pathology in the groin, which could account for pain syndromes. The schema proposed by the authors should serve as a model for the reader.

Neuralgia is perhaps the most troubling of all. I have come to question neurologic syndromes and wonder if they exist in as many patients as we once thought. True genitofemoral, ilioinguinal, etc., neuralgias are probably quite rare, even though the patients commonly come from the neurologists labeled as such. I have always found it peculiar that some surgeons advocate routine division of nerves, whereas others carefully preserve them and yet there does not seem to be an appreciable difference in postoperative pain problems. This has caused some to question whether the way nerves are handled at surgery is of any consequence to postoperative pain. Laparoscopic surgery further calls into question postoperative neuralgia because postoperative pain seen in this group is commonly bilateral. It is inconceivable that the same nerves could be injured symmetrically on either side with staples, dissection or the like. This difficult area remains such. I applaud Dr. Geis and his colleagues for providing us some with guidance in caring for these patients.

R.J.F., Jr.

Nyhus and Condon's Hernia, Fifth Edition, edited by Robert J. Fitzgibbons, Jr. and A. Gerson Greenburg. Lippincott Williams & Wilkins, Philadelphia © 2002.

29

NEURALGIA (INGUINODYNIA) AFTER INGUINAL HERNIORRHAPHY

JAMES R. STARLING

Persistent neuralgia and paresthesia in the inguinal region after inguinal or other lower-abdominal surgery (especially Pfannenstiel's incisions) are uncommon (and frequently denied) complications that may result in severe morbidity in our patients. Most reports suggest the incidence of chronic groin pain (inguinodynia) to be 2% to 5% after inguinal herniorrhaphy and 4% after a Pfannenstiel's incision (6,11,17,25,30,32,35,39,52,56). Surgeons who perform large numbers of inguinal herniorrhaphies per year will attest that neurapraxia and hypoesthesia will occur in upwards of 15% to 20% of their patients following open hernia repair, but these symptoms usually will abate by 3 to 4 months postoperatively. Patients who develop a chronic pain syndrome (neuralgia, inguinodynia) fortunately are few, but when these occur they can be devastating to the patient and extremely frustrating to the surgeon. Compounding the problem is the fact that some of these patients have work-related inguinal hernias and are involved in complex Workman's Compensation issues. There is another subset of patients who are litigious, which further complicates the chronic inguinal pain issue.

The laparoscopic era has created unique neurologic problems not usually seen with the open technique. Specifically these are injuries to the femoral branch of the genitofemoral nerve and lateral femoral cutaneous nerve of the thigh. There has been an occasional report of femoral nerve injury and other rare complications due to the stapled mesh prosthesis (9,28,44,46,55,59).

In the past decade, the use of mesh tension-free hernioplasty has become ubiquitous and perhaps the new gold standard (21,31). The plug technique has additionally resulted in an entirely new frustrating subset of postoperative herniorrhaphy pain syndromes and other complications (42,43,48). Previous algorithms for determining which of the main sensory peripheral nerves were possibly involved (ilioinguinal, iliohypogastric, genitofemoral) no longer apply in the patient with mesh hernioplasty. Physical examination and clinical judgment in these extremely vexing complications are usually all that can be used to render a tentative diagnosis and treatment recommendation.

ANATOMY

Essential to the understanding and possible treatment of these difficult inguinal pain problems after herniorrhaphy is an appreciation of the anatomy. This is further complicated by the fact that the anatomy of the ilioinguinal, iliohypogastric, genitofemoral, and lateral femoral cutaneous nerves not infrequently show marked variation. Moosman and Oelrich reported a typically normal ilioinguinal nerve in only 60% of their dissections (35). The inguinal region, which includes the inguinal canal, spermatic cord, and surrounding skin and subcutaneous tissue (including the femoral Scarpa's triangle), receives sensory innervation from the eleventh and twelfth thoracic nerves and the ventral divisions of the first and second lumbar spinal nerves. The cutaneous branches of the lumbar plexus include the iliohypogastric, ilioinguinal, genitofemoral, lateral femoral cutaneous, and obturator nerves (Fig. 29.1). The spermatic sympathetic plexus contains the sensory fibers for the testes.

The genitofemoral nerve arises from the first and second lumbar vertebral plexus and consists mainly of sensory fibers with a motor component to the cremaster muscle (cremasteric reflex). It lies within the fascial lining of the abdomen by piercing the psoas muscles and psoas fascia near its medial border, opposite the third or fourth lumbar vertebra. It descends under the peritoneum on the surface of the psoas major and crosses obliquely behind the ureter. At a variable distance above the inguinal ligament, the nerve divides into the genital (external spermatic) and femoral (lumboinguinal) branches. The femoral (lumboinguinal) branch is the cutaneous nerve to the femoral triangle. This branch descends laterally to the

J. R. Starling: Department of Surgery, University of Wisconsin–Madison; University of Wisconsin Hospital and Clinics, Madison, Wisconsin.

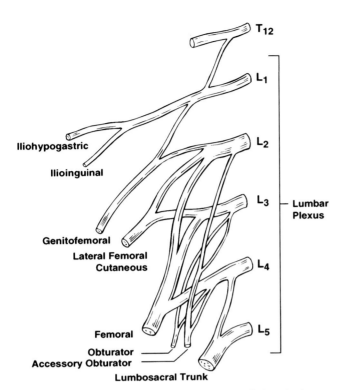

FIGURE 29.1. Origins of the iliohypogastric, ilioinguinal, genitofemoral, and lateral femoral cutaneous nerves.

external iliac artery, behind the inguinal ligament, and through the fascia lata into the femoral sheath. The femoral branch supplies the skin over the upper part of the femoral triangle and communicates with the intermediate cutaneous nerve of the thigh. The genital (external spermatic) branch crosses the lower end of the external iliac artery and enters the inguinal canal through the internal (deep) inguinal ring. It supplies the cremaster muscle and traverses the inguinal canal to the end of the skin of the scrotum. In women, the genital branch accompanies the round ligament of the uterus and ends in the skin of the mons pubis and labia majora (Fig. 29.2).

The ilioinguinal nerve is formed by the first lumbar nerve with contributing filaments from the twelfth thoracic nerve. The ilioinguinal nerve runs subperitoneally and emerges from the lateral border of the psoas major before piercing the transverse abdominal muscle near the anterior part of the iliac crest. It gradually pierces and gives fibers (motor) to the internal oblique muscle and lies between it and the external oblique muscle, close to the internal inguinal ring. Within the inguinal canal, the nerve lies below the spermatic cord and accompanies it through the external inguinal ring. The ilioinguinal nerve is distributed to the skin of the superomedial area of the thigh, to the skin over the root of the penis and anterior of the scrotum, or to the mons pubis and labia majora

(Fig. 29.2). A frequent anatomic variation is an aberrant inguinal sensory trunk of the ilioinguinal nerve, which descends within the genital branch of the genitofemoral nerve. It is also important to recognize that the iliohypogastric nerve is formed from the identical T-12, L-1 nerve roots as the ilioinguinal nerve and has nearly identical sensory innervation (Fig. 29.2). The size of the ilioinguinal nerve is inversely proportional to the iliohypogastric nerve. In some patients, the ilioinguinal nerve joins the iliohypogastric nerve, the latter joins the former, or one of the nerves is entirely absent. As mentioned above, variations in the location and origins of these sensory nerves are frequent. Centrally at the vertebral plexus, as well as in the inguinal region, these nerves *always* interconnect.

The lateral femoral cutaneous nerve is formed at L-1 and L-2; it then passes the psoas muscle at the lateral caudal border and goes on to pass obliquely across the iliacus muscle. Finally, it passes medial to the anterosuperior iliac spine and beneath the iliopubic tract to the abdominal wall, where it supplies sensation to the anterior lateral thigh (Fig. 29.2).

DIAGNOSIS: GENITOFEMORAL–ILIOINGUINAL (ILIOHYPOGASTRIC) NEURALGIA

The main clinical features of genitofemoral entrapment neuralgia consist of intermittent or constant pain and burning sensations in the inguinal region with radiation of pain to the skin of the genitalia and upper medial thigh. The pain can frequently be aggravated by walking, stooping, or hyperextension of the hip, and may be helped by recumbency and flexion of the thigh. Tenderness along the inguinal canal or the inguinal rings may be detected, and hyperesthesia in the distribution of the nerve may be present. The major differential diagnosis of genitofemoral neuropathy is entrapment of the ilioinguinal (iliohypogastric) nerve. The latter condition is characterized by symptoms similar to genitofemoral neuralgia with burning pain over the lower abdomen, which radiates down into the inner portion of the upper thigh and into the scrotum or labia majora. Unlike genitofemoral neuralgia, the pain can occasionally be reproduced by gently tapping over an area of point tenderness (Tinel's sign) or by extending the thigh or hip. Distinguishing genitofemoral neuralgia from the manifestations of ilioinguinal neuralgia can be difficult and can result in misdiagnosis and inappropriate treatment. At times, differentiation is impossible. Both entities must be considered in all instances of inguinal pain, and appropriate evaluations must be performed.

Communication between the genitofemoral–ilioinguinal or iliohypogastric nerve (as well as the lateral femoral

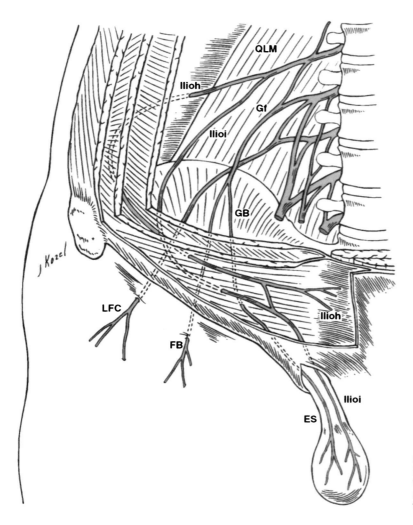

FIGURE 29.2. Course of the genitofemoral (*Gf*), ilio-hypogastric (*Ilioh*), ilioinguinal (*Ilioi*), and lateral femoral cutaneous (*LFC*) nerves. *ES*, external spermatic; *FB*, femoral branch; *GB*, genital branch; *QLM*, quadratus lumborum m.

cutaneous nerve) is common and results in overlap of sensory innervation. Local or specific blocks should therefore be done to determine as accurately as possible whether the ilioinguinal or genitofemoral nerve is involved. If a local entrapment or neuroma is responsible for the pain, a local block of the ilioinguinal nerve through the lower anterior abdominal wall should alleviate the symptoms. If the pain is not relieved the L-1 and L-2 nerve plexus can be blocked through a paravertebral route with 0.5% bupivacaine and 0.75% lidocaine with epinephrine 1:200,000. Recently, we have been attempting to specifically block the main trunk of the genitofemoral nerve with ultrasound-guided transpsoas nerve blocks (19). By performing separate blocks and observing for pain relief, one can make the distinction between genitofemoral and ilioinguinal (iliohypogastric) neuropathy in most but not all patients. This algorithm was developed and followed in all patients prior to the "mesh" era of inguinal herniorrhaphy. Since the late 1980s, almost all patients referred for chronic inguinodynia have had open or laparoscopic mesh herniorrhaphy, and this algorithm has

not helped predict with the same accuracy which of the specific nerves may be entrapped (20,50).

SURGICAL TREATMENT

If an ilioinguinal (iliohypogastric) nerve block provides complete or substantial relief, surgical exploration of the previous inguinal incision and identification of the ilioinguinal and iliohypogastric nerves is initially recommended. The entire nerve as far proximal and distal as possible should be removed, to include the entrapped segment. Both the ilioinguinal and iliohypogastric nerves, if identified, should be removed because of the numerous nerve twigs connecting these main branches. The nerve ends are routinely ligated with an absorbable suture. Some authors recommend folding the cut ends of the nerves back on itself into muscle to prevent neuroma formation (4). Nahabedian and Dellon recommend extending the nerve resection into the preperitoneal fat deep to all muscle (36).

If the ilioinguinal block does not substantially relieve pain, and the L1-2 blocks or transpsoas block result in substantial pain relief, genitofemoral neurectomy should be the initial surgical approach. This is especially true in patients who have previously undergone repeated remedial groin explorations. If pain is partially relieved by both blocks, one should consider staged surgical exploration of these nerves.

Proximal genitofemoral neurectomy is approached through a small transverse flank incision similar to that for lumbar sympathectomy. The oblique and transverse abdominal muscles are divided, if necessary. The retroperitoneum is exposed, and the psoas major muscle and ureter are identified. The genitofemoral nerve can be identified as it penetrates the psoas muscle, usually as a single trunk along the medial edge. A 4- to 5-cm section of the genitofemoral nerve proximal to the assumed site of entrapment is excised to include the bifurcation. Because of frequent variation in the site of nerve bifurcation, both branches of the genitofemoral nerve must be identified to ensure resection of the proximal genitofemoral nerve trunk or both branches in situations when the bifurcation occurs within the substance of the psoas muscle. A segment of the proximal ilioinguinal nerve is also frequently excised during genitofemoral neurectomy. Hypoesthesia of the labia majora and skin over the femoral triangle, and loss of the cremasteric reflex are the only reported side effects of genitofemoral and ilioinguinal neurectomy. There are infrequent reports of laparoscopic retroperitoneal genitofemoral neurectomy and ilioinguinal neurectomy (26,38). Because the open approach is simple, inexpensive, and patient-friendly, the author has not attempted the laparoscopic approach.

LAPAROSCOPIC HERNIORRHAPHY

Anatomy

During the transperitoneal laparoscopic approach to inguinal hernia repair, the femoral branch of the genitofemoral nerve and lateral cutaneous nerve of the thigh are at unique risk. Neither of these two nerves is usually visible during laparoscopic inguinal hernia repair (Fig. 29.3). These nerves, however, can usually be found laparoscopically when dissecting lateral to the "quadrangle of doom" and below the iliopubic tract (27). They become visible as the loose areolar and fatty tissue overlying the psoas and iliacus muscle below the iliopubic tract is pushed aside. The femoral branch of the genitofemoral nerve is usually found first lying directly on the psoas muscle 1 to 2 cm lateral to the iliac artery. There is some variability, and this nerve is not always a single trunk. The lateral femoral cutaneous nerve of the thigh is found laterally to this line on the iliacus muscle beneath its fascial fibers usually 1 to 2 cm medial

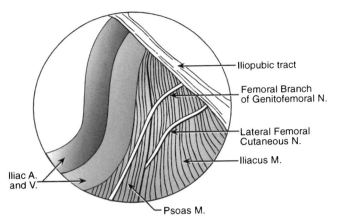

FIGURE 29.3. Preperitoneal course of the lateral femoral cutaneous nerve and femoral branch of the genitofemoral nerve.

to the anterosuperior iliac spine. This bony landmark can be identified by external palpation through the abdominal wall. A discrete fascia overlies the iliacus muscle. The lateral cutaneous nerve of the thigh can often be seen through these fibers, but it may be necessary to cut through the fascia to locate the underlying nerve. Both the femoral branch of the genitofemoral nerve and the lateral cutaneous nerve of the thigh usually pass beneath the iliopubic tract and inguinal ligament but on occasion may pass directly through them as a course to the thigh (3).

Diagnosis/Treatment

The precise mechanism of nerve injury during laparoscopic herniorrhaphy is unknown but presumably due to nerve trauma during dissection, pneumatic compression, or direct injury secondary to staple or mesh placement. If genitofemoral–ilioinguinal (iliohypogastric) or lateral femoral cutaneous (*meralgia paresthetica*) neuropathy is diagnosed, various treatment options are available. Suggestions in patients who have had laparoscopic herniorrhaphy include Seid and Amos's recommendation of treating with local injection based on a 100% success rate in their nine cases (47). Tanner suggested a laparoscopic (transabdominal) approach with staple removal for postlaparoscopy *meralgia paresthetica* (7). Other cases describe operative intervention via an open transabdominal or extraperitoneal approach with mesh removal, neurectomy, or both (9,45). Also described are a retroperitoneal endoscopic technique for treating entrapment neuralgia (26,38). Krahenbuhl and colleagues reported this approach in three patients, of whom two underwent neurectomy of the genitofemoral nerve and one underwent neurectomy of the ilioinguinal nerve (26). Perry reported on three patients with chronic pain and tenderness in the groin, labia majora, and medial thigh caused by genitofemoral neuropathy. These patients underwent laparoscopic genitofemoral neurectomy (38).

DISCUSSION

Operations for entrapment neuropathy in the inguinal region that include the upper thigh are not new. In 1885, Bernhardt (5) and Freud (16), and in 1895, Roth (41), published reports regarding neuropathies of the lateral femoral cutaneous nerve; they called the condition *meralgia paresthetica*. Most of the causes of entrapment of the lateral femoral cutaneous nerve were thought to be anomalous passage of the nerve from the abdomen to the thigh near the inguinal ligament, but previous inguinal operations, blunt trauma, and penetrating trauma were also implicated. Surgical treatment was frequently recommended. Enthusiasm for neurectomy or neurolysis of the lateral femoral cutaneous nerve has decreased, however, because of a reported high incidence of postoperative dysesthesias.

Severe neuralgia and paresthesia in the inguinal region, scrotum, or anterior proximal thigh after an operation are rare. Most general surgeons are familiar with the rare complication of ilioinguinal nerve entrapment. The incidence of neuralgia after herniorrhaphy is probably greater than published. Severe postherniorrhaphy pain can lead to severe drug dependency, family problems, and occupational incapacitation.

Entrapment of the ilioinguinal (iliohypogastric) nerve after open nonmesh herniorrhaphy may be caused by either suture placement (Fig. 29.4), fibrous adhesions, or a cicatricial (traumatic) neuroma. If a local nerve block relieves the pain completely, approximately 85% of patients should have long-term pain relief (50).

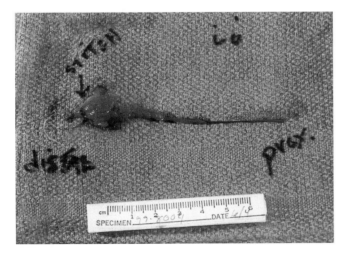

FIGURE 29.4. Ilioinguinal nerve with stitch-induced granuloma/neuroma.

TABLE 29.1. GENITOFEMORAL NEURALGIA: LITERATURE REVIEW

Author, Year (Ref.)	No. of Patients	Presentation (No. of Patients)
Magee, 1942 (39)	7	Postappendectomy (5), blunt trauma (1),[a] psoas abscess–Pott's disease (1)[a]
Lyon, 1945 (40)	3	Postappendectomy (3)
Laha et al., 1977 (3)	1	Bilateral inguinal herniorrhaphy (2)
O'Brien, 1979 (42)	1	Constricting jeans (1)[a]
Kennedy et al., 1994 (43)	23	Inguinal herniorrhaphy (21), appendectomy (2)
Perry, 1997 (27)	3	Gynecologic procedures (3)
Krahenbuhl et al., 1997 (28)	3	Laparoscopic inguinal herniorrhaphy (2), orchidectomy (1)

[a]Patients who did not have surgical treatment.

Before our reports, most surgeons were unaware of the genitofemoral nerve with its resultant neuropathy, and only anecdotal cases were reported (18,51) (Table 29.1). Numerous recent reports have recognized this nerve and its symptom complex when damaged, and suggest ways to prevent inadvertent injury (30). Genitofemoral neuropathy was first described by Magee (34) and Lyon (33), and there are a number of excellent papers advocating genitofemoral neurectomy (29). There are a number of clinicians who are adamant against cutting peripheral nerves, citing the concept of maladaptive neuronal plasticity (10,13,54). This theory postulates that altered pathways in the dorsal horn of the spinal cord maintain the perception of pain, and that long-term neurolytic results are unpredictable at best. Many pain clinics continue to recommend a myriad of pharmacologic treatments rather than neurectomy. In the author's experience with 32 retroperitoneal genitofemoral neurectomies, 65% of patients will have long lasting (greater than 3 years) pain relief. The main factor in failure was in those patients who had testicular pain as a coprimary presenting symptom. If these patients are excluded, the percentage of patients obtaining significant pain relief is 75% to 80%. This number is nearly identical to that for patients after ilioinguinal neurectomy. The author has no experience with testicular denervation for sympathetic control of chronic neuralgia after herniorrhaphy (8). The concept of maladaptive neuronal plasticity does not seem to apply in the majority of our cohort of patients; furthermore, anesthesia dolorosa did not occur in any of our patients.

Two recent publications have proposed a new surgical approach for treating entrapment neuralgia of the genitofemoral nerve. Perry (38) and Krähenbühr (26) et al. have used a retroperitoneal endoscopic technique to excise the genitofemoral nerve successfully in their patients.

Recently, Feinberg and coworkers used a novel approach to ilioinguinal/genitofemoral neuropathy (14). In ten patients, they preoperatively blocked the ilioinguinal nerve and the genital branch of the genitofemoral nerve with bupivacaine (Sensorcaine, AstraZeneca, Westborough, MA, U.S.A.) and a "wash" of methylene blue dye. Postinjection, the patients confirmed complete relief of pain. During surgical exploration, the methylene blue–infiltrated tissue was identified, and patients underwent an en-bloc resection of the previously identified dye-stained tissue. According to the authors, the dye enables removing nerve fibers contained within dense fibrous tissue, which otherwise would be unidentified.

When laparoscopic hernia repair was added to the general surgeon's armamentarium, it was immediately predicted that the number of unfortunate nerve entrapment cases would decrease. Unfortunately, such is not the case, and recent publications document not only the number of genitofemoral–ilioinguinal (iliohypogastric) nerve entrapment, but also injuries to the lateral femoral cutaneous nerve, femoral branch of the genitofemoral nerve, and, rarely, the femoral nerve (15,23,24). Fortunately, most of these injuries are transient and last only a few months.

In patients with pain persisting greater than 3 to 6 months, remedial laparoscopic exploration with staple removal has been reported (15,53). Other authors have recommended transabdominal removal of prosthetic materials and anchoring staples (9,45).

Meralgia paresthetica or damage to the lateral femoral cutaneous nerve has been the most common neurologic injury—both transient and chronic after laparoscopic transabdominal preperitoneal prosthetic (TAPP) repair. Fortunately, with better understanding of the preperitoneal anatomy, injury to this nerve as well as the femoral branch of the genitofemoral nerve is decreasing (12,28). Certainly, surgeons who favor laparoscopic herniorrhaphy are using fewer staples (if any) and are appreciative of the "quadrangle of doom." When chronic *meralgia paresthetica* persists in patients with stapled mesh, the author prefers an open inguinal approach to remove the mesh and staples followed by a conventional herniorrhaphy. For patients with persistent pain after this, the suprainguinal ligament approach to lateral femoral cutaneous neurectomy is very successful (1,58).

The author has found the diagnosis of specific nerve neuralgia to be extremely difficult with the ubiquitous use of mesh for conventional (open), plug, and laparoscopic transabdominal preperitoneal (TAPP) or extraperitoneal (TEP) or extraperitoneal herniorrhaphy. In previous publications, strict criteria were used to attempt to identify with reasonable certainty which nerves were entrapped. Mesh has changed the rules and the previous algorithms are unreliable as reported in our recent publication on mesh inguinodynia (20). In patients with chronic groin pain after herniorrhaphy, our approach is to usually wait

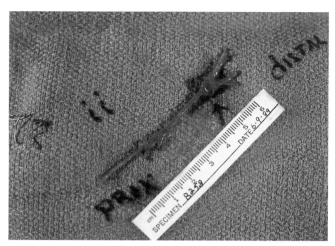

FIGURE 29.5. Ilioinguinal nerve. *Arrow* indicates location of entrapment by an endoscopic tack after laparoscopic herniorrhaphy.

at least 6 months and then operate through an inguinal incision, remove the mesh, remove any obviously entrapped nerves and staples, and perform a "tension-free," "mesh-free" herniorrhaphy (Fig. 29.5). Patients with chronic inguinodynia after the "plug–'stein" repair are no exception. Complications of the "mesh plug–mesh sheet" hernioplasty include not only chronic pain, but also erosion of the colon and small-bowel obstruction. Robbins and Rutkow categorically deny that ilioinguinal or genitofemoral neuralgia has ever occurred in over 3,000 of their plug implants (40). Such is not the case in other experiences. Surgical strategy is simple: anterior remedial approach, and remove plug and any nerves entrapped by the mesh. (Fig. 29.6) Bascom, for obvious reasons, cautions proponents of the plug repair to place them lateral and superior to the cord to avoid the genital branch of the genitofemoral nerve (4).

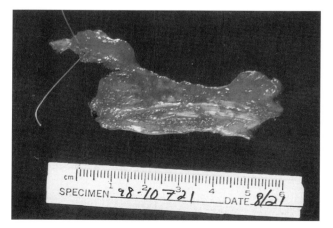

FIGURE 29.6. Portion of removed mesh with genital branch of the genitofemoral nerve incorporated into interstices of contracted mesh.

CONCLUSION

Taking care of patients with chronic groin pain after inguinal herniorrhaphy can be extremely difficult in many instances. Despite large series of senior authors who attest to the rarity of chronic pain (inguinodynia) after inguinal herniorrhaphy [Wantz, 1 of 1,252 patients (57); Skandalakis et al., 0 of 3,000 patients (49); Amid et al., less than 1% in 1,000 patients (2)], the incidence is higher. Because of our mobile society, especially in university communities, long-term critical follow-up is a problem in my patient population and this certainly must be true in other parts of the country. Some of these patients have been treated by many physicians around the country, administered a potpourri of antidepressant drugs, and frequently a wide variety of narcotics. Many have seen their jobs lost and family relationships devastated. Some are aggressively litigious toward their initial surgeon, and they and their attorneys try to involve the treating surgeon using very insidious means. Access to the World Wide Web and Medline by patients and attorneys has resulted in easy access to surgeons who practice and publish their results on groin pain after inguinal herniorrhaphy. Workman's Compensation cases can be extremely difficult and oftentimes annoying. In the state of Wisconsin, there were between 1,053 and 1,270 inguinal hernia claims a year from 1994 to 1998 (totaling 5% of all injury claims per calendar year). This represents an indemnity of approximately $2,000,000 and 45,000 compensable days per year. Not getting involved in Workman's Compensation or insurance issues involving chronic groin pain is not an option after remedial surgical involvement. Disability settlements in some patients have a remarkable therapeutic affect.

REFERENCES

1. Aldrich EF, van den Heever CM. Suprainguinal ligament approach for surgical treatment of meralgia paresthetica. *J Neurosurg* 1989;70:492–494.
2. Amid PK, Shulman AG, Lichtenstein IL. Simultaneous repair of bilateral inguinal hernias under local anesthesia. *Ann Surg* 1996; 223:249–252.
3. Aszmann OC, Dellon ES, Dellon AL. Anatomical course of the lateral femoral cutaneous nerve and its susceptibility to compression and injury. *Plast Reconstr Surg* 1997;100:600–604.
4. Bascom JU. Pelvic pain. *Perspectives in Colon and Rectal Surgery.* 1999;11:21–40.
5. Bernhardt M. Ober isoliert im Gebiete des N. cutaneus femoris externus vorkommende parasthesien. *Neurol Cbl* 1885;14:242–244.
6. Bower S, Moore BB, Weiss SM. Neuralgia after inguinal hernia repair. *Am Surg* 1996;62:664–667.
7. Broin EO, Horner C, Mealy K, et al. Meralgia paraesthetica following laparoscopic inguinal hernia repair. An anatomical analysis. *Surg Endosc* 1995;9:76–78.
8. Choa RG, Swami KS. Testicular denervation: a new surgical procedure for intractable testicular pain. *Br J Urol* 1992;70:417–419.
9. Choi PD, Nath R, Mackinnon SE. Iatrogenic injury to the ilioinguinal and iliohypogastric nerves in the groin: a case report, diagnosis, and management. *Ann Plast Surg* 1996;37:60–65.
10. Coderre TJ, Katz J, Vaccarino AL, et al. Contribution of neuroplasticity to pathological pain: review of clinical and experimental evidence. *Pain* 1993;52:259–285.
11. Cunningham J, Temple WJ, Mitchell P, et al. Cooperative hernia study: pain in the postrepair patient. *Ann Surg* 1996;224:598–602.
12. Dibenedetto LM, Lei Q, Gilroy AM, et al. Variations in the inferior pelvic pathway of the lateral femoral cutaneous nerve: implications for laparoscopic hernia repair. *Clin Anat* 1996;9:232–236.
13. Dubner R. Neuronal plasticity and pain following peripheral tissue inflammation or nerve injury. In: Bond MR, Charlton JE, Woolf CJ, eds. *Proceedings of the Sixth World Congress on Pain.* Amsterdam: Elsevier Science Publishers, 1991:263–276.
14. Feinberg BI, Feinberg RA, Scodary D. Successful surgical treatment for genitofemoral and ilioinguinal neuropathies [abstract]. *Regional Anesthesia and Pain Medicine* 1998;23(Suppl.1):1.
15. Fitzgibbons RJ Jr, Camps J, Cornet DA, et al. Laparoscopic inguinal herniorrhaphy. Results of a multicenter trial. *Ann Surg* 1995;221:3–13.
16. Freud S. Ober die Bernhardt'sche Sensibiliatss-Forung. *Neurol Cbl* 1885;14:491–492.
17. Gilbert AI. Inguinal herniorrhaphy: reduced morbidity, recurrences, and costs. *South Med J* 1979;72:831–834.
18. Harms BA, DeHaas DR Jr, Starling JR. Diagnosis and management of genitofemoral neuralgia. *Arch Surg* 1984;119:339–341.
19. Hartrick CT. Genitofemoral nerve block: a transpsoas technique, *Regional Anesthesia* 1994;19:432–433.
20. Heise CP, Starling JR. Mesh inguinodynia: a new clinical syndrome after inguinal herniorrhaphy? *J Am Coll Surg* 1998;187:514–518.
21. Kark AE, Kurzer MN, Belsham PA. Three thousand one hundred seventy-five primary inguinal hernia repairs: advantages of ambulatory open mesh repair using local anesthesia. *J Am Coll Surg* 1998;186:447–455.
22. Kennedy EM, Harms BA, Starling JR. Absence of maladaptive neuronal plasticity after genitofemoral-ilioinguinal neurectomy. *Surgery* 1994;166:665–670.
23. Keting JP, Morgan A. Femoral nerve palsy following laparoscopic inguinal herniorrhaphy. *J Laparoendosc Surg* 1993;3:557–559.
24. Klaiber CL. Potential risks and complications of laparoscopic hernia repair. *Prog Surg* 1993;3:557–559.
25. Kopel HP, Thompson WA, Postell AM. Entrapment neuropathy of the ilioinguinal nerve. *N Engl J Med* 1962;266:16–19.
26. Krähenbühr L, Striffeler H, Baer HU, et al. Retroperitoneal endoscopic neurectomy for nerve entrapment after hernia repair. *Br J Surg* 1997;84:216–219.
27. Kraus MA. Laparoscopic identification of preperitoneal nerve anatomy in the inguinal area. *Surg Endosc* 1994;8:377–380.
28. Krause MA. Laparoscopic identification of preperitoneal nerve anatomy in the inguinal area. *Surg Endosc* 1994;8:377–381.
29. Laha RK, Rao S, Pidgeon CN, et al. Genito-femoral neuralgia. *Surg Neurol* 1977;8:280–282.
30. Lichtenstein IL, Shulman AG, Amid PK, et al. Cause and prevention of postherniorrhaphy neuralgia: a proposed protocol for treatment. *Am J Surg* 1988;155:786–790.
31. Lichtenstein IL. Herniorrhaphy: a personal experience with 6,321 cases. *Am J Surg* 1987;153:553–559.
32. Luijendijk RW, Jeekel J, Storm RK, et al. The low transverse Pfannenstiel incision and the prevalence of incisional hernia and nerve entrapment. *Ann Surg* 1997;225:365–369.
33. Lyon EK. Genitofemoral causalgia. *Can Med Assoc J* 1945;53:213–216.
34. Magee RK. Genitofemoral causalgia (a new syndrome). *Can Med Assoc J* 1942;46:326–329.
35. Moosman DA, Oelrich TM. Prevention of accidental trauma to the ilioinguinal nerve during inguinal herniorrhaphy. *Am J Surg* 1977;133:146–148.

36. Nahabedian MY, Dellon AL. Outcome of the operative management of nerve injuries in the ilioinguinal region. *J Am Coll Surg* 1997;184:265–268.
37. O'Brien MD. Genitofemoral neuropathy. *Br Med J* 1979;1:1052.
38. Perry CP. Laparoscopic treatment of genitofemoral neuralgia. *J Am Assoc Gynecol Laparosc* 1997;4:231–234.
39. Pollack R, Nyhus LM. Complications of groin hernia repair. *Surg Clin North Am* 1983;63:1363–1371.
40. Robbins AW, Rutkow IM. Mesh plug repair and groin hernia surgery. *Surg Clin North Am* 1998;78:1007–1023.
41. Roth VK. Meralgia paraesthetica. *Med Obozr Moscow* 1895;43:678–688.
42. Rutkow IM, Robbins AW. The mesh plug technique for recurrent groin herniorrhaphy: a nine-year experience of 407 repairs. *Surgery* 1998;124:844–847.
43. Rutkow IM, Robbins AW. "Tension-free" inguinal herniorrhaphy: a preliminary report on the "mesh-plug" technique. *Surgery* 1993;114:3–8.
44. Sampath P, Yeo CJ, Campbell JN. Nerve injuries associated with laparoscopic inguinal herniorrhaphy. *Surgery* 1995;118:823–833.
45. Sampath P, Yeo CJ, Campbell JN. Nerve injury associated with laparoscopic inguinal herniorrhaphy. *Surgery* 1995;118:829–833.
46. Seid AS, Amos E. Entrapment neuropathy in laparoscopic herniorrhaphy. *Surg Endosc* 1994;8:1050–1053.
47. Seid AS, Amos E. Entrapment neuropathy in laparoscopic herniorrhaphy. *Surg Endosc* 1994;8:1050–1053.
48. Shulman AG, Amid PK, Lichtenstein IL. The "plug" repair of 1402 recurrent inguinal hernias. 20-year experience. *Arch Surg* 1990;125:265–267.
49. Skandalakis JE, Skandalakis LJ, Colborn GL. Testicular atrophy and neuropathy in herniorrhaphy. *Am Surg* 1996;62:775–782.
50. Starling JR, Harms BA. Diagnosis and treatment of genitofemoral and ilioinguinal neuralgia. *World J Surg* 1989;13:586–591.
51. Starling JR, Harms BA, Schroeder ME, et al. Diagnosis and treatment of genitofemoral and ilioinguinal entrapment neuralgia. *Surgery* 1987;102:581–586.
52. Stulz P, Pfeiffer KM. Peripheral nerve injuries resulting from common surgical procedures in the lower portion of the abdomen. *Arch Surg* 1982;117:324–327.
53. Tetik C, Arregui ME, Dulucq JL, et al. Complications and recurrences associated with laparoscopic repair of groin hernias. A multi-institutional retrospective analysis. *Surg Endosc* 1994;8:1316–1322.
54. Treede RD, Davis KD, Campbell JN, et al. The plasticity of cutaneous hyperalgesia during sympathetic ganglion blockade in patients with neuropathic pain. *Brain* 1992;115:607–621.
55. Tucker JG, Wilson RA, Ramshaw BJ, et al. Laparoscopic herniorrhaphy: technical concerns in prevention of complications and early recurrence. *Am Surg* 1995;61:36–39.
56. Wantz GE. Complications of inguinal hernia repair. *Surg Clin North Am* 1984;64:287–298.
57. Wantz GE. Testicular atrophy and chronic residual neuralgia as risks of inguinal herniorrhaphy. *Surg Clin North Am* 1993;73:571–581.
58. Williams PH, Trzil KP. Management of meralgia paresthetica. *J Neurosurg* 1991;74:76–80.
59. Woods S, Porglase A. Ilioinguinal nerve entrapment from laparoscopic hernia repair. *Aust N Z J Surg* 1993;69:823–824.

VENTRAL INCISIONAL HERNIAS

30

WOUND FAILURE AND INCISIONAL HERNIA: MECHANISMS AND PREVENTION

LEIF A. ISRAELSSON

Wound failures such as early wound dehiscence, wound infection, and incisional hernia are major sources of morbidity after laparotomies and are also associated with mortality. Considerable effort should be taken to achieve a low rate of such complications. Although the primary operation may have relieved the patient of a disabling or life-threatening condition, he or she may still suffer from early or late effects of a wound complication. The costs for managing wound failures are considerable, frequently requiring medical treatment, surgical intervention, or reoperation and prolonged hospital stay.

Several abdominal surgical procedures are now conducted by a laparoscopic or a laparoscopically assisted technique; wound complications also occur after such operations. Incisional hernia may develop in wounds created for laparoscopic access or in an abdominal incision completing a laparoscopically assisted operation.

Knowledge of etiologic mechanisms may help to lower the rate of wound failures and allow the surgeon to choose an optimal surgical technique for wound closure.

WOUND HEALING

The development of wound complications may be related to functional changes in the wound during the healing process. Wound healing in laparotomy incisions follows the general principles of all tissue healing; the mechanisms are well known.

Principally, wound healing can be divided into three phases: an inflammatory phase, a fibroplastic phase, and a phase of maturation. The inflammatory phase lasts for 4 to 6 days, during which time the wound is prepared for subsequent healing by removal of necrotic tissue and bacteria.

During this period, the wound has no intrinsic strength and its integrity is entirely dependent on the suture and the suture-holding capacity of the tissues. This phase is followed by a fibroplastic phase characterized by collagen synthesis. During this period, the wound rapidly gains in tensile strength by the bridging over of collagen fibers. The fibroplastic phase is gradually succeeded by a prolonged phase of maturation with remodeling of collagen fibers.

The tensile strength of a sutured aponeurosis after 2 to 3 weeks is about 20% of that of unwounded tissue, and after 4 weeks about 50%. After 6 to 12 months, the aponeurosis attains about 80% of its original strength, but complete restitution is never achieved.

WOUND COMPLICATIONS

Wound Dehiscence

Early wound dehiscence with evisceration is reported to occur in 1% to 3% of laparotomies and always requires immediate reoperation (2). Such reoperations are associated with considerable morbidity and incisional hernia develops in a very high proportion. The mortality rates in older series have quoted figures of around 25% (2).

Wound dehiscence usually occurs during the first postoperative week, when the wound is entirely dependent on the suture and the suture-holding capacity of the tissue. Dehiscence occurs if the suture breaks, knots become undone, or the suture cuts completely through the suture-holding tissues.

Mechanisms

Dehiscence is seldom the result of systemic abnormalities, and the causes are almost always found locally in the wound. Early wound dehiscence may occur if wound tension is distributed to the suture line in such a way that the suture-holding capacity of the tissues is exceeded. The

L. A. Israelsson: Department of Surgery, Umeå University, Umeå, Sweden; Department of Surgery, Sundsvall Hospital, Sundsvall, Sweden.

development of wound dehiscence is strongly related to the suturing technique.

The suture-holding capacity of the tissues has been argued to be lower if sutures are placed too close to wound edges. Experimental evidence suggests that the suture pull-out force increases with the distance from the wound edge up to 8 to 9 mm and then reaches a plateau (2). This effect may relate to inflammatory changes within this zone that weakens tissue.

Factors that weaken the aponeurosis and diminish its suture-holding capacity may affect the rate of wound dehiscence. An important risk factor for the development of dehiscence is major wound infection with tissue necrosis and breakdown of aponeurotic tissue.

Inadequate suture technique is probably the main cause of dehiscence during the first 4 to 6 days after laparotomy. After this period and during the fibroplastic phase, the intrinsic strength of the wound increases and the integrity of the wound is less dependent on the suture and suture technique. A major wound infection usually takes several days to develop, and the aponeurosis restrains degradation for some time. A major wound infection is more relevant for wound dehiscence encountered later than 1 week after laparotomy.

Malnourishment, malignant disease, jaundice, old age, and corticosteroid therapy may also be associated with weakening of tissues. A correlation of these factors with an increased rate of dehiscence has been proposed but has not been convincingly substantiated in clinical studies. The choice of suture material is usually not important for the development of wound dehiscence; historically, a high rate of dehiscence has been reported with catgut.

The Tension on the Suture Line

Suture cutting completely through the tissues is probably the main cause of wound dehiscence; a meticulous suture technique is generally regarded as crucial, ensuring that the suture-holding capacity of the tissues is not exceeded. The tension on each stitch is high if wound tension is distributed to only a few stitches; with every stitch added to the suture line, the tension on each stitch decreases (Fig. 30.1).

The suture-holding capacity of the tissues will be exceeded if the tension on the suture line is very high. Obesity, chronic bronchopulmonary disease, postoperative coughing, and abdominal distention causing wound tension are associated with increased wound dehiscence (2). Low tension on the suture line in women with a more relaxed abdomen, especially following pregnancy, and thoracic rather than abdominal breathing may explain their low rate of dehiscence compared with men.

In abdominal distention, elongation of the wound increases the pull on a continuous suture, which may cause the suture to break or the anchor knots to slip. The interval between stitches increases, and abdominal contents may protrude into the wound. Compression of tissue held in the suture may cause necrosis that further augments the risk of the suture cutting through the tissues. The suture technique should be such that the negative effects of abdominal distention are counteracted, and therefore a short stitch interval is of paramount importance (Fig. 30.1).

Certain circumstances indicate the abdominal wound is better left open than sutured with undue tension. Increased tension may cause ischemia of sutured tissue with subsequent risk of wound infection or dehiscence. Such an instance might be when marked bowel distention, massive hemorrhage, or edema is present.

Incisional Hernia

Incisional hernia results in inadequate collagen bridging. It is defined as a palpable defect in the laparotomy wound, often with a protrusion or a visible bulge present. Incisional hernia may cause the patient discomfort or may lead to strangulation of abdominal contents. Bowel may more often incarcerate in small hernias, whereas bowel obstruction due to adhesions in the hernia sac or the hernia orifice is more often encountered with large hernias. Urgent hernia repair is usually required if ulceration of the skin overlying a hernia develops. Most hernias that cause patient discomfort are usually detected within the first 12 months after laparotomy. The hernia rate in midline incisions at 1 year ranges from 9% to more than 20%. The hernia rate is, however, very much related to the definition of incisional hernia used at follow-up.

Mechanisms

There is considerable evidence that incisional hernia develops because aponeurotic edges become separated early in the postoperative period. Separation of aponeurotic edges of 12 mm or more 4 weeks after laparotomy predicts the development of an incisional hernia with great accuracy (18). The regenerative powers of aponeurotic tissue are very limited, and a discontinuity must heal by collagen bridging, which is complicated if the edges are separated.

Aponeurotic edges may be separated after an incomplete early wound dehiscence or after an infection with tissue necrosis. Factors that tend to separate wound edges and increase the tension on the suture line are also associated with an increased rate of incisional hernia as shown in Table 30.1.

As the healing process progresses, increasing in tensile strength, the contribution by suture to wound strength decreases. If wound healing is delayed, then suture contribution to wound strength may be essential for a long period of time. Chemotherapy impairs wound healing and should therefore be postponed, probably for at least 4 weeks after laparotomy.

Incisional hernia probably develops because of a partial separation of wound edges, which makes collagen bridging

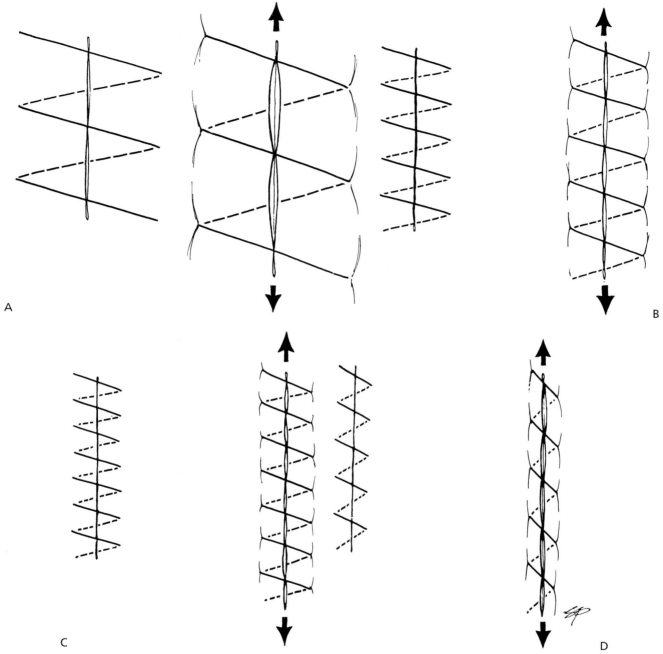

FIGURE 30.1. Diagrams of the effect of 30% wound lengthening in a continuously sutured wound. **(A)**, **(B)**, and **(C)** are closed with a suture length–to–wound length (SL:WL) ratio of 4, and a stitch interval of 20 mm, 10 mm, and 7 mm, respectively. **(D)** is closed with an SL:WL ratio of 2 and a stitch interval of 10 mm. In **(A)** the tension on each stitch is twice as high as in **(B)**, and three times higher than in **(C)**. After wound lengthening, stitch interval is less than 10 mm only in **(C)**. In **(D)**, lengthening of the wound causes marked compression of tissue held in the stitch.

TABLE 30.1. COMPARISON OF PATIENT AND OPERATIVE VARIABLES RELATED TO INCISIONAL HERNIA IN 808 PATIENTS, SUNDSVALL HOSPITAL 1984–93[a]

	Incisional Hernia	
	%	No.
Wound infection		
No	13	94/722
Yes	28	24/86
Overweight		
No	10	42/427
Yes	20	76/381
Age (yr)		
≤45	7	12/172
46–65	17	50/300
>65	17	56/336
Suture length–to–wound length ratio		
<3.5	23	55/242
3.5–3.9	18	18/98
4.0–4.4	7	9/137
4.5–4.9	7	6/84
≥5	12	28/241

[a]Wound infection, overweight, age, and a suture length–to–wound length ratio of less than 4 were significant risk factors.

complicated. The risk factors identified for the development of wound dehiscence and incisional hernia are almost identical. There is one exception, though: the majority of wound dehiscences occur in male patients, but the rate of incisional hernia is usually evenly distributed between the genders (10).

Definition of Incisional Hernia

There is no consistency in clinical studies regarding a definition of incisional hernia at follow-up; this makes comparison of results from different studies very difficult (3,5–7,17,19). It is also difficult to compare the proportion of patients who have incisional hernias repaired, as it may relate more to economic factors and the capacity of the surgical unit than to the actual number of hernias.

Early separation of aponeurotic margins predicts herniation accurately; a defect in the abdominal wound will gradually develop into a protrusion and eventually a visible bulge (18). To allow comparison of results between different clinical studies, patients should be examined for incisional hernia 12 months after index laparotomy. Is any detectable defect in the wound, a palpable defect in combination with protrusion, or only a protrusion regarded as hernia at follow-up? In studies using a broad definition, the hernia rate will most certainly be higher than if only visible bulges are regarded as hernia.

In studies examining patients 5 to 10 years after the index laparotomy, incisional hernias have continued to appear after the first year. It has been speculated that late-appearing her-

nias develop by other mechanisms, for example, by stretching of mature collagen. There is, however, reason to doubt this concept of late development of incisional hernia.

In our series, using a wide definition of incisional hernia and a meticulous examination at follow-up, it was possible to detect practically all hernias at 12 months, and very few appeared within the next 7 years (4). Hernias detected later than after 1 year were very small and had obviously been missed at the first follow-up, often because of patient overweight. There is consequently reason to believe that all incisional hernias develop early during the postoperative period by similar etiologic mechanisms.

Incisional hernia should be defined as any detectable defect in the wound at examination 12 months after the index operation.

Wound Infection

Wound infection in clinical studies is often defined as purulent discharge from the wound and is sometimes divided into minor and major wound infections, with the latter causing general symptoms that prolong hospital stay (1). A wound infection may be subclinical, only presenting with erythema or tenderness.

Mechanisms

The wound is most susceptible to wound infection during the inflammatory phase of healing. Bacterial contamination causes infection, especially in the presence of necrotic tissue or foreign material in the wound. Gastrointestinal surgery, long operation time, emergency operation, reoperation, and inadequate skin preparation have been associated with a high rate of infection (Table 30.2) (1). The risk of developing a wound infection can be reduced if prophylactic antibiotics are administered prior to a contaminated surgical procedure.

Placing high tension on the suture line may cause tissue necrosis and has been associated with an increased rate of wound infection (15). The choice of suture material is important, for the rate of infection is higher with multifilament materials than with the use of monofilaments.

Studies on the effect of surgical technique on wound infection are scarce. In several studies, some surgeons encounter wound infections more often than others, suggesting that the development of wound infection is strongly related to surgical technique. Clearly, a traumatizing technique leaving an abundance of necrotic tissue in the wound will be associated with a high rate of wound infection. Meticulous hemostasis is particularly important.

Age

Data on the importance of patient age for the development of wound infection are contradictory. In some studies, infection has been found to occur more frequently in older

TABLE 30.2. COMPARISON OF PATIENT AND OPERATIVE VARIABLES RELATED TO WOUND INFECTION IN 1,023 PATIENTS, SUNDSVALL HOSPITAL 1989–93[a]

	Wound Infection	
	%	No.
Age (yr)		
≤55	13	43/332
>55	8	54/691
Overweight		
No	7	40/561
Yes	13	57/450
Degree of contamination		
Clean	6	20/333
Contaminated	10	58/579
Dirty	17	19/111
Previous midline laparotomy		
No	9	68/792
More than 14 days ago	10	19/194
Reoperation	27	10/37
Stitch length		
<5 cm	7	21/307
≥5 cm	17	25/150

[a]Age of 55 or less, overweight, degree of contamination, reoperation, and a stitch length of 5 cm or more were significant risk factors.

patients, suggesting that this might correlate to a low host-defense capability in the elderly patient (1). A lower rate of wound infection in elderly patients has also been reported, and this may relate to overweight being uncommon among the elderly (10). Overweight is most common in the middle-aged population, and the proportion is gradually reduced as age increases.

DECISIONS TO BE MADE

Many of the factors identified as being important for the rate of wound complications are not possible to correct preoperatively or cannot be influenced by the surgeon (Tables 30.1 and 30.2). Patient age or overweight cannot, of course, be influenced when an emergent laparotomy of a grossly contaminated abdomen is required. The suture technique is, however, completely in the hands of the surgeon and relates strongly to the rate of wound complications. To reduce the rate of wound failures, we should focus on the suture technique.

During a laparotomy, the surgeon makes several decisions important to the subsequent rate of wound complications. To gain access to the abdominal cavity, he or she can choose a variety of different laparotomy incisions. The surgeon selects the incision for abdominal access, the technique for opening (sharp or electrocautery), and the suture material and technique for closure of the wound.

The Incision

The choice of laparotomy incision is influenced by consideration of the complexity of the incision and the time it takes to open and close the abdomen. The access gained must also be considered. The rate of wound complications is different for midline, paramedian, lateral paramedian, oblique, transverse, and muscle-splitting incisions.

The tension on the suture line is lower in transverse or oblique incisions than in midline incisions. Transverse incisions are thought to be associated with a lower rate of wound dehiscence and incisional hernia than are midline incisions. This has not, however, been convincingly substantiated in clinical studies, and several studies have failed to detect any difference (6). A suggested higher rate of wound dehiscence in incisions in the upper abdomen versus the lower abdomen also has not been verified (2).

Contractions of the abdominal wall will, in muscle-splitting incisions, produce a shutter mechanism that tends to close the wound. This theoretically is the advantage of muscle-splitting incisions. In clinical studies, the rate of wound dehiscence and incisional hernia has indeed been reported to be very low in muscle-splitting incisions (5,14). A very low rate of wound dehiscence and incisional hernia in lateral paramedian incisions, where this shutter mechanism may also be present, has been reported in one study, but the results have not been duplicated (2).

Vertical Midline Incisions

Although muscle-splitting incisions are associated with a lower rate of wound dehiscence and incisional hernia, they are not always feasible because they provide a limited access to the abdominal cavity. Paramedian, lateral paramedian, and oblique incisions provide access that is often more limited than with midline incisions. Vertical midline incisions are preferred when wide or rapid access to the abdomen is required. The high rates of wound complications in midline incisions may be the result of surgeons preferring these incisions for major or emergency abdominal surgery, surgery known to be associated with a high rate of wound failure.

In midline incisions, no major vessels are severed and the risk of entrapping significant nerves with subsequent neuralgia or paralysis of abdominal wall muscles is minimal. Postoperative pain seems to be more pronounced with midline than with transverse or oblique incisions, perhaps due to the fact that more dermatomas are involved.

When restricted access to the abdomen is sufficient, muscle-splitting incisions are preferred as they are associated with a much lower rate of wound complications.

The Suture Material

Basically, the surgeon has to choose between multifilament and monofilament suture materials, and between nonabsorbables and absorbables. An absorbable suture may contribute to the strength of the wound for a various length of time, depending on the material used. Today, the choice is entirely restricted to the group of modern synthetic sutures as materials previously used (e.g., catgut, linen, silk) are associated with a high rate of wound complications.

Monofilaments

Monofilament materials are associated with a lower rate of wound infection than are multifilaments. This may be due to bacteria being enclosed within the interstices of multifilament sutures, where they are protected from phagocytosis. As wound infection is a risk factor for the development of wound dehiscence and incisional hernia, the choice of a monofilament material may also reduce the rate of these complications.

Insufficient strength of the suture material is rarely the cause of wound dehiscence. Generally, larger dimensions than are really necessary to withstand wound tension are used. A suture breaking is more likely to be the result of an inadequate surgical technique than insufficient suture strength. Pinching of the suture with surgical instruments may cause weakening of the material.

With modern suture materials that contribute to the strength of the wound for at least 14 days, no difference has been found in the rate of wound dehiscence. This is to be expected as they all support the wound during the postoperative period, when its intrinsic strength is low and dehiscence usually occurs (2,6,7).

Absorbables

Sir Berkeley G.A. Moynihan in 1920 proposed that the ideal suture should be absorbable, and such materials are commonly used today. The advantage of absorbable suture materials may be mainly theoretic since modern monofilament nonabsorbables do not seem to be associated with any major long-term disadvantages. A reduced risk of suture sinus and "button hole" hernia and a shorter period of postoperative pain have been suggested with absorbable materials. However, sinus formation is encountered with both absorbable and nonabsorbable suture materials, and clinical evidence showing any difference regarding "button hole" hernia or pain is lacking.

It has been proposed that the rate of incisional hernia is similar with all suture materials that contribute to the strength of the wound for at least 14 days. However, this assumption has not been substantiated in clinical studies, probably because wound healing may often be prolonged beyond this time by, for example, a wound infection.

Nonabsorbable suture materials (nylon) allow support of the wound during the entire healing period and have been used with good results. With slowly absorbable monofilament suture materials that retain an acceptable strength for at least 6 weeks (polydioxanone), the rate of incisional hernia has been similar to nonabsorbables (7). With absorbable suture materials that lose 80% of their strength within 14 days, incisional hernia has been shown to be more common.

Comparison of Suture Materials

In studies comparing different suture materials, the suture technique is usually not monitored. Differences in handling properties and color may allow surgeons to recognize individual suture materials and hence unknowingly influence their suture technique. A bias may thus be introduced as both material and technique affect wound healing, and it seems that this bias results in a more meticulous suture technique with a newly introduced suture material (12). A more meticulous technique with a new material may cause a lower rate of incisional hernia. Thus, results of studies comparing suture materials without monitoring the suture technique are difficult to interpret.

Monofilament suture materials should be used to minimize the rate of wound infection. A low hernia rate with nonabsorbable sutures (nylon) is well documented in several clinical studies. Similar results can be produced with absorbable suture materials that retain an acceptable strength for at least 6 weeks (polydioxanone).

The Method of Wound Closure

The surgeon has to choose between different methods for closure of laparotomy wounds. An interrupted or a continuous suture technique can be used, and the wound can be closed in a single layer or in several layers. According to the classic mass closure technique, all layers of the abdominal wall except skin were incorporated in the stitch. The surgeon may feel inclined, however, to include in the stitch only tissue that contributes significantly to the suture-holding capacity of the wound.

The Continuous Suture Line

A continuous suture technique has been shown in several studies to be less time-consuming than an interrupted technique, and the rate of wound dehiscence and incisional hernia is similar with both techniques. With a continuous technique, less foreign material and fewer knots are deposited in the wound, and this may have relevance for the development of wound infection and sinus formation (20).

If a single stitch in an interrupted closure is very tight, ischemia will develop in the tissue enclosed. This is less likely to occur with a running suture, as one of the advantages with a continuous technique is that it allows tension to adjust evenly along the suture line.

The Mass Closure Technique

With a mass closure technique, the tensile strength of the wound is higher during the inflammatory phase of the early postoperative period than with a layered technique. This would be expected to be important for the development of wound dehiscence, and consequently the frequency of this complication has been lower with a mass technique (16). It is not clear why a mass technique is superior to a layered technique, but it might be speculated that a mass technique produces a higher suture length–to–wound length (SL:WL) ratio because more tissue is included in each stitch. Incisional hernia develops with the same frequency whether a layered or a mass closure technique is used.

The original definition of the mass closure technique stated that "all layers of the abdominal wall except skin" were to be included in the stitch. It can be doubted whether this is the common practice for single layer closures today, and its rationale can be questioned. Placing stitches in tissues that do not contribute to wound strength cannot have any positive effect on the rate of wound dehiscence or incisional hernia. Furthermore, circulation is impaired in tissues grasped in a suture, and this causes tissue necrosis that augments the risk of wound infection (18).

Suturing with the Smead–Jones technique by alternating stitches placed far from and near the wound edge is occasionally advised for wound closure. The physical properties of this stitch have not been thoroughly investigated, and clinical data do not support the claim that this technique reduces the rate of wound complications.

Suture-Holding Tissue

Including subcutaneous fat in the suture does not add to the strength of the wound, and the amount of necrotic tissue in the wound is likely to be increased. No evidence available indicates that including muscle in the stitch adds to the strength of the wound, but muscle, as well as subcutaneous fat, is likely to be susceptible to impaired circulation. Including peritoneum in the suture does not contribute to wound strength, and consequently in clinical studies the rate of wound dehiscence is similar whether peritoneum is included in the suture or not. Placing stitches in the peritoneum may even have detrimental effects and, in experimental studies, contributes to the formation of postoperative intraabdominal adhesions.

The tensile strength of a vertical midline incision is related mainly to the strength of the aponeurosis, and consequently the suture technique should primarily aim at holding aponeurotic edges in exact apposition during the early postoperative period in order to permit collagen bridging. From this point of view, it seems rational to suture midline incisions in one layer, including only the aponeurosis but no other layers of the abdominal wall, in the stitch, and this has been done with excellent clinical results in large personal series (11).

The Knot

The knot is always the weakest point of a suture and, in fact, placing a single hitch at the midpoint of a suture reduces its strength by one third. An optimal knot should not weaken the suture or slip, and it should be as small as possible. Differences in physical properties between suture materials cause differences in knot security, and several studies have been carried out on the performance of various knots using different suture materials. The surgeon must therefore be aware of how a particular knot performs with different suture materials and adjust his or her technique accordingly.

Monofilament suture materials have a low surface friction, and knots tend to slip more easily than with multifilaments. To overcome this difficulty with monofilaments, very complex bulky knots are usually created. Bulky knots, especially in superficial sites, may cause the patient discomfort and, particularly in patients with a thin subcutaneous layer, the knots of an abdominal suture line may be palpable and cause discomfort severe enough to motivate their removal.

The size of the knot may also have relevance to the formation of a suture sinus as the volume of the knot is related to the degree of surrounding tissue reaction. Sinus formation is more common after wound infection and is probably related to bacteria retained in knots or in multifilament suture materials.

Anchor Knots

With a continuous suture technique, the anchor knots that start and finish the suture line must be reliable. As monofilament suture materials are preferred for a running suture, complex and bulky knots are often used. The suture loop was designed in an attempt to overcome difficulties with the anchor knots. With this procedure, double the amount of suture material needed is deposited in the wound and, although the starting knot is small and probably reliable, the finishing knot still has to be a bulky conventional knot.

An anchor knot differs from a single stitch knot as it consists of three threads instead of only two. Anchor knots should therefore be tested by applying tension to all three threads. Results from studies of the performance of single-stitch knots should not uncritically be held valid for anchor knots.

Self-Locking Knots

Self-locking knots have been proposed as an alternative for the anchor knots used in a continuous suture (Fig. 30.2). Self-locking knots are formed in such a way that they lock up more tightly when tension is applied to the continuous suture line. Theoretically, this would prevent slipping of the

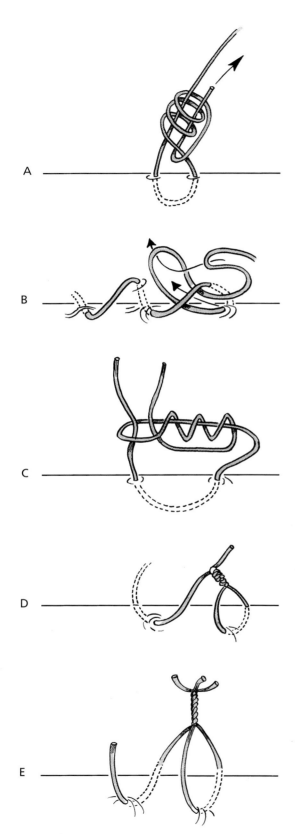

FIGURE 30.2. Types of anchor knots evaluated. Knots **(A)**, **(B)**, and **(C)** are self-locking knots. Knots **(D)** and **(E)** are conventional surgical knots in the configuration 2 × 2 = 1 = 1 = 1 = 1. (From Israelsson LA, Jonsson T. Physical properties of self locking and conventional surgical knots. *Eur J Surg* 1994;160:323–327, with permission.)

knot, and experimental tests and clinical experience have supported this. A self-locking knot can slip neither partially nor totally, whereas conventional anchor knots often slip (Table 30.3).

With self-locking knots, the suture loses less of its strength than with conventional knots. With the large monofilament suture materials used for laparotomy closure, a self-locking knot diminishes the strength of the suture by less than 10%. Thus, a self-locking knot actually reduces the strength of the material less than a single hitch at the midpoint of a suture. This unexpected performance may be due to self-locking knots permitting the end of the continuous suture to slide inside the knot, and this may absorb some of the energy that would otherwise be directly transmitted to the knot.

Self-locking knots are smaller than conventional anchor knots, which may be beneficial in certain situations, and tying them is easy to learn (Figs. 30.3 and 30.4). Self-locking knots have been used in large clinical series with excellent results (9).

The Suture Technique

The choice of suture technique is totally in the hands of the surgeon and is certainly an important factor for the development of wound complications. The purpose of the continuing search for the optimal surgical technique is to reduce the rate of wound complications. That this is possible has also been shown in clinical studies (8).

A surgeon adhering to the principles outlined in the previous discussion may feel inclined to close midline laparotomy incisions by a continuous technique in one layer. The surgeon will also require information about the

TABLE 30.3. PARTIAL AND TOTAL SLIPPAGE OF SELF-LOCKING AND CONVENTIONAL SURGICAL KNOTS OF POLYGLACTIN, POLYDIOXANONE, AND NYLON IN USP SIZES 1, 2-ZERO, AND 4-ZERO

Knot and Suture Material	USP Size		
	1	2-Zero	4-Zero
Self-locking knots (A, B, C)			
Polyglactin	0	0	0
Polydioxanone	0	0	0
Nylon	0	0	0
Conventional starting knot (D)			
Polyglactin	8	4	0
Polydioxanone	4	10	4
Nylon	10	10	0
Conventional finishing knot (E)			
Polyglactin	0	0	0
Polydioxanone	4 total	0	0
Nylon	1 total	2 total	2 total

[a]Ten tests were done for each combination of knot, suture material, and size.
From Israelsson LA, Jonsson T. Physical properties of self locking and conventional surgical knots. *Eur J Surg* 1994;160:323–327, with permission.

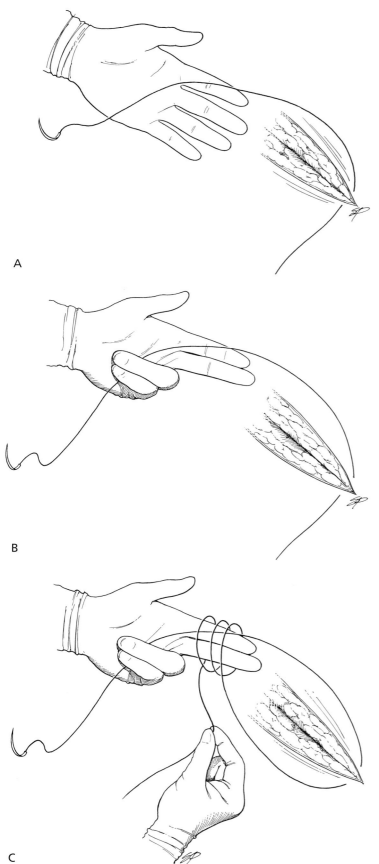

FIGURE 30.3. Technique for hand tie of a self-locking starting knot of a continuous suture. **A:** After placing the first stitch in the wound, the suture attached to the needle is placed along the index/long finger, and over the open palm of the left hand. **B:** Ring and little finger hold the suture in the palm. **C:** With the right hand, the suture is wound three times around the suture attached to the needle and index/long finger.

(Continued)

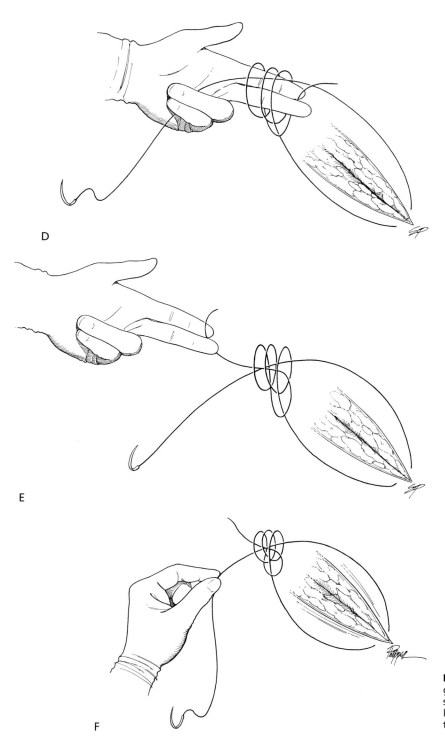

D

E

F

FIGURE 30.3. *(continued)* D: The suture is grasped between index and long finger. **E:** The suture is pulled through the loops. **F:** The knot locks as traction is placed on the suture attached to the needle.

appropriate distance from wound edges to place the stitches, the optimal stitch interval, and the tension that should be applied to the suture. The surgeon might even request a specific measure of the suture technique by which the quality of his or her technique could be evaluated. In continuously closed wounds, such a measure actually exists and is easily achieved.

Monitoring the Suture Technique

In a continuously closed laparotomy incision, the suture technique can be monitored through the SL:WL ratio (7). This ratio between the length of the suture consumed and the length of the wound is easily calculated on a routine basis in the clinical situation.

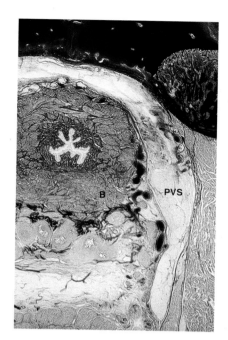

COLOR PLATE 1. Fat configuration of the prevesical space in a newborn boy. *B*, bladder; *PVS*, prevesical space. See Figure 5.2C on page 47. (Courtesy of Prof. Helga Fritsch, Department of Anatomy, University of Innsbruck, Austria.)

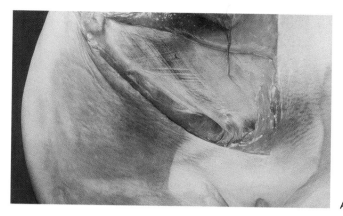

A

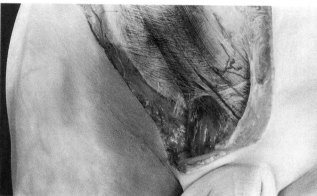

B

COLOR PLATE 2. Gender differences in groin anatomy. **A:** Independently of transversalis fascia strength, direct hernias are rare in women because the direct space is closed hermetically by external oblique aponeurosis. **B:** Holding strength of external oblique aponeurosis is propagated upon inner structures over cord, fat, and fascias. See Figure 5.7 on page 50. (From Thiel W. *Photographischer atlas der praktischen anatomie I*. Heidelberg: Springer Verlag, 1996:19, with permission.)

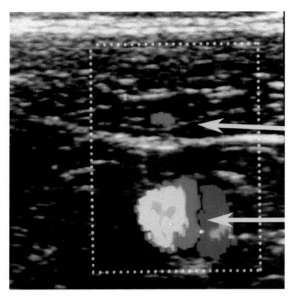

COLOR PLATE 3. Typical findings of epigastric artery in the inguinal region. See Figure 8.5 on page 83.

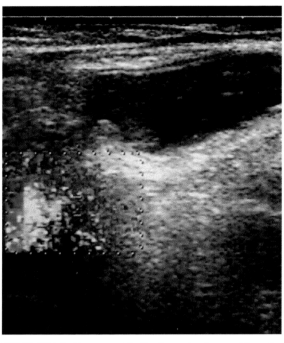

COLOR PLATE 4. Sonographic finding of a femoral hernia. See Figure 8.10 on page 85.

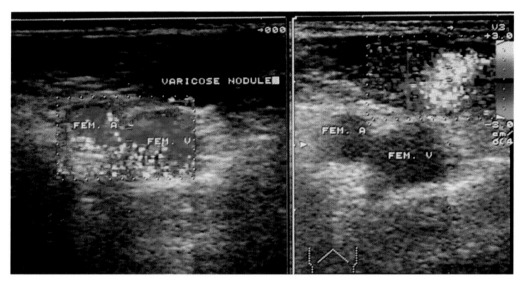

COLOR PLATE 5. Sonographic finding of a varicose nodule. The color-coded duplex sonography shows blood flow inside the nodule. See Figure 8.21 on page 89.

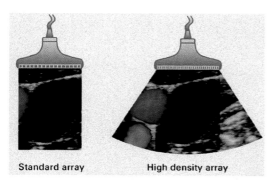

COLOR PLATE 6. Variable format with linear array: standard and high density. See Figure 9.5 on page 97. (Courtesy of Siemens AG, 1999).

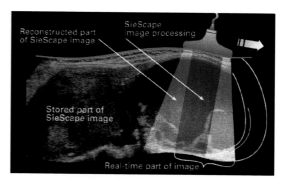

COLOR PLATE 7. SieScape panoramic imaging. See Figure 9.6 on page 97. (Courtesy of Siemens AG, 1999.)

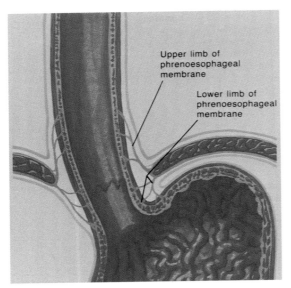

COLOR PLATE 8. The phrenoesophageal ligament, which assists in securing the gastroesophageal junction. See Figure 41.1 on page 479.

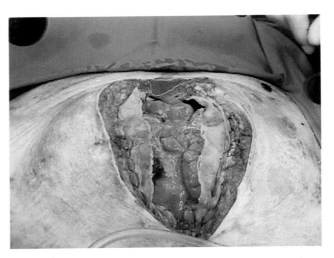

COLOR PLATE 9. Marlex mesh implanted for 6 years. See Figure 47.6 on page 556.

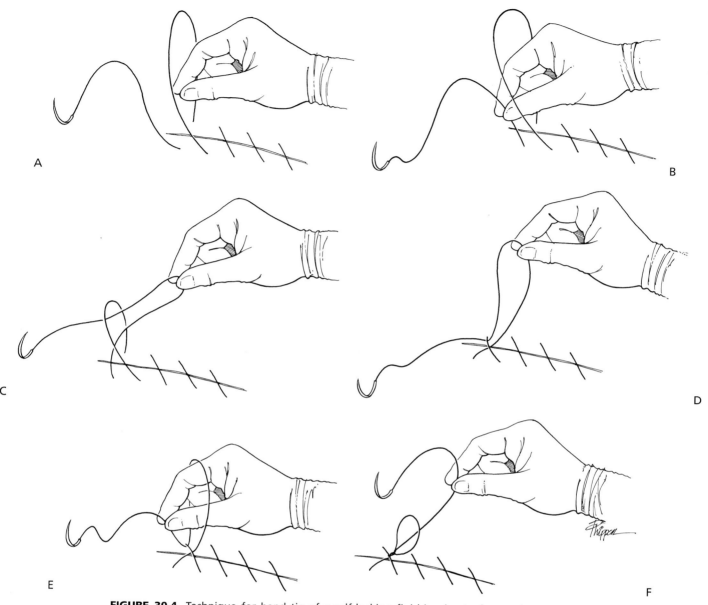

A

B

C

D

E

F

FIGURE 30.4. Technique for hand tie of a self-locking finishing knot of a continuous suture (chain stitch knot or Aberdeen knot). The last stitch placed in the wound is picked up and creates a loop. **A:** Thumb and index finger of the right hand are slipped into the loop. **B:** The suture attached to the needle is grasped close to the wound with thumb and index finger. **C:** The suture is pulled back through the loop. **D:** Traction on the suture tightens the knot and a new loop is formed. **A–D** are repeated three times. Traction on the suture attached to the needle should be avoided. **E** and **F:** The knot locks as the suture with needle is passed completely through the last loop.

The length of the suture material consumed is calculated by subtracting the measured length of suture remnants from the original suture length (SL). Thus, if the original length of the suture is 150 cm and suture remnants are 50 cm, the SL is 100 cm. The wound length (WL) is defined as the length of the skin incision and can be measured during or after closure.

The SL:WL ratio can also be calculated in wounds closed with an interrupted technique, but this is very time-consuming and highly impractical in the clinical situation.

Establishing SL by drying and weighing suture remnants has been performed in some experimental studies.

The importance of suture technique for the development of wound dehiscence or incisional hernia was emphasized by Jenkins (13). He suggested that these complications can be prevented by the use of continuous sutures at 1-cm intervals and by ensuring that the amount of suture consumed was more than four times the length of the wound. Biomechanical studies support the importance of a high SL:WL ratio, as wound bursting strength increases with a higher ratio. With the use of a high SL:WL ratio, wound tension seems to be distributed to the suture line in such a way that the suture-holding capacity of the tissues is not easily exceeded.

The Suture Length–to–Wound Length Ratio

A strong correlation between the SL:WL ratio and the development of incisional hernia has been confirmed in clinical studies. The rate of incisional hernia is lower if the SL:WL ratio is at least 4, and suturing using a lower ratio is associated with a threefold increase in the rate of incisional hernia (Table 30.1) (7–13).

There seems to be no advantage to using an SL:WL ratio higher than 5. In overweight patients, closure with a ratio of more than 5 has been associated with a somewhat higher rate of both wound infection and incisional hernia, probably because a large amount of tissue other than aponeurosis is then included in the suture. The rates of wound infection and incisional hernia may in overweight patients actually be similar to that of others if wounds are closed with an SL:WL ratio of between 4 and 5 (10).

The SL:WL ratio depends on the stitch interval, the size of tissue bites, and the tension on the suture. Wound dehiscence or incisional hernia would, of course, occur with extreme values of stitch interval or size of tissue bites. With a very long stitch interval intestinal contents would protrude into the wound, and with very small tissue bites practically no tissue would be held in the suture (Fig. 30.1). However, within reasonable limits, these factors have separately not been found to be important for the development of incisional hernia (9). Thus, wound closure with small tissue bites placed very closely or with larger tissue bites at greater intervals produces similar hernia rates provided that the SL:WL ratio is 4 or more.

Stitch Length and Tension

The size of tissue bites can be reflected in the stitch length, calculated as the ratio of the SL and the number of stitches. If the stitch length is too long, the rate of wound infection is high. An optimal stitch length is less than 5 cm (Table 30.2). A longer stitch suggests large tissue bites, probably including tissue other than aponeurosis, and poor circulation in such tissue may explain the correlation with infection (9).

Excessive tension should not be placed on the suture since it reduces local blood flow and has been associated with an increased rate of wound infection (15). Furthermore, higher wound strength is achieved during the early postoperative period with a loose suture with just enough tension to approximate fascia edges (2).

"Button hole" hernias at the site of stitches penetrating the aponeurosis have been reported and are probably caused by the suture cutting through the tissue. In my opinion,

"button hole" hernias develop because excessive tension is placed on the suture line, with subsequent tissue necrosis.

The most common mistake made is that too much tension is placed on the suture line. The opposite is hardly possible, as the tension only has to be sufficient for the suture to approximate wound edges, and if this is not fulfilled it will be immediately apparent.

Wound Dehiscence

If wound tension is distributed to the suture line in such a way that the suture-holding capacity of the tissues is exceeded during the early postoperative period, wound dehiscence will occur. The wound bursting strength increases with a higher SL:WL ratio, and it has been found that a high proportion of wound dehiscence occurs in wounds closed using a low ratio (2).

To achieve a low rate of early wound dehiscence then, sutures should be placed at short intervals and at a good distance from wound edges, producing an SL:WL ratio of at least 4. In our series of 577 patients with midline incisions closed with a ratio of more than 4, dehiscence was encountered in only one patient, who developed a major wound infection with total necrosis of abdominal wall tissues.

Repair of the Dehisced Wound

Wound dehiscence requires immediate reoperation, and various methods have been used for this procedure. This reoperation is often difficult as abdominal distention is frequently present and wound tissues are frail due to inflammation or infection.

I have tried closing dehisced wounds by placing stitches 4 to 5 cm from wound edges at an interval of 0.5 cm, producing an SL:WL ratio of about 15. The anatomic layers of the abdominal wall cannot usually be separated, and stitches are therefore placed according to the classic mass closure technique. The skin incision is not sutured, in order to facilitate drainage and reduce the risk of infection.

The rationale for this technique is that wound tension will be distributed to a very large amount of tissue, and the risk of its suture-holding capacity's being exceeded will be low. Satisfactory results have been achieved with this method, and no development of incisional hernia has been noted.

Retention sutures have been suggested for closure of dehisced wounds or when the tension on the suture line is very high, and devices for such sutures are commercially available. With wound tension distributed to only a few retention sutures, the tension on each stitch will be very high, and the risk of the suture-holding capacity of the tissues being exceeded is high. Clinical studies reporting superior results with retention sutures are lacking.

Using a prosthetic mesh with a sublay technique has been proposed for repair of dehisced wounds. No clinical studies reporting results are yet available, but this method should probably be considered when exceptional abdominal distention is present.

PREVENTION OF WOUND COMPLICATIONS

The ultimate purpose of studying wound healing and wound failure is to reduce the risk of patients developing wound complications. To reduce the rate of wound failure, surgeons not only have to be conscious of a possible correlation between the surgical technique and the development of complications, but they also must be able to change their technique. It is possible to reduce the rate of incisional hernia on a large scale and within a short time if surgeons are given instructions and are supplied with adequate feedback concerning their adherence to the instructions (8).

Changing the Suture Technique

In a prospective study, we found that midline incisions were sutured with a mean SL:WL ratio of 3.6. A large proportion of patients were thus sutured with a ratio of less than 4 and subsequently subjected to a high risk of developing incisional hernia.

Surgeons were informed about the low ratio and its correlation with a high hernia rate and urged to suture all wounds with an SL:WL ratio of at least 4. These instructions were followed, and the mean ratio was increased to 4.9 (8). Subsequently, the hernia rate was reduced from 19% to 11%, and the proportion of incisional hernias that required repair within 18 months of the index laparotomy also decreased from 4% to 2%. Wound dehiscence became very rare after the intervention, and the present rate is less than 0.5%.

As demonstrated, it was possible for surgeons to change their suture technique, and this simple adjustment considerably improved late operative results. The change of technique was not expensive and was easy to accomplish: it merely required that the SL:WL ratio be calculated at the completion of every wound closure. The assisting nurse expediently performed this calculation while the surgeon completed the closure of the skin. As the surgeon at every wound closure was made aware of the SL:WL accomplished, adjustment to an adequate suture technique was soon achieved. Surgeons generally chose the easiest and also the most relevant way to increase the SL:WL ratio, by placing more stitches in the wound and thereby reducing the stitch interval (8).

The Length of the Thread

Commercially available suture materials are delivered in fixed lengths, and this will require attention when technique is changed to suturing with a high SL:WL ratio. In our series, some midline incisions were more than 90 cm

long, and suturing with approximately 400 cm of thread was required for an adequate ratio. In such long wounds, suturing with materials that are delivered in short lengths will be inconvenient, as several sutures have to be used. It is also important to note that every suture in a continuous suture line starts and ends with an anchor knot and sutures should not be tied to each other.

We prefer using sutures that are delivered in lengths of 150 cm as these are often sufficient for closing wounds of less than 25 cm. However, in our series, 50% of midline incisions were longer than 25 cm and consequently required several sutures. Loop sutures are delivered in lengths of no more than 75 cm, and surgeons are discouraged from using them (as the length of suture will be sufficient only for the closure of a 15-cm wound) if an SL:WL ratio of more than 4 is to be ascertained.

The Tired Surgeon

Several factors may influence the suture technique, and surgeons must be aware of these as the technique often affects the development of wound complications. When we interpret reports of clinical studies comparing suture materials, it is important to know that the choice of material may affect the technique used, and wound closure may have been more meticulous with a newly introduced material (12). Laparotomy wounds closed after repair of an abdominal aortic aneurysm are less often closed with an SL:WL ratio of more than 4 than after other procedures (11). The higher rate of incisional hernia in aneurysm patients reported in some studies has probably been caused by such a difference in suture technique.

Surgeons tend to close wounds with a lower SL:WL ratio if the laparotomy incision is very long (11). This may relate to surgeons being reluctant to use the number of sutures required to achieve an adequate ratio in long wounds. It may also relate, however, to surgeons being exhausted, since there is a correlation between long incisions and long operation time. Surgeons tend to close wounds using a lower SL:WL ratio if the duration of the operation is over 3 hours.

RECOMMENDATIONS

Wound complications continue to be a major source of morbidity and mortality after laparotomies.

It is recommended that laparotomy incisions be closed by a continuous suture technique in one layer. Self-locking knots should be used for the anchor knots. The suture material should be a monofilament nonabsorbable suture (nylon) or an absorbable material that contributes to the strength of the wound for at least 6 weeks (polydioxanone).

In vertical midline incisions, stitches should mainly include aponeurotic tissue and be placed at least 10 mm from wound edges. The length of each stitch should be less than 5 cm; otherwise, it will be associated with an unnecessary high rate of wound infection. Incorporating peritoneum, muscle, or subcutaneous fat in the suture is not necessary and may have deleterious effects. The surgeon should take care that excessive tension is not placed on the suture.

Under no circumstances should the wound be closed by an SL:WL ratio of less than 4. The only way to ascertain that this does not happen is to calculate the ratio at the end of every laparotomy closure. Suturing with a very high ratio is not necessary, and an optimal SL:WL ratio is between 4 and 5.

REFERENCES

1. Bremmelgaard A, Raahave D, Beier-Holgersen R, et al. Computer-aided surveillance of surgical infections and identification of risk factors. *J Hosp Infect* 1989;13:1–18.
2. Carlson MA. Acute wound failure. *Surg Clin North Am* 1997;77: 607–636.
3. Carlson MA, Condon RE. Polyglyconate (Maxon) versus nylon suture in midline abdominal incision closure: a prospective randomized trial. *Am J Surg* 1995;61:980–983.
4. Cengiz Y, Israelsson LA. Incisional hernias in midline incisions: an eight-year follow up. *Hernia* 1998;2:175–177.
5. Duce AM, Lozano O, Villeta R, et al. Incisional hernia following appendectomy. Surgical experience. *Hernia* 1998;2:169–171.
6. Gislason H, Grønbech JE, Søreide O. Burst abdomen and incisional hernia after major gastrointestinal operations—comparison of three closure techniques. *Eur J Surg* 1995;161:349–354.
7. Israelsson LA, Jonsson T. Closure of midline laparotomy incisions with polydioxanone and nylon: the importance of suture technique. *Br J Surg* 1994;81:1606–1608.
8. Israelsson LA, Jonsson T. Incisional hernia after midline laparotomy; a prospective study. *Eur J Surg* 1996;162:125–129.
9. Israelsson LA, Jonsson T, Knutsson A. Suture technique and healing in midline laparotomy incisions. *Eur J Surg* 1996;162:605–609.
10. Israelsson LA, Jonsson T. Overweight and healing of midline incisions: the importance of suture technique. *Eur J Surg* 1997; 163:175–180.
11. Israelsson LA. Incisional hernias in patients with aortic aneurysmal disease: the importance of suture technique. *Eur J Endovasc Surg* 1999;17:133–135.
12. Israelsson LA. Bias in clinical trials: the importance of suture technique. *Eur J Surg* 1999;165:3–7.
13. Jenkins TP. The burst abdominal wound: a mechanical approach. *Br J Surg* 1976;63:873–876.
14. Luijendijk RW, Jeekel J, Sorm RK, et al. The low transverse Pfannenstiel incision and the prevalence of incisional hernia and nerve entrapment. *Ann Surg* 1997;225:365–369.
15. Mayer AD, Ausobsky JR, Evans M, et al. Compression suture of the abdominal wall: a controlled trial in 302 major laparotomies. *Br J Surg* 1981;68:632–634.
16. Niggebrugge AHP, Hansen BE, Trimbos JB, et al. Mechanical factors influencing the incidence of burst abdomen. *Eur J Surg* 1995;161:655–661.
17. Osther PJ, Gjøde P, Mortensen BB, et al. Randomised comparison of polyglycolic acid and polyglyconate sutures for abdominal fascial closure after laparotomy in patients with suspected impaired wound healing. *Br J Surg* 1995;82:1080–1082.
18. Pollock AV, Evans M. Early prediction of late incisional hernias. *Br J Surg* 1989;76:953–954.
19. Sugerman HJ, Kellum JM, Reines HD, et al. Greater risk of incisional hernia with morbidly obese than steroid-dependent patients and low recurrence with prefascial polypropylene mesh. *Am J Surg* 1996;171:80–84.
20. Trimbos JB, vanRooij J. Amount of suture material needed for continuous or interrupted wound closure: an experimental study. *Eur J Surg* 1993;159:141–143.

31

PROSTHETIC REPAIR OF MASSIVE ABDOMINAL VENTRAL HERNIAS

JEAN B. FLAMENT
JEAN P. PALOT

Incisional hernia is a protrusion, beneath the skin, of intraabdominal viscera through a postoperative defect of the abdominal wall (Fig. 31.1). Progress in surgical techniques, even with laparoscopic surgery, has unfortunately not led to the disappearance of incisional hernia. On the contrary, the frequency of this complication seems to be increasing as major and lengthy operations are performed, especially in elderly patients with concomitant organic disease.

These lesions have a clear tendency to undergo aggravation and recurrence, and thus we often have to treat massive multirecurrent incisional hernias. Surgical repair is very difficult in these cases of large abdominal defect, when the herniated viscera have "lost their right to reside" in the abdominal cavity. Finally, in exceptional cases, incisional herniation is beyond the scope of surgical repair owing to severe deterioration of the patient's condition, notably due to old age, disabling obesity, and grave disturbances of respiratory function.

Closure of an incisional hernia has nothing in common with closure of a laparotomy. Surgical repair must take into account the irremediable weakening of the abdominal wall and the consequences of decreased abdominal pressure on diaphragmatic mobility and respiratory function. It must be considered as a difficult procedure. It begins with careful evaluation of the patient's general health associated with a general preparation that may take several weeks prior to operation. Surgical techniques of

repair should be based largely on the use of prosthetic substitutes; therefore, the precautions that must be taken when artificial material is introduced into the human body should be kept in mind.

A clear definition of these lesions is important: massive incisional hernia, as discussed below, corresponds to cases where the hernial orifice is greater than 10 cm in diameter; often it reaches or exceeds a diameter of 20 cm. In most cases, the tumefaction is of considerable size. The hernial mass is often mushroom-like, and the computed tomography (CT) scan has given us a new vision of the defect, the sac, and its contents (Fig. 31.2). In practically all cases, pruriginous intertrigo is seen at the periphery of the tumefaction. Patients with massive incisional hernia are often obese and in poor general health. These lesions must always be regarded as severe, and the surgical treatment they require may sometimes be a truly "formidable procedure" (52).

In the past, incisional hernias were treated by turndown or overlapping surgery using neighboring aponeurotic structures. These surgical procedures gave manifestly unsatisfactory results (49). However, some of these older techniques (45) should not be forgotten. Judd's technique (39) is one such case: we still use this approach as first-line therapy in minor forms of incisional hernia or when sepsis is present.

Large hernial orifices and recurrent herniation require treatment using replacement material. The failure of autografts naturally led surgeons to investigate the possible usefulness of prosthetic material. Early prostheses were constructed of metal or nylon. The former material was well tolerated, but its rigidity was a major drawback. Early nylon prostheses were also too rigid and led to infection. The advent of Marlex mesh, used in the United States, and later of Dacron–Mersilene (Ethicon, Inc., Somerville, NJ, U.S.A.), widely used in France (41), has clearly meant great progress. We investigated this type of prosthetic material as soon as it was introduced in France in 1966 (41), and used

J. B. Flament and J. P. Palot: Department of Surgery, Reims University; Department of General Surgery, Hôpital Robert Debré, Reims Cédex, France.

This article was written with the participation of C. Avisse, J.F. Delattre, J.P. Concé, and C. Marcus. Their affiliations are as follows: C. Avisse and J.F. Delattre: Department of General and Digestive Surgery, Hôpital Robert Debré, Reims, France. J.P. Concé: Department of Anesthetic Reanimation, Hôpital Robert Debré, Reims, France. C. Marcus: Department of Radiology, Hôpital Robert Debré, Reims, France.

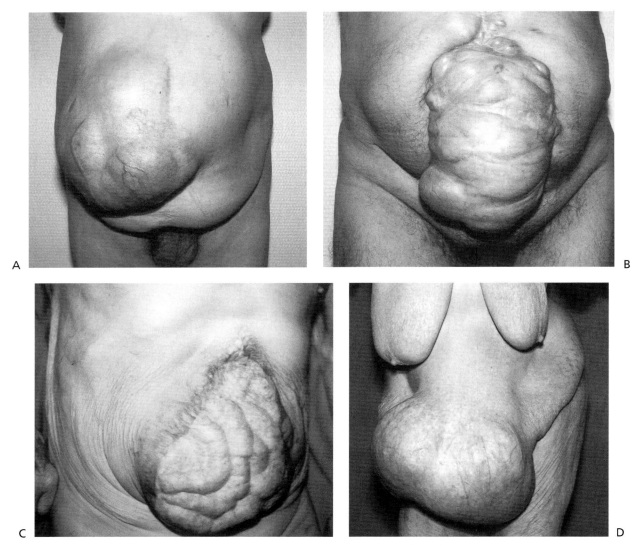

FIGURE 31.1. A–D: Some examples of huge incisional hernias.

at that time large sheets sutured in place to reinforce the abdominal wall.

In the early 1970s, better knowledge was also acquired regarding the serious consequences of respiratory insufficiency, thanks to the important contribution to this field of the work by Goñi Moreno (34), later publications by us on paradoxical abdominal respiration (52), and studies by Italian authors on disturbances of pulmonary compliance (64). The commercial introduction of absorbable prosthetic mesh (Dexon, Davis and Geck, Richmond, Surrey, U.K.; Vicryl, Ethicon) has opened up new therapeutic possibilities in cases of infected lesions. However, the rate

of recurrence of incisional hernia is too high when this material is used, and thus it cannot be used routinely.

ETIOLOGY

Surgical responsibility for the occurrence of incisional hernia may be manifest in cases where laparotomy has been done with disregard of anatomic conditions. In such cases, herniation results from the abusive transection of neurovascular structures and the resulting atrophy of the abdominal wall (Fig. 31.3). The quality of suturing can also be considered

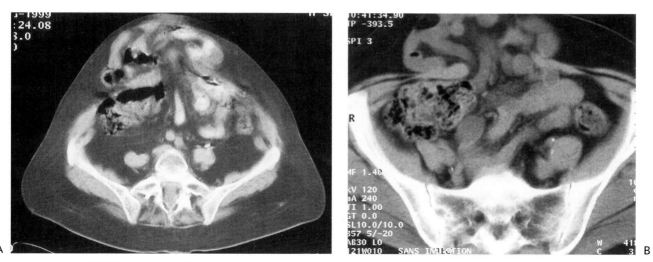

FIGURE 31.2. A and **B:** Computed tomography (CT) scan and incisional hernias. CT has given a new perspective of the sac and its contents.

when incisional hernia occurs rapidly in the absence of infection. In such cases, an obvious cause is poorly fashioned closure, where the spacing and bite of the sutures have been incorrectly evaluated (37, 38).

Incisional hernia may also be a consequence of *infection* along the suture of the operative wound. Such cases can be avoided by withdrawing one or more of the sequestered sutures, which promote infection. The affected zone is a weak point giving rise to a small orifice due to the outward push of abdominal pressure. The orifice continues to

enlarge until a state of equilibrium, i.e., major incisional hernia, is reached.

LOCAL AND GENERAL CONSEQUENCES OF INCISIONAL HERNIAS

The loss of abdominal wall integrity leads to general disturbances, which we have referred to in our earlier publications as "incisional hernia disease" (21–29,48,50,52–55). These

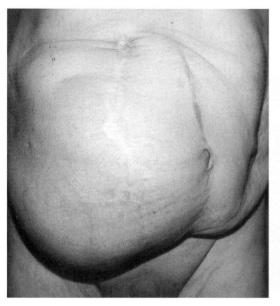
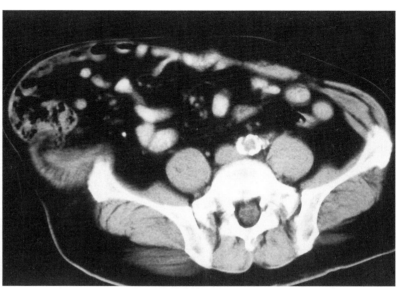

FIGURE 31.3. Complete destruction of the right rectus muscle is shown on the patient **(A)** and the computed tomography scan **(B)**. This patient had been operated on by midline and transrectal incisions and by a horizontal incision.

disturbances are related to a decrease in the intraabdominal pressure resulting from the extraabdominal protrusion of the viscera.

Parietal Disease

The force most frequently involved in incisional hernia is *lateral traction,* dependent mainly upon the contraction of the flat abdominal muscles, i.e., external oblique, internal oblique, and transverse. These lateral forces act particularly in cases of midline laparotomy because of the transverse arrangement of the fibers of these muscles. It should be kept in mind that all midline laparotomies are, in fact, *the equivalent of tendinous detachment of these muscles from the linea alba.*

Muscular Disease

In major incisional hernia, the walls of the abdomen open like sliding doors, giving way to the viscera. The rectus muscles are "sagittalized," and their contraction no longer offers resistance to the protrusion, but pushes the viscera out of the abdominal cavity via a movement of enucleation (Fig. 31.4) (68).

These conditions explain the natural tendency of incisional hernia to progress. The shortening of the muscle fibers reduces their ability to contract. Fatty degeneration of these fibers is often seen, accompanied by retraction of the involved aponeurosis. These lesions are irreversible. The abdominal defect undergoes organization to sharp, resistant sclerotic margins, even in cases where the orifice is apparently subdivided by fibrous bands. It is of interest to note that the circumference of the defect may be partially formed by a bony (pubic symphysis) or cartilaginous structure (chondrocostal margin) (Fig. 31.5).

In some cases, there is only *an apparent loss of abdominal wall tissue.* These patients usually present with a major midline incisional hernia that looks like a pronounced diastasis. Subsequent to appropriate preparation, using the technique of pneumoperitoneum and adequate curarization during anesthesia, it is possible to achieve apposition of the margins of the hernial orifice, although the degree of traction required carries the risk of recurrence. Use of a prosthesis allows the forces of traction to be transferred to the peripheral zone of implantation.

A true loss of abdominal wall tissue, which is related to atrophy or retraction of the recti abdomini, may also be present. Preparation and traction are not enough to close the defect, and a large prosthesis is thus required to replace the missing tissue. We place the prosthesis using transfixing sutures, *under tension*; this procedure of fixation can lead to a recuperation of lateral muscle function, since the physiologic tension lost because of the midline detachment of the muscles is reestablished. Finally, the prosthesis should be solidly fixed in place.

Skin Disease

The skin is also involved in this "abdominal wall disease." Trophic ulcerations are often observed in large tumefactions. These ulcerations are located over the middle and at the apex of the protrusion, and result from the weakening of the subcutaneous cellular tissue and the flattening of blood vessels due to the pressure of the viscera. Our histologic data confirm the thrombosis of small vessels (27). The skin over the apex of the protrusion is thin and poorly vascularized and thus may be the site of circular trophic ulceration. This ulceration, always present as a single lesion, should not be mistaken for erosion due to friction of the

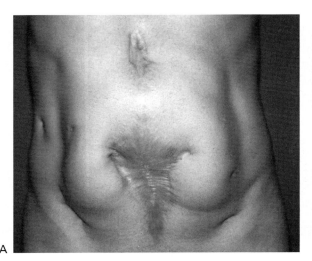
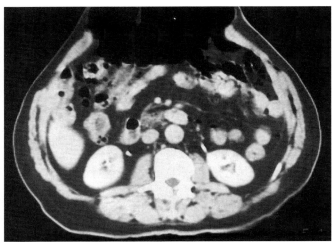

A   B

FIGURE 31.4. Sagittalization of the recti is visible on either the patient **(A)** or the computed tomography scan **(B)**.

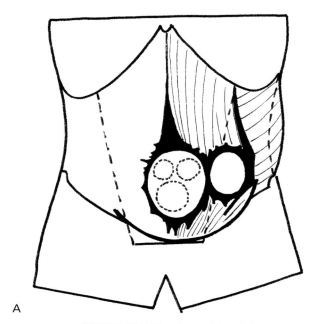
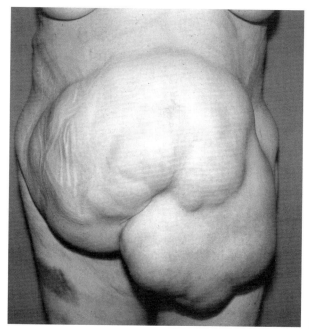

A   B

FIGURE 31.5. True loss of the abdominal wall depicted in an illustration **(A)** and shown on the patient **(B)**.

clothes against the skin. There is a risk of infection, leading secondarily to burst abdomen and fistulization of small bowel or colon (Fig. 31.6) (27).

General Disease

Respiratory Disturbances

Disturbed Respiratory Function

Disturbances of respiratory function are related to the absence of the normal contribution of the abdominal muscles, abdominal pressure, and diaphragm in respiration. These disorders must be evaluated by appropriate respiratory function tests in order to avoid a catastrophic postoperative course. In cases where these functional tests give satisfactory results, emphasis should be given to blood gas levels (O_2, CO_2) (25).

Effects of Reintegration on Respiratory Function

In some cases, voluminous herniation cannot be reintegrated into the abdomen: the herniated organs have lost their "right to reside" in the abdomen. As in the original description of Rives et al. (54), two abdominal cavities can be considered to exist in this situation (Fig. 31.7). The usefulness of CT scan is evident in these cases, to appreciate the volume of bowel to be reintegrated. If specific precautions are not taken, the consequences of hernial reduction are disastrous, because of the increased abdominal pressure and diaphragmatic immobilization. These may be

responsible for postoperative death, due to progressive respiratory insufficiency (29).

Visceral Disturbances

Less study has been devoted to this subject. The pressure within a hollow viscus results from a state of equilibrium. The latter is disrupted when abdominal pressure decreases. We observed a twofold increase in intravesical pressure (measured using a balloon) in cases of subumbilical incisional hernia. It can be deduced that similar modifications occur in the hollow digestive viscera, especially the colon, as evidenced on preoperative examination. Distention of these organs obviously has a negative effect on their vascularization and function, e.g., disturbed intestinal transit and micturition. Trouble with defecation, which is more directly related to the inefficacy of the abdominal wall musculature, is another unpleasant consequence of incisional hernia. Splanchnomegalia is an usual consequence, and sometimes it is necessary to perform a bowel resection to reintegrate the viscera and close the abdominal wall (Fig. 31.8).

Vascular Disturbances

Although we lack precise data on vascular disturbances, it is conceivable that major incisional hernia hinders caval and portal venous return, assuming, as suggested by physiolo-

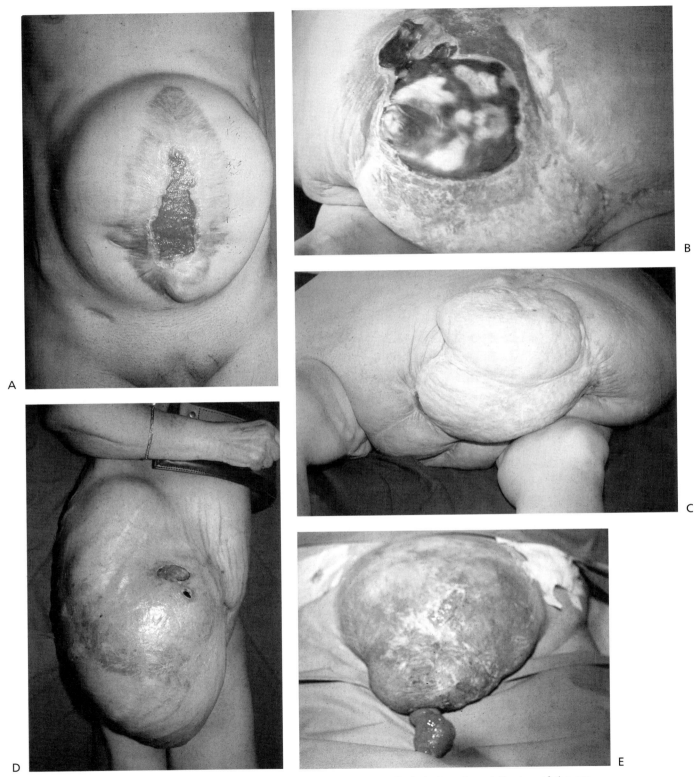

FIGURE 31.6. Some examples of trophic ulceration. **A:** Typical ulceration at the top of the pro-trusion. **B:** Giant ulcer on a giant hernia. **C:** Same patient after grafting on the ulcer. **D:** Ulcera-tion gives way to the omentum. **E:** Giant hernia with ulceration and small-bowel fistula.

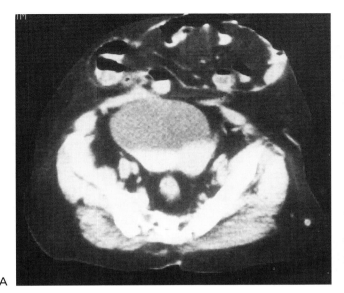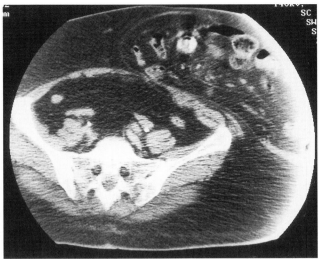

FIGURE 31.7. "A second abdominal cavity." **A:** Original computed tomography scan (1982) that gave Rives the idea of a second abdominal cavity. **B:** A more recent example.

gists, that maintenance of correct abdominal pressure plays a role in normal venous circulation.

Static Disturbances

The abdominal muscles act as anterior braces, for the spine when the subject is standing. Accordingly, weakness of these muscles, especially of the recti abdomini,

will lead to exaggeration of lumbar lordosis. During flexion of the spine, the contraction of the recti muscles relieves the strain on the spine by "the compression of an inflatable structure" created by the closure of the glottis and contraction of the abdominal muscles. This static function is compromised in cases of major incisional hernia, and many of these patients thus suffer from spinal pain.

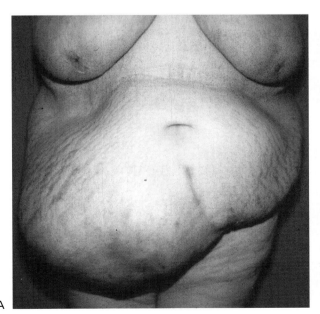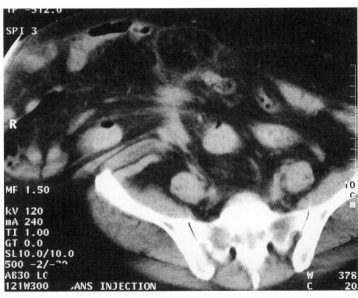

FIGURE 31.8. Splanchnomegalia is visible on the patient **(A)** and the computed tomography scan **(B)**. In these cases, it is sometimes necessary to perform a bowel resection to close the abdominal cavity.

ANATOMICOCLINICAL SUBTYPES

In 1990, we were, with J.P. Chevrel, the editors of the annual monograph (12) of the French Association of Surgery (AFC) dedicated to incisional hernias. We had the opportunity to collect cases from many surgical teams in France. These data are the basis of this anatomicoclinical classification. The number of cases reviewed was high (1,825 cases operated on between January 1988 and July 1989).

Midline

This is the most frequent type of incisional hernia, representing 77.5% of the statistics of the AFC and 79% of our series (574; 71%).

Supraumbilical Incisional Hernia

This type of incisional hernia is equally frequent in both sexes and represents 25.4% of AFC experience. Supraumbilical herniation is seen as a complication of surgery of the stomach and biliary apparatus, and sometimes of the lower part of a sternotomy (9). The hernial orifice undergoes rapid enlargement owing to the contraction of the powerful muscles of this region. The muscle fibers retract in front of and behind the chondrocostal margin, so the "cartilage" forms the upper margin of the hernial orifice. The recti abdomini undergo atrophy in the affected zone of the abdominal wall. A prosthesis is always required.

Infraumbilical Incisional Hernia (Suprapubic)

This type of incisional hernia (26.7% of the AFC experience) is more frequently seen in women as a consequence of one or more gynecologic operations (6). The defect may be very large and the protrusion voluminous. The herniated viscera rest on the pubis like an apron (Fig. 31.9). The hernial sac sometimes contains part of the colon or urinary bladder and almost always omentum and small bowel. Apposition of the wound margins is easier to obtain in this case since instrumental traction involves the longest abdominal muscle fibers. However, the rectus sheath is weakened in this zone owing to the absence of the deep lamina under the arcuate line. In these conditions, the rectus sheath is prone to cicatricial sclerosis and infection, which may lead to atrophy of the inferior fibers of the rectus abdominis near its pubic insertions. Such atrophy may expose much of the bone, especially in cases where previous operative repair has been unsuccessful. As in the preceding case, this evolution may constitute a veritable mass defect of the lower abdominal wall.

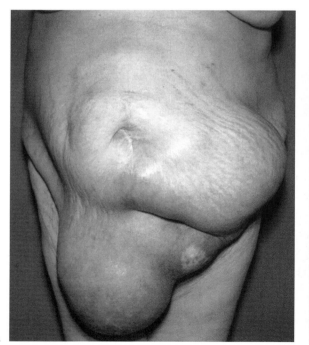

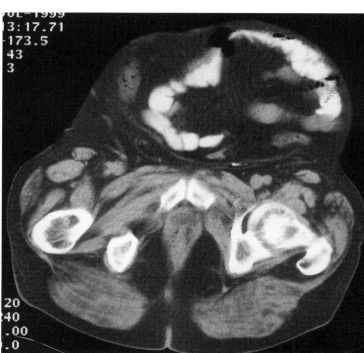

A   B

FIGURE 31.9. Supra pubic hernia shown on the patient **(A)** and the computed tomography scan **(B)**. The sac lies on the pubis like an apron.

Massive Supra- and Subumbilical Midline Incisional Hernia

This type of hernia arises subsequent to single or successive operations involving the supra- and subumbilical regions (24.7% of the AFC experience). We have seen a few cases of such massive hernia after operation on the abdominal aorta. However, most cases are seen in patients who have undergone successive supra- and infraumbilical operations. These hernias may reach monstrous proportions and contain almost all of the abdominal viscera. Complications such as cutaneous erosion and intertrigo are frequent.

Lateral

This type of hernia is less frequent (17% of AFC experience) than that on the midline, but it often raises difficult problems with respect to treatment.

Subchondral Incisional Hernia

These hernias (6.2%) usually lie under the right chondrocostal margin (80% of cases) and are secondary to biliary surgery. The upper muscle flap of the defect undergoes atrophy and retraction, and the upper margin of the hernial orifice is formed by the chondrocostal margin. In some cases,

the linea alba is pulled to the left side by the traction of the muscles that remain intact.

Inguinal Incisional Hernia

Incisional hernia of the inguinal region (7.6%) was seen more often on the right side than on the left, and occurred in patients who had undergone successive major operations for appendicular peritonitis, inguinal hernia, or gynecologic disorders (Fig. 31.10). The inferior margin of the hernial orifice is formed by the psoas major, the vascular pedicle, and the horizontal ramus of the pubis. Repair can be achieved only using prosthetic material.

Incisional Hernia of the Flank

Incisional hernia of the rectus sheath (1.4%) is accompanied by pronounced disruption of the abdominal wall (Fig. 31.11). Retraction and degeneration of the muscle fibers, which are usually free within the sheath, and loss of abdominal wall tissue are seen.

Another type of lateral hernia occurs between the thorax and the iliac crest, in a narrow zone corresponding to the course of the eleventh and twelfth intercostal nerves. Such herniation is often of modest size. Repair is easily achieved

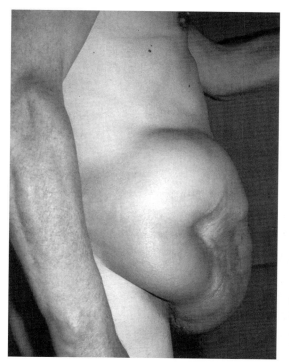
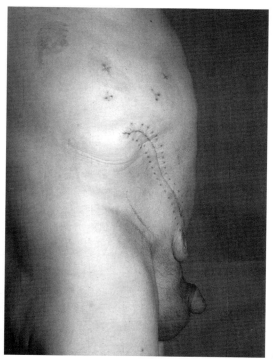

A

B

FIGURE 31.10. Inguinal recurrent incisional hernia. **A:** Preoperative view. **B:** After treatment with a prosthesis.

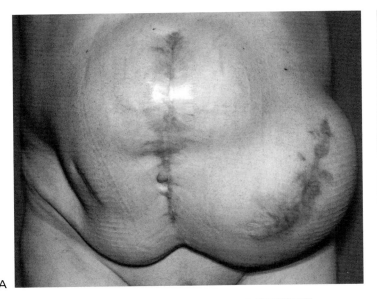

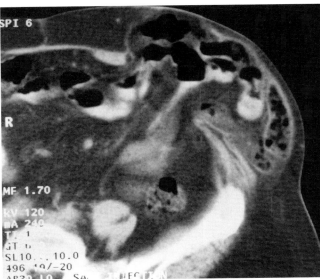

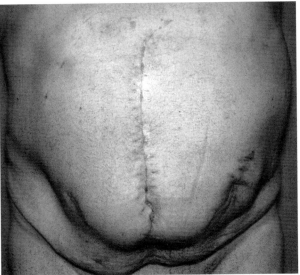

FIGURE 31.11. Midline and lateral incisional hernia. **A:** Preoperatively. **B:** Computed tomography scan. **C:** Postoperatively.

by apposition of the myoaponeurotic flaps, which remain large and supple.

A final type of lateral incisional hernia, seen in the posterior region near the costal ridge, occurs subsequent to urologic surgery. Such herniation may be voluminous. The hernial orifice often shows a margin (tenth and eleventh ribs) constituted by bone.

COMPLICATIONS OF INCISIONAL HERNIAS

Emergency context, septic lesions, or surgical maneuvers in septic conditions contraindicate the use of nonabsorbable prosthetic material.

Strangulation

Strangulation of an incisional hernia is a very serious complication. The situation can be dramatic for elderly patients or in cases of voluminous herniation with intestinal necrosis. We prohibit nonabsorbable prostheses in these cases because of the lack of skin preparation and the almost constant presence of septic fluid within the hernial sac. The use of an absorbable prosthesis may offer an adequate solution to therapeutic management, even if the rate of recurrence is high.

Secondary Burst Abdomen

Neglected trophic ulceration will lead to burst abdomen (Fig. 31.6). We have encountered such a case where, fortunately, the omentum acted as a barrier. In less fortunate cases, jejunal fistulas were found. Treatment requires at least two separate operations.

Associated Forms

Associated Visceral Emergency. The presence of a visceral lesion requiring emergency surgery in a patient with major incisional hernia is not an exceptional situation. Most of these patients present with peritonitis of various origins. Local and general preparation is obviously not possible under these emergency conditions. As in the case of strangulated herniation, the surgeon can do only what is in his or her power; nonabsorbable prostheses are contraindicated because of the risk of septic complications.

Associated Chronic Digestive Tract Disease Requiring Septic Intervention. The accompanying disease involves either the biliary apparatus, the gastrojejunal tract, or the colon. Prudence is mandatory, and it is preferable to use classic treatment procedures and absorbable prosthetic material. A clean recurrence is better than an infected prosthesis.

Incisional Hernia with Colostomy

Incisional hernia that develops around an artificial anus can be of gigantic proportions. The hernia must be surgically approached at a distance from the colostomy and in the midline. In cases where scrupulous preparation has been done and the colostomy has been fully isolated under plastic protectors, a perforated intraabdominal prosthesis can be installed with success.

Incisional hernia that occurs in the midline in proximity to colostomy raises more difficult therapeutic problems. In these cases, where there is only a small distance between the colostomy and the operative site, we prefer not to use prosthetic material. The same difficulties may exist with a urostomy (Fig. 31.12).

TREATMENT

Preoperative Care

Role of the Anesthesiologist–Intensive Care Specialist

On initial contact with the patient, the specialist evaluates respiratory function and notes the existence of cough, expectoration, history of smoking, etc. Respiratory status is then assessed by clinical examination and chest x-ray. A more precise assessment requires study of the minute respiratory volume and the ratio of forced expiratory volume to vital capacity. Blood gas determinations are also of prime importance. Measurements should include Po_2, Pco_2, pH, and oxygen saturation of arterial blood. The results of blood gas measurements are used to evaluate ventilatory efficacy and to identify latent respiratory insufficiency.

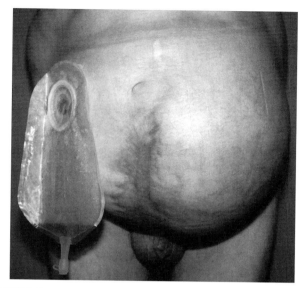

FIGURE 31.12. Huge hernia with urostomy. The problem in these operations is preventing contamination of the prosthesis.

Preparation of the patient is begun on the first day of hospitalization. The results of respiratory exploration on admission are compared with those obtained at regular intervals thereafter. In this way, the course of respiratory status and the efficacy of preparation can be assessed. Electronic spirometry allows daily evaluation of residual volume, forced expiratory volume, and minute volume (25).

Preparation also includes withdrawal of tobacco; respiratory physiotherapy, i.e., costal exercise, diaphragmatic exercise (deep inspiration in different decubital positions), assistance of coughing and expectoration by clapping exercises, and in some cases postural drainage; instrumental physiotherapy using a pressure-relaxation breathing apparatus (Bird Mark 8 or Bennet PRl, PR2, Bird Corporation, Palm Springs, CA, U.S.A.) to facilitate coughing and decrease secretion by increasing alveolar ventilation (the breathing apparatus is driven by pressurized gas and can be used at home); and prescriptions of a mucolytic agent, and antibiotics in case of pulmonary infection. The decision to operate is based in part on the results of preparation. In cases where initial results are satisfactory, the operation need not be further delayed. In other cases, improvement is seen only after several weeks of preparation, in which case the operation should be delayed until this time.

In patients presenting with deteriorated health and showing no improvement after respiratory preparation, the decision to operate must be made with great care, since the postoperative course may have severe complications. In other cases, the results of respiratory function tests lead to a definitive refusal to operate, despite the patient's insistence.

Role of the Nursing Staff

The nursing staff plays a major role in preparation of the patient by ensuring proper hygiene and treatment of skin lesions and by encouraging the patient to ambulate, to use the stairs, etc.

Role of the Surgeon

In cases where the hernia has lost the right to reside in the abdominal cavity, as evaluated by the preoperative CT scan (Fig. 31.13), the technique of pneumoperitoneum according to Goñi Moreno (34) is useful. Sterilized air taken through filter is injected into the peritoneal cavity until the patient feels discomfort (scapular pain). The amount of air that can

be injected during each session varies greatly according to the patient (from a few hundred milliliters to more than a liter). (Fig. 31.14). Sessions of pneumoperitoneum are repeated every 2 to 3 days, and the patient is monitored with x-rays (subdiaphragmatic air shadows). We prefer to use air rather than CO_2, which is more rapidly resorbed, thereby allowing a greater time interval between injections. In some difficult cases, we conduct the pneumoperitoneum in the operative room with the laparoscopic insufflator.

With this technique, we can assess the patient's tolerance to reintegration of the hernial mass. The diaphragm can be readapted to work in physiologic conditions and, according to the author of the technique, dissection of the hernial sac is facilitated. We use a preoperative pneumoperitoneum in 12% of our patients.

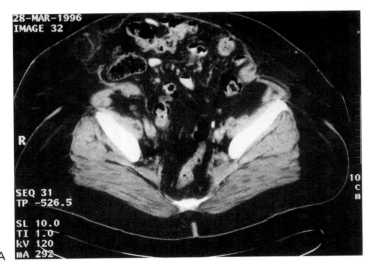

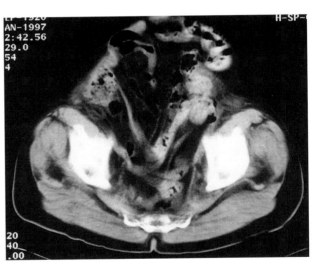

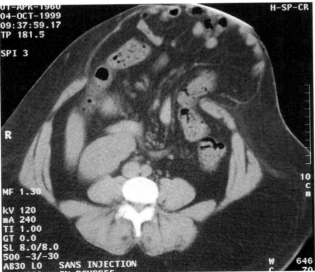

FIGURE 31.13. A–C: Computed tomography gives a good evaluation of the parietal defect and of the quantity of bowel to reintegrate in the abdominal cavity.

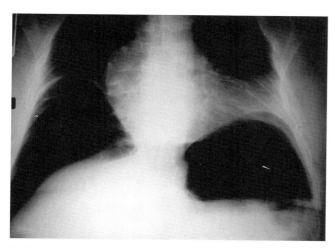

FIGURE 31.14. Chest x-ray shows the volume of air injected at the end of a Goñi Moreno preparation.

Surgical Intervention

Anesthesia

General anesthesia and artificial respiration are used. Operative analgesia is obtained by administration of a morphinomimetic drug. Curarization as required is done with a curarimimetic. The considerable advantages of this technique include its security, reversibility, and controllability, rapid awakening, and early return of intestinal transit.

Exposure and Exploration

Skin Incision. The direction of the incision is chosen according to the previous incision or to the major axis of the tumefaction. Our practice is to resect (at least in cases of major incisional hernia) a fairly large diamond-shaped area of skin, since the hernial sac always adheres to the skin. It is of no use to lose time trying to cut these adhesions to free the overlying skin, which in any case is of no value after reduction of the hernia. The skin over the sac is stretched thin and poorly vascularized and has lost its subcutaneous supportive tissue. Finally, in cases of cutaneous ulceration, the resected area should be as large as possible, extending well beyond the zones of infected lymphatic reticulum.

Dissection of Hernial Sac. As described earlier, the hernial sac is sometimes voluminous and always irregular. Adherent bowel loops are often fixed within the sac, and in some cases septic or aseptic fluid is found. This danger must be kept in mind during dissection of the sac. It is thus preferable to approach the sac by the periphery, beginning the dissection in contact with a solid part of the abdominal wall. Work then progresses from the periphery to the center, and the sac is approached via its neck.

Exploration of Contents of Hernial Sac. Once the periphery of the sac has been well delimited and opened (the peri-

toneum being opened outside the neck or along the convex surface of the sac), exploration of its contents can begin. Different situations can be encountered, and these are discussed below.

In some instances, no adhesions are found within the sac. In this case, the surgeon should simply identify the exact limits of the hernial orifice and then explore the "other side of the coin": search *for secondary orifices must be careful.*

Sometimes a few loose, isolated adhesions are found, and these can easily be broken or sectioned. In some cases, however, major fleshy adhesions are encountered. In the course of these procedures, care should be taken to protect the omentum, which may be needed later on.

Finally, in some cases, the adhesions are major and involve many segments of the intestines. The solution is to perform resections of the omentum and involved bowel. When the resections are done at the proper sites under good conditions, including adequate protection of the abdominal wall, there is less risk of postoperative infection than in case of unexpected opening of either a hollow viscus or a zone of infected epiploic necrosis. Although epiploic necrosis may be aseptic, one should not count on such a situation. Indeed, highly pathogenic organisms can be found; e.g., *Pseudomonas aeruginosa* (pyocyanic bacillus) was noted in one of our patients.

Exposure of Margins of Hernial Orifice. The margins of the orifice must be carefully identified. Secondary orifices should be open: residual aponeurotic bands extending from one margin to another are of no structural significance and cannot be used for repair. The contours of the defect thus identified must be solid, i.e., able to resist the force of strong forceps. Solidity is tested by clamping forceps onto the skin, the margins of the myoaponeurotic orifice, and eventually the peritoneum.

Nonprosthetic Abdominal Wall Repair

Classic methods of repair are based on aponeurotic or muscular reconstructive surgery using the anatomic structures of the abdominal wall. These procedures may still be indicated in some cases. Simple suturing of the aponeurotic margins after reintegration of the herniated viscera and treatment of the hernial sac may be authorized when the hernial orifice is narrow, e.g., in lateral incisional hernia subsequent to drainage. Relaxing incisions of the anterior surface of the recti abdomini (30,69) may be of help; however, we have seen one case of bilateral recurrence on the site of relaxing incision (Fig. 31.15).

Sutures

Suturing by Mayo's (45) or Judd's (39) techniques requires that the aponeuroses be solid. These techniques are mainly applicable to the treatment of lateral incisional hernia, but their long-term results are "unacceptable" (49).

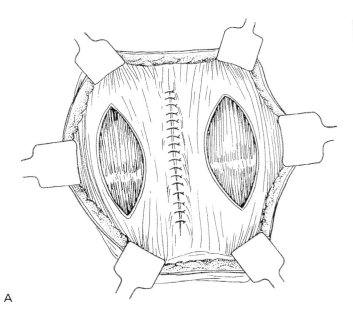

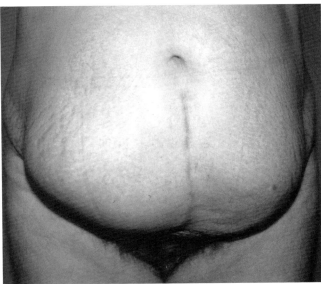

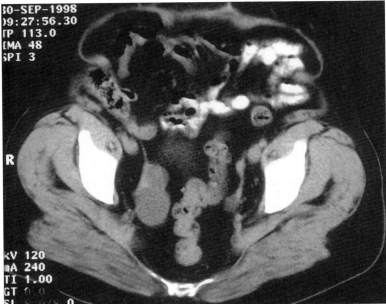

FIGURE 31.15. Nonprosthetic repair. **A:** Gibson's procedure. **B** and **C:** Big recurrence at the level of two relaxing incisions according to Gibson.

Autoplasties—Relaxing Incisions

Reference is often made by French authors to the technique of Welti and Eudel (69). The procedure is used for midline repair and consists of making two lateral incisions (parallel to the midline) through the anterior surface of the recti abdomini. The two resulting aponeurotic flaps are then sutured together over the midline defect. Finally, the medial margins of the recti abdomini are sutured together over the aponeurotic repair.

Autografts

Suturing full-thickness autografted skin bands may be indicated mainly for the repair of midline incisional hernia.

Results published by Banzet (quoted in ref. 12) demonstrate that the strips of skin are not rejected. This procedure of reinforced suturing can be very useful.

Nevertheless, nonprosthetic repair must be done in cases where there is an obvious risk of septic contamination. Under such conditions, we prefer to use Welti–Eudel's procedure with reinforcement of the anterior rectus sheath by an absorbable prosthesis. This technique can be applied to most types of midline incisional hernia. Furthermore, in cases of postoperative recurrence of incisional hernia, a prosthesis can be placed under good conditions since the retromuscular prefascial space has not been opened.

Prosthetic Abdominal Wall Repair

Prosthetic surgery allows repair of massive herniation and can be used to treat formidable lesions, often considered beyond the scope of surgery.

(a) The choice of an appropriate prosthesis is based on the physical and biologic properties of the material to be used (33). The ideal material should be light and solid, with a certain degree of elasticity and suppleness. Elasticity allows the prosthesis to conform freely to the curvatures of the visceral sac. It is also important that the material be a fairly open mesh structure, so a rapid fibroblastic response is able to invest the prosthesis, thereby facilitating its insertion (51,63).

The qualities of the prostheses available have been reported by Amid in 1997, who gives a classification of four types (4):

Type I: totally macroporous (pores greater than 75 μm)
Type II: totally microporous (pores less than 10 μm)
Type III: macroporous with microporous components
Type IV : submicronic pore size

We have used Dacron [Mersuture (Ethicon), polyester Dacron] over the past decades, since it was in our opinion the best material commercially available (21–29,41,56). The results of our long experience with this material in the treatment of inguinal hernia and massive incisional hernia have been confirmed in experimental studies (51). Fibroblastic invasion of the prosthesis is optimal when Mersilene mesh is used: the index of fibroblastic reaction is high, and the index of inflammatory reaction remains low. Furthermore, we have never observed intolerance to this type of prosthetic mesh, and the cases of rejection that have been seen were related to septic contamination during operation. Notaras in England (47), Stoppa in France (60–62), and Wantz in the United States (66–68) have also advocated the use of this mesh.

Thus, we cannot follow the conclusions of Leber et al. (42), who believe that polyester mesh should no longer be used for incisional hernia repair.

Other prostheses are also available on the market. Polypropylene meshes are thought to be very well tolerated by the organism, because they are monofilamented. Marlex (C.R. Bard, Inc., Murray Hill, NJ, U.S.A.) and Prolene (Ethicon) have been studied experimentally by Amid et al. (2). A new prosthesis (Vypro, which is a combination of polypropylene and polyglactin 910) has been studied in experiments by Schumpelick (46). These new prostheses seem very interesting.

(b) The site of prosthetic implantation must be chosen on an anatomic basis.

1. Intraperitoneal positioning of the prosthesis is easy. In a study published in 1997, Arnaud et al. (5) reported the results of this procedure in 210 patients. Good results [two deaths (1%), infection in ten cases (4.8%), and recurrence in eight cases (3.8%)] were obtained in that study, considering the magnitude of the lesions that were seen. Other series have been published (8,43). We do not believe that intraperitoneal implantation has any advantages. Of course, the peritoneum rapidly envelops the prosthesis and offers a good defense against infection without hematoma formation. However, adhesions of the bowel loops to the prosthesis are frequent, thereby hindering intestinal transit and rendering reintervention dangerous (Fig. 31.16). We have even seen a case of intraluminal migration of intraperitoneal prosthesis, and such cases have been reported in the literature (17,36,40,58,59). When possible, interpositioning of the omentum between the viscera and the prosthesis as advocated by Rives et al. in 1973 (52) can afford protection against these complications.

The ideal intraperitoneal prosthesis has not yet been described, even if some partial responses have been found using Gore-Tex (W.L. Gore & Associates, Flagstaff, AZ, U.S.A.) (32) and composite prostheses (3,7,64).

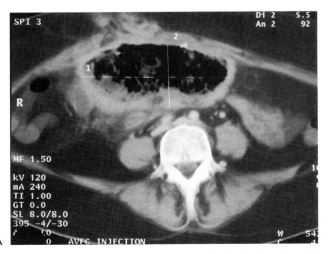

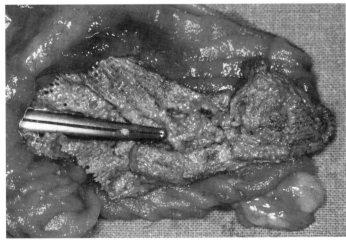

FIGURE 31.16. Intraluminal migration of an intraperitoneal mesh. **A:** Computed tomography scan. **B:** Operative specimen.

Laparoscopic placement of a prosthesis is a variant of intraperitoneal placement (57). We think it is ineffective, because the prosthesis cannot be placed under good tension due to the pneumoperitoneum. This technique is dangerous, because dissection of the intrasaccular adhesions is difficult and may lead to bowel fistulas. Finally, laparoscopic treatment cannot give a good cosmetic result because it does not treat the problem of an excess of skin.

2. Premuscular positioning of the prosthesis was proposed by Chevrel (11) in 1979. The same year, two papers published in the *American Journal of Surgery* described the same techniques (10,18) with very similar pictures. Chevrel's personal experience (14) has now been extended to include over 400 patients. This technique consists of obtaining closure by reflected flaps of the anterior lamina of the rectus sheath with suturing to form a mantle-like covering, reinforced by implantation of a large prosthesis of Mersuture, Prolene, or Marlex over the sutured area (13). Although precautions must be taken when this procedure is used, especially in cases where cutaneous cover is not satisfactory, its major advantage over a deeper implantation is the absence of grave complications for patients with infection, but the prosthesis may be pushed by the abdominal pressure (Fig. 31.17).

3. Retromuscular prefascial placement of the mesh has been proposed by Rives, and has been used in our department since 1966. Described as early as 1973, this technique was clearly demonstrated in 1977 in the *French Encyclopedia of Surgery* (54). The drawings were later reproduced in the first and second editions of *Hernias and Surgery of the Abdominal Wall* by Chevrel (23). They have also been reproduced, with minor modifications, by Wantz (66) and Stoppa et al. (61).

We position the prosthesis in contact with the muscle fibers, i.e., in the space between the rectus abdominis and the posterior lamina of the rectus sheath. This requires opening the rectus sheath near the linea alba to enter the retromuscular space and expose the posterior aspect of the rectus muscle (Fig. 31.18).

- *Closure Posterior to the Prosthesis.* The peritoneal cavity must be closed prior to implantation of the prosthesis. In most cases, suture of the fascial margins can be achieved when the posterior rectus sheath has been correctly and widely freed. When fascial closure cannot be achieved, we close the defect by an absorbable prosthesis. Omentum, when present, can be used to protect viscera from the prosthesis. The posterior surface of the omentum allows good peritonization, while its anterior surface offers a surface of granulation tissue that invests the prosthesis.

- *Placement of the Prosthesis.* The *area of insertion* of the prosthesis must be as large as possible. Our experience has shown that suturing the material to the margins of the defect offered no guarantee of solidity and usually resulted in recurrence of hernia due to lateral detachment (Fig. 31.19). Accordingly, the mesh should extend widely beyond the myoaponeurotic hernial orifice, with intraabdominal pressure being used to ensure its insertion. The upper part of the prosthesis is placed between the rectus abdominis anteriorly and the ribs and internal oblique posteriorly. The lower part of the prosthesis is fixed to Cooper's ligament and extends into the pelvis. The force of abdominal pressure holds the prosthesis against the deep surface of the muscles, thereby achieving a sort of "suture by apposition." However, this pressure-induced apposition is not sufficient to keep the prosthesis correctly positioned during the first few postoperative weeks, and thus it is necessary to ensure solid peripheral suturing of the prosthetic material (Fig. 31.18C–E). Each stitch transfixes the abdominal wall through a cutaneous buttonhole, which is then closed by a single stitch. In cases of midline incisional hernia, the semilunar line (Spieghel's line) is used as the site for peripheral attachment of the prosthesis. Other methods have been described, such as stapling (2,19), using glue (14), etc.

- *Closure Anterior to the Prosthesis.* Due to the tension of the prosthesis, approximation of the musculoaponeurotic layer in front of the prosthesis is always possible. We place two close suction drains in contact with the prosthesis, and two drains beneath the skin. Dermolipectomy in case of obese patients may be an associated procedure. It gives a much better cosmetic result (Fig. 31.20).

- *The conditions for these surgical procedures* should obey the rules of prosthetic implantation. The risk of infection is lowered by operating under conditions of scrupulous asepsis, perfect hemostasis, and absence of direct manipulation of the prosthesis. The overhead light should not be manipulated during operation. Vacuum aspiration should also be proscribed during surgery to avoid the displacement of dust or other air-

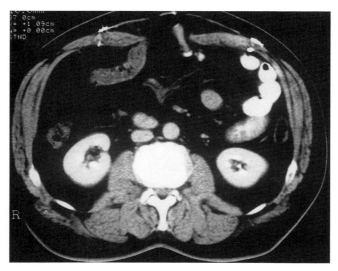

FIGURE 31.17. Premuscular prosthesis is pushed by the intraabdominal pressure.

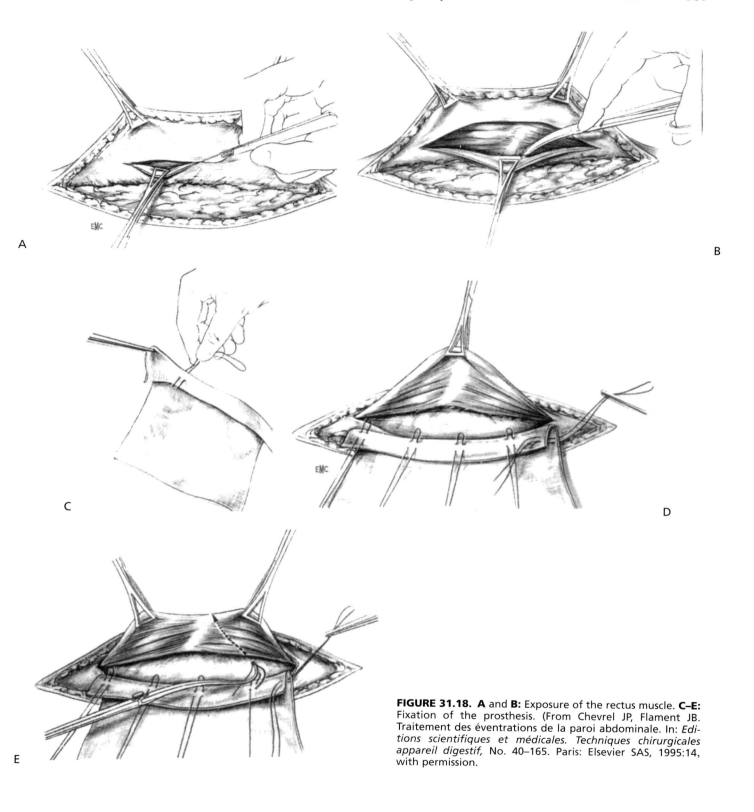

FIGURE 31.18. A and **B:** Exposure of the rectus muscle. **C–E:** Fixation of the prosthesis. (From Chevrel JP, Flament JB. Traitement des éventrations de la paroi abdominale. In: *Editions scientifiques et médicales. Techniques chirurgicales appareil digestif,* No. 40–165. Paris: Elsevier SAS, 1995:14, with permission.

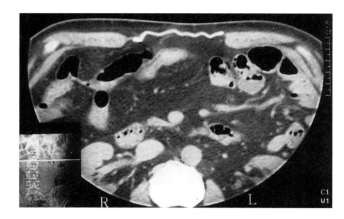

FIGURE 31.19. Recurrence after suture of the prosthesis (Gore-Tex) to the margins of the defect.

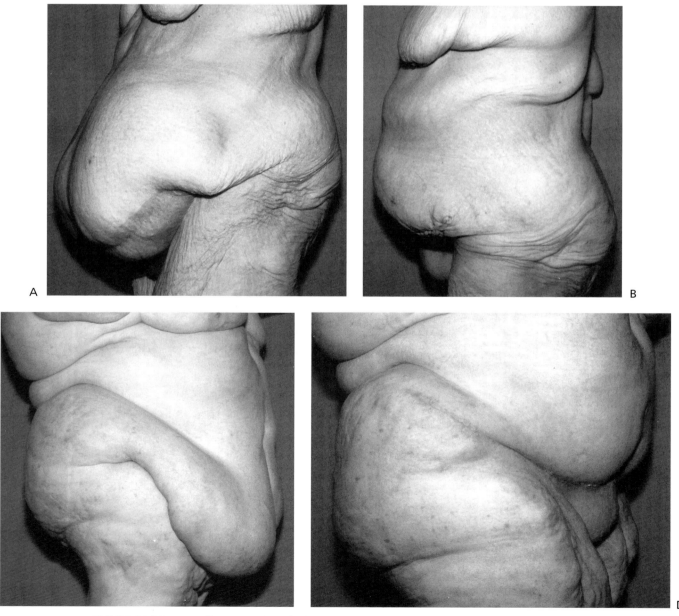

FIGURE 31.20. Dermolipectomy gives the best cosmetic result. Before **(A** and **C)** and after photographs **(B** and **D)** are shown in two respective obese patients.

borne particles that may be contaminated. Antibiotic prophylaxis (1) is recommended.

Postoperative Care

Monitoring of body temperature may demonstrate an initial moderate rise due to inflammatory reaction. However, persistence of fever beyond the fourth postoperative day usually indicates the occurrence of late suppuration.

Aspiration drains should also be monitored. These drains, placed in contact with the prosthesis and/or beneath the skin, are used to evacuate fluid and blood in the areas of dissection, which may be very large. We remove the drains on the sixth postoperative day.

The skin and abdominal cicatrix must be examined, and therefore should be exposed as soon as possible to identify the slightest modification that may reflect the presence of local infection.

Respiratory physiotherapy should resume as soon as the patient leaves the operating room. Early ambulation is recommended in most cases, but precautions should be taken initially. It may be wise to replace early ambulation by mobilization in bed, with guidance by the physiotherapist whenever possible.

Finally, all sports activity and physical stress are contraindicated during the period of connective tissue cicatrization, i.e., for 3 to 6 months after the operation.

RESULTS AND COMPLICATIONS

Immediate Complications

A major source of information is constituted by the investigation that we carried out with Chevrel for the report of the 92nd French Congress on Surgery, which was devoted to incisional hernias of the abdominal wall. A national investigation concerning 1,825 operations carried out between 1 January 1988 and 1 July 1989 gave us a global view of the results of French surgery in the field of large incisional hernias (12).

General Complications

Mortality

The mortality is not insignificant. The investigation carried out by the AFC showed a mortality rate of 1.2% (22 deaths for 1,825 operations). It should be noted that 18 of the 22 deaths were related to postoperative respiratory failure. We must therefore insist on the importance of the respiratory preparation of these patients and the interest of preoperative pneumoperitoneum.

In our personal series (28), the mortality rate was 0.6% (three deaths for 517 operations with a prefascial retromuscular prosthesis). One death of a 71-year-old woman was related to a deep infection of the prosthesis caused by *Staphy-*

lococcus aureus septicemia. The two other deaths were related to a hemodynamic problem (enteritis necroticans confirmed by the autopsy of a 73-year-old man, and cardiac arrest in the recovery room in the case of a 69-year-old woman).

Other Immediate Complications

Respiratory complications have been assessed at 1% by Leber et al. (42). Postoperative ileus occurred in roughly 8% of cases. Finally, vein thrombosis with pulmonary embolism was noted in 1% of the cases.

Local Complications

Hematomas

The occurrence of a hematoma was noted in 4.5% of cases in the AFC investigation (12), with 82 cases of hematoma reported for 1,825 operations. In Chevrel's personal experience (14), this complication was reported in 1.81% of cases. Leber et al. (42) noted a 3% rate of postoperative hematomas. In our own trial (28), the hematoma rate was 0.77% (four cases out of 517 operations with prosthesis placement).

Sepsis

The consequences of sepsis vary according to whether or not it affects the prosthesis.

- Superficial sepsis was noted in 5.1% of cases in the AFC investigation (93 cases out of 1,825 operations). In our series, superficial sepsis occurred in 1% of cases (five of 517). In the series of Leber et al., the rate of superficial infection was estimated at 7% (14 cases for 200 operations) (42).
- Deep sepsis affecting the prosthesis material has more serious consequences. Thus, in our series, there was one death from *S. aureus* septicemia following a deep infection of the prosthesis. The rate of deep infection in the AFC investigation was 0.75%. In Chevrel's recent trial, the rate of deep infection was 2.72% (14). For Leber et al., it was 4% (42). The results published by several French authors at the GREPA (Groupe de Recherche et d'Etude sur la Paroi Abdominale) meeting in 1986 demonstrated a rate of deep suppuration varying from 3% to 21%.

  The treatment of such deep suppuration sometimes requires the ablation of the prosthetic material. We have shown that a large opening, carried out very early, could "save" the prosthesis thanks to the granulation tissue budding through the mesh. Gilbert and Graham arrived at the same conclusion (31).
- The occurrence of cutaneous gangrene can represent a specific cause of infection of the prosthesis. This complication occurred in 1.2% of cases in the AFC study (21 patients) and 0.9% of cases reported by Chevrel.

The prevention of infectious accidents, when prosthetic material is placed, is based on antibioprophylaxis, the effectiveness of which has been demonstrated by Abramov et al. (1).

Late Complications

Recurrences

A recurrence should be considered a late complication of the treatment of large incisional hernias. It must, moreover, be noted that, according to the annual reports of French Insurance, recurrence is the most frequent cause of lawsuits concerning the failures of incisional hernia treatment.

When preparing the report for the AFC, we carried out an investigation on the late results of operations carried out between 1 January 1980 and 1 July 1981 (12). We collected the results of 1,033 operations. The global rate of recurrence was 14%. It was very different depending on whether a prosthesis was used:

- Without prosthesis, the recurrence rate was 24% (100 cases out of 417 operations).
- After prosthetic placement, the recurrence rate was only 16.3% 10 years later (53 cases out of 326 operations).

In the personal experience of Chevrel (14), the results were similar, since the recurrence rate when the operation did not use prosthetic material was 18.3% (28 of 153) while the recurrence rate after prosthesis placement surgery was 4% (13 of 326).

In our personal experience, the data were very similar: the recurrence rate after placement of a prefascial retromuscular prosthesis was 5.7% (27 of 474). Twenty of these recurrences, which were often small at the limits of the prosthesis were treated with success, which brings the final recurrence rate after prosthesis placement down to 2%. On the other hand, in the cases of surgery without prosthesis placement, the recurrence rate was high: 24.9% (45 of 181) (28).

Late Infections

Late complications, in particular infections, depend in large part on the type of prosthetic material used, as Amid has demonstrated (4). This author insisted on the need to differentiate between macroporous and microporous prostheses, and even between multifilament macroporous prostheses.

Polyester Meshes (e.g., Mersilene)

Tardive infection, after the placement of a Mersilene prefascial retromuscular prosthesis, was rare in our experience (0.2%, i.e., one case out of 474 patients followed). We are therefore surprised by the very high figures indicated by Leber et al. (42), who reported rates of 5.9% for late chronic infections and 3.5% for infections related to an enterocutaneous fistula. The participants at a round table organized by Wantz et al., in the framework of the Ameri-

can College of Surgeons (67), reported a substantially lower rate of infection (0.2% to 1%).

Expanded Polytetrafluoroethylene Mesh

Expanded polytetrafluoroethylene (ePTFE) mesh, according to the classification of Amid (4), corresponds to an entirely microporous prosthesis not likely to be colonized by conjunctive tissue. The results with this material were recently published in the journal *Hernia*, in an article by Martinez et al. (44). This author concluded, after reviewing an important number of publications, that the global rate of late suppurations is 4.1%. It was necessary to carry out the ablation of the prosthetic material in 8.2% of cases, and the overall rate of recurrence was 17.5%.

Recurrent Seromas

The appearance of major recurrent seromas on the site of treatment of large incisional hernias is a rare occurrence. Two publications report such cases (20,65). In both publications, these were voluminous multilocular cystic masses that appeared following the treatment of an incisional hernia by the placement of a polypropylene prosthesis. This complication appears more frequently after the placement of an onlay prosthesis according to the Chevrel technique than after the placement of a prefascial retromuscular prosthesis.

We have ourselves observed two cases of recurrent seroma that required further surgery for excision of the voluminous cystic mass.

Digestive Migrations

Late digestive migrations of prosthetic material appear to occur relatively frequently, if we believe the information gathered at congresses devoted to surgery of the abdominal wall. However, they are only reported in literature in the form of isolated cases. They must be differentiated from enterocutaneous fistulas [3.5% of cases for Leber et al. (42)], which appear very often after the occurrence of an unnoticed or sutured injury of the small intestine during the operation.

The digestive migrations of prosthetic material reported in literature occur more often after the placement of the prosthesis in the intraabdominal site than in the prefascial retromuscular site (40,59). The diagnosis can be made by fistulography, by colonoscopy, or during subsequent surgery. The occurrence of this complication has led Kaufman et al. to advise against the placement of prosthetic material in the intraperitoneal site (40).

In our own experience, several cases of intraluminal migration of the parietal prosthesis were observed (12). They must be clearly differentiated from the intestinal fistulas occurring following incisional hernia repair using prosthetic material, with suppuration and postoperative disunion.

COMMENTS

Analysis of Results

Prostheses

The results described above were obtained using our personal procedure, whose principles have been explained and whose technical features have been codified. This technique, which we have used for over 35 years, has given very satisfactory results. Only minor details of the procedure have been modified over the years, e.g., abandonment of the pledgets and use of suction drainage. However, critical analysis of these results, especially of the failures, has led us to reconsider the indications for this procedure. Indeed, the attendant risks of such repair can be decreased by applying more precise, restrictive indications.

A reduction in mortality was achieved by taking into account the fact that many of the patients were elderly and obese and suffered from cardiopulmonary insufficiency. A careful preparation with pneumoperitoneum is therefore mandatory. Aseptic recurrence of incisional hernia (mechanical) was rare (5.2%). These cases seem to be difficult to avoid, at least when the recurrence is due to rupture of the attachment of the prosthesis. Such rupture always occurs at the points of fixation of the prosthetic material. However, prevention of this complication may be possible by placing a larger prosthesis fixed to the ribs or the pubic bone.

The rate of infection was dramatically improved. In ten of our patients, the prosthesis was implanted with accompanying septic procedures. We observed no infections, thanks to vigorous precautions.

Better Selection of Therapeutic Indications

In our department, prostheses are used in most cases of hernia. The main indication is multiple recurrent incisional hernia: special attention must be given to the identification of latent subcutaneous or intraabdominal sources of infection and to disturbances of general health (especially diabetes). We have thus abandoned the use of prosthetic repair in emergency surgery and when operation is indicated primarily for reasons other than incisional hernia. However, in some of these cases, closure cannot be achieved using classic procedures for repair. For such cases, we have adopted the use of resorbable prosthetic material.

Technical Precautions

The need for extreme vigilance in prosthetic surgery cannot be overemphasized. Standard precautions include thorough disinfection of the operating room, prohibiting the use of vacuum aspiration of air and movements of the overhead lights; proper training of all personnel in sound hygienic practice; and "no touch" rules. It can be said that all "unexplained" accidents are caused by the surgeons themselves.

CONCLUSION

Major incisional hernia is a significant lesion affecting general health; in some cases, it is a monstrous disabling lesion that was considered in the past to be beyond the scope of surgical repair. Improved understanding of the physiologic disturbances induced by these lesions, especially respiratory insufficiency, and the judicious use of prostheses offer a reasonable therapeutic solution for these patients. The results obtained reflect the considerable progress that has been made in this domain, since 95% of patients can now be cured. Critical analysis of surgical failures demonstrates that even better results are obtainable by improved definition of operative indications and more precise codifying of surgical techniques.

ACKNOWLEDGMENTS

With the expression of our gratitude to Marie Lise Leglatin for preparing the manuscript, and Denis Germain and Olivier Chauvet for the illustrations.

REFERENCES

1. Abramov D, Jeroukhimow I, Yinnon AM, et al. Antibiotic prophylaxis in umbilical and incisional hernia repair: a prospective randomised study. *Eur J Surg* 1996;162:945–948.
2. Amid PK, Shulman AG, Lichtenstein IL. A simple stapling technique for prosthetic repair of massive incisional hernias. *Am Surg* 1994;60:934–936.
3. Amid PK, Shulman AG, Lichtenstein IL, et al. Experimental evaluation of a new composite mesh with the selective property of incorporation to the abdominal wall without adhering to the intestines. *J Biomed Mater Res* 1994;28:373–375.
4. Amid PK. Classification of biomaterials and their related complications in abdominal wall hernia surgery. *Hernia* 1997;1:15–21.
5. Arnaud JP, Cervi C, Tuech JJ, et al. Surgical treatment of postoperative incisional hernias by intra-peritoneal insertion of a Dacron mesh. *Hernia* 1997;1:97–99.
6. Bendavid R. Incisional parapubic hernias. *Surgery* 1990;108:898–901.
7. Bendavid R. Composite mesh (polypropylene-e-PTFE) in the intraperitoneal position. A report of 30 cases. *Hernia* 1997;1:5–8.
8. Bonnamy C, Samama G, Brefort JL, et al. Résultats à long terme du traitement des éventrations par prothèse non résorbable intrapéritonéale (149 patients). *Ann Chir* 1999;53:571–576.
9. Bouillot JL. Incisional abdominal hernia after median sternotomy. *Hernia* 1997;3:129–130.
10. Browse NL, Hurst P. Repair of long, large midline incisional hernias using reflected flaps of anterior rectus sheath reinforced with Marlex mesh. *Am J Surg* 1979;138:738–740.
11. Chevrel JP. Traitement des grandes éventrations médianes par plastie en paletot et prothèse. *Nouv Presse Med* 1979;8:695–696.
12. Chevrel JP, Flament JB, eds. Les éventrations de la paroi abdominale. In: Association Française de Chirurgie. *92nd French Congress on Surgery*. Paris, France: Masson, 1990.
13. Chevrel JP, Flament JB. Traitement des éventrations de la paroi abdominale. In: *Editions scientifiques et médicales. Techniques chirurgicales—appareil digestif*, No. 40–165. Paris: Elsevier SAS, 1995:14.

14. Chevrel JP, Rath AM. The use of fibrin glues in the surgical treatment of incisional hernias. *Hernia* 1997;1:9–14.

15. Crist D, Gadasz T. Complications of laparoscopic surgery. *Surg Clin North Am* 1993;73:265–289.

16. Marshall JS, DeBord J. Complications of ventral incisional hernia repair. In: Fitzgibbons RJ Jr, Greenburg AG, eds. *Nyhus and Condon's hernia,* 5th ed. Philadelphia: Lippincott Williams & Wilkins, 2002:367–371.

17. DeGutzman LJ, Nyhus LM, Yared G, et al. Colocutaneous fistula formation following polypropylene mesh. Placement for repair of a ventral hernia: diagnosis by colonoscopy. *Endoscopy* 1995;27:459–461.

18. Deitel M, Vasic V. A secure method of repair of large ventral hernias with Marlex mesh to eliminate tension. *Am J Surg* 1979; 137:276–277.

19. d'Oliveira C, Durdon A, Lehn E. Un procédé simple de mise en place et de contention des prothèses pariétales dans les cures d'éventration ou d'éviscération. *Interbloc* 1985;1:10.

20. Fawcett AN, Atherton WG, Balsitis M. A complication of the use of Prolene mesh in the repair of abdominal wall hernias. Hernia 1998;2:173–174.

21. Flament JB, Palot JP. Prostheses and major incisional hernias. In: Bendavid R, ed. *Prostheses and major incisional hernias.* Austin: RG Landes Co, 1994.

22. Flament JB, Palot JP, Burde A, et al. Treatment of major incisional hernias. *Probl Gen Surg* 1995;12:151–158.

23. Flament JB, Rives J, Palot JP, et al. Major incision hernia. In: Chevrel JP, ed. *Hernias and surgery of the abdominal wall.* New York: Springer–Verlag, 1995:116–144.

24. Flament JB, Palot JP. Tratamiento quirurgico de las eventraciones gigantes multirrecidivadas. In: Porrero JL, ed. *Cirugia de la pared abdominal.* Madrid: Masson, 1996:243–248.

25. Flament JB, Palot JP, Avisse C. Massive multi recurrent incisional hernia—prosthetic repair. In: Kurzer M, Kark AE, Wantz GE, eds. *Surgical management of abdominal wall hernias.* London: Martin Dunitz Publishers, 1997:227–240.

26. Flament JB, Rives J, Palot JP, et al. Major incisional hernia. In: Chevrel JP, ed. *Hernia and surgery of the abdominal wall,* 2nd ed. New York: Springer–Verlag, 1997:128–158.

27. Flament JB, Avisse C, Palot JP, et al. Trophic ulcers in giant incisional hernias—pathogenesis and treatment. A report of 33 cases. *Hernia* 1997;1:71–76.

28. Flament JB, Avisse C, Palot JP, et al. Biomaterials. Principles of implantation. In: Schumpelick W, Kingsnorth A, eds. *Incisional hernia.* New York: Springer–Verlag, 1999.

29. Flament JB, Avisse C, Palot JP, et al. Complications in incisional hernia repairs by the placement of retromuscular prostheses. *Hernia* 2000;4 (suppl. 1):25–29.

30. Gibson CL. Operation for cure of large ventral hernias. *Ann Surg* 1920;72:331–333.

31. Gilbert AI, Graham MF. Infected grafts in incisional hernioplasties. *Hernia* 1997;1:77–81.

32. Gillion JF, Begin GF, Marecos C, et al. Expanded polytetrafluorethylene patches used in the intraperitoneal or extraperitoneal position for repair of incisional hernias of anterolateral abdominal wall. *Am J Surg* 1997;174:16–19.

33. Goldstein HS. Selecting the right mesh. *Hernia* 1999;3:23–26.

34. Goñi Moreno I. Chronic eventrations and large hernias. Preoperative treatment by progressive pneumoperitoneum. Original procedure. *Surgery* 1947;22:945–953.

35. Hesselink VJ, Luijendijk RW, de Wilt JHW, et al. A evaluation of risk factors in incisional hernia recurrence. *Surg Gynecol Obstet* 1993;176:228–234.

36. Hume RH, Bour J. Mesh migration following laparoscopic inguinal hernia repair. *J Laparoendosc Surg* 1997;6:333–335.

37. Israelsson LA, Jonsson T. Suture length to wound length ratio and healing of midline laparotomy incisions. *Br J Surg* 1993;80: 1284–1286.

38. Israelsson LA. The surgeon as a risk factor for complications of midline incisions. *Eur J Surg* 1998;164:353–359.

39. Judd ES. The prevention and treatment of ventral hernia. *Surg Gynecol Obstet* 1912;19:175–182.

40. Kaufman Z, Engelberg M, Zager M. Fecal fistula: a late complication of Marlex mesh repair. *Dis Colon Rectum* 1981;24:243–244.

41. Lardennois B, Benoist M, Hibon J, et al. Résultat de l'utilisation d'une étoffe en dacron dans le traitement des grandes éventrations. A propos de 37 cas. *Acta Chir Belg* 1971;70:287–290.

42. Leber GE, Garb JL, Alexander AI, et al. Long-term complications associated with prosthetic repair of incisional hernias. *Arch Surg* 1998;133:378–382.

43. Marchal F, Brunaud L, Sebbag H, et al. Treatment of incisional hernias by placement of an intraperitoneal prosthesis: a series of 128 patients. *Hernia* 1999;3:141–147.

44. Martinez DA, Vasquez JL, Pellicer E, et al. Results of expanded polytetrafluoroethylene patches in moderate and large incisional hernias. *Hernia* 1999;3:149–152.

45. Mayo WJ. An operation for the radical cure of umbilical hernia. *Ann Surg* 1901;34:276–280.

46. Muller M, Klinge U, Conze J, et al. Abdominal wall compliance after Marlex mesh implantation for incisional hernia repair. *Hernia* 1998;21:113–117.

47. Notaras MJ. Experience with Mersilene mesh in abdominal wall repair. *Proc R Soc Med* 1994;67:1187–1190

48. Palot JP, Delattre JF, Burde A, et al. Le traitement des grandes éventrations. *Est-Méd* 1981;1:611–637.

49. Paul A, Korenkov M, Peters S, et al. Unacceptable results of the Mayo procedure for repair of abdominal incisional hernias. *Eur J Surg* 1998;164:361–367.

50. Pire JC, Body C, Flament JB. La capacité vitale, un piège dans le bilan des grandes éventrations. *Nouv Presse Med* 1977;6:36–41.

51. Rath AM, Zhang J, Amouroux J, et al. Les prothèses pariétales abdominales. Etude biomècanique et histologique. *Chirurgie* 1996;121:253–265.

52. Rives J, Lardennois B, Pire JC, et al. Les grandes éventrations. Importance du "volet abdominal" et des troubles respiratoires qui lui sont secondaires. *Chirurgie* 1973;99:547–563.

53. Rives J, Pire JC, Flament JB, et al. Le traitement des grandes éventrations (a propos de 133 cas). *Bordeaux Méd* 1976;9:2115–2120.

54. Rives J, Pire JC, Flament JB, et al. Traitement des éventrations. *Encycl Med Chir Paris* 1977;4.0.07:40–165.

55. Rives J, Pire JC, Flament JB, et al. Le traitement des grandes éventrations. (A propos de 133 cas.) *Min Chir* 1977;32: 749–756.

56. Rives J, Pire JC, Flament JB, et al. Le traitement des grandes éventrations. Nouvelles indications thérapeutiques à propos de 322 cas. *Chirurgie* 1985;3:215–225.

57. Roth JS, Park AE, Witze D, et al. Laparoscopic incisional/ventral herniorrhaphy: a five year experience. *Hernia* 1999;4:209–214.

58. Savioz D, Ludwig C, Leissing C, et al. Repeated macroscopic haematuria caused by intravesical migration of a preperitoneal prosthesis. *Eur J Surg* 1997;163:631–632.

59. Seelig MH, Kaprek R, Tietze L, et al. Enterocutaneous fistula after Marlex net implantation. A rare complication after incisional hernia repair. *Chirurg* 1995;66:739–741.

60. Stoppa RE. The treatment of complicated groin and incisional hernias. *World J Surg* 1989;13:545–554.

61. Stoppa R, Moungar F, Verhaeghe P. Traitement chirurgical des éventrations médianes sus ombilicales. *J Chir* 1992;129:335–343.

62. Stoppa R, Ralaimiaramanana F, Henry X, et al. Evolution of large ventral incisional hernia repair. The French contribution to a difficult problem. Hernia 1999;3:1–3.

63. Trabucchi EE, Corsi FR, Meinardi C, et al. Tissue response to

polyester mesh for hernia repair: an ultramicroscopic study in man. *Hernia* 1998;2:107–112.

64. Trivellini G, Danelli PG. Use of two prostheses in the surgical repair of recurrent hernia. *Postgrad Gen Surg* 1992;4 (theme issue): 136–139.
65. Waldrep DJ, Shabot MM, Hiatt JR. Mature fibrous cyst formation after Marlex mesh ventral herniorrhaphy: a newly described pathological entity. *Am Surg* 1993;59:716–718.
66. Wantz GE. Incisional hernioplasty with Mersilene. *Surgery* 1991;172:129–137.
67. Wantz GE, Chevrel JP, Flament JB, et al. Incisional hernia: the problem and the cure. Symposium. *J Am Coll Surg* 1999;188: 429–447.
68. Wantz GE. Incisional hernia (Reply). *J Am Coll Surg* 1999;188: 635–637.
69. Welti H, Eudel F. Un procédé de cure radicale des éventrations postopératoires par auto-étalement des muscles grand droits, après incision du feuillet antérieur de leurs gaines. *Mem Acad Chir* 1941;28:781–798.

SPECIAL COMMENT

León Herszage

Up to Goñi Moreno's publication in 1940, the operation of a large incisional hernia involved a high risk of respiratory, immune, and hemodynamic complications, which led to death. He presented his works during the XII Argentine Congress of Surgery in October of that year (8). Essentially, it was a description of the advantages of the presurgical treatment of incisional hernias with the intraperitoneal injection of oxygen. But the fast absorption of oxygen lessened the efficiency of the method, and so he changed it to the use of natural air, which we are still using today. He published a lot of papers from then on, with improvements to the method (4,5,6), and so its diffusion allowed other surgeons (2,9,10) to test the benefits in many cases and led to its inevitable use in repairing huge hernias. The simplicity of applying a nonsophisticated apparatus permits the use of this method even in the poorest regions of the world, and so makes it possible to be known worldwide.

TECHNICAL INDICATIONS

There were a few apparatuses created to permit the injection of air, measuring the quantity being introduced. The simplest way was the use of a large syringe (60 cc) (3), but the most common and cheapest was the adaptation of two bitube bottles (Fig. 31.21) of 500 or 1000 cc (one filled with diluted antiseptic solution), joined by a rubber or plastic tube by their depth spouts, and to which we add, to the short spout: in the filled bottle a Richardson pump to push, and in the empty one a tube to be connected to the catheter or needle, put into the abdomen (1). We can introduce air into the abdomen, through a thick needle (Fig. 31.22), being sure that we can reach the abdominal cavity. In this case, we must prick the abdomen each time we decide to add air. Another way is to use a needle through which a small catheter (Fig. 31.22) would be introduced, and

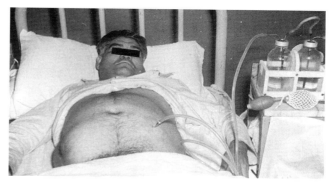

FIGURE 31.21. Air injection through a needle. Apparatus used. Place to prick.

this is fixed to the skin because it will stay in place during the entire procedure. In every case, the puncture should be done under aseptic conditions (gloves, skin antiseptic solutions, etc.) with or without local anesthetic. The place to prick is preferably on the left flank, 3 to 4 cm inner and upper the anterosuperior iliac spine (ASIS) (Figs. 31.21 and 31.22). During the puncture, we always feel two bounces, the first corresponding to the external oblique, and the second when we are going through the peritoneum. Once the needle is in the abdominal cavity, a syringe must be used in order to be sure that no liquid can be aspirated; if liquid can be aspirated, a viscera has been pricked. In that case, the needle must be removed, and the procedure suspended, usually without any complication. It must be proved that the syringe will not aspirate anything and will permit air to be introduced easily; then we can be sure that we are intraperitoneal and in a safe place, between the intestinal loops, ready to begin to introduce air with our apparatus.

It can be done in two ways:

1. ***Continuous injection*** *(Fig. 31.23): The bottles connected are hung one above the other to allow the liquid to drip, owing to the difference in height between the upper bottle*

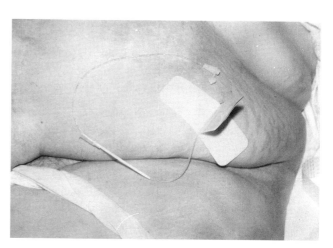

FIGURE 31.22. Catheter fixed in place.

PHYSIOPATHOLOGY

The rise of pressure with injected air into the sac and the abdomen produces the following (3):

1. *The pneumatic detachment of the adhered viscera and the bridles. This will reduce the risk and time of intrasurgical dissection.*
2. *The same as in an inflatable globe, the walls are progressively distended, even more when the patient lies face down.*
3. *The raising of abdominal pressure, gives the diaphragm a floor to support its function and improve breathing.*
4. *The augmented pressure eliminates the edema of the visceral mesos, and the submucous edema of the empty organs.*
5. *The function of large vessels is improved.*
6. *Our laboratory experiments with rats showed that because of the irritation of the peritoneum, a dilation of the capillaries is produced and with that the white cells are increased, which means an improvement in immunity.*
   Length of time used:
   We use this technique to obtain different advantages:

1. *To get the detachment of adhesions: 1 to 7 days.*
2. *The enlargement of the abdominal cavity and the stretching of the wall muscles: for at least 30 days. In this way, we say that the effect of air injection was obtained when by palpation we proved that the flanks were softened, or the spirometric curve was stabilized. More sophisticated methods are not needed in our daily practice.*
3. *From the immunologic point of view (7), we have seen that macrophages accumulated progressively, up to the nineteenth day, and then the quantity was maintained. So we can say that to obtain partial benefits, we can use this method for a few days, but to get all the advantages, it must be applied for not less than 15 days, and usually not more than 30 days.*

ADVANTAGES

With pneumoperitoneum, we are able to regularize the majority of the alterations so well described by Rives and his school (11), in the treatment of large and monstrous hernias:

1. *Breathing insufficiency.*
2. *Large vessels and capillar problems, produced because of lack of pressure.*
3. *Muscle tone.*
4. *The function of abdominal organs.*
5. *The amplitude of the abdominal cavity.*
6. *The reduction of the extruded viscera.*

COMPLICATIONS

As in every invasive technique, there are some complications:

1. *A technical failure provokes subcutaneous or retroperitoneal emphysema. The subcutaneous emphysema can be extended,*

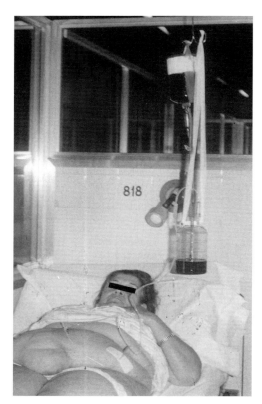

FIGURE 31.23. Continuous pneumoperitoneum through a catheter.

and the lower, permitting the displacement of air from this to the abdominal cavity. We can continue with the procedure for as long as we need, inverting the bottles and the tubes. The only inconvenience is that the patient must remain lying down during the procedure, but the process can be suspended at any moment.

2. ***Fractionated injection:*** *The usual way is to inject a quantity of air each time, through a needle or a catheter. In this case, we begin trying tolerance, injecting only 500 to 1000 cc of air, and the next days, until the patient complains of small pain in the abdomen, subcostal, or in the shoulder, with or without a light sensation of nausea.*

    When the intrasaccular or parietal tension diminishes, we can repeat the procedure (usually in a couple of days). An exaggerated injection of air could bother the patient, and in this case, it would be eliminated with a simple puncture. This form of injecting air could be used in an ambulatory way, thereby reducing the quantity of air injected (usually not more than 500 to 1000 cc each session). It is done in the consulting room, with the same precautions, but resting 20 or 30 minutes afterward, and then allowing a return to normal activity. It must be controlled carefully, because in one case a cardiac complication obliged us to hospitalize the patient, and in another I was informed (by Dr. Juan U. Soto, from Posadas, Misiones) of the death of a cardiac patient.

some times all over the body with crepitation and temporary deformation, without serious consequences.

2. A change of the voice and distention of the neck were seen when air passed to the mediastinum.
3. Sometimes we have seen air cysts among the intestinal loops.
4. A dissection of the gallbladder was reported to us by a colleague.
5. Cardiocirculatory complications had been treated in two cases.

Although these complications are inconvenient, usually they have been temporary, and without major consequences (except one case), but they oblige the surgeon to consider when to use it (12). It is impossible to avoid its use in cases of enormous hernias (Fig. 31.24), in which the advantages are notable. In cases of recently blocked viscera, its use improves this pathology. The socioeconomic cost is a disadvantage, but in these critical cases the advantages outweigh the inconvenience.

FINAL COMMENTS

It is convenient to take the patient to the surgical table with the sac totally inflated and not to deflate it until the end of the dissection time. When we open the sac, we must take care to eliminate all the air among the viscera. The use of pneumoperitoneum improves the intra- and postsurgical times, without doubt. In some of our large operated cases, this is one of the procedures that with other surgical methods (relaxing incisions, use of flaps–sac, meshes) allows us to solve successfully cases that were previously inoperable.

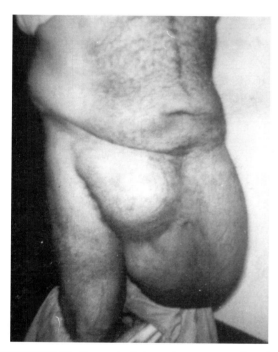

FIGURE 31.24. Presurgical view of a monstrous hernia.

REFERENCES

1. Barroetaveña J, Herszage L, et al. *Cirugia de las eventraciones.* Buenos Aires, Argentina: Ed El Ateneo, 1988.
2. Cady B, Brook Cowden GL. Repair of massive abdominal wall defects. Combined use of pneumoperitoneum and Marlex mesh. *Surg Clin North Am* 1976;56:559–570.
3. Flament JB. Wantz's incisional hernia symposium. *J Am Coll Surg* 1999;188:432.
4. Goñi Moreno I. Eventraciones crónicas y hernias voluminosas. Preparación con el neumoperitoneo progresivo. *Bol Trab Acad Arg Cir* 1946;30:1041.
5. Goñi Moreno I. Tratamiento original de las hernias y eventraciones crónicas voluminosas. *Prensa Med Arg* 1951;38:10.
6. Goñi Moreno I. Preparación pre-quirurgica de las grandes eventracione crónicas. *Bol Trab Acad Arg Cir* 1973;57:93.
7. Herszage L, et al. El incremento de macrófagos con el neumoperitoneo. *J Cient Htal Pirovano* 1988.
8. Jorge JM, Goñi Moreno I. Discusión. Presented at: XII Argentine Congress of Surgery; Buenos Aries, Argentina; 1940.
9. Koontz AR, Graves JW. Preoperative pneumoperitoneum as an aid in handling of giant hernias. *Ann Surg* 1954;140:759.
10. Mason EE. Pneumoperitoneum in the management of giant hernias. *Surgery* 1956;39:143.
11. Rives J, Lardennois B, Pire JC. Physiopathologie des eventrations. Presented at: 75th French Congress on Surgery; Paris, France; 1976.
12. Wantz GE. Incisional hernia symposium. *J Am Coll Surg* 1999; 188:432.

32

COMPLICATIONS OF VENTRAL INCISIONAL HERNIA REPAIR

J. STEPHEN MARSHALL
JAMES R. DEBORD

Ventral or incisional hernias are a common problem in general surgery. It is estimated that the risk of herniation of a midline incision is in the range of 2% to 11% (26). Repair of these hernias can be associated with complications that are common to all types of surgery and those that are specific to hernia repair. This combination can serve to make the repair of ventral hernias challenging.

COMPLICATIONS RELATED TO PRIMARY HERNIA REPAIR

Primary hernia repair (the repair of the ventral hernia without the use of a prosthetic material) can be associated with several complications, such as bleeding, infection, and ileus, that plague every aspect of abdominal surgery. There are also complications that are specifically related to ventral hernia repair itself, including pulmonary complications and hernia recurrence.

The repair of ventral hernias can be expected to be associated with bleeding complications as the repair of these hernias often necessitates much more extensive dissection than we would encounter in a standard midline incision. Prevention of this complication should be proactive, with meticulous hemostasis as the mainstay of prevention. The placement of subcutaneous drains has been used frequently to deal with this problem, but while they may allow identification of a problem, they do not prevent it. White et al. (31) have shown that the use of drains does not appreciably decrease the rate of hematoma formation, and may in fact increase the rate of wound infection. Other measures are helpful in preventing bleeding. A careful history, looking for any signs of bleeding in the past, a family history of

bleeding disorders, or diseases that may predispose the patient to coagulopathies, is mandatory. The preoperative cessation of anticoagulants such as aspirin, coumadin, and heparin is also helpful if possible.

Seromas are also a problem in this type of procedure. These are defined as a collection of serous fluid, not blood, in the subcutaneous space. The extensive dissection that is sometimes necessary to delineate the fascial edges of a hernia defect is a significant predisposing factor in this complication as well. White again showed that drains did not significantly decrease the rate of seroma formation (31), although the judicious use of closed suction drains for short periods of time (2 to 4 days) is still advocated by many surgeons. Careful obliteration of dead space with subcutaneous sutures and compressive dressings or binders may help in the prevention of this complication. Aspiration may become necessary if a seroma persists, but most will resolve over time if the surgeon and the patient can exercise prudence and patience. If aspiration is performed, it should employ strict aseptic technique.

Both of these complications can predispose to the development of a more devastating complication, that of wound infection. Wound infections are the major cause of ventral hernia recurrence. Bucknall et al. (3) demonstrated that a wound that is infected has a fivefold increase in the risk of developing a ventral hernia, and that infection in the surgical wound can prolong inflammation, delay collagen deposition, and cause extrusion of suture material, all of which cause weakening in the wound tensile strength. The edema that occurs with infection causes the tissues to become weakened and allows the sutures to more easily pull through the tissues.

It then follows that prevention of wound infection is very important in the field of ventral hernia repair. Careful skin preparation is essential. A preoperative shower with an antibacterial soap will decrease the risk of infection. If shaving is necessary, this should be done immediately before the procedure. Sterile barriers have not been shown to decrease

J. S. Marshall: Department of Surgery, University of Illinois at Peoria; Department of Surgery, OSF–St. Francis Medical Center, Peoria, Illinois.

J. R. DeBord: Department of Surgery, University of Illinois College of Medicine at Peoria, Peoria, Illinois.

the risk of infection. The use of prophylactic antibiotics in clean wounds is controversial, with concern expressed about the risk of developing resistant organisms with the inappropriate use of antibiotics. However, in the field of ventral hernia repair, prophylactic antibiotic use is warranted. The risk of repair failure increases with infection. The difficulty of every repair cannot be anticipated prior to the operation, so one cannot predict the length of the procedure or the risk of enterotomy. It is also not always possible to predict the need for a prosthetic repair, for which prophylactic antibiotics are indicated. Cefazolin continues to be our prophylactic antibiotic of choice in most patients.

The rate of wound infection can be decreased by careful attention to meticulous surgical technique. This may be quite challenging during the extensive dissection that often occurs during a large incisional hernia repair. The use of gentle tissue handling, sharp dissection, small tissue bites during ligature, and avoidance of tissue dehydration minimizes the trauma to the tissue, resulting in less necrotic tissue. The use of fine suture decreases the amount of foreign material in the wound. Irrigation of the wound at closure decreases the amount of foreign and necrotic debris in the wound. Detailed hemostasis and the obliteration of dead space decrease the rate of formation of hematomas and seromas, which can predispose the wound to infection. However, this must be done judiciously, as improperly placed sutures may cause tissue necrosis, increasing the risk of infection.

Closing the wound under tension or allowing the abdomen to become distended after surgery will increase the pressure on the sutures, thus increasing the damage to the tissue incorporated within these sutures, subsequently increasing the amount of necrotic tissue in the wound. Given the fact that a wound infection may well defeat the purpose of a hernia repair, it should be understood that a hernia repair should not be undertaken in the presence of cellulitis, wound sinuses, or infected foreign material. These situations must be remedied before repair can be safely effected. Scarred or atrophic skin should be excised as this type of skin is prone to ischemia and subsequent infection, and old sutures should be removed completely if at all possible as they may harbor bacteria that could result in wound infection.

Large hernias that are present for a long period of time are often associated with a functional loss of the abdominal wall. The abdominal viscera begin to reside in the hernia defect and the abdominal musculature contracts. The repair of these defects can be quite challenging. Closing these wounds under tension increases the risk of recurrence. Tension also increases the intraabdominal pressure. This has the effect of elevating the diaphragm, thus decreasing respiratory excursion, and consequently increasing the risk of development of pulmonary complications. Venous return to the heart is also decreased, resulting in a degree of the abdominal compartment syndrome. These problems have led to procedures that utilize relaxing incisions in the lateral

abdominal fascia to prevent tension on the wound and the subsequent increased risk of recurrence (19). Progressive pneumoperitoneum was first described to combat this problem in the 1940s, and is still utilized by some authors in certain situations (9,25). Tissue expanders have also been described as a method of trying to regain the abdominal domain (13). The issues of loss of domain and increased wound tension that results from primary repair of large incisional hernias have been best dealt with by the application of modern prosthetic biomaterials to effect a tension-free repair.

Recurrence

The risk of recurrence for those hernias repaired without prostheses can be quite significant—as high as 50% in some reported series (26). Many factors contribute to the recurrence of a hernia. As noted above, the rate of recurrence is felt to be higher in those patients who have infections in their wounds. Recurrence has also been related to the presence of obesity (23). Incisions in the obese abdomen result in significantly more traumatized tissue, predisposing the patient to wound infection. The obese patient also has a high intraabdominal pressure, which increases the tension on the suture line. Stress on the suture line caused by straining under light anesthesia, vomiting, coughing, or gaseous distention of the abdomen can increase the tension on the suture line, resulting in pressure necrosis or tearing of the tissues. Preoperative pulmonary toilet, cessation of smoking, good anesthetic technique, and gastric decompression will help alleviate these problems. The size of the hernia was felt to be important by Hesselink and colleagues, who showed that hernias less than 4 cm had a significantly lower risk of recurrence than those greater than 4 cm (25% versus 41%) (10). Surgical technique is important in the prevention of recurrence of hernias. It is mandatory to use meticulous technique to decrease the rate of hematomas, seromas, and wound infections. It is also very important to use surgical skill and judgment to close these wounds without undue tension, as this tension allows for disruption of the wound. Several techniques have been described to minimize the tension on the wound (16,30), including undermining the fascia, counterincisions, the use of internal retention sutures, the use of a suture–to–wound length ratio of 4:1 to 5:1, and the use of prosthetic material. Hughes and colleagues have suggested that, since the presence of obesity with a large abdominal pannus may contribute to recurrence, panniculectomy should be performed with hernia repair (12). They showed that this procedure decreased the rate of recurrence by allowing better access to the hernia and decreasing postoperative strain on the abdomen, although this study had a relatively short follow-up. We believe panniculectomy may be an important adjunct to ventral hernia repair, especially after massive weight loss resulting from bariatric surgery. It may also be prudent, if the pannus is ulcerated or chronically infected, to excise it at the time of hernia repair. Most hernias recur within 3 years, with about 45% of all recurrences occurring within the first year (17), although they have been described as occurring as late as 10 years after the original surgery (8).

COMPLICATIONS RELATED TO PROSTHETIC HERNIA REPAIR

The closure of wounds under tension will increase the risk of herniation or reherniation. The sutures can saw through the tissues, causing a "button hole" hernia as described by Krukowski and Matheson (15). The tissue that is compressed under a tight primary closure suture will also become necrotic, resulting in both weak fascia, and a nidus for infection. It is also not possible in some patients to find nonattenuated fascia for a secure, tension-free closure of the abdominal defect. For these reasons, the use of a prosthetic biomaterial to close the abdominal wall is necessary.

The use of prosthetic biomaterials to repair ventral incisional hernias has been evolving since the early twentieth century (4,5). Prostheses are attractive because they can bridge gaps, allowing tissues to be closed with minimal tension, and they can reinforce tissues by the process of tissue ingrowth. However, they can also develop complications. These can be the same types of complications seen in the primary repair of hernias, such as hematomas, seromas, and wound infections, as has previously been discussed. A second set of complications can develop secondary to the prosthesis itself, consisting of infection of the prosthetic material, fistulas, and bowel obstructions.

Hematoma/Seroma

Collections of blood or serum in the subcutaneous tissues after a ventral hernia repair are serious complications. These complications are of particular significance in the prosthetic repair of ventral hernias, as they may cause wound breakdown with mesh exposure and resultant prosthetic infection, or become secondarily infected and lead to the same result. Close attention to hemostasis will of course decrease the rate of hematoma formation. Closing the subcutaneous tissue and decreasing the amount of "dead space" may decrease the risk of serous fluid collection. The placement of drains is somewhat controversial, as in primary repair. They remove fluid, but may serve only to increase the rate of infection if they are improperly used or left in place too long. When drains are used in our practice in the presence of a prosthetic repair, they are removed after 2 to 4 days, and antibiotics are continued until the drains are removed. If a fluid collection is noted that is of significant size, or is symptomatic, open drainage in the operating room under sterile conditions should be considered in order to minimize the risk of infection. If aspiration is performed, it should be under formal

surgical skin preparation and antibiotic coverage. Again, many seemingly large seromas will resolve over time if nothing is done except careful observation.

Infection

The development of a wound infection in a hernia that is repaired with a prosthetic material is a grave complication, often requiring removal of the prosthetic material. Therefore, all reasonable measures for preventing wound infection should be taken, including meticulous sterile technique. It is important that any foreign material be removed from the wound prior to surgery. Open sinuses must be excised and healed before placement of prosthetic material. It is also important that a long delay be imposed before prosthetic repair of a hernia that has been infected. No hernia should be repaired in the face of open wounds or distant infections. It may be desirable to use an adhesive skin barrier drape over the exposed abdominal wall to reduce inadvertent contact between the skin and the prosthetic biomaterial. Antibiotic prophylaxis is mandatory, using a broad-spectrum antibiotic effective against skin flora.

Recurrence

Hernias that are repaired with prostheses can recur. However, several studies have shown that the rate of recurrence is lower than those repairs without prosthesis, in the range of about 10%. Care must be taken to ensure that the prosthesis is properly placed, without tension. It is also important to make sure that all hernia defects in the wound are recognized and treated, as untreated defects will recur at a later date. Rarely do recurrent hernias develop in the prosthesis itself. It is much more common for another hernia, which may have been unrecognized at the first operation, to manifest itself, or for an improperly placed prosthesis to pull away from the edge of the repair (32). We feel, therefore, that when using prosthetic biomaterial for hernia repair it is important that wide dissection of the fascia be performed and that the prosthetic material be placed with a generous overlap of the fascia edge with as little tension as possible.

GRAFT COMPLICATIONS

Certain complications can occur due to the presence of the prosthetic material per se. Three different types of prosthetic material are currently used for the repair of ventral hernias. The first of these to be described was Dacron (polyester) (Meadox Medical, Oakland, NJ, U.S.A.) in 1956. Woven polypropylene mesh was introduced in 1958. This has undergone a number of modifications to become the most popular hernia repair mesh in use today. The third type of prosthetic material used today, expanded polytetrafluoroethylene (ePTFE) mesh, was introduced in the 1970s. The mesh prosthetic materials, polypropylene and polyester, create a significant inflammatory reaction with gross tissue ingrowth into the interstices of the mesh. This ingrowth enhances the strength of the repair, and dense scar formation results. The ePTFE biomaterial, however, does not promote such an intense inflammatory reaction, and thus does not form a dense scar. Tissue ingrowth into the ePTFE is demonstrated microscopically, but this tissue incorporation does not enhance the strength of the repair significantly, and this remains dependent on the strength of the surrounding fascia and permanent suture fixation of the patch.

The mesh-type prostheses have been implicated in several types of complications, due in part to the intense inflammatory reaction that they promote. Polypropylene has been reported to create mesh extrusion, wound sepsis, erosion into intraabdominal organs, refractory seromas, and bowel fistulas (18). Other authors feel that polyester is the mesh of choice as it is supple and allows the patient with a large repair much more mobility of the abdomen after repair than if polypropylene had been used (21). Both types of mesh have the limitation of significant adhesion formation. Therefore, the mesh should always be placed in an extraperitoneal position when possible. This has been accomplished by placing it anterior or posterior to the rectus muscles. If intraperitoneal placement cannot be avoided, care should be taken to interpose the omentum between the mesh and the bowel. The placement of a layer of absorbable mesh between the bowel and the non-absorbable mesh has been shown to decrease the rate of adhesion formation (14). It has even been suggested that the use of Seprafilm (Genzyme Corporation, Cambridge, MA, U.S.A.) may decrease adhesions associated with mesh in a hernia model in rats (1). Occasionally, a clinical dilemma will require the use of large pieces of polypropylene mesh that inevitably comes into contact with the viscera. While success may follow such reconstruction, we have had one chronic mesh erosion through the skin and one enterocutaneous fistula in the past several years from this usage.

The third currently popular material for the repair of abdominal wall hernias, ePTFE, has the advantage of forming fewer adhesions to the bowel, and this quality makes ePTFE a good choice for intraperitoneal placement. Repair of ventral incisional hernias with an ePTFE patch can be done with few complications due to adhesions, and with an acceptable recurrence rate (2,20). Our experience has demonstrated that when reexploration is needed in the presence of an ePTFE abdominal wall patch, the adhesions that are present are filmy and easily taken down compared to the often dense adhesions associated with polypropylene and polyester mesh.

The prosthetic material, like any foreign body, can become infected, resulting in a difficult therapeutic dilemma. While an infected patch can occasionally be treated successfully, infection often requires removal of the patch, resulting in a very high rate of recurrent herniation. The coarser mesh types of prosthetic materials may be more resistant to infection due to the fact that the large interstices

do not harbor bacteria. Polypropylene, being monofilament, also eliminates the crevices in the basic mesh material that can harbor bacteria. ePTFE has small (22 to 25 μm) interstices, which may allow bacteria to proliferate, and make eradication of bacteria very difficult. A new antimicrobial impregnated ePTFE patch utilizing silver chlorhexidine may provide some added help in this regard, but clinical studies are not available at this time (7).

The rationale for the selection of a prosthetic biomaterial in hernia repair has been well documented (6). The judgment of the surgeon regarding which available biomaterial to use in which clinical scenario may be a critical decision that impacts the development of postoperative complications. Knowledge of the biologic properties and their appropriate clinical application is the responsibility of all surgeons who undertake these challenging and often underestimated difficult incisional hernia problems. Our current practice has been developed as follows:

1. For preperitoneal and anterior "tension-free" groin hernia repairs, polyester, polypropylene, and ePTFE prostheses are all suitable.
2. For intraperitoneal placement of a biomaterial for groin or ventral hernia repair, by open or laparoscopic technique, ePTFE patches are recommended.
3. For the Stoppa procedure of giant prosthetic reinforcement of the visceral sac (GPRVS), polyester mesh is preferable.
4. For ventral incisional hernia repairs performed extraperitoneally, polyester, polypropylene, and ePTFE prosthetic materials are all satisfactory.
5. For full thickness chest wall or diaphragm defects, ePTFE patches are used.
6. For contaminated or grossly infected abdominal wall defects, polypropylene mesh may be preferable, or absorbable mesh may be utilized to provide adequate temporary closure.

LAPAROSCOPY

Several recent reports have touted the use of laparoscopy as a means of repairing ventral hernias (11,22,24). The laparoscopic approach has several advantages when compared to traditional open ventral incisional hernia repair. These patients are reported to have less time in the hospital than those who undergo an open repair. Due to the technique of using several small incisions to secure the mesh, the risk of wound complications is decreased, and the presence of an infection in one of these incisions does not always lead to infection of the prosthesis. Seromas may also form in the hernia wound, particularly in the area that the hernia contents previously occupied. As these seromas are not in continuity with an open incision, the risk of infection is minimal. A seroma in this position will eventually resorb, although it may take several months. Similarly, the risk of hematoma formation would be expected to be less, as the subcutaneous dissection is less extensive. By examining the hernia defects with the laparoscope after the adhesions have been freed, it is often possible to identify more hernia defects than were suspected. This then allows the placement of a larger patch, which should decrease the rate of late hernia recurrence, or more correctly stated, late hernia expression. Several early studies have also reported that the rate of recurrence is small, in the range of 0% to 11% (24,29,30). Laparoscopic repair may be associated with complications related to laparoscopy, including trocar injuries to bowel or vessels, hernia formation at the trocar sites, and subcutaneous emphysema. This method of repair is a valuable addition to the treatment of ventral incisional hernias as it decreases the rate of both complications and recurrence.

CONCLUSION

The repair of a ventral incisional hernia is a significant operation, not to be taken lightly. Careful preoperative planning combined with meticulous surgical technique and experienced judgment is important in order to minimize the risk of complications and hernia recurrence. The use of prosthetic material has greatly reduced the risk of recurrence, but has introduced additional potential complications. Laparoscopic repair by placement of a prosthetic material may further decrease complications of these formidable operations by reducing the risk of wound complications. Future development of even more biocompatible and infection-resistant prosthetic materials will also have an impact on the future of ventral incisional hernia repair.

REFERENCES

1. Alopant A, Lakshminarasappa SR, Yavuz N, et al. Prevention of adhesions by Seprafilm, an absorbable adhesion barrier: an incisional model in rats. *Am Surg* 1997;63:818.
2. Bauer JJ, Harris MT, Kreel I, et al. Twelve year experience with expanded polytetrafluorethylene in the repair of abdominal wall defects. *Mount Sinai J Med* 1999;66:20.
3. Bucknall TE, Cox PJ, Ellis H. Burst abdomen and incisional hernia: a prospective study of 1129 major laparotomies. *Br Med J* 1987;284:931.
4. Burk GL. Corrosion of metals in tissues and an introduction to tantalum. *Can Med Assoc J* 1940;43:125.
5. DeBord JR. The historical development of prosthetics in hernia surgery. *Surg Clin North Am* 1998;78:973.
6. DeBord JR. The rationale for the selection of a prosthetic biomaterial in hernia repair. *Probl Gen Surg* 1995;12:75.
7. DeBord JR, Bauer JJ, Grischkan DM, et al. Short term study on the safety of antimicrobial agent impregnated ePTFE patches for hernia repair. *Hernia* 1999;3:189.
8. Ellis H. Management of the wound. In: Schwartz SI, Ellis H, eds. *Maingot's abdominal operations,* 9th ed. Norwalk, CT: Appleton & Lange, 1989:195.
9. Harrison D, Taneja R, Kahn D, et al. Repair of a massive ventral hernia in a morbidly obese patient. *N J Med* 1995;92:387.
10. Hesselink VJ, Luijendijk RW, de Wilt JHW, et al. An evaluation of risk factors in incisional hernia recurrence. *Surgery* 1993;176:228.
11. Holzman MD, Purat CM, Reintgen K, et al. Laparoscopic ventral and incisional hernioplasty. *Surg Endosc* 1997;11:32–35.
12. Hughes KC, Weider L, Fischer J, et al. Ventral hernia repair with simultaneous panniculectomy. *Am Surg* 1996;62:678.
13. Jacobsen W, Petty P, Bite U, et al. Massive abdominal wall reconstruction with expanded external/internal oblique and transversalis musculofascia. *Plast Reconstr Surg* 1997;100:326.
14. Kinge U, Klosterhalfen B. Biomaterial—experimental aspects. In: Schumpelick V, Kingsworth A, eds. *Incisional hernia.* New York: Springer-Verlag, 1999:178.
15. Krukowski ZH, Matheson NA. 'Button hole' incisional hernia: a late complication of abdominal wound closure with continuous non-absorbable sutures. *Br J Surg* 1987;74:824.
16. Kuzbari R, Worseg AP, Tairych G. Sliding door technique for the repair of midline incisional hernias. *Plast Reconstr Surg* 1998;101:1235.
17. Langer S, Christiansen J. Long term results after incisional hernia repair. *Acta Chir Scand* 1985;151:217.
18. Leber GE, Garb JL, Alexander AI, et al. Long-term complications associated with prosthetic repair of incisional hernias. *Arch Surg* 1998;133:378.
19. Lucas CE, Ledgerwood AM. Autologous closure of giant abdominal wall defects. *Am Surg* 1998;64:607.
20. Martinez DA, Vazquez JL, Pelliar E, et al. Results of expanded polytetrafluoroethylene patches in moderate and large incisional hernias. *Hernia* 1999;3:149.
21. Muller M, Klinge U, Conze J, et al. Abdominal wall compliance after Marlex mesh implantation for incisional hernia repair. *Hernia* 1998;2:113.
22. Park A, Burch DW, Lovrics P. Laparoscopic and open incisional hernia repair: a comparison study. *Surgury* 1998;24:816.
23. Pitkin RM. Abdominal hysterectomy in obese women. *Surg Gynecol Obstet* 1976;142:532.
24. Ramshaw BJ, Schwab J, Mason EM, et al. Comparison of laparoscopic and open ventral herniorrhaphy. *Am Surg* 1999;177:227.
25. Raynor RW, DelGuerico LR. The place for pneumoperitoneum in the repair of massive hernia. *World J Surg* 1989;13:581.
26. Reed RC, Yoder G. Recent trends in the management of incisional herniation. *Arch Surg* 1989;124:485.
27. Sanders LM, Flint LM, Ferrara JJ. Initial experience with laparoscopic repair of incisional hernias. *Am J Surg* 1999;17:227.
28. Saiz AA, Willis IH, Paul DK, et al. Laparoscopic ventral hernia repair: a community hospital experience. *Am Surg* 1996;62:336.
29. Santora TJ, Roslyn JJ. Incisional hernia. *Surg Clin North Am* 1993;73:557.
30. Wantz GE, Chevrel JP, Flament JB, et al. Incisional hernia: the problem and the cure. *J Am Coll Surg* 1999;188:429.
31. White TJ, Santos MC, Thompson JS. Factors affecting wound complications in repair of ventral hernias. *Am Surg* 1998;64:276.
32. van der Lei B, Bleichrodt RP, Simmermacher RKJ, et al. Expanded polytetrafluoroethylene patch for the repair of large abdominal wall defects. *Br J Surg* 1989;76:803.

33

LAPAROSCOPIC REPAIR OF VENTRAL/INCISIONAL HERNIAS

GUY R. VOELLER
EUGENE C. MANGIANTE

With the resounding success of laparoscopic cholecystectomy, a similar panacea for the difficult problem of ventral/incisional hernias was sought beginning in the early 1990s. Initial attempts to repair this hernia using laparoscopic techniques emerged as little more than a poorly conceived, quick-fix, word-of-mouth approach and several case reports. The stimulus for some success in this area occurred when laparoscopic investigators adopted the sound physiologic principles of the most successful open technique as advocated by Wantz (13). During the ensuing decade, with improved tacking devices and modifications in prosthetic materials, the technique for repair has evolved to a point where a considerable amount of data is now available to assess laparoscopy's role in the repair of ventral/incisional hernias.

Due to the efforts of George Wantz, M.D., surgeons in the United States were made aware of the Rives–Stoppa (6,9) approach for the open repair of ventral/incisional hernias. This technique involves a midline incision and development of a plane behind the rectus muscles as far lateral as possible in order to place a large piece of nonabsorbable mesh. The mesh is held in place by a series of U-stitches placed (in a circumferential manner) through the mesh and the anterior abdominal wall. The prosthesis is behind the hernia defect, and all attempts are made to keep the mesh outside of the peritoneal cavity. While Rives et al. described using Dacron mesh (Ethicon Inc., Somerville, NJ, U.S.A.), polypropylene is frequently used both in Europe and, especially, in the United States. The single most important factor that improved recurrence rates was the sound physiologic principle of diffusing total intraabdominal pressure on each square inch of mesh implantation instead of the tenuous suture line–fascial interface.

The American Hernia Society has declared that this retrorectus repair of ventral/incisional hernias should be considered the standard of care due to the extremely low recurrence rates. While many have noted similar very low recurrence rates, a few drawbacks to this repair have emerged. The operation requires a significant soft tissue dissection in tissues that already may be of poor quality. This has led to a complication rate of up to 20% involving the wound, exposure and infection of the mesh, fistula formation, and other problems (8). There is a lengthy hospital stay and recovery time of 6 to 8 weeks. Several investigators have recently shown that when polypropylene mesh is used, the compliance of the abdominal wall is altered significantly and this can lead to patients complaining of discomfort and restriction of movement of their abdominal wall (3). A number of investigators believed that the Rives–Stoppa approach was sound and that modification in techniques and not principles could permit laparoscopic mesh placement with fewer side effects.

The author's first attempt at laparoscopic repair of a ventral/incisional hernia involved a Spigelian hernia. This was prior to the development of automatic hernia staplers, and a reloadable hernia stapler was used to affix a piece of mesh to the peritoneum. While aesthetically pleasing, the hernia soon recurred, and when evaluated laparoscopically it could be seen that the prosthetic had simply migrated with the peritoneum into the hernia defect. We thus realized that suture fixation as in the Rives–Stoppa approach would be critical to long-term success in these oftentimes large patients. Several other investigators (Toy, Smoot, Park, Gagner) (4,11) were evaluating laparoscopic repair of ventral/incisional hernias at the same time. The ability to mimic the Rives–Stoppa approach laparoscopically (a large piece of nonabsorbable mesh is placed behind the hernia defect and sutured to the entire thickness of the abdominal wall) is now a viable alternative.

EQUIPMENT

As with all advanced laparoscopic procedures, a three-chip videoendoscopic camera and an up-to-date light source are

G. R. Voeller: Department of Surgery, University of Tennessee at Memphis, Memphis, Tennessee.

E. C. Mangiante: Department of Surgery, University of Tennessee; Department of Surgery, VAMC, Memphis, Tennessee.

critical for performance of laparoscopic repair of ventral/incisional hernias. Because one must be able to view the anterior abdominal wall and the mesh as it is placed into the abdominal cavity, a 45-degree angle telescope (both 5 mm and 10 mm) is used. Five-millimeter working ports for the laparoscopic repair of ventral/incisional hernias are used, and atraumatic bowel graspers are needed to reduce incarcerated intestines. The 2- to 3-mm needlescopic instruments may also be beneficial.

Monopolar cautery is beneficial as long as appropriate visceral precautions are taken. If the dissection remains in a plane close to the abdominal wall and hernia sac, minimal bleeding occurs. Even though the harmonic scalpel has less current spread than monopolar cautery, the tip of the device gets tremendously hot and can burn viscera, which can be difficult to detect at the time of surgery. This may lead to "delayed" intestinal necrosis, perforation, and disaster.

The strength of the repair is due to the transabdominal sutures and not the spiral tacks. Although nonabsorbable, monofilament polypropylene sutures inhibit bacterial migration onto the mesh, and suture memory makes manipulation tedious. A CV-zero polytetrafluoroethylene (PTFE) suture by W.L. Gore (Flagstaff, AZ, U.S.A.) is nonabsorbable and has no memory, which makes it very easy to manipulate laparoscopically. While many things can be used to pass the sutures through the entire thickness of the abdominal wall, the Toy–Smoot suture passer is made specifically for this purpose (Fig. 33.1).

The 5-mm spiral-tacking device for repair of ventral/incisional hernias is of benefit because the device allows the use of all 5-mm working ports, thus reducing pain, and in addition provides better penetration of the mesh and the abdominal wall. The tacks allow strong apposition of the mesh to the peritoneum to prevent intestines from slipping between the two and thus internal hernia formation.

Finally, it is now clear that any mesh placed laparoscopically for ventral/incisional hernia repair will have to be placed intraperitoneally for technical reasons. While some

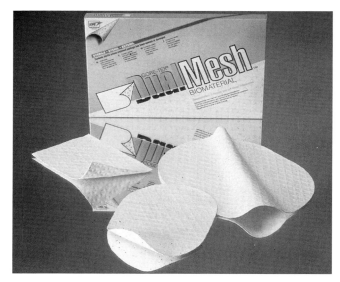

FIGURE 33.2. W.L. Gore Dual-Mesh Plus.

investigators have used polypropylene and Dacron mesh, it is well documented that these meshes create an intense inflammatory response that leads to dense scarring with fibrosis. This may result in bowel obstruction, fistula formation, and technically difficult surgery if reoperation is required. The majority of laparoscopic ventral/incisional hernia work has been with PTFE mesh, especially the dual-sided mesh from W.L. Gore (Fig. 33.2). This mesh is well suited for laparoscopic repair since the pore size on one side is so small as to inhibit tissue ingrowth (visceral side), while the pore size on the opposite side is large enough to allow fibroblastic ingrowth (peritoneal side). In addition, silver salts and chlorhexidine are impregnated into the Dual-Mesh Plus (W. L. Gore) for antimicrobial reasons.

PATIENT PREPARATION AND SELECTION

Hesselink et al. (1) have shown that any ventral/incisional hernia greater than 4 cm and recurrent hernias have a high rate of recurrence if not repaired with mesh. The obese patient, regardless of size, would also benefit from mesh repair. Obviously, if the viscera have lost the right-of-domain, then the laparoscopic approach is not indicated. As the surgeon undertakes this method of treatment, initial repairs should be on "easier" hernias like epigastric, umbilical, or first-time small incisional hernias. Surgeons in Europe often recommend weight loss prior to open ventral/incisional hernia repair. While this would be advantageous, it is often not practical. Fortunately, it may be less important in the laparoscopic approach since wound problems are fewer. A formal bowel preparation is used if the colon is incarcerated to a significant degree. The patient is always told that if a safe and secure repair cannot be accomplished laparoscopically, an open

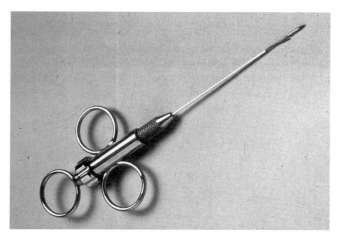

FIGURE 33.1. Toy–Smoot suture passer.

repair will be performed, and that if an enterotomy occurs the hernia may not be repaired at that time.

TECHNIQUE

A Foley catheter is placed if the hernia is a low hernia that will require fixation to Cooper's ligament or if the repair will take a prolonged amount of time. A nasogastric tube is not routinely placed. As for all prolonged laparoscopic procedures, sequential pneumatic compression devices are placed at the time of surgery and are left on the patient until he or she is ambulating. The laparoscopic monitors can be positioned similarly to laparoscopic cholecystectomy for most midline hernias but will have to be moved toward the feet for lower hernias. It will be necessary to operate from all angles, and if the patient's size allows, one or both arms should be "tucked" at the side of the patient. In the case of the very large patient where it is not possible to tuck the arm, the surgeon should move the operating room table away from anesthesia and drape out, so that the surgeon can stand cephalad to the arm boards. The patient should be prepared and draped very far laterally since trocars will have to be placed very lateral to avoid interfering with the mesh. An Ioban protective drape (3M Company, St. Paul, MN, U.S.A.) is used to avoid any contamination of the mesh.

A cogent concern of laparoscopic repair of ventral/incisional hernia is how to safely gain access to the abdomen operated upon previously. A helpful technique is the placement of a balloon-tipped blunt Hasson trocar at either costal margin as far lateral as possible, while staying superior to the colon (Fig. 33.3). This requires the use of S-shaped retractors to visualize each fascial and muscle layer as it is separated. When the peritoneum is visualized, it is incised and the balloon-tipped Hasson trocar inserted.

It is important to limit accessory trocars to 5-mm sizes or less. These patients are usually large and have already proven that they are prone to hernia formation. The use of a 5-mm telescope and 5-mm tacker along with the one Hasson port allows one to avoid using 10-mm working ports, large-diameter mesh spreaders as described by Toy and Smoot, and large holes in the abdominal wall. While accessory trocar placement can be variable depending on the hernia location, most midline hernias can be repaired with one or two 5-mm ports on the same side as the Hasson port. Due to the patient's size, it is often advantageous to use one 5-mm port for dissection and use the nondominant hand to compress the abdominal wall to "push" the tissues down, so that dissection can take place. Always try to operate in the direction the camera is viewing—this usually means placing two additional 5-mm ports opposite the original ports for dissection and, later, use of the tacking device.

Adhesiolysis is the first step and should be done very carefully (Fig. 33.4). It must be remembered that depth perception is lost laparoscopically, and bowel and hernia sac can look very similar. The surgeon should try to "uncover" the entire peritoneal surface since this will make mesh placement easier and oftentimes uncovers occult hernias. It is critical that if safe adhesiolysis cannot be done, then the procedure should be converted to an open case. In addition, if the surgeon cannot determine if a bowel injury has occurred, an incision should be made to evaluate the bowel. A missed bowel injury can be a deadly complication. While *not* recommended to beginners, the author has on two or three occasions recognized small bowel enterotomies, repaired them laparoscopically, and placed the Dual-Mesh Plus. All of these patients recovered uneventfully. A small limited incision to reduce densely incarcerated viscera may be used, and following closure of that wound, the hernia repair may be performed laparoscopically. This allows less tissue dissection, less morbidity and quicker recovery than an open Stoppa repair.

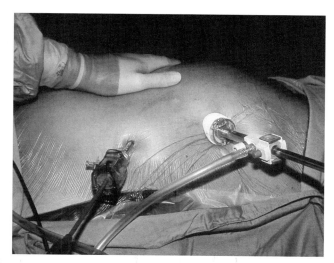

FIGURE 33.3. Initial access with balloon-tipped Hasson cannula.

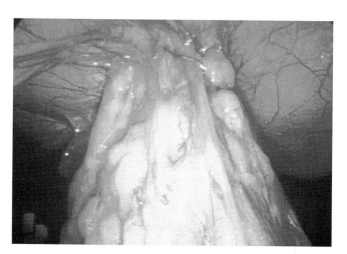

FIGURE 33.4. Adhesiolysis.

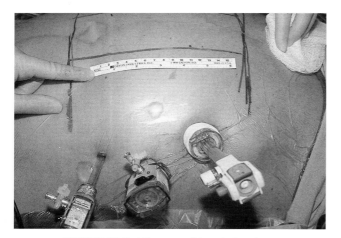

FIGURE 33.5. Diagram of hernia borders.

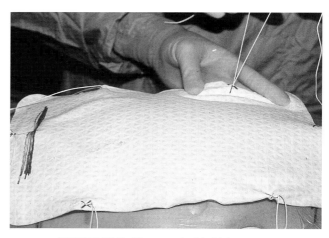

FIGURE 33.7. Placement of initial sutures.

Once all of the adhesions are removed, the borders of the fascial defect(s) are determined and diagrammed on the skin of the anterior abdominal wall (Fig. 33.5). If the surgeon can palpate the fascial defect preoperatively, then it should be diagrammed on the skin at this time. Toy and Smoot have described a technique using a spinal needle passed through the abdominal wall and then viewed with the laparoscope to aid in determining fascial borders of the defect. Once the "fascial hernia" is drawn on the abdominal wall, 3 to 5 cm is added to this, and this is diagrammed on the skin with the abdomen deflated (Fig. 33.6). This is the size of the prosthetic that will be required. This is measured and the appropriate size of Dual-Mesh Plus selected. The cephalad end of the mesh is marked and "Xs" are placed at four to six equidistant points at the perimeter of the mesh, as well as on the corresponding site on the skin. The "Xs" indicate where the initial stay sutures will be placed. These U-stitches of W.L. Gore CV-zero are placed through and through the mesh, tied (leaving the ends long enough to tie

again), and clipped together with a hemoclip (Fig. 33.7). One suture is left a little longer than the other to facilitate grasping the sutures with the Toy–Smoot suture passer (Fig. 33.8). The number of initial U-stitches is four for small patches and five to six for larger pieces.

While larger trocars and tissue spreaders have been described for intraabdominal mesh placement, the mesh can be rolled from two opposite edges to the middle, compressed (Fig. 33.9), and passed through the Hasson port's wound. A laparoscopic grasper is placed through a 5-mm port opposite the Hasson cannula, directed out through the Hasson, and the Hasson cannula removed. The pneumoperitoneum evacuates and the tip of the grasper is seen coming out through the skin. The rolled mesh is placed into the grasper and the mesh pulled into the abdominal cavity (Fig. 33.10). The balloon-tipped Hasson cannula is easily replaced and pneumoperitoneum reestablished. Two laparoscopic graspers are then used to unfurl the mesh by placing them in the middle of the mesh and pushing in opposite directions. Turning the angled telescope over to look down onto the mesh is very helpful at this point.

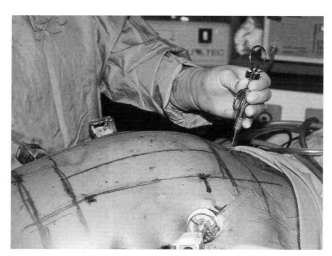

FIGURE 33.6. Size of mesh required.

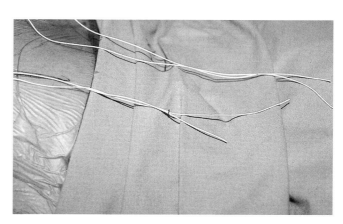

FIGURE 33.8. Clip suture pair.

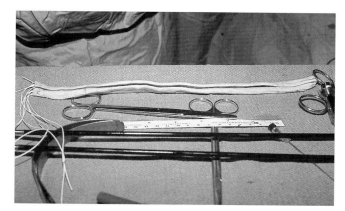

FIGURE 33.9. Dual-Mesh Plus rolled.

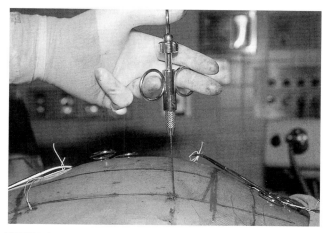

FIGURE 33.11. Sutures brought out through entire thickness of abdominal wall.

The No. 11 scalpel blade is then used to make a small puncture at each of the "Xs" marked on the skin. A hemostat is used to spread the fat down to the level of the fascia, so that the knots of the suture will tie down onto the fascia. The suture passer is inserted through these punctures and each suture brought out through the entire thickness of the abdominal wall (Fig. 33.11). Each skin puncture has a pair of sutures coming through it, but each suture passes through a separate fascial puncture such that there is a 1-cm fascial bridge between each suture of a pair. Each suture is tied down with the knots in the subcutaneous layer. Thus, a large piece of mesh is anchored to the *entire* thickness of the abdominal wall behind the hernia defect (Fig. 33.12).

The spiral-tacking device is then used to affix the mesh 360 degrees to the peritoneal surface. This prevents internal hernia formation between the mesh and the peritoneum. It is important to stretch the mesh as tightly as possible, so that when the pneumoperitoneum is evacuated there is a good tension-free repair (Fig. 33.13). Skin punctures are then made at 5- to 7-cm intervals (or more frequent in large defects) and the suture passer used to place additional U-stitches at these points. The sutures are the key to the

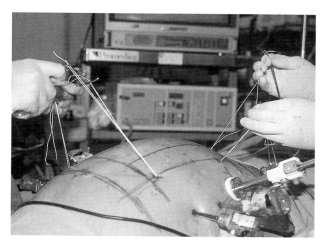

FIGURE 33.12. Mesh anchored with initial stay sutures

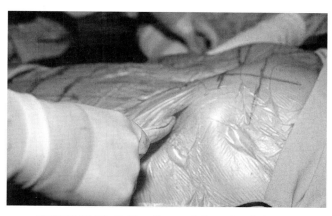

FIGURE 33.10. Pulling the mesh into the abdomen.

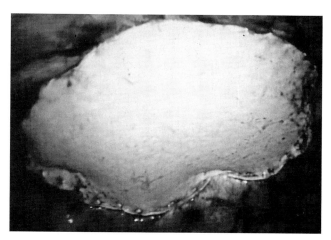

FIGURE 33.13. Tacking mesh in between stay sutures.

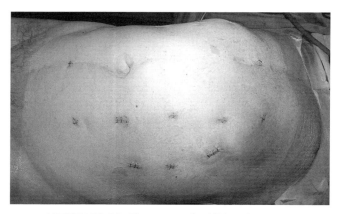

FIGURE 33.14. Placement of additional sutures.

strength of the repair, not the tacks (Fig. 33.14). No drains are placed.

POSTOPERATIVE CARE

The surgeon should be prepared for much more pain in the ventral/incisional hernia patient compared to the laparoscopic cholecystectomy patient. Narcotic analgesia is usually required due to all of the peritoneal tacking and U-stitches. The pain decreases rapidly; however, an oral pain medication is usually used after the first day. We place a compression bandage and abdominal binder over large defects or defects with a lot of stretched soft tissue. With time, redundant skin and fat will contract, and concomitant or subsequent excision is rarely needed. Most patients will limit their activities for 2 weeks due to discomfort, etc. We give them no limitations postoperatively with regard to physical activity.

The surgeon must prepare each patient for the possibility of seroma formation. Not everyone will have a clinically apparent seroma, but when they occur it causes patient concern that the hernia has recurred. Large seromas should be aspirated to put the patient at ease. When performed using sterile technique, infection of the mesh is not a concern. In addition, we take a laparoscopic picture of the hernia defect and then another picture once the mesh is in place. This will help the patient understand what a seroma is and how it will be handled.

DISCUSSION

The author is involved in a multicenter study of laparoscopic ventral/incisional hernia repair that reported preliminary results in 1998 (11). There were 144 patients, and all

TABLE 33.1. RESULTS

	Average	Range
Hernia size	100.1 cm^2	1–480 cm^2
Mesh size	287 cm^2	24–924 cm^2
Operative time	97 min	11–270 min

types of ventral hernias were repaired (92 being incisional) using the technique described above. The mean defect size was 98 cm^2, with a mean operating time of 2 hours and a mean length of stay (including Canadian sites) of 2.3 days. The recurrence rate was 4%, and two patches were removed due to infection. In total, 200 patients have been enrolled in this study and the 5-year data will soon be available.

There have been three studies (2,5,7) that compared laparoscopic repair of ventral/incisional hernias to open repair. While the open approach was usually not a Rives–Stoppa approach, the hernias were similar in size in both groups, with the laparoscopic group having more failed prior open repairs. Complications, hospitalizations, costs, and recurrences were all lower in the laparoscopic groups.

Voeller et al. recently presented 407 laparoscopic ventral/incisional hernia repairs at the October 1999 American College of Surgeons Meeting (12). The patients were large, with a mean body mass index of 32 kg^2, and 90% had previous abdominal surgery, with 136 of the hernias being recurrent. The average hernia size was 100 cm^2 (Table 33.1). Length of stay was short, with few serious complications and no mortality (Table 33.2). The mean follow-up has been approximately 2 years, with a range of up to 5 years. There were six bowel injuries and four mesh infections (Table 33.3). The 14 recurrences (3.4%) compares favorably to the 10% to 36% described in the literature for open ventral/incisional hernia repair (Table 33.4). The majority of recurrences were from mesh removal due to infection.

The laparoscopic technique described above has been used to repair lumbar hernias as well as parastomal hernias as described via an incision by Sugarbaker (10). The high coronary artery bypass graft ("CABG") epigastric hernia and the low juxtapubic bone hernia can present many chal-

TABLE 33.2. POSTOPERATIVE RESULTS

Length of Stay		
Average	1.8 d	
Range	0–17 d	
Complications		53 (13%)
Mortality		0
Follow-up		
Average	23 mo	
Range	1–60 mo	

TABLE 33.3. COMPLICATIONS

	No.	Percent
Prolonged ileus	9	2.21
Seroma (>6 wk)	8	1.97
Suture pain (>8 wk)	8	1.97
Intestinal injury	6	1.47
Trocar cellulitis	5	1.23
Mesh infection	4	0.98
Hematoma/bleeding	3	0.75
Urinary retention	3	0.75
Fever of unknown origin	3	0.74
Respiratory distress	2	0.49
Intraabdominal abscess	1	0.25
Trocar site hernia	1	0.25

lenging aspects laparoscopically. The mesh in the low hernia must be sutured to Cooper's ligament, and in the high epigastric hernia sutured to any available tissues around the sternum and ribs.

The author has laparoscopically reoperated upon several patients who have had a prior laparoscopic ventral/incisional hernia repair and found any adhesions to be filmy and readily taken down when PTFE mesh, especially the dual-sided mesh from W. L. Gore, is used. There is a "pseudoperitoneum" covering the mesh, and if one dissects between this and the mesh the adhesions are quickly lysed much more readily than the dense adhesions seen with polypropylene mesh. Thus, laparoscopic repair of ventral/incisional hernias now appears to be a very safe technique that can give a very low recurrence rate. It is absolutely essential that suture fixation of the prosthesis be a part of the procedure to continue to yield low recurrence rates. A long-term follow-up will certainly be necessary to further evaluate the procedure.

TABLE 33.4. RECURRENCES

14 Patients with recurrences—3.4%
    4 infected meshes removed
    1 unsuspected bowel injury—reoperated
    6 not enough sutures used
    1 MVA with mesh disruption
6 recurrences in nonmidline hernias

MVA, motor vehicle accident.

REFERENCES

1. Hesselink VJ, Luijendijk RW, de Wilt JHW, et al. An evaluation of risk factors in incisional hernia recurrence. *Surg Gynecol Obstet* 1993;176:228–234.
2. Holzman MD, Purut CM, Reintgen K, et al. Laparoscopic ventral and incisional hernioplasty. *Surg Endosc* 1997;11:32–35.
3. Klinge U, Muller M, Brucker C, et al. Application of three-dimensional stereography to assess abdominal wall mobility. *Hernia* 1998;2:11–14.
4. Park A, Birch DW, Lovrics P. Laparoscopic and open incisional hernia repair: a comparison study. *Surgery* 1998;124:816–822.
5. Ramshaw BJ, Schwab J, Mason EM, et al. Comparison of laparoscopic and open ventral herniorrhaphy. Abstract presented at: Southeastern Surgical Congress, February 1999, Orlando, FL.
6. Rives J, Pire JC, Flament JB, et al. Traitement des eventration. *Encycl Med Chir* 1977;4.0.07,40165.
7. Rives J, Pire JC, Flament JB, et al. Treatment of large eventrations. New therapeutic indications apropos of 322 cases. *Chirurgie* 1985;111:215–225.
8. Sampsel J. Delayed and recurring infection in postoperative abdominal wounds. *Am J Surg* 1976;132:316–319.
9. Stoppa RE. The treatment of complicated groin and incisional hernias. *World J Surg* 1989;13:545–554.
10. Sugarbaker PH. Peritoneal approach to prosthetic mesh repair of paraostomy hernias. *Ann Surg* 1985;201:344–346.
11. Toy FK, Bailey RW, Carey S, et al. Multicenter prospective study of laparoscopic ventral hernioplasty: preliminary results. *Surg Endosc* 1998;12:955–959.
12. Voeller G, Park A, Heniford T, et al. Laparoscopic repair of ventral and incisional hernias. Paper presented at: American College of Surgeons, October 1999, San Francisco, CA.
13. Wantz GE. Incisional hernioplasty with Mersilene. *Surg Gynecol Obstet* 1991;172:129–137.

EDITOR'S COMMENT

Dr. Voeller has done an excellent job of bringing us up-to-date on the currently evolving techniques for repair of ventral/incisional hernias laparoscopically. There is increasing interest among laparoscopic surgeons about the use of laparoscopy for repair of incisional hernias as it becomes obvious that the results using most of the conventional techniques are grossly overestimated. In other words, the recurrence rates are much higher than most surgeons dream exist in their own practices. In the end, it may be that a laparoscopic ventral herniorrhaphy will be the big winner, despite what one would have thought several years ago when it appeared that laparoscopic inguinal herniorrhaphy was going to become such an important player.

The biggest drawback to laparoscopic ventral herniorrhaphy is the placement of a prosthesis in the peritoneal cavity in contact with intraabdominal viscera. Although techniques have been described to try to cover the prosthesis with peritoneum, they are very cumbersome and usually compromise the ability to obtain a wide overlap of the defect. For the most part, they are not practical. To my knowledge, there has never been a report of fistula formation or erosion into intraabdominal viscera associated with the placement of an expanded polytetrafluoroethylene prosthesis (ePTFE) in the peritoneal cavity. If it proves to be true that ePTFE can be placed in the abdomen without fear of the complications associated with polypropylene, I believe that the incidence of laparoscopic ventral herniorrhaphy will increase dramatically. The only thing holding it back then will be expense, which is especially significant because of larger sheets required for ventral hernia repair.

R.J.F., Jr.

34

VISCERAL INJURY ASSOCIATED WITH PNEUMOPERITONEUM IN THE REPAIR OF ABDOMINAL WALL HERNIAS

JOSEPH F. AMARAL

The creation of a pneumoperitoneum carries a finite risk of visceral injury. Although a pneumoperitoneum is created most commonly for the performance of transabdominal laparoscopic surgery, it may also be used in the management of massive ventral hernias in which the right of abdominal domain has been lost. Visceral injury, in its broadest sense, during pneumoperitoneum is divisible into injuries of blood vessels, gastrointestinal organs, and the genitourinary system. Although these catastrophic injuries are rare, they represent a major cause of mortality from laparoscopic procedures, a major reason for conversion to open procedures, and a significant source of the morbidity associated with any laparoscopic procedure.

Despite the rapid evolution and adoption of laparoscopic surgery in the past decade by general surgeons, most case reports and large series reporting these injuries are derived from older gynecologic literature. Although one may argue that newer instrumentation and knowledge should reduce the risk of these complications, reports from the general surgical literature suggest this not to be the case. In fact, these injures often occur with greater frequency. In part, this relates to the well-defined learning curve associated with the adoption of laparoscopic surgery. Additional factors include a lack of understanding of the mechanisms involved in creating these injuries and a lack of appreciation for the proximity of important visceral structures to the anterior abdominal wall.

The following discussion will draw heavily upon the gynecologic literature since, to date, it provides the most comprehensive area of study of these injuries. It will be assumed that findings in the gynecologic literature are transferable to general surgery because gynecologic and hernia repair are both pelvic procedures. Reference will be made to the general surgical literature in general and laparo-

scopic hernia repair in particular when possible. An attempt will be made not only to define the injuries and their incidence, but more importantly to provide methods to prevent their occurrence.

MAJOR VASCULAR INJURY DURING THE INITIATION OF LAPAROSCOPY

Major vascular injury during the initiation of pneumoperitoneum is a well-recognized and extremely feared complication of laparoscopic procedures, not only because of its dramatic nature, but more importantly because of the significant mortality associated with it. Vascular injury is a major cause of death from laparoscopy, second only to anesthesia, with a reported mortality rate of 15% (41).

Major retroperitoneal vascular injury can occur when the Veress needle is inserted prior to insufflation, when a trocar is inserted prior to insufflation, or when a trocar is inserted after insufflation (29,30,35,39,41,46,49,50,56,72). The reason for these injuries is the close proximity of the anterior abdominal wall to the retroperitoneal vascular structures. In thin patients, this distance can be as little as 2 cm (31). The distal aorta and right common iliac artery are particularly prone to injury. This is not surprising, given the fact that the takeoff of the right common iliac artery lies directly below the umbilicus (Table 34.1).

Major vascular injuries may be recognized either by direct visualization of free blood in the abdominal cavity or, more commonly, by a retroperitoneal hematoma. Since these injuries most often occur with a Veress needle, the hole is not large and the only visual indication of injury may be a hematoma. The view on initiation of laparoscopy may be reduced or poor because the red pigment in blood absorbs light. This can be used as a clue to an occult injury. Other factors that may indicate injury are hypotension and a rise in end tidal CO_2 from embolization of carbon dioxide gas.

J. F. Amaral: Department of Surgery, Brown University School of Medicine; Rhode Island Hospital, Providence, Rhode Island.

TABLE 34.1. FACTORS RESPONSIBLE FOR LARGE VESSEL INJURY

Inexperienced or unskilled surgeon
Failure to sharpen the trocar
Failure to place the patient in Trendelenburg position
Failure to elevate or stabilize the abdominal wall
Perpendicular insertion of the needle or trocar
Lateral deviation of the needle or trocar
Inadequate pneumoperitoneum
Forceful thrust
Failure to note anatomic landmarks

The first report to bring to light the complication of major vascular injury during laparoscopy was by Levinson in 1974 (31). The first significant review of the problem was by McDonald et al. in 1978 (35). In that report, two cases of major retroperitoneal vascular injury occurring with a Touhey needle in a series of 400 laparoscopies (0.5% incidence) were noted. An earlier survey of the American Association of Gynecologic Laparoscopists cited an incidence of hemorrhage following diagnostic laparoscopy requiring conversion to laparotomy of 4.1% and following tubal sterilization of 1.8%, but did not specify the site or cause of bleeding (50). Thus, the report by McDonald et al. in 1978 is the first to call attention to this significant and potentially catastrophic complication (35).

A German series of gynecologic laparoscopy gave a detailed analysis of information with respect to major vascular injury, noting a 0.07% incidence (56). A large survey of nearly 37,000 gynecologic laparoscopies in the United States revealed a 0.26% incidence of major vascular injury (46), and similar incidences among gynecologic laparoscopies for major vascular injury were noted in a large study from Canada (72). Based on information gathered in the Canadian survey, 39.8% of vascular and intestinal injuries were caused by the Veress needle, 37.9% by insertion of the primary trocar, and 22% by the secondary trocar (72). A large series from France involving 100,000 laparoscopies detected major vascular injury by Veress needle in 0.03% and by trocar in 0.01%, for a total incidence of 0.04% (39). The finding that the Veress needle is the cause of more vascular accidents is confirmed in other studies (2).

The most recent series to report on these injuries also comes from France (7). In this retrospective review of 29,966 gynecologic patients, 0.02% sustained a major vascular injury (7). Importantly, these investigators noted the experience of the surgeons was an important factor in the overall complication rate in this group of patients, but not in the incidence of major vascular injury (7).

The introduction of laparoscopic cholecystectomy in 1989 to the United States marked the beginning of widespread use of laparoscopy in general surgery. In subsequent years, there have been numerous reports in the literature regarding results and complications of laparoscopic procedures, many of which note major vascular injury. The incidence of major vascular injury following laparoscopic cholecystectomy is reported to vary between 0.03% and 0.3% (6,12,29,64).

Only three cases of major vascular injury were identified in a review of 54 reports on laparoscopic hernia in the English literature (51,58,71). In total, there were 10,837 patients who were operated on, for an incidence of 0.03% of major vascular injury during laparoscopic transabdominal hernia repair. It is important to note that the true incidence of visceral and vascular injury is unknown and probably higher than the literature suggests because most injuries are not reported in the literature. Others may be inadvertently omitted from retrospective data collections. Furthermore, reported series usually come from surgeons with greater experience, whose technical complications may be less. Finally, the exact reason of the injury may be erroneously attributed to the wrong etiology. For example, until the landmark paper by Levy et al. (32) in 1985, most intestinal injuries during laparoscopy that actually were the result of needles and trocars were incorrectly attributed to electrosurgery.

MINOR VASCULAR INJURIES

Minor vascular injuries are so named because they are injuries to vessels of lesser importance than the aorta, inferior vena cava, and iliac vessels. It is not because these injuries are minor in nature. Indeed, these minor vascular injuries are often the reason for reoperation, conversion, and transfusion. Although injuries of mesenteric and omental vessels are reported following laparoscopic hernia repair, by far the most common minor vascular injury is to the inferior epigastric vessels. Injury to these vessels is reported to occur in up to 2.5% of laparoscopic hernia repairs (53). There were 76 cases of minor vascular injuries involving principally the epigastric vessels identified in a review of 54 reports on laparoscopic hernia in the English literature. In total, there were 10,837 patients who were operated on for an incidence of 0.7% of minor vascular injury during laparoscopic transabdominal hernia repair.

In part, an injury to the inferior epigastric artery and/or vein during laparoscopic hernia repair or gynecologic procedures relates to the anatomy of these vessels. In the upper abdominal wall, there is usually a plexus of arteries rather than a single large vessel that is present in the lower abdominal wall. As a result, this injury is much more common in lower abdominal procedures than in those of the upper abdomen. It is important to remember that the inferior epigastric vessels lie at the lateral-most portion of the rectus sheath. Thus, even if a secondary cannula is placed lateral to the sheath, it can still injure the vessel as it enters the abdomen if the cannula is placed obliquely toward the midline (Table 34.2).

TABLE 34.2. SAFE PLACEMENT OF LATERAL TROCARS

Avoid abdominal wall vessels by transillumination
Use the smallest diameter cannula possible
Make incision larger than trocar to avoid excessive force
Do not angle trocar towards the midline
Observe penetration of abdominal wall through laparoscope

Injuries to the inferior epigastric vessels during laparoscopic hernia repair are also related to the type of trocar used. Cutting trocars with sharp blades are more likely to injure the vessels than smooth, conical-tip trocars that tend to push the vessels away without injury (66). Furthermore, partial lacerations of the inferior epigastric artery or vein are unlikely to stop on their own. This occurs because the entire vessel cannot go into spasm if it is tethered at some point.

Finally, injuries of the epigastric vessels can be related to carelessness during the operative procedure. These injuries invariably occur during placement of secondary cannulas, which should be placed under direct vision and with prior transillumination of the abdominal wall. Although injury of the epigastric vessels is still possible if these measures are taken, the incidence should be dramatically reduced.

It is important to inspect all cannula sites at the end of the procedure after the cannulas have been removed since there may be no appreciable bleeding during the procedure from these sites despite injury to the epigastric vessels. This occurs from the tamponade effect provided by the cannula when in place.

Epigastric vascular injuries can be treated with placement of a Foley catheter in the cannula site, the balloon inflated intraabdominally and pulled up against the abdominal wall. Alternatively, the bleeding can be dealt with by cut-down over the area to identify and ligate the vessels, or by blind suture ligation of the bleeding site. The latter is often most successful when horizontal mattress sutures are placed full thickness through the anterior abdominal wall above and below the cannula site. Either the Foley catheter or the sutures can be removed the next day.

BOWEL INJURY

Bowel injury is the third leading cause of death from a laparoscopic procedure following major vascular injury and anesthesia (41). Unlike major vascular injury, where the risk and presentation are immediate, many bowel injuries go unrecognized at the time of the procedure. Consequently, patients present postoperatively, often after discharge, with peritonitis. This delay makes it a significant cause of morbidity and mortality as well as a major reason for medicolegal action in the United States following laparoscopic procedures in general (63).

A German series of gynecologic laparoscopy (56) gave a detailed analysis of information with respect to intestinal injury, noting a 0.05% incidence, and a large survey of nearly 37,000 gynecologic laparoscopies in the United States revealed a 0.16% incidence of bowel injury (46). In Canada, a 0.18% incidence among gynecologic laparoscopies was noted for bowel injury (72). Based on information gathered in this survey, 39.8% of vascular and intestinal injuries were caused by the Veress needle, 37.9% by insertion of the primary trocar, and 22% by the secondary trocar (72). A large series from France involving 100,000 laparoscopies detected bowel injury by Veress needle in 0.01% and by trocar in 0.03%, for a total incidence of 0.04% (39).

The most recent series to report on these injuries also comes from France (8). In this retrospective review of 29,966 gynecologic patients, 0.16% sustained an intestinal injury (8). Overall, one third (32.1%) of the bowel injuries detected during this review occurred during the initiation phase of laparoscopy (7). Furthermore, 33% occurred during the insertion of a pneumoperitoneum needle, 50% during placement of the umbilical trocar, and 17% during placement of a secondary trocar (7). The remaining two thirds of gastrointestinal injuries resulted during dissection, electrocoagulation, or grasping.

Importantly, these investigators noted the experience of the surgeons was an important factor in the overall complication rate and in the incidence of intestinal injury (8). This is consistent with the work of Phillips, in which complications decreased with experience, notably after performance of 250 diagnostic and 500 operative procedures (48).

The incidence of intestinal injury following laparoscopic cholecystectomy is reported to vary between 0.05% and 0.3% (12,29,64). Five cases of intestinal perforation due to a pneumoperitoneum needle or cannula were identified in a review of 54 reports on laparoscopic hernia in the English literature. In total, there were 10,837 patients who were operated on, for an incidence of 0.05%. One case involved the colon (30), three the small bowel (17,44), and one the stomach (14). There was no mortality from these injuries.

Postoperative Bowel Obstruction

A remarkable complication of laparoscopic hernia repair is the development of a postoperative bowel obstruction and cannula site hernia. Most large, multiinstitutional series note this complication (17,18,51,54). There are at least 14 case reports in the world literature to date documenting 17 cases of postoperative small-bowel obstruction following laparoscopic hernia (3,11,15,16,24,25,36,43,47,57,62,65, 67,68,70,71). Eight of these cases occurred at the peritoneal site of hernia repair and nine at a lateral cannula site. The former cases do not appear related to the pneumoperitoneum since reports exist of similar complications following totally extraperitoneal repair in which a peritoneal rent

TABLE 34.3. MEASURES TO PREVENT POSTOPERATIVE RICHTER'S HERNIA

Do not remove cannulas with their valves open
Use the smallest diameter cannula possible
Visualize removal of the cannula
Close the fascia at all cannula sites
Shake the abdominal wall after the cannulas are removed
Close the peritoneum tightly or not at all

occurred (34). However, the latter cases appear related to the pneumoperitoneum. An outward pressure is produced as cannulas are removed, which fosters entrapment of the small bowel at a cannula site to produce a Richter's type hernia. This is even more likely if the flapper valve is held open during cannula removal. In this situation, suction is created between the lower atmospheric pressure and the higher intraabdominal pressure, which causes the bowel to be sucked up into the wound. Furthermore, trocar-site hernias are reported to occur in 0.77% to 3% of all types of laparoscopic procedures (1,20).

Measures can be taken to minimize this complication. The two most important measures noted in Table 34.3 are not removing cannulas with their valves open and closing the fascia at all cannula sites. Numerous devices have been manufactured to aid surgeons in this closure. To date, there is no convincing evidence in the literature to support or refute the benefit of these devices. Although careful adherence to both of these measures should limit this complication, reports exist documenting a high incidence of trocar site hernias despite primary fascial closure of port sites of 10 mm or greater (1).

BLADDER INJURY

Bladder injury is a rare but reported injury during the initiation of the pneumoperitoneum. In a survey of 407 obstetrician–gynecologists in Canada, accounting for 136,997 laparoscopies, there were eight bladder injuries (73). Four occurred with the pneumoperitoneum needle, two with the primary trocar, and two with the secondary trocar. Although there are at least nine reports of bladder injury during laparoscopic herniorrhaphy in the literature, these seem to all have resulted from dissection or electrocoagulation and not during the initiation of laparoscopy (27,28,30,33,51,54,58,69,71). Nonetheless, this remains a potential complication of the procedure.

In general, puncture of the bladder results when a midline, suprapubic trocar is placed in a patient with an overdistended bladder. Previous pelvic surgery places the patient at further risk (21). A small, 3-mm or 5-mm puncture in the dome of the bladder should resolve spontaneously with indwelling bladder catheter for 7 to 10 days (21). Large or irregular defects will require a two-layer suture closure with absorbable sutures either through an open or laparoscopic approach (52). A bladder catheter should be left in place for 4 to 10 days, depending on the location and size of the puncture or tear.

The diagnosis of injury to the bladder is often made by distention of the urinary drainage bag during the procedure (60). Alternatively, instillation of indigo carmine into the bladder may aid in identifying an injury. The major step in preventing this complication is ensuring adequate drainage of the bladder prior to the procedure. Although it is commonplace for patients to void immediately prior to the procedure, it is safer to drain the bladder with a catheter after the induction of anesthesia. This ensures that dystonic bladders will be completely emptied. Furthermore, it allows for easy recognition of the complication when it occurs if the catheter is left in place for the duration of the operative procedure.

PREVENTION OF MAJOR VISCERAL AND VASCULAR INJURIES DURING INITIATION OF PNEUMOPERITONEUM

There are three basic techniques used to create the pneumoperitoneum: blind Veress needle insertion followed by blind trocar insertion, blind direct trocar insertion without Veress needle or pneumoperitoneum, and open visualized trocar insertion without pneumoperitoneum. Blind situations are classified as closed laparoscopy, whereas visualized placement is generally referred to as open laparoscopy. In addition, there are many other techniques that will not be commented on, because limited numbers of surgeons use them (38,59).

Each of these techniques has proponents to recommend its use. Nonetheless, major vascular and visceral injuries have been reported with all of these techniques (4,5,19,23,37,42,45). This includes the open technique, which should theoretically carry the least risk. Indeed, proponents of the open technique often cite a lack of major vascular injuries with this technique reported in the literature. However, a recent report notes two cases of aortic injury using the open laparoscopy (22). In this regard, it is important to note that the injuries result from a faulty cannula and not from the cannula itself. Nonetheless, injuries can and do occur. Measures must be taken to prevent or minimize this risk.

Veress Needle Technique

Veress needle insertion and insufflation followed by blind trocar insertion is the most widely used technique by gynecologists and general surgeons. For example, the 1982 American Association of Gynecologic Laparoscopists survey noted that 96% of gynecologists surveyed used the Veress needle technique, whereas only 4% used the open technique (49).

The Veress needle consists of a blunt-tipped, spring-loaded inner stylet and a sharp outer needle. The stylet retracts during passage of the needle through the abdominal layers to allow penetration. Once the peritoneum is entered, the lack of tissue resistance allows the blunt stylet to protrude. This theoretically should prevent perforation of intraabdominal structures. However, it is important to note that the stylet does not lock once it protrudes. Therefore, it can penetrate an intraabdominal structure because the stylet will again retract on contact with an intraabdominal structure. Important procedural steps during insertion of the Veress needle are the Trendelenburg position, elevation of the abdominal wall, and direction of the needle at 45 degrees to the spine and aimed toward the pelvis in the midline (Table 34.4).

The needle is aspirated for blood, bowel contents, or urine once it is thought to be in the abdominal cavity. That is, aspiration is used to determine if there is an injury to a vessel or hollow viscus. Next, a saline drop is placed on the end of the needle. This should easily enter the abdominal cavity because the intraabdominal pressure is less than atmospheric when the abdominal wall is elevated. In addition, the forces of gravity should direct the fluid to enter the free peritoneal space. Finally, the needle is attached to an insufflator that measures the pressure at the tip. The pressure will be low (less than 5 mm Hg) if it is appropriately placed. Insufflation to 12 to 15 mm Hg with carbon dioxide gas follows. Once this pressure is achieved, a 10-mm trocar with or without a safety shield (discussed later) is placed blindly into the abdomen. It must be emphasized that a full pneumoperitoneum should be established prior to insertion of the blind umbilical trocar. Once again, care must be taken to ensure that the trocar is inserted in the midline and at 45 degrees to the spine, aimed toward the pelvis.

Proponents of this technique state that the pressure of a pneumoperitoneum by Veress needle will reduce the likelihood that there will be injury to underlying organs by creating a space between the organs and the abdominal wall

(8,49). Interestingly, one third to one half of major intraabdominal vascular and intestinal injuries occur from the Veress needle itself (49). In addition, the presence of the pneumoperitoneum does not prevent major vascular or intestinal injury (73). For example, Sigman et al. (61) reported a 0.1% incidence of major vascular injuries and a 0.3% incidence of bowel injuries in a series of 781 laparoscopies. In part, this occurs because the distended abdomen is difficult to grasp and elevate. Furthermore, the pressure of the pneumoperitoneum is not sufficient to resist the forces applied by the surgeon to insert the trocar. As a result, the pneumoperitoneum does not prevent contact of the abdominal viscera and vessels with the anterior abdominal wall. For this reason, Reich (55) and others have advocated inflation of the abdominal cavity to a pressure of 25 to 30 mm Hg prior to insertion of the umbilical trocar. This transient increase in intraabdominal pressure is well tolerated if brief. Once the cannula is in place, the pressure is restored to the usual 12 to 15 mm Hg.

Direct Trocar Insertion without Pneumoperitoneum

The rationale for the direct insertion of a cannula without pneumoperitoneum is based on the difficulty in grasping and elevating an abdomen that is distended by gas. In addition, many of the complications noted with laparoscopy, such as subcutaneous emphysema, were directly related to the Veress needle (13). Furthermore, the pressure required to insert a trocar even in the presence of a pneumoperitoneum brings the abdominal wall in contact with the viscera if the abdominal wall is not held and elevated (9). Copeland and colleagues (9) stressed key points for safe direct trocar insertion, including adequate abdominal wall relaxation, a sharp trocar, and an adequate skin incision (Table 34.5).

An important concept in the application of the direct insertion techniques is the use of a safety shield trocar (26). The disposable safety shield trocar has the sharp tip of the trocar shielded by a plastic sheath. This spring-loaded plastic sheath retracts into the cannula when it meets tissue

TABLE 34.4. SAFE NEEDLE AND CANNULA INSERTION WITH PNEUMOPERITONEUM

Place patient in Trendelenburg position
Elevate the abdominal wall
Insert needle and cannula at 45 degrees to the spine and toward the pelvis
Stay in the midline during insertion
Aspirate needle, looking for blood, urine, or intestinal contents
Perform the saline drop test
Ensure intraabdominal pressure is low when connected to insufflator
Place cannula only after an intraabdominal pressure of 15 to 30 mm Hg is reached
Visually inspect abdomen for injury

TABLE 34.5. SAFE DIRECT CANNULA INSERTION WITHOUT PNEUMOPERITONEUM

Avoid in patients with previous surgery
Do not use on a thin patient
Make an adequate-sized incision
Be sure the patient is relaxed
Elevate the abdominal wall with the left hand midway between the umbilicus and pubis
Use a sharp trocar
Use constant pressure

resistance on insertion, thus exposing the sharp tip. Once the tip enters the peritoneal cavity, the shield automatically protrudes and locks. This is an important theoretic advantage over the Veress needle, in which the stylet does not lock.

Theoretically, the disposable safety shield trocar should minimize injury because of the locking mechanism. Furthermore, because it is disposable, the trocar is always sharp and not dull, as is the case with reusable trocars, which on average are sharpened once in 16 uses (10). To date, there is no experimental or randomized study that proves the safety of the safety shield. In the only comparison study, Nezhat et al. (40) failed to show statistical significance between the two types of trocars. As a result of the lack of evidence in favor of these trocars, the U.S. Food and Drug Administration has prohibited the use of the term "safety shield" by device manufactures because there is no evidence in the literature to support the alleged safety of these devices.

Open Laparoscopy

The concept in the open technique is to create a tiny incision or minilaparotomy of approximately 10 to 15 mm, directly incise the layers of the abdominal wall, directly cut the peritoneum, and enter the abdomen (Table 34.6). Since gas can escape around the incision, an olive tip is placed over the end of the trocar to occlude the incision and sutures that are placed on the abdominal fascia and attached to the cannula. Proposed advantages for the open technique are avoidance of blind puncture with a needle and subsequent trocar, certainty of establishing a pneumoperitoneum, and correct anatomic repair of the abdominal wall incision. In general, widespread use of this technique has been limited to patients with previous lower abdominal surgery, pregnant patients, children, and very thin patients where little space exists between the abdominal wall and the spine. Reasons for limiting the use of the open technique include greater time needed to perform, difficulty with the technique, obesity, difficulty maintaining the pneumoperitoneum, and definite incidence of major intraabdominal injury.

TABLE 34.6. SAFE OPEN LAPAROSCOPY

Make a small incision in the umbilicus (12 to 15 mm)
Grasp the fascia with Kocher clamps
Divide fascia longitudinally in the midline
Identify and grasp peritoneum
Divide peritoneum sharply
Ensure there is an intraabdominal space
Insert cannula
Visually inspect abdomen with scope prior to insufflation

CONCLUSION

Laparoscopic procedures of any type, including laparoscopic transabdominal preperitoneal hernia repairs, carry with them a small but definite risk of visceral and vascular injury. The incidence of these dramatic and often life-threatening complications can be minimized by attention to meticulous surgical technique. However, they cannot be eliminated, given the limits of current instrumentation and techniques. Finally, open laparoscopy has the best support in the literature for safety and should be strongly considered in the future as the standard means for establishment of the pneumoperitoneum.

REFERENCES

1. Azurin DJ, Go LS, Arryo LR, et al. Trocar site herniation following laparoscopic cholecystectomy and the significance of incidental preexisting umbilical hernia. *Am Surg* 1995;5:419–421.
2. Baadsgaard SE, Bille S, Egeblad K. Major vascular injury during gynecologic laparoscopy. *Acta Obstet Gynecol Scand* 1989;68:283–285.
3. Bendsen AK, Bauer T, Johansen TP. Richter hernia in trocar site after laparoscopic herniotomy. *Ugeskr Laeger* 1995;157:6438–6439.
4. Borgatta L, Gruss L, Barad D, et al. Direct trocar insertion versus Veress needle use for laparoscopic sterilization. *J Reprod Med* 1990;35:891–894.
5. Byron J, Markenson G. A randomized comparison of Veress needle and direct trocar insertion for laparoscopy. *Surg Gynecol Obstet* 1993;177:259–262.
6. Campault G, Cazacu F. Les accidents des trocarts: etude multicentrique de 65,000 interventions par laparoscopie. In: *96me Congres de l'Association Francaise de Chirurgie*, 1994;6–82.
7. Chapron C, Pierre F, Harchaoui Y, et al. Gastrointestinal injuries during gynaecological laparoscopy. *Hum Reprod* 1999;14:333–337.
8. Chapron C, Querleu D, Bruhat MA, et al. Surgical complications of diagnostic and operative gynaecological laparoscopy: a series of 29,966 cases. *Hum Reprod* 1998;13:867–872.
9. Copeland C, Wing R, Hulka JF. Direct trocar insertion at laparoscopy: an evaluation. *Obstet Gynecol* 1983;62:655–659.
10. Corson SL, Batzer FR, Gocial B, et al. Measurement of the force necessary for laparoscopic trocar entry. *J Reprod Med* 1989;34:282–284.
11. Cueto J, Vazquez JA, Solis MA, et al. Bowel obstruction in the postoperative period of laparoscopic inguinal hernia repair (TAPP): review of the literature. *J Soc Laparoendosc Surg* 1998;2:277–280.
12. Deziel D, Millikan KW, Economou SG, et al. Complications of laparoscopic cholecystectomy: a national survey of 4,292 hospitals and an analysis of 77,604 cases. *Am J Surg* 1993;165:9–14.
13. Dingfelder J. Direct laparoscope trocar insertion without prior pneumoperitoneum. *J Reprod Med* 1978;21:45–47.
14. Dirksen CD, Beets GL, Go P, et al. Bassini repair compared with laparoscopic repair for primary inguinal hernia: a randomized controlled trial. *Eur J Surg* 1998;164:439–447.
15. Esteve C, Tolck P. Incarcerated hernia following laparoscopic surgery. A complication to be avoided. Case presentation and literature review [in French]. *Rev Med Suisse Romande* 1997;117:25–28.

16. Evans DS, Ganeh P, Khan IM. Day-case laparoscopic hernia repair. *Br J Surg* 1996;83:1361–1363.
17. Felix EL, Harbertson N, Vartanian S. Laparoscopic hernioplasty: significant complications. *Surg Endosc* 1999;13:328–331.
18. Fitzgibbons RJ Jr, Camps J, Cornet DA, et al. Laparoscopic inguinal herniorrhaphy. Results of a multicenter trial. *Ann Surg* 1995;221:3–13.
19. Fitzgibbons R, Schmid S, Santoscoy R, et al. Open laparoscopy for laparoscopic cholecystectomy. *Surg Laparosc Endosc* 1991;1: 216–222.
20. George JP. Presentation and management of laparoscopic incisional hernias. *J Am Assoc Gynecol Laparosc* 1994;1[Suppl]:S12.
21. Georgy FM, Fetterman HH, Chefetz MD. Complications of laparoscopy: two cases of perforated urinary bladder. *Am J Obstet Gynecol* 1974;120:1121–1124.
22. Hanney RM, Carmalt HL, Merrett N, et al. Vascular injuries during laparoscopy associated with the Hasson technique. *J Am Coll Surg* 1999;188:337–338.
23. Hasson H. Open laparoscopy: a report of 150 cases. *J Reprod Med* 1974;12:234–238.
24. Hendrickse CW, Evans DS. Intestinal obstruction following laparoscopic inguinal hernia repair. *Br J Surg* 1993;80:1432.
25. Huang SM, Wu CW, Lui WY. Intestinal obstruction after laparoscopic herniorrhaphy. *Surg Laparosc Endosc* 1997;7:288–290.
26. Jarrett J. Laparoscopy: direct trocar insertion without pneumoperitoneum. *Obstet Gynecol* 1990;75:725–727.
27. Kald A, Smedh K, Anderberg B. Laparoscopic groin hernia repair: results of 200 consecutive herniorrhaphies. *Br J Surg* 1995;82:618–620.
28. Kiruparan P, Pettit SH. Prospective audit of 200 patients undergoing laparoscopic inguinal hernia repair with follow-up from 1 to 4 years. *J R Coll Surg Edinb* 1998;43:13–16.
29. Larson G, Vitale GC, Casey J, et al. Multipractice analysis of laparoscopic cholecystectomy in 1,983 patients. *Am J Surg* 1992; 163:221–226.
30. Leibel BJ, Schmedt CG, Schwarz J, et al. A single institution's experience with transperitoneal laparoscopic hernia repair. *Am J Surg* 1998;175:446–452.
31. Levinson C. Laparoscopy is easy—except for the complications: a review with suggestions. *J Reprod Med* 1974;5:187–194.
32. Levy BS, Soderstrom RM, Dail DH. Bowel injuries during laparoscopy: gross anatomy and histology. *J Reprod Med* 1985;30: 168–175.
33. Litwin DEM, Pham QN, Oleniuk FH, et al. Laparoscopic groin hernia surgery: the TAPP approach. *Can J Surg* 1997;40: 192–198.
34. Lodha K, Deans A, Bhattacharya P, et al. Obstructing internal hernia complicating totally extraperitoneal inguinal hernia repair. *J Laparoendosc Adv Surg Tech A* 1998;7:167–168.
35. McDonald P, Rich NM, Collins GJ, et al. Vascular trauma secondary to diagnostic and therapeutic procedures: laparoscopy. *Am J Surg* 1978;135:651–655.
36. McDonald D, Chung D. Large bowel obstruction: a postoperative complication after laparoscopic bilateral inguinal hernia repair. *J Laparoendosc Adv Surg Tech A.* 1997;7:187–189.
37. McKernan JB, Champion JK. Access techniques: Veress needle—initial blind trocar insertion versus open laparoscopy with the Hasson trocar. *Endosc Surg Allied Technol.* 1995;3:35–38.
38. Melzer A, Riek S, Roth K, et al. Endoscopically controlled trocar and cannula insertion. *Endos Surg Allied Technol* 1995;3:63–68.
39. Mintz M. Risks and prophylaxis in laparoscopy: a survey of 100,000 cases. *J Reprod Med* 1977;5:269–272.
40. Nezhat F, Silfen SL, Evans D, et al. Comparison of direct insertion of disposable and standard reusable laparoscopic trocars and previous pneumoperitoneum with Veress needle. *Obstet Gynecol* 1991;78:148–150.
41. Nordestgaard AG, Bodily KC, Osborne RW, et al. Major vascular injuries during laparoscopic procedures. *Am J Surg* 1995;169: 543–545.
42. Nuzzo G, Guilliante F, Tebala GD, et al. Routine use of open technique in laparoscopic operations. *J Am Coll Surg* 1997;184: 58–62.
43. Ohta J, Yamuchi Y, Yoshida S, et al. Laparoscopic intervention to relieve small bowel obstruction following laparoscopic herniorrhaphy. *Surg Laparosc Endosc* 1997;7:464–468.
44. Paget GW. Laparoscopic inguinal herniorrhaphy: a personal audit of 222 hernia repairs. *Med J Aust* 1994;161:249–253.
45. Penfield A. How to prevent complications of open laparoscopy. *J Reprod Med* 1985;30:660–663.
46. Peterson HB, Hulka JF, Phillips JM. American Association of Gynecologic Laparoscopists' 1988 membership survey on operative laparoscopy. *J Reprod Med* 1990;35:587–589.
47. Petersen TI, Qvist N, Wara P. Intestinal obstruction—a procedure-related complication of laparoscopic inguinal hernia repair. *Surg Laparosc Endosc* 1995;5:214–216.
48. Phillips JM. Complications in laparoscopy. *Int J Gynaecol Obstet* 1977;15:157–162.
49. Phillips JM, Hulka JF, Peterson HB. American Association of Gynecologic Laparoscopists' 1982 membership survey. *J Reprod Med* 1984;29:592–594.
50. Phillips J, Keith D, Hulka J, et al. Gynecologic laparoscopy in 1975. *J Reprod Med* 1976;3:105–117.
51. Phillips EH, Arregui M, Carroll BJ, et al. Incidence of complications following laparoscopic hernioplasty. *Surg Endosc* 1995;9: 16–21.
52. Poffenberger RJ. Laparoscopic repair of intraperitoneal bladder injury. *Urology* 1996;47:248–249.
53. Quilici PJ, Greanery EM, Quilici J, et al. Transabdominal preperitoneal laparoscopic herniorrhaphy: results of 509 repairs. *Am Surg* 1996;62:849–852.
54. Ramshaw BJ, Tucker JG, Conner T, et al. A comparison of the approaches to laparoscopic herniorrhaphy. *Surg Endosc* 1996;10: 29–32.
55. Reich H. High-pressure trocar insertion technique. *JSLS* 1999;3: 45–48.
56. Riedel HH, Lehmann-Willenbrock E, Conrad P, et al. German pelviscopic statistics for the years 1978–1982. *Endoscopy* 1986; 18:219–222.
57. Rodda DJ, Otto GM, Pese KE. Intestinal obstruction following transabdominal preperitoneal laparoscopic inguinal hernia repair. *Aust N Z J Surg* 1997;67:142–143.
58. Sandbichler P, Draxl H, Gstir H, et al. Laparoscopic repair of recurrent inguinal hernias. *Am J Surg* 1996;171:366–368.
59. Schaller G, Kuenkel M, Manegold BC. The "optical-Veress needle"—initial puncture with a miniopti. *Endosc Surg Allied Technol* 1995;3:55–57.
60. Sia-Kho E, Kelly RE. Urinary drainage by distention: an indication of bladder injury during laparoscopy. *J Clin Anesth* 1992;4:346–347.
61. Sigman H, Fried GM, Garzon J, et al. Risks of blind versus open approach to celiotomy for laparoscopic surgery. *Surg Laparosc Endosc* 1993;3:296–299.
62. Sioris T, Perhoneime V, Schroeder T. Peritoneal herniation and intestinal obstruction: a complication of laparoscopic inguinal herniorrhaphy. *Eur J Surg* 1995;161:533–534.
63. Soderstrom R. Bowel injury litigation after laparoscopy. *J Am Assoc Gynecol Laparosc* 1993;1:74–77.
64. Southern Surgeons Club. A prospective analysis of 1518 laparoscopic cholecystectomies. *N Engl J Med* 1991;324:1073–1078.
65. Spier LN, Lazzaro RS, Procaccino A, et al. Entrapment of small bowel after laparoscopic herniorrhaphy. *Surg Endosc* 1993;7: 535–536.

66. Rioux JE, Yuzpe AA. Gynecologic endoscopic equipment. *Curr Probl Gynecol* 1981;5:13–41.

67. Tews G, Arzt W, Bohaumilitzy T, et al. Significant reduction of operational risk in laparoscopy through the use of a new blunt trocar. *Surg Gynecol Obstet* 1991;173;67–68.

68. Tsang S, Normand R, Karlin R. Small bowel obstruction: a morbid complication after laparoscopic herniorrhaphy. *Am Surg* 1994;60:332–334.

69. Vanclooster P, Meersman A, de Gheldere C. Small bowel obstruction after laparoscopic inguinal hernia repair: a case report. *Acta Chir Belg* 1995;95[Suppl 4]:199–200.

70. Voitk AJ. The learning curve in laparoscopic inguinal hernia repair for the community general surgeon. *Can J Surg* 1998;41:446–450.

71. Wegener ME, Chung D, Crans C, et al. Small bowel obstruction secondary to incarcerated Richter's hernia from laparoscopic hernia repair. *J Laparoendosc Surg* 1993;3:173–176.

72. Wheeler KH. Laparoscopic inguinal herniorrhaphy with mesh: an 18-month experience. *J Laparoendosc Surg* 1993;3:345–350.

73. Yuzpe A. Pneumoperitoneum needle and trocar injuries in laparoscopy: a survey on possible contributing factors and prevention. *J Reprod Med* 1990;35:485–490.

35

INCIDENCE AND MANAGEMENT OF PRIMARY ABDOMINAL WALL HERNIAS: UMBILICAL, EPIGASTRIC, AND SPIGELIAN

DAVID BENNETT

35A

UMBILICAL HERNIA

Umbilical hernias are the most common type of midline fascial defect and may be classified as (a) infantile umbilical hernia, (b) acquired umbilical hernia, (c) paraumbilical hernia (supraumbilical or infraumbilical), or (d) umbilical hernia in adults. Umbilical hernias occur in both children and adults, but the mode of presentation, natural history, and treatment strategy are different in the two groups.

HISTORY

The first references to umbilical hernia were recorded in the *Egyptian Papyrus of Ebers* (circa 1552 B.C.), but the first formal description of umbilical hernias comes from the Hindu physician Charaka in his writings dated A.D. 1 or earlier. The ancient Jews also recognized umbilical hernias and treated them conservatively (19). Celsus, in the first century A.D., treated umbilical hernias with an elastic suture, and Soranus (A.D. 98–117) described a technique of strapping (25).

The first recorded description of umbilical hernia repair comes from Albucasis, Abul Qasim al-Zahrawi, the great Moorish surgeon (A.D. 1013–1106) (1). Antonio Benivieni (1443–1502) probably was the first to treat an incarcerated hernia in a child; he ligated the hernia. Once the mortified flesh fell off, the child "regained perfect health" (7). In 1737, Queen Caroline of England had an incarcerated hernia that eventually was lanced to permit drainage of intestinal matter. She succumbed to her illness, however, because surgical treatment had been delayed for 3 days while she was treated with polypharmacy, enemas, eperients, and bleeding (7), illustrating the need for timely surgical intervention. In his *Anatomy of the Human Body,* published in 1740, William Cheselden describes a patient with an incarcerated hernia in whom he amputated the protruding mass of "mortified bowel and left the end of the sound gut hanging out of the navel to which it afterwards adhered: she recovered and lived many years after, voiding excrement through the intestine at the navel" (7). Credit for the modern surgical treatment of umbilical hernias is given to William J. Mayo (17), who repaired these defects by overlapping fascia downward from above ("vest-over-pants").

EMBRYOLOGY AND ANATOMY OF THE UMBILICUS

Embryologically, the fascial margins of the umbilical defect are formed by the third week of fetal life when the four folds of the somatopleure tend to fold inward. An umbilical cord is produced in the fifth week. By the tenth week of embryonic life, abdominal contents return from their location outside the coelom into the developing abdominal cavity. The vitelline duct and the allantois regress by the fifteenth to sixteenth week. If any of these processes are defective, umbilical malformations occur (6).

D. Bennett: Department of Surgery, Derriford Hospital, Plymouth, United Kingdom.

At birth, the umbilical arteries and the umbilical vein become thrombosed, and the vitelline duct and the allantois have already been obliterated. The umbilical ring then scars and contracts. The obliterated umbilical vein (round ligament) is usually attached to the inferior border of the umbilical ring along with remnants of the urachus and the two obliterated umbilical arteries. The round ligament, by crossing and partially covering the umbilical ring, may protect against herniation. In instances where the ligament divides and inserts in the upper part of the umbilical ring without crossing it, a potential weakness is present. The umbilical Richet's fascia also reinforces the umbilical ring. If Richet's fascia is absent, located outside the limits of the umbilical ring, or only partially covers the ring, the area appears much weaker (20). Askar (2) believes that variations in decussation of aponeurotic fibers in the midline have a role in the occurrence of umbilical and paraumbilical hernias.

INFANTILE UMBILICAL HERNIA

In children, umbilical hernias are the third most common surgical disorder after hydroceles and inguinal hernias. The incidence is one in every five live births (26). The incidence is much higher in Afro-Caribbean infants than in whites. James (13) reported from Capetown, South Africa, that 61.8% of Xhosa infants and children had umbilical hernias. Several reports from the United States suggest that the incidence of umbilical hernia is as much as eight times higher in black infants than in white infants (5,22,26). Jeliffe (14), reporting from the West Indies, found that 58.5% of children of African origin had umbilical hernias compared to 8% of white children. In East Africa, 60% of black infants have umbilical hernias compared to only 4% of Asian infants (16). In the United States, 32% to 42% of black infants have umbilical hernias (5,26). There is no clear explanation for the higher incidence in Afro-Caribbean children.

Prematurity and low birth weight are known to predispose to umbilical hernias (5). Vohr et al. (24) studied a group composed almost entirely of white infants at age 3 months and found umbilical hernias in 75% of those who weighed less than 1,500 g at birth; all of the hernias resolved spontaneously by age 12 months. Vohr et al. described an association between the diagnosis of respiratory distress syndrome in the immediate postnatal period and the development of umbilical hernias, possibly related to the effect of increased intraabdominal pressure associated with the respiratory distress syndrome on inadequately developed anterior abdominal muscle and fascia. Evans (8) reported the incidence of umbilical hernias to be 84% in babies weighing between 1,000 and 1,500 g, 38% in those weighing between 1,500 and 2,000 g, and 20.5% in those weighing between 2,000 and 2,500 g at birth. Umbilical hernias are also common in children with Down syndrome, hypothyroidism, mucopolysaccharidosis (particularly Hurler's

syndrome), Beckwith–Wiedemann syndrome, and trisomy 13 and 18 (6,26). The tendency to spontaneous resolution is maintained in patients with Down syndrome. There also appears to be a 9% to 12% familial predisposition to umbilical hernias (5,22), but no genetic pattern of inheritance has been identified. In sets of identical twins, both children are invariably affected (12,26).

Diagnosis

The most common reason for a child's referral with an umbilical hernia is the cosmetic appearance. The hernia results in a cone-like protrusion at the umbilicus that bulges every time the child cries or strains (Fig. 35.1). There may also be a history of vague abdominal pain or pain on pressure over the umbilicus. The size of the fascial defect must be evaluated, a collar of fibrous tissue typically being found at the neck of the sac. The reducibility of the hernia should also be evaluated, incarceration being extremely rare. The whole length of the linea alba above the umbilicus should also be evaluated to identify a coexisting paraumbilical or epigastric hernia, or diastasis recti.

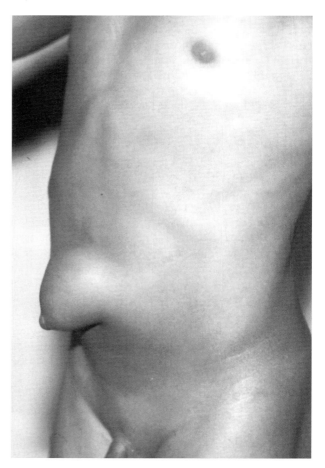

FIGURE 35.1. A 6-year-old black male patient with a large infantile umbilical hernia. The typical conical shape is maintained, although it is starting to droop downward.

If the diagnosis is in doubt, dynamic ultrasound can be useful in clarifying the situation (Fig. 35.2).

Differential Diagnosis

The most common differential diagnoses relate to other developmental abnormalities. The most important of these is an omphalocele. In this condition, the umbilical cord is at the apex of a thinned, avascular, two-layer translucent sac. The sac itself is not covered by skin, but the surrounding skin may be seen to advance upward on the sac for a short distance. The intestine lies freely mobile within the intact sac without evidence of adhesions or inflammation. When the fascial defect is less than 4 cm, the omphalocele is termed a herniation of the umbilical cord. The importance of identifying this defect at birth is to avoid inadver-

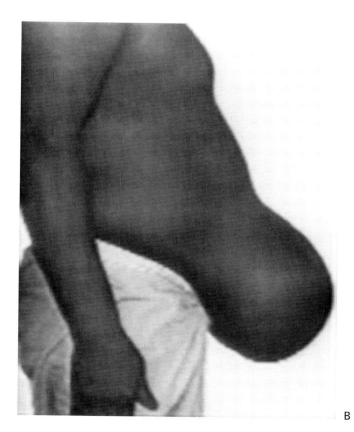

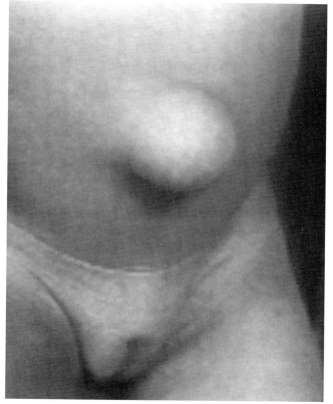

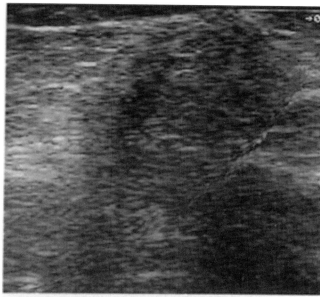

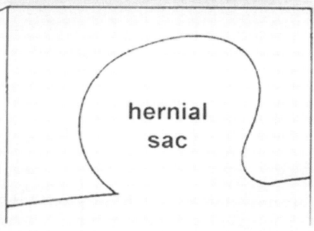

hernial
sac

A

B

C

FIGURE 35.2. A: Typical sonographic findings of an umbilical hernia. **B:** Example of a periumbilical hernia. **C:** Example of an umbilical hernia. *(continued on next page)*

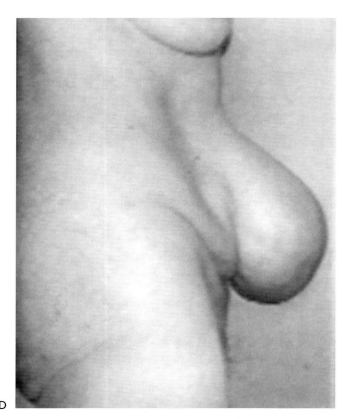

D

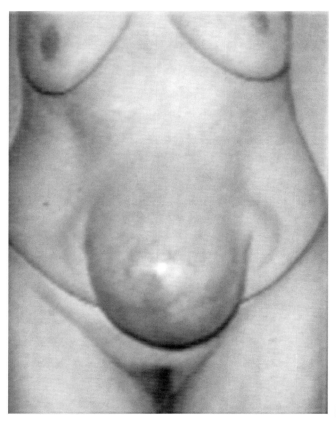

E

FIGURE 35.2. (***continued***) **D** and **E:** Examples of paraumbilical hernias. (Part **A** reproduced from Truong SN, Muller M. Diagnosis of abdominal wall defects. In: Schumpelick V, Kingsnorth AN, eds. *Incisional hernia.* Berlin: Springer–Verlag, 1999:117–135. Parts **B–E** reproduced from Wellcome Centre Medical Photographic Library, with permission.)

tently clamping the sac or dividing the wide base of the cord, which results in enterectomy. The management of these defects is discussed further in Chapter 37.

An umbilical granuloma is a subacute infection at the umbilicus that is treated with the application of silver nitrate. If two or three applications do not result in resolution of the problem, an umbilical polyp (which is covered with pinched-off intestinal mucosa), an omphalomesenteric duct, or a urachus must be considered. Remnants of the omphalomesenteric duct and urachus can also produce cystic masses within the umbilicus. In addition, the fact that metastatic tumor nodules (Sister Joseph's nodules) occur at the umbilicus should be kept in mind, although this is rare in the pediatric age range. An incarcerated umbilical hernia may be simulated by an abscess of the obliterated umbilical vessels or by primary bacterial peritonitis. Patients with bowel obstruction from other causes not related to the umbilicus may have an irreducible umbilical hernia that is not truly incarcerated.

Natural History

The majority of infantile umbilical hernias resolve spontaneously. However, there are no prospective, longitudinal studies of infants followed to adulthood to provide absolute evi-

dence that this is the case. Blumberg (4) states that all true infantile umbilical hernias close by age 3 to 4 years. In his opinion, only paraumbilical or adult-type umbilical hernias do not resolve spontaneously. Several other reports (22,24,26) suggest that umbilical hernias persisting after age 5 to 6 years are unlikely to close spontaneously, while Crump (5) found no cases of umbilical hernia in children older than 7 years. A study of black children between ages 4 and 11 years estimated that half of the hernias present at 4 to 5 years closed spontaneously by 11 years (11). Mack (16) has reported healing of umbilical hernias until puberty, but not after. There is therefore some indirect evidence that spontaneous closure of umbilical hernias continues, even after age 5 years.

The size of the umbilical ring appears to be an important determinant of the spontaneous resolution of umbilical hernias. Walker (25) observed 314 black children over a 6-year period and found that 96% of hernias with a fascial ring defect of less than 5 mm at age 3 months healed spontaneously, usually within 2 years. If the ring had a diameter greater than 1 cm, it did not close spontaneously until after age 4 years, and none of the defects that had a ring diameter greater than 1.5 cm closed spontaneously by age 6 years. A retrospective review (12) also suggested those fascial defects greater than 1.5 cm persisted into adult life. In a fur-

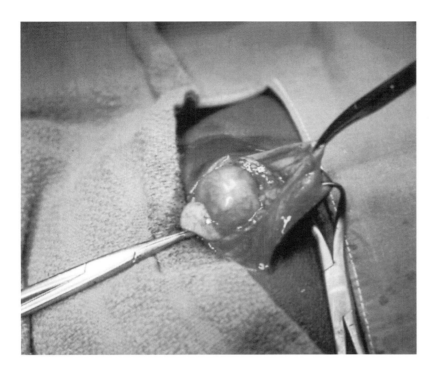

FIGURE 35.3. Incarcerated but viable transverse colon in an infantile umbilical hernia resulting from inspissated feces.

ther prospective study, 78 infants with umbilical hernias who had a fascial ring greater than 5 mm in diameter were observed over a 4-year period. Seventy-two hernias (92%) closed spontaneously: 31 in the first year of life, 20 in the second year, 16 in the third year, and five more after 3 years. The hernias disappeared by gradual contraction of the ring until there was no longer room for intraabdominal contents to protrude, larger defects therefore taking longer to close than smaller ones.

Complications of infantile umbilical hernias are extremely uncommon, incarceration being estimated to occur in 1:1,500 cases (20). In one series of 590 children (14), the incidence of complications was 5.1%, the complications including incarceration, strangulation, and evisceration. Radhakrishnan (22) reported three cases of umbilical hernia requiring emergency surgery over a 15-year period, two for incarceration of the transverse colon caused by inspissated feces (Fig. 35.3) and one for strangulated omentum (Fig. 35.4).

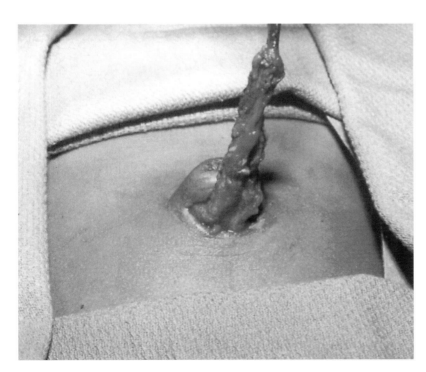

FIGURE 35.4. Incarcerated infantile umbilical hernia with strangulated omentum that was adherent to the undersurface of the cicatrix.

Treatment

The treatment options are observation and operative repair. Unless complicated by pain, incarceration, or strangulation, there is no indication for surgical intervention before age 2 years. If the fascial defect is less than 1.5 cm, there is a high likelihood of spontaneous resolution. After age 2 years, there is debate about the need for and timing of surgical repair. There is no doubt that the child with a protuberant hernia is teased when at school, and the British Society of Paediatric Surgeons (personal communication, 1999) recommends repair prior to the child commencing school (age 3 to 4 years). Similarly, if the fascial defect is greater than 1.5 cm, there is probably no more than a 50% chance of spontaneous resolution and surgical repair is indicated. Any child with a tender hernia, even if it is reducible, warrants early surgical intervention. Patients who have a defect in the ring but no protuberance can be observed for longer, per-haps until age 9 or 10 years, but the surgeon should have a low threshold for intervening.

There is no place in the treatment of umbilical hernias for strapping, and the definitive treatment of umbilical hernias is surgical repair.

Operative Technique

Elective repair of umbilical hernias in children is performed as a day-case procedure under general anesthetic. The patient is positioned in the supine position on the operating table and prepared appropriately. A curvilinear "smile" incision is made within a skin fold on the inferior aspect of the hernia. The apex of the umbilicus may be elevated with a tissue holding forceps to aid the placement of the incision if necessary (Fig. 35.5B). The incision is carried through the subcutaneous fat to expose the caudal aspect of the sac. The sac neck

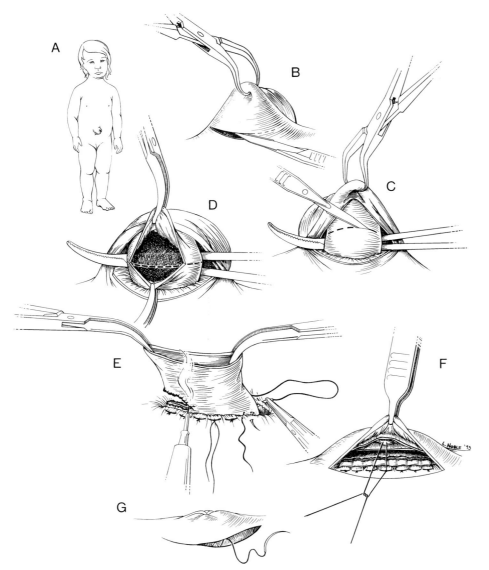

FIGURE 35.5. A: The typical infantile umbilical hernia. **B:** The hernia is held at the cicatrix with a towel clip and elevated. A subumbilical "smile" incision is made in a skin fold. **C:** The hernia sac is encircled completely by a clamp and opened on its caudal aspect. **D:** The sac is entered and the contents are reduced. The cephalad aspect of the sac then is incised. **E:** After the fascial defect is repaired with horizontal mattress sutures, the redundant part of the sac is excised using electrocautery. **F:** The button of sac left on the undersurface of the umbilicus is tacked down to the repaired fascia. **G:** The subcutaneous tissues are repaired with interrupted sutures of chromic catgut, and the skin is closed with a running subcuticular suture of chromic catgut.

is then encircled by blunt dissection with a hemostat. The apex of the sac is dissected off the undersurface of the umbilicus and the edges of the sac adherent to the fascial defect mobilized. Once the sac is completely mobile, it is reduced by inversion into the abdominal cavity. The fascial defect is repaired by interrupted mattress sutures, using a nonabsorbable suture of appropriate size. Extensive extraperitoneal dissection is unnecessary as, once the sac has been inverted, the fascial edges become clear and mattress sutures may be safely positioned. It is not necessary to "double-breast" the repair. Occasionally, umbilical vessels may require ligation. It is usually easier to obtain a tension-free repair in the transverse direction. If the defect is larger vertically or if there is an associated supraumbilical defect, a longitudinal closure is more appropriate. The inner surface of the cicatrix is tacked down to the area of the fascial repair with one or two nonabsorbable sutures. After meticulous hemostasis has been secured, the subcutaneous tissues are approximated with interrupted absorbable sutures and a subcuticular skin closure is performed, also with an absorbable suture.

Other techniques of managing the sac include incising the sac on its caudad aspect (Fig. 35.5C). Abdominal contents may adhere to the fundus of the sac, and such an incision avoids inadvertent damage to them. Once the sac has been entered, the contents are reduced and the incision is carried around to the cephalad aspect of the sac (Fig. 35.5D). The cut edges of the sac are held up to permit abdominal contents to fall back into the peritoneal cavity. Horizontal mattress sutures may then be placed at the edges of the fascial defect and the defect repaired.

Complications of umbilical herniorrhaphy are extremely uncommon as long as meticulous surgical technique is employed. The formation of a seroma or hematoma occurs in a small minority of patients (1% to 2%), and secondary infection is rare. Recurrence is possible if a large defect is closed under tension, if an associated paraumbilical hernia is overlooked, or if the wound becomes infected. The undersurface of the linea alba and rectus sheath should be palpated through the umbilical defect to identify any coexisting fascial defects.

Concern regarding redundancy of periumbilical skin exists if the umbilical hernia is large. If it is tacked down properly, the skin will shrink down to a normal appearance over time. The use of pressure by placing a compression dressing is advocated by some surgeons. A cotton wool ball may be placed over the umbilicus and retained in place with an Elastoplast dressing (Smith & Nephew Healthcare Ltd., Hull, U.K.) for 4 to 7 days. On rare occasions, it may be worthwhile to excise the redundant skin.

ACQUIRED UMBILICAL HERNIA

Patients with acute abdominal distention (e.g., intestinal obstruction) often have a partially unfolded umbilicus. If the raised intraabdominal pressure persists, the umbilical cicatrix gives way, resulting in an acquired umbilical hernia. Acquired hernias may be noted in patients who have ascites resulting from cirrhosis, congestive heart failure, or nephrosis. Patients undergoing peritoneal dialysis also have a higher incidence of acquired umbilical hernias. Patients with serious underlying problems should not undergo operative repair unless the hernia incarcerates or the overlying skin is thinned down to such an extent that spontaneous rupture is possible. If surgical intervention is required, the fascial defect is often too large to be closed primarily with sutures without the repair being under excessive tension. In these cases, the defect is best closed with prosthetic mesh, preferably with the mesh sited in the preperitoneal plane.

PARAUMBILICAL HERNIA

Paraumbilical hernias occur in all age groups, but are more common after age 35 years and are five times more common in women than in men. These lesions are the result of defects in the linea alba and the umbilical fascia, the latter being a direct extension of the transversalis fascia. The most common site is in the supraumbilical linea alba, but defects can also occur below the umbilicus. They may occur in association with umbilical hernias and can be multiple, especially when associated with diastasis recti.

Paraumbilical hernias do not resolve spontaneously. The most common presenting symptom is pain (possibly caused by dragging on the fat and peritoneum of the falciform ligament), with or without a lump being present. The incidence of complications, such as incarceration, inflammation and gangrene, is much higher than for true umbilical hernias.

Diagnosis

Due the difference in natural history, these hernias must be distinguished from umbilical hernias. In the supraumbilical hernia, about half of the fundus of the sac is covered by the umbilicus, and the skin of the abdomen immediately above the umbilicus (Fig. 35.6) covers the remainder. This is in contrast to the umbilical hernia, in which the protrusion is directly under the umbilicus with a circumferentially symmetric bulge (Fig. 35.7). In addition, paraumbilical hernias have no collar of fibrous tissue at the neck. If the hernia is small, the diagnosis may be aided by standing the patient erect and tracing the line of the linea alba with the pulp of one finger. The paraumbilical hernia may be felt as a small, palpable nodule, often tender, just above or below the umbilicus.

Operative Technique

Surgical repair is always indicated because these hernias do not resolve spontaneously. If the defect is difficult to feel

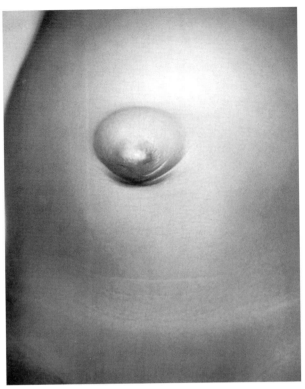

FIGURE 35.6. Paraumbilical (supraumbilical) hernia in a child. Note that the lower half of the fundus is covered by the cicatrix, whereas the upper half is covered by supraumbilical skin. This is in contrast to Fig. 35.7.

with the patient supine, the position of the hernia should be marked preoperatively with the patient standing. For solitary lesions separated from the umbilicus, the traditional incision is horizontal directly over the hernia. The incision is carried down through the subcutaneous fat and the fas-

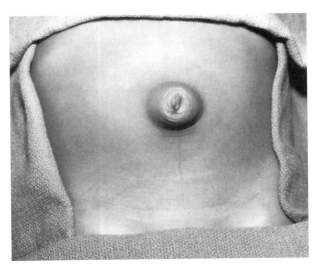

FIGURE 35.7. A typical umbilical hernia in a child, with the cicatrix in the center of the protrusion and symmetric swelling circumferentially.

cial margins dissected out circumferentially around the protruding fat. If the fat is viable, it is reduced into the preperitoneal plane; if ischemic or gangrenous, it is best excised. The fascial defect is then closed either horizontally or vertically, depending on the orientation of the defect and the direction that produces least tension. Mattress sutures of nonabsorbable material of appropriate size are used. The subcutaneous tissues are then opposed with absorbable sutures and the skin closed with a subcuticular suture.

In patients with a paraumbilical hernia associated with an umbilical hernia, the incision can be made curvilinear in the same fashion as for an infantile umbilical hernia, except that it is made supraumbilically. In such cases, the fascial defect is best closed in a vertical direction. It is important to examine the whole of the linea alba from within by placing a finger through the defect and palpating the fascia up to the xiphoid process. If multiple fascial defects are present, a vertical midline incision encompassing all of the defects is advised.

With the increasing role of laparoscopic surgical techniques, both occult umbilical and paraumbilical hernias are being encountered more frequently. If present at the time of laparoscopy, it is important to repair the fascial defect of the hernia in addition to the fascial defect created by the 10-mm trocar.

UMBILICAL HERNIA IN ADULTS

The pathophysiology of umbilical hernia in adults is disputed. It is generally believed that these hernias do not represent persistence from childhood but arise *de novo* in adult life. A retrospective review of adults with umbilical hernias (12) found that only 10.9% recalled having hernias from childhood. In a separate series of 71 women and 82 men (23), it was noted that only two women had recurrence of their infantile umbilical hernias and this occurred during pregnancy. In both cases, the hernia resolved completely after delivery. None of the men followed developed a recurrence.

While the infantile umbilical hernia is a direct hernia, umbilical hernias in adults are indirect herniations through an umbilical canal that is bordered by umbilical fascia posteriorly, the linea alba anteriorly, and the medial edges of the two rectus sheaths on each side. Therefore, these hernias tend to incarcerate and strangulate, and do not resolve spontaneously. Askar (2) suggests that they are really paraumbilical hernias that occur just above and laterally to the umbilicus. Their clinical behavior is certainly more akin to paraumbilical hernias. The incidence of incarceration of umbilical hernias in adults is 14 times that in children. In addition there is a high associated morbidity and mortality. There is a large sex difference with over 90% occurring in women, and almost all are obese and multiparous. In this patient population, umbilical hernias incarcerate half as often as inguinal hernias and three times more often than femoral hernias (17). There is no racial difference in incidence.

As for the acquired umbilical hernias, which are direct hernias, umbilical hernias in adults are also common in cirrhotic patients with ascites (a reported incidence of 24%). It appears that a persistent increase in intraabdominal pressure exerted against a thinned-out umbilical ring and fascia is the cause of herniation in both the cirrhotic patients with ascites and the obese multipara. The factors that determine whether the hernia occurs through the umbilical cicatrix or through a paraumbilical canal are not known.

Diagnosis

The diagnosis of umbilical hernia in adults is usually obvious (Fig. 35.8). In large hernias, reduction is often impossible because omentum becomes adherent to the sac. In addition, if the hernia is long-standing, there are often multiple fascial defects. As the hernia enlarges, it becomes oval and has a tendency to drag downward. These hernias are very symptomatic. Patients complain of a local dragging pain, due to the weight of the lesion; gastrointestinal symptoms, probably due to traction on the stomach or transverse colon; and intermittent colicky pain, due to partial intestinal obstruction. In long-standing cases, maceration of adjacent skin surfaces by the panniculus and chronic infection can be noted.

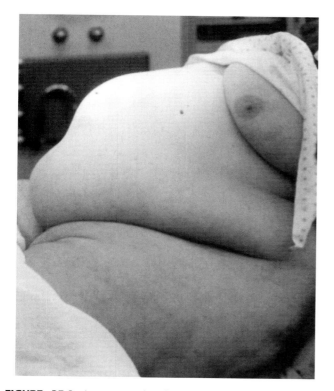

FIGURE 35.8. An extremely obese, multiparous middle-aged woman with a large incarcerated adult type of umbilical hernia. The fatty panniculus hangs down to the pubis. She had to be anesthetized in the upright position because she was unable to breathe when supine. Strangulated cecum was found in the hernia. Postoperatively, the patient required prolonged ventilatory support, tracheostomy, and a 3-week intensive care unit stay. She finally recovered and was discharged after 6 weeks in the hospital.

Operative Technique

Nonoperative therapy of any sort is uniformly unsuccessful. In elective cases, it is important to identify any underlying associated pathology and try to improve the general condition of the patient before undertaking surgical correction. Unfortunately, these patients often have incarcerated hernias, and prolonged preoperative therapy is not possible. Large adult umbilical hernias are difficult operations, and their technical difficulty should not be underestimated.

The appropriate anesthetic technique should be discussed with the anesthetist prior to arrival in the operating department. General anesthesia with full muscle relaxation aids the surgeon but, frequently, the patient is not deemed fit for general anesthesia and the procedure is performed using regional or local anesthetic techniques. In smaller adult umbilical hernias, a subumbilical incision can be used, but large hernias, and particularly incarcerated hernias, often require a large incision that may be either transverse or vertical. Dissection is carried around the hernia sac through the subcutaneous tissue down to the aponeurotic layer above, below and on the sides of the sac. The entire mass of skin, fat, and hernia is elevated while the neck of the sac is incised because adhesions of the underlying omentum or bowel are more likely at the fundus. The incarcerated contents must be evaluated and treated as required. Richter's hernia occurs not uncommonly and must be actively sought. Concomitant buttonhole defects are also frequently present and the fascial bridges should be divided to create a single fascial defect. After the contents are dealt with and reduced, the redundant sac should be excised and, if possible, the peritoneum closed with absorbable sutures. Ideally, the fascial defect should be repaired by primary suture with nonabsorbable sutures and edge-to-edge closure performed in either the transverse or the vertical direction, whichever is appropriate. The classic Mayo "vest-over-pants" operation has been discarded since Farris (9) demonstrated that the bursting strength of the wound did not improve by imbrication and actually was impaired to a degree that was proportional to the amount of overlapping and tension.

The overlying umbilical skin usually should not be excised unless it is macerated or infected. In such cases, a new umbilicus could be created. However, this increases the risk of recurrence (2) at the point where the new umbilicus is created. The patient should therefore be advised preoperatively that the umbilicus will be excised and a new umbilicus not created. It may not be possible to oppose the fascial edges in large hernias without undue tension, and in these cases the defect should be repaired with a prosthetic mesh (4a) placed anchored circumferentially beneath the aponeurotic layer. If the site of operation is infected, it is acceptable to leave the subcutaneous fat and skin open and plan for delayed primary closure when the infection has settled.

Complications include the development of seroma (especially when prosthetic mesh is used), hematoma, and infection. Meticulous attention to hemostasis and the use of suction drains may help to reduce these complications. In addition to local problems, these patients often have respiratory and cardiovascular complications and may require prolonged hospitalization. The true incidence of recurrence of these hernias is unknown, but there appears to be an increase in the number of incisional hernias presenting to surgical clinics.

REFERENCES

1. Albucasis. *On surgery and instruments. A definitive edition of the Arabic text with English translation and commentary by MS Spink and GL Lewis.* London: The Wellcome Institute of the History of Medicine, and Oxford: The University Press, 1973.
2. Askar OM. Aponeurotic hernias. Recent observations upon epigastric and paraumbilical hernias. *Surg Clin North Am* 1984;64:315.
3. Bergsman D, ed. *Birth defects compendium,* 2nd ed. New York: Alan R. Liss, 1979.
4. Blumberg NA. Infantile umbilical hernia. *Surg Gynecol Obstet* 1980;150:187.
4a. Condon RE. Incisional hernia. In: Nyhus LM, Condon RE, eds. *Hernia.* 4th ed. Philadelphia: JB Lippincott Co., 1995:319.
5. Crump EP. Umbilical hernia. I. Occurrence of the infantile type in Negro infants and children. *J Paediatr* 1952;40:214.
6. Cullen TS. *Embryology, anatomy and diseases of the umbilicus together with diseases of the urachus.* Philadelphia: WB Saunders, 1916:1.
7. Ellis H. The umbilical hernia of Queen Caroline. *Contemp Surg* 1980;17:83.
8. Evans AG. The comparative incidence of umbilical hernias in coloured and white infants. *J Natl Med Assoc* 1941;33:158.
9. Farris JM. Umbilical hernia. In: Nyhus LM, Harkins HN, eds. *Hernia.* Philadelphia: JB Lippincott Co., 1964:315.
10. Farris JM, Smith GK, Beattie AS. Umbilical hernia: an inquiry into the principle of imbrication and a note on the preservation of the umbilical dimple. *Am J Surg* 1959;98:236.
11. Hall DE, Roberts KB, Charnley E. Umbilical hernia: what happens after age 5 years? *J Paediatr* 1981;98:415.
12. Jackson OJ, Moglen LH. Umbilical hernia: a retrospective study. *Calif Med* 1970;113:8.
13. James T. Umbilical hernia in Xhosa infants and children. *J R Soc Med* 1982;75:537.
14. Jeliffe DB. The racial incidence of umbilical hernia. *J Trop Med Hyg* 1954;57:270.
15. Lassaletta L, Fonkalsrud EW, Tovar JA, et al. The management of umbilical hernias in infancy and childhood. *J Paediatr Surg* 1975;10:405.
16. Mack NK. The incidence of umbilical herniae in Africans. *East Afr Med J* 1945;22:369.
17. Mayo WJ. An operation for the radical cure of umbilical hernia. *Ann Surg* 1901;34:276.
18. Morgan WW, White JJ, Stumbaugh S, et al. Prophylactic umbilical hernia repair in childhood to prevent adult incarceration. *Surg Clin North Am* 1970;50:839.
19. Olch PD, Harkins HN. Historical survey of treatment of inguinal hernia. In: Nyhus LM, Harkins HN, eds. *Hernia.* Philadelphia: JB Lippincott Co., 1964:1.
20. Orda R, Nathan H. Surgical anatomy of the umbilical structures. *Int Surg* 1973;58:458.
21. Papagrigoriadis S, Browse DJ, Howard ER. Incarceration of umbilical hernias in children: a rare but important complication. *Paed Surg Int* 1998;14:231.
22. Radhakrishnan J. Umbilical Hernia. In: Nyhus LM, Condon RE, eds. *Hernia,* 4th ed. Philadelphia: JB Lippincott Co., 1995:361.
23. Sibley WL III, Lynn HB, Harris LE. A 25-year study of infantile umbilical hernia. *Surgery* 1964;55:462.
24. Vohr BR, Rosenfield AG, Oh W. Umbilical hernia in the low-birth-weight infant (less than 1,500 gm). *J Pediatr* 1977;90:807–808.
25. Walker SH. The natural history of umbilical hernia. A six-year follow-up of 314 negro children with this defect. *Clin Pediatr (Phila)* 1967;6:29–32.
26. Woods GE. Some observations on umbilical hernia in infants. *Arch Dis Child* 1953;28:450.

35B

EPIGASTRIC HERNIA

An epigastric hernia (fatty hernia of the linea alba) may be defined as a fascial defect in the linea alba between the xiphoid process and the umbilicus (Fig. 35.9). It is the second most common location of a defect in the aponeurotic–fascial layer in the midline, the most common being an umbilical hernia.

HISTORIC PERSPECTIVE

The entity of epigastric hernia was first recorded by Arnauld de Villeneuve in 1285, but it was not until 1743 that De-Garengeot first ascribed vague abdominal symptoms to this condition. In 1744, based on his finding of

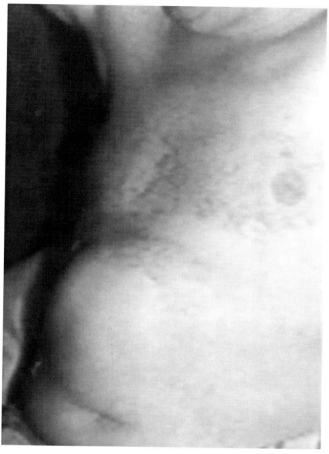

FIGURE 35.9. Epigastric hernia. (Reproduced from Wellcome Centre Medical Photographic Library, with permission.)

commonly noted gastric symptoms, Gunz referred to the lesion as a gastrocele, promoting the concept that the stomach was always contained in the protuberant sac. Richter discounted this concept in 1884, and Leville coined the term "epigastric hernia" in 1812. Bernitz in 1848 and Cruveilhier in 1849 provided further detailed anatomic descriptions.

Maunior reported the first successful epigastric hernia repair in 1802, but it was not until Terrier's (15) report in 1886 that the operation gained acceptance. Prior to this, the procedure had been shunned because of the frequent complication of peritonitis. In 1887, Luecke (7) described two patients in whom epigastric hernia repair was followed by the disappearance of chronic gastric symptoms. Perhaps as a result, undue enthusiasm was attached to the operation and epigastric symptoms stemming from intraabdominal pathology were overlooked or attributed erroneously to the hernia. The result was numerous reports of epigastric hernias occurring with coexisting intraabdominal disease.

Capelle (5) reported on 31 cases of epigastric hernia repair: four patients later died of gastric carcinoma, 12 continued to have gastric symptoms, and 6 developed recurrent hernias. It became clear that, while an epigastric hernia may potentially contribute to symptoms, concurrent intraabdominal pathology could coexist and be responsible for the majority of the symptoms experienced. Indeed, Lewisohn (7) recommended that any patient with an epigastric hernia and associated gastrointestinal symptoms should undergo a thorough laparotomy at the time of hernia repair.

In the early twentieth century, epigastric hernias were implicated in the underlying etiology of gastric ulcers, the theory being that incarcerated omentum exerted traction on the stomach (14). This theory was simulated experimentally in dogs by Meyer and Ivy (9), who, although they were able to demonstrate deformities of the greater curvature, could not produce gastric ulcer formation. The accepted current approach acknowledges that epigastric hernia is an important clinical entity that in and of itself may produce a variety of clinical symptoms. However, the presence of gastrointestinal symptoms should never be wholly attributed to an epigastric hernia until thorough investigation has excluded an alternative intraabdominal pathology.

DEMOGRAPHICS

As many epigastric hernias are asymptomatic, they remain undiagnosed, and the actual incidence of epigastric hernia is therefore difficult to determine. Autopsy studies suggest a prevalence of 0.5% to 10% in the general population. Epigastric hernias are seldom seen in infants and children, and congenital epigastric hernias are rare. There is a male predominance, with a male-to-female ratio of at least 3:1. The diagnosis is usually made in the third to fifth decade. The hernia occurs with extraordinary frequency among the sepoys of India (6).

ANATOMY AND PATHOLOGY

The linea alba is the midline raphe formed by the junction of the rectus sheaths. It extends from the xiphoid process to the symphysis pubis. Superficial to the linea alba lies only skin and subcutaneous adipose tissue. Deep to the linea alba in the epigastric region is found transversalis fascia, preperitoneal fat, fat of the falciform ligament, and peritoneum. The rectus muscles diverge as they proceed superiorly to insert on the fifth, sixth, and seventh ribs and on the costal cartilage. Although the linea alba is narrow below the umbilicus, it may be as much as 2.5 cm wide above it, this anatomic feature possibly accounting for the rarity of midline hernias below the umbilicus.

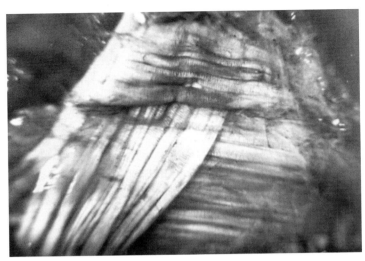

FIGURE 35.10. Anterior rectus sheath seen under the dissecting microscope. Note fine tendinous fibers arranged as interwoven sheets. (From Askar OM. Surgical anatomy of the aponeurotic expansions of the anterior abdominal wall. *Ann R Coll Surg Engl* 1977;59:313–321, with permission.)

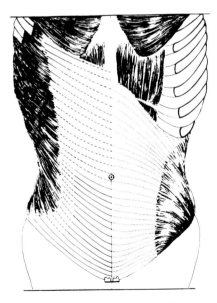

FIGURE 35.11. Digastric pattern between the external oblique aponeurosis **(right)** and the anterior lamina of the internal oblique aponeurosis **(left)**. (From Askar OM. Surgical anatomy of the aponeurotic expansions of the anterior abdominal wall. *Ann R Coll Surg Engl* 1977;59:313–321, with permission.)

The anterior abdominal wall aponeurosis consists of fine tendinous fibers invested in loose areolar tissue and arranged as interwoven sheets (Fig. 35.10). This arrangement results in a triple layer criss-cross pattern in the anterior and posterior rectus sheaths and contributes to the anatomic functional linkage of the muscles of the anterior abdominal wall, allowing them to work in concert (Figs. 35.11 and 35.12). Askar (1) reported a detailed anatomic study of the anterior abdominal wall and demonstrated that these tendinous fibers do not stop in the midline but decussate, creating an intricate interwoven pattern that links all layers of the abdominal wall with those of the other side. Decussation above the umbilicus may appear as a single line in the midline (30%), or, more commonly, as a triple decussation pattern (70%). Below the umbilicus, a single line of decussation is always seen.

Fascial defects may vary in diameter from a few millimeters to several centimeters. Smaller ones are often incarcerated, whereas larger ones are usually readily reducible. Most commonly, a preperitoneal mass of fat attached to the peritoneum by a pedicle is herniated. The other variety is a true hernia with a peritoneal sac. Peters and Nesselrode (12), Pollack (13), and Wilkinson (16) found a sac to be present in 17 of 28 (61%), 26 of 45 (58%), and 2 of 16 (12.5%), respectively. The sac usually contains omentum, with intestinal contents being rare and only occasional reports of strangulation. In about 20% of patients, multiple fascial defects are present.

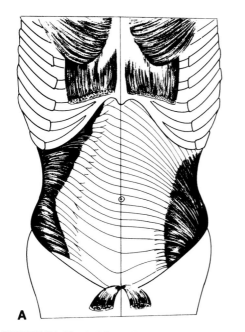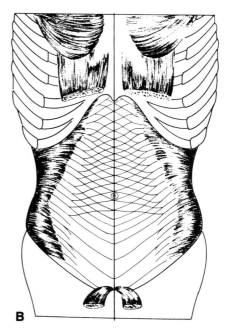

FIGURE 35.12. A: Digastric pattern between the transversus **(right)** and the posterior lamina of the internal oblique aponeurosis **(left)**. **B:** Digastric pattern between the two transversi. (From Askar OM. Surgical anatomy of the aponeurotic expansions of the anterior abdominal wall. *Ann R Coll Surg Engl* 1977;59:313–321, with permission.)

ETIOLOGY AND PATHOGENESIS

It was originally considered that an epigastric hernia was a congenital defect. Moschowitz (10) noted that the transversalis fascia was prolonged at the points in the linea alba where blood vessel perforated the fascia layer, and suggested that preperitoneal fat enclosed in the falciform ligament would insinuate itself into the fascial foramen created by the vessel, enlarge it, and result in an epigastric hernia. He argued that this explanation accounted for the uniform absence of a peritoneal sac and the consistent presence of a vessel in his experience. This theory has, however, been universally challenged, and only rarely have isolated vessels been identified accompanying the hernial mass.

Current opinion is that an epigastric hernia is an acquired lesion, probably related to excessive strain on the anterior abdominal wall aponeurosis. Askar (2,3) applied his studies of the anatomy and function of the anterior abdominal wall to the problem and emphasized the importance of the pattern of aponeurotic decussation in the pathogenesis of an epigastric hernia. He observed epigastric hernias exclusively in patients who had a single midline pattern of decussation (Figs. 35.13 and 35.14).

The pathogenesis of epigastric hernia can be related to the structural–functional relations of the anterior abdominal wall. The midline aponeurotic area may be divided functionally into an upper abdominal "parachute" area, allowing respiratory motion, and a lower "belly support" area, divided by the lowest tendinous intersection. The tendinous fibers are situated obliquely in the aponeurotic sheets, allowing for changes in the shape of the abdominal wall such as would be required during respiration. The midline raphe, however, can change only in length and breadth, with an increase in one necessitating a decrease in the other. During abdominal distention, the linea alba must increase in both dimensions. The resultant tearing of fibers or stretching of spaces between fibers may play a role in the development of an epigastric hernia.

The origin of fibers may also play a role in the development of epigastric hernias. Askar demonstrated that fibers originating from the diaphragm traverse the upper midline aponeurosis posteriorly and join with fibers of the posterior rectus sheath and middle tendinous intersection. They attach to the linea alba at a site midway between the xiphoid and the umbilicus. These fibers may coordinate respiratory movements of the diaphragm and upper abdomen. Uncoordinated, vigorous, synchronous contractions of the diaphragm and upper abdomen may occur during events such as straining and coughing. The force caused by upward traction on the diaphragm and lateral traction on the tendinous intersection would be maximal at this point of attachment midway between the xiphoid and the umbilicus, the most common site of epigastric herniation.

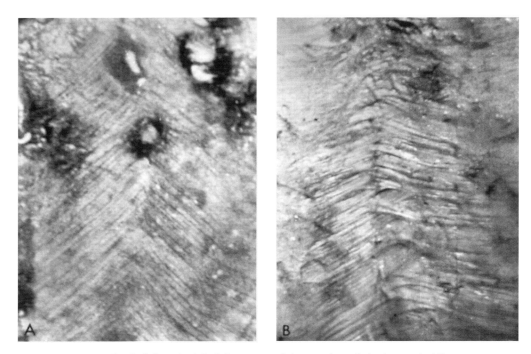

FIGURE 35.13. Single **(A)** and triple **(B)** pattern of decussation of the internal oblique aponeurosis seen in a midline epigastric incision. (From Askar OM. Surgical anatomy of the aponeurotic expansions of the anterior abdominal wall. *Ann R Coll Surg Engl* 1977;59:313–321, with permission.)

CLINICAL PRESENTATION

The majority of epigastric hernias, up to 75%, are asymptomatic. The most common presenting feature is a lump that the patient has noticed but that is not causing any symptoms. Alternatively, a lump may be felt during examination of the abdomen for another reason. Smaller hernias, even when they are not incarcerated, tend to cause more symptoms than do larger ones. Symptomatic hernias present with a wide variety of complaints, many of which are

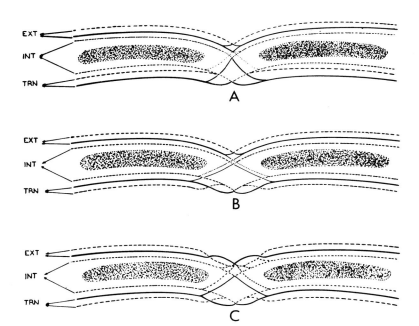

FIGURE 35.14. A: Single anterior and single posterior lines of decussation (30%). **B:** Single anterior and triple posterior lines of decussation (10%). **C:** Triple anterior and triple posterior lines of decussation (60%). *ext,* external oblique; *int,* internal oblique; *trn,* transversus. (From Askar OM. Surgical anatomy of the aponeurotic expansions of the anterior abdominal wall. *Ann R Coll Surg Engl* 1977;59:313–321, with permission.)

seemingly unrelated to the hernia. Common symptoms include epigastric pain that is dull, burning, or colicky and sometimes radiates to the lower abdomen, back, or chest; this may occasionally be accompanied by abdominal distention, dyspepsia, nausea, and vomiting. The typical pain of an epigastric hernia is epigastric pain on exertion. The pain is often exacerbated by bending or standing and relieved by reclining in the supine or prone position.

Incarceration is common, especially in smaller hernias, probably occurring in over 50% of cases, but strangulation is rare. Strangulation of preperitoneal fat or omentum results in localized pain and tenderness. Incarceration and strangulation of intraabdominal viscera are extremely rare, with the symptoms produced related to the organ incarcerated.

DIAGNOSIS

The diagnosis is usually made by clinical examination, a palpable midline mass being present. Additional aids are performing the examination with the patient standing or in tangential light. Occasionally, palpation of the mass can be difficult, especially in obese patients. A local area of tenderness in the linea alba is usually present, however, even in reducible hernias. The presence of a mass and/or tenderness, combined with typical symptoms, is sufficient to justify surgical exploration. However, the caveat noted previously should be remembered—it is dangerous to assume atypical symptoms are solely due to the presence of a hernia, and relevant investigations should be performed prior to hernia repair to exclude an intraabdominal cause for their symptoms.

The diagnosis of an epigastric hernia can be confirmed as the mass becomes more obvious when the patient strains, coughs, or raises the head in the supine position. Despite these maneuvers, differentiating this condition from subcutaneous tumors may be difficult. Further investigation includes imaging of the abdominal wall by either ultrasound or computed tomography (CT). The characteristic appearances have been documented by Yeh et al. (17). Intestine in a sac may be detected by the demonstration of peristalsis on real-time ultrasonography or by the delineation of contrast medium or air in the loop of intestine on CT scan. These modalities may prove useful in the occasional hernia that escapes clinical diagnosis. The diagnosis is made definitively by surgical exploration.

TREATMENT

An operation offers the only chance of permanent cure for these defects in adults. However, epigastric hernias are unusual in children. In a series of patients aged 2 to 7 years

with asymptomatic epigastric or paraumbilical hernias, most of the hernias resolved spontaneously with time (11). Therefore, expectant management in children is not unreasonable. The decision for surgical intervention should be based on the child's age and type and severity of symptoms.

There has been considerable debate over the last hundred years as to the best technique for surgical repair. In the majority of cases, a small hernia traversed by preperitoneal fat is encountered. After the fat has been resected/reduced, in most defects less than 2.5 cm in diameter simple suture closure suffices. The orientation of suture closure remains a matter of controversy. Some surgeons claim that a transverse closure is more sound, while others prefer a vertical closure because of the frequency of multiple defects and of recurrence adjacent to the transverse hernioplasty (although many of these "recurrences" are probably missed primary defects at the time of original surgery). A third group of surgeons prefers an oblique orientation of sutures, claiming it to be more anatomic. The important principle is to do no harm, and for small defects, elaborate procedures that violate normal surrounding fascia are meddlesome and unnecessary and should be avoided.

For larger hernias, enlarging the defect transversely and performing a vest-over-pants Mayo-type repair has been advocated. This technique adds nothing to the strength of a simple primary suture closure and may create undue tension in an unanatomic plane. There is no documented evidence to support its use in epigastric hernia repairs.

In the 1940s, Berman (4) advocated a vertical "Mayo-type" repair in which the rectus sheath is opened anteriorly, on one side, near the line of fusion. The contralateral posterior rectus sheath is incised near its line of fusion, thus creating a short anterior and long posterior fascial flap on one side and the reverse on the other. The vertical defect is then closed in three layers, using imbricated mattress sutures for the fascial flaps and approximating the rectus muscles in the midline as a middle layer.

Askar (2) described a method of dealing with larger defects (greater than 2.5 cm) based on bridging the fascial defect with strips of autograft fascia lata. Using the strips, an interwoven mesh is created that is orientated obliquely in line with the native aponeurotic fibers. Contemporary practice would employ a prosthetic polypropylene mesh that should be fixed in the preperitoneal, retromuscular plane as for incisional hernias (5a).

While there is room for flexibility within the exact technique employed, several principles should be adhered to:

1. Adequate exposure of the hernial defect by sharp dissection and debridement if necessary (Fig. 35.15).
2. Preparation of the defect for closure. The sac may be either excised or reduced. It is not essential to close the peritoneum as a separate layer prior to repair.
3. Anatomic repair without tension.

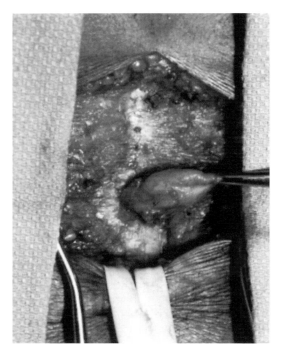

FIGURE 35.15. The linea alba has been exposed from xiphoid to umbilicus. Preperitoneal fat can be seen exiting from the fascial defect about 3 cm above the umbilicus. A Penrose drain encircles an associated umbilical hernia.

The size of the midline incision is debatable. It has been recommended that the whole of the midline be exposed from xiphoid to umbilicus to avoid missing multiple defects. An alternative approach is simply to expose the defect itself with an approximately 2-cm diameter ring of normal fascia. Once the hernia has been reduced/excised, a finger is inserted through the defect and searches superiorly and inferiorly to define any further defects that may not have been obvious on examination. If other defects are palpable, the skin incision can then be extended to visualize those defects and the incision in the linea alba subsequently extended to combine all the defects into one. An effective primary suture closure can be achieved by placing nonabsorbable sutures 1 cm apart, taking 1.5-cm bites on either side of the defect.

RESULTS

The majority of complications are not unique to this operation, the common ones being wound infection and wound hematoma, and their rate should be low. Wound infection is a cause for concern because it greatly increases the rate of recurrence.

There have been very few reported series of recurrence rates, presumably because the recurrence rate is very low with modern sutures and aseptic techniques.

Obesity and infection are the main risk factors leading to a high recurrence rate. In up to half of the patients, however, the recurrence actually represents persistence of a second defect or an area of weakness that was overlooked at the time of the initial procedure. This emphasizes the importance of careful palpation of the whole length of the supraumbilical linea alba during the primary repair.

REFERENCES

1. Askar OM. Surgical anatomy of the aponeurotic expansions of the anterior abdominal wall. *Ann R Coll Surg Engl* 1977; 59: 313.
2. Askar OM. A new concept of the aetiology and surgical repair of paraumbilical and epigastric hernias. *Ann R Coll Surg Engl* 1978; 60: 42.
3. Askar OM. Aponeurotic hernias: Recent observations upon paraumbilical and epigastric hernias. *Surg Clin North Am* 1984; 64: 315.
4. Berman EF. Epigastric hernia: an improved method of repair. *Am J Surg* 1945; 68: 84.
5. Capelle. Dauerresultate mach operationen der hernia epigastrica. *Beitr Klin Chir* 1909; 63: 264.
5a. Condon RE. Incisional hernia. In: Nyhus LM, Condon RE, eds. *Hernia.* 4th ed. Philadelphia: JB Lippincott Co., 1995:319.
6. Iason AH. Hernia. Philadelphia, Blakiston, 1941.
7. Lewisohn R. The importance of a thorough exploration of the intra-abdominal organs in operations for epigastric hernia. *Surg Gynecol Obstet* 1921; 32: 546.
8. Luecke. Operative beseitigungvon sog. Fetternien wegen gastralgie. *Zentrabl Chir* 1887; 14: 68.
9. Meyer J, Ivy AC. Studies on gastric and duodenal ulcer: the relation of epigastric hernia to gastric ulcer—a clinical and experimental study. *J Lab Clin Med* 1922; 8: 37.
10. Moschowitz AV. The pathogenesis and treatment of hernia of the linea alba. *Surg Gynecol Obstet* 1914; 18: 504.
11. Pentney BH. Small ventral hernias in children. *Practitioner* 1960; 184: 779.
12. Peters GR, Nesselrode CC. Epigastric hernia: a factor in upper abdominal diagnosis. *J Kansas Med Soc* 1945; 46: 289.
13. Pollack LH. Epigastric hernia. *Am J Surg* 1936; 34: 376.
14. Soper HW. A case of concomitant epigastric hernia and gastric ulcer. *N Y Med J* 1910; 92: 259.
15. Terrier F. Hernias epigastriques et ad-umbilicales. *Rev Chir* 1886; 6: 985.
16. Wilkinson WR. Epigastric hernia. *W V Med J* 1949; 45: 328.
17. Yeh H-C, Lehr-Janus C, Cohen BA, Rabinowitz JG. Ultrasonography and CT of abdominal and inguinal hernias. *J Clin Ultrasound* 1984; 12: 479.

35C

SPIGELIAN HERNIA

Spigelian hernias are rare and generally difficult to diagnose because of their often intramural location and vague and nonspecific symptoms. The diagnosis has been considerably aided by the introduction of real-time ultrasonographic scanning and computed tomography (CT), and the number of proven spigelian hernias has increased dramatically during the last 20 years.

HISTORIC REVIEW

Adriaan van der Spieghel (25) (1578–1625) was born in Brussels and studied first in Leiden and later in Padua, where he subsequently held the chair of anatomy and surgery. He did not diagnose spigelian hernia, but was the first to describe the semilunar line; therefore, it is also known as the linea semilunaris Spigeli or the linea Spigeli (*Adrianus Spigelius* being the Latin form of his name). Spontaneous rupture along the semilunar line was first described by Henry-Francois Le Dran (16) in 1742, but Josef T. Klinkosch (14) was the first to refer to this condition as hernia in the linea semilunaris. While many articles on spigelian hernias have been published, most authors report only a few cases of their own. Some of the larger series are listed in Table 35.1.

A total of 979 cases of spigelian hernia treated surgically have been reported in the literature. Most have been diag-

nosed in patients between 40 and 70 years of age (mean age in the compiled series, 51 years). The sex ratio is 4:3 female to male, with both sides being equally affected. Less than 5% were bilateral and less than 5% occurred in children younger than 16 years. The reported incidence of incarceration is 27%.

ANATOMY

The semilunar line (Figs. 35.16–35.18) forms and marks the transition from muscle to aponeurosis in the transversus abdominis muscle of the abdomen (25). It is a lateral convex line between the costal arch and the pubic tubercle. The part of the aponeurosis that lies between the semilunar line and the lateral edge of the rectus muscle is often called the spigelian fascia or zone.

Spigelian aponeurosis is a more accurate anatomic designation. Protrusion of a peritoneal sac, an organ, or preperitoneal fat from its normal position through a congenital or acquired defect in the spigelian aponeurosis is referred to as hernia Spigeli or spigelian hernia. Hernias that penetrate the aponeurosis more medially and protrude into the rectus sheath are referred to as intravaginal hernias (Fig. 35.17).

Hernias that have arisen within the spigelian aponeurosis after either surgery or direct trauma should not be considered spigelian hernias. The term "spigelian hernia" usually refers to defects that are located above the inferior epigastric vessels. Hernias that penetrate the spigelian aponeurosis within Hesselbach's triangle (i.e., caudal and medial to the inferior epigastric vessels) are called low spigelian hernias (Fig. 35.18). A spigelian hernia is usually located between the different muscle layers of the abdominal wall and therefore is called interparietal, interstitial, intermuscular, intramuscular, or intramural (Fig. 35.17). In this location, a small hernia is especially difficult to detect by palpation and often is referred to as occult or masked.

The spigelian hernia belt (Fig. 35.19) is a transverse belt lying 0 to 6 cm cranial to the interspinal plane (i.e., the horizontal plane through both the anterosuperior iliac spines). The spigelian aponeurosis is widest here, and up to 90% of spigelian hernias arise in this location.

Below the umbilicus, there are considerable structural variations in both muscle and aponeurotic tissue within both the internal oblique and transversus abdominis muscles. Both present finger-like bands and varying numbers of slit-like gaps (30). The fibers of the two muscles run almost parallel here, so that the gaps in the muscles may coincide. In such circumstances, the fibers can be separated easily,

TABLE 35.1. LARGE SERIES OF SPIGELIAN HERNIAS

Author	Year	No. of Hernias
Spangen	1984	45[a]
Stuckej et al.	1973	43[b]
Houlihan	1976	31[c]
Persson et al.	1975	19
Ponka	1980	19[d]
Artioukh and Walker	1996	19
Guivarc'h et al.	1988, 1989	16
Gullmo et al.	1980, 1984	13
Lindholm and Hulin	1969	12
Kienzle and Staemmler	1978	12
Stirnemann	1982	12
Rodighiero et al.	1996	11

[a]Includes 12 low spigelian hernias.
[b]Compilation of all spigelian hernias from a single department, 1951–1971.
[c]Compilation of all spigelian hernias from a single department, 1963–1971.
[d]Includes two low spigelian hernias.

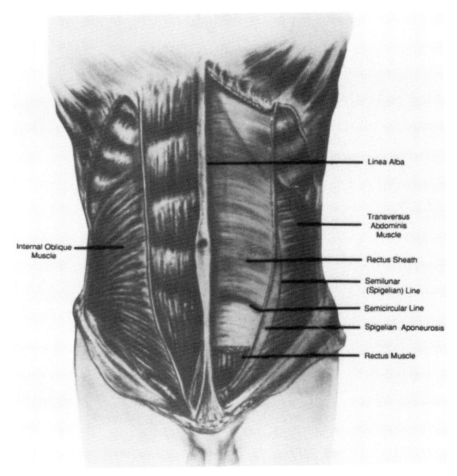

Linea Alba

Transversus Abdominis Muscle

Rectus Sheath

Semilunar (Spigelian) Line

Semicircular Line

Spigelian Aponeurosis

Rectus Muscle

Internal Oblique Muscle

FIGURE 35.16. Ventral view of the abdominal wall shows the topographic anatomy. **Right:** the external oblique muscle and the ventral lamella of the rectus sheath are cut away. **Left:** the internal oblique and rectus abdominis muscles are removed. [From Spangen L. Spigelian hernia. *Acta Chir Scand* 1976;462(Suppl):7, with permission.]

creating a risk of herniation. Above the umbilicus, the fibers cross one another at angles, making herniation less likely.

Above the semicircular line, the aponeurosis of the transversus abdominis muscle divides into two layers, which blend with the anterior and posterior lamellae of the rectus sheath (18). This division occurs within the spigelian aponeurosis, which therefore consists of two lamellae. The posterior lamella becomes thinner as it approaches the semicircular line. The medial part of the spigelian aponeurosis is weakest within the last few centimeters above the semicircular line, and this is probably one of the most important reasons that most spigelian hernias are located in the vicinity of this line. Caudal to the line, all fibers from the transversus aponeurosis run to the anterior lamella of the rectus sheath, and the spigelian aponeurosis consists of a single layer again.

Spigelian hernia is rare in the most cranial part of the abdomen. The muscle belly of the transversus abdominis muscle here reaches to and behind the lateral edge of the rectus muscle. The semilunar line lies dorsal to the rectus

muscle, and there is accordingly no spigelian aponeurosis in this area (Figs. 35.16 and 35.19). As a result, herniation through the transversus aponeurosis at this level is intravaginal. This is another reason why so few spigelian hernias have been found above the umbilicus.

The external oblique muscle, which is the most stable structure in the anterolateral part of the abdominal wall, is aponeurotic ventral to the spigelian aponeurosis throughout its length and prevents the hernia from entering the subcutaneous tissue, which explains why the hernial sac was located subcutaneously in only 18 reported cases. In most instances, the hernia is located between the musculoaponeurotic layers of the anterior abdominal wall.

The internal oblique muscle consists of muscle fibers ventral to the spigelian fascia more often in patients with spigelian hernias than in others (Fig. 35.17). The width of the spigelian aponeurosis in patients with a hernia does not differ from that in other people. A hernia usually penetrates both the transversus abdominis and the internal oblique muscles. The layer between the two oblique muscles is loose

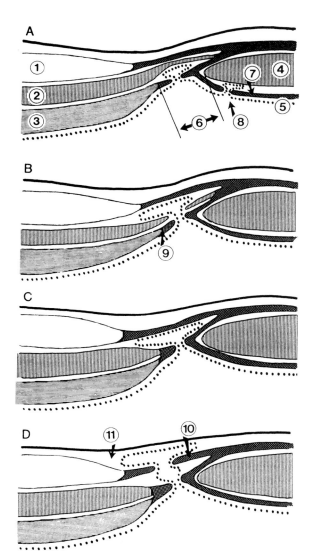

FIGURE 35.17. A–D: Schematic cross section of ventral abdominal wall cranial to the semicircular line, indicating the possible location of the hernial sac in spigelian hernias. *1,* external oblique muscle; *2,* internal oblique muscle; *3,* transversus abdominis muscle; *4,* rectus abdominis muscle; *5,* peritoneum; *6,* spigelian aponeurosis; *7,* dorsal lamella of the rectus sheath; *8,* intravaginal hernia; *9,* semilunar line (linea Spigeli); *10,* external oblique aponeurosis; *11,* subcutaneous tissue.

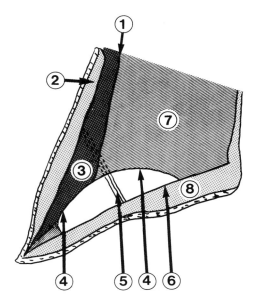

FIGURE 35.18. Schematic presentation of the anatomy in Hesselbach's triangle. *1,* semilunar line; *2,* internal oblique muscle; *3,* spigelian aponeurosis; *4,* arch of transversus abdominis aponeurosis; *5,* inferior epigastric vessels; *6,* inguinal ligament; *7,* transversus abdominis muscle; *8,* external oblique aponeurosis.

hernia grows, it probably dissects the muscle fibers, so that the sac penetrates the glide layer between the two oblique muscles. The hernial orifice is usually oval, although some are more triangular or round, and the edges are well defined and rigid. Most hernias are small, the diameter of the orifice usually ranging from 0.5 to 2.0 cm (although diameters of 8 cm have been reported). In hernias of this size, the orifice is limited to the spigelian aponeurosis.

and normally acts as a glide layer. The hernial sac can expand easily in this space and therefore adopts the typical T- or mushroom-shaped appearance. The hernia expands laterally where more space is present, usually toward the anterosuperior iliac spine and the groin. The medial progress of a spigelian hernia is arrested by the fusion of the external oblique aponeurosis with the deeper layers to form the rectus sheath. Occasionally, however, the hernia may protrude intravaginally. It is unusual for the hernia to extend between the transversus abdominis and internal oblique muscles (Fig. 35.17). This is possible if the internal oblique muscle consists of muscle fibers that are elevated by a small hernia. When the

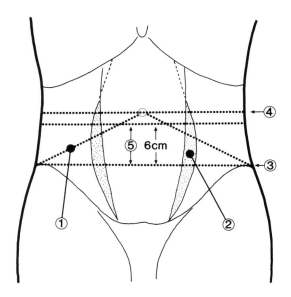

FIGURE 35.19. Location of spigelian hernia belt in relation to the umbilical plane, the interspinal plane, and Monro's line. *1,* Monro's line; *2,* spigelian aponeurosis; *3,* interspinal plane; *4,* umbilical plane; *5,* spigelian hernia belt.

ETIOLOGY

Congenital spigelian hernias are rare, and the lesion is acquired in most cases. The musculoaponeurotic structure within and ventral to the spigelian aponeurosis generally is considered to be the most important contributing factor. The spigelian aponeurosis is one of the congenital weak areas in the ventral abdominal wall. Other predisposing factors are the same as for other types of hernias (e.g., collagen disorders, increased intraabdominal pressure of any cause). Spigelian hernia has been observed in patients treated with continuous ambulatory peritoneal dialysis. In the upright position, the intraabdominal pressure is greatest in the lower part of the abdomen. This means that the pressure on the abdominal wall is greatest below the navel, which could be another reason spigelian hernias occur most often in this region. Aging and weight loss generally are regarded as important causative factors. Paralysis of the abdominal wall muscles may also contribute. Fat apparently can force its way between the fibers of the spigelian aponeurosis, paving the way for herniation (15,22). A spigelian hernia may consist of preperitoneal fat alone, and the fact that the hernial sac is always surrounded by prolapsing preperitoneal fat, being thickest at the top (prehernial lipoma), supports this theory.

It was previously believed that neurovascular openings in the spigelian aponeurosis might become enlarged, permitting herniation (5), but this is now considered to be of minor importance. Spigelian hernia is associated with a high incidence of incarceration, which probably can be explained by the combination of a small hernial opening with rigid edges and the fact that the hernia is often diagnosed when symptoms consistent with incarceration are apparent.

DIAGNOSIS

Symptoms

A spigelian hernia in its earliest form is often simply a protrusion of preperitoneal fat through the spigelian aponeurosis—a condition similar to fatty herniation of the linea alba. The hernia can also be part of an extraperitoneal organ, but a peritoneal sac is found in most cases. If the peritoneal sac has content, it is usually greater omentum, small intestine, or part of the colon, although the majority of intraabdominal organs have been reported within the sac on at least one occasion. Richter-type hernias have also been reported. The symptoms vary considerably, probably because so many different organs can be included in the hernia, resulting in diagnostic confusion.

The symptoms that cause a patient to consult a physician are usually abdominal pain, a mass in the anterior abdominal wall, or signs of incarceration with or without intestinal obstruction. The pain varies in type, severity, and location, and depends on the content of the hernia. Abdominal pain of uncharacteristic type, not typical of a hernia, is common. Pain can often be provoked or aggravated by maneuvers that increase intraabdominal pressure and is relieved by rest. Intense pain occurs if the hernia is incarcerated, and if intestine is present in the hernial sac at the same time, symptoms of intestinal obstruction may ensue.

Physical Examination

If the hernia produces a palpable mass along the spigelian aponeurosis, the diagnosis is generally easy to make, provided the possibility of this hernia is considered. If the contents of an abdominal mass can be reduced, a spigelian hernia is highly probable. The same applies if the hernia appears when the patient is upright and reduces spontaneously when the patient lies down, or if it appears when the patient strains or lifts heavy loads. The clinical diagnosis of a palpable hernia is complicated by the fact that the defect often continues to develop laterally and caudally between the two oblique muscles. The palpable mass, therefore, is most prominent lateral to the spigelian aponeurosis.

Patients who complain of pain but have no visible or palpable mass present the greatest difficulty in diagnosis. This condition exists when the hernial sac content is reduced at the time of examination, or when a small interparietal hernia cannot be detected on palpation.

The hernial orifice, while not often palpable, may be palpated through the external aponeurosis in some cases if the patient is examined with a tense abdominal wall. Physical examination should be carried out while the patient alternately tenses and relaxes the abdominal muscles. When the abdominal muscles are tensed, all patients with spigelian hernias have a tender spot over the hernial orifice in the spigelian aponeurosis. On palpation, the hernia is pressed against the hernial ring, which is firm during Valsalva's maneuver. This finding is not pathognomonic of spigelian hernia, but offers a useful method for screening: patients without distinct tenderness in the spigelian aponeurosis on palpation do not have spigelian hernia, whereas those with positive findings may have.

Diagnostic Procedures

Radiologic procedures in the diagnostic evaluation of spigelian hernias are aimed at demonstrating a hernial orifice or sac and obtaining information regarding sac contents.

Plain abdominal x-rays are not particularly sensitive in diagnosing spigelian hernias. Herniography with contrast medium injected into the peritoneal cavity may be attempted, but the diagnostic accuracy of this procedure is also low and it carries some complications (9,10). Large hernias can usually be detected (Fig. 35.20), but the diagnosis is frequently clear after the physical examination.

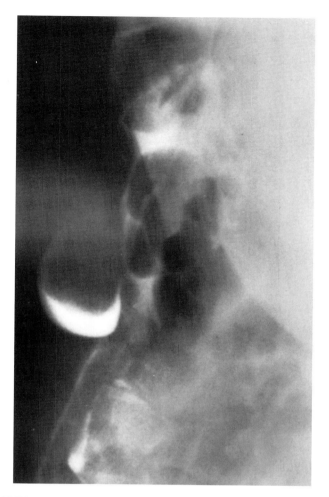

FIGURE 35.20. Spigelian hernia diagnosed by herniography. Horizontal supine oblique (45 degrees) position; anteroposterior projection.

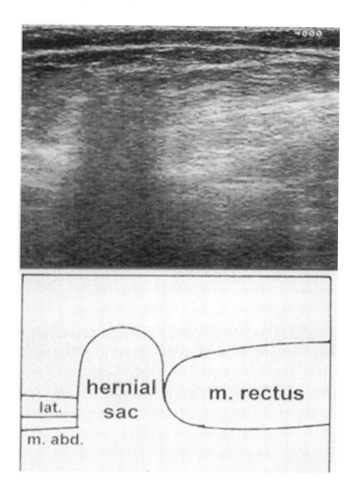

FIGURE 35.21. Typical sonographic findings of a spigelian hernia.

Ultrasonic scanning is now a valuable diagnostic tool in both palpable and nonpalpable spigelian hernias (3,4,19,28,29). It is rapid, accurate, noninvasive, and easy to perform, and the abdominal wall layers can be clearly delineated. The diagnosis is based on demonstration of a hernial orifice in the spigelian aponeurosis, on an interparietally located hernial sac, and on sac content in the form of intestine or omentum.

In the scans (Fig. 35.21), echogenic stripes can be seen below the subcutaneous fat, running almost parallel to the outline of the skin. The hernial orifice is visualized as a defect in the echo line from the aponeurosis. Due to the presence of air-containing intestine, the hernial sac often casts an acoustic shadow.

Preperitoneal fat and omentum are highly echogenic, more so than the adjacent subcutaneous fat. Patients with spigelian hernias always have a distinct tenderness over the hernial orifice and an ultrasound probe positioned over this point makes it possible to determine with certainty whether there is a defect in the spigelian aponeurosis.

Computed tomography (CT) is a good alternative to ultrasound and is able to clearly delineate the abdominal wall layers (3,4,29). CT provides information about the hernial orifice, the sac and the sac contents (Fig. 35.22A and B). Scanning must include the abdominal wall defect, and the distance between cross-sectional scans must be short.

Ultrasound and CT are probably equally effective in demonstrating the hernial orifice, but CT may provide more information regarding hernial sac contents. To identify bowel loops, Yeh and colleagues (29) recommend the routine use of oral contrast medium in CT scanning of the abdominal wall when a hernia is suspected.

Ultrasound and CT may prove helpful to the surgeon by demonstrating the precise location and extent of the musculoaponeurotic defect. The examinations also provide useful information regarding the thickness of the abdominal musculature. By performing the tests in conjunction with Valsalva's maneuver, the contractility of the abdominal muscles and possible muscle paresis can also be assessed. As a result, those patients in whom a synthetic prosthesis may be indicated can be identified.

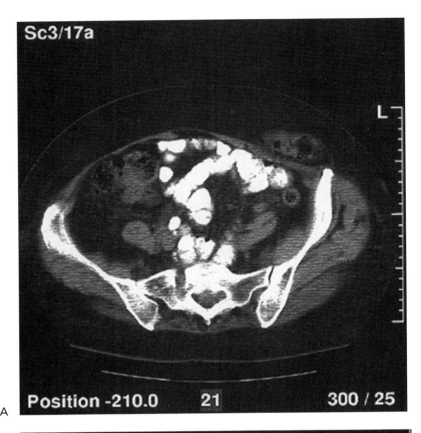

A

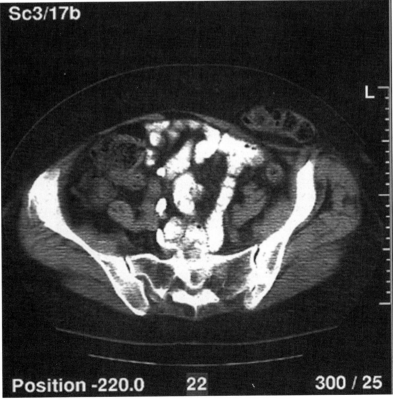

B

FIGURE 35.22 A and **B:** Computed tomographic appearance of a spigelian hernia. Spigelian hernia protruding through the spigelian aponeurosis.

SURGICAL TREATMENT

Spigelian hernia should be treated by surgical repair. Traditionally, different incisions have been recommended for palpable and nonpalpable hernias. In palpable hernias, a gridiron incision is excellent. After the external aponeurosis is split, it is usually easy to locate the hernia (Fig. 35.23). The simplest form of hernioplasty is usually sufficient. As a rule, the hernial orifice is so small that the repair will be tension free. If not, relaxing incisions should probably not be employed and the defect should be repaired with prosthetic mesh.

If a gridiron incision is used, a short incision in the anterior lamella of the rectus sheath should also be made. This provides better exposure of the spigelian aponeurosis, reducing the risk of an undetected intravaginal hernial offshoot. Defects in the posterior lamella of the rectus sheath are common and should be closed. A gridiron incision may also be used in patients without a palpable hernia in whom CT or ultrasound has shown that the hernial sac lies between the two oblique muscles. The hernial sac is then visible when the external aponeurosis is split.

If no palpable hernia or hernial orifice is detected preoperatively, a preperitoneal exploration through a paramedian incision provides good exposure (Fig. 35.24). The paramedian incision is made through the anterior lamella of the rectus sheath and the rectus muscle retracted medially so that the posterior lamella can be split longitudinally. Preperitoneal dissection is then carried out down to the spigelian aponeurosis. This enables easy inspection of a large part of the spigelian aponeurosis and the posterior lamella of the rectus sheath. The hernial orifice and additional aponeurotic defects can be exposed without difficulty and repaired without cutting muscles and aponeuroses ventral to the spigelian aponeurosis.

The advent of laparoscopic hernia repair has made these approaches obsolete in the hands of experienced laparoscopists (1,6,12). Spigelian hernias are ideally suited to preperitoneal laparoscopic repair because the defect in the spigelian aponeurosis is more clearly identifiable in the preperitoneal plane. A vertical incision is made next to the umbilicus on the contralateral side to the spigelian hernia and the anterior lamella of the rectus sheath opened. The rectus muscle is retracted laterally and a hemostat introduced into the preperitoneal plane and opened to create a pocket in the preperitoneal plane. The plane can then be further developed infraumbilically either by gentle dissection with the laparoscope or by the use of balloon dissectors. Once the plane has been opened, gas is insufflated and a further port positioned in the midline approximately halfway between the pubis and the umbilicus. An additional port is inserted laterally as close to the anterosuperior iliac spine as possible. The preperitoneal plane may then be dissected, the hernia reduced (if it has not reduced spontaneously), and the defect in the spigelian aponeurosis identified. A prosthetic mesh is then inserted in the preperitoneal plane and fixed in position covering the defect.

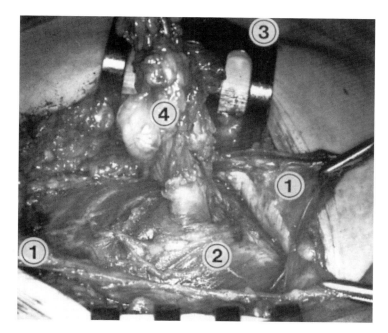

FIGURE 35.23. A typical spigelian hernia shown through a gridiron incision. The orifice measured 1.5 × 1.0 cm, and the sac was 5 cm long and surrounded by preperitoneal fat. *1,* external oblique aponeurosis; *2,* internal oblique aponeurosis; *3,* umbilicus; *4,* hernial sac enclosed in preperitoneal fat.

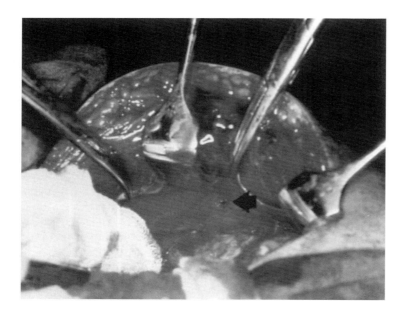

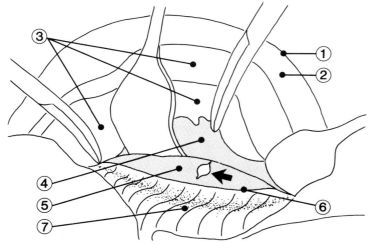

FIGURE 35.24. Spigelian hernia exposed by preperitoneal dissection. *1,* skin; *2,* subcutaneous fat; *3,* rectus abdominis muscle; *4,* dorsal lamella of rectus sheath; *5,* spigelian aponeurosis; *6,* semilunar line; *7,* peritoneum. The *arrow* marks the hernial orifice, which measured 0.4 × 0.3 cm. The hernia consisted of preperitoneal fat only.

RESULTS

The results of open operations for spigelian hernia are excellent and the risk of recurrence low (only six reported to date). The follow-up for the laparoscopic technique is still too short to be able to compare it with the open procedures. Indications for the use of prosthetic mesh in the open techniques include multiple defects within the spigelian aponeurosis, recurrent herniation, atrophy of the abdominal wall musculature due to nerve injury, and large hernial orifices.

LOW SPIGELIAN HERNIA

Hesselbach's triangle includes part of the spigelian aponeurosis caudal and medial to the inferior epigastric vessels.

Therefore, both direct inguinal hernias and low spigelian hernias may occur within the triangle. Indeed, the infrequently reported incidence of low spigelian hernias may be due to these hernias being inappropriately labeled direct inguinal hernias.

Low spigelian hernia is difficult to diagnose preoperatively, and the diagnosis is often established at the time of surgery for inguinal hernia. It is easier to treat than is a direct inguinal hernia because the hernial orifice is usually small, and the risk of recurrence is lower.

REFERENCES

1. Amendolara M. Videolaparoscopic treatment of Spigelian hernias. *Surg Lap End* 1998; 8: 136.
2. Artioukh DY, Walker SJ. Spigelian herniae: presentation, diag-

nosis and treatment. *Journal Royal Coll Surgeons Edinburgh* 1996; 41: 241.

3. Balthazar EJ, Subramanyam BR, Megibow A. Spigelian hernia: CT and ultrasonography diagnosis. *Gastrointest Radiol* 1984; 9: 81.

4. Campos SM, Walden T. Images in clinical medicine: Spigelian hernia. *N Eng J Med* 1997; 336: 1149.

5. Cooper A. *The anatomy and surgical treatment of crural and umbilical hernia, part II.* London, T Cox, T Bensley, 1807: 58.

6. Gedebou TM, Neubauer W. Laparoscopic repair of bilateral spigelian and inguinal hernias. *Surg End* 1998; 12: 1424.

7. Guivarc'h M, Fonteny R, Boche O, Roullet-Audy JC. Hernies ventrles antero-laterales dites de Spiegel. 16 cas et revue de la literature. *Chirugie* 1988:114: 572.

8. Guivarc'h M. Traitment chirugical des hernies anterior-laterales dites de Spiegel. *Presse Med* 1989; 18: 177.

9. Gullmo A. Herniography. The diagnosis of hernia in the groin and incompetence of the pouch of Douglas and pelvic floor. *Acta Radiol Scand* Suppl 1980; 361.

10. Gullmo A, Bromee A, Smedberg S. Herniography. *Surg Clin North Am* 1984; 64: 229.

11. Houlihan TJ. A review of spigelian hernias. *Am J Surg* 1976; 131: 734.

12. Kasirajan K, Lopez J, Lopez R. Laparoscopic technique in the management of Spigelian hernia. *J Laparoendosc Adv Surg Tech* 1997; 7: 385.

13. Kienzle HF, Staemmler S. Die Spighel-Hernie und ihre Behandlung. *Fortschr Med* 1978; 96: 876.

14. Klinkosch JT. Divisionem Herniarum Novamgue Herniae Ventralis Speciem Proponit. *Dissertationum Medicorum* 1764: 184.

15. Koljubakin SL. Hernia linea Spigeli. *Arch Klin Chir* 1925; 136: 739.

16. Le Dran H-F. *Traite des operations de chirurgic.* Paris, 1742: 142

17. Lindholm A, Hulin E. Hernia Spigelii-ett vanligt forekommande brack? *Nord Med* 1969; 39: 1225.

18. McVay CB, Anson BJ. Composition of the rectus sheath. *Anat Rec* 1940; 77: 213.

19. Mufid MM, Abu-Yousef MM, Kakish ME et al. Spigelian hernia: diagnosis by high-resolution real-time ultrasonography. *J Ultrasound Med* 1997; 16: 183.

20. Persson PH, Grennert L, Jogi P, Pallin B. Diagnos och operativ teknik vid hernia Spigelii. *Acta Soc Med Suecanae* 1975; 84: 213.

21. Ponka JL. Spigelian hernias. In: Joseph K, Ponka MD, eds. *Hernias of the abdominal wall.* Philadelphia, WB Saunders, 1980: 478.

22. Read RC. Spigelian hernia. In: Nyhus LM, Condon RE, eds. *Hernia,* ed 2. Philadelphia, JB Lippincott, 1978:375.

23. Rodighiero D, Fusato G, Omodei Sale S et al. Surgical anatomy, diagnosis and treatment of spigelian hernia. *Giornale di Chirurgia* 1996; 17: 485.

24. Spangen L. Spigelian hernia. *Surg Clin North Am* 1984; 64: 351.

25. Spieghel A. *Opera Quae Extant Omnia.* Amsterdam, John Bloew, 1645:103.

26. Stirnemann H. Die Spigelische Hernie: Verpasst? Selten? Verlegenheitsdiagnose? *Der Chirurg* 1982; 53: 314.

27. Stuckej AL, Lutjko GD, Tivarovskij VI. Hernias of the Spigeli line. *Tsitologiia* 1973; 15: 10.

28. Torzilli G, Carmana G, Lumachi V et al. The usefulness of ultrasonography in the diagnosis of the spigelian hernia. *Int Surg* 1995; 80: 280.

29. Yeh H-C, Lehr-Janus C, Cohen BA, Rabinowitz JG. Ultrasonography and CT of abdominal and inguinal hernias. *JCU* 1984; 12: 479.

30. Zimmerman LM, Anson BJ, Morgan EH, McVay CB. Ventral hernia due to normal banding of the abdominal muscles. *Surg Gynecol Obstet* 1944; 78: 535.

Nyhus and Condon's Hernia, Fifth Edition, edited by Robert J. Fitzgibbons, Jr. and A. Gerson Greenburg. Lippincott Williams & Wilkins, Philadelphia © 2002.

36

MANAGEMENT OF PERISTOMAL HERNIA: TECHNIQUES OF REPAIR

RUSSELL K. PEARL
JULIA H. SONE

Peristomal hernia is an incisional hernia that develops at the site of a colostomy or ileostomy, and is among the more common complications of intestinal stomas. The hernia sac usually lies within the attenuated layers of the abdominal wall, but in some instances may tract subcutaneously adjacent to the stoma.

Like many stomal complications, formation of a hernia often results from one or more technical errors, which underscores the importance of proper preoperative planning and close attention to detail in the operating room. Other factors that may contribute to the development of peristomal hernias include obesity, advanced age, malignancy, malnutrition, steroid use, and increased abdominal pressure from ascites, chronic pulmonary disease, or obstructive uropathy.

Most of these hernias should be managed conservatively, with only 10% to 20% of patients eventually needing operative intervention (11). However, a peristomal hernia may become more than a slight inconvenience for a patient already trying to cope with basic stoma care, especially if it becomes painful or precludes the adherence of a collecting pouch around the ostomy, resulting in leakage. Furthermore, a hernia sac with a narrow neck may even precipitate obstruction or strangulation of an intestinal loop, necessitating urgent laparotomy.

This chapter presents an overview of the incidence, diagnosis, and guidelines for the prevention of this complication. In addition, the indications for operation as well as the spectrum of operative repairs and corresponding outcomes are reviewed.

R. K. Pearl: Department of Surgery, University of Illinois at Chicago; Division of Colon and Rectal Surgery, Cook County Hospital, Chicago, Illinois.

J. H. Sone: Department of Surgery, Rush–Presbyterian St. Luke's Medical Center; Department of Surgery, Cook County Hospital, Chicago, Illinois.

INCIDENCE

The reported incidence of peristomal hernia varies considerably, because the data presented in many studies are not always comparable. For example, in one review, almost 1% of patients developed peristomal hernias during the same hospitalization in which the stoma was constructed (12). However, with long-term follow-up, as many as 50% of all ostomies may eventually develop this problem. Also, hernias that are included in most studies are clinically symptomatic and cannot be compared legitimately with those detected on physical examination in an asymptomatic patient, or found incidentally by computed tomography (CT).

There appears to be a stratification of hernia incidence with respect to stoma type. Pericolostomy hernias occur in 1% to 50% of patients, the most realistic estimate being 5% to 10%. The incidence of periileostomy hernia ranges from 1% to 10%, but the morbidity is higher because of the consistency and caustic nature of ileal effluent as well as the tendency for the neck of the hernia sac to be narrow (7). Cheung reviewed 322 stomas, of which 156 (48.5%) were end-sigmoid colostomies (4). The risk of a peristomal hernia in this series was 36%. The median time for appearance of a peristomal hernia associated with an end-sigmoid colostomy was 15 months. Within the first 2 years after creation of an end-sigmoid colostomy, 62% of peristomal hernias appeared.

SYMPTOMS

The majority of peristomal hernias are minimally symptomatic, with patients usually complaining only of an unsightly bulge or occasional leakage from around the stoma. Sometimes, the hernia may grow to such proportions that it becomes cosmetically unacceptable and a source of considerable psychological stress when it can no longer be concealed under loose-fitting clothing. However, the symptoms become severe enough to warrant operative correction in only 10% to 20% of patients.

Pain is a common symptom in patients with peristomal hernias. This usually results from stretching of the abdominal wall and adjacent skin by the underlying distended hernia sac. In cases where the history suggests but the physical examination does not reveal the presence of a hernia, an abdominal ultrasound or CT scan may be helpful to confirm the diagnosis. As in most abdominal hernias, a loop of intestine may become entrapped within the sac, resulting in obstructive symptoms that may progress to strangulation of the bowel. Fortunately, the necks of most peristomal hernia sacs are generally broader than those associated with inguinal hernias, accounting for the lower incidence of strangulation and obstruction among peristomal hernias.

Peristomal skin irritation is a common complaint among patients with hernias because it precludes the proper adherence of a stoma appliance to the skin. This can lead to leakage of stoma effluent, which often results in peristomal dermatitis. In some instances, the contents of a large hernia sac recede into the peritoneal cavity when the patient is recumbent and then abruptly return into the sac when the patient stands or strains. This alternating cycle of extreme stretch followed by relaxation of the abdominal skin disrupts the seal around the stoma and may result in dermatitis severe enough to necessitate operative repair.

ETIOLOGY AND PREVENTION

The development of most peristomal hernias is attributable either to inadequate preoperative preparation, such as neglecting to mark a stoma site in an emergent situation, or to one or more technical errors committed in the operating room. Other contributing factors include obesity, malnutrition, postoperative sepsis with abdominal distention, long-term steroid use, and chronic cough or obstructive uropathy, which tends to aggravate this condition.

Ideally, all patients should be evaluated preoperatively by a surgeon and an enterostomal therapist. The stoma site should be placed away from any bony prominence such as the costal margin or iliac crest; it should not be near skin folds, scars, or belt lines; nor should it be brought out through an operative incision. A small paper disc or ostomy appliance should be affixed to the abdominal skin at the desired site with the patient assuming standing, sitting, and lying positions. Ideally, two or

more alternate stoma sites should be marked for operative contingencies.

Placement of an ostomy lateral to the rectus muscle or through an operative incision is among the more common technical errors that contribute to formation of a parastomal hernia. In a study by Sjodahl and associates, the stoma was brought out through the rectus abdominis muscle in 107 patients and lateral to it in 23 patients in a standardized manner. The respective prevalence of parastomal hernia in these groups was 2.8% and 21.6% (17). Marks and Ritchie advocate tunneling the end of the intestine extraperitoneally before exteriorizing it (8). Goligher, however, is not convinced that this technique is effective (5). Furthermore, tunneling a stoma in this manner angulates the intestinal lumen at the fascial level, complicating routine stomal irrigation and follow-up colonoscopy.

Pearl and associates polled 245 practicing surgeons to determine which techniques of stomal construction are commonly in use (13). For end colostomy, 85% of surgeons routinely bring the stoma through the rectus muscle and 15% tunnel the colostomy extraperitoneally. Only 8% bring it out through the main laparotomy incision. When forming an ileostomy, 80% bring it through the rectus muscle, 12% tunnel it extraperitoneally, and 7% deliver it through the main laparotomy incision.

Fashioning the proper size opening in the abdominal wall in cases of obstruction where the proximal bowel is markedly distended is a common operative dilemma. Too large an aperture will most certainly result in a peristomal hernia, whereas too small an opening may compromise the blood supply to the stoma or obstruct the lumen. Since there is no definitive method to resolve this issue, care should be taken to avoid either extreme.

MANAGEMENT GUIDELINES AND INDICATIONS FOR OPERATION

The initial management of peristomal hernias should, with few exceptions, be nonsurgical. Most patients are willing to accept the inconvenience of a small bulge or the minimal discomfort associated with a hernia provided stoma function is satisfactory. In some instances, these symptoms can be controlled with a suitable abdominal binder fitted with a plastic ring over the stoma device, which may help keep the hernia reduced and the patient comfortable. In patients with temporary stomas, the problem is self-limited because hernia repair is accomplished in conjunction with stoma closure.

Emergency surgical intervention is indicated for intestinal obstruction or perforation occurring during colostomy irrigation. Among the most common indications for surgical treatment is failure of nonsurgical therapy, such as difficulty maintaining an adequate seal around the stoma, resulting in intractable dermatitis. Other indications include a hernia so large that it becomes cosmetically unacceptable, persistently painful, or renders stoma care practically impossible.

Contraindications to revision are factors that would probably lead to early hernia recurrence, such as severe cardiopulmonary distress and extreme obesity. Also, it would probably not be wise to operate on a patient with a limited life expectancy because of widespread metastatic disease.

Prior to surgery, a standard mechanical and antibiotic bowel preparation plus perioperative antibiotics are recommended. As stated above, evaluation of the patient by an enterostomal therapist for preoperative stoma teaching and marking is important. It is generally best to have at least two alternative stoma sites marked.

OPERATIVE STRATEGIES AND TECHNIQUES

There are two conceptual surgical approaches to peristomal hernias. The first involves moving the stoma to another preselected location on the abdominal wall and repairing the original defect. This can be accomplished either by a formal laparotomy or by locally resiting the stoma to a fresh adjacent location by gaining access to the peritoneal cavity directly through the hernial orifice after the stoma has been mobilized (Figs. 36.1 and 36.2). In the second technique, the hernia is repaired locally without changing the site of the stoma (Figs. 36.3 and 36.4). This can be carried out either by directly approximating the fascial defect with nonabsorbable sutures alone or by concomitantly reinforcing the repair with prosthetic mesh, which can be applied intraperitoneally or extrafascially. A variation of this method involves occlusion of large hernia defects with a sheet of synthetic mesh, without attempting primary fascial repair either by formal laparotomy or laparoscopy (14).

The concept of local repair seems attractive because it avoids formal laparotomy. However, the placement of prosthetic mesh adjacent to bowel with the potential for erosion and subsequent sepsis raises serious concerns. In contrast, stoma relocation has a lower recurrence rate than do any of the local repairs (with or without mesh) but requires a more extensive operation.

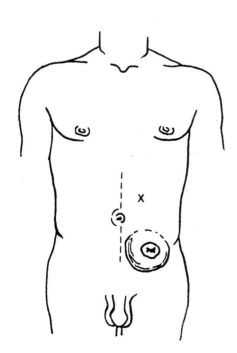
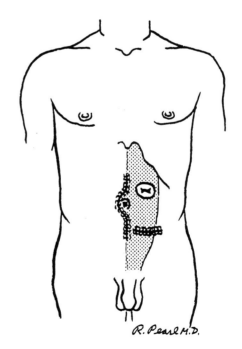

A

B

FIGURE 36.1. Relocation of colostomy for repair of peristomal hernia by formal laparotomy. **A:** A midline incision is used to take down the colostomy and repair the hernia with nonabsorbable sutures. The *X* marks the preselected stoma site. **B:** The new colostomy is brought through the rectus abdominis muscle far enough away from the costal margin and incision for secure placement of a collecting pouch. (From Pearl RK. Parastomal hernias. *World J Surg* 1989;13:569, with permission.)

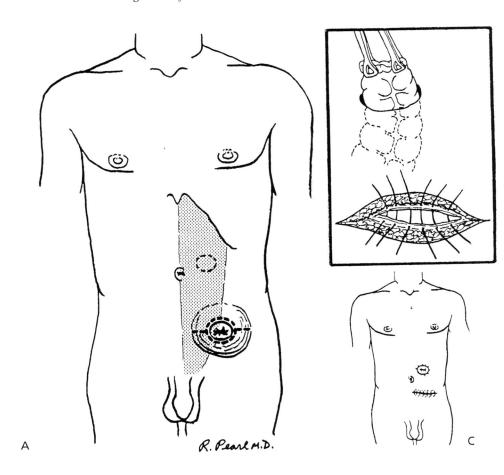

A

B

C

R. Pearl M.D.

FIGURE 36.2. Relocation of a colostomy and repair of hernia without formal laparotomy. **A:** A circumferential incision is made at the mucocutaneous junction and extended laterally. The stoma is mobilized, and the abdomen is entered via the hernia sac through this incision. The shaded area delineates the location of the rectus abdominis muscle, and the dashed circle indicates the intended stoma site. **B:** The hernia sac is excised and the fascial defect at the primary stoma site closed with interrupted sutures that are pulled up and not tied. The new stoma site is made, and the mobilized colostomy is drawn through it and matured. The sutures at the primary stoma site are now tied. This method ensures a large separation between both fascial sheath incisions and closure of the primary stoma site without tension. The skin is closed or packed open, depending upon surgeon preference. **C:** Overview of completed local stoma relocation. (From Botet X, Boldo E, Llaurado JM. Colonic parastomal hernia repair by translocation without formal laparotomy. *Br J Surg* 1996;83:981; and Stephenson BM, Phillips RKS. Parastomal hernia: local resiting and mesh repair. *Br J Surg* 1995;82:1395, with permission.)

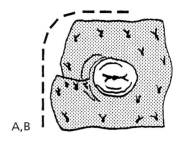
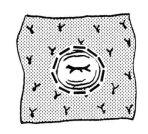

A,B

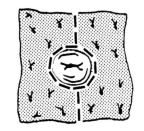
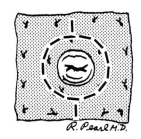

C,D

R. Pearl M.D.

FIGURE 36.3. Local peristomal hernia repair using prosthetic mesh applied extrafascially, "onlay" mesh repair. In each case, a wide area around the stoma and hernia are undermined in the subcutaneous plane. The sac is entered, its contents are reduced, and the fascial edges are reapproximated to fashion a stomal orifice of the proper size. The mesh is then sutured to the fascia to reinforce the repair in an "onlay" fashion. **A:** Curved or "hockey-stick" incision 4 to 5 cm from the edges of the stoma to preserve a zone of smooth intact peristomal skin to facilitate adherence of a collecting pouch. **B:** Incision made at the mucocutaneous junction. **C:** Extended excision at the mucocutaneous junction. **D:** Incision with 2 to 3 cm skin island around the stoma with extensions to facilitate placement of mesh. [From Pearl RK. Parastomal hernias. *World J Surg* 1989;13:569 **(A)**; Condon RE, ed. *Hernia*, 4th ed. Philadelphia, JB Lippincott Co, 1995 **(B)**; Rosin JD, Bonardi RA. Paracolostomy hernia repair with Marlex mesh: a new technique. *Dis Colon Rectum* 1977;20:299 **(C)**; and Abdu RA. Repair of paracolostomy hernias with Marlex mesh. *Dis Colon Rectum* 1982;25:529 **(D)**, with permission.]

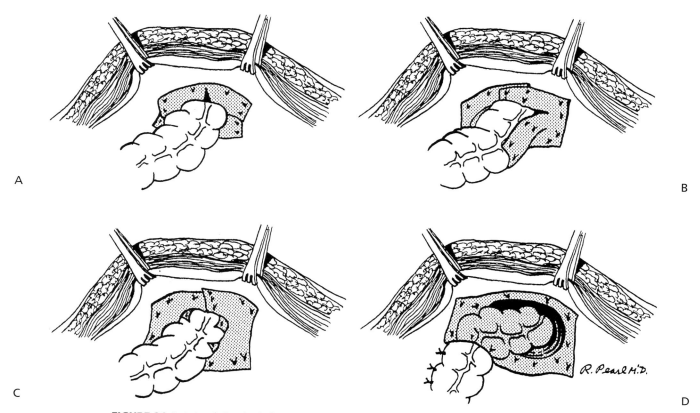

FIGURE 36.4. Intraabdominal placement of prosthetic mesh for repair of peristomal hernia via a midline laparotomy, "inlay" mesh repair. Prior to the placement of prosthetic mesh, the contents of the hernia sac are reduced and the stomal orifice is tightened with interrupted sutures. **A:** Two strips of mesh (3 cm wide and of appropriate length) are sutured lateral to the stoma overlying the hernia repair. A small slit is made in one piece of mesh to accommodate expansion of the bowel. **B:** Two pieces of rectangular mesh are cut so that each has three "fingers." The central fingers are sutured to the bowel wall. The outer fingers are passed around the bowel and overlapped to strengthen the abdominal wall. The bulk of the mesh is sutured to the abdominal wall using interrupted nonabsorbable sutures to ensure coverage well beyond the hernia repair. **C:** A stellate-shaped incision is made in a large sheet of polytetrafluoroethylene material and fixed to the fascia and bowel wall. **D:** In this instance, the fascia is not repaired primarily, but after the hernia has been reduced, a large sheet of mesh is placed over the defect and sutured to the edges of the fascia as well as the bowel wall. [From Byers JM, Steinberg JB, Postier RG. Repair of parastomal hernias using polypropylene mesh. *Arch Surg* 1992;127:1246 **(A)**; Morris-Stiff G, Hughes LE. The continuing challenge of parastomal hernia: failure of a novel polypropylene mesh repair. *Ann R Coll Surg Engl* 1998;80:184, **(B)**; Hofstetter WL, Vukasin P, Ortega A, et al. New technique for mesh repair of paracolostomy hernia. *Dis Colon Rectum* 1998;41:1054; and **(C)** Sugarbaker PH. Peritoneal approach to prosthetic mesh repair of paraostomy hernias. *Ann Surg* 1985;201:344 **(D)**, with permission.]

OUTCOMES AND RECOMMENDATIONS

Most of the literature on the surgical repair of peristomal hernias consists of small anecdotal retrospective series. The fact that no definitive prospective randomized studies have been carried out make it difficult to draw meaningful conclusions as to which procedure consistently results in the most favorable outcome.

For example, in a large published series, Rubin and associates reviewed the outcomes of 68 peristomal hernia repairs in 55 patients with a median follow-up of 31 months (16). Of these cases, 36 (53%) underwent a local

fascial repair only, 25 (37%) had the stomas relocated, and the remaining 7 (10%) had a fascial repair reinforced with mesh. Overall, 63% of patients developed a recurrent peristomal hernia. For first-time repairs, hernias recurred in 76% of patients following local repairs and in 33% of the relocation group. However, the incidence of incisional hernias was 52% in patients following stoma relocation and only 3% of patients following fascial repair. For recurrent peristomal hernias, local repair with prosthetic mesh was successful in two out of three patients studied (67%), whereas only two of seven (29%) stoma relocations yielded satisfactory results (16). These disappointing data suggest that there is no optimal technique for peristomal hernia repair, and that each method seems to be associated with substantial morbidity.

The best way of dealing with peristomal hernias is preventing them from occurring. This can be facilitated by proper preoperative planning and close attention to detail in the operating room, especially with respect to the size of the stomal aperture in the abdominal wall. When assessing a patient for potential operative repair, it is important to remember that the majority of peristomal hernias are well tolerated and can usually be managed conservatively. When surgery is indicated, it has been our preference to relocate the stoma to another quadrant of the abdominal wall after an optimal site has been selected in conjunction with an enterostomal therapist. For recurrent hernias, it may be worthwhile to reinforce the repair with prosthetic mesh using one of the techniques outlined above.

REFERENCES

1. Abdu RA. Repair of paracolostomy hernias with Marlex mesh. *Dis Colon Rectum* 1982;25:529.
2. Botet X, Boldo E, Llaurado JM. Colonic parastomal hernia repair by translocation without formal laparotomy. *Br J Surg* 1996;83:981.
3. Byers JM, Steinberg JB, Postier RG. Repair of parastomal hernias using polypropylene mesh. *Arch Surg* 1992;127:1246.
4. Cheung MT. Complications of an abdominal stoma: an analysis of 322 stomas. *Aust NZ J Surg* 1995;65:808.
5. Goligher JC, ed. *Surgery of the anus, rectum and colon,* 4th ed. London: Bailliere Tindall, 1980.
6. Hofstetter WL, Vukasin P, Ortega A, et al. New technique for mesh repair of paracolostomy hernia. *Dis Colon Rectum* 1998;41:1054.
7. Horgan K, Hughes LE. Para-ileostomy hernia: failure of a local repair technique. *Br J Surg* 1986;73:439.
8. Marks CG, Ritchie JK. The complications of synchronous combined excision for adenocarcinoma of the rectum at St. Mark's Hospital. *Br J Surg* 1975;62:901.
9. Morris-Stiff G, Hughes LE. The continuing challenge of parastomal hernia: failure of a novel polypropylene mesh repair. *Ann R Coll Surg Engl* 1998;80:184–187.
10. Nyhus LM, Condon RE, eds. *Hernia,* 4th ed. Philadelphia: JB Lippincott Co, 1995.
11. Pearl RK. Parastomal hernias. *World J Surg* 1989;13:569.
12. Pearl RK, Prasad ML, Orsay CP, et al. Early local complications from intestinal stomas. *Arch Surg* 1985;120:1145.
13. Pearl RK, Prasad ML, Orsay CP, et al. A survey of technical considerations in the construction of intestinal stomas. *Am Surg* 1988;51:462.
14. Porcheron J, Payan B, Balique JG. Mesh repair of paracolostomal hernia by laparoscopy. *Surg Endosc* 1998;12:1281.
15. Rosin JD, Bonardi RA. Paracolostomy hernia repair with Marlex mesh: a new technique. *Dis Colon Rectum* 1977;20:299.
16. Rubin MS, Schoetz DJ, Matthews JB. Parastomal hernia: is stoma relocation superior to fascial repair? *Arch Surg* 1994;129:413.
17. Sjödahl R, Anderberg B, Bolin T. Parastomal hernia in relation to the site of the abdominal stoma. *Br J Surg* 1988;75:339–341.
18. Stephenson BM, Phillips RKS. Parastomal hernia: local resiting and mesh repair. *Br J Surg* 1995;82:1395.
19. Sugarbaker PH. Peritoneal approach to prosthetic mesh repair of paraostomy hernias. *Ann Surg* 1985;201:344.

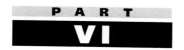

PEDIATRIC HERNIAS

37

OMPHALOCELE AND GASTROSCHISIS: PEDIATRIC SURGERY

JOHN J. AIKEN

Omphalocele and gastroschisis are two common congenital abdominal wall defects. Although an understanding of the etiology of these defects remains incomplete, most pediatric surgeons consider them as distinct embryologic and developmental malformations. The prenatal and newborn management of these disorders remains a major challenge in modern pediatric surgical practice (12). Similar to other congenital disorders, they represent defects in development linked to either chromosomal abnormalities or environmental and teratogenic effects. This chapter examines briefly the embryology of normal abdominal wall development and specific fetal events believed to lead to the newborn presentation of either omphalocele or gastroschisis, and describes the current diagnostic and therapeutic management of infants with these congenital abdominal wall malformations.

EMBRYOLOGY

During the third and fourth weeks of fetal life, the midgut grows and elongates more rapidly than the embryo and becomes housed in the yolk sac outside the embryonic coelom. The primitive gut of the embryo is already partitioned into foregut, midgut, and hindgut. By the fourth week, as the abdominal cavity enlarges, the midgut returns into the embryo and undergoes rotation and fixation. The integrity of the abdominal wall and the development of the peritoneal cavity are dependent on the return of the midgut along with proper development and fusion of cephalic, caudal, and lateral embryonic folds as they come together at the umbilicus. Omphalocele is thought to result from partial or complete arrest in the development of one or more of these embryonic folds (10,31). Cephalic fold arrest leads to varying degrees of "epigastric omphalocele," which is fre-

quently associated with lower thoracic wall malformations such as sternal cleft, and diaphragmatic, pericardial, and cardiac anomalies. The consistent association of defects of the abdominal wall, lower sternum, ventral diaphragm, pericardium, and heart is referred to as "Cantrell's pentalogy" (5). Caudal fold arrest leads to "hypogastric omphalocele" and abnormalities of the hindgut (imperforate anus) or lower abdominal wall defects such as bladder exstrophy or cloacal exstrophy. The most common condition is lateral fold arrest, leading to "midabdominal omphalocele" and varying degrees of extrusion of the intraabdominal contents, including liver, spleen, stomach, and intestines. As a consequence of these different forms of developmental arrest and failure of midgut return, omphalocele is always characterized by failure of normal formation of the umbilical ring and nonrotation of the intestines (31).

The developmental anatomy of gastroschisis is controversial, and the research lacks the study of early fetal specimens that was done with omphalocele. In 1953, Moore and Stokes reviewed the literature and "redefined" gastroschisis as an "extraumbilical abdominal wall defect with a large extracorporeal mass of discolored intestines of leathery consistency often embedded in a rather dense gelatinous matrix" (24). The eviscerated intestines are not covered by a sac, and the insertion of the umbilical cord into the abdominal wall is normal. The hernia defect is to the right of the umbilical cord insertion, and small and large intestine are herniated, but rarely is there herniation of a portion of the liver. The herniated loops of bowel are thickened, adherent, and frequently covered with an inflammatory "peel." The herniated bowel is more frequently infarcted or associated with atresia than in omphalocele. There is obligate malrotation of the intestines, but other major congenital malformations are infrequent. Gastroschisis is believed to represent rupture of the umbilical cord at a site of failure of vascularization of the abdominal wall, likely secondary to complete dissolution of the right umbilical vein at a time before collateral circulation can maintain integrity of the mesenchyme (9,17).

J. J. Aiken: Division of Pediatric Surgery, Medical College of Wisconsin; Division of Pediatric Surgery, Children's Hospital of Wisconsin, Milwaukee, Wisconsin.

DEFINITION

Omphalocele is a central abdominal wall defect through which both solid and hollow abdominal viscera may pass. The defect is covered by a membrane consisting of amnion externally and peritoneum internally. The umbilical cord inserts onto this membrane unless there has been prenatal rupture and dissolution of the membrane (rare). The omphalocele defect can vary considerably in size, from only a few centimeters allowing herniation into the base of the umbilical cord to large defects extending to the lower costal margins and pelvis. These large defects, known as "giant omphalocele," may be associated with complex malformations of the lower thorax, diaphragm, pericardium, and heart (Cantrell's pentalogy) or pelvic viscera with bladder or cloacal exstrophy (Figs. 37.1 and 37.2) (25).

In gastroschisis, the abdominal wall defect is uniformly small (4 cm or less) and is located to the right of the umbilical cord, which has a normal insertion into the abdominal wall. There may be a patch of skin between the umbilical cord and the defect. There is no membrane covering the eviscerated intestines, which typically include the entire small intestine and colon down to the sigmoid and may also

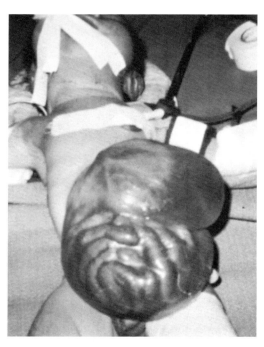

FIGURE 37.2. Giant omphalocele that contained the entire liver, spleen, gonads, and gastrointestinal tract. The abdominal wall defect extends from the flank to flank and from xiphoid to pubis. With the staged method, using silicone rubber sheets that were sewn to the skin flaps, after 4 weeks it finally was possible to make a ventral hernia covered with the patient's own skin.

involve extruded stomach, internal genitalia, undescended testis, and bladder. The bowel serosa is thickened and covered with an inflammatory "peel," presumably as a result of exposure to amniotic fluid. Individual loops of bowel are often matted together by dense, fibrinous adhesions, and

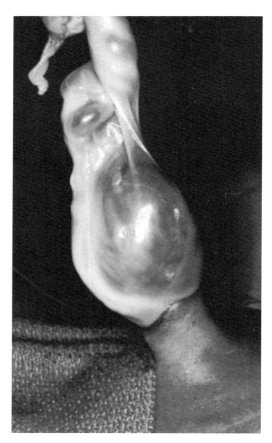

FIGURE 37.1. Small intact omphalocele (hernia into the umbilical cord) was repaired with one-stage primary closure of the abdominal wall defect.

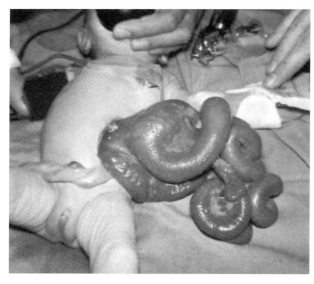

FIGURE 37.3. Newborn infant with gastroschisis showing moderate visceroabdominal disproportion. The intestine is thick and edematous, and it appears shortened as a result of exposure to amniotic fluid.

there is frequently associated intestinal atresia, stenosis, or infarction (15%) (Fig. 37.3) (13,22).

INCIDENCE AND EPIDEMIOLOGY

In the United States, the combined incidence of omphalocele and gastroschisis is approximately 1 in 2,000 to 3,000 live births. It is difficult to determine the relative incidence of the individual defects because most earlier series lack precise classification, with cases of gastroschisis being included as ruptured omphalocele. Interestingly, in earlier reports omphalocele was the more common condition, but in the past 2 decades there seems to be a significant increase in the incidence of gastroschisis, with the incidence of omphalocele being unchanged during the same period (12,21,22). Epidemiologic studies have also demonstrated the incidence of gastroschisis to be increased in association with young maternal age and low gravidity. No geographic or racial predilections have been observed for either condition. Both conditions occur in males and females equally.

ASSOCIATED MALFORMATIONS

Associated malformations occur more frequently with omphalocele than with gastroschisis, and an incidence greater than 50% is reported in most series. More than 40% of fetuses with omphalocele have chromosomal abnormalities, including trisomy 13, 18, and 21, as well as Turner's syndrome and Klinefelter's syndrome (12,31). Gastrointestinal, cardiac, central nervous system, genitourinary, and skeletal abnormalities are also common in association with omphalocele. Clustering of anomalies including omphalocele occurs as part of three syndromes: (a) the lower midline syndrome with vesicointestinal fistula, imperforate anus, colonic agenesis, and bladder exstrophy; (b) the upper midline syndrome described by Cantrell, Haller, and Ravitch, which includes sternal, diaphragmatic, pericardial, and cardiac defects; and (c) the Beckwith–Wiedemann syndrome with macroglossia, hypoglycemia, and gigantism (31). Cardiovascular malformations are reported in 10% to 25% of the cases, with the most common lesions being Fallot's tetralogy and atrial septal defects (secundum). It is the high incidence of these severe associated cardiac and chromosomal anomalies that explains the high mortality rates for many infants with omphalocele.

In contrast, gastroschisis is rarely associated with other serious malformations. Chromosomal abnormalities are so infrequently reported that it is not routine to recommend amniocentesis in infants diagnosed prenatally. The most serious associated malformations are intestinal atresia, stenosis, and infarction presumably related to ischemia of the eviscerated intestines (Fig. 37.4) (28). Other associated abnormalities include malrotation, Meckel's diverticulum,

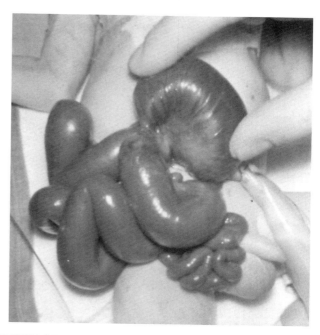

FIGURE 37.4. Newborn male infant with gastroschisis defect and low jejunal atresia.

growth retardation, and cryptorchidism in males (19,31). Occasionally, infants have suffered volvulus or extensive intestinal infarction *in utero* and at the time of birth have extremely short length of intestine and short bowel syndrome. The overall mortality rate for gastroschisis is approximately 5% to 10% and is related to the complications of sepsis or prolonged intestinal dysfunction.

PRENATAL DIAGNOSIS AND MANAGEMENT

The diagnosis of omphalocele or gastroschisis is often made on *in utero* ultrasound after 14 weeks of gestation, when the fetal midgut has normally returned to the abdominal cavity. Differentiation between omphalocele and gastroschisis can be made by the identification of liver outside the abdomen or the presence of a sac or sac remnant (Fig. 37.5) (2,18). When an abdominal wall defect is identified on screening maternal ultrasound, a follow-up examination should be performed with a detailed anatomic survey for associated malformations, especially in cases of omphalocele. Assessment of fetal growth parameters by measurement of biparietal skull diameter and femur length should be performed. The size of the defect and the volume of eviscerated intestine can be estimated as well as the presence of a covering and the umbilical cord insertion site. Careful survey for possible associated heart, central nervous system, or genitourinary abnormalities is performed. Patients believed to have omphalocele should have karyotype analysis by amniocentesis. Prenatal diagnosis allows for delivery in a

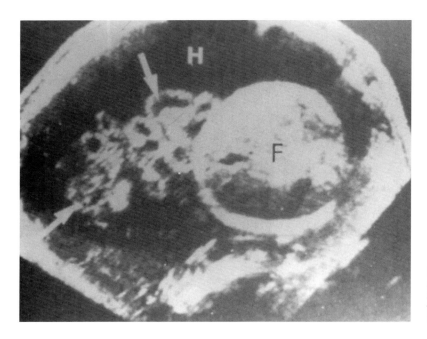

FIGURE 37.5. Maternal ultrasound study performed at 30 weeks of gestation, shows appearance of characteristic gastroschisis abdominal wall defect. *F,* fetus; *H,* amniotic fluid. *Arrows* point to eviscerated intestine.

perinatal center able to provide both high-risk obstetric care and early pediatric surgical evaluation after delivery. Most infants can be delivered vaginally, but in infants with giant omphalocele cesarean section may be necessary (34). Recent reports have demonstrated that immediate repair of gastroschisis after delivery may increase the percentage of infants able to have primary abdominal wall closure, and also improve outcome variables such as time on mechanical ventilation, time to enteral feedings, and total length of hospitalization (6,7,34). In gastroschisis, timing of delivery is controversial. There is a significant incidence of late fetal demise in cases of gastroschisis, and present studies are investigating the importance of progressive bowel dilation on serial ultrasound examinations. At present, some perinatologists and pediatric surgeons favor induced delivery in cases of gastroschisis at a point after 36 weeks of gestation, once fetal lung maturity has been demonstrated.

NEWBORN MANAGEMENT

The physiologic impact of omphalocele is related to its size and, more significantly, to the presence of associated anomalies. In cases of giant omphalocele, there may be significant pulmonary hypoplasia and a globular central liver, which can compromise venous return to the heart and cardiac output. Generally, with omphalocele the intestinal length is normal and there is no thickening or inflammation unless there has been *in utero* rupture of the membrane (rare). Normal intestinal motility and absorptive function have been almost universally observed. In contrast, gastroschisis typically results in severe abnormalities of bowel function. A spectrum of changes is seen involving intestinal length, motility, and nutrient absorption. These changes are presumably related to vascular compromise, volvulus, partial or complete bowel obstruction leading to dilation, and exposure to amniotic fluid, particularly amniotic fluid containing urine, which exists after 30 weeks of gestation (27).

Common principles of newborn resuscitation and preoperative management apply to infants with omphalocele and gastroschisis. The immediate management of the newborn with an abdominal wall defect involves nasogastric decompression, ventilatory support if necessary, and systemic antibiotics. Masked ventilation should be avoided because it is likely to contribute to distention of the intestines. A careful examination is made for associated malformations. All infants require aggressive fluid resuscitation and careful attention to avoid hypothermia. In cases of omphalocele, specific evaluation for macroglossia and craniofacial abnormalities characteristic of Beckwith–Wiedemann syndrome must be identified as these infants are at risk of hypoglycemia and seizures, which can lead to permanent neurologic injury (12,26). In omphalocele, the intestines and viscera are covered and protected by the membrane and an optimum dressing is saline-moistened gauze and plastic wrap to prevent heat loss. In omphalocele, the careful evaluation for associated anomalies should have priority over concern for surgical repair, provided the membrane is intact. Severe mechanical problems can also occur due to the weight of the intestinal mass and liver, and can result in volvulus, caval compression, and hepatic vein kinking. These problems are avoided by placing the infant on his or her side and supporting the intestinal mass. Palpation of the sternum for a sternal cleft, a chest radiograph, echocardiogram, and renal ultrasound are all important in the early evaluation of infants with omphalocele.

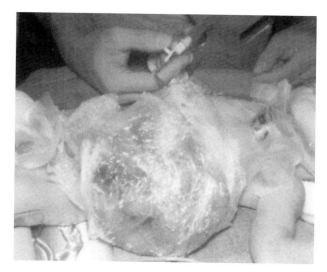

FIGURE 37.6. Newborn infant with gastroschisis abdominal defect showing Silastic sheet over viscera to maintain body heat and prevent injury to intestine as the infant is transported to the operating room.

The initial approach to gastroschisis is different because of the relative freedom from associated anomalies and the urgency created due to the exposure of the bowel. In cases of gastroschisis, the intestine is uniformly associated with malrotation and a narrow vascular pedicle supplying the entire midgut. A preeminent concern in management is to avoid torsion or kinking of the vascular pedicle, leading to intestinal ischemia and possible infarction. The infant should be positioned on his or her side with the bowel mass carefully supported to prevent torsion or kinking of the vascular pedicle. The exposed bowel in gastroschisis should be covered with a transparent dressing, allowing for frequent assessment of bowel perfusion. This can be accomplished using transparent surgical bowel bags, which also aid in maintaining warmth of the infant (Fig. 37.6). The infant with gastroschisis is at much greater risk for fluid losses from the exposed bowel, hypothermia, and sepsis. Aggressive fluid administration, warming measures, and broad-spectrum antibiotics should be instituted immediately after delivery (23).

DEFINITIVE MANAGEMENT

Nonoperative Treatment

Nonoperative treatment is rarely indicated. Nonoperative management consists of using topical agents, which initially provide desiccation of the intact membrane and a bacteriostatic eschar, followed by progressive epithelialization, creating a large ventral hernia. This treatment plan requires an intact sac and therefore is not applicable in cases of gastroschisis or ruptured omphalocele. Select patients with giant omphalocele, and premature infants with omphalocele and acute respiratory distress syndrome, and omphalo-

cele associated with major anomalies such as complex heart disease or lethal chromosomal abnormalities may be managed nonoperatively (1,38). Alcohol was first used, and subsequently a wide variety of agents have been tried, including Mercurochrome (Purepac, Elizabeth, NJ, U.S.A.) (mercury levels must be monitored), silver sulfadiazine (Silvadene, Hoescht–Marion–Roussel, Kansas City, MO, U.S.A.), 0.5% silver nitrate solution, povidone–iodine solution (Betadine, The Purdue Frederick Company, Norwalk, CT, U.S.A.), and Xeroform (Kendall Healthcare Products, Manfield, MA, U.S.A.) gauze. It must be remembered that any prolonged use of iodinated compounds is accompanied by the risk of thyroid suppression. Problems encountered with nonoperative management include a significant risk of infection and possible sepsis, rupture of the sac during the dressing and epithelialization phase, and the resultant large ventral hernia, which may eventually require repair (34). Improved surgical measures in conjunction with advances in respiratory support and neonatal intensive care have relegated topical therapy to a secondary role that is employed only in highly selected cases.

Surgical Treatment

The goal of surgical management of abdominal wall defects is to accomplish skin, fascia, and muscle closure of the abdominal wall, which ultimately restores the form and normal muscular function of the anterior abdominal wall. Most cases of omphalocele and gastroschisis are managed operatively with either primary or staged abdominal wall closure. Surgical management and decision-making of omphalocele and gastroschisis is similar, and must take into account the size of the defect, the volume of eviscerated mass, gestational age and birthweight of the infant, and the presence of other severe anomalies. The decision to perform skin flap closure (Fig. 37.7), primary abdominal wall closure, or staged reduction followed by delayed closure requires significant surgical experience and judgment in conjunction with quantitative measures of physiologic parameters. The major complications of overzealous attempts at primary closure are due to the attendant marked increase in intraabdominal pressure resulting in respiratory compromise from elevated diaphragms, cardiovascular compromise from caval compression, and decreased venous return and intestinal and renal compromise from hypoperfusion and ischemia (37).

Omphalocele

The major advance in the surgical management of infants with omphalocele came in 1948, when Gross described a technique for repairing the abdominal wall in two stages (14). The essential feature of the first stage was the preservation of the amniotic membrane and coverage with widely mobilized skin flaps. The skin flaps were raised laterally off the fascial edges and approximated in the midline over the

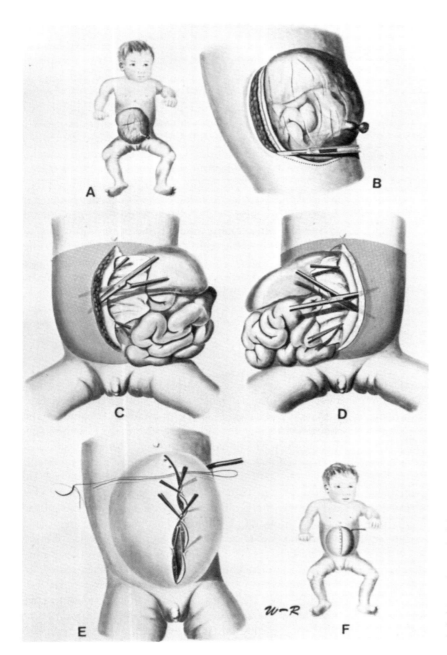

FIGURE 37.7. Operative technique for skin closure over the omphalocele (**A**). The cuff of skin at the base of the sac is incised circumferentially (**B**). The umbilical vein and arteries are ligated, and the sac with the attached small rim of skin is removed. After a thorough abdominal exploration, the skin and subcutaneous tissues are cut free on both sides and sufficiently undermined into each flank over the lower abdomen, but not above the level of the xiphoid (**C** and **D**). Then the cutaneous flaps are approximated without tension over the exposed viscera (**E**) to create a ventral hernia covered with skin (**F**).

viscera with simple sutures. After a period of growth and enlargement of the abdominal cavity, the second stage was repair of the massive ventral hernia. The problem realized with this technique was that the intestines and often the liver simply lay under the skin flaps but over the muscles of the anterior abdominal wall and even the lower ribs, so that growth of the viscera merely stretched the skin but did not enlarge the abdominal cavity. Also, the separation of the fascial edges from the skin permitted retraction of the muscle and fascia posteriorly, creating a massive ventral hernia that was later difficult to close. In modern practice, skin flap closure is most often employed in patients with major associ-

ated anomalies, in conjunction with primary closure when there is a small residual area of muscular defect and as a secondary measure when a planned staged closure using a silo fails due to separation or dislodgement.

Small and medium-sized omphalocele defects can usually be managed with primary closure of all layers (muscle, fascia, and skin) with appropriate monitoring of ventilatory changes and intraabdominal pressure. Primary closure is the ideal treatment as it accomplishes definitive treatment of the abdominal wall defect with a single operation and eliminates the potential problems of infection and sac disruption. After initial stabilization and completion of the preoperative evaluation, including chest x-ray and cardiac and renal ultrasound, the infant is brought to the operating room in a warm, sterile environment, with the sac covered with warm dressings and plastic sheeting. Surgery is performed with the infant under general endotracheal anesthesia, including maximal paralysis with muscle relaxants. Once anesthesia has been induced and stabilized, the dressings are removed and the skin prepared using warm povidone–iodine solution. The infant is particularly prone to hypothermia during skin preparation, and prior to removal of the dressings appropriate measures to avoid hypothermia include ensuring a warm operating room, wrapping of the extremities, a warming pad beneath the infant, and warmed intravenous fluids. Arterial and central venous lines, if not already present, are placed to be used in assessment of ventilatory status and intraabdominal pressure when the abdomen is closed. Nasogastric tubes and Foley catheters can be transduced to quantitatively measure intraabdominal pressure (36).

Controversy exists regarding the removal of the membrane in the operative management of omphalocele. In cases of small or medium-sized defects, without evisceration of the liver, removal of the sac facilitates delineation of the fascial edges and either primary closure or securing a silo to the fascial edges. With larger defects, the sac is attached to larger areas of the liver, and removal of the sac can be attended by significant laceration of the newborn liver and hemodynamic instability due to difficulty controlling the position of the liver and the large volume of eviscerated intestines. If the sac is removed, the umbilical vessels are individually identified and ligated. Alternatively, one umbilical artery may be cannulated and transplanted to the lower abdomen through a stab wound and used as an arterial line. If the sac is removed, care is taken to avoid injury to the liver capsule in areas of adherence as liver lacerations or capsular tears can be life threatening in the newborn. Portions of the sac may be left attached to the liver capsule if they cannot be detached safely. If the sac is removed, the intestines and remainder of the abdomen should be inspected for other anomalies. Because most of these infants exhibit various degrees of nonrotation of the intestine, the area of the duodenum is inspected carefully for obstructive bands and kinks that may require correction. Skin flaps are raised using sharp dissection to delineate the fascial edges. The intestines are decompressed of fluid and meconium both proximally, with a nasogastric or orogastric tube, and distally by "milking" the meconium through the anus. It is important during this time to ensure that the infant does not receive excessive intravenous fluids, which can lead to marked swelling and engorgement of the liver and the possibility of spontaneous rupture of the liver capsule. The abdominal wall may be stretched manually in all quadrants to enlarge the abdominal domain. Most often, the muscle and fascia are closed as a single layer closure, employing simple or figure-of-eight dissolvable sutures. Some pediatric surgeons prefer a musculofascial closure using a series of far-near/near-far "pulley"

stitches of absorbable suture with simple stitches placed between them. This method helps overcome excess tension without tearing through the fascia. The sutures are all placed prior to tying any, in accordance with traditional principle of closure without tension. When the pulley stitches are pulled up gradually, the fascial edges will approximate, allowing the simple sutures to be tied without tension followed by the pulley stitches. The previously described pressure monitoring is employed to guide the closure and ensure the abdomen is not "too tight" (37). Assessment must be made of airway compliance, peak ventilatory pressure, and perfusion. Optimum results are obtained when the abdominal compartment pressure and central venous pressure do not exceed 20 mm Hg, and peak ventilatory pressures do not exceed 30 cm H_2O. At the completion of the fascial closure, there commonly is excess skin with ragged edges. Nonviable skin edges are trimmed and the skin is typically closed using a dissolvable subcuticular dermal suture. A purse-string suture may be used to recreate an umbilical site.

If a staged silo reduction is used, a Dacron (Meadox Medical, Oakland, N.J., U.S.A.)-reinforced Silastic (Dow Corning, Midland, MI, U.S.A.) membrane is attached to the full thickness of the musculofascial abdominal wall on both sides of the abdominal defect after delineating the fascial edges by raising small skin flaps (3,30,32). The silo is attached to the musculofascial abdominal wall using either interrupted or continuous nonabsorbable sutures (Fig. 37.8). Aggressive skin flap formation should be avoided because it leads to skin retraction, which is detrimental to subsequent skin closure. The walls of the prosthetic silo should be constructed parallel to each other as a straight-walled structure so that the base is as wide as the top, preventing a conical narrow entry into the abdominal cavity. The Silastic sheets are sutured or stapled closed along the sides and along the top (Fig. 37.9). Preformed silos are also available in various sizes. These typically have a compressible ring, which is inserted beneath the fascia and then expands, and are secured to the full thickness abdominal wall and skin with interrupted nonabsorbable sutures. Antibiotic ointment is applied along the skin edges and the suture line attaching the silo to the fascia. The silastic sheeting is wrapped with sterile gauze wrap (Kerlix Soft Band, Ethicon, Inc., Somerville, NJ, U.S.A.), which can also be moistened with a dilute povidone–iodine solution. Plastic wrap is then generally used as a final layer around the silo to minimize heat loss. Once the infant is returned to the neonatal intensive care unit, the silo is stabilized and supported to the heating element of the warming table over the infant, using heavy suture material or an umbilical tape.

At daily intervals, staged reduction is accomplished in the neonatal intensive care unit (Fig. 37.8). Mild sedation is administered, and the silo is unwrapped under aseptic conditions. Careful inspection is performed for signs of sepsis or dehiscence. The viscera are reduced into the abdomen by gently squeezing down from the top portion of the silo

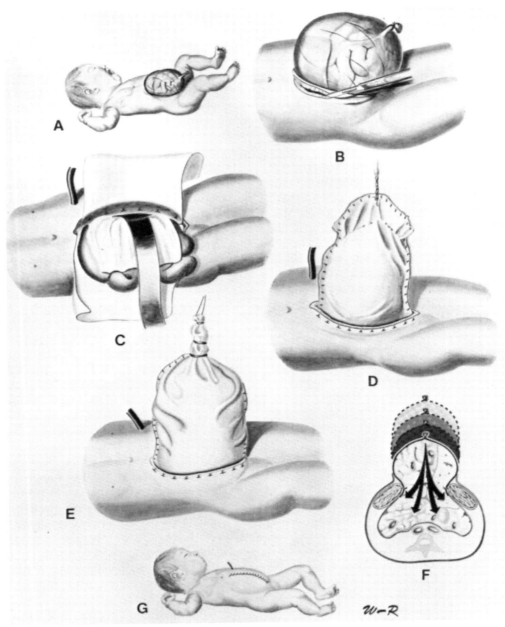

FIGURE 37.8. Method for the staged primary repair of a large omphalocele **(A)**. A circumferential incision is made around the base of the omphalocele sac **(B)**, the umbilical vein and arteries are ligated, and the sac with a small rim of the adjacent skin is removed. After abdominal exploration and performance of gastrostomy, two silicone rubber sheets are sewn to the full thickness of the abdominal wall around the margins of the defect **(C)**. The sheets are approximated over the viscera as the excess sheeting is removed **(D)**. Postoperatively, the size of the prosthesis is reduced progressively at intervals of 1 to 3 days. This is done by squeezing off and tying the sac **(E)** to reduce its size and to increase the size of the true intraabdominal space **(F)**. At the final stage, all remaining excess sheeting is removed and the abdominal wall is closed anatomically **(G)** without producing excessive intraabdominal pressure.

while the infant is observed for signs of respiratory distress or excessive increase in intraabdominal pressure. The sac is tied or sutured at the reduced level and covered with a sterile dressing and plastic wrap as before. Experience with the staged reduction technique has demonstrated that closure usually can be accomplished within 5 to 7 days, and this is attended with reduced morbidity and mortality compared to earlier experience, when often the reduction process was protracted over several weeks (21). Once the silo has been in place for 7 days, there is significant increase in the inci-

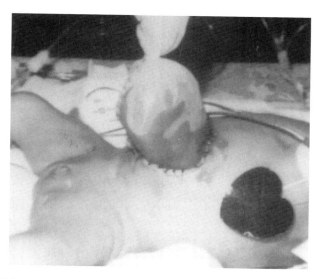

FIGURE 37.9. Prosthetic Silastic chimney attached to skin and muscle to contain eviscerated intestine until edema subsides and the abdomen enlarges.

dence of sepsis and dehiscence. When the sac is flush or nearly flush with the abdominal wall without tension, the infant is returned to the operating room and placed under general endotracheal anesthesia. After skin preparation as previously described, the silo is removed and fascial closure is performed with interrupted absorbable sutures in identical fashion as was described for primary closure. The infant is returned to the neonatal intensive care unit and typically is maintained sedated and even paralyzed for 24 to 48 hours to permit an initial period of healing before straining against the closure. Intestinal decompression with a nasogastric or orogastric tube is continued until there is return of bowel function. Systemic antibiotics are continued typically for 24 to 48 hours.

Considerable experience and judgment are required in the management of larger defects and giant omphaloceles. Management options include staged reduction using a silo followed by delayed primary closure, or staged reduction followed by delayed partial musculofascial closure and the use of prosthetic material to complete the musculofascial closure (14). Alternatively, in difficult cases, primary coverage with skin flaps may be used. In any of the described abdominal wall closure techniques, either closed suction or passive drains may be used if large flaps are raised.

GASTROSCHISIS

In infants with gastroschisis, the focus of the newborn evaluation is not on associated anomalies but on the recognition of possible *in utero* complications, including prematurity; initial infant growth retardation; malrotation and midgut volvulus; and segmental bowel infarction, perfora-

tion, and atresia (27). Resuscitation has previously been discussed, including aggressive intravenous fluids, nasogastric decompression, and systemic antibiotics. Hypothermia and dehydration are immediate primary concerns because exposure of the intestines to the ambient environment results in rapid heat and fluid losses. All efforts to prevent hypothermia are employed, including a warming pad, wrapping of extremities, and warming of intravenous fluids. The intestine should be wrapped with thin plastic sheeting and the infant placed in either an incubator or a plastic bag up to the axilla. The placement of warm, moist gauze to the intestines should be avoided as it leads to rapid cooling of the infant, and the gauze may become adherent to the inflamed intestine, making it difficult to remove without causing injury. A nasogastric or orogastric tube is inserted for intestinal decompression, and systemic antibiotics are initiated. Fluid requirements in a newborn with gastroschisis are typically 175 to 225 mL/kg/day (or two and one half to three times the normal requirement) in the first 24 hours of life (23). After initial resuscitation and stabilization, and typically within hours of birth, the infant is taken to the operating room for repair. Under general endotracheal anesthesia, careful evaluation of the eviscerated intestine is performed, looking for necrotic tissue, perforations, or atresias. Intestinal atresia and perforation are seen in approximately 10% to 15% and 6% of cases, respectively (Fig. 37.9). Any manipulation of the bowel is performed with attention to the narrow vascular pedicle to avoid torsion or injury. The abdominal wall defect is enlarged either vertically or transversely to improve the ability to inspect the viscera and proceed with reduction and closure. Because the umbilical cord has a normal insertion into the abdominal wall, it may be preserved or removed after ligation of the individual vessels. Attempts to evacuate the bowel by gentle "milking" of the meconium out through the anus or warm saline rectal irrigations may be helpful, but care must be taken to avoid injury to the intestine or mesentery. If a Meckel's diverticulum is present, it should be left in place and not excised. The abdominal wall may be manually stretched to enlarge the abdominal domain. Once the abdominal contents—which may include small and large bowel, stomach, bladder, ovaries, uterine tubes, and undescended testis—have been reduced, interrupted absorbable suture closure of the musculofascial layer is performed as previously detailed for primary closure of omphalocele. Skin closure is typically with absorbable subcuticular sutures. Decisions regarding staged silo reduction versus primary closure are guided by assessment and measurement of peak ventilatory pressures, central venous pressure, and intraabdominal pressure as previously discussed. Safe reference guides are maximum ventilatory pressure not higher than 30 cm H_2O and central venous and intraabdominal pressure not higher than 20 mm Hg. Most modern series report primary closure rates for gastroschisis in excess of 70% (2). If the infant requires staged reduction, a silo is secured in identical manner to that described for staged reduction of omphalocele. Because there is not a need for detailed evaluation prior to surgery, some centers are presently performing resuscitation and repair in the delivery room or immediately in an adjoining operating room (6). Postoperative care includes continued nasogastric or orogastric decompression of the intestines, 24 to 48 hours of sedation and muscle relaxation, and systemic antibiotics. Most infants with gastroschisis will have 2 to 4 weeks of adynamic ileus as well as decreased absorption of carbohydrates, protein, and fat, and require total parenteral nutrition during this period.

A major challenge in newborns with gastroschisis is the management of infarcted bowel and intestinal atresia (34). Definitively necrotic tissue should be debrided or resected, and if there is discontinuity of the bowel the open bowel ends should be oversewn. Sites of bowel perforation may be repaired or imbricated with interrupted nonabsorbable sutures. Generally, no attempt should be made for primary anastomosis in areas of infarction or atresia as experience has demonstrated that the inflamed character of the bowel and hypomotility at the time of delivery is likely to result in an unacceptably high rate of anastomotic leak or stricture. Previously, many pediatric surgeons performed proximal decompression with an enterostomy in cases of atresia, followed by delayed anastomosis 2 to 6 weeks later after resolution of the inflammatory reaction. Recent experience indicates that decompressive enterostomies are not required. Bowel atresia is optimally managed by nasogastric tube decompression for 2 to 4 weeks after abdominal wall closure, allowing for the edema and inflammation of the matted bowel to subside. Following this period, the infant can be returned to the operating room for precise anastomosis of even multiple atretic segments. Tapering enteroplasty to narrow a significantly dilated segment of bowel proximal to an atresia may also be performed at the time of anastomosis. Parenteral nutrition is critical during this time for growth and nutritional optimization for the next surgery.

POSTOPERATIVE MANAGEMENT AND COMPLICATIONS

In the immediate postoperative period, care is focused on respiratory support, nutritional support, and wound care. For both omphalocele and gastroschisis, full parenteral nutrition via a central line should be initiated immediately. Infants are often sedated and paralyzed for 24 to 48 hours to allow an initial period of healing before there is significant straining against the closure, but prolonged use will lead to peripheral and abdominal wall edema. The wound and flaps should be frequently assessed for signs of ischemia, cellulites, or fasciitis. Oral or nasogastric tube decompression is continued until there is return of bowel function. Infants following repair of gastroschisis should be expected to have a prolonged period of adynamic ileus and malabsorption.

In addition, other postoperative complications following repair of gastroschisis include sepsis, aspiration pneumonia, abdominal wall cellulitis, temporary groin and lower-extremity edema, necrotizing enterocolitis, and total parenteral nutrition–related cholestasis. Symptomatic gastroesophageal reflux and inguinal hernia are common problems due to increased intraabdominal pressure. Generally, bowel function permitting initiation of enteral feedings should return in 4 to 5 weeks, and prolonged signs of obstruction should prompt intestinal contrast studies in an attempt to identify a mechanical cause of obstruction, such as a missed atresia or stricture.

An association of abdominal wall defects, particularly gastroschisis, with necrotizing enterocolitis following repair has been demonstrated. Most series report successful management with nasogastric or orogastric tube decompression, systemic broad-spectrum antibiotics, and physiologic support. Serial evaluation of the infant should be performed for signs of intestinal perforation or infarction. Progression to these complications seems to occur infrequently in this setting.

OUTCOME

The past 3 decades have seen a dramatic increase in survival of infants with congenital abdominal wall defects. This improvement in survival is mostly related to the advent of parenteral nutrition and the introduction of staged methods of closure. Most modern series report survival of infants with omphalocele in the 60% to 70% range, with the majority of deaths related to lethal chromosomal abnormalities or major associated malformations. Survival of infants with gastroschisis is typically in excess of 90%, with deaths most often related to sepsis associated with parenteral nutrition and prolonged intestinal dysfunction (12).

REFERENCES

1. Adam AS, Corbally MT, Fitzgerl RJ. Evaluation of conservative therapy for exomphalos. *Surg Gynecol Obstet* 1991;172:394.
2. Adzick NS, Flake AW, Harrison MR. Recent advances in prenatal diagnosis and treatment. *Pediatr Clin North Am* 1985;32:1103.
3. Allen RG, Wrenn EL. Silon as a sac in the treatment of omphalocele and gastroschisis. *J Pediatr Surg* 1969;4:3.
4. Bernstein P. Gastroschisis: a rare teratological condition in the newborn. *Arch Pediatr* 1940;57:505.
5. Cantrell JR, Haller JA, Ravitch MM. A syndrome of congenital defects involving the abdominal wall, sternum, diaphragm, pericardium and heart. *Surg Gynecol Obstet* 1958;107:602.
6. Coughlin JP, Drucker DE, Jewell MR, et al. Delivery room repair of gastroschisis. *Surgery* 1993;114:822.
7. Canty TG, Collins DL. Primary fascial closure in infants with gastroschisis and omphalocele: a superior approach. *J Pediatr Surg* 1983;18:707.

8. DeLorimer AA, Adzick NS, Harrison MM. Amnion inversion in the treatment of giant omphalocele. *J Pediatr Surg* 1991;26:804.

9. DeVries PA. The pathogenesis of gastroschisis and omphalocele. *J Pediatr Surg* 1980;15:245.

10. Duhamel B. Embryology of exomphalos and allied malformations. *Arch Dis Child* 1963;38:142.

11. Glick PL, Harrison MR, Adzick NS, et al. The missing link in the pathogenesis of gastroschisis. *J Pediatr Surg* 1985;20:406.

12. Grosfeld JL, Dawes I, Weber TR. Congenital abdominal wall defects: current management and survival. *Surg Clin North Am* 1981;61:1037.

13. Grosfeld JL, Weber TR. Congenital abdominal wall defects: gastroschisis and omphalocele. *Curr Probl Surg* 1982;19:159.

14. Gross RE. A new method for surgical treatment of large omphaloceles. *Surgery* 1948;24:277.

15. Hadziselimovic F, Duckett JW, Snyder HM III. Omphalocele, cryptorchidism and brain malformations. *J Pediatr Surg* 1987;22:854.

16. Hatch EI, Baxter R. Surgical options in the management of large omphaloceles. *Am J Surg* 1987;153:449.

17. Hoyne HE, Jones MC, Jones KL. Gastroschisis: abdominal wall disruption secondary to early gestational interruption of the omphalomesenteric artery. *Sem Perinatol* 1983;7:294.

18. Langer JC, Khanna J, Caco C, et al. Prenatal diagnosis of gastroschisis: development of objective sonographic criteria for predicting outcome. *Obstet Gynecol* 1993;81:53.

19. Lewis BE Jr, Kraege RR, Danis RK. Gastroschisis. Ten year review. *Arch Surg* 1973;107:218.

20. Loder RT, Guiboux JP. Musculoskeletal involvement in children with gastroschisis and omphalocele. *J Pediatr Surg* 1993;28:584.

21. Mabogunje OA, Mahour GH. Omphalocele and gastroschisis. Trends in survival across two decades. *Am J Surg* 1984;148:679.

22. Martin LW, Torres AM. Omphalocele and gastroschisis. *Surg Clin North Am* 1985;65:1235.

23. Mollitt DL, Ballantine TV, Grosfeld JL, et al. A critical assessment of fluid requirements in gastroschisis. *J Pediatr Surg* 1978;13:217.

24. Moore TC, Stokes GE. Gastroschisis: report of two cases treated by a modification of Gross' operation for omphalocele. *Surgery* 1953;33:112.

25. Moore TC. Gastroschisis and omphalocele: clinical differences. *Surgery* 1977;82:561.

26. Nakayama DK, Harrison MR, Gross BH, et al. Management of the fetus with an abdominal wall defect. *J Pediatr Surg* 1984;19:408.

27. Novotny DA, Klein RL, Boeckman CR. Gastroschisis: an 18 year review. *J Pediatr Surg* 1993;28:650.

28. Pokorny WJ, Harberg FJ, McGill CW. Gastroschisis complicated by intestinal atresia. *J Pediatr Surg* 1981;16:261.

29. Rickham PP, Johnston JH, eds. *Neonatal surgery*. New York: Appleton–Century–Croft, 1969:254.

30. Schuster SR. A new method for staged repair of large omphaloceles. *Surg Gynecol Obstet* 1967;125:837

31. Schuster SR. Omphalocele and gastroschisis. In: Welch KJ, Randolph JG, Ravitch MM, et al., eds. *Pediatric surgery*, 4th ed. Chicago: Year Book Medical, 1986:740.

32. Schwartz MZ, Tyson KRT, Millioron K, et al. Staged reduction using a silastic sac is the treatment of choice for large congenital abdominal wall defects. *J Pediatr Surg* 1983;18:713.

33. Sipes SL, Weiner CP, Sipes DR II, et al. Gastroschisis and omphalocele: does either antenatal diagnosis or route of delivery make a difference in perinatal outcome? *Obstet Gynecol* 1990;76:195.

34. Stringer MD, Brereton RJ, Wright VM. Controversies in the management of gastroschisis: a study of 40 patients. *Arch Dis Child* 1991;66:34.

35. Towne BH, Peters G, Chang JHT. The problem of giant omphalocele. *J Pediatr Surg* 1980;15:543.

36. Wesley JR, Drongowski R, Coran AG. Intragastric pressure measurement: a guide for reduction and closure of the silastic chimney in omphalocele and gastroschisis. *J Pediatr Surg* 1981;16:264.

37. Yaster M, Buck JR, Dudgeon DL, et al. Hemodynamic effects of primary closure of omphalocele/gastroschisis in human newborns. *Anesthesiology* 1988;69:84.

38. Yazbeck S, Ndoye M, Khan KH. Omphalocele: a 25 year experience. *J Pediatr Surg* 1986;21:761.

UNIQUE FEATURES OF GROIN HERNIA REPAIR IN INFANTS AND CHILDREN

ARLET G. KURKCHUBASCHE
THOMAS F. TRACY, JR.

Although the surgical techniques in the repair of inguinal hernia in adults and children share common features, there are unique aspects to the childhood hernia that merit specific consideration. These relate to the pathophysiologic processes leading to the manifestation of a hernia, the differential diagnosis to be considered, and the potential for incarceration and strangulation. This chapter presents the current concepts of the embryology of childhood hernia, tools for clinical diagnosis, and techniques for operative management, as well as a discussion of the age-specific anesthetic risks and options for postoperative pain control.

DEFINITION AND INCIDENCE

As in the adult, the occurrence of a groin hernia in the infant or child is based on the protuberance of intraabdominal contents beyond the confines of the abdominal wall. In the child, this is most commonly related to persistent patency of the processus vaginalis, although direct, femoral, and obturator hernia can occur in this population as well. For the purposes of this chapter, hernia will refer to an indirect inguinal hernia unless otherwise specified.

The overall incidence of childhood hernia is estimated at between 1% and 5%. While the incidence of a true congenital hernia (present at birth) is low, the incidence of developing a hernia is related to both gestational and postnatal age. The incidence of hernia in preterm infants is particularly high. Thirteen percent of those infants born before 32 weeks of gestation will present with hernia, and the incidence approaches 30% in those with a birth weight of less than 1,000 g (29).

Childhood hernias occur predominantly on the right (60%), and 10% of hernias will be present bilaterally. These overall incidences must be adjusted to age, particularly in the preterm infant, where the incidence of bilateral hernias has been reported as high as 40% to 60%. Although girls were more often subjected to bilateral operations because of the perceived lesser risk with operation, the actual incidence of bilateral hernia is likely no different from boys (see later discussions). Factors other than prematurity associated with the occurrence of hernia include a positive family history in 20% of patients, with the highest relative risk (17.8) in sisters of female hernia patients (15). Other predisposing conditions include the presence of cryptorchidism, abdominal wall defects, cystic fibrosis, increased peritoneal fluid volume, connective tissue disorders, and intersex conditions.

ANATOMY AND EMBRYOLOGY

The occurrence of an inguinal hernia during infancy and childhood is related to the persistent patency of the processus vaginalis, an embryologic structure that accompanies testicular descent in the male and is alternatively termed the *canal of Nuck* in female patients. While patency of this peritoneal diverticulum is a prerequisite for forming an indirect hernia, it is not sufficient to predict the inevitable occurrence of a subsequent hernia. The events regulating closure of the processus are complex and under neurohormonal control. By assimilating evidence from clinical observations, autopsy studies, and experimental models, an embryologic sequence can be proposed.

The processus vaginalis first appears in the 12th week of gestation as it protrudes into the abdominal wall and through the inguinal canal, evaginating the muscular layers to eventually form the scrotal coverings. Within the inguinal canal and adjacent to the processus vaginalis, the gubernaculum develops as a thick mesenchymal structure that extends cephalad into the retroperitoneum and toward

A. G. Kurkchubasche and T. F. Tracy, Jr.: Department of Surgery and Pediatrics, Brown Medical School; Division of Pediatric Surgery, Rhode Island Hospital/Hasbro Children's Hospital, Providence, Rhode Island.

the caudal end of the testis, which at this point in development is located at the level of the internal ring. Although the progressive separation between testis and mesonephros is referred to as the internal descent of the testis, it is actually the result of longitudinal mesonephric growth in the lumbar region, moving the mesonephros cephalad. The actual descent of the testis through the inguinal canal occurs after the 28th week of gestation and has been speculated to result from the progressive shortening of the gubernaculum to two thirds of its length.

The mediators of testicular descent appear to segregate between the abdominal (first) and inguinoscrotal (second) phases of descent. Androgen presence and receptor sensitivity are essential to the second stage of descent (13). Experimental inhibition of androgen activity (i.e., flutamide) results in bilateral cryptorchidism as is seen clinically in testicular feminization (androgen insensitivity syndrome). Excess androgen activity, in contrast, is not sufficient to control gonadal descent alone. The role of müllerian-inhibiting substance (MIS) in this process is thought to be limited to the abdominal phase of descent and to specifically control the swelling of the gubernaculum in preparation for inguinoscrotal descent. In the absence of MIS, the gubernaculum remains thin and elongated (feminized) and the testis remains above the level of the internal ring. One of the critical mediators for inguinoscrotal descent is known to be calcitonin gene-related peptide (CGRP) elaborated from the genitofemoral nerve whose sensory spinal cord nucleus exhibits androgen receptors (12). Experimental division of the nerve results in unilateral cryptorchidism. Epidermal growth factor has recently been proposed as another integral regulator of descent. Removal of maternal rodent salivary glands, a major source of fetal epidermal growth factor, can inhibit testicular descent in the offspring (37).

It remains completely open to question whether all of these growth factors and hormones are required to act in concert or in a specific sequence to achieve inguinoscrotal descent. To further increase speculation regarding the molecular effectors of descent, there is even some suggestion that contraction of the gubernaculum would not generate sufficient force to bring the testis into the scrotum. Interestingly, infants born at various gestational periods demonstrate that progressive gubernacular shortening cannot be documented. Furthermore, the consequences of these mediators on the obliteration of the processus vaginalis have not been defined. There has been recent data, however, to suggest that hepatocyte growth factor and CGRP may act in concert to induce fusion of the processus vaginalis (4).

The processus vaginalis, which establishes its presence in the inguinal canal early in development, retains an anterior and medial position in relation to the testis and cord structures emanating from the retroperitoneum. It initially nearly completely envelops the testis and cord structures,

having preceded them into the scrotum. Although the testis traverses the short inguinal canal in a matter of days (internal and external rings are nearly superimposed), full descent into the base of the scrotum may take another 4 weeks. Once full testicular descent has been accomplished, the processus vaginalis narrows to a tubular structure on the anteromedial aspect of the cord structures. It eventually undergoes obliteration above the testis, leaving a partial investment around the testis that subsequently is referred to as the tunica vaginalis.

Studies have shown obliteration of the processus on the right side prior to the left. This has led to the unsubstantiated claim that, when a right-sided hernia occurs as failure of closure, a left-sided hernia may follow. This is based on the incorrect assumption that closure of the processus vaginalis is sequential and codependent on events occurring on the contralateral side. Defects in obliteration of the processus vaginalis result in the spectrum of inguinal disorders from hydrocele to hernia as depicted in Fig. 38.1.

In the female embryo, the events leading to closure of the processus vaginalis and resulting in ligamentous fixation are not well delineated. The processus vaginalis in the female, also referred to as Nuck's canal, never becomes as large as in the male, and typically obliterates by the seventh month of gestation. Incomplete obliteration results in either a cystic fluid collection (cyst of Nuck's canal) or an indirect inguinal hernia. In 20% of girls with hernia, the fallopian tube, ovary, or part of the uterus resides within the sac, constituting a sliding hernia.

On exploration, the hernia sac ends in a fibrovascular bundle (gubernacular attachment) that does not completely extend to the labia majora. Examination of the posterolateral surface of the lumen of the hernia sac reveals a fold of peritoneum or ligamentous structure that extends proximally to the midlateral portion of the fallopian tube. Although this has been referred to as the round ligament, a wolffian duct remnant corresponding to the vas deferens, it has recently been suggested that it actually represents the suspensory ligament of the ovary (cranial suspensory ligament) (Fig. 38.2) (2). The presence of this attachment explains the facility with which either the fallopian tube or the ovary can enter the hernia sac. Reevaluation of the anatomy has resulted in speculation regarding whether the ovaries of patients with hernia are "descended ovaries" rather than simply prolapsed structures (27).

The natural history of the processus vaginalis is relevant to the pediatric surgeon in many clinical instances. These include the timing of hernia repair in an infant with undescended testes, the management of hydroceles, and impact on the management of the contralateral inguinal canal in the patient presenting with a unilateral hernia. An appreciation of the fact that bilateral hernia in girls is actually an infrequent occurrence will prompt consideration of underlying etiologies, such as testicular feminization (androgen

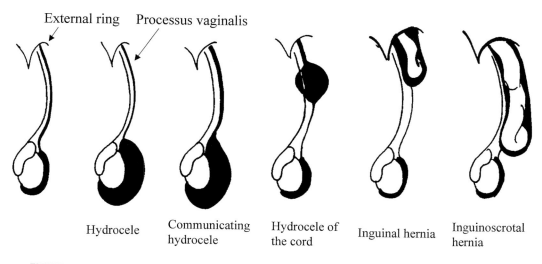

External ring   Processus vaginalis

Hydrocele   Communicating hydrocele   Hydrocele of the cord   Inguinal hernia   Inguinoscrotal hernia

FIGURE 38.1. Variants of closure of the processus vaginalis, resulting in clinical variants of inguinal anatomy (from left to right): normal anatomy with obliterated processus vaginalis with tunica vaginalis, noncommunicating hydrocele, communicating hydrocele, hydrocele of the cord, inguinal hernia, and inguinoscrotal hernia.

insensitivity) syndrome. Clearly, patency of the processus vaginalis and inguinal hernia are parallel conditions. It is evident, however, that not every patent processus vaginalis will become clinically apparent as an inguinal hernia. With further understanding of the processes that regulate gonadal descent and closure of the processus, options may become apparent to reduce the incidence of these pediatric problems.

CLINICAL PRESENTATION AND DIAGNOSIS

The clinical presentation of a hernia in a boy is that of an intermittent groin bulge. This is typically located over the external ring and may extend toward the top of the scrotum or into the scrotum. In girls, this groin bulge presents immediately superolateral to the mons pubis. The bulge is most evident when the child generates increased intraab-

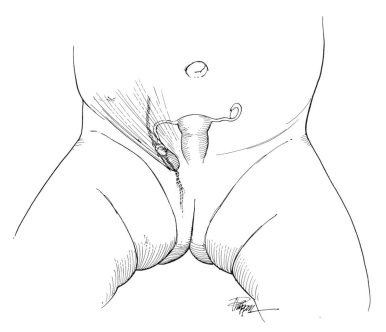

FIGURE 38.2. Anatomy of the female inguinal canal in inguinal hernia. Note the ligamentous attachment from the fallopian tube extending on the posteromedial surface of the hernia sac. Excessive traction and twisting of the hernia sac can result in injury to the fallopian tube.

dominal pressure, such as when crying, laughing, or straining. It may also be easily evident when the patient is standing, as opposed to being recumbent. Not uncommonly, the first presentation in infants and children may be that of an incarcerated hernia (to be discussed subsequently).

The examination of a child with a history of a groin bulge is best begun with simple inspection. In infants, the bulge often is present when the diaper is first opened (Fig. 38.3). Children who are able to stand can initially be examined in this position, while remaining with their parent. In the absence of evident asymmetry, inspection still yields valuable and necessary information regarding the development of the external genitalia and descent of the testes. The parents can then be asked to indicate where they have visualized the bulge.

In boys, the physical examination starts with the verification of the descent of the testes and the presence or absence of fluid around it (hydrocele). The inguinal canal is then palpated. Occasionally, one can feel a small hernia reducing its contents with minimal manipulation, despite not being able to see a contour change. The inguinal canals are compared side to side for the relative thickness of the cord structures and the presence of a "silk glove (string) sign." Whereas rolling the cord structures over the pubic tubercle allows an assessment of the thickness of the cord, the "silk glove sign" is the result of two smooth/frictionless surfaces gliding past each other, which is relevant in both boys and girls. The two surfaces represent the patent or enlarged processus vaginalis, with its potential space available for abdominal contents or peritoneal fluid. The accuracy of this sign or the appreciation of cord thickening frequently depends on the experience of the examiner.

If palpation is insufficient to render the diagnosis, efforts to provoke the child to increase the intraabdominal pressure are reasonable. When the hernia cannot be confirmed by examination, but was identified by an experienced referring physician or is accurately described by the parents, many pediatric surgeons will proceed with exploration for hernia repair to avoid the risk of an intercurrent incarceration (48). If significant doubt exists, the parents are instructed to watch for specific evidence of an inguinal hernia and the child is reexamined within several weeks.

Occasionally, a hernia will be detected as an incidental finding on radiographic studies such as ultrasound or computerized tomography (CT) performed for other urologic or gastrointestinal reasons. Apart from these unusual circumstances, these imaging modalities generally do not supplement the physical examination.

The clinical presentation of a hydrocele in boys is significantly different from that of a hernia. Although parents may not recognize the significance of their own observations, they will indicate that the swelling is limited to the scrotum (Fig. 38.4). It may be unilateral or bilateral, and may be either constant in size or fluctuate in volume during the course of the day. On inspection, the inguinal canal appears normal, but the scrotum is typically more full on one side compared with the other. Palpation confirms that the fullness surrounding the testicle ends superiorly before reaching the inguinal canal. Transillumination confirms the fluid-filled cystic nature and helps exclude the differential diagnosis of a testicular malignancy, which would present as a solid testicular mass. This easy technique is not, however, designed to clearly and reliably differentiate between paratesticular fluid and a fluid-filled, paratesticular viscus indicating an incarcerated hernia. Therefore, with the demonstration of paratesticular fluid, the remainder of the examination is crucial. Extension of the fullness through the inguinal canal is a key indication of an inguinal hernia. Occasionally, in infants a rectal examination can be extremely helpful to bimanually demonstrate the passage of small or large bowel through the internal ring in order to

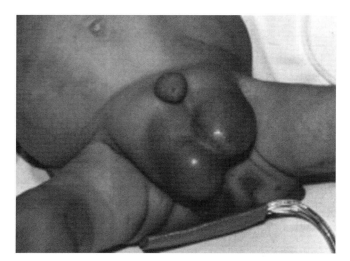

FIGURE 38.3. Bilateral inguinal hernia in a preterm infant. Note extension of bulge bilaterally to the level of external ring.

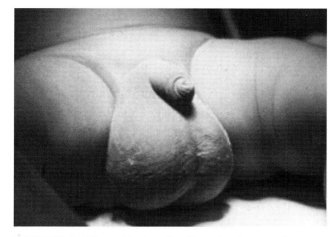

FIGURE 38.4. Bilateral hydroceles. Note the absence of any protuberance on the abdominal wall.

differentiate an incarcerated hernia from an extensive hydrocele. The management of the incarcerated hernia is further discussed in a separate section.

Between the ends of the spectrum of hernia and hydrocele, a number of variants can occur. Communicating hydroceles present the most frequent diagnostic challenges. The differentiation of a communicating from a noncommunicating hydrocele is based on the history and can only occasionally be verified on examination. The history of a uni- or bilateral scrotal swelling that comes and goes with some definite periodicity, i.e., after crying or at the end of the day with resolution overnight, prompts the consideration of a communicating hydrocele. The ability to partially or completely decompress a hydrocele with persistent gentle pressure is infrequently possible, but would constitute a definite sign of communication.

Since hernia and hydrocele are not mutually exclusive, one must take care not to dismiss patients presenting with history of a groin bulge, but with only a large hydrocele on initial inspection. Another source of confusion is provided by hydroceles that extend from the scrotum through the inguinal canal into the abdomen. They are referred to as abdominoscrotal hydroceles and are fascinating occurrences, which extend through the internal ring and into the retroperitoneum rather than into the peritoneal cavity (19).

Hernia and Cryptorchidism, Other Variants

Masses seen at the level of the external ring do not always have to come from within the canal. Highly retractile or incompletely descended testes can be mistaken for a hernia, and the examiner therefore must be sure that the testis is accounted for when such a mass is noted. Underdevelopment of the ipsilateral hemiscrotum is a very sensitive indicator for the likelihood of undescended testis. Occasionally, incomplete obliteration of the processus vaginalis in its midportion results in a cystic enlargement completely separate from the testes and a normal cord that is palpated above. This represents a hydrocele of the cord. The counterpart in girls is the cyst of Nuck's canal.

In considering differential diagnoses, thickening of the cord with symptoms of pain or heaviness without a discretely visible hernia in a teenager may represent a varicocele. Other groin bulges that constitute the differential diagnosis include direct and femoral hernias. Their location, as in the adult, should provide the basis for diagnosis. Suppurative lymphadenopathy or presentation of a retroperitoneal abscess on the medial thigh is occasionally referred for evaluation of an incarcerated hernia due to the generalized tenderness and erythema. Even simple lymphadenitis, common in infants and children, can present a confounding picture. Careful examination should be able to differentiate these entities on the basis of the findings in the inguinal canal. Acute scrotal conditions such as testicu-

lar torsion or torsion of the appendix testes can present with an initially similar physical presentation. Historic details and an expert physical examination can reduce the difficulty in discriminating these from an incarcerated hernia. Ancillary use of Doppler ultrasound or testicular perfusion scans is encouraged if necessary for rapid diagnosis and repair or relief of torsion.

The Incarcerated Hernia

The primary indication for early repair of infant hernias is the relatively high (30%) likelihood for incarceration in the first months of life. This is accompanied by the attendant morbidities of strangulation of the herniated intestine or vascular compromise to the testicular blood supply. The latter complication has a subsequent risk of necrosis or atrophy in a reported 15% to 20% of boys. In girls beyond infancy, the risk of incarceration appears to be greater than in boys (21% versus 17%), with a low but potential risk to the tuboovarian structures.

Infants typically present due to inconsolable crying, poor feeding, and eventually bilious emesis. Older children present with complaints of sudden and severe pain in the groin. Examination reveals a tender mass at the level of the external ring. The reduction of an incarcerated hernia requires a three-dimensional understanding of the anatomic features of the inguinal canal. The edematous hernia sac with its contents is situated at the external ring as a knoblike protuberance. Gentle and consistent circumferential pressure on the knob end while pulling it away from the external ring may allow for evacuation of some intestinal contents and reduction of some of the edema resultant from venous congestion. Alignment of the incarceration with the inguinal canal, gentle traction, and subsequent guidance into the external ring is achieved by creating a channel in line with the external ring, using the contralateral hand. This technique prevents the intestine from simple folding over the top of the inguinal canal. This usually results in reduction of the incarcerated intestine. This process is referred to as reduction by taxis (Fig. 38.5). Certainly, attempting to calm or sedate the child before the procedure is reasonable, although this should not include feeding the infant. Some physicians use narcotics and sedatives to relax the infant sufficiently to allow for reduction of the hernia. This is not universally endorsed for fear of reduction of bowel with impending ischemic injury. This theoretic complication has not been reported, and a "best-case," optimized manual reduction should be attempted. If a hernia cannot be reduced, operative intervention is necessary on an urgent basis. The exception to this may be the incarcerated ovary without associated incarcerated bowel. In this instance, the risk to the gonad is not as extreme (21) and is related to the possibility of torsion rather than vascular compression. As long as the child is asymptomatic, operation can safely be delayed. The presence of discomfort may

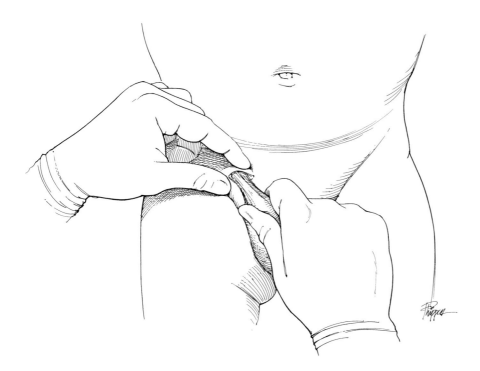

FIGURE 38.5. Reduction of incarcerated hernia by taxis. Note gentle compression of eviscerated material and redirection into external ring.

provide sufficient indication to proceed with immediate exploration for a potentially ischemic ovary.

TIMING OF OPERATION

The urgency with which a child who has been diagnosed with a hernia is scheduled for operation is based on the child's medical condition, the perceived risk of incarceration, and the potential for avoiding hospitalization. Healthy term infants are generally scheduled within several weeks of diagnosis to minimize the risk of incarceration. When an acute respiratory illness occurs, a period of 2 to 4 weeks is generally allowed to elapse prior to operation. This allows for the resolution of bronchiolitis and microalveolar collapse, and minimizes the anesthetic risk related to residual bronchospasm. This period of delay is cautiously extended in the face of infection with respiratory syncytial virus.

Premature infants diagnosed with inguinal hernia while still hospitalized generally are observed until they meet medical criteria for discharge home. Numerous studies indicate that repair is safe immediately prior to their discharge from the hospital (24,32,33). Exceptions are made if the infant has underlying medical problems, remains exceedingly small, or has an incompletely descended testis. In these cases, the infant is followed closely on an outpatient basis until the operative risk is considered acceptable and orchiopexy can be performed simultaneously. Premature infants who are diagnosed after discharge from the hospital are generally repaired promptly since it is this population who appears to have the highest risk of incarceration. Whether the size of the hernia sac has any correlation to likelihood for incarceration has not been independently evaluated.

Management of the infant who presents with an incarcerated hernia that is successfully reduced is more controversial. The basis for overnight hospitalization and prompt repair within 48 hours is established based primarily on the high incidence of recurrent incarceration events. These repeat incarcerations are less likely to be reduced preoperatively (50% versus 80% in first-time incarcerations) (9,36). Since patients with an incarcerated hernia have a 13-fold higher incidence of complications (22.1% versus 1.8%) when the operation is performed under emergency rather than semielective circumstances, this justifies observation and operation at the next available time point. In a recent report by Stylianos et al. (43), the incidence of complications associated with emergency repair was reported to be as high as 31%, supporting early semielective repair to reduce complications and length of hospital stay. Demographic factors have identified right-sided hernias, hernias in girls, and patients under age 1 year as being at highest risk of incarceration (36).

OPERATIVE REPAIR
History/Background

The management and repair of the childhood hernia has had a remarkable history. An excellent synopsis has been presented in the chapter by Jay Grosfeld, in the previous

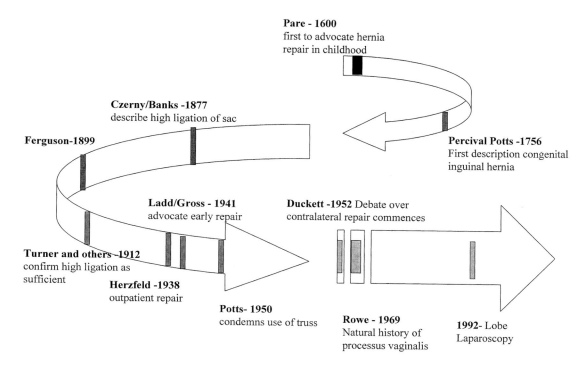

FIGURE 38.6. Historic synopsis of key events in infant hernia repair.

edition of this book. We provide a graphic representation of the cardinal events as documented by landmark publications and events in Fig. 38.6.

Technique

Palpation of the inguinal canal and cord structures with the patient under anesthesia allows determination of the location for the incision, which is placed in the vicinity of the external ring. The inferior skin crease of the lower abdomen provides a suitable topographic landmark that also helps hide the incision in both boys and girls (Fig. 38.7A). An incision adequate in length to allow for visualization of the necessary structures is made. Most pediatric surgeons will utilize magnifying operating glasses or loupes for infant operations. The subcutaneous tissues are bluntly separated to expose Scarpa's fascia, which is grasped and incised with scissors, exposing a variable amount of subfascial fat directly over the external oblique fascia. Scarpa's fascia is separated by spreading the scissors at first perpendicular and then parallel to the incision, thereby clearly exposing the external oblique. Staying on the surface of the external oblique, the blunt spreading dissection is carried laterally to lift the fascia and subcutaneous tissues off the lateral-most external oblique in an avascular plane. By following this clear lateral line of the plane inferiorly, an acute lateral turn of the medial tissues is encountered (Fig.

38.7B). This denotes the level of the external ring, as the canal contents are no longer contained in the canal and exit into the scrotum or labia. The arch of the external ring can be demonstrated by pushing the rounded tips of Metzenbaum scissors underneath the external oblique at this point. The external oblique is then opened by making a small incision over the midportion of the canal. The scissors is inserted closed tip and pushed distally to demonstrate extension into the scrotum or top of the labia. This is a valuable maneuver in a small child, where it is conceivable to mistake the rounded belly of the rectus muscle for the inguinal canal. It also serves as a double check on the visual identification of the external ring by the angulation of the cord structures as they exit the canal. This step also bluntly moves the ilioinguinal nerve from the path of the projected incision. The external oblique incision can then be extended through the external ring as well as proximally, if necessary (older child or adolescent, during orchiopexy), to the level of the internal ring.

The inguinal canal length is quite short in a premature newborn and in infants less than 6 months old. This may justify why some surgeons do not believe it necessary to open the external oblique as the external ring is dilated and essentially superimposed on the internal ring. The edges of the external oblique are dissected from the underlying tissues sufficiently to identify the ilioinguinal nerve and to prepare them for the final closure (Fig. 38.7C).

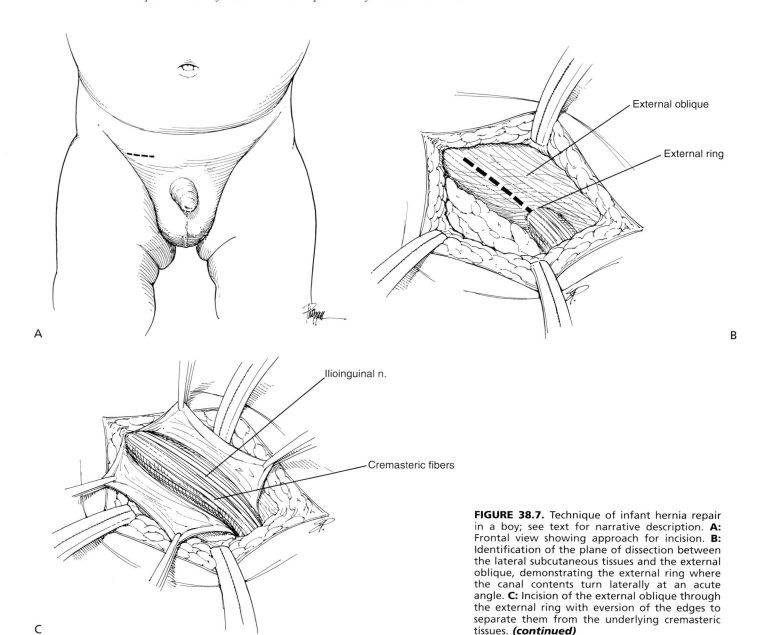

A

B

External oblique

External ring

C

Ilioinguinal n.

Cremasteric fibers

FIGURE 38.7. Technique of infant hernia repair in a boy; see text for narrative description. **A:** Frontal view showing approach for incision. **B:** Identification of the plane of dissection between the lateral subcutaneous tissues and the external oblique, demonstrating the external ring where the canal contents turn laterally at an acute angle. **C:** Incision of the external oblique through the external ring with eversion of the edges to separate them from the underlying cremasteric tissues. *(continued)*

The dissection for boys then follows a series of distinctive and critical steps. The cremasteric fibers are visualized encasing the sac and cord structures. They are separated at a convenient site distal to the internal ring and safely proximal to the testicle. The sac should be visible on the anteromedial aspect as a white, pearlescent structure. The sac can be grasped with two forceps, distributing this force over a generous area so as not to tear the sac. It should then easily lift with cord structures from the floor of the canal, raising the testicle out of the scrotum slightly. By staying on the anteromedial aspect of the contents of the canal, it is unlikely that the initial grasp will include important cord components, which are posterolateral.

The residual cremasteric fibers are bluntly pushed posteriorly on the medial and lateral side along with the nerve if it is attached. This exposes the bottom of the complex of hernia and cord structures allowing an inverted V-shaped opening bounded anteriorly by the vas, vessels, and hernia sac and posteriorly by the dissected cremasteric fibers. An instrument is passed underneath the cord, now fully elevating the complex to the surface of the incision (Figs. 38.7D and 38.8). On careful inspection, with the assistant holding the medial sac, the surgeon pushes overlying tissues posteriorly and hands newly exposed sac to the assistant, thereby rolling it progressively toward the assistant (Fig. 38.7E). At one point, a small mound of fatty tissue is visible with the

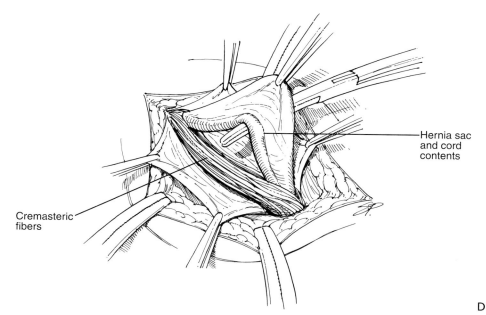

FIGURE 38.7 (continued). D: Elevation of the canal structures after dissection through cremasteric fibers. Note the inverted V seen subjacent to the hernia sac, **(E)** rolling of the sac sequentially to the medial aspect so as to expose **(F)** the fatty tissue identifying the investing fascia of the cord structures, **(G)** separation of sac from the cord structures which are now retracted with a vessel loop, and **(H and I)** application of gentle traction on the vessel loop toward the ipsilateral knee and dissection of the sac to the level of the internal ring, identified by the appearance of properitoneal fat. *(continued on next page)*

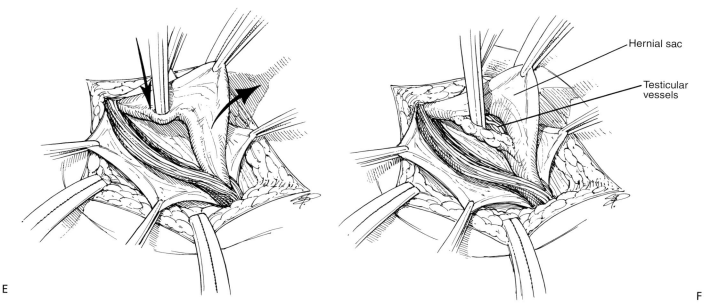

vessels of the cord inferior to it. This is the site to open the spermatic cord fascial investment and tease the cord structures inferiorly and away from the hernia sac (Fig. 38.7F). One must remember to stay perpendicular to the sac rather than getting into an oblique plane. In sequence, the fat pad is lifted, the vessels appear, and lastly the vas is mobilized off the sac. By sliding a blunt forceps from top to bottom in the visual field of the surgeon and on the surface of the sac, these structures can be lifted away and a vessel loop or fine Allis clamp placed around them for the purpose of isolation and gentle retraction (Fig. 38.7G). The assistant is left holding the sac, which can now be clamped in the midportion after meticulously verifying that the cord structures are

safely retracted. There is no specific reason to place two clamps to isolate proximal and distal sac. An extra, errant clamp in this small space compounds the risk of injury to the vas and vessels. Some surgeons, however, feel that the double-clamp technique allows for greater stability prior to division if the vas and vessels are clearly dissected proximally and distally.

If, in the process of the dissection, the testis has been pulled up and out of the scrotum, there will be a tendency to dissect obliquely along the sac toward the testis, thereby complicating the dissection. It is ideal to keep the upward traction on the sac at the minimal level or have another assistant providing some counter-traction on the testis. If

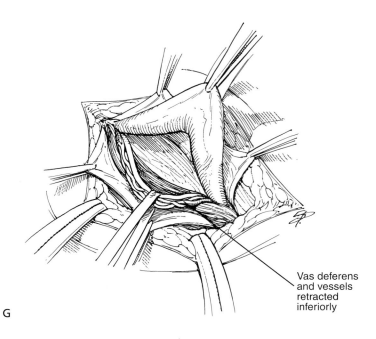

Vas deferens
and vessels
retracted
inferiorly

G

FIGURE 38.7 *(continued).*

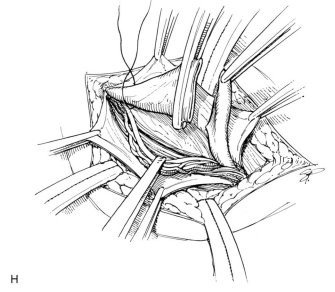

H

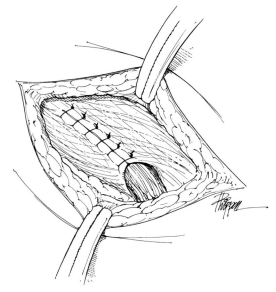

I

the sac has been singly clamped, scissors divide the sac along the clamp as the cord is carefully retracted from the area. With double clamps, division is performed between clamps.

The proximal portion of the sac now must be dissected fully to the level of the internal ring. The surgeon holds the clamp with this end of the sac, and the assistant keeps the cord structures retracted inferiorly to the ipsilateral knee of the patient (Fig. 38.7H and I). This creates enough angulation between the cord and the sac that one can spatially separate these structures from each other. The same investing fascia that had to be entered to move the cord structures off the sac initially now sometimes needs to be incised with Stevens/fine-tipped scissors. This allows for full separation,

which can be achieved with downward pressure along the sac with either a forceps, a cotton swab, or a sponge since the remaining structures do not have as much tensile strength as this fascia. Simply pushing the vas and vessels away from the sac without cutting the spermatic fascia can result in either a tear in the thin-walled sac or an avulsion injury to the cord. Once properitoneal fat is visible at the proximal end of the sac, the level of the internal ring has been reached and the sac can be ligated.

Many surgeons at this point twist the sac to keep abdominal contents reduced or to seal any microtears from the dissection. It must be recognized that this maneuver, if not carefully performed, has the potential for binding up the

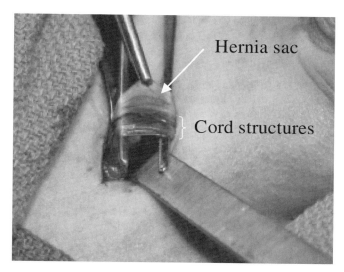

FIGURE 38.8. Right inguinal canal contents elevated out of cremasteric sheath and elevated to surface of wound. Note the sac is clearly located medially.

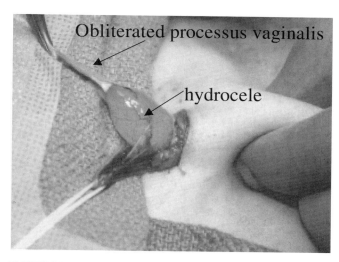

FIGURE 38.9. Distal dissection of hydrocele after proximal ligation of processus vaginalis. The hydrocele can be decompressed with needle aspiration to allow its full length to be brought into the wound.

vas and thereby exposing it to ligation and transection. Generally, the sac is ligated with nonabsorbable suture, although with a sufficiently high ligation and retraction into the peritoneal cavity, any type of ligature is equally effective. Just as when ligating a vessel such as a high flow/fragile vein, the most proximal ligature is often a tie, and the more distal one a suture ligature so as not to create a rent in the most proximal portion of the sac.

If a hole in the sac has to be chased proximal into the internal ring, it is important to remember the direction from which the cord components approach the ring. The vessels come from the posterolateral/retroperitoneal location, whereas the vas is posterior but joins the vessel from a medial origin. Once the proximal sac is controlled and ligated, only the extremely redundant sac distal to the ligature is removed. The distal sac is of no consequence except as a potential space for collection of edema fluid or hematoma. Distal dissection puts the vas and vessels again at risk. If the sac extends to the testis, it is sufficient to open it to prevent closure and formation of a distal fluid-filled space analogous to a hydrocele. Any bleeding from the cut edge of the sac usually ceases on its own. Again, recognizing possible thermal injury to the cord, one can carefully cauterize the edges in older boys. Decisions as to whether to fully visually evaluate the testis depend on the concern for a residual hydrocele (Fig. 38.9) and the risk of injury to the testis. In the repair of an incarcerated hernia, the testis must be assessed for viability.

The testis is lastly returned to the base of the scrotum by pulling on the scrotal ligament/gubernaculum. The cord structures are aligned within the canal, which is then closed with interrupted absorbable stitches along the edges of the prepared external oblique, taking care not to incorporate the ilioinguinal nerve. The wound is then closed with a subcuticular closure. An occlusive dressing is applied.

Laparoscopic techniques have been employed for primary repair of inguinal hernia in infants and children. Although they can be safely performed (25) with no apparent increased risk of recurrence or cord injury, they do not appear to provide substantial benefit in this setting.

Female Repair

In girls, the basic steps of repair are identical. The same landmarks need to be identified prior to opening the external oblique. The hernia sac is also invested in some fine muscular fibers and can be lifted from the inguinal floor, demonstrating the V-shaped aperture through which an instrument is passed. The distal end of the hernia is controlled with a clamp, and the tissues distal to it are transected with electrocautery. Consistently, there are several substantial vessels accompanying the hernia sac on its posterior surface. Care must be taken not to injure these in dissecting the sac to the internal ring, since they may retract into the retroperitoneum. All vessels in this area must be cauterized as they are dissected off the hernia sac. Although no contents may be evident in the sac, it should not be placed on so much traction that it risks exposing the midportion of the fallopian tube, which is usually attached via a ligamentous structure (either the round ligament or suspensory ligament of the ovary). Opening the sac avoids potential injury to the fallopian tube, which presents as a sliding hernia in up to 20% of girls (10). It also allows for verification of female gonadal structures since an occasional patient with testicular feminization will present with hernias (unilateral as well as bilateral) (46). An alternative method, short of genetic analysis, for evaluating the patient for müllerian-derived structures is to perform a rectal examination under anesthesia, which allows palpation of the cervix. If an abnormal gonad is unexpectedly encountered, biopsy is indicated and definitive procedures are deferred until full evaluation has been accomplished.

Repair of the Incarcerated Hernia

Repair of the incarcerated inguinal hernia remains a challenge in the infant. If spontaneous reduction does not occur with induction of anesthesia, many surgeons will not attempt further reduction, so as to be able to view the involved segment of intestine in order to determine viability. Exposure of the inguinal canal is obtained in the manner described above. In this instance, opening the external oblique fascia through the external ring is essential. With an open external ring, the sac and its contents are often easily visualized. Ischemic or necrotic bowel can then be identified. In the absence of ischemia, gentle manual reduction of the bowel is usually feasible. With the presence of ischemic bowel, the hernia sac and cord must be carefully isolated and controlled. The sac may then be opened in order to examine the intestine and perform reduction if viable or resection if necrotic. A primary anastomosis may be performed at this point and gently reduced into the abdomen through an expanded internal ring. In infants and children, reduction of incarcerated bowel does not require other peritoneal approaches that have occasionally been advocated for adults.

If the intestine reduces before it can be examined, the nature of the peritoneal fluid may provide relevant information. The presence of cloudy fluid that resembles purulent material is often encountered as a result of chylous obstruction and does not require exploration. The presence of serosanguinous fluid is more concerning, but often the patient is managed expectantly to determine whether signs of peritonitis develop. Only in the event of frank perforation with inadvertent reduction into the abdomen is laparotomy instituted. Control and secure ligation of the hernia sac may be difficult due to its edematous and fragile state. Since the testis is as much at risk of ischemic necrosis, it must be examined prior to closure. Unless total and irreversible necrosis is evident, orchiectomy is avoided and the testis is returned to the scrotum and followed postoperatively by serial examinations, which may include Doppler ultrasound and perfusion scans. Although infants who undergo emergency repair of an incarcerated hernia have an increased incidence of developing a metachronous hernia (44), most surgeons will avoid contralateral exploration in the acute setting. Alternatives to standard inguinal exploration include a properitoneal approach as described by Kamaledeen and Shanbhogue (16).

CONTRALATERAL EXPLORATION

The rationale for exploration of the contralateral inguinal canal in a patient presenting with a unilateral hernia (subsequently referred to as contralateral exploration) is to avoid the morbidity of a second hernia (discomfort, potential for incarceration) as well as a second operation with all its attendant risks and inconveniences. The decision to proceed with contralateral exploration depends on a risk/benefit analysis that has been most heavily weighted by the likelihood of encountering a patent processus vaginalis versus the risk of injury to the inguinal canal structures. Patency of the processus is defined as a patent tubular structure extending at least 2 cm from the internal ring. Routine contralateral exploration was adopted by many in the 1950s, after Duckett and subsequently Rothenburg published the frequency with which a contralateral patent processus was encountered (34). In 1969, Rowe and colleagues published the largest analysis of infants and children presenting with a unilateral hernia who underwent routine contralateral exploration (35). The authors attempted to identify predictive factors for contralateral patency of the processus vaginalis (positive exploration). Age below 2 months was associated with a 63% positive exploration rate, which declined to and leveled off at 40% by age 2 years. Contralateral exploration to age 2 years and exploration beyond this age, if the hernia presented on the left or in a girl, were adopted into subsequent practice.

Any uniformity in surgical practice that may have been perceived in the past was no longer discernible by the time the 1996 survey by the Surgical Section of the American Academy of Pediatrics was performed (48). The concern that patients were being exposed to unnecessary morbidity by contralateral exploration was readdressed using new operative tools. Laparoscopy had been introduced into common practice by 1992, and variations in laparoscopic technique were applied and published to determine patency of the processus by other than open exploration. The premise of these techniques was that observation of an obliterated canal should completely obviate the need for exploration or subsequent metachronous hernia repair. Visualization of a patent processus vaginalis still resulted in exploration and allowed for an assessment of the sensitivity and specificity of the various endoscopic techniques. In most studies, those that did not undergo open exploration (had obliterated processus by laparoscopic evaluation) were followed for the subsequent presentation of a hernia. In the metaanalysis of 13 studies reporting on laparoscopic evaluation of the contralateral canal by Miltenburg et al. (22), the incidence of encountering a patent processus vaginalis or hernia in children over a large range of ages was 39% (376 of 964 patients) prompting contralateral exploration. False-positive and false-negative rates were very low on subsequent open exploration. Only one of 526 patients reported to have an obliterated canal subsequently developed a hernia. Laparoscopy has therefore provided a good technique for rapid and sensitive assessment of the contralateral groin, but has not answered the fundamental question of which patent processus vaginalis will progress to clinical hernia, still resulting in potentially unnecessary explorations.

Rather than speculating on the basis of circumstantial evidence, the most direct approach is to determine what the incidence of metachronous hernia actually is. Although this does not help determine the risk to the individual patient, it allows decisions to be made regarding the risk/benefit relationship for exploration versus expectant management. From this information, a population should be identified that would benefit from primary contralateral exploration. Whereas multiple studies have evaluated this issue retrospectively, a recent study from this institution approached the question prospectively (44). Between 1995 and 1998, only patients presenting with bilateral hernia underwent bilateral operations, whereas all others were followed prospectively after unilateral repair for an average period of 2 years. This period of follow-up is sufficient to capture the vast majority (more than 90%) of metachronous hernias that will develop. Of 656 patients, 108 (16.5%) presented with bialteral inguinal hernia, and 48 patients (7.3%) who underwent unilateral repair developed a metachronous hernia. Only premature infants and children who underwent repair of an incarcerated hernia (which may actually be a subset of the first group) had a significantly higher incidence of metachronous hernia than other groups. Interestingly, a girl was no more likely than a boy to develop a metachronous hernia.

Given the relatively low incidence of metachronous hernia, as evidenced in this study as well as numerous retrospective studies best summarized in the metaanalysis by Miltenburg et al. (23), support has significantly declined for routine contralateral exploration. Contralateral exploration remains appropriate in the instance of a child with risk factors for anesthesia or with a predisposing condition for the development of bilateral hernias.

COMPLICATIONS OF HERNIA REPAIR

As in any operation, the incidence of complications after hernia repair, whether anesthetic or technical, are related to the risk classification of the patient [American Society of Anesthesiologists (ASA) class] and the conditions under which the operation is performed (elective; semielective, i.e., after reduction of an incarceration; or emergent). Premature infants and young infants (younger than 3 months) warrant a separate discussion of their complications and particularly anesthetic management, given the implications for potential respiratory complications and how this affects their outpatient status (30). Operative and late operative complications include wound infections, bleeding (scrotal hematoma), persistent or reactive hydrocele, gonadal

ischemia, injury to the vas deferens, iatrogenic cryptorchidism, and recurrent hernia.

Under elective circumstances, wound infection is expected to occur less than 1% of the time, with the exception of premature infants with very large hernias or on high-dose steroids. The presence of a perineal rash or distant concomitant infections (otitis media, urinary tract infection) increases the risk of infection and therefore presents relative contraindications to operation. The use of prophylactic antibiotics is not warranted unless congenital heart disease or a ventriculoperitoneal shunt is present. One clinical scenario in which there may be a relative indication for the use of antibiotics against gram-positive organisms is in the preterm/former preterm infant with a very large hernia. These hernias require prolonged dissection and create large potential spaces that have been associated with postoperative hematoma and abscess, which may jeopardize testicular viability.

It is not unusual for the scrotum to be edematous and even ecchymotic in the immediate postoperative period, raising concerns for bleeding, infection, a residual hydrocele, or even a recurrent hernia. In premature infants, this swelling normally takes months to resolve. When erythema constitutes a prominent component of this examination, the clinical dilemma arises of whether infection or even acute testicular necrosis may account for this finding. Ultrasound examination can be helpful in this setting.

Although care is taken not to injure the vessels in the process of dissection, the subsequent identification of poor testicular growth and atrophy suggests that subacute injuries occur even in elective hernia repair. Long-term studies of testicular size demonstrate atrophy in 1%, with diminution in size of the testes in an additional 2.7% of boys who underwent hernia repair (7). Factors leading to these complications are believed to include excessive traction on the vessels, excessive dissection, and thermal injury following use of an electrocautery device. Acute testicular loss is more commonly suspected and identified after operation for incarcerated hernia (31).

Potential injury to the vas deferens is one of the primary concerns in inguinal hernia repair and has been one of the reasons for reevaluating the risks of contralateral exploration. Even in the absence of transection, the vas is susceptible to injury. In animal experiments, it has been shown that even simple, gentle grasping with a forceps results in obliterative pathology (14). This is clinically correlated with the documented greater incidence of infertility in men who underwent herniorrhaphy in childhood. If transection of the vas is recognized at operation in an infant, marking the vas with permanent suture is the most appropriate intervention. The current evidence for successful vasovasostomy indicates that repair should be attempted using microsurgical techniques in children just before puberty. Vasal structures are larger, and a more precise anastomosis can be accomplished at that time.

The microscopic evaluation of hernia sacs for potential occult injury to the vas is still routinely performed at many institutions. This practice has been questioned in this era of cost containment, especially since transection of the vas is typically recognized in the operating room, independent of the microscopic examination (47). In reviews of large series, the incidence of microscopically identifying the vas deferens varies between 0.13% and 0.23% (28), and not all of these cases were occult injuries. Other gonadal structures such as the epididymis were encountered in 0.3% of cases and embryonal rests in 0.41% (41). Not every histologic specimen appearing to be a segment of vas deferens is necessarily the result of an operative injury, as müllerian duct remnants can be mistaken for the vas deferens.

The overall incidence of hernia recurrence is estimated to be 1% to 3%. A higher incidence (20%) is quoted for preterm infants (30). Technical reasons predominate and include failure to achieve ligation at the level of the internal ring, an unrecognized tear on the posterior aspect of the sac, damage to the floor of the canal resulting in a direct hernia, infection, and increased intraabdominal pressure (11). A recurrent hernia may present in the immediate postoperative period or generally within 2 months. Alternatives available for the management of recurrent hernia include the standard transinguinal approach, the properitoneal approach, and laparoscopic surgery. The use of mesh is based on the nature of the recurrence and the quality of the native tissues. In a recent report on 225 patients who underwent laparoscopic hernia repair, 10 were performed for recurrences after standard open repair (6). The benefits of this approach were that the nature of the defect (direct versus indirect) could be identified without dissecting scar tissue, avoiding manipulation and potential injury to the cord structures. In eight cases, recurrence was due to simple patency of the processus vaginalis. These hernias were amenable to laparoscopic closure, and none of these cases have since recurred.

Other complications encountered in the postoperative period include iatrogenic cryptorchidism, which is best avoided by assuring that the testes are returned to and extend into the scrotum at conclusion of the operation. The premature infant in particular appears to be at significant risk of this complication. Nerve entrapment and neuromas are not frequently reported conditions in infants.

An extraordinary difference in complication rates has been documented between emergent repair and semielective repair after reduction of an incarceration. Rowe and Clatworthy, reporting on children of all ages, encountered complications in 1.7% of semielective operations versus 22% of emergent procedures (36). These remarkable differences are further amplified when infant (less than 2 months of age) statistics are specifically examined. Rescorla and Grosfeld reported overall complication rates of 4.5% and 33%, respectively (33). Gonadal loss in infant incarcerated hernia repair was particularly high (more than 20%) in this

as well as other series as compared to a 7% to 14% incidence in older patients with irreducible incarceration. Uemura and colleagues investigated postponing the operation in order to minimize anesthetic risks in very-low-birth-weight infants (45). As a result of the long wait, the hernia sac was found to have become large and thick, with fibrous adhesions that made repair difficult and actually increased the risk of gonadal ischemia. This further supports the practice of repairing infant hernias soon after diagnosis, avoiding more complicated repairs and incarceration (18).

ANESTHESIA AND ANALGESIA

Anesthetic management should facilitate operative repair, while not exposing the infant to excessive risk of postoperative respiratory and cardiovascular complications. The anesthetic management of the term infant and child has evolved into less invasive techniques, even circumventing intubation and using laryngeal mask airways in the young child. In contrast, management of the immature respiratory responses and mechanics in the premature infant's upper and lower respiratory tract remains a challenge even to the pediatric anesthesiologist. An excellent discussion of the factors involved in anesthesia for newborn infants is presented by Spaeth et al. (39).

Postoperative apnea is one of the significant events for which infants are monitored after a general anesthesic. One important factor to remember is that the absence of preoperative apnea does not imply that postoperative apnea will not occur. Postoperative apnea is defined as an episode lasting longer than 15 seconds, which typically occurs in clusters and is not always accompanied by bradycardia. The apnea events do not always result in arterial desaturation, and the bradycardia that occurs is therefore not in response to hypoxia. Apnea can occur on the basis of central and obstructive components. The central components that place the preterm infant at risk include a biphasic ventilatory response to hypoxia and an immature response to carbon dioxide (further blunted in those with underlying apnea). Both responses are exacerbated by hypoxia and anesthetic gases. Obstructive components to postoperative apnea are related to the decrease in pharyngeal muscle tone resulting in collapse at the level of the hypopharynx and larynx. How aggressively to monitor and protect infants from these adverse events has significant implications for the economics of health care, given that 10% to 20% of inguinal hernia repairs are performed in former preterm infants. As in decision-making regarding contralateral exploration, the management of the former preterm infant after hernia repair should be based on a risk/benefit analysis rather than a cost analysis alone.

After demonstrating that preterm infants are more prone to respiratory complications following minor surgery than are term infants, Steward (42) advised that preterm infants should be continuously observed for 24 hours postoperatively and should not be operated upon as outpatients in the first 3 months of life. His study was based on 33 infants less than 38 weeks of estimated gestational age (EGA) with an average birthweight (BW) of 1.4 kg. These infants underwent operation between 3 and 28 weeks postnatally. Outcomes were compared to 38 full-term infants with a minimum BW of 2.5 kg, who underwent repair between 1 and 36 weeks postnatally. Eleven of the 33 preterm infants had complications (six episodes of apnea; two patients with atelectasis; two patients with aspiration pneumonia; and one patient each with excessive secretions, extubation stridor, and coughing with cyanosis). Only one full-term infant had problems with a breath-holding episode.

Subsequent studies have sought to determine whether this risk to preterm infants can be modulated by altering anesthetic techniques (i.e., spinal versus general), avoiding longer-acting paralytics, or avoiding narcotics. Efforts have also been made to identify age or other physiologic criteria that correlate with a lower incidence of complications, sufficient not to warrant inpatient observation. These efforts have been hampered because of the lack of uniformity in categorizing patients in terms of demographics, as well as variance in the sophistication of monitoring and even in the definition of what constitutes a clinically significant event (20). The authors defined risk as being less than 5% when corrected gestational age [(CGA) = EGA + postnatal age] exceeded 43 weeks, and concluded that outpatient surgery is safe after CGA 50 weeks. Numerous other guidelines based on different thresholds were proposed, ranging from CGA 44 weeks if there was no history of apnea or lung disease to CGA 60 weeks. Allen concluded that CGA 45 weeks was a safe age on the basis of 57 former preterm infants (EGA less than 36 weeks) who underwent hernia repair at CGA less than 60 weeks. Five required prolonged ventilation (mean CGA, 41 weeks) while 52 remained extubated (mean CGA, 47 weeks). No respiratory complications occurred in those with ASA class 1 after 6 hours. ASA class 2 and class 3 patients have a 10% risk of anesthetic complications, and surgery should be delayed if improvement in ASA class is possible (1).

In a combined analysis, Cote et al. in 1995 attempted to bring some uniformity to the subject (5). Their study derived patient data from eight published prospective studies, including only those infants who underwent general anesthesia (specifically excluding those infants operated on under regional anesthesia, having additional procedures, or receiving xanthine stimulants such as caffeine). Their findings were that apnea was strongly and inversely related to both EGA and CGA, with an associated risk factor being apnea episodes at home (not simply being monitored for apnea at home). Anemia (hematocrit less than 30) was a risk factor for those older than CGA 43 weeks. No relationship was determined to a previous history of necrotizing enterocolitis, neonatal apnea, respiratory distress syn-

drome, bronchopulmonary dysplasia, or the operative use of opioids or muscle relaxants. Based on this stratification, they were able to define probability intervals that allow the practitioner to decide what level of risk is acceptable. In infants (EGA 35 weeks) without episodes of apnea while in the recovery room and without anemia, the probability of subsequent apnea did not become less than 5% until after CGA 48 weeks. The probability of apnea did not become less than 1% for the same 35-week EGA infant until CGA 54 weeks or, for a 32-week premature infant, until CGA 56 weeks. Despite this venerable attempt at establishing common practice guidelines, some reservations remain regarding the statistical power of the study that enabled the authors to make these recommendations (8).

The alternative to general anesthesia is regional anesthesia (either spinal or epidural). In a prospective study of high-risk infants (ASA class 2 or greater), Somri et al. (38) concluded that the risk of postoperative respiratory complications, and therefore the need for mechanical ventilation and length of the hospital stay, could be reduced by providing spinal anesthesia. As the authors point out, spinal anesthetics are not without risks, the principal disadvantage being technical difficulties for both the anesthesiologist and the surgeon. Bloody taps are not infrequent, and there is the potential for total spinal anesthesia as a result of lifting the infant for placement of the cautery grounding pad. The limited duration of the spinal anesthetic and restlessness of the infant may have an impact on the surgeon's ability to achieve a secure repair. Although supplemental ketamine or other sedatives can be given to the infant, these generally eliminate the benefit that spinal anesthesia provided over a general anesthetic. Furthermore, the availability of newer volatile agents such as sevoflurane and desflurane, which have rapid recovery characteristics when used for maintenance of anesthesia, may obviate the benefit provided by spinal anesthesia, since there is less residual volatile agent to affect the respiratory center (26). Spinal anesthesia is thus generally reserved for the infant with severe pulmonary disease in whom extubation may be difficult postoperatively.

Analgesia for the Nonpremature Infant

Methods for providing postoperative analgesia that have shown efficacy over placebo include the following:

1. Opioids such as codeine
2. Nonsteroidal antiinflammatory agents such as ketorolac tromethamine (1 mg/kg intravenously)
3. Regional anesthesia/ilioinguinal block (0.25% bupivacaine 1 mL/kg)
4. Regional anesthesia/caudal (0.25% bupivacaine with 1:200,000 epinephrine, 1 mL/kg)

Individual studies that have examined the relative merits and adverse effects of these interventions include a study by Splinter et al. (40), which demonstrated that inguinal nerve block was equivalent in providing postoperative analgesia to a caudal block. When ketorolac was used in addition to ilioinguinal block and compared to caudal as a supplement to block, it was associated with decreased pain, decreased emesis, earlier ambulation and earlier micturition. Although ketorolac has been associated with complications including bleeding, acute renal failure, and bronchospasm, these were not encountered in the study. In a randomized trial of 10% lidocaine aerosol applied to the wound, only short and clinically insignificant pain relief was afforded (17).

One of the most powerful tools for managing pain and anxiety is the provision of information to the parent and the child. "Postop pain is negatively related to the parent's provision of surgery-relevant information to the child in the preop period" (3). This has been incorporated in our institution as the "preop program," in which families are acquainted with the events that will occur when the child enters the operating room. Parents are encouraged to be present until the child undergoes induction of anesthesia and are involved in the immediate postoperative period. The use of preoperative anxiolytics and postoperative narcotics was reduced, along with enhanced satisfaction with this otherwise stressful event in the parents' and child's life.

The postoperative analgesia regimen at our institution usually involves either caudal injection of bupivacaine or direct ilioinguinal nerve block, either administered preoperatively or by the surgeon under direct vision. Postoperative analgesics are provided on a routine basis and can consist of either acetaminophen (10mg/kg every 4 hours for 24 hours, then as needed) or acetaminophen with codeine in those in whom there is expected to be greater discomfort (i.e., older kids with a more extensive dissection, or boys undergoing concurrent orchiopexy).

Most operations are performed on an outpatient basis, reserving overnight hospitalization for those with underlying medical problems that require postoperative monitoring. Former premature infants younger than CGA 50 weeks either undergo an extended period of observation in the recovery room phase or are admitted for overnight heart rate and apnea monitoring.

REFERENCES

1. Allen GS, Cox CS Jr, White N, et al. Postoperative respiratory complications in ex-premature infants after inguinal herniorrhaphy. *J Pediatr Surg* 1998;33:1095–1098.
2. Ando H, Kaneko K, Ito F, et al. Anatomy of the round ligament in female infants and children with an inguinal hernia. *Br J Surg* 1997;84:404–405.
3. Christiano B, Tarbell SE. Brief report: behavioral correlates of postoperative pain in toddlers and preschoolers. *J Pediatr Psychol* 1998;23:149–154.
4. Cook BJ, Hasthorpe S, Hutson JM. Fusion of childhood inguinal hernia induced by HGF and CGRP via an epithelial transition. *J Pediatr Surg* 2000;35:77–81.
5. Cote CJ, Zaslavsky A, Downes JJ, et al. Postoperative apnea in former preterm infants after inguinal herniorrhaphy. A combined analysis [see comments]. *Anesthesiology* 1995;82:809–822.
6. Esposito C, Montupet P. Laparoscopic treatment of recurrent inguinal hernia in children. *Pediatr Surg Int* 1998;14:182–184.
7. Fischer R, Mumenthaler A. Ist bilaterale Herniotomie bei Sauglingen und Kleinkindern mit einseitiger Leistenhernie angezeigt? *Helv Chir Acta* 1957;24:346–350.
8. Fisher DM. When is the ex-premature infant no longer at risk for apnea [Editorial; Comment]? *Anesthesiology* 1995;82:807–808.
9. Gahukamble DB, Khamage AS. Early versus delayed repair of reduced incarcerated inguinal hernias in the pediatric population. *J Pediatr Surg* 1996;31:1218–1220.
10. Goldstein IR, Potts WJ. Inguinal hernia in female infants and children. *Ann Surg* 1958;148:819–822.
11. Grosfeld JL, Minnick K, Shedd F, et al. Inguinal hernia in children: factors affecting recurrence in 62 cases. *J Pediatr Surg* 1991; 26:283–287.
12. Hrabovszky Z, Farmer PJ, Hutson JM. Does the sensory nucleus of the genitofemoral nerve have a role in testicular descent? *J Pediatr Surg* 2000;35:96–100.
13. Hutson JM. Testicular feminization: a model for testicular descent in mice and men. *J Pediatr Surg* 1986;21:195–198.
14. Janik JS, Shandling B. The vulnerability of the vas deferens (II): the case against routine bilateral inguinal exploration. *J Pediatr Surg* 1982;17:585–588.
15. Jones ME, Swerdlow AJ, Griffith M, et al. Risk of congenital inguinal hernia in siblings: a record linkage study. *Paediatr Perinat Epidemiol* 1998;12:288–296.
16. Kamaledeen SA, Shanbhogue LK. Preperitoneal approach for incarcerated inguinal hernia in children. *J Pediatr Surg* 1997;32: 1715–1716.
17. Kokinsky E, Cassuto J, Sinclair R, et al. Topical wound anaesthesia in children—a temporary postoperative pain relief. *Acta Anaesthesiol Scand* 1999;43:225–229.
18. Krieger NR, Shochat SJ, McGowan V, et al. Early hernia repair in the premature infant: long-term follow-up. *J Pediatr Surg* 1994;29:978–981; discussion 981–982.
19. Luks FI, Yazbeck S, Homsy Y, et al. The abdominoscrotal hydrocele. *Eur J Pediatr Surg* 1993;3:176–178.
20. Malviya S, Swartz J, Lerman J. Are all preterm infants younger than 60 weeks postconceptual age at risk for postanesthetic apnea? *Anesthesiology* 1993;78:1076–1081.
21. Marinkovic S, Kantardzic M, Bukarica S, et al. When to operate nonreducible ovary? *Med Pregled* 1998;51:537–540.
22. Miltenburg DM, Nuchtern JG, Jaksic T, et al. Laparoscopic evaluation of the pediatric inguinal hernia—a meta-analysis. *J Pediatr Surg* 1998;33:874–879.
23. Miltenburg DM, Nuchtern JG, Jaksic T, et al. Meta-analysis of the risk of metachronous hernia in infants and children. *Am J Surg* 1997;174:741–744.
24. Misra D, Hewitt G, Potts SR, et al. Inguinal herniotomy in young infants, with emphasis on premature neonates. *J Pediatr Surg* 1994;29:1496–1498.
25. Montupet P, Esposito C. Laparoscopic treatment of congenital inguinal hernia in children. *J Pediatr Surg* 1999;34:420–423.
26. O'Brien K, Robinson DN, Morton NS. Induction and emergence in infants less than 60 weeks post-conceptual age: comparison of thiopental, halothane, sevoflurane and desflurane. *Br J Anaesth* 1998;80:456–459.
27. Ozbey H, Ratschek M, Schimpl G, et al. Ovary in hernia sac: prolapsed or a descended gonad? *J Pediatr Surg* 1999;34: 977–980.
28. Partrick DA, Bensard DD, Karrer FM, et al. Is routine pathological evaluation of pediatric hernia sacs justified? *J Pediatr Surg* 1998;33:1090–1092; discussion 1093–1094.

29. Peevy KJ, Speed FA, Hoff CJ. Epidemiology of inguinal hernia in preterm neonates. *Pediatrics* 1986;77:246–247.
30. Phelps S, Agrawal M. Morbidity after neonatal inguinal herniotomy. *J Pediatr Surg* 1997;32:445–447.
31. Puri P, Guiney EJ, O'Donnell B. Inguinal hernia in infants: the fate of the testis following incarceration. *J Pediatr Surg* 1984;19:44–46.
32. Rajput A, Gauderer MW, Hack M. Inguinal hernias in very low birth weight infants: incidence and timing of repair. *J Pediatr Surg* 1992;27:1322–1324.
33. Rescorla FJ, Grosfeld JL. Inguinal hernia repair in the perinatal period and early infancy: clinical considerations. *J Pediatr Surg* 1984;19:832–837.
34. Rothenburg RE, Barnett T. Bilateral herniotomy in infants and children. *Surgery* 1955;37:947–950.
35. Rowe M, Copelson L, Clatworthy H. The patent processus and the inguinal hernia. *J Pediatr Surg* 1969;4:102–107.
36. Rowe MI, Clatworthy HW. Incarcerated and strangulated hernias in children. A statistical study of high-risk factors. *Arch Surg* 1970;101:136–139.
37. Siow Y, Fallat ME. Testicular descent—a proposed interaction between mullerian inhibiting substance and epidermal growth factor [Editorial; Comment] [see comments]. *J Urol* 1997;158:613–614.
38. Somri M, Gaitini L, Vaida S, et al. Postoperative outcome in high-risk infants undergoing herniorrhaphy: comparison between spinal and general anaesthesia. *Anaesthesia* 1998;53:762–766.
39. Spaeth JP, O'Hara IB, Kurth CD. Anesthesia for the micro-premie. *Semin Perinatol* 1998;22:390–401.
40. Splinter WM, Reid CW, Roberts DJ, et al. Reducing pain after inguinal hernia repair in children: caudal anesthesia versus ketorolac tromethamine. *Anesthesiology* 1997;87:542–546.
41. Steigman CK, Sotelo-Avila C, Weber TR. The incidence of spermatic cord structures in inguinal hernia sacs from male children [see comments]. *Am J Surg Pathol* 1999;23:880–885.
42. Steward DJ. Preterm infants are more prone to complications following minor surgery than are term infants. *Anesthesiology* 1982;56:304–306.
43. Stylianos S, Jacir NN, Harris BH. Incarceration of inguinal hernia in infants prior to elective repair. *J Pediatr Surg* 1993;28:582–583.
44. Tackett LD, Breuer CK, Luks FI, et al. Incidence of contralateral inguinal hernia: a prospective analysis. *J Pediatr Surg* 1999;34:684–687; discussion 687–688.
45. Uemura S, Woodward AA, Amerena R, et al. Early repair of inguinal hernia in premature babies. *Pediatr Surg Int* 1999;15:36–39.
46. Viner RM, Teoh Y, Williams DM, et al. Androgen insensitivity syndrome: a survey of diagnostic procedures and management in the UK. *Arch Dis Child* 1997;77:305–309.
47. Wenner WJ Jr, Gutenberg M, Crombleholme T, et al. The pathological evaluation of the pediatric inguinal hernia sac [see comments]. *J Pediatr Surg* 1998;33:717–718.
48. Wiener ES, Touloukian RJ, Rodgers BM, et al. Hernia survey of the Section on Surgery of the American Academy of Pediatrics. *J Pediatr Surg* 1996;31:1166–1169.

39

CONGENITAL INTERNAL ABDOMINAL HERNIAS: INCIDENCE AND MANAGEMENT

LAWRENCE E. STERN
BRAD W. WARNER

Internal hernia is defined as a fossa, fovea, or defect of unusual size within a body cavity, into which intestines may intrude and become incarcerated or strangulated (48). The hernia orifice is usually a preexisting anatomic structure; however, abnormalities of intestinal rotation and peritoneal attachment are common causes of congenital internal hernia (25). Unlike the classic external hernia, the internal hernia does not require a peritoneal sac or membrane to surround its contents. The origins of the internal hernias are multiple and include congenital defects, inflammation, infectious processes affecting the peritoneal cavity, trauma, and postoperative defects. This review will focus on hernias that are of congenital origin.

At autopsy, the incidence of internal hernia ranges from 0.2% to 0.9% (11,25,40). In patients presenting with intestinal obstruction, internal hernia is cited as the cause in 4.1% (25,62). This incidence may vary with the patient population studied as some series have shown rates as low as 0.8% while White has reported an incidence as high as 13% in Africans (15,61,72). The majority of patients will have small, easily reducible hernias that remain asymptomatic. The typical clinical presentation of an internal hernia is as an acute intestinal obstructive event, although many patients describe a history of chronic, vague abdominal pain (58). The classification of internal hernias has been complicated by a difficult nomenclature identifying hernias by location of their orifice and not by the eventual position of the viscera (25). Gullino et al. (27) have differentiated normal and paranormal hernias from abnormal hernias. Normal hernias leave the peritoneal cavity through a physio-

logic foramen (e.g., Winslow's foramen), while paranormal hernias pass through a peritoneal orifice, which expands with age (e.g., paraduodenal hernias through Landzert's foramen). Abnormal hernias, unlike normal and paranormal hernias, lack a true peritoneal sac. Perhaps the easiest way to discuss the various hernias is to categorize them into two broad groups: retroperitoneal hernias and those formed from congenital anomalous openings (Table 39.1). The vast majority of internal abdominal hernias fall into the categories of paraduodenal, Winslow's foramen, transmesenteric, and broad ligament hernias, and will be discussed in this order (58).

PARADUODENAL HERNIA

History

Although rare, the paraduodenal hernia is the most common of the internal abdominal hernias, accounting for 30% to 53% of these hernias (3). The history of this hernia variant extends back to 1786, when Neubauer first described a paraduodenal hernia during an autopsy (49). He felt this anomaly represented a defect in peritoneal development. In 1857, Treitz described numerous folds and fossa that he believed represented areas permitting the intestine to herniate into the retroperitoneum and thus coined the term "hernia retroperitonealis" (66). In 1899, Moynihan described nine paraduodenal peritoneal pockets or fossa located near the fourth portion of the duodenum (46). He attributed their creation to physiologic adhesions occurring during embryologic development. He concluded the gradual enlargement of the fossa allowed herniation of the intestine. Landzert's fossa was implicated in the development of the left paraduodenal hernia, while the mesentericoparietal or Waldeyer's fossa formed the right paraduodenal hernia.

Moynihan's theory of paraduodenal hernia development remained intact until 1923, when Andrews proposed an

L.E. Stern and **B.W. Warner:** Department of Surgery, University of Cincinnati College of Medicine; Division of Pediatric Surgery, Children's Hospital Medical Center, Cincinnati, Ohio.

TABLE 39.1. CATEGORIES AND TYPES OF INTERNAL ABDOMINAL HERNIAS

Retroperitoneal
Paraduodenal
Winslow's foramen
Paracecal
Intersigmoid
Congenital Anomalous Openings
Transmesenteric
Broad ligament
Transomental

embryologic basis for the formation of the paraduodenal hernia. He put forth the notion that congenital anomalies of intestinal rotation caused the small bowel to become entrapped behind the peritoneum (1). Although there has been continued debate as to the exact development of these hernias, Andrews' theory is generally accepted as correct (4,9,10,12,21,29,45,53).

Normal Embryology

Early in fetal development, the intestinal midgut, a straight tube, is suspended from the dorsal abdominal wall by a short mesentery and communicates with the yolk sac by way of the vitelline duct. At about the fourth week of development, the rate of growth of the midgut exceeds the rate of growth of the body stalk and rapidly elongates, forming the primary intestinal loop. The cephalic limb, or prearterial segment, develops into the distal duodenum and jejunum. The caudal limb, or postarterial segment, becomes the ileum, cecum, appendix, ascending colon, and the proximal two thirds of the transverse colon. Due to this rapid elongation, as well as the increasing size of the liver, a physiologic herniation at the umbilical ring occurs and the intestinal loops enter the extraembryonic coelom (Fig. 39.1).

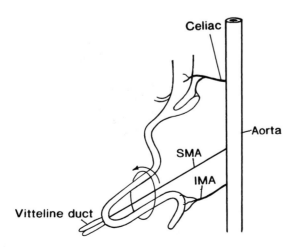

FIGURE 39.1. Rapid enlargement of the midgut results in physiologic herniation through the umbilical ring.

At about the eleventh to twelfth week postconception, the intestine begins to return to the abdominal cavity and rotates around the superior mesenteric artery (SMA). The prearterial segment rotates in a counterclockwise rotation, first inferior and then to the left of the SMA, completing a total of 270 degrees of rotation around the SMA axis, forming the normal duodenal C-loop (Fig. 39.2). Simultaneously, the postarterial segment completes a 270-degree counterclockwise rotation, superior and to the right of the SMA (Fig. 39.3). At the completion of intestinal growth, return to the abdominal cavity, and normal rotation and fixation, the mesentery is attached to the posterior abdominal wall. This extends from Treitz's ligament in the left upper quadrant to the cecum in the right lower quadrant. The ascending and descending colon fuse with the retroperitoneum (56,73).

Embryology of the Paraduodenal Hernia

A right paraduodenal hernia is formed when the prearterial limb fails to rotate around the SMA, and a portion of the small bowel remains to the right of the artery. The postarterial segment continues its normal rotation; fusion of the ascending colonic mesentery to the retroperitoneum causes entrapment of the bowel within the primitive coelom (Fig. 39.4) (21,73). The extent of entrapment can vary from a single loop to the entirety of the intestine becoming encased (69). The anatomic result is a hernia orifice that is always to the right of midline and usually faces medially and slightly downward. The mesentery of the ascending colon and a portion of the transverse colon make up the anterior wall of the sac, while the SMA and ileocolic artery lie in the free edge of the sac (5,24).

Andrews suggested that the left paraduodenal hernia resulted from "reversed" rotation of the midgut loop, and the small bowel was "covered up" by the left mesocolon (1). However, the fact that the duodenum sits posterior to the SMA argues against the "reversed" rotation theory (73). Callander et al. proposed that during migration to the left superior portion of the abdominal cavity, the small intestine invaginates into the unsupported area of the descending mesocolon between the inferior mesenteric vein and the posterior attachment (10). This theory is supported by the following facts: The inferior mesenteric artery and vein and the left colic artery with their branches are integral parts of the hernia sac. The anterior wall of the sac is composed of the descending colonic mesentery. The cecum has completely rotated and sits in its normal anatomic position. The duodenum is rarely visible at the neck of the sac, and the ileum exits the sac at a variable distance from the ileocecal valve (Fig. 39.5) (5,73).

Incidence

The asymptomatic nature of many paraduodenal hernias makes the precise incidence unknown; however, they are

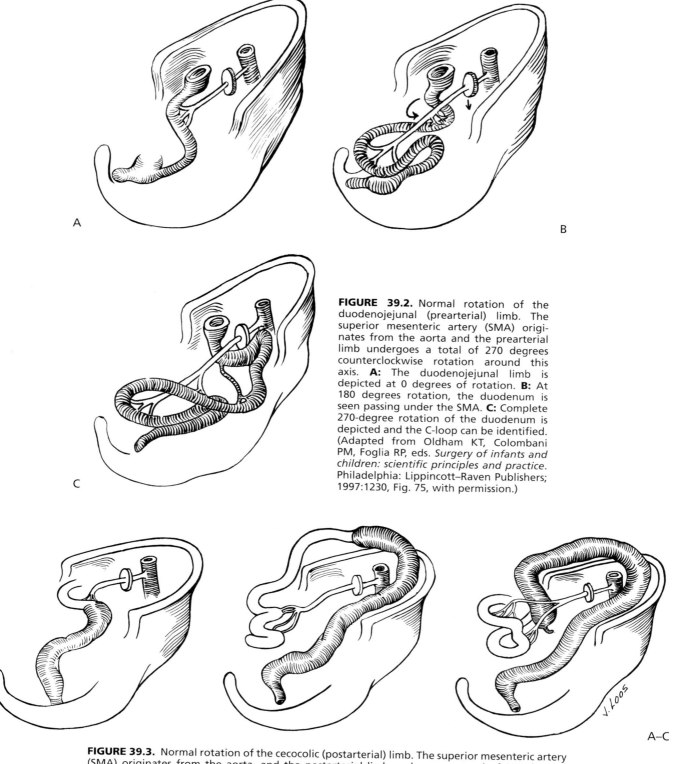

FIGURE 39.2. Normal rotation of the duodenojejunal (prearterial) limb. The superior mesenteric artery (SMA) originates from the aorta and the prearterial limb undergoes a total of 270 degrees counterclockwise rotation around this axis. **A:** The duodenojejunal limb is depicted at 0 degrees of rotation. **B:** At 180 degrees rotation, the duodenum is seen passing under the SMA. **C:** Complete 270-degree rotation of the duodenum is depicted and the C-loop can be identified. (Adapted from Oldham KT, Colombani PM, Foglia RP, eds. *Surgery of infants and children: scientific principles and practice.* Philadelphia: Lippincott–Raven Publishers; 1997:1230, Fig. 75, with permission.)

FIGURE 39.3. Normal rotation of the cecocolic (postarterial) limb. The superior mesenteric artery (SMA) originates from the aorta, and the postarterial limb undergoes a total of 270 degrees counterclockwise rotation around this axis. **A:** The cecum is depicted at 0 degrees rotation relative to the SMA. **B:** 180 degrees rotation has occurred and the cecum is identified directly above the SMA. **C:** Complete 270-degree rotation of the cecocolic limb is depicted and the cecum is located in the right lower quadrant. (Adapted from Oldham KT, Colombani PM, Foglia RP, eds. *Surgery of infants and children: scientific principles and practice.* Philadelphia: Lippincott–Raven Publishers; 1997:1230, Fig. 75, with permission.)

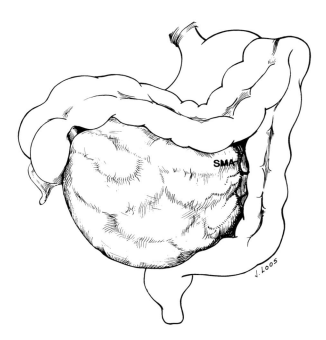

FIGURE 39.4. Right paraduodenal hernia. The hernia sac is identified to the right of the superior mesenteric artery *(SMA)*, which lies along the free edge of the hernia sac. The anterior wall of the sac is composed of the ascending colonic mesentery and the transverse colon.

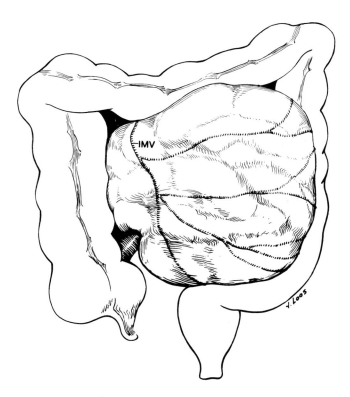

FIGURE 39.5. Left paraduodenal hernia. The hernia sac is seen protruding to the left of the inferior mesenteric vein *(IMV)*. The anterior wall of the sac is composed of the descending colonic mesentery.

the most common of all internal hernias, accounting for 53% of these hernias (5). The male-to-female ratio is approximately 3:1, and the average age at diagnosis is 38.5 years (36). The left variant is three to six times more common than the right (18,69).

Clinical Presentation and Diagnosis

Internal hernias represent only a small fraction of the patients presenting with intestinal obstruction; however, 50% of paraduodenal hernias present as an acute intestinal obstruction. The signs and symptoms of obstruction secondary to a paraduodenal hernia are similar to obstructive symptoms from other causes. Approximately 70% to 80% of patients have a history of chronic or intermittent abdominal pain with the associated symptoms of nausea, vomiting, bloating after meals, and episodic abdominal discomfort and resultant weight loss (36,43,69). The diagnosis is often confused with peptic ulcer, cholecystitis, pancreatitis, and gastritis.

Physical examination during symptom-free periods is usually normal. When incarceration or strangulation occurs, the examination is usually nondiagnostic unless the hernia is large enough to be palpated as an abdominal mass (17,38). Incarceration and strangulation can quickly progress to necrosis as this represents a closed-loop bowel obstruction. Classic signs and symptoms of the acute abdomen may be present, i.e., fever, leukocytosis, abdominal pain with rebound, and guarding, all of which suggest intestinal necrosis.

The preoperative diagnosis of an internal hernia is extremely difficult and is rarely reported in the surgical and radiologic literature. The majority of paraduodenal hernias are discovered during exploration for other presumed causes of intestinal obstruction or are found incidentally during laparotomy for other disease. The initial radiographic study usually includes standard flat and upright abdominal radiographs. Occasionally, this will demonstrate several dilated loops of small bowel in a laterally situated ovoid mass (30). However, the majority of plain films will be nondiagnostic, and other imaging modalities may therefore prove useful.

Kummer (37a) was the first to describe a paraduodenal hernia via a radiographic study, and his description remains the standard for the diagnosis using a small-bowel contrast follow-through series: "There is total absence of small intestine in the true pelvis in the upright position; the small intestine is confined in a smooth, sharply circumscribed mass" (Fig. 39.6). The right and left variants can be distinguished by the position of the intestinal mass (8). The small-bowel series is limited due to its inability to demonstrate the hernia sac and its anatomic relationship to surrounding organs and vascular structures.

Computed tomography (CT) scanning has been used to evaluate patients with paraduodenal hernias and is now the study of choice. Left paraduodenal hernias will demonstrate a hernia sac located behind the body of the pancreas, displacement of the duodenal–jejunal junction medially, dilated air- and fluid-filled small bowel proximal to and/or in the hernia sac, and small-bowel herniation into the transverse mesocolon or into the ascending mesocolon (65). The right hernia will show grouping of the small bowel in the right midabdomen with looping of arterial and venous jejunal branches behind the SMA (Fig. 39.7) (36).

Angiography has been successfully used to evaluate the paraduodenal hernia and has the added benefit of demonstrating the aberrant vascular anatomy. In the right paraduodenal hernia, the jejunal arteries arise normally from the left of the SMA but reverse direction and flow behind the parent vessel toward the right (Fig. 39.8). In the left paraduodenal hernia, the SMA is normally situated, but the jejunal arteries will flow behind the inferior mesenteric vessels into the descending colon and are directed medially and posteriorly (8). Due to the invasive nature of the procedure and its own accompanying morbidity, it is less often used as a primary diagnostic modality.

Magnetic resonance (MR) imaging and ultrasound scanning of a paraduodenal hernia have been reported. These modalities offer the noninvasive advantage of CT scanning but do not require the use of intravenous contrast in a potentially hypovolemic patient. Visualization of the arterial system via MR angiography and of the hernia sac proper via ultrasound has been described (51,70).

Treatment

The most important regimen for an incarcerated or strangulated paraduodenal hernia is prompt operative intervention. The mortality of an obstructed internal hernia exceeds 50% (2,48,76). The operative treatment of the left and

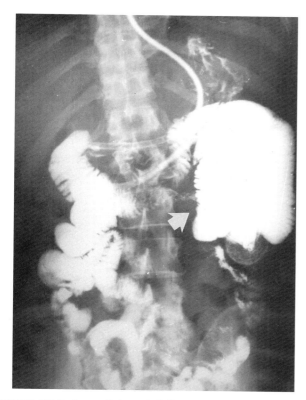

FIGURE 39.6. A small bowel follow-through series demonstrates a left paraduodenal hernia. Note the circumscribed mass of small intestine located within the left-upper quadrant *(arrow).*

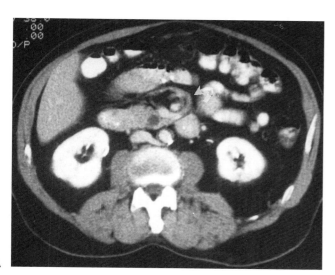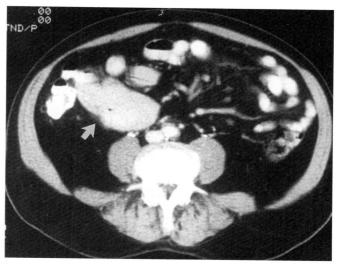

A B

FIGURE 39.7. An abdominal computed tomography scan demonstrates a right paraduodenal hernia. **A:** The jejunal vessels are noted to be looping behind the superior mesenteric artery *(arrow).* **B:** The herniated bowel is identified as a right-sided opacified mass *(arrow).*

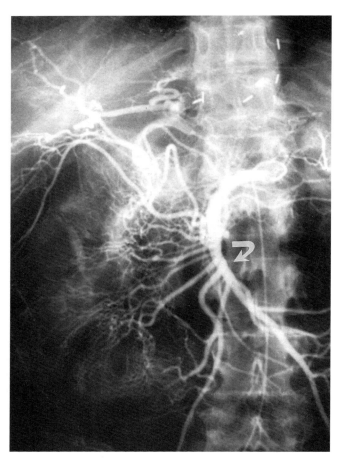

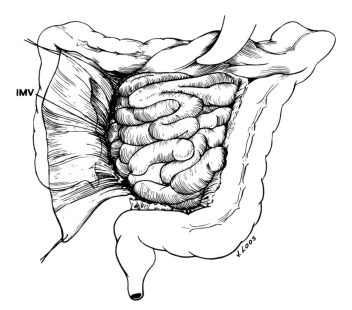

FIGURE 39.9. Repair of a left paraduodenal hernia via Bartlett's technique. The hernia sac is opened and the inferior mesenteric vein *(IMV)* and artery are divided in order to free the terminal ileum.

FIGURE 39.8. A superior mesenteric arteriogram demonstrates a right paraduodenal hernia. The jejunal branches are seen turning to the right *(arrow)* and pass behind the superior mesenteric artery. (From Ghahremani GG. Internal abdominal hernias. *Surg Clin North Am* 1984;64:393–406, with permission.)

right hernias is distinct owing to the differences in embryologic origin.

The left hernia can frequently be reduced by gentle traction on the efferent loop as it exits the hernia sac orifice. If reduction is successfully achieved, the remnant orifice should be permanently closed. This is accomplished by suturing the peritoneal folds to the intestine or its mesentery at the duodenojejunal junction. During both traction and closure, the surgeon must be constantly aware of the inferior mesenteric vein (IMV) as it makes up the anterior wall of the hernia sac (5,16). Failure of simple traction to reduce the hernia requires a more drastic operative approach. Bartlett et al. have advocated making an incision into an avascular plane of the descending colonic mesentery, thereby delivering the intestine into the peritoneal cavity (Fig. 39.9) (3). This requires division of the inferior mesenteric artery (IMA) and vein in order to abolish the ring encompassing the terminal ileum. Many other surgeons have advocated preservation of the IMA and IMV, fearing ischemia of the intestine. Willwerth et al. success-

fully reduced a left paraduodenal hernia with preservation of its vasculature (Fig. 39.10) (73). The IMV was identified on the right side of the sac; an incision was made to the right of the vein and carried inferiorly. The bowel was reduced beneath the IMV and the vein was then returned to its normal position on the left side of the small intestinal mesentery. The peritoneum adjacent to the vein was sutured to the posterior abdominal peritoneum to achieve closure of the sac (73). A variety of other surgical techniques have been described, allowing for the preservation of the IMV; however, the key surgical principle is identification of the vessels within the anterior wall of the sac prior to any attempt at reduction (5).

Operative management of the right paraduodenal hernia is less controversial. Due to the abnormal intestinal rotation, the small bowel is located behind the ascending colon. The ascending colon and cecum are mobilized and transferred to the left side of the abdomen, and the small intestine is freed from the hernia sac. This maneuver allows for placement of the duodenum, jejunum, and the majority of the ileum on the right side of the abdominal cavity, and the terminal ileum, cecum, and colon on the left side (Fig. 39.11). The appendix should be removed to avoid future potential diagnostic confusion. This is the same anatomic orientation that results from operative correction of a midgut volvulus (Ladd's procedure). As the SMA is part of the anterior wall of the hernia sac, care should be taken to avoid incision into this area of the sac (3,5,69).

The management of an incidentally discovered paraduodenal hernia remains controversial. Bartlett et al. have

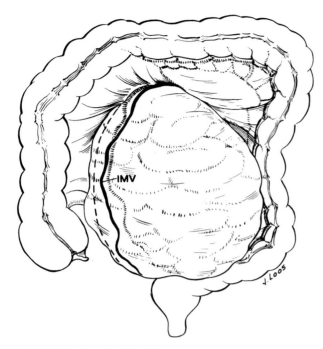

FIGURE 39.10. Repair of a left paraduodenal hernia via Will-werth's technique. The inferior mesenteric vein *(IMV)* is identified, and an incision is made to the right of the vein and carried inferiorly *(dashed line)*. The bowel can then be reduced beneath the IMV.

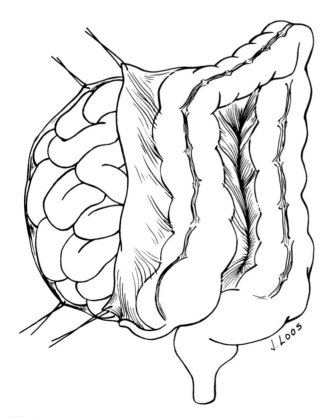

FIGURE 39.11. Repair of a right paraduodenal hernia. The hernia sac is divided and the terminal ileum, ascending colon, and cecum are transposed to the left side of the abdominal cavity.

stated that "all paraduodenal hernias should be considered potentially lethal and capable of causing strangulating obstruction" (2). However, the low incidence of obstruction secondary to paraduodenal hernia makes empiric treatment less clear.

WINSLOW'S FORAMEN HERNIA

Winslow's foramen is an opening that allows communication between the greater and lesser omental sacs. Its anatomic boundaries are composed of the caudate lobe of the liver superiorly, the duodenum inferiorly, the lesser omentum that surrounds the hepatic artery, portal vein and bile ducts anteriorly, and the peritoneum overlying the inferior vena cava posteriorly. The normal aperture will allow the surgeon to pass one or two fingers. Due to the small aperture and the natural barrier created by the hepatic flexure and transverse colon, herniation through Winslow's foramen is rare, accounting for only 8% of all internal hernias (19,22). The first reported surgical procedure for this hernia was by Treves in 1888 (67). He was unable to reduce the intestine through the foramen, and the patient expired shortly after operation.

Pathogenesis

The segments of intestine that pass through Winslow's foramen and their frequencies of occurrence can be divided into three categories: (a) small intestine (63%), (b) cecum and right colon (30%), and (c) transverse colon (7%) (19). Moynihan concluded that a congenital abnormality was prerequisite and described several variations that he felt could lead to this situation (46). It is currently felt that a very long mesentery, a large foramen, and absence of the attachment of the ascending colon to the posterior abdominal wall are the major factors predisposing to herniation (74). An additional precipitating factor is increased intraabdominal pressure. Sudden increased pressure as seen during strenuous lifting may induce a pressure gradient between the greater and lesser sacs and thereby allow herniation through the foramen (13).

Clinical Presentation and Diagnosis

The most common complaint of patients with an incarcerated Winslow's foramen hernia is pain; however, its location may be referred to the actual organ that has become entrapped and thus may mislead the physician (74). The pain is worse when the trunk and legs are extended or when the patient is standing straight up. The position that produces the least discomfort has been described as sitting or bending forward, or lying with the trunk and hips flexed (20,67). It is postulated that the aperture of the foramen opens and closes in response to body positioning, and the fluctuations in pain experienced by the patient are related to the change in compression of the herniated organ. Similar to the paraduodenal hernia, there may be a history of chronic abdominal pain, but this is less common in the foramen hernia variant. The quality of pain varies from patient to patient and may begin as mild cramping and become progressively more severe. The use of nasogastric decompression has allowed for resolution of the pain and can thereby cloud the diagnosis. While nausea and vomiting may occur, it is not a prominent component of this condition (19).

Physical examination can reveal an epigastric mass that may be palpable or visualized. Epigastric tenderness is not always elicited by examination, and rebound tenderness is only rarely encountered. The stomach and surrounding structures act as buffer between the involved intestinal segment and the parietal peritoneum, and the classic signs of peritoneal irritation are therefore frequently absent. Clinical and laboratory evidence of jaundice may be discovered preoperatively. Stretching or compression of the common bile duct as the herniated intestine passes through the foramen is the likely cause for this finding (19).

The first preoperative diagnosis of Winslow's foramen hernia via radiographic study was by Hollenberg in 1945 (31). The difficulty in preoperative diagnosis is exemplified by the study of Ohkuma and Miyazaki, in which less than 10% of 115 cases of herniation through Winslow's foramen were correctly diagnosed preoperatively (50). On plain abdominal radiographs, a distended loop of bowel located near the lesser sac can be indicative of this hernia. As the stomach is displaced anteriorly and to the left, placement of a nasogastric tube can aid in differentiating between distended intestine and the stomach.

Contrast enema can provide an image that is often confused with cecal volvulus as the right colic gutter may be empty if the cecum and ascending colon are involved in the hernia (Fig. 39.12). Ultrasound evaluation may demonstrate a mass located in the lesser sac (22). The results of CT scanning for herniation of the cecum through Winslow's foramen have been described. The herniated bowel is identified within the lesser sac by its retrogastric position with anterior and lateral displacement of the stomach. Air- and/or fluid-filled intestine will extend to the foramen, which is located posterior to the portal structures and anterior to the inferior vena cava. The mesenteric vessels and surrounding fat may be seen passing through the foramen and thereby confirm the herniation (74).

Treatment

Similar to the left paraduodenal hernia, gentle traction on the herniated intestine can often reduce the incarceration. This method will be most efficacious in situations where the aperture is not excessively tight. If the surgeon is unable to achieve reduction by traction, the lesser sac should be

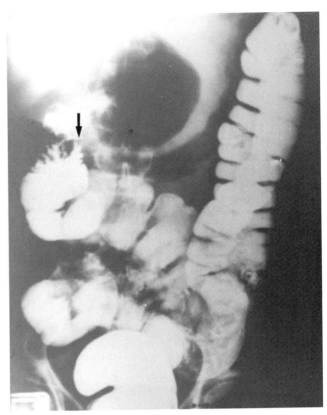

FIGURE 39.12. Contrast enema demonstrates Winslow's foramen hernia. The cecum has become incarcerated within the lesser sac *(arrow)*, thus causing the appearance of an empty right colic gutter. (With thanks to Joel Lichtenstein, M.D.)

entered via the gastrocolic ligament or the gastrohepatic ligament. Pressure can be applied to the incarcerated segment from within the lesser sac, while traction is applied from outside the foramen. This will often allow for reduction; however, if continued difficulties arise, Kocher's maneuver of the duodenum should be performed. This will allow mobilization of the duodenum and the head of the pancreas with subsequent enlargement of the foramen. Reports of needle decompression of the incarcerated region have been described but should be avoided if possible due to the increased risk of peritoneal soilage (52). Once reduction has been achieved, careful inspection of the bowel, liver, and gallbladder for signs of ischemia or necrosis should be performed. Resection of necrotic or ischemic structures should be performed, as the surgeon deems necessary. If the ascending colon has been involved in the hernia, fixation to the right colic gutter may prevent volvulus (22).

Surgical closure of the foramen entails significant risk to the portal structures. There have been no reported recurrences of Winslow's foramen hernia despite numerous cases in which the foramen was left open. Therefore, it would seem prudent to allow the natural inflammatory response to seal the foramen.

TRANSMESENTERIC HERNIA

History

Transmesenteric hernias occur when a loop of intestine protrudes through a defect in the intestinal mesentery or omentum. Like many other internal hernias, there is no true peritoneal sac (Fig. 39.13) (75). Numerous anatomists and pathologists have described defects of the mesentery, with a reported incidence of one in 400 cadavers (34). In 1885, Treves provided a detailed account of the occurrence of ileal mesenteric defects. He described an area that was thin and contained no fat, visible blood vessels, or lymph nodes (28,68). Herniation through this defect has been classically referred to as a hernia of Treves' fold. Marsh described the first successful operative procedure for a transmesenteric hernia in 1888 (41).

Pathogenesis

The etiology for congenital mesenteric defects is unclear, and multiple hypotheses have been put forward: partial regression of the dorsal mesentery, fenestration of poorly vascularized areas, "rupture" of the colon through the mesentery, and defective stromal development are a few of the noteworthy theories (23,61). The aperture of the mesenteric defect is always solitary and circular, and ranges from 1 to 3 cm in diameter (75). As a result of intestinal peristalsis, a loop of bowel migrates through the defect and becomes incarcerated. The trapped loop fills with gas, distends and continues to drag additional intestine through the defect. The increase in intestinal distention and quan-

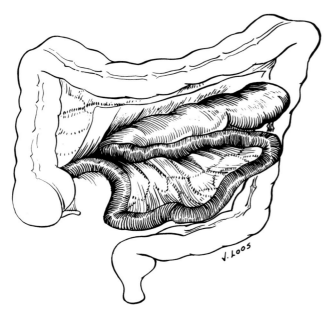

FIGURE 39.13. Transmesenteric hernia. The distal ileum is seen passing into an ileocolic defect with a resulting proximal bowel obstruction.

tity of intestine involved causes compression of the vascular supply and can result in rapid gangrene (61).

Incidence

Transmesenteric hernias comprise approximately 5% to 10% of all internal hernias. Interestingly, 35% of transmesenteric hernias occur in the pediatric population, representing the most common type of internal hernia in this age group (47,71). This increased frequency in the pediatric population may have an association with intestinal ischemic accidents as mesenteric defects are found with a significantly increased incidence in infants with intestinal atresia (47). A reported 71% of defects occur through openings in the small bowel, with ileocecal defects accounting for 54% of these occurrences. Mesocolic defects represent 26% of the transmesenteric hernias, and transverse mesocolic defects make up 59% of this variant (61).

Clinical Presentation and Diagnosis

The most common presenting complaint of patients with mesenteric hernias is pain. The pain is typically sudden in onset and severe in intensity. Its location is frequently epigastric and periumbilical. Vomiting is present in over half of the patients. Similar to the paraduodenal hernia, a history of prior intermittent abdominal pain may be seen in almost 20% of patients (34).

Physical examination consistently reveals abdominal tenderness that is most frequently right sided. A palpable abdominal mass representing the Gordian knot of herniated intestine may be present in a minority of patients; however, this mass may not represent incarcerated bowel (25). A previous report has detailed an obstruction of the stomach caused by herniation of the small bowel through the transverse mesocolon into the lesser sac and then through the gastrohepatic omentum (34). The mass palpated was actually the two halves of the distended stomach.

While the diagnosis is most often made during exploration for presumed intestinal obstruction or appendicitis, preoperative radiographic studies may suggest the diagnosis. In the absence of small-bowel obstruction, plain abdominal films are nonspecific. The use of contrast medium may demonstrate a constriction of the intestine at the point of passage through the mesenteric aperture (35). Arteriography may provide the best means of making a preoperative diagnosis; however the patient's condition may limit its therapeutic use. The mesenteric arteriogram may reveal an abrupt change in the course of the SMA with displacement of the visceral branches (Fig. 39.14). With incarceration, the blood vessels will taper at the site of obstruction, and delays in both arterial and venous flow would be expected. Volvulus may be demonstrated by abrupt tapering or termination of the mesenteric vessels at the site of mesenteric twist, abnormal course and whirlpool arrange-

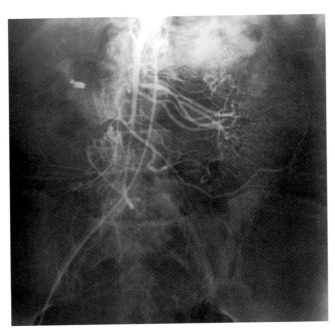

FIGURE 39.14. A superior mesenteric arteriogram demonstrates a transmesenteric hernia. The superior mesenteric artery is seen folding back upon itself, and the terminal ileal and ileocolic branches twist toward the left-upper quadrant. (From Cohen AM, Patel S. Arteriographic findings in congenital transmesenteric internal hernia. *AJR Am J Roentgenol* 1979;133:541–543, with permission.)

ment of the arteries at the point of mesenteric twist, and delayed arterial and venous filling and emptying (14).

Treatment

Early operation is the key to successful treatment of the transmesenteric hernia. In a review of 150 patients with transmesenteric hernia, 13 patients were not operated upon and the resultant mortality was 100% (34). During laparotomy, the viability of the incarcerated bowel must be determined. If the intestine is deemed viable, simple reduction of the incarcerated loop and closure of the defect with nonabsorbable sutures is the recommended treatment modality. If the bowel is nonviable, then a resection with end-to-end anastomosis is the most sensible course. Incidentally discovered mesenteric defects should be closed to protect against future intestinal herniation (61).

HERNIATION THROUGH THE BROAD LIGAMENT

Protrusion of an intraabdominal viscus through or into a defect of the supporting structures of the uterus is extremely rare. The first description of an incarcerated hernia of the

broad ligament was by Quain in 1861 (54). As of 1972, only 81 additional cases had been documented in the French or English literature (7). The actual incidence is difficult to ascertain but has been suggested to range from 4% to 7% of all internal hernias. The average patient age is 47 years; however, this number represents all reported broad ligament hernias, which includes those of noncongenital origin (60).

Anatomy and Embryology

The female paramesonephric duct develops into the main genital duct. As the ovary descends, the first two parts of the genital duct form the uterine tube, while the caudal portion becomes the uterine canal. The second part of the paramesonephric duct moves in a mediocaudal direction, allowing the urogenital ridges to lie in a transverse plane. Fusion of the ducts at the midline forms a transverse pelvic fold. This fold or broad ligament extends laterally in a tripod fashion and attaches to the pelvic sidewalls. The superior margin of the broad ligament is delineated by the fallopian tube. The mesosalpinx is formed from the anterior and posterior peritoneal folds and is bounded by the fallopian tube superiorly, the uterus medially, and the ovarian ligament inferiorly. The anterior leaf of the broad ligament covers the round ligament and forms the mesoligament teres. The lateral extent of the broad ligament covers the ovarian vessels and forms the infundibulopelvic ligament (56,60).

Pathogenesis

Until recently, herniation through the broad ligament was felt to occur secondary to trauma, pregnancy, childbirth, and inflammation. However, 19% of the hernias described fall into the category of bilateral defects or defects in a nulliparous woman with no antecedent history of abdominal surgery, trauma, or pelvic infection. A congenital origin would therefore appear to be necessary to account for these hernias. Additional evidence for a congenital origin was provided by Gray's and Skandalakis' description of cystic structures of the broad ligament, which they believed were remnants of the mesonephric or müllerian ducts (26). Rupture of these cysts may lead to defects within the broad ligament, thereby allowing herniation through the defect (59).

Broad ligament hernias occur with equal frequency on the left and right sides and occasionally occur bilaterally. Bowel may pass through both layers of the broad ligament or may enter into the mesometrium through the posterior leaf (Fig. 39.15). Other potential sites include the mesosalpinx and the round ligament. The small intestine is involved in 90% of cases, with sigmoid colon, ovary, cecum, omentum, appendix, and ureter being described in a few case reports (42,44,60).

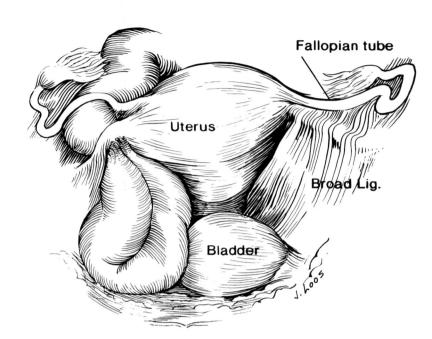

FIGURE 39.15. Broad ligament hernia. A loop of small intestine is seen passing to the right of the uterus through the broad ligament.

Clinical Presentation and Diagnosis

Similar to most internal hernias, the presenting symptoms are those of acute intestinal obstruction: cramping abdominal pain, nausea, vomiting, distention, and abdominal tenderness. The preoperative diagnosis remains elusive and has rarely been made. Plain films of the abdomen are usually not helpful but may demonstrate dilated loops of bowel with or without a pelvic mass. CT scanning has been able to detect a dilated loop of small bowel with an air–fluid level in the pelvic cavity (63). Ultrasound may provide confirmatory evidence if the diagnosis is suspected (32).

Treatment

The majority of broad ligament hernias can be treated by simple surgical reduction of the incarcerated loop followed by closure of the defect with nonabsorbable sutures. On occasion, division of the superior margin of the aperture is necessary to reduce the incarceration. Some surgeons perform salpingo-oophorectomy in menopausal women; however, a hysterectomy is rarely required. It is important to examine the contralateral broad ligament for defects prior to completion of the surgical procedure (7,44,59,60).

OTHER HERNIA

A variety of other internal hernias have been described in the literature; however, they account for only a small percentage of these hernias. Paracecal hernia accounts for approximately 6% of abdominal hernias and has two proposed origins. Andrews believed it was the result of intestinal malrotation with subsequent trapping of the small bowel behind the transverse mesocolon (1). More recent proponents feel herniation is the result of progressive entry of a small bowel loop into the peritoneal fossa (55).

Hernias involving the sigmoid colon represent 5% of all internal hernias. Intersigmoid herniation is extremely rare, with less than 40 reported cases. It arises in the congenital fossa present at the attachment of the lateral aspect of the sigmoid mesocolon to the posterior abdominal wall. An intrasigmoid hernia has a defect with only the left leaf of the peritoneum involved. The hernia sac resides within the sigmoid mesocolon proper (6). Recently, the first case of herniation through a colonic epiploica has been described (37).

Transomental herniation has been postulated to occur secondary to trauma, inflammation, arteriosclerosis, and congenital causes. Treves postulated that two overlapping omental defects would exist and thus allow passage of the intestine through the omentum (39). Transomental herniation is rare, representing only 1% to 4% of internal hernias. It presents as an intestinal obstruction and can be diagnosed preoperatively with the use of CT scanning (33,64).

Herniations through congenital defects of the falciform ligament have been described in isolated case reports. The opening may represent failure of the peritoneum to fuse with the ventral abdominal wall or may be a congenital area of weakness in the ligament, which leads to disruption (57).

CONCLUSION

Internal hernias are a rare cause of intestinal obstruction, accounting for less than 5% of such cases. The diagnosis is seldom made preoperatively as it is rarely considered in the differential diagnosis. The patient's condition and physical findings may preclude extensive testing as operative therapy in an unstable patient should never be delayed in pursuit of a radiographic diagnosis. The mortality of nonoperative therapy for incarcerated or strangulated internal hernia approaches 100%, and delay in surgical therapy can lead to undue morbidity.

The surgical approach to internal hernia repair is usually straightforward and often requires no more than simple manual reduction. More complicated repair necessitates an adequate understanding of the embryologic basis of the particular hernia variant encountered. The surgeon must always exercise extreme care when working near the hernia sac as major vascular structures are frequently found in close proximity.

REFERENCES

1. Andrews E. Duodenal hernia—a misnomer. *Surg Gynecol Obstet* 1923;37:740.
2. Bartlett JDJ, Martel W, Lindenauer SM. Right paraduodenal internal hernia. *Surg Gynecol Obstet* 1971;132:443–449.
3. Bartlett MK, Wang CA, Williams WH. The surgical management of paraduodenal hernia. *Ann Surg* 1968;168:249–254.
4. Batson OV. Anatomic variations in the abdomen. *Surg Clin North Am* 1955;35:1527.
5. Berardi RS. Paraduodenal hernias. *Surg Gynecol Obstet* 1981;152:99–110.
6. Bircher MD, Stuart AE. Internal herniation involving the sigmoid mesocolon. *Dis Colon Rectum* 1981;24:404–406.
7. Bolin TE. Internal herniation through the broad ligament. Case report. *Acta Chir Scand* 1987;153:691–693.
8. Brigham RA. Paraduodenal hernia. In: Nyhus L, Condon R, eds. *Hernia*, 4th ed. Philadelphia: JB Lippincott Co, 1995:485–490.
9. Burnham PJ. Retromesocolic hernia; development and treatment. *J Int Coll Surg* 1953;20:753.
10. Callander CL, Rusk GY, Nemir A. Mechanism, symptoms and treatment of hernia into the descending mesocolon (left duodenal hernia): a plea for a change in nomenclature. *Surg Gynecol Obstet* 1935;60:1052.
11. Carlisle BB, Killen DA. Spontaneous transverse mesocolic hernia with re-entry into the greater peritoneal cavity: report of a case with review of the literature. *Surgery* 1967;62:268–273.
12. Chaurasia BD, Kanhere MH, Dharker RS. Exocoelomic internal hernia: elucidation of Papez's concept. *Acta Anat* 1975;91:305–312.
13. Chung CC, Leung KL, Lau WY, et al. Spontaneous internal herniation through the foramen of Winslow: a case report. *Can J Surg* 1997;40:64–65.
14. Cohen AM, Patel S. Arteriographic findings in congenital transmesenteric internal hernia. *AJR Am J Roentgenol* 1979;133:541–543.
15. Corberi O, Crespi G, Deho E. Le ernie interne addominali: prezentazione di 10 casi trattadi. *Minerva Chir* 1980;35:1685.
16. Davis R. Surgery of left paraduodenal hernia. *Am J Surg* 1975;129:570–573.
17. Dengler WC, Reddy PP. Right paraduodenal hernia in childhood: a case report. *J Pediatr Surg* 1989;24:1153–1154.
18. Donnelly LF, Rencken IO, deLorimier AA, et al. Left paraduodenal hernia leading to ileal obstruction. *Pediatr Radiol* 1996;26:534–536.
19. Erskine JM. Hernia through the foramen of Winslow. *Surg Gynecol Obstet* 1967;125:1093–1109.
20. Erskine JM. Hernia through the foramen of Winslow. A case report of the cecum incarcerated in the lesser omental cavity. *Am J Surg* 1967;114:941–947.
21. Estrada RL. *Anomalies of intestinal rotation and fixation.* Springfield: Thomas, 1958.
22. Evrard V, Vielle G, Buyck A, et al. Herniation through the foramen of Winslow. Report of two cases. *Dis Colon Rectum* 1996;39:1055–1057.
23. Federschmidt F. Embryonal origin of lacunae in mesenteric tissue; the pathologic changes resulting there from. *Deutsche Ztschr f Chir* 1920;158:205.
24. Freund H, Berlatzky Y. Small paraduodenal hernias. *Arch Surg* 1977;112:1180–1183.
25. Ghahremani GG. Internal abdominal hernias. *Surg Clin North Am* 1984;64:393–406.
26. Gray SW, Skandalakis JE. *Embryology for surgeons.* Philadelphia: WB Saunders, 1972.
27. Gullino D, Giodano O, Gullino E. Les hernies internes de l'abdomen. *J Chir* 1993;130:179–195.
28. Harbin WP, Andres J, Kim SH, et al. Internal hernia into Treves' field pouch. Case report and review of the literature. *Radiology* 1979;130:71–72.
29. Haymond HE, Dragstedt LR. Anomalies of intestinal rotation; review of literature with report of two cases. *Surg Gynecol Obstet* 1931;53:316.
30. Hirasaki S, Koide N, Shima Y, et al. Unusual variant of left paraduodenal hernia herniated into the mesocolic fossa leading to jejunal strangulation. *J Gastroenterol* 1998;33:734–738.
31. Hollenberg MS. Radiographic diagnosis of hernia into lesser peritoneal sac through foramen of Winslow: report of a case. *Surgery* 1945;18:498.
32. Ishihara H, Terahara M, Kigawa J, et al. Strangulated herniation through a defect of the broad ligament of the uterus. *Gynecol Obstet Invest* 1993;35:187–189.
33. Iuchtman M, Berant M, Assa J. Transomental strangulation. *J Pediatr Surg* 1978;13:439–440.
34. Janin Y, Stone AM, Wise L. Mesenteric hernia. *Surg Gynecol Obstet* 1980;150:747–754.
35. Judd JR. Mesenteric defects with special reference to their etiology and report of rare case of colonic obstruction. *Surg Gynecol Obstet* 1929;48:264.
36. Khan MA, Lo AY, Vande MD. Paraduodenal hernia. *Am Surg* 1998;64:1218–1222.
37. Krijgsman B, Salter MC. Internal herniation through a colonic epiploica [Letter]. *Surgery* 1997;122:643.
37a. Kummer E. Signes radiologiques de la hernie interne duodenojejunale. *J Radiol Electrol* 1921;5:362.
38. Lee TK, Voon FC, Chow KW, et al. Unusual variant of right paraduodenal hernia. *Aust N Z J Surg* 1990;60:483–485.
39. Leissner KH. Transomental strangulation. A rare case of an internal hernia. *Acta Chir Scand* 1976;142:483–485.
40. Liakakos T, Liatas AC, Kakoulides D, et al. Multiple congenital internal hernias as a cause of acute abdominal symptoms in late adult life. *Eur J Surg* 1992;158:561–562.
41. Marsh H. Case of intestinal obstruction treated by laparotomy; recovery, remarks. *Br Med J* 1888;1:1157.
42. Mathieson AM, Miller WG. Ileovaginal fistula. Complicating internal hernia strangulation through a broad ligament defect. *Br J Surg* 1971;58:353–355.
43. McDonagh T, Jelinek GA. Two cases of paraduodenal hernia, a rare internal hernia. *J Accid Emerg Med* 1996;13:64–68.
44. Mersheimer WL, Kazarian KK, Roeder WJ. Internal hernia due to defects in the broad ligament: report of two cases. *Rev Surg* 1973;30:241–245.

45. Miller JM, Wakefield EG. Congenital anomalies of the primary midgut loop. *Am J Dig Dis* 1942;9:383.

46. Moynihan BGA. *On retroperitoneal hernia.* London: Balliere, Tindall and Cox, 1899.

47. Murphy DA. Internal hernias in infancy and childhood. *Surgery* 1964;55:311–316.

48. Nathan H. Internal hernia. *J Int Coll Surg* 1960;34:563–571.

49. Neubauer JE. Descripto anatomica parissimi peritonaei conceptaculi tenuia intestine a reliquis abdominis sedusa tenentis. In: Hinder G, ed. *Opera Anatomica Collecta.* Francofurti, 1786.

50. Ohkuma R, Miyazaki K. Hernia through the foramen of Winslow. *Jpn J Surg* 1977;7:151–157.

51. Oriuchi T, Kinouchi Y, Hiwatashi N, et al. Bilateral paraduodenal hernias: computed tomography and magnetic resonance imaging appearance. *Abdom Imaging* 1998;23:278–280.

52. Panula HE, Alhava E. Internal hernia of foramen of Winslow: a rare congenital condition. *Eur J Surg* 1995;161:695–696.

53. Papez JW. Rare intestinal anomaly of embryonic origin. *Anat Rec* 1932;54:197.

54. Quain. Case of internal strangulation of a large portion of the ileum. *Trans Pathol Soc Lond* 1861;7:103.

55. Rosen L, Woldenberg D, Friedman IH. Small-bowel obstruction secondary to pericecal hernia. *Dis Colon Rectum* 1981;24:45–46.

56. Sadler TW, ed. *Langman's medical embryology,* 6th ed. Baltimore: Williams & Wilkins, 1990.

57. Sampliner JE, Lee YC. Small-bowel obstruction due to congenital anomaly of the falciform ligament. *Arch.Surg* 1976;111:200.

58. Shaffner LD, Pennell TC. Congenital internal hernia. *Surg Clin North Am* 1971;51:1355–1359.

59. Simstein NL. Internal herniation through a defect in the broad ligament. *Am Surg* 1987;53:258–259.

60. Slezak FA, Schneider TJ. Hernia of the broad ligament. In: Nyhus L, Condon R, eds. *Hernia,* 4th ed. Philadelphia: JB Lippincott Co, 1995:491–497.

61. Stone AM, Janin Y, Wise L. Mesenteric hernia. In: Nyhus L, Condon R, eds. *Hernia,* 4th ed. Philadelphia: JB Lippincott Co, 1995:467–474.

62. Sufian S, Matsumoto T. Intestinal obstruction. *Am J Surg* 1975; 130:9–14.

63. Suzuki M, Takashima T, Funaki H, et al. Radiologic imaging of herniation of the small bowel through a defect in the broad ligament. *Gastrointest Radiol* 1986;11:102–104.

64. Takagi Y, Yasuda K, Nakada T, et al. A case of strangulated transomental hernia diagnosed preoperatively. *Am J Gastroenterol* 1996;91:1659–1660.

65. Toppins AC, Ford KL. Aunt Minnie's corner. Left paraduodenal internal hernia. *J Comput Assist Tomogr* 1998;22:844.

66. Treitz W. *Hernia retroperitonealis: Ein Beitrag zur gesichte innerer hernies.* Prague: Credner, 1857.

67. Treves F. Clinical lecture on hernia into the foramen of Winslow. *Lancet* 1888;2:701.

68. Treves F. Lectures on the anatomy of the intestinal canal and peritoneum in man. *Br Med J* 1885;1:470–474.

69. Turley K. Right paraduodenal hernia: a source of chronic abdominal pain in the adult. *Arch Surg* 1979;114:1072–1074.

70. Wachsberg RH, Helinek TG, Merton DA. Internal abdominal hernia: diagnosis with ultrasonography. *Can Assoc Radiol J* 1994;45:223–224.

71. Weber P, Von LH, Oleszczuk-Rascke K, et al. Internal abdominal hernias in childhood. *J Pediatr Gastroenterol Nutr* 1997;25: 358–362.

72. White A. Mesenteric hernia and double volvulus in Africa and Rhodesia. *J R Coll Surg Edinb* 1962;7:138.

73. Willwerth BM, Zollinger RMJ, Izant RJJ. Congenital mesocolic (paraduodenal) hernia. Embryologic basis of repair. *Am J Surg* 1974;128:358–361.

74. Wojtasek DA, Codner MA, Nowak EJ. CT diagnosis of cecal herniation through the foramen of Winslow. *Gastrointest Radiol* 1991;16:77–79.

75. Yip AW, Tong KK, Choi TK. Mesenteric hernias through defects of the mesosigmoid. *Aust N Z J Surg* 1990;60:396–399.

76. Zimmerman LM, Laufman HL. Intra-abdominal hernias due to developmental and rotational anomalies. *Ann Surg* 1953; 138:82.

40

CONGENITAL DIAPHRAGMATIC HERNIA

RONALD K. WOODS
KEITH W. ASHCRAFT

Congenital diaphragmatic hernia (CDH) has an appreciable morbidity and mortality secondary to its unique pathophysiology. Unlike all other hernias occurring in humans, the classical therapy of content reduction and defect closure does not cure the patient with CDH. Although the hernia is held ultimately accountable for initiating the pathophysiology of pulmonary hypoplasia and pulmonary artery hypertension, postnatal correction of the anatomic hernia defect does not reverse this process or eliminate the problems initiated by the hernia.

As an anatomic boundary with multiple embryologic origins, the diaphragm contains various sites where defects can occur. The anterior foramen of Morgagni's hernia and diffuse eventration are well-known examples for which treatment is not controversial. Hiatal hernia and paraesophageal hernias are also quite common and merit detailed attention provided by other chapters in this book. This chapter will therefore focus exclusively on Bochdalek's posterolateral CDH (Fig. 40.1).

EMBRYOLOGY

An understanding of the embryology of the diaphragm, normal intestinal midgut herniation, and normal lung development provides the basis for understanding the physiologic derangements associated with CDH (26). In humans, week 4 marks the initial event with formation of the septum transversum, the component of the diaphragm that ultimately gives rise to the central tendon. The septum transversum partially separates the thoracic and abdominal cavities, leaving paired dorsolaterally located canals. Pleuroperitoneal folds from the lateral body wall grow ventrally and medially, and eventually fuse with the septum transversum and the mesentery of the esophagus (the origin of the

crura) during week 7. The process of muscularization of the diaphragm is believed to occur by migration of myoblasts from cervical myotomes and fusion of lumbar and costal muscle groups.

The normal process of midgut herniation through the abdominal wall occurs concurrent with formation of the diaphragm. During weeks 9 and 10, the return of the midgut to the abdominal cavity should occur after closure of the pleuroperitoneal canals. Herniation of viscera into the chest of the baby with CDH may therefore occur via three possible mechanisms: (a) incomplete closure of the pleuroperitoneal canal; (b) early return of the midgut preceding closure of the canal; or (c) the midgut undergoing primary herniation into the chest, rather than through the anterior body wall.

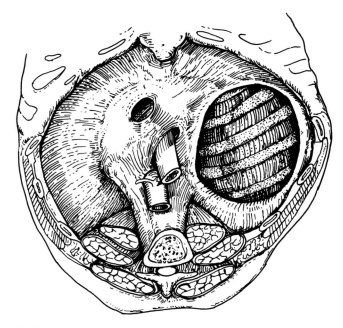

FIGURE 40.1. Depiction of left-sided congenital diaphragmatic defect.

R. K. Woods: Department of Surgery, Division of Cardiothoracic Surgery, University of Washington, Seattle, Washington.

K. Ashcraft: Department of Surgery, University of Missouri at Kansas City; Children's Mercy Hospital, Kansas City, Missouri.

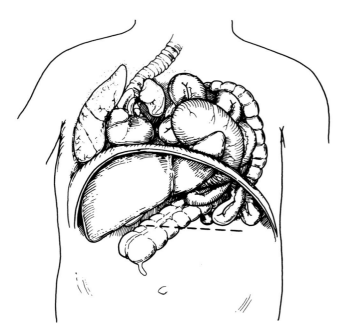

FIGURE 40.2. Herniation of abdominal viscera associated with hypoplasia of the lung and mediastinal shift to the contralateral side. *Dashed line* indicates the location of the incision for a subcostal approach.

The abdominal viscera in the chest either cause or are associated with diminished growth of the ipsilateral lung. Associated mediastinal shift produces less severe effects on the contralateral lung (Fig. 40.2) (28,37). Impairment of bronchial subdivision causes a decrease in the total number of alveoli. In addition, pulmonary vasculature is concurrently altered (28,41). The pulmonary intravascular space is reduced, and the arterial system is more reactive, demonstrating medial hyperplasia and an increase in adventitial thickness. The reactivity of the arterioles leads to pulmonary hypertensive crises that may be impossible to mitigate.

HISTORY

The first written record of this condition dates to the 17th century with Lazarus Riverius' report of a postmortem analysis of a 24-year-old man (24). The anatomist Vincent Alexander Bochdalek reported two cases and an anatomic description of CDH in 1848 (5). Despite incorrectly assigning significance to rupture of a membrane of the lumbocostal triangle, his name has persisted in the designation of the foramen classically associated with CDH.

Heidenhain performed the first successful repair in a 9-year-old boy (11). Although Bettman and Hess performed the first repair in an infant in 1928, Ladd and Gross in the 1940s were the first to direct surgical attention to the newborn (4,16). Nine of their first 16 patients survived. Over

the next 3 decades, the regard for CDH became one of a surgical emergency—unless the bowel is removed from the chest, the baby will die of respiratory failure. Success of the neonatal intensive care and anesthetic efforts in the 1970s facilitated an apparent initial improvement in the outcome of immediate surgical intervention, further fostering its popularity. The state of the art in the mid-1970s was conceptually clear—surgery allowed those who could survive to do so with the viscera in the correct compartment of the body.

Subsequent capability for early recognition of the defect and support of the infant for transport to a facility providing definitive care did not improve surgical outcome, however. Patients formerly dying at delivery or during transport were now dying postoperatively in pediatric surgical units. The impetus to reevaluate the role of early surgery was further motivated by the early results of using extracorporeal membrane oxygenation (ECMO). This technology was first used successfully in the neonate in 1975 and subsequently used for the infant with CDH in 1982 (2). Although there were spurious reports of increased survival, the significance of ECMO was based more on its impact on our understanding of the underlying disease process. In many cases, it allowed life to continue without surgical intervention for an extended time. This permitted more extensive observation of the underlying pathophysiology of pulmonary hypertension and relegated surgical intervention to a less significant and certainly less emergent realm.

Extracorporeal support and lung rest also contributed to our understanding of iatrogenic lung injury. Prior to ECMO, babies' lungs were severely damaged by the use of ventilatory peak pressures often exceeding 50 or 60 cm H_2O needed to keep the babies alive. Research performed in the 1980s and early 1990s demonstrated the capability of inducing acute lung injury, histologically indistinguishable from that of adult or infant respiratory distress syndrome, with the use of mechanical ventilation and volutrauma (12,15). This led to the use of limited pressure ventilation, which, if not adequate, was supplanted by ECMO to rescue the case and allow minor degrees of lung injury to heal. With management based on this philosophy, some centers are now reporting survivals in excess of 80% (7,23,31,40). More widespread confirmation of the reality of this improvement is eagerly awaited.

The most recent step in the history of CDH is the understanding of the true natural history of this condition afforded by *in utero* intervention studies. Attention to early diagnosis and careful followup has shown that mortality for all fetuses diagnosed early in gestation remains a prohibitive 40% to 50%, despite optimal *in utero* and postnatal intervention (9,10,32). The discrepancy in mortality rates at various centers is probably based in part on variations in referral patterns and patient populations. Although most authors would agree that we have improved the outcome for babies with CDH in the past decade, the incremental increase in survival compared to the invested effort has been disappointingly small.

EPIDEMIOLOGY

CDH occurs in approximately one in every 2,000 gestations (30). There is no obvious correlation with maternal age or ethnicity. The male-to-female ratio is approximately 1.25. Although cases occurring in twins have been reported, there is currently no evidence for a genetic predisposition to CDH. The posterolateral defect accounts for greater than 95% of cases. Approximately 80% to 90% of CDHs occur on the left side, and 10% to 15% are bilateral.

ASSOCIATED ANOMALIES

Approximately 30% to 50% of newborn infants have associated anomalies (6). This incidence exceeds 90% in stillborns with CDH. The range of anomalies and syndromes is extensive. Cardiovascular anomalies account for over 50% of associated abnormalities, with cardiac hypoplasia predominating. Atrial septal defect and ventricular septal defect each accounts for approximately 10% to 12% of cardiac anomalies. Genitourinary malformations, mostly hydronephrosis and cystic dysplasia, account for approximately 25% of anomalies. Other less frequently occurring abnormalities include spina bifida, hydrocephalus, cleft palate, gastroschisis, and Meckel's diverticulum. Known chromosomal aberrations associated with CDH include trisomies of chromosomes 5, 13, 18, 20, and 21, and tetraploidy of chromosome 21. The presence of associated anomalies in the newborn increases the mortality to approximately 90% to 100%.

DIAGNOSIS

Diagnosis of CDH is confirmed prenatally or immediately postnatally in the majority of cases. A prenatal diagnosis, although theoretically possible, is not obtained in many cases. In fact, a recent multicenter survey reported a mean prenatal diagnosis rate of 37%; the highest rate in this survey was 66% (23). Failure to achieve higher rates is based on the lack of use of prenatal ultrasonography and the limitations inherent to the technology. Sensitivity for the ultrasonographic diagnosis of CDH ranges from 40% to 90%. Diagnosis at 15 weeks of gestation is possible; however, the majority of prenatal diagnoses are made later in the second trimester. Typical diagnostic findings include absence of intraabdominal gastric bubble, thoracic gastric bubble, presence of liver in the thorax, polyhydramnios, mediastinal and cardiac shift from the side of herniation, and, in extreme cases, hydrops. If the diagnosis is made *in utero*, it is appropriate to obtain a high level ultrasound study and to evaluate the fetal karyotype using amniocentesis, chorionic villus sampling, or cord blood sampling. Such information is obviously relevant to the potential decision about termination of pregnancy.

Postnatal diagnosis is usually confirmed in the first 24 hours of life. The physical examination may demonstrate asymmetry of the chest, a scaphoid abdomen, decreased breath sounds, or the presence of bowel sounds with auscultation of the affected chest. The classic presentation is respiratory distress, for which a chest radiograph is obtained, revealing loops of bowel in the chest or the tip of a nasogastric tube turned upward into the chest (Fig. 40.3). Any ambiguity in diagnosis can usually be eliminated by passage of a nasogastric tube and a limited upper gastrointestinal contrast study. The differential diagnostic possibilities include congenital cystic lung anomalies, eventration of the diaphragm, Morgagni's hernia, pulmonary agenesis, Cantrell's pentalogy, and hiatal or paraesophageal hernia. After confirming the diagnosis, further evaluation should proceed to rule out

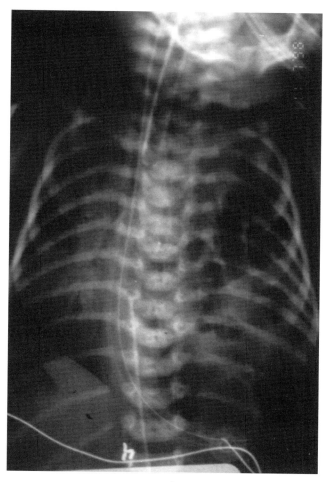

FIGURE 40.3. Chest radiograph of an infant with left-sided congenital diaphragmatic hernia showing multiple loops of bowel in the left chest.

anomalies of the cardiovascular, renal, and central nervous systems. A combination of abdominal and cranial ultrasonography and echocardiography is usually sufficient.

Presentation of CDH beyond the neonatal period is uncommon, estimated to occur in 5% to 20% of babies born with CDH. A report of 20 years of experience at a single institution estimated a frequency of 10% (3). The late presentation is sometimes mistaken for pulmonary infection, reactive airway disease, empyema, or effusion, for which several children have undergone inappropriate thoracentesis. Repair is indicated in all cases. In general, patients with a delayed presentation do not manifest problems with pulmonary hypertension and tend to have a more benign postoperative course.

TREATMENT

Prenatal Management

The natural history of prenatally diagnosed CDH has been well defined. Eighty-three fetuses diagnosed before 25 weeks of gestation, with no other anatomic or chromosomal abnormalities, were followed for anticipated conventional care after planned delivery at a tertiary neonatal center (9). Fifty-eight percent did not survive, with seven fetuses dying *in utero*. Immediate, severe respiratory distress precluded use of ECMO in 16 babies. An additional 20 babies died despite what was considered optimally sequenced management of conventional ventilation, ECMO, and surgical intervention.

There are potentially useful prognostic factors relevant to decisions about *in utero* intervention or termination of pregnancy. Chromosomal analysis and fetal echocardiography should be performed. The relevance of karyotyping is clear. Some authors advocate the use of echocardiographic findings for survival prediction. While it is true that fetuses with CDH have reduced left heart dimensions, discriminant predictive power is not uniformly supported by the data. There are several general ultrasound findings that relate to pulmonary hypoplasia and are associated with a lower survival (20). Polyhydramnios implies displacement of the stomach into the chest. Occurrence early in gestation is more predictive of a negative outcome. Liver in the chest with the umbilical vein above the diaphragm ("liver-up" CDH), detectable by color flow Doppler, signifies a larger volume of herniated viscera and likely a greater degree of pulmonary hypoplasia. Moreover, *in utero* reduction of the liver is technically difficult, with a propensity to cause severe problems secondary to kinking and obstruction of the umbilical vein.

Another useful ultrasound measurement is the contralateral lung area–to–head circumference ratio (assuming head circumference is grossly normal for gestational age). Values less than 0.6 indicate a very low to zero chance of survival, whereas a value greater than 1.35 predicts greater than 95% survival (20).

Results of a comparison of *in utero* diaphragm repair and conventional postnatal repair were reported in 1997 (8). Criteria for enrollment in this study included "liver-down" CDH and no associated anatomic or genetic abnormalities. There was no difference in survival, length of ventilator support, requirement for ECMO, or length of hospital stay. Cost for the *in utero* intervention group was insignificantly higher. The authors of this study currently consider fetuses for *in utero* diaphragm closure if they demonstrate "liver-down" anatomy and (a) hydrops or (b) polyhydramnios to a severe degree or occurring very early. *In utero* repair is not strongly recommended for otherwise uncomplicated "liver-down" CDH as this form of disease often demonstrates a more benign natural history.

The presently recommended *in utero* intervention is tracheal occlusion (10,32). Occlusion of the trachea impedes egress of amniotic fluid from the lung, thereby effecting a tremendous improvement of the growth of both lungs and a concomitant slow gentle reduction of herniated viscera. This approach showed great promise in the lamb model. It has been applied selectively in human fetuses, initially with open *in utero* surgery using tracheal plugs or externally applied occlusion, and more recently with fetoscopic clipping of the trachea. Recent findings suggest that lungs subjected to tracheal occlusion have altered surfactant production and decreased blood flow and oxygenation, despite the tremendous size of the affected lung (21). Although surfactant and steroids may diminish this effect, details about optimal timing and dosage as well as the outcome of the lungs accordingly treated are not known. The technique is therefore still considered highly experimental.

Obviously, *in utero* intervention can and will be performed in only a few centers with extensive experience. For the general community, referral to such a center can be considered; however, in most cases, prenatal management will focus on the detection of lethal anomalies and reliable prognostic factors, optimum care of the mother, multidisciplinary counseling, and arrangement for delivery at an appropriate tertiary neonatal center.

Postnatal Management

Evolution of our understanding of CDH has introduced substantial change to the philosophy of postnatal management. Emphasis is currently placed on pulmonary hypertension and emergent nonsurgical management, relegating the timing of surgical intervention to a secondary consideration (7,25,28,40,41). The therapeutic spectrum includes a variety of ventilation techniques, pharmacologic therapy, and ECMO, and optimal combinations thereof. Our discussion of therapeutic strategies will emphasize the more general, relevant points.

Initial postnatal management should focus on a timely response to respiratory distress with tracheal intubation and appropriate ventilator support. Subsequent management should allow or facilitate the resolution of pulmonary hypertension with a minimum degree of iatrogenic insult. It is important to recognize the case of the "living nonsurvivor." This is the infant who presents certain findings that almost certainly indicate a fatal outcome. One such indicator is the inability to achieve full saturation of preductal blood or a $Paco_2$ less than 50 mm Hg on maximal conventional ventilator support (18,40). Although postductal sampling assesses the extent of any right-to-left shunting and therefore potentially assesses the effects of pulmonary hypertension, preductal analysis is a more pure measure of the oxygenating capability of the collective alveolar capillary interface. Moreover, increasing the airway pressure to achieve an adequate postductal Pao_2 intensifies the degree of iatrogenic lung injury. A relevant fact is that the Registry of the Extracorporeal Life Support Organization contains no survivors who failed to meet the aforementioned preductal measures of the gas exchange surface (22).

After intubation, an orogastric or nasogastric tube is placed and the bowel decompressed. Umbilical artery and venous lines are placed as indicated. Attempting to pass a line through an umbilical vein kinked by "liver-up" anatomy is impractical and unwise. Sedation is important and safely accomplished with midazolam (Versed) and morphine. The adequately sedated infant may benefit from initial temporary paralysis to prevent air swallowing and resistance to assisted ventilation. The "uncomfortable" infant may simply need an adjustment in ventilator settings and should not be paralyzed in the absence of this consideration.

Hypoxia and/or acidosis exacerbate pulmonary hypertension. Metabolic acidosis is typically due to decreased cardiac function secondary to an underdeveloped left ventricle and poor diastolic myocardial perfusion. It is best treated by establishing euvolemia and providing inotropic support, usually with dopamine (beginning at a dose of 5 to 7.5 μg/kg/min), although dobutamine or epinephrine is a reasonable alternative. Maintaining a normal to supranormal (e.g., 50 to 55 mm Hg) mean arterial pressure is beneficial to systemic perfusion as well as minimizing right-to-left shunting. Every effort is made to establish an initial Pao_2 of greater than 60 mm Hg or a preductal oxygen saturation greater than 88% to 90%. The initial $Paco_2$ should be less than 55 mm Hg. In many infants, such values are attainable with pressure-controlled ventilation using peak inspiratory pressures (PIP) of 25 cm H_2O or less and a positive end expiratory pressure (PEEP) of 5 cm H_2O or less. Pneumothorax is not uncommon, occurring with greater frequency on the contralateral side. It should be a consideration in any instance of clinical instability or failure to improve. Chest tube thoracostomy is definitive care.

At some point early in the initial management, cranial ultrasound should be obtained, because grade II to IV intracranial hemorrhage (ICH) precludes use of ECMO in most centers. Echocardiography is likewise indicated to both assess pulmonary hypertension and diagnose structural anomalies that may preclude use of ECMO or significantly alter the evaluation of survivability. Because ECMO is regarded as a potential requirement for any infant with CDH, arrangements should be made early for transfer to a center with ECMO capability.

Postnatal Management

Mechanical Ventilation

The optimum ventilation strategy remains to be defined, but high airway pressures and prolonged use of high concentrations of oxygen are known to be detrimental (15). In general, PIP should be limited to 25 cm H_2O and PEEP limited to 5 to 6 cm H_2O. Rates can vary from 30 to 60 breaths per minute, depending on the amount of ventilation required and the degree of acceptable auto-PEEP. Inspired oxygen concentration should be reduced to approximately 50% in the first 2 to 3 days. Goals for oxygenation include a preductal saturation of approximately 90% or a Pao_2 of no less than 60 mm Hg. The initial pH should be normal to slightly alkalotic, if possible, using intravenous sodium bicarbonate in a judicious manner. Over the first 24 hours, ventilation can be reduced to allow the $Paco_2$ to rise to as high as 55 to 60 mm Hg, if necessary, while allowing adequate time for renal regulation of bicarbonate. Some infants quickly demonstrate a capability of maintaining adequate oxygenation with inspired oxygen at less than 50%. Such infants are rarely a problem and can be subjected, with near uniform success, to a variety of ventilator strategies.

A variant of customary ventilatory management has been reported in 63 infants who required mechanical support within 2 hours of birth (40). Ventilator settings included PIP limited to 20 to 25 cm, PEEP of 5 cm, and rates of 20 to 40 breaths per minute. Oxygen was administered to maintain preductal saturation at approximately 90%. Infants with labile oxygenation or with $Paco_2$ greater than 60 mm Hg were switched to an unconventional high-frequency pressure-control intermittent mandatory ventilation (PC-IMV) mode using PIP of 18 to 20 cm, PEEP of 0 cm, and a rate of 100 breaths per minute. In this mode, supplemental oxygen was administered to achieve a preductal saturation of greater than 80%. Narcotic sedation was used as needed, and muscle paralysis was uniformly excluded (except during surgery), allowing infants to breathe spontaneously. The primary goal, stated by the authors, was avoidance of hyperinflation and iatrogenic lung injury. Persistent hypoxemia was treated with pulmonary vasodilators (tolazoline or dobutamine). Using this strategy, they reported a survival of greater than 90%, with use of ECMO in less than 10% of infants. This study demonstrated several important points, the most significant of which was the ability to achieve an excellent outcome without using hyperoxia or hypocarbia. Other authors have reported similar findings (7,39).

The "difficult-to-ventilate" infant can usually be recognized in the first few hours and almost uniformly by 24 hours. If the infant remains hypoxic with an Fio_2 of 0.6 or above at 24 hours, or remains hypercarbic to the point of pulmonary hypertensive crises, the conventional mode should be abandoned. Options include rapid-rate PC-IMV or standard high-frequency oscillation ventilation (HFOV). Both techniques strive to minimize cyclic overdistention of the lung and to provide the mean airway pressure requisite for oxygenation with less barotrauma and oxygen toxicity. HFOV is particularly effective at controlling CO_2. Reasonable goals while on HFOV include adequate arterial blood gas values with mean airway pressures less than 10 cm and an inspired oxygen concentration of approximately 50% or less. There is no uniformly accepted limit on the duration of effort required to achieve a satisfactory status on HFOV. Once HFOV is assessed to be inadequate, the next echelon of management is ECMO. The use of inhaled nitric oxide (NO), in our experience, has not eliminated the need for ECMO in the majority of patients.

Extracorporeal Membrane Oxygenation

Understanding the true role of ECMO is paramount to the process of patient selection. It does not cure pulmonary hypertension. It does not cure cardiogenic shock. It does minimize iatrogenic lung injury and provide a surrogate gas exchange surface while providing optimal conditions for the natural maturation of the pulmonary vasculature and parenchyma to the point of sustaining life.

The decision to employ ECMO and the appropriate time to do so are both important decisions with significant implications. ECMO subjects the patient to a new set of risks with potential lifelong implications. It also subjects the family to a potentially lengthy and emotionally burdensome process, perhaps to the point of caring for a neurologically severely challenged child. The financial considerations are likewise significant. On the other hand, it may be an effective intervention that allows the child to recover and live a meaningful life. The complex heterogeneity of the population of infants with CDH precludes uniform application of a single set of criteria. In general, infants who fail maximal conventional support and who are (a) at least 34 weeks of postconceptual age, (b) do not have grade II to IV ICH, and (c) do not have cardiac or other congenital anomalies incompatible with life are considered for ECMO.

An unclearly defined issue is the duration of conventional therapy defining failure and the most appropriate time for initiating ECMO. The pulmonary vasculature is known to mature in the first few days of life, albeit at a slower rate in the baby with CDH than that of a normal newborn. Experience at the authors' institution suggests little benefit in persisting beyond 2 or 3 days of HFOV if hypoxia and hypercarbia remain uncontrollable with safe ventilator settings (28,29). Progressive dysfunction in an

even shorter period of time would likewise be an appropriate indication. Information obtained from echocardiography is relevant to this decision. Failure of pulmonary artery pressure to decrease from systemic levels in the first 2 to 3 days of HFOV is a reasonable adjunctive criterion. Prolonged postponement of ECMO is generally not in the interest of the patient, as it increases the degree of iatrogenic lung injury and increases the cost of hospitalization.

The initiation and daily management of ECMO are conducted according to well-established guidelines (34). Certain points specific to the infant with CDH are noteworthy. Although venoarterial (VA) and venovenous (VV) ECMO are valid options, VA ECMO is indicated for the infant requiring cardiac support. In addition to routine chest films and head ultrasounds, serial echocardiograms (every 3 to 5 days) may be obtained to assess pulmonary artery pressure. Infants with CDH requiring ECMO experience resolution of pulmonary hypertension over a period of 7 to 14 days. A third week of ECMO is usually not beneficial and exposes the infant to an increased risk of complications. Traditional guidelines for weaning and discontinuing ECMO apply to the infant with CDH and are based on the demonstration of acceptable physiology with diminishing ECMO support and "low-trauma" ventilator settings. The ratio of mean pulmonary artery pressure to mean systemic arterial pressure is a more quantitative assessment. Values of 0.5 or less usually indicate the infant can safely tolerate physiologic stress, such as rapid weaning from ECMO or surgical repair. This guideline is consistent with the growing recognition of the importance of stabilization of the pulmonary vasculature.

Despite its widespread use in CDH, ECMO has never been adequately evaluated in a prospective, randomized trial. Results from a forthcoming prospective study are anticipated. Many centers have, however, reported retrospective studies showing improved survival. One study reported a survival of 92% using prolonged preoperative stabilization and ECMO, citing much lower survivals from other locations and eras not relying so heavily on ECMO (7). Another recent study reported a survival of 96%, compared to a survival of 57% in the 1970s, when ECMO was not used (35). In contrast, one investigation demonstrated no difference in survival between a recent study group and a group of historic controls (27). One probable explanation offered by the authors of this paper was the inclusion of a larger percentage of patients with more severe disease in the study group. In an attempt to avoid the bias inherent to the use of historic controls, results using ECMO in Boston were compared to those in Toronto, where ECMO is not used. There was no significant survival advantage of ECMO, but there was a survival advantage associated with the use of "low-trauma" ventilation (1,38).

It is difficult to offer a thoroughly satisfactory explanation for the discrepancies in the results of clinical trials. It is quite possible that ECMO allows the salvage of a certain percentage of babies residing in a delicate balance that would otherwise be easily swayed to mortality from the iatrogenic insult of mechanical ventilation. Babies residing at one of the two extremes of presentation, however, may not derive a significant benefit from ECMO. Obviously, the demand placed on a study designed to discern these and other subtle differences is tremendous. Given the estimated increase in cost due to ECMO—approximately $130,000 without ECMO versus $360,000 with ECMO—there is ample financial motivation, not to mention a desire to simply know the truth (19).

Pharmacologic and Other Adjuncts to Management

As is often the case with challenging clinical problems, several adjunctive measures have been attempted. While many of these interventions have demonstrated efficacy in respiratory failure in the non-CDH context, none of them have been clearly beneficial in patients with CDH. Surfactant is offered to patients at many centers, on the belief that babies with CDH either are deficient in surfactant or produce an ineffective surfactant. Although one study reported inadequate levels of surfactant, a more recent study reported similar amounts and relative contributions of the various phospholipids in ventilated CDH infants and ventilated non-CDH infants (13,36). A prospective evaluation of clinical efficacy has not been reported to date.

Perfluorocarbon liquid ventilation, with or without NO, has also been evaluated at various centers, again in a nonrandomized manner. There are reproducible improvements in oxygenation that do not translate into meaningful differences in survival. Specifically, NO often improves pulmonary artery pressure and oxygenation, but the effect is usually transient. Its utility is likely limited to that of a short-lived (less than 24 hours) rescue agent, while other more definitive strategies are being employed. Other agents with potential efficacy, such as selective β-agonists, are used in some centers, but have never been adequately evaluated in a controlled study.

Repair of the Defect

Although the defect must eventually be repaired, surgical repair almost invariably causes an immediate decline in physiologic status—it never improves it. The most significant factor determining the appropriate time for operation is the degree to which pulmonary hypertension has diminished and stabilized. The criteria discussed previously, especially echocardiographic demonstration of a pulmonary-to-systemic pressure ratio of 0.5 or less, are reasonable guidelines for timing the repair.

Conduct of the operation should be consistent with minimizing operative time, stress, tissue trauma, and excessive fluid shifts. Anesthesia is best conducted with an infant

ventilator or an oscillator and avoidance of overdistention. The anesthetic is typically based on narcotics and muscle relaxants. Repair can be performed via a thoracotomy; however, most surgeons approach the defect via a subcostal incision. All viscera are carefully reduced and any membrane or sac excised. The anterior leaflet of the diaphragm is readily apparent; however, the posterior leaflet must usually be carefully dissected and unrolled from the posterior wall. The medial-most aspect of the anticipated repair site must be assessed for adequate integrity, as this is the most common site for recurrence. If necessary, the left crus can be reconstructed to provide an adequate base for sutures. If primary repair requires undue tension, repair with a prosthetic patch is indicated. Polytetrafluoroethylene is a preferred material (Fig. 40.4). The development of chest wall flaps is less practical as it adds considerable operative time and bleeding and increases the risk for subsequent bleeding should the infant require ECMO postoperatively. Although surgeon preference varies, interrupted repair with braided, permanent suture is appropriate.

Once the diaphragm is repaired, attention is directed to the disposition of the bowel and the abdominal wall. The bowel is usually based on a narrow mesentery. Torsion with reduction must obviously be avoided. Ladd's bands, if present, should be divided. Widening of the mesentery and appendectomy are not indicated, despite the intuitive inclination to do so. Further dissection simply increases time

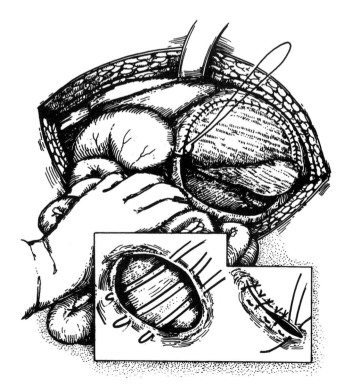

FIGURE 40.4. Primary repair **(inset)** and prosthetic repair as viewed from the subcostal approach.

and bleeding. There are no reported experiences of reducing the risk of volvulus by widening the base of the mesentery. In a series of 24 patients with CDH, all with various anomalies of fixation, there were no subsequent cases of volvulus (17). Once the bowel is properly reduced, an attempt is made to primarily close the abdomen. In most cases, this can be accomplished without difficulty. For difficult primary closures, adjuncts include stretching the abdominal wall, inserting a prosthetic mesh or silo, or simply closing the skin and planning a second operation after the child has improved and the abdomen has undergone accommodation. There is no indication for insertion of chest tubes, except in the context of bleeding, air leak, or some other specific indication. Pleural space mechanics will fill the unoccupied area with fluid and accommodate subsequent expansion of the lung (Fig. 40.5). If a tube is placed, negative pressure should be avoided, at least while the patient is being ventilated with positive pressure.

The potential merits of repairing a patient while on ECMO are not obvious. Criteria guiding the decision to

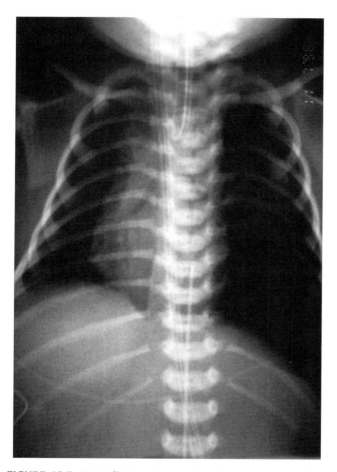

FIGURE 40.5. Immediate postoperative chest radiograph of an infant (corresponding to Fig. 40.3) with left-sided congenital diaphragmatic hernia demonstrating a small hypoplastic left lung and a predominantly air-filled pleural space.

discontinue ECMO apply equally to the selection of an appropriate time for repair. In the unusual context of strangulation or another absolute indication for an unrelated procedure, operative technique obviously must be meticulous, employing liberal use of electrocautery, minimal dissection, and possibly pharmacologic adjuncts to reduce the risk of bleeding.

Postoperative Care

Some degree of postoperative decline in clinical status should be anticipated. Principles guiding the care are the same as those outlined for preoperative management. Although unproven, HFOV may be more appropriate immediately postoperatively. If the patient demonstrates ongoing deterioration manifested by increasing needs for oxygenation and ventilation, early consideration for ECMO is appropriate. Many infants have been "rescued" by a second course of ECMO. Criteria guiding this decision are essentially the same as those described previously, although less time should be spent maximizing less aggressive interventions. The postoperative patient has already experienced a period of iatrogenic ventilator injury and has less reserve to tolerate further injury. In most uncomplicated cases, slow deliberate weaning of ventilator support allows extubation in 5 to 10 days. The complicated case may require ventilator support for up to 3 to 4 weeks.

Transpyloric feeding may begin during the second postoperative day. Feedings are subsequently transitioned to bolus gastric feeding and oral feeding after extubation. Foregut dysmotility and gastroesophageal reflux are common, occurring in as many as two thirds of patients. Conventional conservative measures are helpful and obviate the need for surgical intervention in most infants. One study documented a need for antireflux surgery in 20% of patients (14). The authors of this study suggest the degree of stomach herniation correlates with the incidence of reflux. They also recommend more liberal use of prosthetic closure of the diaphragm and abdominal wall to reduce distortion of the crus and intragastric pressure, respectively. Although not well documented in the literature, these babies can have substantial problems with intake and growth and mandate careful long-term follow-up.

Bronchopulmonary dysplasia is common in CDH babies. Usually, only babies recovering from a prolonged, severe course require ongoing supplemental oxygen. Another complication is pneumonia, occurring more frequently in babies requiring prolonged ECMO (greater than 2 weeks). Aggressive surveillance and antibiotic therapy are the basics of management. Pleural effusions occur on the ipsilateral side in most babies and less commonly on the contralateral side. Ipsilateral fluid is a necessary component of the natural history of the involved hemithorax. Infection and excessive mass effect are indications for drainage. Transient reactive airway disease is also common and readily managed with inhaled bronchodilators. Inhaled or systemic pulsed steroid therapy is infrequently required. Most babies eventually achieve quite satisfactory pulmonary function.

OUTCOMES

Variation in patient population accounts for a wide range of reported survivals, approximately 50% to 95%. Evaluating the impact of recent changes in management on mortality is understandably difficult. It is estimated that overall survival has increased from approximately 50% to 65% (29).

Results of pulmonary function testing vary, depending on the age of the child. Infants less than 1 month of age typically demonstrate restrictive disease. With time, the forced vital capacity improves more rapidly than maximal expiratory flow (MEF), consistent with the development of lower airway obstruction that is usually bronchodilator responsive. Longer-term follow-up is more limited; however, one study evaluating patients aged 7 to 18 years revealed overall function to be quite good, with near-normal lung volume, diffusion capacity, and MEF, but persistence of mild obstruction and airway responsiveness. Evaluation of cardiac function is even more limited. One study reported electrocardiographic evidence of right ventricular hypertrophy in toddlers but normal echocardiographic estimates of pulmonary artery pressure (33).

Neurocognitive outcome generally parallels that of infants with other diagnoses requiring prolonged intensive care and ECMO. One study of 30 infants revealed similar neurologic outcome, but decreased cognitive function. Another study comparing only ECMO-treated infants showed no difference in Bayley or Stanford–Binet scale values between CDH and non-CDH children between 1 and 4 years of age (33). Overall neurodevelopmental status has been estimated to be normal in approximately 60% of children. Abnormalities, when they exist, range from severe quadriparesis to subtle abnormalities of muscle tone. Scheduled long-term multidisciplinary follow-up is indicated to help these children achieve their best possible outcome.

Postnatal management unfortunately cannot significantly alter the underlying pathophysiology of CDH. It can, however, impose a host of additional insults that increase morbidity and mortality. With this understanding, the surgeon and intensivist should focus on detection of the unsalvageable infant, early detection of the salvageable but difficult case, and rapid advancement through progressive echelons of intervention that provide adequate cardiopulmonary support and yet maintain the balance of risk of iatrogenic injury and anticipated benefit in the favor of the child.

REFERENCES

1. Azarow K, Messineo A, Pearl R, et al. Congenital diaphragmatic hernia—a tale of two cities: the Toronto experience. *J Pediatr Surg* 1997;32:395–400.
2. Bartlett RH, Toomasian J, Roloff D, et al. Extracorporeal membrane oxygenation (ECMO) in neonatal respiratory failure: 100 cases. *Ann Surg* 1986;204:236–245.
3. Berman L, Stringer D, Ein SH, et al. The late-presenting pediatric Bochdalek hernia: a 20-year review. *J Pediatr Surg* 1988;23:735–739.
4. Bettman RB, Hess JH. Incarcerated diaphragmatic hernia in an infant, with operation and recovery. *JAMA* 1929;92:2014–2016.
5. Bochdalek VA. Einige Betrachtungen uber die Entstehung des angeborenen Zwerchfellbruches. Als Beitrag zur pathologischen Anatomie der Ilernien. *Vierteljahrschrift fur die praktische Heilkunde* 1848;19:89–97.
6. Fauza DO, Wilson JM. Congenital diaphragmatic hernia and associated anomalies: their incidence, identification, and impact on prognosis. *J Pediatr Surg* 1994;29:1113–1117.
7. Frenckner HE, Granholm T, Linden V, et al. Improved results in patients who have congenital diaphragmatic hernia using preoperative stabilization, extracorporeal membrane oxygenation, and delayed surgery. *J Pediatr Surg* 1997;32:1185–1189.
8. Harrison MR, Adzick NS, Bullard KM, et al. Correction of congenital diaphragmatic hernia in utero VII: a prospective trial. *J Pediatr Surg* 1997;32:1637–1642.
9. Harrison MR, Adzick NS, Estes JM, et al. A prospective study of the outcome for fetuses with diaphragmatic hernia. *JAMA* 1994;271:382–384.
10. Hedrick MH, Estes JM, Sullivan KM, et al. Plug the lung until it grows (PLUG): a new method to treat congenital diaphragmatic hernia in utero. *J Pediatr Surg* 1994;29:612–617.
11. Heidenhain L. Geschichte eines Falles von chronischer Inkarzeration des Magnes in einer angeborenen Zwerchfellhernie, welcher durch Laparotomie geheilt wurde, mit anschliessenden Bemerkungen uber die Moglichkeit, das Cardiacarcinom der Peiserohre zu reseziren. *Deutsche Zeitschrift fur Mund Kiefer and Gesichts Chirurgie* 1905;76:394–403.
12. Hernandez LA, Peevy KJ, Moise AA, et al. Chest wall restriction limits high airway pressure-induced lung injury in young rabbits. *J Appl Physiol* 1989;66:2364–2368.
13. Ijsselstijn H, Zimmermann LJ, Bunt JE, et al. Prospective evaluation of surfactant composition in bronchoalveolar lavage fluid of infants with congenital diaphragmatic hernia and of age-matched controls. *Crit Care Med (United States)* 1998;26:573–580.
14. Kieffer J, Sapin E, Berg A, et al. Gastroesophageal reflux after repair of congenital diaphragmatic hernia. *J Pediatr Surg* 1995;30:1330–1333.
15. Kolobov T, Gattinoni L, Moretti MP, et al. Mechanical pulmonary ventilation at high airway pressures: is it safe? *Int J Artif Organs (Italy)* 1984;7:315–316.
16. Ladd W, Gross RE. Congenital diaphragmatic hernia. *N Engl J Med* 1940;223:917–925.
17. Levin TL, Liebling MS, Ruzal-Shapiro C, et al. Midgut fixation in patients with congenital diaphragmatic hernia: what is the risk of midgut volvulus? *Pediatr Radiol* 1995;25:259–261.
18. Lloret J, Boix-Ochoa J, Marhuenda C, et al. Prognostic factors in congenital diaphragmatic hernia. Can they modify our therapeutic approach? *Cir Pediatr (Spain)* 1993;6:108–110.
19. Metkus AP, Esserman L, Sola A, et al. Cost per anomaly: what does a diaphragmatic hernia cost? *J Pediatr Surg* 1995;30:226–230.
20. Metkus AP, Filly RA, Stringer MD, et al. Sonographic predictors of survival in fetal diaphragmatic hernia. *J Pediatr Surg* 1996;31:148–151.
21. O'Toole SJ, Karamanoukian HL, Glick PL, et al. Tracheal ligation: the dark side of in utero congenital diaphragmatic hernia treatment. *J Pediatr Surg* 1997;32:407–410.
22. Price MR, Galantowicz ME, Stolar CJH. Congenital diaphrag-

matic hernia, extracorporeal membrane oxygenation, and death: a spectrum of etiologies. *J Pediatr Surg* 1991;26:1023–1026.

23. Reickert CA, Hirschl RB, Atkinson JB, et al. Congenital diaphragmatic hernia survival and use of extracorporeal life support at selected level III nurseries with multimodality support. *Surgery* 1998;123:305–310.

24. Riverius L. Opera medica universa. *Observation* 1679;67.

25. Sakai H, Tamura M, Hosokowa Y, et al. Effect of surgical repair on respiratory mechanics in congenital diaphragmatic hernia. *J Pediatr* 1987;111:432–438.

26. Skandalakis JE, Gray SW, Ricketts RR. The diaphragm. In: Skandalakis JE, Gray SW, eds. *Embryology for surgeons*. Baltimore: Williams & Wilkins, 1994.

27. Steimle CN, Meric F, Hirschl RB, et al. Effect of extracorporeal life support on survival when applied to all patients with congenital diaphragmatic hernia. *J Pediatr Surg* 1994;29:997–1001.

28. Thibeault DW, Haney B. Lung volume, pulmonary vasculature, and factors affecting survival in congenital diaphragmatic hernia. *Pediatrics* 1998;101:289–295.

29. Thibeault DW, Sigalet DL. Congenital diaphragmatic hernia from the womb to childhood. *Curr Probl Pediatr* 1998;28:1–25.

30. Torfs CD, Curry CJR, Bateson TF, et al. A population based study of congenital diaphragmatic hernia. *Teratology* 1992;46:555–565.

31. Vanamo K. A 45-year perspective of congenital diaphragmatic hernia. *Br J Surg* 1996;83:1758–1762.

32. VanderWall KJ, Skarsgard ED, Harrison MR, et al. Fetendo-clip: a fetal endoscopic tracheal clip procedure in a human fetus. *J Pediatr Surg* 1997;32:970–972.

33. Van Meurs KP, Robbins ST, Reed VL, et al. Congenital diaphragmatic hernia: long-term outcome in neonates treated with extracorporeal membrane oxygenation. *J Pediatr* 1993;122:893–899.

34. von Allmen D. Extracorporeal membrane oxygenation. In: Nakayama DK, Bose CL, Chescheir NC, et al., eds. *Critical care of the surgical newborn*. Armonk, NY: Futura Publishers, 1997.

35. Weber TR, Kountzman B, Dillon PA, et al. Improved survival in congenital diaphragmatic hernia with evolving therapeutic strategies. *Arch Surg* 1998;133:498–502.

36. Wilcox DT, Glick PL, Karamanoukian HL, et al. Pathophysiology of congenital diaphragmatic hernia. XII: amniotic fluid lecithin/sphingomyelin ratio and phosphatidylglycerol concentrations do not predict surfactant status in congenital diaphragmatic hernia. *J Pediatr Surg* 1995;30:410–412.

37. Wilcox DT, Irish MS, Holm BA, et al. Pulmonary parenchymal abnormalities in congenital diaphragmatic hernia. *Clin Perinatol (United States)* 1996;23:771–779.

38. Wilson JM, Lund DP, Lillihei CW, et al. Congenital diaphragmatic hernia—a tale of two cities: the Boston experience. *J Pediatr Surg* 1997;32:401–405.

39. Wung JT, James LS, Kilchevsky E, et al. Management of infants with severe respiratory failure and persistence of the fetal circulation without hyperventilation. *Pediatrics* 1985;76:488–494.

40. Wung JT, Sahni R, Stolar CJH, et al. Congenital diaphragmatic hernia: survival treated with very delayed surgery, spontaneous respiration, and no chest tube. *J Pediatr Surg* 1995;30:406–409.

41. Yamataka T, Puri P. Pulmonary artery structural changes in pulmonary hypertension complicating congenital diaphragmatic hernia. *J Pediatr Surg* 1997;32:387–390.

DIAPHRAGMATIC HERNIAS

41

SLIDING HIATAL HERNIA

ROBERT E. MARSH
CHARLES J. FILIPI
FRANCISCO TERCERO

Hiatal hernia, a common finding at radiography, was first diagnosed at autopsy and was considered a congenital defect. Occasionally trauma was the causative factor, but hiatal hernia formation and its high incidence of occurrence was not appreciated until the technology of radiographic imaging was refined. By 1926, it was reported that hiatal hernia was found in 2.6% of all upper gastrointestinal examinations, and now with provocative tests some have found the entity present in up to 55% of patients examined. The association of sliding hiatal hernia with gastroesophageal reflux disease (GERD) was first noted by Allison in the late 1940s. The controversy concerning the cause-and-effect relationship of the two remains today.

Consequently, in this chapter, the pathogenesis of GERD as it relates to hiatal hernia will be covered. Laparoscopic surgery has irreversibly altered the therapeutic approach to GERD. Currently, over 50,000 laparoscopic operations are being performed in the United States, and it is expected this number will continue to increase. Approximately 28,000 operations were performed for GERD in 1992. Thus, diagnosis of hiatal hernia will be covered, but most importantly the laparoscopic surgical treatment of hiatal hernia and its causes of recurrence will be emphasized.

ANATOMY AND PHYSIOLOGY

The esophagus, diaphragmatic crus, and stomach all play an important role in the physiology of swallowing. The diaphragm and its attachments (in particular, the phrenoesophageal ligament) are critical in separating the negative pressure in the thorax from the positive pressure of the abdomen. The ligament acts as a tether for the dynamic gastroesophageal junction, which moves with bending, Valsalva maneuvers, and each respiration and heartbeat, plus esophageal gastric peristalsis (Fig. 41.1). Attaching the distal esophagus to the diaphragm, the phrenoesophageal ligament is a membranous continuation of the endoabdominal fascia (4). Recoil of this membrane pulls the gastroesophageal junction back to its intraabdominal position (30). This, in turn, creates a hydrostatic force sufficient to overcome the thoracoabdominal pressure gradient. Fykes in 1956 first described the evidence for an antireflux sphincter. Since that description, mounting evidence has established a role for both the intrinsic musculature of the distal esophagus (lower esophageal sphincter) and the diaphragm in maintaining that sphincter. While its individual physiology is beyond the scope of this chapter, the lower esophageal sphincter maintains a resting pressure that disallows the reflux of gastric contents at end-expiration.

The role of the diaphragm has been largely speculative until recently. The fibers of the crus contract momentarily

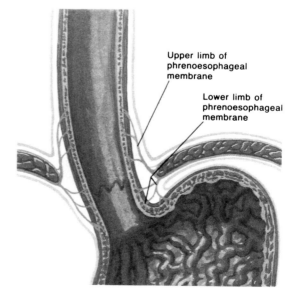

Upper limb of phrenoesophageal membrane

Lower limb of phrenoesophageal membrane

FIGURE 41.1. The phrenoesophageal ligament, which assists in securing the gastroesophageal junction. See Color Plate 8.

R.E. Marsh, C.J. Filipi, and F. Tercero: Department of Surgery, Creighton University, Omaha, Nebraska.

before the rest of the diaphragm, causing an increase in pressure on the distal esophagus. An augmentation of the resting pressure has been shown in manometric studies concurrent with electromyographic activity of the diaphragm (16). There remains a sphincter-like mechanism when the lower esophageal sphincter is removed *en bloc* with the distal esophagus and proximal stomach. The only structure remaining that could generate such a pressure is the diaphragmatic crus.

A review of the normal swallowing mechanism elucidates the role of the diaphragm and its attachments. On initiation of a swallow, the upper and lower esophageal sphincters of the esophagus immediately relax but do not open. A peristaltic wave proceeds down the length of the esophagus due to contraction of the circular fibers. Concomitantly, the longitudinal muscles of the esophagus contract, physiologically shortening the esophagus (30). Each segment of the esophagus is returned to its original length by the contraction of the segment immediately distal. At the level of the gastroesophageal junction, a phrenic ampulla is created by the distal muscular shortening of the esophagus (Fig. 41.2). This phrenic ampulla, in essence, is a herniation of the proximal stomach upward through the esophageal hiatus (13). The pressure relationships are such that the pressure in the ampulla is less than either the distal esophageal pressure or the pressure brought to bear by the contraction of the diaphragmatic crus. This physiologic shortening of the esophagus, and thus the size of the phrenic ampulla, is limited by the phrenoesophageal ligament (30).

The crus has a second role in the propagation of a swallow. The pressure differences between the thorax and abdomen are such that reflux is promoted with an increase in abdominal pressure unless a process is in place to stop it. The phrenoesophageal ligament, by virtue of its insertion on the proximal lower esophageal sphincter, serves to impart the positive pressure of the abdomen across the sphincter (4). Similarly, the

diaphragm serves as a "one-way valve" in the act of swallowing. The esophageal ampulla fills from above as the bolus is propelled ahead of the peristaltic wave. As the wave reaches the phrenic ampulla, intraampullary pressure increases and emptying begins with the relengthening of the esophagus. At expiration, the intraabdominal pressure diminishes and flow is forward into the stomach. The crus at this point is in a relaxed position. The opposite is true with inspiration: the intraabdominal pressure increases and antegrade flow is stopped because of this pressure head. Contraction of the crus imparts a further pressure across the gastroesophageal junction such that backward flow is also impaired. This relationship relies on the proper positioning of the phrenoesophageal ligament.

The physiology of the structures surrounding and within the esophageal hiatus is complex and incompletely understood. Nevertheless, it is helpful to think of the lower esophageal sphincter as the internal sphincter of the gastroesophageal junction and the crus as the external sphincter.

PATHOPHYSIOLOGY

To adequately understand the contributions of a hiatal hernia to gastroesophageal reflux, an understanding of the various mediators for reflux control is needed. Esophageal clearance of acid via chemical and peristaltic clearance, as well as gravity, are essential in limiting both the contact time of acid and subsequent injury due to that contact. The "pinchcock" effect of the diaphragm is also important in the maintenance of a sphincter pressure to inhibit aboral movement of refluxate. Anatomic factors such as the position of the phrenoesophageal ligament, His' angle, and the size of hiatal hernia have been shown to correlate with esophageal acid exposure. Similarly, the lower esophageal sphincter length, pressure, position, and transient relaxation rate all influence the rate of reflux. In order to facilitate or promote GERD, a hiatal hernia must disrupt the control of reflux via the above-mentioned mechanisms (4).

The presence of a phrenic ampulla that either does not reduce or reduces minimally has repeatedly been demonstrated to delay esophageal clearance (14,28). Esophagitis is a very common finding in hiatal hernia and vice versa. In fact, the size of a hiatal hernia has been directly correlated with the severity of esophagitis (28). There are many theories as to how a hiatal hernia may promote or facilitate reflux. Due to the multifactorial nature of the disease, however, direct evidence of the causative role of a hiatal hernia has been limited.

The presence of a hiatal hernia decreases forward bolus flow by disrupting the normal emptying mechanism of the distal esophagus (17). A "common channel" is formed between the proximal stomach and the distal esophagus, allowing the free transfer of acid. This occurs after the start of a swallow and with the relaxation of the lower esophageal sphincter. Under normal conditions, the lower esophageal sphincter does not open because the pressure within the ampulla is less than the pressure of the lower esophageal sphincter. In the presence of a hiatal hernia, however, the pressure of the phrenic ampulla

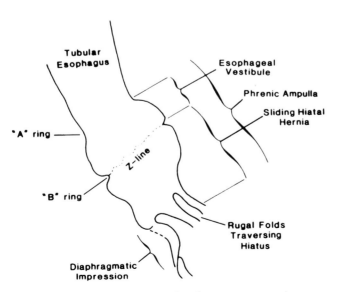

FIGURE 41.2. The phrenic ampulla often seen on esophagography.

exceeds that within the lower esophageal sphincter (with a larger radius, more tension is placed across the wall as dictated by Laplace's law), and the lower esophageal sphincter is opened prematurely. This not only creates a common channel, but also disrupts the fundamental method for esophageal emptying. The lack of compartmentalized pressures in the distal esophagus disables the action of relengthening of the esophagus. This, in turn, impairs the normal emptying of the esophagus (14). In fact, complete emptying of the esophagus occurs in less than a third of swallows when a nonreducing hiatal hernia is present (28). The presence of a phrenic ampulla that is not maximally reduced with each swallow (a reducing hiatal hernia) is also associated with impairment of esophageal clearance. Even when the common channel is transient, as in the case of a partially reducing hiatal hernia, multiple concurrent episodes of reflux occur, increasing the percentage of time that the esophagus is exposed to an acidic environment (28). This repeated "backwash" of acid, coupled with the inherent delay in esophageal clearance, causes repetitive injury to the esophageal mucosa (17).

The presence of a hiatal hernia may further promote reflux by augmenting the pressure within the phrenic ampulla. Laplace's law states that the force [or tension (T)] generating a pressure (P) is directly proportional to the radius (R) of the lumen (T = PR/2). The radius of the lower esophageal sphincter lumen is much less than that of the lumen of the stomach, and therefore much less force is required to maintain its occlusion. However, in the presence of a persistent phrenic ampulla (i.e., a hiatal hernia), this relationship is changed. The lumen of the stomach is now split in two by the constrictive effects of the diaphragm, the lumen of the ampulla, and the lumen of the stomach. With this larger radius, the amount of tension across the ampulla is increased over that of the stomach and approaches that of the lower esophageal sphincter, tending to open it. Reflux is the result.

There is a respiratory dependent emptying of the distal esophagus presumably aided by gravity (28). With inspiration, the lower esophageal sphincter is occluded at maximal pressure regardless of peristalsis. The converse is true with expiration. In the presence of a hiatal hernia, the augmentation of the lower esophageal sphincter is lost as is respiration-dependent emptying. The result is an opening of the lower esophageal sphincter with inspiration, allowing any contents of the proximal stomach lying above the diaphragm to reflux (28). This is further complicated by ineffective emptying of the esophagus when relengthening, as mentioned above.

The presence of a hiatal hernia disrupts the normal spatial relationships of the lower esophageal sphincter and proximal stomach. The His' angle formed by the cardia of the stomach has been shown to be important to the integrity of the lower esophageal sphincter. When made more obtuse, this angle changes the effect that increasing gastric tension has on the lower esophageal sphincter. At the more normal angle, an increase in gastric pressure would serve to push the cardia against the lower esophageal sphincter and maintain its occlusion. Flattening this angle, on the other hand, has the opposite effect. Because the stomach lies freely below the diaphragm, this angle is easily maintained in normal patients. The migration of the stomach above the diaphragm occurs in such a way that the lower esophageal sphincter is pulled through the hiatus first, then the cardia. Thus, the angle is increased and any distention of the cardia serves to pull the walls of the lower esophageal sphincter apart.

The phrenoesophageal ligament is an important component in the prevention of reflux. Because of its insertion, any increase in abdominal pressure increases the pressure across the lower esophageal sphincter as well. When this ligament is transected experimentally, the pressure of the lower esophageal sphincter drastically diminishes. Its reanastomosis results in a return of normal lower esophageal sphincter pressures. There are three conditions in which the phrenoesophageal ligament could theoretically promote reflux: (a) the ligament inserts too low on the lower esophageal sphincter; (b) it is attenuated; or (c) it is absent altogether (4).

Normally, the augmentation of the lower esophageal sphincter is maintained due to an increase in the circumferential pressure to the walls of the distal esophagus and stomach. If the insertion of the phrenoesophageal ligament is too low, not only is this augmentation lost, but the relationships are such that the tension on the stomach is much greater than that across the lower esophageal sphincter, which now lies in the relatively negative environment of the chest. The lower esophageal sphincter is then "pulled open" by the increase in tension, and reflux results.

An attenuation of the phrenoesophageal ligament promotes reflux in four separate ways. First, serving as an anchor holding the lower esophageal sphincter in the abdominal cavity, attenuation of this ligament would allow the migration of the lower esophageal sphincter into the chest. As mentioned previously, this changes the His' angle, thereby promoting reflux. Concomitantly, the elastic recoil necessary for esophageal clearance is severely diminished. Relengthening of the esophagus is impaired, and reflux-induced injury is much more likely (30). Third, in the absence of a phrenoesophageal ligament, free oral migration of the lower esophageal sphincter is possible with its attendant complications. Instead of augmentation of sphincter pressure with an increase in abdominal pressure, distraction results. Finally, the pinchcock effect of the diaphragm is no longer imparted on the lower esophageal sphincter but rather on the nonreduced stomach (4). This increases the wall tension at the junction of the lower esophageal sphincter and stomach (4).

The size of the hiatus itself may increase the likelihood of reflux. As stated previously, evidence correlating the size of a hiatal hernia with severity of esophagitis exists (28). By increasing the distance between the two limbs of the crus, the amount of force necessary to increase the pressure at the lower esophageal sphincter increases. This would result in a decrease in pressure conferred across the lower esophageal sphincter, especially in the presence of provocative maneuvers (Fig. 41.3). The relatively low pressure of the lower esophageal sphincter then would be easily overcome, and reflux would result.

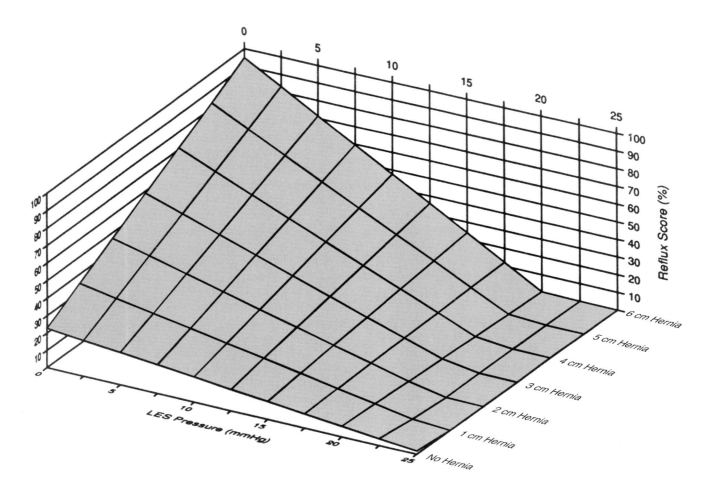

FIGURE 41.3. Representation of the relationship between lower esophageal sphincter pressure (*x axis*), the size of a hiatal hernia (*y axis*), and the susceptibility to gastroesophageal reflux disease caused by provocative maneuvers that increase intraabdominal pressure as shown by reflux score (*z axis*). The equation used (based on 50 subject data) indicates that 75% of the observed variance in susceptibility to stress reflux among individuals is accounted for by the size of the hiatal hernia and the instantaneous value of lower esophageal sphincter pressure.

Indirect evidence for this phenomenon exists in the form of transient lower esophageal sphincter relaxations, which are thought by many to be a key component in the etiology of GERD and esophagitis. These relaxations are accompanied by a marked inhibition of the crural diaphragm, diminishing the contraction across the hiatus (16). Transient lower esophageal sphincter relaxations have been shown to be more common in patients with reflux disease, suggesting that the lack of augmentation of the lower esophageal sphincter by the crus is at least partially responsible for GERD.

CLINICAL PRESENTATION

Ten percent of the North American population is found to have a hiatal hernia, the most common disorder of the foregut (27). It is rare for type I hernias to present before age 30. The typical onset is in the fifth decade of life. Up to 90% of patients with GERD have a concomitant sliding type I hernia; however, only 5% of radiographically demonstrated hiatal hernias have associated reflux symptoms. The symptomatic patients present with the typical symptoms of heartburn, regurgitation, dysphagia with or without stricture formation, and respiratory disorders such as asthma or chronic cough. The cause of dysphagia may simply be diaphragmatic impingement on the gastric fundus. Kaul et al. demonstrated that 91% of patients presenting with dysphagia and a hiatal hernia had complete resolution of their swallowing difficulty with hiatal hernia repair (15). The larger sliding hiatal hernias often have a shorter and weaker lower esophageal sphincter, the amount of reflux is greater, and esophageal acid clearance is ineffective (23). Pulmonary function may be compromised by the larger hernias, especially in the elderly.

A less commonly recognized complication of hiatal hernia is chronic gastrointestinal bleeding. In a report by Boyd et al. (5), 55% of 49 patients with an endoscopically proven hiatal hernia ulcer were found to have either chronic or acute gastrointestinal bleeding. The ulcers were slow to heal with traditional medical therapy, and surgery was often required. Chronic tissue ischemia secondary to the fundus intermittently being compressed by the diaphragmatic crus is the likely cause, the so-called Cameron's ulcer. The symptoms of GERD are most common, bleeding is rare, and the incidence of strangulation in type I hernias, even in the irreducible type I hernias, is zero.

Radiology

Radiography of hiatal hernia formation is usually not difficult for large hernias. They may be noticed on chest x-ray and an esophagram will readily show gastric mucosa above the diaphragm. However, smaller hernias are not always easy to detect and often require the prone or anterior oblique position at esophagography. Small hiatal hernias constitute 90% of all radiographically demonstrated hiatal hernias.

The exact position of the gastroesophageal junction and the diaphragmatic hiatus are difficult to discern. Criteria for small sliding hernias include the presence of gastric folds, an A-ring (a mucosal indentation denoting the squamocolumnar junction) seen in some patients above the diaphragm, a vestibule or outpouching above the diaphragm in which a B-ring (a mucosal fold at the gastroesophageal junction) is seen distally, and the absence of esophageal peristalsis in the vestibule (Fig. 41.2) (9,25). These criteria become germane to the surgeon when preoperatively determining the presence or absence of a short esophagus.

A computed tomography (CT) scan will demonstrate hiatal hernias and will show the relationship of the herniated stomach to mediastinal structures. Experienced surgeons have long recognized that increased scarring occurs overlying the left limb of the right diaphragmatic crus in patients with large hiatal hernias as the stomach rides up and over this structure. Therefore, this limb is more difficult to dissect. The CT scan shows the predominant left-sided stomach in type I hernias (Fig. 41.4). It also demonstrates the intimate relationship of the stomach to the pleura, the underlying aorta, and the left atrium, all of which are important when performing laparoscopic surgery for hiatal hernia formation.

Smaller hiatal hernias usually cannot be demonstrated in the upright position but, in fact, are of little significance from a surgical perspective. They are easily repaired and often make the laparoscopic antireflux operation easier. The large type I hernia, however, may be associated with a short esophagus, and thus its diagnosis and size become important. We have demonstrated that an irreducible hiatal hernia with the patient in the upright position (type I, II, or III) larger than 5 cm in length is a risk factor for a short esophagus (18). The esophagram is performed using both single- and double-con-

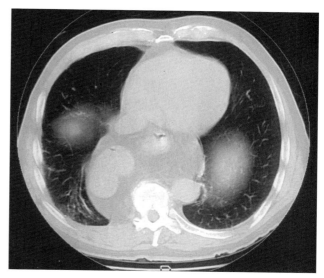

FIGURE 41.4. Computed tomography of a hiatal hernia in the lower mediastinum.

trast techniques. Initially, the patient is placed in the upright position and swallows effervescent crystals to help distend the esophagus, stomach, and any hiatal hernia. The patient then drinks high-density barium to coat the esophagus for double-contrast images that show mucosal details. The patient is next placed in the prone, right anterior oblique position and given thin barium to drink, which distends the esophagus for single-contrast images that most sensitively demonstrate hernias and strictures. Finally, a standard upright posterior–anterior and lateral chest x-ray is obtained while the patient swallows barium, and any hernia seen on these upright films is measured (directly off the film) from the gastroesophageal junction to the level of the hemidiaphragmatic esophageal hiatus (Fig. 41.5). It is apparent that this measurement is affected by

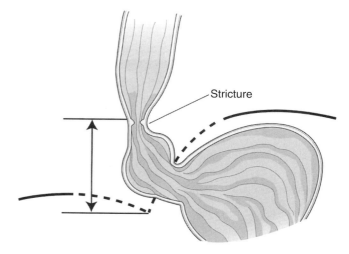

FIGURE 41.5. The method by which an irreducible hiatal hernia is measured on upright esophagogram.

peristalsis, magnification, and an indistinct midline diaphragm image. Nevertheless, a 5-cm or larger irreducible hiatal hernia, utilizing the above technique, should alert the surgeon to the 37% chance that the patient has a short esophagus (18).

Endoscopy

It is often difficult to differentiate a small type I hiatal hernia from Barrett's mucosa at antegrade endoscopy. A biopsy is mandatory. On endoscopic retroflexion with the stomach distended, the diaphragmatic crural impression can be determined by asking the patient to sniff. A fold of gastric fundus, more often seen in patients previously operated upon, can be confused with the diaphragmatic crus impression. Radiographic confirmation of the hiatal hernia is advisable in this circumstance. If eructations repeatedly occur with gastric distention secondary to an incompetent lower esophageal sphincter, the endoscopic diagnosis of a hiatal hernia may be difficult, but with patience and good sedation, this view, with photograph confirmation, is almost always obtainable. Hiatal hernia size can be measured at endoscopy, but the patient is flat and the hernia is artificially enlarged. For this reason, endoscopic hiatal hernia size measurement has not proven greatly helpful. Close examination for a "riding ulcer" at the crura during retroflexion is appropriate. The size of the hiatus is worth noting as well. If a large irreducible hernia is associated with a small diaphragmatic defect, the chances of incarceration and resultant strangulation are increased.

The type I hernia and valvular appearance is represented in Fig. 41.6. In a study by Hill and Kozarek (11), the grade of the valve correlated better with gastroesophageal reflux than lower esophageal sphincter manometry. In a similar study, using the Hill Endoscopic Valve classification, Ober et al. (20) determined that the endoscopic appearance of the gastroesophageal junction is a useful predictor of GERD. In 268 patients who underwent endoscopy, manometry, and 24-hour pH monitoring, a Hill grade IV valve predicted increased acid exposure in 75% of patients. The predictive value of the Hill grading system was of equal value to that of manometry but not as good as the presence of Barrett's esophagus or esophagitis. Therefore, the grading of the valve in conjunction with a careful inspection of the hiatal hernia can be helpful to the clinician and, in turn, the patient.

Manometry

Manometry is required preoperatively for all patients undergoing Nissen fundoplication. If a hiatal hernia is present, the double-hump phenomenon will often be observed manometrically (26). In the normal patient, when utilizing the station pull-through manometric technique, the lower esophageal sphincter high-pressure zone (HPZ) overlaps with the crural component. In hiatal hernia patients, the lower esophageal sphincter migrates into the chest and thus the two HPZs do not overlap. A near baseline tracing intervenes between the two HPZs as seen in (Fig. 41.7). In this study, 46 patients with a hiatal hernia proven by endoscopy or esophagography were also studied by pH monitoring as well as station pull-through manometry (26). Seventeen of the 46 patients with a hiatal hernia demonstrated a double hump for a sensitivity of 37%, but of those patients with a hiatal hernia of 5 cm or larger (n = 15), 14 had a double-hump configuration for a specificity of 95%. Patients without reflux on pH monitoring had a higher distal pressure than those with a positive score, but the proximal pressures showed no difference between groups. This study supports the concept that crural pressure is an important component of the antireflux barrier.

The size of the hiatal hernia can be correlated by manometry with the strength of the lower esophageal sphincter as well as esophageal body function (23). Hypomotility of the esophageal body was demonstrated to be a causative factor of GERD in patients with a hiatal hernia by Benz et al. (3). Ninety-two patients with hiatal hernia underwent pH monitoring and manometry. A motility problem in patients with GERD and hiatal hernia was significantly more common than in those with a hernia but no GERD. The lower esophageal sphincter pressure was not different between groups.

pH Monitoring

Thirty-one percent of patients with hiatal hernia will have positive pH monitoring scores, as opposed to only 18% of patients without a hiatal hernia. Larger hiatal hernias do have an increase (35%) of acid reflux as evidenced by 24-hour pH monitoring data, in comparison to 27% of patients with a minimal hiatal hernia (22). Patients with a hiatal hernia also are more likely to have higher reflux scores (14). Significantly higher reflux times in both the upright and supine positions, and more reflux episodes lasting longer than 5 minutes were found in patients with hiatal hernia as compared to those without. Acid clearance times were also prolonged. These major predictors of GERD are indicative of the key role that the proper position of the lower esophageal sphincter in relation to the diaphragmatic crus and phrenoesophageal ligament has in the prevention of pathologic reflux. In another study by Mittal et al., acid clearance was tested using a combination of pH monitoring and radioisotope clearance (17). The authors demonstrated that acid is trapped in the hernia and often refluxes back into the esophagus as the lower esophageal sphincter relaxes with swallows.

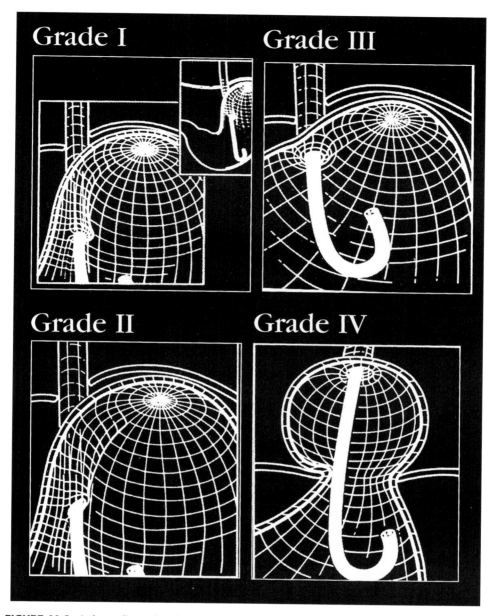

FIGURE 41.6. A three-dimensional representation of the gastroesophageal junction as seen with the endoscope in the "J'ed" position. Grade I valves **(left upper corner)** show a normal ridge of tissue with the squamocolumnar junction approximately at the level of the lower edge of the flap valve. Grade II valves **(left lower corner)** show a slight deterioration of the ridge with a widening of the His' angle and a slight orad migration of the squamocolumnar junction. In grade III **(right upper corner)**, the ridge of tissue is barely visible and there is often incomplete closure of the gastroesophageal junction with air insufflation and complete gastric distention. This valve is almost always accompanied by a small type I hiatal hernia. In the grade IV valve **(right lower corner)** a hiatal hernia is always present, the squamocolumnar valve is easily seen and effaced on the gastric mucosa, and the distal esophageal mucosa is often visible with gastric distention. There is no identifiable ridge of muscle seen.

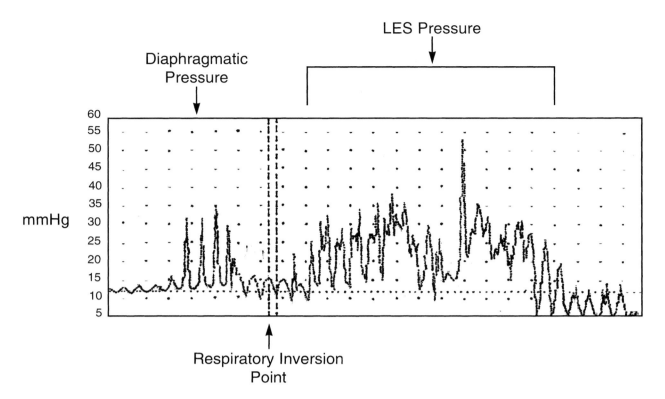

FIGURE 41.7. Manometric double-hump configuration often seen with hiatal hernia.

TREATMENT

In 1951, Allison first reported success with hiatal hernia surgery using a transthoracic approach (1). He then reported 332 cases in which he simply closed the hiatus and reduced the stomach back into the abdomen (2). Immediate relief of symptoms such as pain and regurgitation was noted, but persistent heartburn and anatomic recurrence (54% and 39%, respectively) occurred. Others avoided fundoplication by performing gastropexies alone or adding vagotomy and pyloroplasty to the crural closure. These, too, met with a high symptom recurrence rate.

Currently, medical management for the associated acid reflux disease is of the first order. Three to 6 months of proton pump inhibitor therapy will successfully heal esophagitis secondary to GERD, but approximately 5% of patients on long-term therapy will have breakthrough symptoms or an early recurrence of symptoms if medication is stopped. After physiologic testing, surgery may be appropriate.

Surgical Indications

Surgical therapy for an asymptomatic type I hernia is inappropriate. Dysphagia may be associated with a pure type I hernia, but this is rarely severe enough to warrant surgery. Relative indications for surgical intervention include (a)

type III hernias (the combined sliding and paraesophageal hernia) that with time become exceedingly large and create a multitude of symptoms, including those associated with GERD and the intrathoracic position; and (b) the complications of reflux disease. Patients with peptic stricture formation are often treated with acid reduction therapy and repeated dilations but are often best served with an antireflux operation. One must be cognizant of a possible short esophagus in this circumstance. Esophageal mobilization may provide adequate length for a tension-free repair; if not, a Collis lengthening repair in conjunction with the hiatal herniorrhaphy is necessary. Upper airway disease and Barrett's esophagus are frequently associated with a hiatal hernia. A judicious preoperative evaluation followed by surgery is often appropriate. Finally, most agree that fit patients with uncomplicated reflux disease refractory to high-dose proton pump inhibitor therapy are candidates for antireflux surgery and a concomitant hernia repair.

Absolute indications for surgical intervention include perforation of a hernia secondary to instrumentation, a Barrett's ulcer, and an intrathoracic peptic ulcer. Perforations are life threatening and there is no one operative approach that will serve all. The intervention must be individualized on the basis of the location and duration of the perforation. Drainage and some type of closure must be accomplished. A nondilatable distal stricture with weight loss necessitates resection of the proximal stomach and esophagus. Uncontrolled bleeding from a peptic or Barrett's ulcer is a rare occurrence, but if bleeding cannot be managed by conservative endoscopic therapeutic maneuvers, surgery is required. The underlying hernia must be dealt with at the time of surgery if possible. Surgery for gastric necrosis and volvulus in type III combined hernias is the only method by which the patient's life may be saved. The prevention of gangrene and perforation is required as the mortality rate with surgical correction for this disorder is 50%. The key technical features of a successful hiatal hernia repair, be it for reflux disease, bleeding, or the prevention of hernia strangulation, remain the same.

Laparoscopic Technique

The hiatal opening is easily seen at laparoscopy or at open surgery with the liver retracted anteriorly. Other diaphragmatic defects, especially the small defect lateral to the left limb of the right crus (type IV hernia), and the troublesome left phrenoesophageal artery should be looked for. The artery, if present, can be seen on the undersurface of the left hemidiaphragm coursing toward the hiatus. The size of the hiatal defect and patient age correspond with attenuation of the right and left limb of the right diaphragmatic crus but not necessarily with the amount of viscera within the mediastinum.

The peritoneal sac is divided at the diaphragm and initially separated from the thoracic extension of the phrenoesophageal ligament (endothoracic fascia), thus preventing entry into the pleural cavities. This plane of dissection may be difficult to find. If necessary, the dissection can be performed external to the phrenoesophageal ligament, but pneumothoraces are more common with this approach. In obese patients, the dissection plane is more difficult to find. The entire sac must be stripped from the mediastinum to assist in preventing hernia recurrence.

To facilitate sac excision and gastric intraabdominal positioning, the short gastrics should be ligated and the posterior aspect of the left limb of the right crus entirely separated from the sac and exposed. This maneuver guarantees that all anterior and posterior short gastric vessels have been divided, and enables creation of the posterior gastroesophageal window. The crus of the diaphragm is then closed (Fig. 41.8). We are convinced that inclusion of the subdiaphragmatic fascia in these sutures is important. Data provided by inguinal hernia surgeons demonstrate that muscle-to-muscle apposition by suture is likely to fail. Therefore, care must be taken to avoid cutting the subdiaphragmatic fascia, which overlies the left hemidiaphragm, as it will slide to the left if divided, making suture inclusion difficult. Crus closure calibration with a 60-F dilator follows.

A fundoplication is then performed. There are two types: (a) the tethered fundoplication to either retroperitoneal structures (Hill) or the diaphragm (Belsey or Toupet), and (b) the untethered fundoplications (Nissen and Collis–Nissen). The untethered are most dependent on the quality of the diaphragmatic crural closure. The fundoplication and the abdominal esophagus should be maintained in the increased pressure environment of the abdomen. The added pressure of the abdominal cavity is one of the mechanisms by which acid reflux is prevented. The Nissen fundoplication has a proven track record of success and is the most commonly performed antireflux procedure. Thus, the quality of diaphragm closure is of utmost importance.

HIATAL HERNIA RECURRENCE

Laparoscopic surgery of the foregut has emerged. Improved instrumentation, numerous large series with good early results, and technical modifications have made laparoscopic

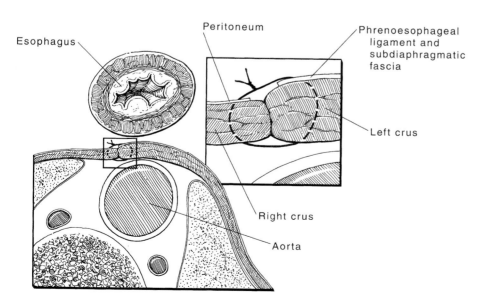

FIGURE 41.8. Subdiaphragmatic fascia is shown in cross section. *Dashed line* indicates the plane of section. **Inset** demonstrates the fascia and other diaphragmatic structures that should be included in the crus closure to ensure a secure closure.

Nissen fundoplication for GERD commonplace; in fact, the incidence of surgery for this condition has multiplied four-fold in recent years. The incidence of death has decreased, and the complication of splenic bleeding with resultant splenectomy has almost disappeared. The problem of long-term dysphagia and the gas bloat syndrome is unchanged from that of open surgery. However, the hiatal hernia recurrence rate after laparoscopic hernia repair has been reported to be as high as 24% to 42% (Table 41.1) (10,31).

In a recent article presented at the American College of Surgeons meeting in 1999, the University of Southern California surgical group reported their laparoscopic experience with 54 patients undergoing surgery for type III hernias between 1985 and 1998 (10). An open laparotomy was performed in 13, thoracotomy in 14, and laparoscopic repair in 27. Videoesophagram was performed in 75% of patients. Forty-two percent of patients with the laparoscopic approach as opposed to 15% of the open group demonstrated a recurrent hernia (*p* <0.001). Over half of the recurrences were asymptomatic. Posterior crural repair was accompanied by fundoplication in all patients. No mesh was utilized for reinforcement. Speculation on the reason for the high laparoscopic recurrence rate included lower esophageal sphincter adhesion formation, difficult identification of anatomy, and excessive redundant sac making fundoplication difficult. This group now recommends open thoracotomy rather than laparoscopy for patients with type III hernias.

There are additional explanations for this increase of hiatal hernia recurrence: technical error, operator experience, decreased adhesion formation, the unrecognized short esophagus, an older higher risk-patient population, more rigorous follow-up, fewer postoperative restrictions, and deviation from the established technique of open repair. There is, of course, also the causative factor of early postoperative vomiting, and severe intraperitoneal pressure rises as related to falls, car accidents, and heavy lifting. In a recent publication (19), their temporal relationship to recurrence was demonstrated. The authors suggested prophylactic antiemetics, patient awareness, and postoperative restricted activity. There are other causative factors for hiatal hernia recurrence.

Short Esophagus

The enigmatic short esophagus is a known cause of hernia recurrence. The foreshortened esophagus literally pulls the fundoplication into the chest with time. Recurrent heartburn and regurgitation plus dysphagia and even strangulation of the incarcerated paraesophageal hernia (fundoplication) can result. Preoperative testing can help delineate patients with a short esophagus (18) and allow the surgeon to plan for an alternative: the lengthening procedure. Further studies to more accurately identify these patients are in progress.

The key issues currently are the lack of a single accurate preoperative test for short esophagus patients and the

TABLE 41.1. LAPAROSCOPIC WITHOUT MESH

Source	No. of Patients	Mean Age (Yr)	Recurrence Rate (%)	Length of F/U (Mo)	F/U Type	Surgery[a]	Mortality (%)
Basso et al. *Surg Laparosc Endosc Percutan Tech* 1999;9:257	65	47.8	13.8	48.3	Early—esophagogram Late—symptoms	Lap	0
Edye et al. *Ann Surg* 1998;228:528	49	68	4	29	Symptoms	Lap	0
Frantzides et al., 1999 (8)	18	55	16.6	36	Esophagogram	Lap	0
Gantert et al. *J Am Coll Surg* 1998;186:428	55	67	5	11	Not reported	Lap	1.8
Hashemi, 2000 (10)	27	68	42	17	Esophagogram	Lap	0
Horgan et al. *Am J Surg* 1999;177:354	41	67	4.9	36	Symptoms	Lap	2.4
Perdikis et al., 1997 (24)	65	63.6	15	18	Esophagogram	Lap	0
Schauer et al. *Am J Surg* 1998;176:659	70	65.2	0	13	Symptoms	Lap	1.4
Swanstrom et al. *Am J Surg* 1999;177:359	52	63	8	18	Symptoms	Lap	0
Watson et al. *Arch Surg* 1999;134:1069	86	63	2.3	24	Early—esophagogram Late—symptoms	Lap	0
Wu et al., 1999 (31)[a]	28	67	24	>12	Early—esophagogram Late—symptoms	Lap	5
Wu et al., 1999 (31)[a]	33	67	6	24	Esophagogram	Lap	0

F/U, follow-up; Lap, laparoscopy.
[a]Subpopulation of a larger study.
Total no. of patients: 589
Mean age: 63
Total recurrence rate: 9.3

importance of a scientifically established intraoperative assessment method against which the preoperative tests can be measured. Surgeon awareness of a possible short esophagus and familiarity with the surgical methods by which it can be corrected are both necessary. Lack of experience with the lengthening procedures should stimulate referral to a center performing these procedures, as the morbidities associated with reoperative surgery are significant.

Follow-up

Symptoms associated with hiatal hernia recurrence include dysphagia, postprandial fullness (the most reliable symptom), shortness of breath with large hernias, recurrent symptoms of GERD, and, most important, intermittent severe chest pain caused by hernia strangulation. Many have assumed that symptomatic follow-up is adequate for recurrent hiatal hernias and that asymptomatic hernias are not clinically significant. Nevertheless, the best method of assessment of hiatal repair adequacy is an esophagram. If an asymptomatic hernia is present, it is appropriate for the clinician to explain the potential of strangulation and related symptoms that should direct the patient back to physician care. In addition, an "asymptomatic" large recurrence may represent a significant problem that, on further patient questioning, has associated symptoms. Thus, the recurrence rate differs greatly between series on the basis of the method of follow-up. An esophagram on a regular basis is recommended.

Mesh Repair

In a report by Frantzides et al. (8), 33 patients underwent repair of a large sliding or paraesophageal hernia, and patients were randomly selected to have crural closure with or without a polytetrafluoroethylene (PTFE) mesh onlay. A radial slit was placed in the patch, and a keyhole was made. The prosthesis was positioned around the esophagus and stapled to the diaphragm. Patients were followed with an esophagram at 6-month intervals. The group without the PTFE prosthesis experienced a 16.7% recurrence rate at 6-month follow-up.

From the same institutions, Carlson et al. reported their results of open hiatal hernia repair for large hernias utilizing a polypropylene prosthetic patch configured in the same fashion (6). Concomitant gastrostomy was performed in 38 patients. All operations were performed between 1976 and 1991, and all patients were followed by telephone interview. Those patients experiencing recurrent symptoms underwent endoscopy and/or esophagography. Asymptomatic patients were not studied. The mean follow-up was 52 months. No significant postoperative complications were reported, and there were no clinical recurrent hernias. One patient did experience a gastric cancer, and in this same patient mesh was found in the bed of a chronic benign ulcer.

Huntington reported in 1997 his tension-free technique for laparoscopic hiatal hernia repair (12). The technique is reserved for patients in whom sutures tear tissue or require excessive tension to approximate the crura. An incision is made to the right of the right limb of the right crus, and muscle and fascia are split to the level of the pericardium (Fig. 41.9). A patch of polypropylene mesh is then stapled in place. Eight patients had this technique applied, and at a mean follow-up of 8 months no recurrences had been observed. This technique is analogous to the Lichtenstein repair for inguinal hernia, and has the advantage of displacing the mesh from the esophagus and thus reducing the threat of erosion.

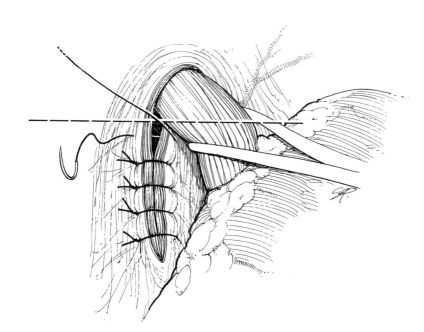

FIGURE 41.9. The tension-free mesh repair—a technique similar in principle to the inguinal hernia repair of Lichtenstein.

TABLE 41.2. LAPAROSCOPIC WITH MESH

Source	No. of Patients	Mean Age (Yr)	Recurrence Rate (%)	Length of F/U (Mo)	F/U Type	Surgery	Mortality (%)
Basso et al. *Surg Endosc* 2000;14:164	70	47.38	0	22.5	Early—esophagogram Late—symptoms	Lap—mesh	0
Carlson et al., 1998 (6)	44	60	0	52	Symptoms	Lap—mesh	2.3
Frantzides et al., 1999 (8)	17	53	0	36	Esophagogram	Lap—mesh	0
Huntington, 1997 (12)	58	67.36	0	12	Symptoms	Lap—mesh	0

F/U, follow-up; Lap—mesh, laparoscopy with mesh.
Total no. of patients: 189
Mean age: 57
Total recurrence rate: 0.0

The overall benefit of mesh repair in terms of recurrence rate is shown in Table 41.2. The long-term results of mesh repair would best be determined by comparing in a prospective fashion a control group without suture tearing to patients with mesh buttressing, and a third group with a relaxing incision, mesh bridging, and primary hiatal suture repair. Anecdotal reports of mesh migration with resultant esophagectomy make many surgeons reluctant to utilize mesh repair. A scientific trial is needed to determine not only recurrence rates for various techniques, but also the long-term complications of mesh repair.

Technical Considerations

Techniques of laparoscopic crural closure have changed, and multiple techniques have been proposed. Cuschieri first utilized a continuous suture and his Dundee knot (7). This was reported in 1993 in four patients, all of whom had early good results. Subsequently, we successfully used interrupted polypropylene sutures placed approximately 1 cm apart in patients with large hiatal hernias (24). Others have used a similar technique with a variety of suture materials. The use of silk sutures may be contraindicated as there is evidence that silk deteriorates with time. A truly nonabsorbable synthetic suture and a figure-of-eight configuration rather than a simple suture may be preferable.

Clearly, the absence of diaphragmatic crus closure will result in recurrent hiatal hernia formation. There are still a few surgeons who deny the need for fundoplication placement in the abdominal environment. Surgeon inexperience in knot tying and deep accurate suture placement has been established as a cause of hernia recurrence following open surgery (21). In a series recently reported, 38 patients with type II or III hiatal hernias were repaired laparoscopically (31). A variety of techniques were used for hiatal closure in the first 12 patients, "depending on hiatal width." These included no closure, placement of polypropylene mesh anterior to the hiatus, anterior hiatal closure with interrupted sutures, posterior and anterior hiatal closure with interrupted suture, and posterior closure with interrupted

sutures. In the initial patients, the hernia sac was variably excised. In the last 25 patients, the closure was performed posteriorly and the sac was excised. A barium swallow was obtained 3 to 5 months postoperatively in all patients. A 24% hiatal hernia recurrence rate was noted, but there was no statistical relationship between recurrence rate and the technical form of repair. It is probable, however, that inexperience and a nonstandardized approach contributed to the high recurrence rate.

The magnification provided with laparoscopy is a double-edged sword in this respect. It will allow you to see that the knot is tied securely, but the crural size may be exaggerated and thus the deep inclusion of muscle and adjacent fascia is ignored. Large needles with strong nonabsorbable suture material are necessary. The early division of short gastric vessels allows the stomach to be easily reduced into the abdomen, thus avoiding excessive tension and gastric perforations. Complete excision of the sac is easily performed after gastric reduction but can be ignored by the inexperienced. Sac excision has been shown to prevent recurrent hernia formation and must be included in all repairs. The presumed mechanism for prevention of hernia formation is increased mediastinal adhesion formation with obliteration of the dead space above the diaphragm.

The subdiaphragmatic fascia, a derivative of transversalis fascia, must be differentiated from the phrenoesophageal ligament. The latter structure anchors the gastroesophageal junction and extends up into the chest as the endothoracic fascia. Underlying the left hemidiaphragm and intimately attached to it is the subdiaphragmatic fascia. This structure is often divided by sharp dissection during laparoscopic hiatal hernia repair, but was rarely injured during open hiatal dissection as only blunt finger dissection was used to create the window behind the esophagus. The satisfactory long-term results of open hernia repair (Table 41.3) may be related to this difference in technique. Division of the subdiaphragmatic fascia occurs in the process of dividing the sac at the hiatal rim if the incision is too deep. The fascia, when divided, slides laterally toward the spleen, thus making suture inclusion during hiatal closure difficult. The ideal

TABLE 41.3. OPEN PROCEDURES

Source	No. of Patients	Mean Age (Yr)	Recurrence Rate (%)	Length of F/U (Mo)	F/U Type	Surgery	Mortality (%)
Ellis et al. *Arch Surg* 1986; 121:416	51	60.6	8	59	Symptoms	A + T	2
Gardner et al. *Am J Surg* 1977;133:554	42	53.9	0	38.5	Early—esophagogram Late—symptoms	A	0
Gatzinsky et al. *Acta Chir Scand* 1979;145:45	105	52	9.5	48	Symptoms/ esophagogram	A + T	1.4
Mokka et al. *Acta Chir Scand* 1977;143:265	50	50	12	60	Esophagogram	A	0
Nicholson/Nohl-Oser. *J Thorac Cardiovasc Surg* 1976;72:938[a]	283	0–80+	13.1	12+	Symptoms/ esophagogram	T	3.4
Orringer et al., 1972 (21)[a]	892	Not reported	14.5	120–180	Early—esophagogram Late—symptoms	T	1
Pearson et al. *Ann Thorac Surg* 1983;35:45	53	62	17	74.4	Symptoms/ esophagogram	A + T	0
Refsum/Nygaard. *Acta Chir Scand* 1979;145:39	43	59	16.3	35	Symptoms	A	0
Schauer et al. *Am J Surg* 1998;176:659	25	64	8	48	Symptoms	A + T	0
Singh. *Scand J Thorac Cardiovasc Surg* 1980;14:311[a]	238	18–73	8.4	84–120	Symptoms	T	0
Weissberg/Refaely. *Scand J Thorac Cardiovasc Surg* 1995;29:201[a]	55	9–68	5.5	108	Symptoms	A + T	1.8
Williamson et al. *Ann Thorac Surg* 1993;56:447	119	64	10	61.5	Symptoms	A	13

+, plus; A, abdominal; T, thoracic.
[a]Not included in mean age calculations.
Total no. of patients: 1956
Mean age: 58
Total recurrence rate: 12.2

method is to avoid its division and then include it in the interrupted crus closure suture line as shown in Fig. 41.8.

The results shown in Tables 41.1 to 41.3 (tables include only series with greater than 30 patients, follow-up length greater than 1 year, and a stated recurrence rate) reveal several interesting findings. The incidence of recurrence is higher with esophagram follow-up. The mortality rates were low for both the open and laparoscopic repairs. The laparoscopic repair has a higher incidence of recurrence at early follow-up, and laparoscopic mesh repair results are promising but long-term follow-up is needed to rule out the feared complication of mesh erosion and resultant esophagectomy.

CONCLUSION

Hiatal hernia formation is important. It influences the incidence of GERD, and occasionally hiatal hernias can be life threatening. The diagnosis of hiatal hernia is usually straightforward, but the optimal method of repair is yet to be determined as hernia recurrence rates are high. Further innovation to obtain a biocompatible material that would strengthen the

repair without injuring adjacent viscera is needed. Scientific investigation to determine the benefit and safety of the mesh buttressing and tension-free repair is required.

REFERENCES

1. Allison PR. Reflux esophagitis, sliding hiatal hernia and the anatomy of repair. *Surg Gynecol Obstet* 1951;92:419.
2. Allison PR. Hiatus hernia: (a 20-year retrospective survey). *Ann Surg* 1973;178:273–276.
3. Benz C, Jakobs R, Riemann JF. [Axial hiatal hernia—correlation of motility disorders and pathological reflux in the esophagus in patients with and without reflux esophagitis.] *Z Gastroenterol* 1994;32:12–15.
4. Bombeck CT, Dillard DH, Nyhus LM. Muscular anatomy of the gastroesophageal junction and role of phrenoesophageal ligament; autopsy study of sphincter mechanism. *Ann Surg* 1966; 164:643–654.
5. Boyd EJ, Penston JG, Russell RI, et al. Hiatal hernial ulcers: clinical features and follow-up. *Postgrad Med J* 1991;67:900–903.
6. Carlson MA, Condon RE, Ludwig KA, et al. Management of intrathoracic stomach with polypropylene mesh prosthesis reinforced transabdominal hiatus hernia repair [see comments]. *J Am Coll Surg* 1998;187:227–230.

7. Cuschieri A. Laparoscopic antireflux surgery and repair of hiatal hernia. *World J Surg* 1993;17:40–45.

8. Frantzides CT, Richards CG, Carlson MA. Laparoscopic repair of large hiatal hernia with polytetrafluoroethylene. *Surg Endosc* 1999;13:906–908.

9. Gore RM, Levine MS, Laufer I. Esophagus. In: *Textbook of gastrointestinal radiology*. Philadelphia: WB Saunders; 1994.

10. Hashemi M, Peters JH, DeMeester TR, et al. Laparoscopic repair of large type III hiatal hernia: objective follow-up reveals high recurrence rate. *J Am Coll Surg* 2000;190:553–560.

11. Hill LD, Kozarek RA. The gastroesophageal flap valve [Editorial; Comment]. *J Clin Gastroenterol* 1999;28:194–197.

12. Huntington TR. Laparoscopic mesh repair of the esophageal hiatus. *J Am Coll Surg* 1997;184:399–400.

13. Kahrilas PJ. Anatomy and physiology of the gastroesophageal junction. *Gastroenterol Clin North Am* 1997;26:467–486.

14. Kasapidis P, Vassilakis JS, Tzovaras G, et al. Effect of hiatal hernia on esophageal manometry and pH-metry in gastroesophageal reflux disease. *Dig Dis Sci* 1995;40:2724–2730.

15. Kaul BK, DeMeester TR, Oka M, et al. The cause of dysphagia in uncomplicated sliding hiatal hernia and its relief by hiatal herniorrhaphy. A roentgenographic, manometric, and clinical study. *Ann Surg* 1990;211:406–410.

16. Mittal RK, Fisher MJ. Electrical and mechanical inhibition of the crural diaphragm during transient relaxation of the lower esophageal sphincter. *Gastroenterology* 1990;99:1265–1268.

17. Mittal RK, Lange RC, McCallum RW. Identification and mechanism of delayed esophageal acid clearance in subjects with hiatus hernia. *Gastroenterology* 1987;92:130–135.

18. Mittal SK, Awad ZT, Tasset M, et al. The preoperative predictability of the short esophagus in patients with stricture or paraesophageal hernia. *Surg Endosc* 2000 *(in press)*.

19. Mittal SK, Filipi CJ, Anderson PJ, et al. Additional mechanisms of hiatal hernia recurrence and its prevention. *Hernia* 1999;3: 215–220.

20. Oberg S, Peters JH, DeMeester TR, et al. Endoscopic grading of the gastroesophageal valve in patients with symptoms of gastroesophageal reflux disease (GERD). *Surg Endosc* 1999;13: 1184–1188.

21. Orringer MB, Skinner DB, Belsey RH. Long-term results of the Mark IV operation for hiatal hernia and analyses of recurrences and their treatment. *J Thorac Cardiovasc Surg* 1972;63: 25–33.

22. Ott DJ, Glauser SJ, Ledbetter MS, et al. Association of hiatal hernia and gastroesophageal reflux: correlation between presence and size of hiatal hernia and 24-hour pH monitoring of the esophagus. *AJR Am J Roentgenol* 1995;165:557–559.

23. Patti MG, Goldberg HI, Arcerito M, et al. Hiatal hernia size affects lower esophageal sphincter function, esophageal acid exposure, and the degree of mucosal injury. *Am J Surg* 1996;171: 182–186.

24. Perdikis G, Hinder RA, Filipi CJ, et al. Laparoscopic paraesophageal hernia repair. *Arch Surg* 1997;132:586–589.

25. Putman CE, Ravin CE, eds. The gastrointestinal system—the esophagus. In: *Textbook of diagnostic imaging*. Philadelphia: WB Saunders, 1994.

26. Klaus A, Raiser F, Swain JM, et al. Manometric components of the lower esophageal double hump. *Dig Dis* 2000;18:172–177.

27. Skinner DB. Esophageal hiatal hernia. The condition: clinical manifestations and diagnosis. In: Sabiston DC Jr, Spencer FC, eds. *Surgery of the chest*. Philadelphia: WB Saunders, 1990: 890–902.

28. Sloan S, Kahrilas PJ. Impairment of esophageal emptying with hiatal hernia. *Gastroenterology* 1991;100:596–605.

29. Soper NJ, Dunnegan D. Anatomic fundoplication failure after laparoscopic antireflux surgery. *Ann Surg* 1999;229:669–676.

30. Sugarbaker DJ, Rattan S, Goyal RK. Swallowing induces sequential activation of esophageal longitudinal smooth muscle. *Am J Physiol* 1984;247:G515–G519.

31. Wu JS, Dunnegan DL, Soper NJ. Clinical and radiologic assessment of laparoscopic paraesophageal hernia repair. *Surg Endosc* 1999;13:497–502.

42

PARAESOPHAGEAL HIATAL HERNIA

DAVID A. NAPOLIELLO
RONALD A. HINDER
NEIL R. FLOCH
GALEN PERDIKIS

Hiatal herniation was a recognized condition prior to Postempski completing the first successful surgical repair in 1889 (30). Abdominal visceral herniation through an associated diaphragmatic hiatal defect can be categorized into four subtypes. Type 1, or "sliding" hiatal hernia, involves herniation of the gastroesophageal junction into the chest through the esophageal hiatus (Fig. 42.1). Type 2, or "rolling hernia" is considered to be the "true" paraesophageal hernia, having an anatomically correctly positioned gastroesophageal junction with herniation of the fundus of the stomach through the hiatus (Fig. 42.2). Type 3 is a "mixed" hiatal hernia, combining both a displaced gastroesophageal junction seen with type 1 hernias and an associated portion of stomach into the chest as in type 2 (Fig. 42.3). By convention, type 3 has also been accepted as a paraesophageal hernia. Type 4 hiatal gastric herniation is associated with visceral herniation of other organs into the chest through a very large defect (Fig. 42.4). A lesser-known defect is the parahiatal hernia. This rare entity occurs through a congenital defect in the diaphragm immediately to the left of the hiatus known as the canalis paraesophagalis diaphragmatis. This can be differentiated from a true paraesophageal hernia by the presence of a fibrous strand of diaphragmatic tissue between the esophagus and the hernia sac. If subsequent loss of this strand occurs, it is difficult to differentiate between these two types of hernia.

INCIDENCE

The overall incidence of hiatal hernias has been reported to be anywhere from 10% to 50% of the general population.

D. A. Napoliello: Surgical Associates of Venice and Engelwood, Venice, Florida.

R. A. Hinder: Department of Surgery, Mayo Clinic, Jacksonville, Florida.

N. R. Floch: Department of Surgery, Norwalk Hospital, Floch Surgical Associates, Norwalk, Connecticut.

G. Perdikis: Department of Plastic Surgery, Mayo Clinic, Jacksonville, Florida.

The most common are type 1 hernias, seen in more than 85% of cases, while paraesophageal hernias make up the minority of approximately 5% to 15% of hiatal hernias. There is a median age of 61 for patients with paraesophageal hernias and a median age of 48 for patients with sliding hernias, with a higher prevalence in women, who have a 2:1 incidence over men (6,10,22).

PATHOGENESIS

Sliding and paraesophageal hiatal hernias are the result of both anatomic weakness and pressure differentials. Negative pressure created intermittently within the chest with respiration has a resultant action on the abdominal viscera by drawing the stomach through the esophageal hiatus. As the stomach is drawn towards the hiatus, attachments to the preaortic fascia, median arcuate ligament, and the phrenoesophageal membrane begin to weaken and stretch. Further weakening of the gastrocolic, gastrosplenic, and gastrohepatic ligaments occurs with herniation through the hiatus. Maziak et al. believe that esophageal shortening may pull the stomach into the chest as the esophageal tissue fibroses and shortens secondary to reflux esophagitis (21).

A widened hiatus anterior to the esophagus is a consistent finding in patients with a paraesophageal hernia. Occasionally, the left bundle of the right crus is absent and the defect extends into the left leaf of the diaphragm. The defect tends to have a firm fibrous rim (22). This lateral defect may be caused by pressure on the left bundle of the right crus by the stomach, resulting in atrophy and extension of the defect to the left. The gastroesophageal junction remains fixed to the preaortic fascia and the median arcuate ligament. The fundus acts as the lead point and herniates first. The greater curvature is then able to roll into the thorax in front of and to the left of the fixed gastroesophageal junction. Due to this fixation, the stomach tends to rotate around its longitudinal axis,

(continued on page 496)

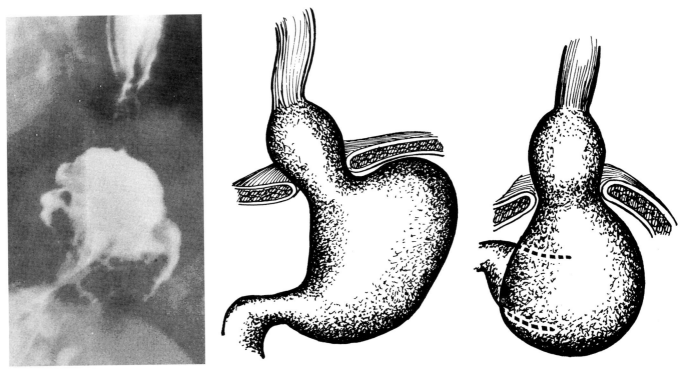

A–C

FIGURE 42.1. A sliding hiatal hernia demonstrated by contrast radiography **(A)**, anterior schematic diagram and **(B)**, lateral schematic diagram **(C)**.

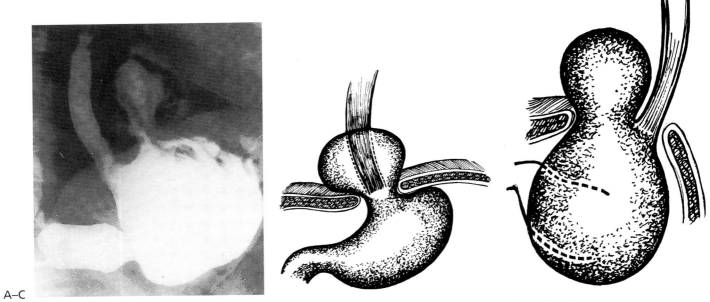

A–C

FIGURE 42.2. A paraesophageal hiatal hernia demonstrated by contrast radiography **(A)**, anterior schematic diagram **(B)**, and lateral schematic diagram **(C)**.

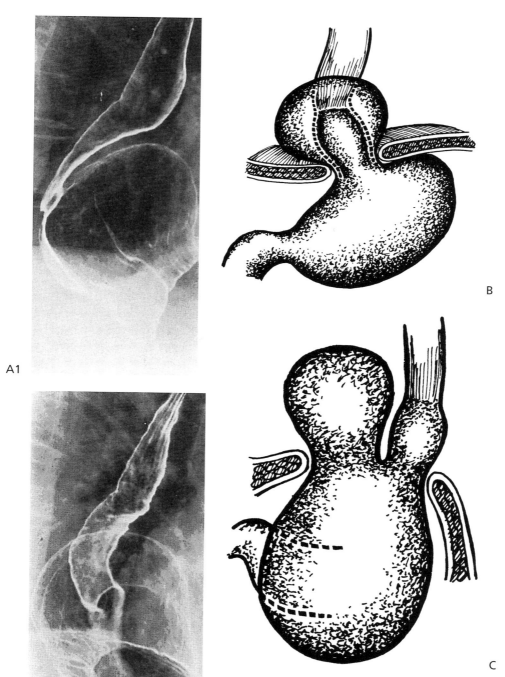

FIGURE 42.3. A mixed hiatal hernia demonstrated by **(A)** contrast radiography, **(B)** anterior schematic diagram, and **(C)** lateral schematic diagram.

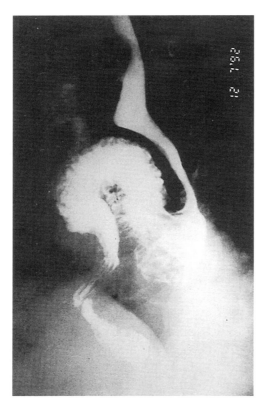

FIGURE 42.4. This large type 4 hiatal hernia demonstrates a completely intrathoracic stomach that was associated with herniation of the transverse colon into the chest.

(continued from page 493)

creating an organoaxial volvulus (Fig. 42.5). A less frequent occurrence is a mesentericoaxial volvulus which occurs with rotation around the transverse axis (Fig. 42.6).

Iatrogenic paraesophageal hernias have occurred after antireflux procedures, esophagomyotomy, esophagogastrectomy, gastric distention, and the use of the Angelchik prosthesis (35). Disruption of the phrenoesophageal membrane due to operative dissection or endoscopic dilation, and failure or lack of a crural repair after surgical dissection have been cited as causative agents. A study in children showed the paraesophageal hernia rate to be 16.8% after Nissen fundoplication (2). The lack of a crural repair was common, with patients under age 1 year at highest risk. Failure to notice a shortened esophagus, and existing hernia defects have also been implicated.

CLINICAL PRESENTATION

The symptoms associated with paraesophageal hernias are variable. Dysphagia, chest pain, regurgitation, and postprandial fullness are common complaints. These complaints are representative of the physiologic sequelae of the mechanical defect. Dysphagia is believed to be related to the axial rotation of the stomach. It is an intermittent phenomenon and usually is more severe when it is associated with gastroesophageal reflux. Progression to gastric volvulus with strangulation is rarely seen. Heartburn is less common than in a sliding hernia due to the nature of the anatomic defect (Fig. 42.7). The fixed gastroesophageal junction associated with type 2 paraesophageal hernias acts to provide an adequate lower esophageal sphincter (LES) mechanism, whereas type 1 and type 3 hernias can have significant reflux symptoms. Current

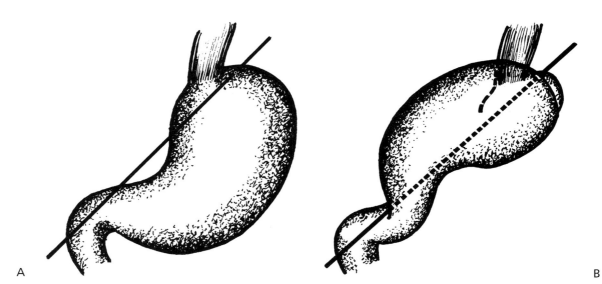

A   B

FIGURE 42.5. Organoaxial volvulus of the stomach before **(A)** and after volvulus **(B)**. The stomach may obstruct at the gastroesophageal junction or in the pyloroduodenal region.

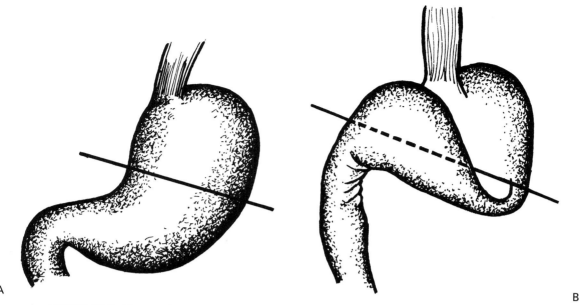

A

B

FIGURE 42.6. Mesentericoaxial volvulus of the stomach before **(A)** and after volvulus **(B)**. The stomach may obstruct in the fixed pyloroantral region.

theories on the etiology of reflux include a defective LES or, more infrequently, pressure associated with diaphragmatic obstruction overwhelming an otherwise competent LES.

Pulmonary complications include dyspnea, coughing, pneumonia, and chronic bronchitis. These occur as a result of both aspiration and decreased lung volume associated with a large paraesophageal hernia. This can be quite significant with type 4 hernias, in which the colon and spleen may be located within the thorax. Symptoms of asthma may also be present, with bronchodilator therapy being required in up to 35% of the cases (19).

Chest pain associated with paraesophageal hernias is often confused with angina. Careful cardiac evaluation is required. The chest pain may be repetitive before a gastrointestinal source is identified. Chronic anemia due to bleeding is an occult sign associated with paraesophageal hiatal hernias. This has been reported in up to 38% of patients (1,19,22,38,41). A large hematemesis rarely occurs. Cameron's ulcers are associated with a sliding hiatal hernia and are related to mucosal injury from friction of the stomach and the underlying mucosa against the hiatal defect. Venous obstruction causing hemorrhage also occurs with a paraesophageal hernia. Vascular engorgement results in slow oozing of blood from the mucosa. Peptic ulceration associated with paraesophageal hernias was found in 23% of patients in the series of 34 by Rakic et al. (32). In 66%

Nonrefluxers

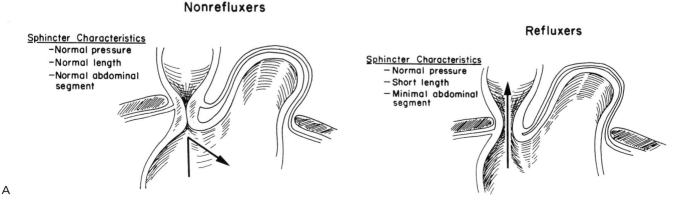

Sphincter Characteristics
  −Normal pressure
  −Normal length
  −Normal abdominal
    segment

Refluxers

Sphincter Characteristics
  − Normal pressure
  − Short length
  − Minimal abdominal
    segment

A

B

FIGURE 42.7. A schematic diagram of the anatomic and manometric differences in patients with normal LES pressure and a paraesophageal hernia without **(A)** and with reflux **(B)** as defined by 24-hour pH monitoring.

of the cases, they are multiple (4). Larger hernias have a higher incidence of ulcers.

In 11% of patients, there are no symptoms (39). The hernia in these individuals is identified during routine chest radiography or endoscopy (Fig. 42.8). This is more frequent when a large hiatus is present as the stomach is able to move into the mediastinum without obstruction. In some patients, the initial presentation is as a surgical emergency. Acute strangulation, volvulus, massive hemorrhage, and perforation all can occur with paraesophageal hernias (39,40). Recent reports reveal that 2% to 17% will need

emergent surgical management for acute obstruction or volvulus (23,28). Volvulus is usually associated with acute pain and obstructive symptoms. Associated compromise of the vascular supply will lead to necrosis and perforation. Resultant peritonitis and sepsis has a mortality rate of 17% to 50% (15,40). Huntington reported that in 10 of 58 patients with paraesophageal hernias who were operated on emergently there was a complication rate of 40% (16). The mortality was higher than for elective treatment. This has caused surgeons to recommend elective repair of all symptomatic paraesophageal hernias.

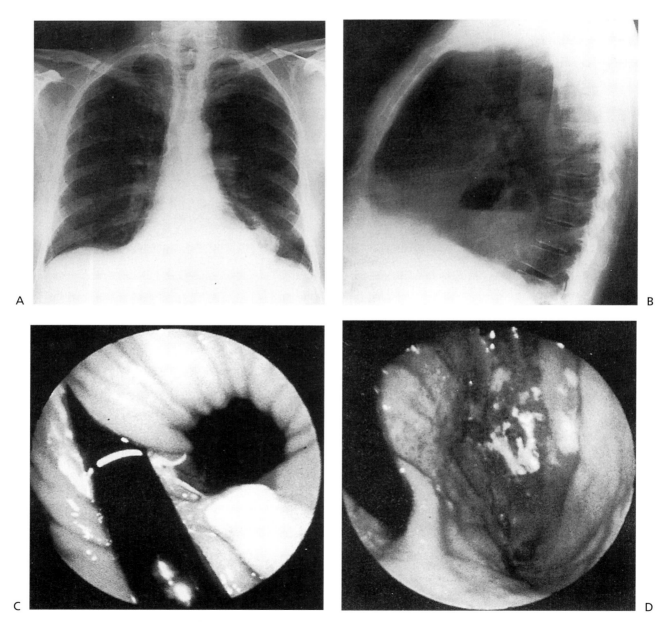

FIGURE 42.8. A and **B:** Anteroposterior and lateral chest radiograph demonstrating a gastric air–fluid level in the chest characteristic of a hiatal hernia. **C:** A retroflexed endoscopic view of a paraesophageal hiatal hernia. Note the gastric rugal folds ascending into the orifice to the side of the gastroesophageal junction. **D:** A retroflexed view of a mixed hiatal hernia.

DIAGNOSTIC STUDIES

An upright chest radiograph establishes the diagnosis with the finding of an air–fluid level behind the heart in 95% of patients (21). If the location of the stomach is not clearly defined, confirmation may be made by passing a nasogastric tube into the intrathoracic stomach. Failure to pass the tube below the hiatus may further support the diagnosis. Although not a common mode of diagnosis, a paraesophageal hernia can also be detected on computed tomography (CT).

An upper gastrointestinal series can establish the diagnosis in up to 100% of patients and can define the type of hiatal hernia and any concomitant esophagogastric pathology (23). In our series of 65 patients, 56 (86%) were found on barium swallow or esophagogastroduodenoscopy to have a type 3 paraesophageal hernia (28). The remaining nine (14%) had a type 2 paraesophageal hernia. Twenty-one percent had greater than 50% of their stomach in the chest. Four percent had a gastric volvulus. Controversy exists concerning the accuracy of determining the location of the LES by barium swallow. Some believe that endoscopy is more sensitive in determining the LES location to differentiate between a type 2 and type 3 hernia. The technique of "sniffing" or performing Valsalva's maneuver with the endoscope at the distal esophagus has been used to aid in identifying the location of the crura (23). Manometry and 24-hour esophageal pH studies can also be helpful adjuncts to assess the status of the LES and the degree of reflux. Technical difficulty in passing the diagnostic catheters may occur, limiting its usefulness. Manometry will evaluate esophageal body motility and identify concurrent motility disorders, as well as aid in defining the level, resting pressure, and length of the LES.

INDICATIONS FOR SURGERY

The presence of symptoms is an indication for elective surgical repair. Asymptomatic patients do not require surgery, particularly if they are a poor surgical risk. They must be followed closely because the appearance of symptoms may warrant urgent surgical intervention. In the past, all patients were advised to have a surgical repair since nonoperative management resulted in a high mortality. This was mainly as a result of the previously noted complications associated with the her-

nia. Elective surgery had a 1% mortality rate (34). Current evidence that asymptomatic patients have a lower risk of complications supports a nonoperative approach in these patients (23,28). Allen et al. showed that in 23 patients followed for up to 20 years, only four eventually developed symptoms with one mortality associated with aspiration pneumonia (1).

The recent use of laparoscopy for the repair of paraesophageal hernias shows that patients with comorbidities can undergo surgery with fewer complications and shorter postoperative recovery when operated on by experienced surgeons (17). In our series of 65 patients, there was no mortality and a low morbidity (28). Laparoscopic repair had a 15% recurrent hernia rate. Most were small asymptomatic hernias. Similar findings have also been reported by Eyde (11) and Schauer (33) et al. This is a similar recurrence rate to that seen after the open repair. The recurrence rate for the laparoscopic may reach 45% (DeMeester et al., unpublished data). It should be noted that the radiographic recurrence of a hiatal hernia does not usually correlate with recurrence of symptoms.

SURGICAL MANAGEMENT

The operative steps of performing a paraesophageal herniorrhaphy include reduction of the hernia content, excision of the hernia sac, and repair of the hiatal defect. The addition of an antireflux procedure or gastropexy remains controversial. Removal of the hernia sac from the chest is important since remnants of the sac may produce a seroma or fever and are associated with an increased hernia recurrence rate. The hiatal repair can usually be performed by simple suture; however, larger defects may require the addition of prosthetic material to complete the repair. The surgical approach may be by laparotomy, thoracotomy, or laparoscopy.

Paraesophageal hernias have in the past been repaired using a thoracotomy or laparotomy, with high mortality, long hospitalization, prolonged recovery times, and associated morbidity (Table 42.1). Open paraesophageal hernia repair has an average morbidity rate of 14% and a mortality rate of 3%. Complications include pneumonia, sepsis, postoperative bowel obstruction, and bowel or splenic injury (10,22,27,38). Williamson et al. reported a recurrence rate of 11% within a median period of 2 years after open abdominal repair (42). Eight patients underwent reoperation.

TABLE 42.1. RESULTS OF LAPAROTOMY AND THORACOTOMY FOR PARAESOPHAGEAL HERNIA REPAIRS

Author	No. of Patients	Complications (%)	Recurrence (%)	Reoperative Rate (%)	Mortality (%)
Menguy (22)	30	7	—	—	0
Harriss et al. (14)	29	13	—	—	13
Williamson et al. (42)	119	11.8	11	7.0	1.7
Maziak et al. (21)	94	19	2.1	5.3	2.1
Allen et al. (1)	124	29	2	1	1
Martin et al. (20)	51	29	—	—	0

Thoracotomy has been indicated for concomitant chest pathology, obesity, shortened esophagus, and reexplorations. Morbidity rates of 19% have been reported in these high-risk patients. Excellent results can be seen in some series, with reoperation required in only 5% (23). Maziak et al. describe reoperation for recurrent reflux, delayed esophageal perforation, and esophagectomy for malignancy (21).

The benefits of laparoscopy include the advantages of the minimally invasive approach, shorter hospitalization, less blood loss, and better cosmesis. Technical advantages include superior visibility, with the laparoscope creating magnification and a direct view of the hernia sac in the thorax (17). The procedure can be performed by experienced surgeons with similar or better results and less morbidity and mortality than the open procedure (7,8,25,29). We have had no deaths in over 100 consecutive procedures, and the average hospital stay is only 2 days. This is most significant for older patients with multiple medical problems, who would not have tolerated a thoracotomy or laparotomy.

LAPAROSCOPIC TECHNIQUE

The laparoscopic approach is performed through five trocar ports in similar position to that used for the Nissen fundoplication (Fig. 42.9). The viscera are reduced from the chest by gently grasping the stomach with a Babcock instrument and reducing the contents into the abdomen. This allows for exposure of the free edges of the hiatus. Care must be taken not to be too forceful to avoid perforation of the stomach. Similar caution should be followed when other organs are reduced. The spleen may be at risk of injury if it is covered by the colon.

The initial dissection begins by dividing the gastrohepatic ligament into the hiatus. This may contain an aberrant left hepatic artery in up to 17% of patients in our experience. In most cases, we attempt to leave this artery intact; however, it can usually be sacrificed without complication. The usual position of the left gastric artery may be distorted by the herniation. With the hiatus exposed, the peritoneal sac is divided along the free edge of the hiatus. This allows for careful stripping of the hernia sac from the thorax. It can usually be reduced with gentle tugging without the need for sharp dissection or electrocautery. Care must be taken not to breach the pleura and to avoid injury to the pericardium. This dissection is continued in a clockwise fashion around the entire border of the hiatus, so that all of the sac can be removed from the mediastinum. Once the sac is reduced from the chest, it remains adherent to the anterior cardia. We do not excise the sac since this avoids unnecessary bleeding or damage to the anterior vagus nerve. The esophagus can now be identified lying in the mediastinum. It should be carefully mobilized from the surrounding tissues and a window created behind it. This requires great care as esophageal and gastric injury are not uncommonly reported during this part of the procedure. The position of the left crus and posterior vagus nerve behind the esophagus are useful in deciding where the window should be created. The hiatal defect is then closed behind the esophagus using simple interrupted nonabsorbable sutures. If the defect is very large, prosthetic mesh may be used to further reinforce the closure (Fig. 42.10). The fundus of the stomach is then inspected to identify its usefulness for the wrap. Due to the chronic herniation of the stomach, the gastrolienal ligament is stretched and short gastric vessels do not usually have to be divided.

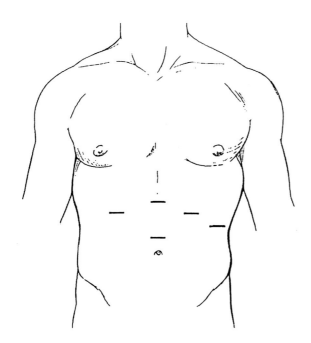

FIGURE 42.9. Five small abdominal incisions are used for the laparoscopic repair. Each incision is 0.5 to 1 cm long.

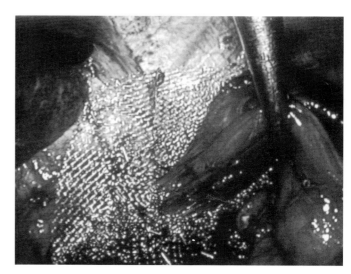

FIGURE 42.10. Partial sutured approximation of the crus followed by mesh reinforcement of the hiatus. The esophagus is elevated by the grasper.

The fundus may then be pulled through the window. The fundoplication is fashioned with a pledgeted polypropylene suture to create a "floppy" Nissen fundoplication.

Failure to perform a concomitant antireflux procedure has resulted in postoperative reflux in 20% to 40% of patients. Reflux has been reported in 27% of type 3 and 19% of type 2 hernia repairs (3,5,24,28,40). This difference has been attributed to the sliding component associated with type 3 hernias. An antireflux procedure may not be necessary in a type 2 hernia; however, mobilization of the LES may lead to reflux, which occurs in 18% to 65% of patients with no symptoms before surgery (42). Extensive dissection, which involves detaching the LES from the phrenoesophageal membrane and the preaortic fascia, is implicated (28). Another theory is that LES incompetence may be masked by a paraesophageal hernia (13). After reduction of the hernia, a resultant loss of LES pressure may occur. It is our opinion that a fundoplication is always required with paraesophageal hernia repair. A "floppy" Nissen fundoplication is our procedure of choice, with a partial fundoplication being applied in those patients with poor esophageal body motility or in emergent cases when preoperative motility studies are not possible.

Avoidance of tension is the hallmark of a good crural repair because it directly correlates with the potential for hernia recurrence. If a tension-free repair is not possible after an attempted crural closure, then a mesh repair is indicated (26). Ellis et al. found a 10% recurrence rate after primary repair without the use of mesh (10). Frantzides and Carlson reported the use of mesh placed over a crural repair using sutures to first approximate the muscle (12). Current materials available include polypropylene and commercially treated pigskin. Many do not encourage the use of mesh because of the risk of erosion into the esophagus (8,36,39). Huntington suggests a relaxing muscle incision lateral to the right crus, which is closed with mesh followed by primary closure of the hiatus (17). Although migration, adhesions, infection, and fistulas have been reported, mesh remains a viable resource to reinforce a large defect.

A Collis–Belsey procedure has been recommended for the treatment of the 15% of patients with a short esophagus in the presence of a type 3 paraesophageal hernia (28). Preoperative indicators of short esophagus include paraesophageal hernias greater than 5 cm, severe esophagitis with fibrosis and stricturing, and poor esophageal body motility (31). A short esophagus can be diagnosed intraoperatively by the presence of fibrosis, and difficulty with mobilization of the LES and replacement in the abdomen. Some feel that extensive transhiatal mediastinal dissection will allow for mobilization of the esophagus; however, others feel that it is best managed with a thoracic approach (23). Swanstrom et al. described a technique for a combined laparoscopic and thoracoscopic Collis gastroplasty (37). Three patients who underwent this procedure had no postoperative dysphagia or symptoms of reflux at 8 months.

A laparoscopic gastrostomy or anterior gastropexy has been suggested as an addition to a paraesophageal hernia repair that is not combined with an antireflux procedure (18,19). The gastrostomy is felt to secure the stomach in the abdomen, preventing future herniation. Proponents believe that a chronically incarcerated stomach may have impaired peristalsis and be prone to stasis and delayed gastric emptying. Subsequent gastric decompression would allow the stomach to regain its motility. However, experience indicates that a gastrostomy may not always adequately secure the stomach in the abdomen. A report of four patients who underwent an associated gastropexy found recurrence of the hernia and severe reflux in two patients. These procedures should be considered only in elderly patients with comorbid conditions.

COMPLICATIONS

Our conversion rate of laparoscopic repair to an open procedure for paraesophageal hernias is 3%. A slipped Nissen, small-bowel obstruction, and gastric volvulus resulted in a 5% early reoperation rate. Trus et al. had an 11% incidence of bowel perforation (39). There were three gastric lacerations, two esophageal lacerations, and three esophageal perforations secondary to the use of a bougie. Also described was a 4% incidence of delayed perforations, all of which were repaired by an open procedure. Hemorrhage can occur from liver and splenic capsule tears, as well as from the short gastric vessels. Pleural entry with subsequent pneumothorax is another potential hazard.

The extensive dissection in the chest may lead to tracking of air through the mediastinum. Crepitus may be present in the neck, shoulders, and chest. This problem has no postoperative sequelae and resolves without intervention. Another benign condition is shoulder pain. This occurs as a result of diaphragmatic irritation and also resolves without incident.

Late sequelae are rare. In our series of 65 patients, four experienced dysphagia, three had a slipped Nissen, one had a disrupted fundoplication, and one had a gastric volvulus. Other complications included pneumonia, deep vein thrombosis, pulmonary embolus, urinary retention, atrial fibrillation, and wound infection. Gas bloat syndrome, chronic cough, and weight loss were also observed. Although some believe that recurrence is secondary to the presence of an undiagnosed short esophagus, this is more likely due to a technically poor crural repair, with most patients presenting with either a sliding herniation of the wrap or a recurrent paraesophageal hernia. The overall recurrence rate of hiatal herniation is about 15% with the laparoscopic technique (11,28,33) and 2% to 11% with the open technique (1,21,42). Most are asymptomatic. This rate of recurrence was found by us in patients who did or did not have the fundoplication fixed to the crura at the end of the procedure. De Meester et al. have recently reported a 45% recurrent hernia rate after the laparoscopic technique compared to 15% after thoracotomy (personal communication, 2000).

CONCLUSION

Symptomatic patients are candidates for paraesophageal hernia repair after careful evaluation. Although laparotomy and thoracotomy are successful approaches, laparoscopy is favored by experienced laparoscopic surgeons due to the short length of hospitalization and low complication rate and mortality. On average, patients return to normal activities within 2 to 3 weeks. The laparoscopic technique combined with an antireflux procedure is our recommended surgical approach.

REFERENCES

1. Allen MS, Trastek VF, Deschamps C, et al. Intrathoracic stomach. Presentation and results of operation. *J Thorac Cardiovasc Surg* 1993;105:253.
2. Alrabeeah A, Giacomantonio M, Gillis DA. Paraesophageal hernia after Nissen fundoplication: a real complication in pediatric patients. *J Pediatr Surg* 1988;23:766.
3. Behrns KE, Schlinkert RT. Laparoscopic management of paraesophageal hernia: early results. *J Laparoendosc Surg* 1996;6:311.
4. Cameron AJ, Higgins JA. Linear gastric erosion. A lesion associated with large diaphragmatic hernia and chronic blood loss anemia. *Gastroenterology* 1986;91:338.
5. Casabella F, Sinanan M, Horgan S, et al. Systematic use of gastric fundoplication in laparoscopic repair of paraesophageal hernias. *Am J Surg* 1996;171:485–489.
6. Chapman JE, Kamath MV, Wilson BW. Combined paraesophageal and sliding hiatal hernia. *South Med J* 1988;81:1177.
7. Cloyd DW. Laparoscopic repair of incarcerated paraesophageal hernias. *Surg Endosc* 1994;8:893.
8. Congreve DP. Laparoscopic paraesophageal hernia repair. *J Laparoendosc Surg* 1992;2:45.
9. Curley SA, Weaver W, Wilkinson LH, et al. Late complications after gastric reservoir reduction with external wrap. *Arch Surg* 1987;122:781.
10. Ellis FH Jr, Crozier RE, Shea JA. Paraesophageal hiatus hernia. *Arch Surg* 1986;121:416.
11. Eyde MB, Canin-Endres J, Gattorno F, et al. Durability of laparoscopic repair of paraesophageal hernias. *Ann Surg* 1998;228:528.
12. Frantzides CT, Carlson MA. Prosthetic reinforcement of posterior cruroplasty during laparoscopic hiatal herniorrhaphy. *Surg Endosc* 1997;11:769.
13. Fuller CB, Hagen JA, DeMeester TR, et al. The role of fundoplication in the treatment of type II paraesophageal hernia. *J Thorac Cardiovasc Surg* 1996;111:655.
14. Harriss DR, Graham TR, Galea M, et al. Paraoesophageal hiatal hernias: when to operate. *J R Coll Surg Edinb* 1992;37:97.
15. Hill LD. Incarcerated paraesophageal hernia. A surgical emergency. *Am J Surg* 1973;126:286–291.
16. Huntington TR. Short-term outcome of laparoscopic paraesophageal hernia repair. A case series of 58 consecutive patients. *Surg Endosc* 1997;11:894.
17. Huntington TR. Laparoscopic mesh repair of the esophageal hiatus. *J Am Coll Surg* 1997;184:399–400.
18. Johnson PE, Persuad M, Mitchell T. Laparoscopic anterior gastropexy for treatment of paraesophageal hernias. *Surg Laparosc Endosc* 1994;4:152.
19. Landreneau RJ, Johnson JA, Marshall JB, et al. Clinical spectrum of paraesophageal herniation. *Dig Dis Sci* 1992;37:537.
20. Martin TR, Ferguson MK, Naunheim KS. Management of giant paraesophageal hernia. *Dis Esophagus* 1997;10:47.
21. Maziak DE, Todd TR, Pearson FG. Massive hiatus hernia: evaluation and surgical management. *J Thorac Cardiovasc Surg* 1998;115:53.
22. Menguy R. Surgical management of large paraesophageal hernia with complete intrathoracic stomach. *World J Surg* 1988;12:415.
23. Mittal RK. Hiatal hernia: myth or reality? *Am J Med* 1997;103[Suppl]:33S.
24. Myers GA, Harms BA, Starling JR. Management of paraesophageal hernia with a selective approach to antireflux surgery. *Am J Surg* 1995;170:375.
25. Oddsdottir M, Franco AL, Laycock WS, et al. Laparoscopic repair of paraesophageal hernia. New access, old technique. *Surg Endosc* 1995;9:164.
26. Paul MG, DeRosa RP, Petrucci PE, et al. Laparoscopic tension-free repair of large paraesophageal hernias. *Surg Endosc* 1997;11:303.
27. Pearson FG, Cooper JD, Ilves R, et al. Massive hiatal hernia with incarceration: a report of 53 cases. *Ann Thorac Surg* 1983;35:45.
28. Perdikis G, Hinder RA, Filipi CJ, et al. Laparoscopic paraesophageal hernia repair. *Arch Surg* 1997;132:586.
29. Pitcher DE, Curet MJ, Martin DT, et al. Successful laparoscopic repair of paraesophageal hernia. *Arch Surg* 1995;130:590.
30. Postempski P. Nuovo processo operativo per la riduzione cruenta delle ernie diaframmatiche da trauma e per la sutura delle ferite del diaframma. *Bull Reale Accad Med Roma* 1889;15:191.
31. Raiser F, Hinder RA, McBride P, et al. Laparoscopic antireflux surgery in complicated gastroesophageal reflux disease. *Sem Lap Surg* 1995;2:45.
32. Rakic SR, Pesko P, Dunjic M, et al. Healing of gastric ulcer associated with paraesophageal hernia after hernial reduction. *Am J Surg* 1992;163:443.
33. Schauer PR, Ikramudden S, McLaughlin RH, et al. Comparison of laparoscopic versus open repair of paraesophageal hernia—new access, old technique. *Am J Surg* 1998;176:659.
34. Skinner DB, Belsey RH. Surgical management of esophageal reflux and hiatus hernia. Long-term results with 1,030 patients. *J Thorac Cardiovasc Surg* 1967;53:33.
35. Streitz JM, Ellis FH Jr. Iatrogenic paraesophageal hiatus hernia. *Ann Thorac Surg* 1990;50:446.
36. Subramanyam K, Robbins HT. Erosion of Marlex band and silastic ring into the stomach after gastroplasty: endoscopic recognition and management. *Am J Gastroenterol* 1989;84:1319.
37. Swanstrom LL, Marcus DR, Galloway GQ. Laparoscopic Collis gastroplasty is the treatment of choice for the shortened esophagus. *Am J Surg* 1996;171:477.
38. Treacy PJ, Jamieson GG. An approach to the management of para-oesophageal hiatus hernias. *Aust N Z J Surg* 1987;57:813.
39. Trus TL, Bax T, Richardson WS, et al. Complications of laparoscopic periesophageal hernia repair. *J Gastrointest Surg* 1997;1:221.
40. Walther B, DeMeester TR, Lafontaine E, et al. Effect of paraesophageal hernia on sphincter function and its implication on surgical therapy. *Am J Surg* 1984;147:111.
41. Wichterman K, Geha AS, Cahow CE, et al. Giant paraesophageal hiatus hernia with intrathoracic stomach and colon: the case for early repair. *Surgery* 1979;86:497.
42. Williamson WA, Ellis FH Jr, Streitz JM Jr, et al. Paraesophageal hiatal hernia: is an antireflux procedure necessary? *Ann Thorac Surg* 1993;56:447.

43

TRAUMATIC DIAPHRAGMATIC HERNIAS

DEMETRIOS DEMETRIADES
JAMES A. MURRAY

Migration of abdominal viscera through traumatic defects in the diaphragm was first described in the 16th century. During a postmortem examination in 1541, Sennertus described a strangulated diaphragmatic hernia that followed a penetrating injury 7 months previously. Subsequently, Ambroise Paré described patients with diaphragmatic hernias from both penetrating and blunt injuries diagnosed at autopsy (15). Bowditch in 1853 made the first antemortem diagnosis of diaphragm herniation (8). The first successful repair of a diaphragmatic injury was reported by Riolfi in 1886. Naumann (23) reported in 1888 repair of a diaphragmatic hernia with gastric herniation.

Many centuries later, the diagnosis of diaphragmatic injury is still often delayed and diaphragmatic hernias are still associated with significant morbidity and mortality. Early diagnosis and repair of diaphragmatic injuries remain the cornerstone for optimal results.

SURGICAL ANATOMY AND PHYSIOLOGY OF THE DIAPHRAGM

The diaphragm is a dome-shaped muscular sheet with a central tendinous portion that fuses with the pericardium. The anterior portion of the diaphragm attaches to the lowermost aspect of the sternum and xiphoid process. Laterally, it attaches to the lower six ribs and costal cartilages. This lateral attachment extends from the six ribs anteriorly to the 12th rib posteriorly. The first three lumbar vertebrae secure the diaphragm posteriorly.

The diaphragm is innervated by the phrenic nerves, which arise from the third through fifth cervical roots. Each

branch divides into four rami: a sternal (anterior), an anterolateral, a posterolateral, and a crural (posterior) ramus. This branching pattern must be appreciated when incising the diaphragm. Radial incisions run the risk of transecting the major branches of the phrenic nerves with the resultant paralysis.

During exhalation, the diaphragm may rise to the level of the nipples anteriorly (fourth to fifth intercostal spaces). Posteriorly, it rises to the level of the eighth intercostal space. This is important to remember because of the potential for injury to the diaphragm and intraabdominal organs during the evaluation of patients with penetrating injuries to the lower chest. Also, insertion of thoracostomy tubes should be performed above this level to avoid injury to the diaphragm and underlying abdominal viscera.

A resting intrathoracic pressure is between -5 and -10 cm H_2O, and the intraabdominal pressure is between 0 and 10 cm H_2O. In the supine resting position, there is a pressure gradient of up to 20 cm H_2O. This pressure gradient between the thoracic cavity and the abdomen may reach levels of 100 cm H_2O during forced inspiration or Valsalva's maneuver. This pressure gradient predisposes the displacement of fluids and abdominal viscera into the chest through traumatic defects in the diaphragm.

EPIDEMIOLOGY OF DIAPHRAGM INJURIES
Blunt Trauma

The reported incidence of diaphragmatic injuries in blunt trauma patients undergoing laparotomy or thoracotomy is between 4% and 6% (27). In severe traffic accidents with seat belt wearers, diaphragmatic rupture was found in 9.5% of the victims with abdominal injuries (1). Abdominal trauma is much more important in diaphragmatic rupture than chest trauma. There is a higher incidence of diaphragmatic rupture in patients wearing a seat belt during high-speed accidents. Also, front-seat passengers wearing a seat belt are at greater risk of diaphragm rupture than rear-seat passengers. It has been suggested that awareness of the

D. Demetriades: Department of Surgery, Division of Trauma and Critical Care, University of Southern California School of Medicine; Department of Surgery, Division of Trauma and Critical Care, LAC+USC Medical Center, Los Angeles, California.

J. A. Murray: Department of Surgery, University of Southern California, Keck School of Medicine; Division of Trauma, LAC+USC Medical Center, Los Angeles, California.

TABLE 43.1. COLLECTIVE REVIEW OF 514 PATIENTS WITH DIAPHRAGM RUPTURE DUE TO BLUNT TRAUMA—SITE OF RUPTURE

	%
Right diaphragm	25
Left diaphragm	75
Both sides of diaphragm	1.9
Pericardium	1.6

Data based on references 2, 4, 9, 10, 11, 16, 18, 19, 26, 30, 33, and 36.

TABLE 43.2. COLLECTIVE REVIEW OF 514 PATIENTS WITH DIAPHRAGM RUPTURE DUE TO BLUNT TRAUMA—ASSOCIATED INJURIES

Associated Injury	Incidence
Chest trauma	58%
Long bone fracture	38%
Pelvic fractures	34%
Head trauma	29%
Splenic rupture	44%
Liver rupture	28%

Data based on references 2, 4, 9, 10, 11, 16, 18, 19, 26, 30, 33, and 36.

impending collision may provide the ideal situation for diaphragmatic rupture. A voluntary inspiration is initiated, tensing the thoracoabdominal muscles. The diaphragm becomes contracted and tense. The intraabdominal pressure is elevated, and the intraabdominal volume is decreased. A further increase in abdominal pressure due to direct trauma causes a rupture of the diaphragm, the weakest structural point. High placement of the seat belt, over the trunk, especially in short individuals may also play a role (6). Lateral impacts with shearing forces, may result in avulsion of the diaphragm from its points of attachment. Rib fractures can also account for diaphragmatic injuries sustained during blunt trauma.

Review of 514 patients from 12 studies in the English literature showed that 75% of blunt diaphragmatic ruptures occur in the left diaphragm, 25% in the right, 1.9% bilaterally, and 1.6% intrapericardially (Table 43.1) (2,4,9–11,16,18,19,26,30,33,36). The protective mechanism of the liver and a greater inherent strength may account for the lesser frequency of rupture to the right hemidiaphragm.

Blunt diaphragmatic injuries are associated with a high incidence of other major injuries. In a collective review of 514 patients with diaphragmatic rupture due to blunt trauma, 58% had chest trauma, 38% long bone fractures, 34% pelvic fractures, and 29% head injuries. The most common intraabdominal injury was the spleen (44%) followed by the liver (28%) (Table 43.2) (2,4, 9–11,16,18,19,26,30,33,36). Rupture of the right

diaphragm requires a major external force to the abdomen, and in nearly all cases there is an associated intraabdominal injury. In left diaphragmatic ruptures, there is an associated intraabdominal injury in about 80% of the patients.

Penetrating Trauma

The reported incidence of diaphragmatic injuries following penetrating trauma to the thoracoabdominal area varies significantly and depends on the wounding mechanism (gunshot versus stab wounds), the anatomic area of the wound entry or exit, and, most importantly, the methods used to diagnose the diaphragmatic injury (Table 43.3). In a prospective study of 107 patients with penetrating left thoracoabdominal injuries (the area between the nipple and the tip of the scapula superiorly and the costal margin inferiorly), Murray et al. (20) performed laparotomy in the presence of an acute abdomen or laparoscopy in asymptomatic patients. Diaphragmatic injury was found in 42% of the patients (59% of gunshot wounds and 32% of stab wounds). There was no significant difference between anterior, lateral, and posterior thoracoabdominal injuries (22%, 27%, and 22% respectively) (21). Uribe et al. (34) performed routine laparoscopy in 28 patients with penetrating thoracoabdominal trauma and identified diaphragmatic injuries in

TABLE 43.3. INCIDENCE OF DIAPHRAGMATIC INJURIES IN PENETRATING TRAUMA TO THE LEFT THORACOABDOMINAL AREA: PROSPECTIVE STUDIES WITH ROUTINE LAPAROSCOPY OR LAPAROTOMY IN ALL PATIENTS

Reference	Stab Wounds		Gunshot Wounds	
	No. of Patients	Incidence of Diaphragm Injury	No. of Patients	Incidence of Diaphragm Injury
Murray et al. (20)	68	32%	39	59%
Uribe et al. (34)	28	32%	—	—
Madden et al. (17)	95	18.9%	—	—
Stylianos and King (32)	20	50%	—	—
Murray et al. (21)[a]	94	26%	16	13%

[a]All patients in this study were asymptomatic and were evaluated laparoscopically.

32%. Madden et al. (17) performed routine laparotomy in 95 patients with stab wounds to the lower chest and abdomen and found diaphragmatic injuries in 18.9%. In a similar study with 20 patients, Stylianos and King reported diaphragmatic injuries in 50% (32).

SURGICAL PATHOLOGY

The size of the defect in the diaphragm is dependent upon the mechanism of injury. Blunt ruptures of the diaphragm are usually long radial lacerations extending 7 to 10 cm in length. Typically, large defects in the diaphragm allow herniation to occur immediately or soon after the injury. In deceleration injuries, the diaphragm may become detached from its points of attachment on the ribs. Injuries associated with penetrating trauma are an average of 2 to 4 cm in length. Typically, it is these smaller defects that go undetected during the initial evaluation of the patient and may become complicated with herniation occurring hours to years after the injury.

The natural history of unrepaired diaphragmatic injuries is not known. It is possible that many small injuries heal without problems. However, many, especially the larger ones, fail to heal and may result in late diaphragmatic hernias. It has been suggested that the thinness of the diaphragm and the constant motion may impede healing. Another possible mechanism is the early herniation of omentum through the diaphragmatic wound, which prevents healing (foot in the door).

CLINICAL PRESENTATION

Uncomplicated Diaphragmatic Injuries

In the presence of associated significant intraabdominal injuries, the diagnosis of diaphragmatic injury is made intraoperatively. It is essential that during an exploratory laparotomy for trauma the diaphragm be carefully inspected.

Isolated injuries occur in 25% to 33% of patients with penetrating trauma to the diaphragm (13,17,20). These patients may be completely asymptomatic or have minor abdominal tenderness or usually a hemothorax. In a series of 41 patients with isolated diaphragmatic injuries, 10 (24%) were completely asymptomatic on admission (13). In another prospective study of 45 patients with diaphragmatic injuries, 31% had no abdominal tenderness (20). The diagnosis in this group of patients may be missed. A high index of suspicion remains the cornerstone of early diagnosis. Every asymptomatic patient with penetrating trauma in the left thoracoabdominal area should be aggressively investigated for diaphragmatic injury. Injuries to the right thoracoabdominal region are of lesser importance because the risk of visceral herniation is very small, due to the protective presence of the liver. However, anterior injuries to the right diaphragm may result in herniation, and we recom-

mend evaluation of these wounds as in the left side. The importance of aggressive evaluation of asymptomatic patients cannot be overemphasized. In a prospective study of 110 asymptomatic patients with penetrating left thoracoabdominal injuries, Murray et al. (21) performed routine laparoscopy, and in 26 patients (24%) there was a diaphragmatic injury.

In blunt trauma, 82% to 90% of diaphragmatic injuries have significant associated intraabdominal injuries and 54% to 97% of patients present with shock in the emergency room (5,26,35). These conditions are usually indications for laparotomy, and the diagnosis of diaphragmatic rupture is made intraoperatively. However, in the small group of patients with isolated blunt diaphragmatic rupture, the symptoms may be unremarkable and the diagnosis may be delayed. The reported delayed diagnosis ranges from 8% to 12% (14,30).

Diaphragmatic Hernias

A diaphragmatic hernia may be completely asymptomatic for many years and be discovered on a routine chest film. In a study by Degiannis et al. (12) of 45 patients with diaphragmatic hernias due to penetrating trauma, only 29 (64.4%) were diagnosed during the first admission. The other 35.6% of cases were diagnosed at a subsequent admission. Other patients may complain of nonspecific upper abdominal pain, which is the most common symptom and is often attributed to peptic ulcer disease, pancreatitis, or gallstone disease. In complicated cases, the patient may present with intestinal obstruction or respiratory distress. In neglected, strangulated hernias, the patient may be septic and in shock. On physical examination, the affected hemithorax may be prominent and immobile, breath sounds may be absent, bowel sounds may be heard in the chest, and tympany to percussion may be elicited. The abdominal findings are often unremarkable. The diagnosis is not infrequently missed, especially if the physician does not suspect the pathology, or fails to see a small scar in the lower chest or obtain a history of injury that could have happened many years previously. These patients are often treated for pneumonia, lung abscess, pleural effusion, and spontaneous pneumothorax.

INVESTIGATIONS

The initial investigation for a suspected diaphragmatic injury is a chest film. Suspicious radiologic findings include an elevated diaphragm, an irregular diaphragmatic contour, abnormal radiolucencies at the base of lung, air–fluid levels at the basal lung fields, and the combination of pneumothorax with free air under the diaphragm. A nasogastric tube curling up in the chest is diagnostic of gastric herniation.

Unfortunately, in uncomplicated diaphragmatic injuries, the initial chest films have a very low sensitivity and fail to

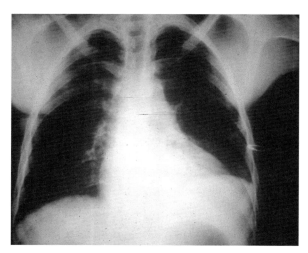

FIGURE 43.1. Elevation of the left diaphragm due to diaphragmatic injury. Only about 14% of penetrating trauma patients with an elevated diaphragm have a diaphragmatic injury.

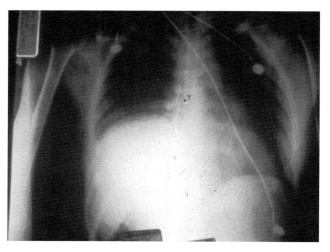

FIGURE 43.2. Elevation of the right diaphragm. Ruptured diaphragm with liver in the chest.

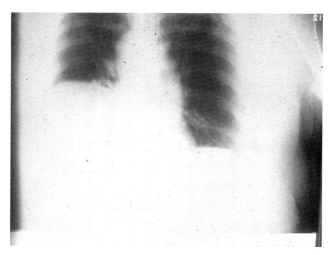

FIGURE 43.3. Elevation of the right diaphragm due to eventration. The differential diagnosis is often not possible without laparoscopy.

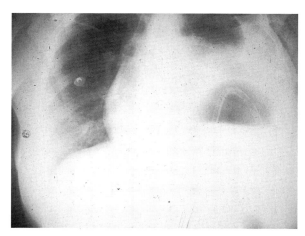

FIGURE 43.4. Diaphragmatic hernia due to blunt trauma. Notice nasogastric tube in the chest.

identify or even suspect the majority of injuries. In a prospective study of 45 cases with diaphragmatic injuries, the initial chest film was normal in 40%, showed a hemopneumothorax in 49%, and was suspicious for diaphragmatic injury in only 11% (20). Furthermore, an elevated diaphragm, which is considered by many authors as highly suspicious for diaphragmatic injury, had a low specificity. Of seven patients with an elevated left diaphragm following penetrating trauma, only one (14%) had a diaphragmatic injury (21). Traumatic conditions that may result in or mimic diaphragmatic elevation include diaphragmatic injury, subpulmonary hemothorax, atelectasis, lung contusion, phrenic nerve injury, fractures of the lower ribs, splenic hematoma, a dilated stomach, and congenital eventration (Figs. 43.1–43.3).

In the presence of a diaphragmatic hernia, the chest film is abnormal in most cases (Figs. 43.4–43.6). A film showing a nasogastric tube curling up in the left chest is diagnostic of

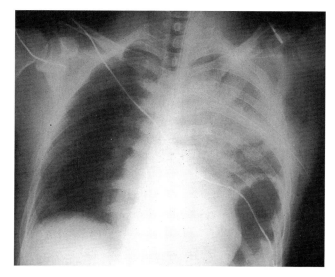

FIGURE 43.5. Diaphragmatic hernia due to penetrating trauma. Colon in the chest.

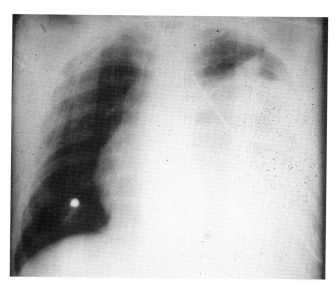

FIGURE 43.6. Tension diaphragmatic hernia following a stab wound 2 weeks previously.

gastric herniation. However, it is possible to have a normal film with omental or small gastric or intestinal herniations. If a patient with diaphragmatic hernia presents to the emergency room long after the initial injury, the chest film may be misread as atelectasis, pleural effusion, encysted pneumothorax, bronchopneumonia, or lung abscess (Fig. 43.7). It is not infrequent that these patients are not initially referred to surgeons.

Barium meal with follow-through or barium enema studies may be valuable investigations for suspected gas-

trointestinal herniation. In a small number of patients, the above studies may be not definitive and laparoscopy may be necessary. In our experience, the differential diagnosis between a diaphragmatic eventration and a hernia may be impossible with conventional noninvasive studies, and laparoscopic evaluation is necessary.

Many other investigations have been used to detect occult diaphragmatic injuries. Diagnostic peritoneal lavage has been one of the most extensively used investigations. In order to increase its sensitivity, the criteria for positive lavage have been lowered from 100,000 red cells per mm³ to 10,000 or even 5,000. With the strict criteria of 10,000 red cells, up to 25% of diaphragmatic injuries may be missed, and with the loose criteria of 100,000 red cells there is a high incidence of negative laparotomies (3). We believe that diagnostic peritoneal lavage has little or no role in the evaluation of suspected diaphragmatic injuries in a modern trauma center.

Diagnostic laparoscopy is currently the most valuable investigation for the detection of occult diaphragmatic injuries and has become the standard of practice in many trauma centers (Fig. 43.8). About 24% of patients with left thoracoabdominal penetrating injuries and no clinical symptoms have an occult diaphragmatic injury (21). We also advocate laparoscopy for anterior right thoracoabdominal injuries because in our experience they may develop late diaphragmatic hernias.

The timing for laparoscopic evaluation is controversial. Many authors advocate laparoscopy as soon as possible. The drawback of this early approach is that if not enough time has elapsed since injury, the presence of a diaphragmatic injury or peritoneal violation precludes laparoscopic repair and should be an indication for laparotomy. Laparoscopic evaluation of the bowel is not reliable, and small perforations may be missed (24). We prefer to observe these patients for peritoneal signs for 6 to 8 hours before we perform laparoscopy. With this policy, laparoscopic repair may be done without risking the possibility of missing an associated hollow viscus perforation.

During insufflation of the abdomen in the presence of a diaphragmatic perforation, there is the risk of tension pneu-

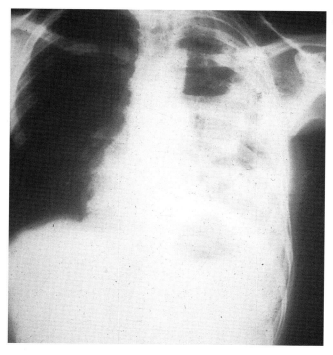

FIGURE 43.7. Complicated diaphragmatic hernia with colon and small bowel in the chest. The case was initially treated as bronchopneumonia.

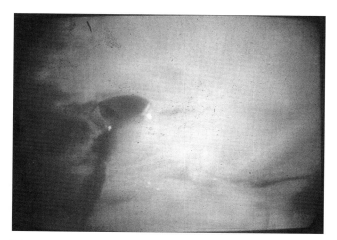

FIGURE 43.8. Laparoscopic appearance of penetrating diaphragmatic injury.

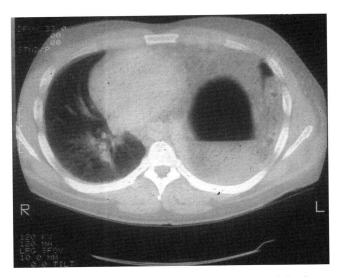

FIGURE 43.9. Computed tomography appearance of diaphragmatic hernia with stomach in the chest.

mothorax if the patient does not have a thoracostomy tube. It is essential that the patient be monitored closely, and with any persistent tachycardia, hypotension, or low oxygen saturation, the abdomen should be deflated and a thoracostomy tube inserted.

The laparoscopic evaluation is done in the operating room with the patient under general anesthesia. Attempts to perform the procedure with sedation and local anesthesia and using small-caliber scopes (3 mm or 5 mm) have been unsuccessful in our hands. The patient usually experiences severe pain, and the view through a small scope is not satisfactory.

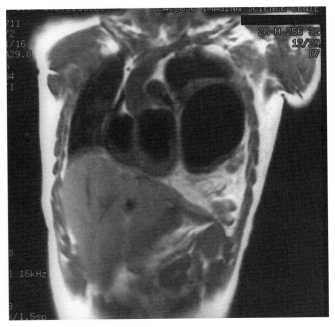

FIGURE 43.10. Magnetic resonance imaging appearance of diaphragmatic hernia with stomach in the chest.

Thoracoscopy has also been successfully used for evaluation of the diaphragm (31,34). It has the advantage of better visualization of the diaphragm, especially the posterior part, which is not easily seen laparoscopically. However, thoracoscopy requires double-lumen endotracheal intubation and collapsing of the lung, procedures associated with significant problems. We reserve thoracoscopy for diaphragmatic evaluation only for patients with residual hemothorax requiring evacuation.

Computed tomography (CT) evaluation is not sensitive enough in identifying uncomplicated small diaphragmatic injuries without herniation and should not be used for this purpose. Suspicious CT findings include diaphragmatic discontinuity, intrathoracic abdominal contents, and waist-like constriction of bowel (collar sign). CT scans and magnetic resonance imaging (MRI) investigations have a high sensitivity in diagnosing diaphragmatic hernias (7,37) (Figs. 43.9 and 43.10). However, their role in detecting small, uncomplicated diaphragmatic tears is questionable, and the existing experience is very limited. Figure 43.11 shows an algorithm for evaluation of penetrating thoracoabdominal injuries.

MANAGEMENT

Most patients with diaphragmatic injuries require an emergency laparotomy for associated intraabdominal injuries. Closure of the defect can be performed with one layer, figure-of-eight, interrupted, nonabsorbable sutures. Access to posterior diaphragmatic defects can be significantly facilitated by applying a tissue forceps on the edge of the defect and delivering it by traction into the abdominal wound. It is extremely rare that primary closure is not feasible and a prosthetic material required. Detachment of the diaphragm from the chest wall can be repaired by reattachment with pericostal sutures around the corresponding rib or higher than its original attachment.

Injuries identified during laparoscopic evaluation can be easily repaired with additional properly placed ports. The wound can be repaired with laparoscopically placed sutures or hernia clips. Experimental work at our center has shown that healing following laparoscopic repair (sutures or clips) is as good as with open repair. In some cases, laparoscopic repair may not be possible because of loss of the pneumoperitoneum through the diaphragmatic defect. In these cases, an open repair is indicated. Following diaphragmatic repair, a thoracostomy tube should always be placed, even after complete evacuation of any blood or air through the diaphragmatic defect. Failure to place a thoracostomy tube will result in a residual hemothorax in most of the cases.

Diaphragmatic hernias diagnosed soon after the injury should be managed with a laparotomy because of the possibility of other associated injuries. The most common herniating viscera are the omentum, stomach, and colon. However, small bowel, spleen, liver, and tail of the pancreas may also be found in the chest. Usually, the hernia is reduced and the defect repaired as previously described.

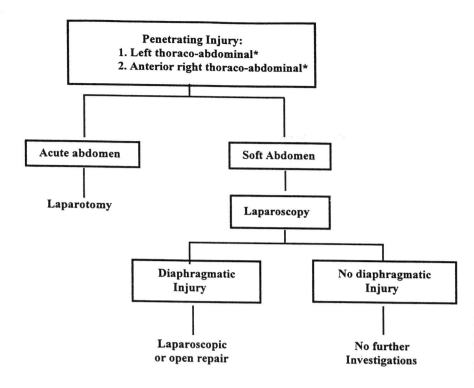

FIGURE 43.11. Algorithm for evaluation of penetrating thoracoabdominal injuries. The *asterisk* refers to the thoraco-abdominal area between the nipple and tip of the scapula superiorly and the costal margin inferiorly.

In chronic diaphragmatic hernias, the repair may be performed through a laparotomy or a thoracotomy or laparoscopically. Many surgeons prefer a thoracotomy because it might be easier to divide any adhesions between the abdominal viscera and the lung, and possibly avoid inadvertent perforations of the herniating viscus (27). However, other surgeons, including ourselves, prefer an abdominal approach, with equally good results. Enlargement of the diaphragmatic defect may be necessary to reduce the hernia or divide any adhesions under direct view.

In complicated hernias presenting with gastrointestinal obstruction or suspected strangulation with visceral necrosis, a laparotomy is the approach of choice because resections may be necessary.

Laparoscopic repair of uncomplicated late diaphragmatic hernias is possible, and small series have been reported in the literature (Fig. 43.12) (25,29). In most chronic cases, there is a hernia sac, which prevents loss of the pneumoperitoneum after reduction of the contents of the hernia. In the absence of a sac or if the sac is perforated

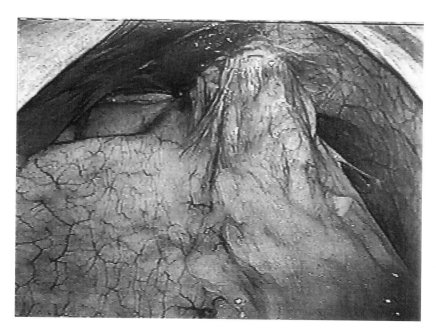

FIGURE 43.12. Laparoscopic appearance of a late diaphragmatic hernia containing stomach. The hernia was successfully repaired laparoscopically.

TABLE 43.4. DIAPHRAGMATIC INJURIES: OUTCOME

	No.	Mortality (%)	Morbidity (%)	Hospital Stay
No hernia	139	2.9%	12.6%	6 d
Early diaphragmatic hernia	14	7.1%	35.7%	11.6 d
Late diaphragmatic hernia	10	30.0%	60.0%	29.0 d

From Demetriades D, Kakoyannis S, Parekh D, et al. Penetrating injuries of the diaphragm. *Br J Surg* 1988;75:824–826, with permission.

during the operation, laparoscopic repair may not be possible because of loss of the pneumoperitoneum. In these cases, gasless laparoscopic repair may be possible. The diaphragmatic defect can be closed primarily in the vast majority of late hernias. In rare cases with massive defects, a nonabsorbable mesh may be necessary.

The prognosis and outcome of surgical treatment in diaphragmatic hernias depend on the presence or absence of ischemia or necrosis of the herniating viscus, the timing of the operation, and the contents of the hernia. Early diagnosis and operation during the first hospitalization for the initial injury are associated with the best results (12,13). Any mortality during this period is usually due to associated injuries. In late, complicated hernias, the mortality and morbidity increase significantly (Table 43.4). In the presence of gangrenous contents in the hernia, the prognosis is grave; about 30% of these patients die of uncontrollable sepsis and multiorgan failure (12,13). Colon herniation is associated with the worst prognosis because of its contents; thin wall, which perforates early; and inferior blood supply, which results in earlier ischemic necrosis than stomach or small bowel.

CONCLUSIONS

1. Diaphragmatic injuries occur very commonly with penetrating trauma to the thoracoabdominal area.
2. Many isolated diaphragmatic injuries remain asymptomatic, and the diagnosis can be easily missed. Laparoscopy remains the more reliable investigation for the detection of occult diaphragmatic injuries and should be used in all asymptomatic patients with penetrating trauma to the left thoracoabdominal or the right anterior thoracoabdominal area.
3. Laparoscopic repair of diaphragmatic injuries or diaphragmatic hernias is safe and effective in the appropriate cases.

REFERENCES

1. Arayarvi E, Santavirta S, Toloren J. Abdominal injuries sustained in severe traffic accidents by seatbelt wearers. *J Trauma* 1987;27:393–397.
2. Arendrup HC, Jensen BS. Traumatic rupture of the diaphragm. *Surg Gynecol Obstet* 1982;154:526–530.
3. Asensio JA, Demetriades D, Rodriguez A. Injury to the diaphragm. In: Feliciano DV, Moore EE, Mattox KL, eds. *Trauma*. Stamford, CT: Appleton & Lange, 1996:461–485.
4. Bauchamp G, Khalfallah A, Girard R, et al. Blunt diaphragmatic rupture. *Am J Surg* 1984;148:292–295.
5. Beal SL, McKennan M. Blunt diaphragm rupture. A morbid injury. *Arch Surg* 1988;123:828–832.
6. Bergqvist D, Dahlgren S, Hedelin H. Rupture of the diaphragm in patients wearing seatbelts. *J Trauma* 1978;18:781–783.
7. Boulanger BR, Mirvis SE, Rodriguez A. Magnetic resonance imaging in traumatic diaphragmatic rupture: case reports. *J Trauma* 1992;32:89–93.
8. Bowditch HI. Diaphragmatic hernia. *Buffalo Med J* 1853;9:65–94.
9. Brown GL, Richardson JD. Traumatic diaphragmatic hernia: a continuing challenge. *Ann Thorac Surg* 1985;39:170–173.
10. Carter JW. Diaphragmatic trauma in southern Saskatchewan—an 11 year review. *J Trauma* 1987;27:987–993.
11. Christophi C. Diagnosis of traumatic diaphragmatic hernia: analysis of 63 cases. *World J Surg* 1983;7:277–280.
12. Degiannis E, Levy RD, Sofianes C, et al. Diaphragmatic herniation after penetrating trauma. *Br J Surg* 1966;83:88–91.
13. Demetriades D, Kakoyannis S, Parekh D, et al. Penetrating injuries of the diaphragm. *Br J Surg* 1988;75:824–826.
14. Guth AA, Pachter HL, Kim U. Pitfalls in the diagnosis of blunt diaphragmatic injury. *Am J Surg* 1995;170:5–9.
15. Hanby WB, ed. *The case reports and autopsy records of Ambroise Paré*. Springfield, IL: Thomas, 1968:50–51.
16. Ilgrenfritz FM, Stewart DE. Blunt trauma of the diaphragm. *Am J Surg* 1992;58:334–339.
17. Madden MR, Paull DE, Finkelstein JL, et al. Occult diaphragmatic injury from stab wounds to the lower chest and abdomen. *J Trauma* 1989;29:292–298.
18. McCune RP, Roda CP, Eckert C. Rupture of the diaphragm caused by blunt trauma. *J Trauma* 1976;16:531–537.
19. Morgan AS, Flancbaum L, Esposito T, et al. Blunt injury of the diaphragm: an analysis of 44 patients. *J Trauma* 1986;26:565–567.
20. Murray JA, Demetriades D, Cornwell EE, et al. Penetrating left thoracoabdominal trauma: the incidence and clinical presentation of diaphragm injuries. *J Trauma*, 1997;43:624–626.
21. Murray JA, Demetriades D, Asensio JA, et al. Occult injuries to the diaphragm: prospective evaluation of laparoscopy in penetrating injuries to the left lower chest. *J Am Coll Surg* 1998;187:626–630.
22. Murray JG, Caoili E, Gruden JF, et al. Acute rupture of the diaphragm due to blunt trauma: diagnostic sensitivity and specificity of CT. *Am J Roentgenol* 1996;166:1035–1039.
23. Naumann G. Diaphragmatic hernia. *Hygica* 1888;5:524–530.
24. Ortega AE, Tang E, Froes ET, et al. Laparoscopic evaluation of penetrating thoracoabdominal traumatic injuries. *Surg Endosc* 1996;10:19–22.

25. Rasiah KK, Crone BJ. Laparoscopic repair of a traumatic diaphragmatic hernia. *J Laparoendosc Surg* 1995;5:405–407.

26. Rodriguez Morales G, Rodriguez A, Shatney CH. Acute rupture of diaphragm in blunt trauma. Analysis of 60 cases. *J Trauma* 1986;26:438–444.

27. Shah R, Sabanathan S, Mearus AJ, et al. Traumatic rupture of the diaphragm. *Ann Thorac Surg* 1995;60:1444–1449.

28. Shanmuganathan K, Mirvis SE, White CS, et al. MR imaging evaluation of hemidiaphragms in acute blunt trauma: experience with 16 patients. *Am J Roentgenol* 1996;167:397–402.

29. Slim K, Bousquet J, Chipponi J. Laparoscopic repair of missed blunt diaphragmatic rupture using a prosthesis. *Surg Endosc* 1998;12:1358–1360.

30. Smithers BM, Loughlin O, Strong RW. Diagnosis of ruptured diaphragm following blunt trauma: results from 85 cases. *Aust N Z J Surg* 1991;61:737–741.

31. Spann JC, Nwariaku FE, Wait M. Evaluation of video-assisted thoracoscopic surgery in the diagnosis of diaphragmatic injuries. *Am J Surg* 1995;170:628–630.

32. Stylianos S, King TC. Occult diaphragm injuries at celiotomy for left chest stab wounds. *Am Surg* 1992;58:364–368.

33. Troop B, Myers RM, Agarwal N. Early recognition of diaphragmatic injuries from blunt trauma. *Ann Emerg Med* 1985;14:97–101.

34. Uribe RA, Pachon CE, Frame SB, et al. A prospective evaluation of thoracoscopy for the diagnosis of penetrating thoracoabdominal trauma. *J Trauma* 1994;37:650–654.

35. Voeller GR, Reisser JR, Fabian TC, et al. Blunt diaphragmatic injuries. A five-year experience. *Am Surg* 1990;56:28–31.

36. Ward RE, Flynn TC, Clark WP. Diaphragmatic disruption due to blunt abdominal trauma. *J Trauma* 1981;21:35–38.

37. Worthy SA, Kang EY, Hartman TE, et al. Diaphragmatic rupture: CT findings in 11 patients. *Radiology*, 1995;194:885–888.

Nyhus and Condon's Hernia, Fifth Edition, edited by Robert J. Fitzgibbons, Jr. and A. Gerson Greenburg. Lippincott Williams & Wilkins, Philadelphia © 2002.

MISCELLANEOUS CONSIDERATIONS IN HERNIA REPAIR

44

ANESTHETIC CONSIDERATIONS IN THE MANAGEMENT OF ABDOMINAL WALL HERNIA

HUGH P. COWDIN, JR.
ANDREW S. TRIEBWASSER

The perioperative anesthetic management of abdominal wall herniorrhaphy is somewhat unique in its heavy reliance on the surgeon. The emergence of local anesthetic infiltration as the preferred technique for herniorrhaphy has required the surgeon to shoulder his/her share of the responsibility for anesthetic delivery, thus redefining anesthesia in this setting as a truly collaborative effort. This responsibility extends beyond the practical acquisition of technical expertise and mandates a more academic understanding of the rationale underlying the anesthetic management of hernia repair. Therefore, this chapter reviews available anesthetic options for herniorrhaphy, emphasizing the surgeon's role, and addressing the anesthesiologic consideration of the complex weave of patient variables and surgical requirements in the construct of a safe and effective perioperative anesthetic plan.

PREOPERATIVE CONSIDERATIONS

Physical Status

The American Society for Anesthesiologists (ASA) classification of physical status is especially helpful in evaluating outpatient suitability. Traditionally, patients bearing the designation class I to III are considered appropriate outpatients. It is the ASA class IV patient, defined as having severe systemic disease with a threat to life (12), who may be considered more appropriate for the inpatient setting. These patients may require invasive monitoring and/or sophisticated pharmaceutic adjuncts intraoperatively. All realistic comorbid contingencies should be addressed. The mistake

to be avoided is minimization of the surgical intervention. The contribution of a thorough preanesthetic evaluation to patient care as well as surgical scheduling is obvious.

Age

Although aging progressively alters the pharmacokinetic parameters of distribution, metabolism, and excretion, clinically salient pharmacodynamic alterations are generally reserved for the extremes of the age spectrum.

Body Habitus

Morbid obesity may limit anesthetic options. Expanded tissue mass may impair adequate local infiltration necessary to achieve surgical analgesia. Further, local anesthetic requirements may exceed dosage limitations calculated on the basis of lean body weight (4). Regional anesthetic techniques may be compromised by the obscurity of key physical landmarks. Likewise, morbid obesity may challenge general anesthetic techniques in regard to airway management, aspiration prophylaxis, and intraoperative ventilation (4,42).

Mental Status

Application of local infiltration or regional anesthetic techniques may be inappropriate in the severely anxious or significantly demented patient because the depth of requisite sedation may approach general anesthetic levels.

Pulmonary Disease

Coexisting pulmonary disease will have significant bearing on the choice of anesthesia for herniorrhaphy, and must be considered in relation to the size and location of the defect to be repaired. In general, local infiltration techniques are preferable for inguinal, umbilical, and small ventral hernior-

H.P. Cowdin, Jr.: Department of Anesthesiology, Brown University; Department of Anesthesia, The Miriam Hospital, Providence, Rhode Island.

A. S. Triebwasser: Department of Medicine, Brown University; Department of Anesthesiology, Rhode Island Hospital, Providence, Rhode Island.

rhaphy in patients suffering from ventilatory impairment. This technique allows for the intra- and postoperative maintenance of near-normal respiratory mechanics (19,43), depending on the degree of concomitant sedation.

Spinal or epidural anesthesia may be a reasonable alternative for inguinal herniorrhaphy in patients whose ventilatory capacity is not so severely impaired as to render the patient incapable of tolerating midthoracic anesthetic levels. Physical examination, arterial blood gases, and pulmonary function testing may help guide this decision. Regional anesthetics are generally inappropriate, however, for umbilical and supraumbilical ventral herniorrhaphy in any patient, regardless of ventilatory status, given the unacceptably high level of block necessary to provide relaxation and analgesia sufficient for surgical repair. General anesthesia is preferable in these cases, unless the umbilical or ventral defect is small enough to lend itself to local infiltration.

Preoperative chest x-ray, arterial blood gases, and pulmonary function testing are not routinely requisite for those surgical candidates with mild or well-controlled asthma or chronic obstructive pulmonary disease. Rather, such testing should be reserved for those more severely afflicted or overtly symptomatic patients in whom this additional data will be instrumental in gauging risk and guiding anesthetic choice, postoperative disposition, and pain management. Daily maintenance medications (e.g., β-agonists, theophylline derivatives, steroids) and inhalers should be continued perioperatively. Patients taking steroids during the 2 months prior to surgery should receive stress doses perioperatively (16). Elective herniorrhaphy should be postponed for those patients suffering acute lower respiratory tract infections (7) and rescheduled no sooner than 2 to 4 weeks after symptom resolution (57).

Difficult Airway

Anesthetic management of the difficult airway has surgical implications insofar as it affects the choice of anesthetic technique. It is preferable to manage and secure the difficult airway unhurried by the pain of incision. Although not unreasonable to employ local infiltration techniques (in the appropriate patient) to circumvent airway management entirely, it is inadvisable to rely on regional anesthesia techniques to accomplish this goal. The dermatomal level, anesthetic duration, and surgical adequacy of spinal or epidural block can, on occasion, be difficult to control or predict. Subsequent incision may then impose a potentially disastrous urgency on the management of a difficult airway during intraoperative conversion to a general anesthetic.

Cardiovascular Disease

Coexisting cardiovascular disease will also have significant bearing on the choice of anesthesia for herniorrhaphy. Arguably, local infiltration techniques (in lieu of general

anesthesia) reduce perioperative risk in patients with significant cardiovascular disease (47). This may be true only if performed meticulously with sufficient concomitant sedation. Several studies have also implied that regional anesthesia reduces perioperative risk in patients with significant cardiovascular disease (48). Confirmation studies have not been uniformly supportive, however, and it has been argued that a well-managed general anesthetic allows a degree of hemodynamic control superior to other techniques. Parenthetically, anticoagulated patients by reason of valvular disease/repair, atrial dysrhythmia, or cerebrovascular event may not be candidates for regional anesthesia without documented return of coagulation parameters to normalcy.

The emergence of new angina symptoms, the progression of existing anginal patterns, or a recent history of congestive heart failure all mandate medical evaluation and optimization prior to elective herniorrhaphy (44,47). Recently documented myocardial infarction should also delay elective surgery since the incidence of repeated infarction and subsequent mortality is increased during the first 6 months after the initial event (20). Preoperative evaluation of the patient with known coronary disease should include (a) a recent baseline 12-lead electrocardiogram; (b) some estimate of global left ventricular function (especially if the patient is otherwise limited in exercise capability); and (c) some indication of the nature and location of ischemic myocardium in relation to stress (37,56). Intraoperative monitoring may include an arterial line in those with more severe disease, but a pulmonary artery catheter is rarely required for herniorrhaphy. The value of perioperative nitroglycerin administration is controversial (56), although it may be considered in patients with unstable angina or in those reliant on cutaneous nitrates.

Severe, uncontrolled hypertension can be problematic intraoperatively, and ideally should be managed preoperatively. The pathologic combination of chronic intravascular volume depletion and diminished vascular bed compliance contributes to potentially dangerous intraoperative hemodynamic volatility in response to regional or general anesthetic administration. Furthermore, preoperative uncontrolled hypertension is generally considered predictive of perioperative cardiac morbidity (37). It must be emphasized that the physiologic stress and thus the inherent risk of herniorrhaphy to the hypertensive patient, and likewise to the patient with coronary disease, stems as much from the anesthetic as from the surgical repair.

ANESTHESIA FOR ABDOMINAL WALL HERNIORRHAPHY

Table 44.1 reviews the basic anesthesiologic considerations for each anesthetic technique available for abdominal wall herniorrhaphy. Table 44.2 organizes the anesthetic options in accordance with patient and procedural variables.

TABLE 44.1. ANESTHETIC CONSIDERATIONS FOR ABDOMINAL WALL HERNIORRHAPHY

Technique	Advantages	Disadvantages
Local anesthetic infiltration	• Minimal postop pain and n/v • Minimal postop sedation • Rapid PACU discharge • Unimpaired pulmonary function • Preemptive analgesia	• Time and dosage are limited • No muscle relaxation • No visceral analgesia • Tissue distortion • More time-consuming
Paravertebral block	• Rapid PACU discharge • Unimpaired pulmonary function • Muscle relaxation • No tissue distortion	• High failure rate • Poor patient acceptance • Need identifiable landmarks • Not for bilateral repair
Subarachnoid block	• Muscle relaxation • Visceral analgesia • Preemptive analgesia	• Headache (PDPH) • Hypotension • Time limited • Possible impaired pulm fxn • Normal coags required
Epidural block	• Same as SAB • Intraop redosing capable • Postop pain management	• Same as SAB
General anesthesia	• Muscle relaxation • No time limitations • Comprehensive patient control (a) Hemodynamics (b) Ventilation (c) Mental status	• Slower PACU discharge • Airway management • Coughing/Valsalva's maneuver • Postop pain management

coags, coagulation parameters; intraop, intraoperative; n/v, nausea/vomiting; PACU, postanesthesia care unit; PDPH, postdural puncture headache; postop, postoperative; pulm fxn, pulmonary function; SAB, subarachnoid block.

TABLE 44.2. ANESTHETIC OPTIONS FOR ABDOMINAL WALL HERNIORRHAPHY

	Inguinal				Ventral			
	LA	PVB	RA	GA	LA	PVB/IC	RA	GA
Procedural								
• Conventional	X	X	X	X	X	X	X	X
• Redo	X	X	X	X		X	X	X
• Relaxation		X	X	X		X	X	X
• Prolonged				X				X
• Incarcerated	X	X	X	X			X	X
• Strangulated				X				X
• Bilateral	X		X	X				
• Laparoscopic				X				
• Umbilical					X		X	X
• Supraumbilical					X			X
Comorbidity								
• Anxiety/dementia				X				X
• Pulmonary	X	X	X	X	X			X
• Cardiovascular	X	X	X	X	X	X	X	X
• Obesity			X	X			X	X
• Difficult A/W	X			X	X			X
• Anticoagulation	X			X	X			X

A/W, airway; GA, general anesthesia; IC, intercostal LA, local anesthesia; PVB, paravertebral block; RA, regional anesthesia.

Choice of Technique

The demands of the outpatient setting have driven the evolution of anesthesia for herniorrhaphy (51). The rapid achievement of hospital discharge criteria regarding pain, nausea, and sedation are the most critical of these demands (61). Local anesthetic infiltration, by minimizing intraoperative anesthetic and postoperative analgesic requirements, has emerged as the most effective anesthetic technique in this regard (43,50,72). The refinement of a complementary sedative regimen has facilitated its implementation. Propofol, for example, offers a more titratable sedative than benzodiazepines or narcotics by virtue of its shorter duration of action and elimination half-times (70). Furthermore, the absence of active metabolites as well as the suspected antiemetic effect of propofol yield a postoperative patient with less sedation and nausea (67). Not surprisingly, patients with comorbidity are often best served by this technique (72).

But not all patients are candidates for local infiltration with sedation. Strangulated and large incarcerated hernias are more appropriately repaired under general anesthesia because of the nature of the visceral involvement. Bilateral and redo herniorrhaphy may be constrained by local anesthetic dosage limitations as well as duration of procedure. Certain surgical approaches, especially laparoscopic and preperitoneal repairs, require more muscle relaxation than local anesthetic infiltration can provide [although a recent study reports on the feasibility of laparoscopic extraperitoneal herniorrhaphy under local anesthesia with sedation (17)]. Finally, patient temperament, anxiety, and mental status may render all techniques but general anesthesia unrealistic.

Fortunately, the recent technical, pharmacologic, and strategic advances in general anesthetic delivery have allowed these postsurgical patients to achieve hospital discharge criteria much more rapidly as well. The laryngeal mask airway (LMA), for example, provides an adequate airway without tracheal stimulation, thereby reducing anesthetic requirement and obviating the need for muscle relaxant (68). The newest inhalation agents [e.g., desflurane (Suprane; Baxter Pharmaceutical Products Inc., Liberty Corner, NJ, U.S.A.) and ultane (Sevoflurane, Abbott Laboratories, Abbott Park, IL, U.S.A.)] have shortened emergence times by virtue of their lower blood:gas partition coefficients, which speeds molecular recoupment by and exhalation from the lungs (68). The practice of infiltrating soft tissue with local anesthetic during herniorrhaphy under general anesthesia, often with parenteral nonsteroidal antiinflammatory as adjunct, has been shown to diminish analgesic requirement in the immediate postoperative period (5,15,39,40,60). Each of these advances facilitates early hospital discharge of patients recovering from herniorrhaphy performed under general anesthesia.

Preemptive Analgesia

The burgeoning concept of preemptive analgesia has found application to anesthetic choice for abdominal wall herniorrhaphy. There is a growing body of evidence, albeit not uniformly supportive (5,21), to indicate that local or regional preincision analgesia, alone or in concert with general anesthesia, significantly decreases the intensity of postoperative pain (2,15,34,60). It is postulated that this preemptive analgesia results from the prevention of nociceptive impulses entering the central nervous system (CNS) during and immediately after surgery, suppressing the formation of the sustained hyperexcitable state in the CNS that is thought to be responsible for the maintenance of postoperative pain (45). This concept argues for the utility of concomitant local anesthetic infiltration during general anesthesia for herniorrhaphy.

Local Anesthetic Infiltration

Pharmacology

Although a half dozen local anesthetics are available for infiltration, lidocaine and bupivacaine are used most frequently. Table 44.3 outlines physicochemical properties and dosage recommendations. Lidocaine offers the advantage of rapid onset by virtue of its lower pK_a, allowing a greater percentage of the injected drug to exist in the nonionized, membrane-transmissible form at physiologic pH. Its disadvantage is its limited duration of action without epinephrine. Bupivacaine offers the advantage of a more prolonged duration of action by virtue of its greater lipid solubility and high degree of protein binding. Its disadvantage is its slower onset of action. Some practitioners mix the two in an effort to reap the cumulative benefits while limiting the total dosage and toxicity of each drug (2). Mepivacaine is an attractive alternative for local infiltration when epinephrine is contraindicated, given its rapid onset and longer duration of action than plain lidocaine. If not contraindicated by the presence of underlying coronary artery disease, the addition of 1:200,000 epinephrine is beneficial regardless of the local anesthetic chosen. The localized vasoconstriction and decreased tissue pH effected by epinephrine serve to intensify and prolong the block while retarding systemic absorption, thereby reducing local anesthetic toxicity (59).

Anatomy

The course and distribution of four nerves must be addressed to ensure the success of local anesthetic infiltration for inguinal herniorrhaphy (Table 44.4). The *subcostal nerve* (T-12) contributes to the innervation of all muscle layers of the abdominal wall in the inguinal region. It courses medially deep to the internal oblique muscle, eventually innervating the rectus abdominus and pyramidalis muscles, and finally ending as anterior cutaneous branches sensory to the suprapubic skin. The *iliohypogastric nerve* (L-1) also contributes to the innervation of all muscle layers of the lower abdominal wall. It pierces the internal oblique muscle several centimeters in front of the anterosuperior iliac spine and

TABLE 44.3. LOCAL ANESTHETIC PROPERTIES AND CHARACTERISTICS

	Lidocaine	Mepivacaine	Bupivacaine	Tetracaine
Trade name	Xylocaine[a]	Carbocaine[b], Polocaine[a]	Marcaine[b], Sensorcaine[a]	Pontocaine[c]
pKa	7.9	7.6	8.1	8.5
% Nonionized	25	39	15	7
Lipid solubility	2.9	0.8	27.5	4.1
Protein binding	64%	78%	96%	76%
Infiltration				
• Concentration	0.5%–1.0%	0.5%–1.0%	0.125%–0.25%	
• Maximum dosage	5 mg/kg (plain) 7 mg/kg (+epi)	5 mg/kg (plain) 7 mg/kg (+epi)	2 mg/kg (plain) 3 mg/kg (+epi)	
• Onset (min)	<1	<1	1–5	
• Duration (min)	75–120	90–180	120–240	
Nerve Block				
• Concentration	1.0%–2.0%	1.0%–1.5%	0.25%–0.5%	
• Maximum dosage	As above	As above	As above	
• Onset (min)	1–5	1–5	5–20	
• Duration (h)	1–3	2–3	4–12	
Spinal				
• Concentration	5%		0.75%	1.0%
• Dosage (mg)	50–100		10–20	6–12
• Onset (min)	2–5		5–15	5–15
• Duration (h)	0.5–1.5		2–4	2–4
Epidural				
• Concentration	2%		0.5%	
• Dosage (mg)	200–400		50–100	
• Onset (min)	5–10		10–30	
• Duration (h)	0.75–2.0		1.5–4.0	

+epi, plus epinephrine; pKa, pH at which 50% ionized.
[a]Astra Pharmaceuticals, L.P.; Wayne, PA, U.S.A.
[b]AstraZeneca, Wilmington, DE, U.S.A.
[c]Abbott Laboratories, Abbott Park, IL, U.S.A.

continues medial-ward deep to the external oblique. Sometimes it gives off an inguinal branch that joins the ilioinguinal nerve passing into the inguinal canal. The iliohypogastric nerve ends as an anterior cutaneous branch that penetrates the aponeurosis of the external oblique several centimeters above the superficial inguinal ring, providing sensation to the suprapubic skin. The *ilioinguinal nerve* (L-1) pierces the internal oblique muscle near the deep inguinal ring, and courses medial-ward (together with the inguinal branch of the hypogastric nerve, when it exists) through the inguinal canal. At the superficial inguinal ring, the ilioinguinal nerve becomes subcutaneous, offering sensory branches to the skin overlying the pubis, and ending in the anterior scrotal (or labial) nerve, supplying sensation to the root of the penis and anterior scrotum (or labia majora). Along its course, the ilioinguinal nerve contributes motor fibers to the abdominal wall musculature. The genital branch of the *genitofemoral nerve* (L1-2) perforates the iliopubic tract just lateral to the deep inguinal ring, entering the inguinal canal and passing medially on the posterior aspect

TABLE 44.4. LOWER ABDOMINAL WALL INNERVATION

Nerve	Origin	Course	Branch	Sensory	Motor
Subcostal	T-12	Deep to internal oblique		Suprapubic skin	• Rectus abdominus • Pyramidalis
Iliohypogastric	L-1	Deep to external oblique	• Inguinal • Anterior cutaneous	Suprapubic skin	• External oblique • Internal oblique • Transversus abdominis
Ilioinguinal	L-1	Inguinal canal	• Anterior scrotal • Anterior labial	Suprapubic skin Root of penis Anterior scrotum Labia majora	• External oblique • Internal oblique • Transversus abdominis
Genitofemoral	L1–2	Spermatic cord	• Genital	Scrotum Medial thigh	• Cremaster

of the spermatic cord, emerging through the superficial inguinal ring. It is sensory to the scrotum and medial thigh and motor to the cremaster muscle.

Technique

After the surgical field has been prepared, a series of intracutaneous injections is made with a 25-gauge needle along the course of the contemplated incision using about *10 mL* of local anesthetic solution (Fig. 44.1A). Subcutaneous

infiltration is performed next with a 22-gauge needle, injecting *10 to 15 mL* of solution along the line of incision (Fig. 44.1B and C). Analgesia may be expected within 1 minute after injection. After analgesic adequacy has been confirmed, the incision is made through the skin down to the aponeurosis of the external oblique muscle. Infiltration is then carried out along the line of the next incision through this aponeurosis using another *10 mL* of local anesthetic solution (Fig. 44.1D). Once the external oblique is divided and retracted, the ilioinguinal and iliohypogastric

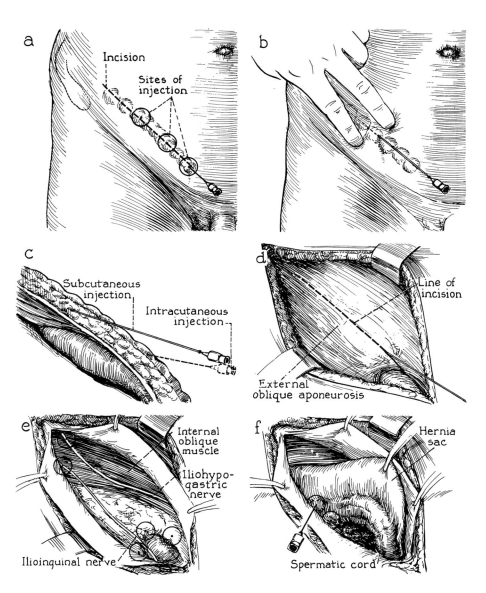

FIGURE 44.1. Technique of local infiltration of anesthetic solution for inguinal hernia repair. **A:** A series of intracutaneous injections are made along the proposed line of the incision. **B:** Subcutaneous injection using an 8-cm, 22-gauge needle guided by the fingers of the left hand. **C:** Cross section of the injection site showing the relationship between the intracutaneous and subcutaneous injections. **D:** Injection of the aponeurosis of the external oblique muscle along the line of incision. **E:** Injection of the ilioinguinal and inguinal branches of the iliohypogastric nerves and the peritoneum of the hernial sac. **F:** Injection of the spermatic cord.

nerves are identified coursing along the surface of the internal oblique musculature. *Two to 3 mL* of solution is infiltrated around each of these nerves, taking care to avoid intraneural injection (Fig. 44.1E). If the internal oblique muscle is to be incised, it is first infiltrated with *8 to 10 mL* of local anesthetic. The genital branch of the genitofemoral nerve is effectively blocked by injecting *5 to 10 mL* of solution into the region of the internal inguinal ring (Fig. 44.1F). No attempt should be made to infiltrate the sensory fibers of the spermatic plexus directly because injury to cord vessels can result in serious hematoma. If the repair involves suture of the lacunar or pectineal ligaments, these structures should be infiltrated beforehand. Finally, it is advisable to infiltrate over the pillars of the external ring since branches of the subcostal nerve often reach this point (Fig. 44.1E). The technique of infiltration described herein entails the use of *50 to 60 mL* of solution, less than the maximum recommended dosage of any local anesthetic agent.

Patience and anticipation are key to the successful implementation of this technique. The onset of infiltrated analgesia is rapid, but not instantaneous, and care must be taken not to outrun one's blockers. Likewise, the scope of infiltrated analgesia is thorough but not boundless, and care must be taken not to operate outside its limits without further injection. The amnestic quality of benzodiazepines should not be relied on to make up for a lack of patience and/or anticipation.

Sedation

It should be noted that adequate intravenous (i.v.) sedation is also critical to the success of any local anesthetic infiltra-

tion technique for herniorrhaphy. The fidgety, talkative, hyperresponsive patient may well render the operating conditions suboptimal—and justifiably so. The operating room is bright. The scrub solution is cold. The local anesthetic hurts. Bovied tissue smells bad. Cord manipulation aches. Fear turns pressure into pain, and magnifies every spoken word. In general, this sensory overload is counterproductive, and for many, the unfiltered patient experience may approach the intolerable.

Table 44.5 describes the pharmacologic characteristics and dosage recommendations for various sedative options. An effective sedative regimen includes a baseline benzodiazepine (usually midazolam), with or without concomitant narcotic (usually fentanyl), supplemented by propofol as a bolus during initial local infiltration and as a continuous infusion throughout the remainder of the procedure. This regimen is titratable, amnestic, and (without narcotic) arguably antiemetic. It is not, however, a quasigeneral anesthetic designed to compensate for inadequate local analgesia. More local anesthetic will compensate for inadequate analgesia. More sedation will eventually constitute a general anesthetic, which, with its attendant concerns for airway management, hemodynamic monitoring, and physiologic manipulation, is most efficiently and safely performed when planned.

Complications

The most important complication of local anesthetic infiltration arises from its systemic toxicity involving primarily the central nervous and cardiovascular systems. Toxicity may be induced by direct intravascular injection or by tissue infiltration of an excessive dosage.

TABLE 44.5. INTRAVENOUS SEDATIVE OPTIONS

Drug	Dosage	Onset	Distribution Half-life	Elimination Half-life	Metabolites
Benzodiazepine					
• Midazolam (Versed)	1 mg IVB 1–5 mg total	Rapid	6–30 min	1.7–4.0 h	1′-hydroxymidazolam (inactive)
• Diazepam (Valium)	1 mg IVB 1–5 mg total	Rapid	30–40 min	24–57 h	Desmethyldiazepam (+ active)
Narcotic					
• Fentanyl (Sublimaze)	25–50 µg IVB 50–250 µg total	Rapid	13 min	3.6 h	Norfentanyl (inactive)
• Remifentanil	0.05–0.1 µg/kg/min	Rapid	3.5 min[a]	8–48 min	Demethylated acid (inactive)
Propofol					
• Bolus	5–20 mg IVB	Rapid	2–8 min	1–3 h	Glucuronide (inactive)
• Infusion	25–100 µg/kg/min	Rapid	2–8 min	1–3 h	Glucuronide (inactive)
Ketamine	5–10 mg IVB 10–50 mg total	Rapid	11–17 min	2.5–3.1 h	Norketamine (+ active)

IVB, intravenous bolus.
[a]Context-sensitive half-life.

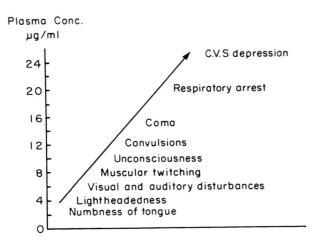

FIGURE 44.2. Relationship of signs and symptoms of local anesthetic toxicity to plasma concentrations of lidocaine.

Most toxic reactions to local anesthetics involve the CNS. Premonitory signs and symptoms are usually excitatory in nature (Fig. 44.2). Lightheadedness and dizziness are followed by auditory and visual disturbances such as tinnitus and difficulty focusing. Circumoral numbness is followed by shivering, twitching, and tremors. Ultimately, generalized convulsions of a tonic–clonic nature occur. Further local anesthetic administration leads to CNS depression with subsequent respiratory and cardiovascular collapse (CC). CNS excitation involves the selective blockade of cortical inhibitory pathways, allowing unopposed facilitatory neuronal imbalance. Further local anesthetic inhibits all pathways, both inhibitory and facilitatory, resulting in generalized CNS depression.

Also noteworthy is that local anesthetic convulsive threshold is related directly to arterial pH and inversely to arterial Pco_2 (9). This relationship is salient because of the propensity for i.v. sedation to induce hypoventilation, resulting in hypercarbia and respiratory acidosis. An elevation of Pco_2 will increase cerebral blood flow, so that more local anesthetic is delivered to the brain. Acidosis will decrease the plasma protein binding of local anesthetic agents, thereby increasing the portion of free drug available for diffusion into the brain. Thus, the sedation concomitant to and requisite for local anesthetic infiltration can, in fact, generate physiologic conditions more favorable for the development of neurologic toxic reactions.

Local anesthetic–induced cardiovascular depression occurs less frequently than CNS toxicity, but tends to be more serious and more difficult to manage. All local anesthetics exert a dose-dependent negative inotropic action. The relative negative inotropic effect is directly proportional to each agent's relative *in vivo* anesthetic potency (9). That is, the more potent local anesthetic agents tend to depress cardiac contractility at lower doses and concentrations than do the less potent agents. Notably, this negative

TABLE 44.6. TREATMENT OF ACUTE LOCAL ANESTHETIC TOXICITY

Airway
Establish clear airway; suction, if required
Breathing
Oxygen with face mask
Encourage adequate ventilation (prevent cycle of acidosis, increased uptake of local anesthetic into CNS, and lowered seizure threshold)
Artificial ventilation, if required
Circulation
Elevate legs
Increase i.v. fluids if ↓ blood pressure
CVS support drug if ↓ blood pressure persists (see below) or ↓ heart rate
Cardioversion if ventricular arrhythmias occur
Drugs
CNS depressant
   Diazepam 5–10 mg, i.v.
   Thiopental 50 mg, i.v., incremental doses until seizures cease
Muscle relaxant
   Succinylcholine 1 mg/kg, if inadequate control of ventilation with above measures (requires artificial ventilation and may necessitate intubation)
CVS support
   Atropine 0.6 mg, i.v., if ↓ heart rate
   Ephedrine, 12.5–25 mg, i.v., to restore adequate blood pressure
   Epinephrine for profound cardiovascular collapse

↓, decreased; CNS, central nervous system; CVS, cardiovascular system; i.v., intravenous, intravenously.
From Covino B. Clinical pharmacology of local anesthetic agents. IN: Cousins M, Brigenbaugh D, eds. *Neural blockade.* Philadelphia: JB Lippincott Co, 1988:135, with permission.

inotropism is potentiated by hypercarbia, acidosis, and hypoxia. Furthermore, all local anesthetics except cocaine exert a dose-dependent peripheral vasodilatory effect. Cocaine vasoconstricts indirectly by virtue of its unique inhibition of norepinephrine reuptake by tissue-binding sites, resulting in increased concentrations of this profound vasoconstrictor. Ultimately, the combined peripheral vasodilation, decreased myocardial contractility, and depressant effects on cardiac rate and conductivity will lead to circulatory collapse and cardiac arrest.

It should be emphasized that bupivacaine is especially cardiotoxic in its ability to induce ventricular dysrhythmia and fibrillation, from which resuscitation is notoriously difficult. Furthermore, the ratio of the dosage required for irreversible CC and the dosage that will produce CNS toxicity, the CC:CNS ratio, is much lower for bupivacaine than for other local anesthetic agents (9). All this points to the need for care in avoiding intravascular injection and respect for recommended dosage limitations.

Table 44.6 outlines the treatment of acute local anesthetic toxicity. Early signs and symptoms may not require pharmacologic intervention, but certainly warrant constant verbal contact, cardiovascular monitoring, oxygen administration, and ventilatory encouragement. Given that hypercarbia, acidosis, and hypoxia lower convulsive threshold and potentiate myocardial depression by local anesthetic agents, normalization of these physiologic parameters is helpful. Convulsions should be terminated by the i.v. injection of diazepam or thiopental and accompanied by ventilation with 100% oxygen. Succinylcholine may be required to facilitate adequate ventilation and intubation. Hypotension is due to a combination of myocardial depression and vasodilation, making it preferable to treat with an agent that stimulates both α- and β-adrenergic receptors, like ephedrine or norepinephrine. Anticholinergics may be required to reverse bradycardia. Cardiopulmonary resuscitation, defibrillation, and epinephrine may ultimately be required to effect resuscitation.

Subarachnoid Block

Rarely is subarachnoid block considered the first-line choice of anesthesia for inguinal herniorrhaphy. In general, local anesthetic infiltration is less invasive with fewer side effects and faster recovery, while general anesthesia tends to be more tactically precise. Rather, subarachnoid block is considered a reasonable alternative to general anesthesia for surgical repairs requiring profound muscle relaxation, and for surgical candidates suffering from significant cardiovascular or pulmonary disease. Here, patient or anesthesiologist preference often comes in to play. Subarachnoid block is not considered a reasonable strategy to circumvent the management of a difficult airway, nor is it recommended for patients with sliding or strangulated hernias. It is cer-

tainly not an anesthetic option for laparoscopic herniorrhaphy or for the anticoagulated patient.

Several basic disadvantages of subarachnoid block limit its utility. First, although the hypotension caused by sympathetic blockade can be minimized by crystalloid preload or countered in part by parenteral vasopressors (e.g., intramuscular ephedrine or i.v. phenylephrine), it is not well tolerated by patients with ischemic cardiomyopathy or stenotic valvular disease. Secondly, patient selection and small-caliber needles can reduce the incidence of postdural puncture headache to less than 10%, but not eliminate it (10). The headache can be intolerable, necessitating an epidural blood patch as definitive treatment. Finally, clinical experience can only partly overcome the difficulty controlling the dermatomal spread of anesthetic or predicting its duration.

Epidural Block

Those aforementioned issues of invasiveness, recovery time, side effects, and tactical precision with bearing on subarachnoid block as an anesthetic choice for inguinal herniorrhaphy in general apply to epidural blockade as well. However, the presence of an indwelling catheter enhances the utility of the epidural technique. The ability to redose intraoperatively eliminates the concern for the duration of a single-shot anesthetic. Furthermore, the ability to use the indwelling epidural catheter to manage postoperative pain is the signature characteristic of this technique, and is most useful for inpatients suffering from significant cardiopulmonary disease or obesity (4,71). Postoperative analgesia may be provided by a continuous infusion of local anesthetic and narcotic in combination, or by intermittent morphine injection.

Paravertebral Block

In theory, the paravertebral block is designed to offer the advantages of both the local infiltration and subarachnoid techniques without the disadvantages of either (30,63). Unilateral blockade of T10-L2 provides the intraoperative and immediate postoperative analgesia of local infiltration without the tissue distortion, as well as the segmental muscle relaxation of subarachnoid block without instrumenting the neuraxis and without sympathectomy-induced hypotension. In practice, however, the paravertebral block is flawed, and has therefore failed to gain wide acceptance and implementation. First and foremost, the technique is difficult and unpleasant for the patient because it requires multiple "needle sticks" and paresthesias. Secondly, identifiable landmarks are requisite for the performance of this block. Finally, because accurate placement of the needle at each of the five nerve roots is essential for optimal anesthesia, the failure rate for this technique is higher than for the other anesthetic alternatives.

General Anesthesia

As previously discussed, and as summarized in Tables 44.1 and 44.2, it is reasonable to consider general anesthesia for inguinal herniorrhaphy in a variety of clinical situations. Absolute indications for general anesthesia include educated patient preference and hernia strangulation. Strong consideration of general anesthesia should be given to patients undergoing bilateral, redo, or laparoscopic repair. General anesthesia should also be strongly considered for severely anxious and demented patients, and for those with a difficult airway when local infiltration techniques are deemed inappropriate. Reasonable consideration of general anesthesia may be given to patients with morbid obesity, severe cardiovascular disease, and for prolonged repairs and those requiring significant muscle relaxation.

The LMA is a useful tool in the effort to shorten recovery time after general anesthesia. Unlike the endotracheal tube, the LMA does not pass through the vocal cords into the trachea, but is inflated in the hypopharynx. It is therefore less stimulating, and a lighter anesthetic plane is tolerated. Furthermore, emergence is usually unaccompanied by the potentially disruptive coughing and Valsalva's maneuver attributable to the endotracheal tube. The LMA technique is appropriately employed for herniorrhaphy under general anesthesia except in those patients with reflux, and for those repairs requiring muscle relaxation. Reflux may be considered inherent in diabetics and the morbidly obese. The peritoneal insufflation requisite for laparoscopic repair mandates general anesthesia with an endotracheal tube.

Soft tissue infiltration with local anesthetic is another useful tool in the effort to hasten the achievement of discharge criteria after general anesthesia for herniorrhaphy (40). The minimal investment of time and effort spent injecting local anesthetic around the nerves and into the subcutaneous tissue yields substantial reduction in immediate postoperative pain, promoting early ambulation and discharge (5,15,34,39,60).

Femoral Hernia

Femoral hernias are considered with direct and indirect inguinal hernias in the overall classification of groin hernias. Anesthetic considerations for inguinal herniorrhaphy apply to femoral repair as well. Anesthetic options for femoral herniorrhaphy include local infiltration, paravertebral block of the first through third lumbar nerves, subarachnoid or segmental epidural block involving the twelfth thoracic to the third lumbar dermatomes, and, of course, general anesthesia.

Ventral Hernia

Anesthetic considerations for ventral herniorrhaphy do not mirror those for inguinal herniorrhaphy. Several characteristics of the ventral hernia distance it from the groin. First,

many ventral hernias are peri- or supraumbilical, putting them in the T8-10 dermatomes. This cephalad location significantly affects the utility of regional anesthesia for ventral hernia repair. Effective surgical analgesia as high as the requisite T6-8 level begins to impair respiration intraoperatively. Furthermore, the proximity of the surgical repair to the diaphragm has a negative impact on the immediate postoperative course regarding pain and atelectasis, especially for those patients with preexisting ventilatory impairment (45).

The second characteristic distinguishing ventral hernias is that many are, in fact, larger and require more extensive fascial resection than initially thought based on preoperative examination. This tendency, especially troubling in its difficulty to predict, significantly affects the utility of local anesthetic infiltration for ventral herniorrhaphy. A more extensive repair may exceed anesthetic dosage limitations. Furthermore, it may introduce the need for muscle relaxation not afforded by this technique. Although it is certainly possible to convert a local infiltration technique to a general anesthetic intraoperatively, this is considered a suboptimal anesthetic strategy.

In line with previous recommendations for inguinal herniorrhaphy, repair of small ventral hernias is best performed under local anesthetic infiltration when possible. However, surgical repair of larger, especially supraumbilical, defects is best performed under general anesthesia with muscle relaxation and an endotracheal tube. Strong consideration of general anesthesia should also be given for the morbidly obese, the redo and/or mesh repair, and incarceration. Strangulation mandates this technique. Postoperative pain management with a continuous epidural infusion is especially useful for patients with significant cardiovascular and pulmonary comorbidity. Soft tissue injection of local anesthetic during closure is a sound pain management alternative.

Umbilical Hernia

Anesthetic considerations for ventral herniorrhaphy apply to umbilical hernia repair as well. Anesthetic options for umbilical herniorrhaphy include local anesthetic infiltration, subarachnoid and epidural block, and general anesthesia. Notably, surgical repair of defects in the T-10 dermatome are more amenable to regional techniques than ventral hernias more cephalad. Further discussion of umbilical herniorrhaphy in infants and children will follow.

ANESTHESIA FOR INGUINAL HERNIORRHAPHY IN CHILDREN

Inguinal herniorrhaphy is the most frequently performed operation in infancy, with an overall incidence from 4.8% to as high as 30% in former preterm infants. Male-to-female ratio is approximately 5:1. Incarceration may occur in up to 31% of inguinal hernias (46), more commonly in premature infants, so repair is performed soon after diagnosis. Other complications from inguinal hernia in infants include intestinal obstruction and cryptorchidism. Bilateral hernias are common in children younger than 2 years of age; if contralateral exploration is planned, the obvious hernia should be repaired first in the event of an unexpected occurrence that requires cessation of surgery.

Preoperative Preparation

The perioperative care of children requires both medical and psychological preparation. Despite the prevalence of inguinal hernias in premature infants, the most common pediatric patient presenting for inguinal herniorrhaphy is an otherwise healthy child in the first 2 to 3 years of life. Preoperative medical evaluation is accomplished ideally in a preoperative clinic but commonly is deferred until the day of surgery. The child's pediatrician should help clarify and/or optimize any chronic medical conditions, such as asthma, heart murmurs, etc. Most institutions no longer require routine laboratory evaluation for healthy children undergoing peripheral outpatient surgery, such as herniorrhaphy.

Nearly half a century ago, Eckenhoff described "stormy" induction of anesthesia as a significant risk factor for behavioral changes in hospitalized children (14). There is evidence that children as young as 2 years of age gain benefit from preoperative psychological preparation, as exhibited by reduced anxiety (62), more cooperative anesthetic induction, and fewer postoperative behavioral changes. Preoperative programs range from simple information-based programs to those in which information is coupled with modeling behavior and coping strategies. Age-specific aids, such as coloring books, puppet shows, and videotapes, might be utilized. Although programs that teach coping skills are more effective anxiolytics, these benefits appear limited to the preoperative area (23). Ideally, preoperative preparation should include the family unit as a whole, with careful attention to the developmental stage of the child, and avoidance of inappropriate phraseology, for example, harsh phrases (*"cut you open"*), medical jargon (*"IV"*), or phrases that can be misconstrued by the concrete mind of a young child (*"put you to sleep"*). The preschool child is likely to exhibit severe separation trauma, fear of the unknown, and fear of pain and needles. The school-aged child is mature enough to participate in the preoperative discussion, which can focus on issues such as separation anxiety, fear of needles, fear of punishment, and reassurances that he or she is not being lied to. The older child and adolescent are concerned about pain and loss of autonomy, and must be reassured regarding fears of mutilation, death, and/or awakening during the procedure. In any case, it is imperative that the anesthesiologist approach the family with warmth and tactful honesty, making concessions when able, but employing a gentle firmness about issues over which the child (or parent) cannot exercise control.

Studies suggest that parents want full risk disclosure during the preoperative anesthesia interview (35), and that hearing of risks, including the risk of death, does not increase parental anxiety (24). Educational materials such as videotapes (6) are valuable and appreciated tools (38).

The premature infant must be evaluated for specific underlying problems. These might include chronic respiratory disease related to lung immaturity and prolonged mechanical ventilation and/or oxygen therapy. Increased pulmonary vascular resistance and reduced functional residual volume might necessitate chronic oxygen therapy. Subglottic stenosis is a potential consequence of endotracheal intubation. Intrinsic lung disease might require diuretic therapy, with decreased intravascular volume and potential electrolyte abnormalities. Neurologic consequences of prematurity include seizures, intraventricular hemorrhage, and prolonged apnea. Anemia is common in former premature infants and increases the risk of postoperative apnea (65).

Anesthetic Management

The successful anesthetic management of small children requires an appreciation for the anatomic and physiologic differences that exist between children and adults, and familiarity with specific equipment and techniques that are useful in the care of smaller patients. It is worthwhile noting that most anesthetics administered to children are not administered by pediatric anesthesiologists (36). Although it is unclear whether this has implications in "routine" cases, nonpediatric anesthesiologists have been shown to have a higher complication rate in high-risk situations, including the care of infants (27,28).

As noted above, the anesthetic care of children begins with preoperative assessment and preparation. Recent studies have allowed anesthesiologists to liberalize preoperative fluids (53); this is especially important in small children, who are at particular risk for dehydration, hypoglycemia, and emotional distress. Most institutions allow clear fluids up to 2 to 3 hours prior to surgery, and solid food 6 to 8 hours prior to surgery.

It is important to reassess children prior to induction of anesthesia, including confirmation of preoperative information, review of laboratory data (if any), and evaluation of temperament and level of anxiety. Some children will have new or worsened "cold" symptoms, occasionally necessitating postponement of elective surgery.

Premedication may be used to alleviate anxiety in the preoperative holding unit and facilitate separation from parents. The most common premedication is midazolam, administered either orally (0.5 to 0.7 mg/kg) or nasally (0.2 to 0.4 mg/kg). Some studies suggest that premedication with midazolam attenuates acute postoperative behavioral changes (25); this complication, however, is multifactorial and quite dependent on the child's underlying temperament and support system. Premedication should be used to complement, rather than replace, psychological coping mechanisms. An active child-life program can be instrumental in alleviating anxiety through age-appropriate diversions, including arts and crafts, video games, and movies.

In all but a very few instances, general anesthesia is utilized. The actual induction of anesthesia is usually via the inhalation technique, with either halothane or sevoflurane in an oxygen and nitrous oxide gas mixture. Sevoflurane is a relatively new agent, which offers the advantages of speedier onset and low incidence of cardiovascular complications. Its major drawback is high cost. Pitfalls of inhalation induction include combativeness, airway obstruction, emesis, and hemodynamic effects, such as hypotension and arrhythmias. Alternatives to inhalation induction include i.v. (usually with either thiopental or propofol), rectal (usually with methohexital), and intramuscular ketamine. Nitrous oxide analgesia and/or application of eutectic mixture of local anesthetics cream may facilitate i.v. insertion. Older children should be encouraged to participate in the choice of induction technique. Many institutions permit a parent to remain with the child through induction; most studies suggest that this practice, while endorsed by parents, may actually increase anxiety in certain situations. It is crucial, therefore, to institute a program that provides emotional preparation for parents who plan to participate in the induction process. Parents should be counseled that turbulent induction might predict negative behavioral changes in the immediate postoperative period (26).

Maintenance of anesthesia for pediatric herniorrhaphy proceeds in a fairly routine manner. Standard noninvasive monitoring is employed. Blood loss and third-space fluid losses are minimal. In most cases, a single 22-gauge peripheral i.v. catheter is inserted after inhalation induction. If the child is older than 1 year, and without confounding risk factors, mask anesthesia (either with face mask or LMA) is appropriate. Endotracheal intubation is preferred in infants, often facilitated with an intermediate-acting muscle relaxant. Although most pediatric anesthesiologists use uncuffed endotracheal tubes in children younger than 8 to 10 years, recent evidence suggests that cuffed endotracheal tubes may reduce operating room contamination without an increase in complications (29).

Pain Control Strategies in Pediatric Patients Undergoing Herniorrhaphy

Postoperative pain is mild to moderate after herniorrhaphy; the cornerstone of pain management is a peripheral-acting analgesic, such as acetaminophen (40 mg/kg rectal loading dose, followed by 10 to 20 mg/kg orally every 4 hours) or ketorolac (0.5 mg/kg i.v. loading dose), in combination with local anesthesia. Small doses of opioids, such as morphine, may be utilized to supplement analgesia, but side effects such as sedation, pruritus, and nausea and vomiting (64), which occur in a dose-dependent manner, make opioid-sparing strategies preferable, especially in outpatients. Several regional techniques are effective, including ilioinguinal/iliohypogastric nerve block, local wound infiltration by the surgeon prior to closure, and caudal blockade.

Ilioinguinal nerve block is preferred by many clinicians due to safety and efficiency. It is not, however, entirely without side effects, such as transient femoral nerve block with quadriceps weakness (49), and rare complications, such as local anesthetic toxicity and colonic puncture (22). Generally, 1 mg/kg of 0.25% bupivacaine is deposited on each operative side, using a 22-gauge, slightly dulled needle and a two-pop technique (after skin, the needle must penetrate the fascia of the external and internal oblique muscles). Unless the child weighs less than 10 kg, this block can be placed after induction and prior to incision, allowing for the theoretic advantage of preemptive analgesia. In smaller children, the volume of local anesthetic deposited near the operative site may distort surgical planes of dissection. In these patients, the surgeon might prefer direct infiltration. An alternative technique in this situation is caudal blockade.

Advocates of caudal blockade cite its ease, familiarity, and high safety profile. The caudal space is well identified in young children, and the sacrococcygeal ligament is entered with a 22- or 20-gauge needle or i.v. catheter. A single injection of 1 ml/kg of 0.25% bupivacaine will provide excellent anesthesia (T-10 level) within 15 minutes. Epinephrine (1:200,000) or clonidine (31) may be added to prolong the blockade. In mask cases, preemptive caudal analgesia has the advantage of preventing laryngospasm in response to surgical manipulation, thus reducing intraoperative requirements for volatile anesthetic or opioids. Potential complications such as nerve injury, local anesthetic toxicity, and dural puncture are rare (3). Delayed micturition has been shown to be an overstated concern, as 92% of children will void within 8 hours of surgery, regardless of anesthesia (18). Lower extremity weakness is uncommon, and can be avoided entirely by using 0.125% bupivacaine, which has similar efficacy to 0.25% bupivacaine for postoperative analgesia (69). Despite the excellent operative anesthesia provided by caudal block, most studies find no postoperative advantage to caudal blockade versus local anesthetic infiltration (11,52).

Primary regional anesthesia is an uncommon technique in small children, although there have been recent advocates for spinal anesthesia during herniorrhaphy for high-risk neonates with respiratory disease and/or apnea of prematurity (1). The usual approach is L4-5 in the midline, keeping in mind that the subarachnoid space is only 1 to 1.5 cm from the skin in these infants. Generally, a 25-gauge, 1.5-inch spinal needle is used, often with the infant in the sitting position. Care must be taken not to overflex the neck, as this may result in airway obstruction and hypoxemia. Tetracaine 1% will provide approximately 60 minutes of anesthesia, slightly more with the use of epinephrine "wash." The usual dose is 0.8 to 1.0 mg/kg. Raising the legs to place an electrocautery pad has resulted in a "high" spinal block and respiratory insufficiency. Hypotension is rare, and some practitioners will place an i.v. in the lower extremity after the block is in place. During the procedure, blood pressure should be obtained in the lower extremity, lest the intermittent cuff inflation cause distress.

Spinal anesthesia may reduce postoperative oxygen desaturation and bradycardia in this patient population (32), although evidence is lacking that the risk of postoperative apnea is decreased (see Postoperative Apnea in Premature Infants, below). Furthermore, unique complications may occur, such as recently documented aseptic meningitis in an infant who underwent spinal anesthesia for herniorrhaphy (13). Overall, despite the potential advantages of regional anesthesia, most clinicians would argue that it remains an unfamiliar technique and should not be rolled out on an infrequent basis for the most high-risk patients. Certainly, to ensure the success of spinal anesthesia, the surgeon should be comfortable (if not enthusiastic) with its use.

Postoperative Apnea in Premature Infants

In 1982, Steward described the risk of postoperative apnea in the former premature infant (less than 37 weeks of gestation) recovering from general anesthesia (55). Risk factors include postconceptual age less than 60 weeks (33), particularly in the face of severe prematurity, and ongoing apnea or anemia (8). Postoperative apnea monitoring is mandatory, usually necessitating overnight hospitalization. Over the years, investigators have sought to determine whether specific strategies could eliminate the need for overnight monitoring; these include the perioperative administration of caffeine (66) and use of regional anesthesia. Case reports of life-threatening apnea following spinal or caudal anesthesia for inguinal herniorrhaphy alerted anesthesiologists that regional anesthesia did not obviate the risk of postoperative apnea. Many of these infants, however, had received supplemental sedation, such as ketamine or nitrous oxide. A recent case report described two former preterm infants (38 weeks postconception) who had perioperative apnea and bradycardia after spinal anesthesia with tetracaine (58). No additional anesthetic agents were administered. In one case, apneic episodes occurred as late as 8 hours following the procedure. Neither of these infants had a history of apnea during the preceding 4 weeks. The authors concluded that apnea remains a risk in former preterm infants who undergo spinal anesthesia without sedation, and perioperative monitoring is still required.

Other Postoperative Considerations

Outpatients will typically spend 1 to 1.5 hours in the postanesthesia care unit (PACU) prior to discharge. Preparation for this recovery phase should ideally begin during the preoperative preparation. Parents are often included in recovery room care; in fact, immediate presence in the PACU has been noted as a parent's single most important perioperative concern (41). However, parents must be attuned to potential postanesthesia problems, and their presence must not interfere with patient care.

Potential PACU issues include respiratory compromise (apnea, airway obstruction, postintubation croup), nausea and vomiting, pain, and emergence delirium. Discharge criteria are institution specific, but generally entail a return to baseline level, including awareness, and the ability to manage any complications on an outpatient basis. This would imply the presence of a responsible adult who receives and understands written postoperative instructions. Mandatory fluid intake is no longer required for most outpatient surgery in children, as it has been shown to be associated with an increased incidence of emesis, and nondrinkers are no more likely to be readmitted for dehydration (54). In an uncomplicated herniorrhaphy, where the risk of bladder injury is low, postoperative voiding is generally not a requirement for discharge, but surgical considerations may warrant longer observation in certain cases.

As is the case during the preoperative period, providing a "kid-friendly" environment that maintains positive family dynamics is crucial during the recovery period. Parents should be reunited with children early in the postoperative period and receive clear instructions regarding postoperative care.

REFERENCES

1. Abajain JC, et al. Spinal anesthesia for surgery in the high-risk infant. *Anesth Analg* 1984;63:359–362.
2. Amid PK, Shulman AG, Lichtenstein IL. Local anesthesia for inguinal hernia repair step-by-step procedure. *Ann Surg* 1994; 220:735–737.
3. Broadman LM, et al. "Kiddie caudals": experience with 1154 consecutive cases without complications. *Anesth Analg* 1987;66 [Suppl]:S18.
4. Buckley FP, et al. Anesthesia in the morbidly obese. *Anesthesia* 1983;38:840–851.
5. Callesen T, Kehlet H. Postherniorrhaphy pain. *Anesthesiology* 1997;87:1219–1230.
6. Cassady JF, et al. Use of a preanesthetic video for facilitation of parental education and anxiolysis before pediatric ambulatory surgery. *Anesth Analg* 1999;88:246–250.
7. Cohen MM, Cameron CB. Should you cancel the operation when a child has an upper respiratory tract infection? *Anesth Analg* 1991;72:282–288.
8. Cote CJ, et al. Postoperative apnea in former preterm infants after inguinal herniorrhaphy: a combined analysis. *Anesthesiology* 1995;82:809–822.
9. Covino BG. Clinical pharmacology of local anesthetic agents. In:

Cousins MJ, Bridenbaugh PO, eds. *Neural blockade*. Philadelphia: JB Lippincott Co, 1988:111–144.

10. Covino BG, Lambert DH. Epidural and spinal anesthesia. In: Barash PG, Cullen BF, Stoelting RK, eds. *Clinical anesthesia*. Philadelphia: JB Lippincott Co, 1992:809–840.

11. Cross GD, Barrett RF. Comparison of two regional techniques for postoperative analgesia in children following herniotomy and orchiopexy. *Anesthesia* 1987;42:845–849.

12. Dripps RD. Preanesthetic consultation and choice of anesthesia. In: Dripps RD, Eckenhoff JE, Vandam LD, eds. *Introduction to anesthesia: the principles of safe practice*. Philadelphia: WB Saunders, 1988:13–21.

13. Easley RB, et al. Aseptic meningitis after spinal anesthesia in an infant. *Anesthesiology* 1999;91:305–307.

14. Eckenhoff JE. Relationship of anesthesia to postoperative personality changes in children. *Am J Dis Child* 1953;86:587.

15. Ejlersen E, et al. A comparison between preincisional and postincisional lidocaine infiltration and postoperative pain. *Anesth Analg* 1992;74:495–498.

16. Feely J. Drugs and the endocrine system. In: Wood M, Wood AJJ, eds. *Drugs and anesthesia*. Baltimore: Williams & Wilkins, 1990:553–569.

17. Ferzli G, Sayad P, Vasisht B. The feasibility of laparoscopic extraperitoneal hernia repair under local anesthesia. *Surg Endosc* 1999;13:588–590.

18. Fisher QA, et al. Postoperative voiding interval and duration of analgesia following peripheral or caudal nerve blocks in children. *Anesth Analg* 1993;76:173–177.

19. Godfrey PJ, et al. Ventilatory capacity after three methods of anesthesia for inguinal hernia repair: a randomized controlled trial. *Br J Surg* 1981;68:587–589.

20. Goldman L, et al. Multifactorial index of cardiac risk in noncardiac surgical procedures. *N Engl J Med* 1977;297:845–850.

21. Johansson B, et al. Preoperative local infiltration with ropivacaine for postoperative pain relief after inguinal hernia repair. *Eur J Surg* 1997;163:371–378.

22. Johr M, Sossai R. Colonic puncture during ilioinguinal nerve block in a child. *Anesth Analg* 1999;88:1051–1052.

23. Kain ZN. Preoperative preparation programs in children: a comparative examination. *Anesth Analg* 1998;87:1249–1255.

24. Kain ZN, et al. Parental desire for perioperative information and informed consent: a two-phased study. *Anesth Analg* 1997;84:299–306.

25. Kain ZN. Postoperative behavioral outcomes in children: effects of sedative premedication. *Anesthesiology* 1999;90:758–765.

26. Kain ZN, et al. Distress during the induction of anesthesia and postoperative behavioral outcomes. *Anesth Analg* 1999;88:1042–1047.

27. Keenan RL. Frequency of anesthetic cardiac arrests in infants: effects of pediatric anesthesiologists. *J Clin Anesth* 1991;3:433–437.

28. Keenan RL, et al. Bradycardia during anesthesia in infants: an epidemiologic study. *Anesthesiology* 1994;80:976–982.

29. Khine HH, et al. Comparison of cuffed and uncuffed endotracheal tubes in young children during general anesthesia. *Anesthesiology* 1997;86:627–631.

30. Klein SM, et al. Paravertebral somatic nerve block for outpatient inguinal herniorrhaphy: an expanded case report of 22 patients. *Reg Anesth Pain Med* 1998;23:306–310.

31. Klimscha W, et al. The efficacy and safety of a clonidine/bupivacaine combination in caudal blockade for pediatric hernia repair. *Anesth Analg* 1999;86:54–61.

32. Krane EJ, et al. Postoperative apnea, bradycardia and oxygen desaturation in formerly premature infants: prospective comparison of spinal and general anesthesia. *Anesth Analg* 1995;80:7–13.

33. Kurth CD, et al. Postoperative apnea in preterm infants. *Anesthesiology* 1987;66:483–488.

34. Langer JC, et al. Intraoperative bupivacaine during outpatient hernia repair in children: a randomized double blind trial. *J Ped Surg* 1987;22:267–270.

35. Litman RS. Parental knowledge and attitudes toward discussing the risk of death from anesthesia. *Anesth Analg* 1993;77:256–260.

36. Macario A, et al. The demographics of inpatient pediatric anesthesia: implications for credentialing policy. *J Clin Anesth* 1995;7:507–511.

37. Mangano DT. Perioperative cardiac morbidity. *Anesthesiology* 1990;72:153–184.

38. Margolis JO. Pediatric preoperative teaching: effects at induction and postoperatively. *Pediatr Anesth* 1998;8:17–23.

39. Moiniche S, et al. A qualitative systematic review of incisional local anesthesia for postoperative pain relief after abdominal operations. *Br J Anesth* 1998;81:377–383.

40. O'Riordain DS, et al. A randomized controlled trial of extraperitoneal bupivacaine analgesia in laparoscopic hernia repair. *Am J Surg* 1998;176:254–257.

41. Parnass SM, et al. A survey of parental attitudes following pediatric anesthesia at a community hospital. *Anesthesiology* 1988;89:A1156(abst).

42. Passannante AN. Anesthesia for the morbidly obese patient. *Wellcome Trends in Anesthesiology* 1993;11:3.

43. Peiper C, et al. Local versus general anesthesia for Shouldice repair of the inguinal hernia. *World J Surg* 1994;18:912–916.

44. Rao TLK, et al. Reinfarction following anesthesia in patients with myocardial infarction. *Anesthesiology* 1983;59:499–505.

45. Ready LB. Acute postoperative pain. In: Miller RD, ed. *Anesthesia*. New York: Churchill Livingstone, 1994:2327–2344.

46. Rescorla FG, Grosfeld JL. Inguinal hernia in the perinatal period and early infancy: clinical considerations. *J Pediatr Surg* 1984;19:332–837.

47. Roizen MF. Anesthetic implications of concurrent diseases. In: Miller RD, ed. *Anesthesia*. New York: Churchill Livingstone, 1994:903–1014.

48. Ross AF, Tinker JH. Anesthesia risk. In: Miller RD, ed. *Anesthesia*. New York: Churchill Livingstone, 1994:791–825.

49. Roy-Shapira A, et al. Transient quadriceps paresis following local inguinal block for postoperative pain control. *J Pediatr Surg* 1985;20:554–555.

50. Rudkin GE, Maddern GJ. Peri-operative outcome for day-case laparoscopic and open inguinal hernia repair. *Anesthesia* 1995;50:586–589.

51. Ryan JA, et al. Outpatient inguinal herniorrhaphy with both regional and local anesthesia. *Am J Surg* 1984;148:313–316.

52. Schindler M, et al. A comparison of postoperative analgesia provided by wound infiltration or caudal anesthesia. *Anesth Intensive Care* 1991;19:46–49.

53. Schreiner MS, et al. Ingestion of liquids compared with preoperative fasting in pediatric outpatients. *Anesthesiology* 1990;72:593–597.

54. Schreiner MS, et al. Should children drink before discharge from day surgery? *Anesthesiology* 1992;76:528–533.

55. Steward DJ. Preterm infants are more prone to complications following minor surgery than term infants. *Anesthesiology* 1982;56:304–306.

56. Stoelting RK, Dierdorf SF, McCammon RL, eds. *Anesthesia and co-existing disease*. New York: Churchill Livingstone, 1988:1–36.

57. Tait AR, Knight PR. Intraoperative respiratory complications in patients with upper respiratory tract infections. *Can J Anesth* 1987;34:300–303.

58. Tobias JD, et al. Apnea following spinal anesthesia in two former preterm infants. *Can J Anesth* 1998;45:985–989.

59. Tucker GT, Mather LE. Properties, absorption and disposition of local anesthetic agents. In: Cousins MJ, Bridenbaugh PO, eds. *Neural blockade*. Philadelphia: JB Lippincott Co, 1988: 47–110.

60. Tverskoy M, et al. Postoperative pain after inguinal herniorrhaphy with different types of anesthesia. *Anesth Analg* 1990;70:29–35.

61. Twersky RS. Recovery and discharge of the ambulatory anesthesia patient. In: ASA Annual Refresher Course Lectures, 1998: 232:1–7.

62. Vetter TR. The epidemiology and selective identification of children at risk for preoperative anxiety reactions. *Anesth Analg* 1993; 77:96–99.

63. Wassef MR, et al. The paravertebral nerve root block for inguinal herniorrhaphy—a comparison with the field block approach. *Reg Anesth Pain Med* 1998;23:451–456.

64. Weinstein MS, et al. A single dose of morphine sulfate increases the incidence of vomiting after outpatient inguinal surgery in children. *Anesthesiology* 1994;81:572–577.

65. Welborn LG, et al. Anemia and postoperative apnea in former preterm infants. *Anesthesiology* 1991;74:1003–1006.

66. Welborn LG, et al. The use of caffeine in the control of postanesthetic apnea in former preterm infants. *Anesthesiology* 1988;68:796–798.

67. White PF. Propofol: pharmacokinetics and pharmacodynamics. *Semin Anesth* 1988;7:4.

68. White PF. What is new in ambulatory anesthesia techniques. In: ASA Annual Refresher Course Lectures, 1998:231:1–7.

69. Wolf A, et al. Bupivacaine for caudal analgesia in infants and children: the optimal effective concentration. *Anesthesiology* 1988;69:102–106.

70. Wood M. Intravenous anesthetic agents. In: Wood M, Wood AJJ, eds. *Drugs and anesthesia*. Baltimore: Williams & Wilkins, 1990:179–223.

71. Yeager MP, et al: Epidural anesthesia and analgesia in high-risk surgical patients. *Anesthesiology* 1987;66:729–736.

72. Young DV. Comparison of local, spinal and general anesthesia for inguinal herniorrhaphy. *Am J Surg* 1987;153:560–563.

Nyhus and Condon's Hernia, Fifth Edition, edited by Robert J. Fitzgibbons, Jr. and A. Gerson Greenburg. Lippincott Williams & Wilkins, Philadelphia © 2002.

45

PAIN MANAGEMENT FOR INGUINAL HERNIORRHAPHY

HENRIK KEHLET
TORBEN CALLESEN

Inguinal herniorrhaphy is a relatively small operation and often performed on an outpatient basis with little intra- or postoperative morbidity. Postherniorrhaphy pain, however, may be a significant problem with socioeconomic implications since pain may contribute to prolonged convalescence (4). Furthermore, early postherniorrhaphy pain may continue in some patients into a long-lasting chronic pain state that may severely impair level of function and quality of life (4,12,19). In this chapter, we review the time course and consequences of early postherniorrhaphy pain, and discuss the effects of different surgical techniques, local anesthetic techniques, and other treatment modalities on early postherniorrhaphy pain. Finally, we consider future strategies to improve postherniorrhaphy pain relief and thereby reduce the potential risk for development of a chronic pain state.

TIME COURSE AND CONSEQUENCES OF EARLY POSTHERNIORRHAPHY PAIN

Like other operations, inguinal herniorrhaphy is followed by pain, which may subsequently diminish or disappear during the following weeks. Most data are available from randomized trials to compare different types of surgical technique, and relatively little data are available from large, consecutive series (4,6). The typical average time course of pain during rest and mobilization is shown in Fig. 45.1, and emphasizes a significant postoperative pain problem during the first week. After 4 weeks, pain remains a problem in only about 5% of patients (6). However, when assessing

pain during function (coughing or mobilization), a higher number of patients report clinically significant pain, amounting to about 30% after 1 week and about 10% after 1 month (6).

The clinical consequences of early postherniorrhaphy pain are related to duration of convalescence (time to return to work or leisure activities). Thus, detailed studies where standard recommendations for short convalescence have been applied have demonstrated pain to be the most significant factor for prolonged convalescence, other factors being fear of recurrence, and counteradvice from other physicians (7).

Predictive factors of early postherniorrhaphy pain have not been evaluated in detail. In a large prospective consecutive study of 500 patients, young age was predictive for a higher intensity of early postoperative pain compared to elderly patients (6). The role of other factors, such as intensity of preoperative pain, psychological factors, insurance status, and so on, has not been evaluated.

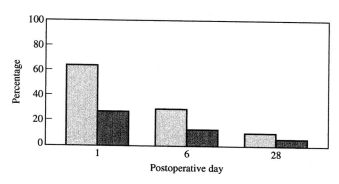

FIGURE 45.1. Percentage of patients having moderate or severe pain during rest (*dark bars*) and activity (*light bars*) after open herniorrhaphy. (From Callesen T, Bech K, Nielsen R, et al. Pain after groin hernia repair. *Br J Surg* 1998;85:1412–1414, with permission.)

H. Kehlet: Department of Surgical Gastroenterology, Hvidovre University Hospital, Hvidovre, Denmark.
T. Callesen: University of Copenhagen; Department of Anesthesia, Rigshospitalet, Copenhagen, Denmark.

The intensity of early postoperative pain may have long-term consequences since large consecutive studies have demonstrated initial high pain scores to be related to an increased risk of late or chronic pain 1 year or later after the operation (9).

In summary, existing data suggest that increased attention should be paid toward effective treatment of early post herniorrhaphy pain because of its consequences on convalescence and the risk of developing chronic pain.

EFFECT OF SURGICAL TECHNIQUE ON EARLY POSTHERNIORRHAPHY PAIN

The use of tension-free mesh implants instead of other types of open herniorrhaphy was hypothesized to reduce early pain intensity. However, this assumption has not been confirmed in randomized studies (Table 45.1). Also, there has been no difference in early postherniorrhaphy pain pattern between other types of open, sutured herniorrhaphy (annuloplasty, Shouldice technique, etc.) (Table 45.1). The use of plugs and unsutured patches versus the sutured techniques on postherniorrhaphy pain remains to be evaluated in well-designed randomized studies.

Much attention has been paid to comparing the laparoscopic repair techniques to the open herniorrhaphy techniques, and most randomized studies have demonstrated reduced pain and convalescence with laparoscopic repair (Fig. 45.2 and Table 45.1). However, interpretation of these studies is difficult since the type of postoperative pain treatment is rarely described in detail, and optimal local and systemic anesthetic and analgesic therapy rarely have been applied, especially in the "open" repair groups.

Regarding convalescence, this may merely depend on traditions and recommendations, which are extremely variable (7). In large consecutive series from hernia centers where specific short-term reconvalescence recommendations have been given, the convalescence period usually amounted to 5 to 7 days (7), which is less than the 2 to 3 weeks of convalescence observed in randomized studies comparing laparoscopic and open techniques, but without specific and/or shortened convalescence recommendations.

In summary, the specific role of surgical techniques on early postherniorrhaphy pain remains to be determined when well-defined and optimal analgesic therapy is provided in all groups, and with shortened convalescence recommendations in all patients.

TREATMENT OF EARLY POSTHERNIORRHAPHY PAIN

The different strategies and target points of pain treatment are outlined in Fig. 45.3.

Local Anesthetic Techniques

Techniques of Administration

Local anesthesia represents the most commonly used analgesic technique for inguinal herniorrhaphy, and the favorable effect of several techniques has been documented in randomized controlled clinical trials (Table 45.2). Furthermore, the regional anesthetic techniques are often used for intraoperative anesthesia, and inguinal field block (IFB) and wound infiltration (WIF) represent the most attractive anesthetic methods because of their simplicity, safety, and low cost.

The effect of spinal or epidural anesthesia on postherniorrhaphy pain compared with general anesthesia has not been sufficiently evaluated in well-designed clinical studies, but no clinically relevant analgesic effects may be expected beyond the few hours of duration of the block.

The analgesic effects of local anesthetics for IFB, WIF, or wound instillation (WIS) are well documented and probably without differences in efficacy and duration (Table 45.3). No comparative studies of these techniques are

TABLE 45.1. EFFECT OF SURGICAL TECHNIQUES ON EARLY POSTHERNIORRHAPHY PAIN

References	Surgical Technique	Pain/Convalescence
2,8,13,35,39	Tension-free vs. sutured repair	No difference in pain scores in most studies
4,10,15,22, 39	Laparoscopic vs. sutured repair	Less pain and shortened convalescence after laparoscopic surgery
4,10,39	Laparoscopic vs. open, tension-free	Less pain and shortened convalescence after laparoscopic surgery
4	TAPP vs. TEPP	Lower pain scores with TAPP? (too few data)

TAPP, transabdominal preperitoneal prosthetic; TEPP, totally extraperitoneal prosthetic.

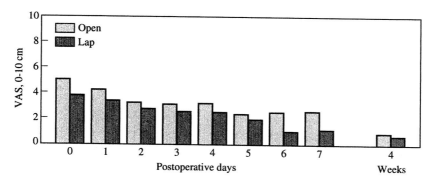

FIGURE 45.2. Average pain course after open (*light bars*) and laparoscopic inguinal herniorrhaphy (*dark bars*). (Data from Callesen T, Kehlet H. Postherniorrhaphy pain. *Anesthesiology* 1997;87:1219–1230; Kawji R, Feichter A, Fuchsjäger N, et al. Postoperative pain and return to activity after five different types of inguinal herniorrhaphy. *Hernia* 1999;3:31; and Liem MSL, van der Graaf Y, van Steensel CJ, et al. Comparison of conventional anterior surgery and laparoscopic surgery for inguinal hernia repair. *N Engl J Med* 1997;336:1541–1547, with permission.)

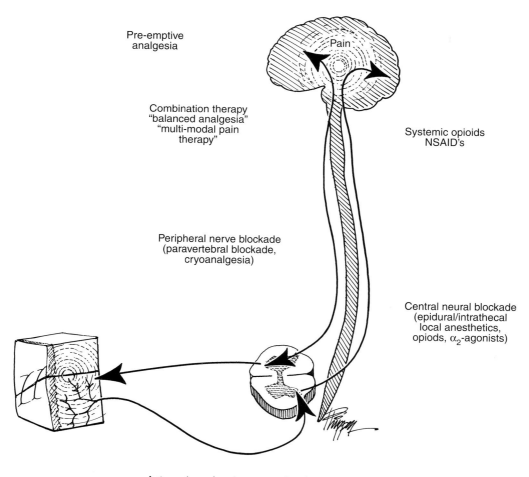

FIGURE 45.3. Measures to provide pain relief after inguinal herniorrhaphy.

TABLE 45.2. EFFECT OF LOCAL ANESTHETIC TECHNIQUES ON POSTHERNIORRHAPHY PAIN (RANDOMIZED STUDIES VS. PLACEBO OR VS. NO TREATMENT)

		Effective on Pain	Duration
Open herniorrhaphy	Spinal anesthesia	—	—
	Epidural anesthesia	—	—
	Inguinal field block	Yes	~6 hr
	Wound infiltration	Yes	~6 hr
	Wound instillation	Yes	~6 hr
	Paravertebral block	—	—
Laparoscopic herniorrhaphy	Preperitoneal instillation	No	—

—, no or insufficient data.
Data from reviews (4,27) and single studies (14,20,33).

available in adults, but no differences in analgesic efficacy or duration have been demonstrated between IFB and WIF in children (Table 45.3). A drawback of the local anesthetic techniques with the presently available local anesthetic preparations is the relatively short duration of effective analgesia (approximately 6 hours). The use of a paravertebral local anesthetic block, which is simple and with few side effects, may be a promising technique, although little data are available from herniorrhaphy. One randomized study has shown a paravertebral block to be more effective compared with IFB with regard to intraoperative quality of analgesia (38), but no data are available on potential differences in duration of analgesia between these techniques. The effect of combined local anesthetic techniques (IFB + WIF or WIS compared with either technique alone) has not been evaluated, but a placebo-controlled study with the combination of IFB and WIF showed an effect for only 6 hours (20), which is comparable to other studies using single site administration (27).

The use of local anesthetic techniques in laparoscopic herniorrhaphy has not been evaluated as regards infiltration in port sites. Preperitoneal local anesthetic instillation in extraperitoneal laparoscopic herniorrhaphy is ineffective (14,33).

Choice of Local Anesthetic

Although a short-acting local anesthetic (lidocaine) is often included for *intraoperative* analgesia because of early onset,

TABLE 45.3. COMPARISON OF DIFFERENT LOCAL ANESTHETIC TECHNIQUES ON POSTHERNIORRHAPHY PAIN RELIEF (RANDOMIZED STUDIES)

Inguinal field block = wound infiltration
Inguinal field block = wound instillation
Inguinal field block < paravertebral block
Wound infiltration > spinal and general anesthesia

<, shorter duration of analgesia; >, longer duration of analgesia.
Data from refs. 1, 4, 11, 31, and 38.

the choice of local anesthetic for *postoperative* analgesia should be a long-acting local anesthetic. So far, only bupivacaine, ropivacaine, and levobupivacaine are available, and the few comparative randomized studies have not demonstrated any differences in efficacy or duration of analgesia (3,18). The choice of local anesthetic therefore does not depend on efficacy, but use of ropivacaine and levobupivacaine may be preferable because of the documented lower toxicity, thereby increasing the safety margin in case larger doses are needed or warranted.

Dose–Response Relationships

Few well-designed studies have evaluated the optimal volume versus concentration relationship. In a comparative study, 30 mL ropivacaine 0.25% and 0.5% were more effective than 0.125% (28). In a large placebo-controlled study comparing 0.5% ropivacaine (40 mL) and 0.25% ropivacaine (40 mL), 0.5% ropivacaine was more effective (20). Therefore, about 30 to 40 mL of 0.25% to 0.5% of the long-acting local anesthetic preparations are recommended for early postoperative analgesia.

Continuous Wound Administration of Local Anesthetic and Ultralong-Acting Preparations

Because of the relatively short effect (approximately 6 hours) of the available local anesthetics, various techniques for continuous local anesthetic wound perfusion have been investigated. In the only placebo-controlled randomized trial, continuous infusion (which has no side effects) reduced pain for the 48 hours of administration compared with saline perfusion (29). Further studies are needed before general recommendations can be made.

In order to increase the duration of action of local anesthetics, various agents have been added, such as dextrane (to delay absorption) or triamcinolone (to reduce tissue inflammation). However, such efforts have not been demonstrated to prolong analgesia or reduce the need for analgesics (4). Slow-release preparations by incorporation of local anesthetics into microspheres, liposomes, and so on, may significantly prolong the duration of analgesia in experimental studies (16). If confirmed in clinical studies, these results may have a major impact for the treatment of early post-herniorrhaphy pain.

Site of Administration

The exact anatomic origin of postherniorrhaphy pain has not been clarified, and therefore the optimal site of local anesthetic administration is not known. There seems to be no difference in analgesic efficacy or duration between IFB and WIF. However, most studies have used subcutaneous local anesthetic infiltration, which may be less effective than infiltration into deeper layers (27). Based upon results from recent studies, where detailed description of the infiltration technique into the various layers has been given (3,20,28), the potential advantageous effect of combined deep and superficial infiltration may not be of clinical significance compared with single-site administration. Future well-designed, comparative studies of different sites of local anesthetic instillation are necessary before final recommendations can be made.

In conclusion, local anesthetic techniques with IFB or WIF are simple, cheap, and safe, provide effective analgesia for up to 6 hours, and should therefore be used routinely. There seems to be no difference in efficacy and duration between the long-acting local anesthetic preparations (bupivacaine, ropivacaine, levobupivacaine), and choice of preparation therefore depends on safety aspects (risk of toxicity). Proper dose–response relationships have not been performed, but 30 to 40 mL of a 0.25% to 0.5% local anesthetic preparation may be effective and sufficient, and should include administration into the deeper muscular layers. The effect of combined techniques (IFB, WIF, etc.) remains to be evaluated compared to either technique alone. The use of continuous WIS of local anesthetics and paravertebral block also needs further evaluation before recommendations for routine use can be made.

Opioids

Opioids represent the classic analgesics in moderate-to-severe postoperative pain, but side effects such as nausea, vomiting, drowsiness, bladder dysfunction, and so on, after *systemic* administration may make them less ideal in outpatient operations such as inguinal herniorrhaphy. The routine use of opioids for inguinal herniorrhaphy therefore cannot be recommended, except for short-acting opioids (alfentanil, remifentanil, etc.) used *intraoperatively* together with general anesthesia. However, opioids should be used as a rescue analgesic, in case of insufficient analgesia by other techniques [local anesthesia, nonsteroidal antiinflammatory drugs (NSAIDs), etc.].

The demonstration in experimental studies of a postinjury increase in peripheral opioid receptors has led to the concept of *peripheral* opioid analgesia. Most clinical experience comes from arthroscopic knee procedures where the analgesic effect is debatable, and peripheral (incisional) application of opioid in other operations has not proven to be clinically effective (30). In accordance with these findings, the effect of incisional morphine or fentanyl after inguinal herniorrhaphy is debatable (32,37). Incisional opioid cannot be recommended for analgesia after inguinal herniorrhaphy before further conclusive data are available.

Nonsteroidal Antiinflammatory Agents

It is well documented that NSAIDs have clinical significant analgesic effects in various surgical procedures, including inguinal herniorrhaphy. The analgesic effect is mediated at the peripheral wound site, as well as at the spinal cord level. There seem to be no clinically relevant differences between the NSAIDs regarding analgesia and potential early side effects (wound bleeding, gastrointestinal side effects, renal dysfunction). Since herniorrhaphy patients are able to take oral medications, oral NSAIDs are recommended routinely, starting immediately postoperatively (when the local anesthetic block is still effective) and continuing for 2 to 5 days.

NSAIDs are more potent analgesics than acetaminophen or acetaminophen–codeine preparations. Combined use of NSAIDs and acetaminophen may potentially increase analgesia (24), but more data on potential side effects are needed before recommendations for routine use can be made.

Since arachidonic cascade metabolites participate in the inflammatory response at the wound site, peripheral (wound) administration of NSAIDs has been compared with intramuscular or intravenous administration in several studies (4,23). Although local incisional administration of NSAIDs has been shown to improve analgesic efficacy, the advantages have been small compared to the potential risk of wound complications (impaired wound healing and bleeding). Therefore, incisional administration of NSAIDs cannot be recommended for inguinal herniorrhaphy until further safety and efficacy data are available.

In summary, oral administration of NSAIDs is recommended routinely for analgesia after inguinal herniorrhaphy. No interdrug differences in analgesic efficacy or side effects have been demonstrated.

Other Analgesics

Since acute postoperative pain is mediated by several analgesic substances (bradykinin, serotonin, arachidonic cascade metabolites, nerve growth factor, etc.) that participate in the inflammatory response in the wound, several possibilities exist for improvement of acute pain control by inhibition of the release and/or effect of these mediators. In addition, the postinjury central nervous system activation may amplify the intensity and duration of acute pain, thereby providing several potential targets for drugs to improve postoperative pain control (Fig. 45.3). However, at present, few drug classes have been investigated to improve pain control after surgery.

Glucocorticoids applied peripherally or systemically have been demonstrated to improve pain relief in dental and orthopedic procedures, but addition of glucocorticoid to a local anesthetic block did not reduce pain after hernia surgery (4). The use of peripheral glucocorticoid administration in hernia surgery therefore cannot be recommended.

The anesthetic agent ketamine may have both central and peripheral analgesic effects. To date, the effect of pre- or intraoperative use of ketamine has not been evaluated in inguinal herniorrhaphy, but it may prolong analgesia by several hours in other procedures (34). The effect of peripheral (wound site) administration of ketamine is debatable, but one study has shown a prolongation of analgesia when ketamine is added to local anesthetic block (36). Further studies are needed before recommendations for use of ketamine in inguinal herniorrhaphy can be made.

The α2-agonist clonidine has been shown to have central and peripheral analgesic effects, but in the only inguinal herniorrhaphy study, addition of clonidine did not increase duration of analgesia after WIF with bupivacaine (17). The effect of other potential new analgesics (bradykinin and neurokinin antagonists, leukotriene synthetase inhibitors, etc.) or central-acting drugs has not been sufficiently evaluated, and they therefore cannot be recommended for routine clinical use.

Cryoanalgesia

Application of extreme coldness to sensory nerves and nerve endings provides analgesia (cryoanalgesia). Cryoanalgesia has been used for decades, topically for cutaneous procedures and for intercostal nerve blockade after thoracotomy. Since the iliohypogastric and ilioinguinal nerves are normally identified during hernia surgery, cryoanalgesia is a logical approach for supplementary analgesia. To date, three controlled studies are available (4,5), but only one study was of sufficient size and with cryoanalgesia of both nerves, and demonstrated no significant effects on pain patterns (less than 30 days) during rest or function (5). Cryoanalgesia cannot be recommended in connection with inguinal herniorrhaphy.

Balanced Analgesia

The concept of multimodal or balanced analgesia is based on improvement of analgesia through additive or synergistic effects of different analgesics, with a concomitant reduction of side effects due to the resulting lower doses of indi-

vidual drugs and differences in side effect profiles (24). Although limited data exist from inguinal herniorrhaphy, results from other postoperative studies may be applicable for herniorrhaphy. Such results have demonstrated improved analgesia with combined NSAID–opioid, acetaminophen–codeine, and probably NSAID–acetaminophen combinations. Other rational approaches, although less well documented, are local anesthetic infiltration plus NSAID or acetaminophen. Multimodal (balanced) analgesic treatment should be used whenever possible (24).

Preemptive Analgesia

Surgical injury induces sensitization of peripheral nociceptors as well as neuroplastic changes in the central nervous system, which may amplify the intensity and duration of postoperative pain. Based upon experimental studies, it was therefore hypothesized that preemptive analgesia (pain treatment before the nociceptive stimulus) could reduce the intensity and duration of postoperative pain. Although still an important working hypothesis, the documentation of its clinical implications from several randomized clinical studies in different surgical procedures and with different types of preemptive analgesic techniques has been disappointing (25). The discrepancy between the experimental and clinical studies is probably explained by the more pronounced and prolonged afferent neural input following surgery, insufficient blockade/inhibition of afferent stimuli and central neuroplastic changes with the applied analgesic techniques, and a too short duration of "preemptive" treatment in the clinical studies (25). So far, randomized controlled trials comparing pre- versus postoperative local anesthetic infiltration and NSAIDs have not demonstrated improved analgesic efficacy or duration after inguinal herniorrhaphy (4). The timing of local anesthetic treatment may therefore merely depend on the advantageous use of *intraoperative* anesthesia than on assumed improved analgesia by "preemptive" analgesia per se.

CONCLUSIONS AND FUTURE DEVELOPMENTS

Since postherniorrhaphy pain may cause significant discomfort and contribute to prolonged convalescence, increased efforts should be made for effective treatment. Routine use of local anesthetic techniques (IFB, WIF) is recommended in combination with oral NSAID therapy. Use of opioids should be restricted for rescue analgesia when other techniques provide insufficient pain relief.

An increased attention to the pathogenesis of early postherniorrhaphy pain (obligatory inflammatory response, activation of nociceptors and central neuroplastic changes, risk of intraoperative nerve injury) is needed since prospective studies have shown the intensity of early postherniorrhaphy pain to predict the risk for transition to a chronic postherniorrhaphy pain state (9). However, the effect of vigorous early postherniorrhaphy pain treatment in decreasing the risk of chronic postherniorrhaphy pain remains to be confirmed.

Although available techniques have been proven to be efficient, there is a demand for improvement of postherniorrhaphy analgesic treatment in order to reduce the discomfort and shorten convalescence, as pain is the most important factor to prolong postherniorrhaphy convalescence (7). Several new analgesics are undergoing clinical evaluation, but the development of very long-acting local anesthetics (2 to 4 days) will probably represent the most important breakthrough in improving postherniorrhaphy pain relief since such preparations are simple to administer and probably without side effects. The most promising ultralong-acting local anesthetic preparations are based upon slow-release preparations with conventional local anesthetics (bupivacaine) incorporated into liposomes or polyglycolic lactic microspheres (16).

In summary, increased attention to improving early postherniorrhaphy pain relief is important among surgeons since inadequate pain relief may prolong convalescence and potentially increase the risk of developing a chronic pain state.

REFERENCES

1. Anatol TI, Pitt-Miller P, Holder Y. Trial of three methods of intraoperative bupivacaine analgesia for pain after paediatric groin surgery. *Can J Anaesth* 1997;44:1053–1059.
2. Barth RJ, Burchard KW, Tosteson A, et al. Short-term outcome after mesh or Shouldice herniorrhaphy: a randomized prospective study. *Surgery* 1998;123:121–126.
3. Bay-Nielsen M, Klarskov B, Bech K, et al. Levobupivacaine vs bupivacaine as infiltration anaesthesia in inguinal herniorrhaphy. *Br J Anaesth* 1999;82:280–282.
4. Callesen T, Kehlet H. Postherniorrhaphy pain. *Anesthesiology* 1997;87:1219–1230.
5. Callesen T, Bech K, Thorup J, et al. Cryoanalgesia: effects on postherniorrhaphy pain. *Anesth Analg* 1998;87:896–899.
6. Callesen T, Bech K, Nielsen R, et al. Pain after groin hernia repair. *Br J Surg* 1998;85:1412–1414.
7. Callesen T, Klarskov B, Bech K, et al. Short convalescence after inguinal herniorrhaphy with standardised recommendations: duration and reasons for delayed return to work. *Eur J Surg* 1999;165:236–241.
8. Callesen T, Beck K, Andersen J, et al. Pain after primary inguinal herniorrhaphy: influence of surgical technique. *J Am Coll Surg* 1999;188:355–359.
9. Callesen T, Beck K, Kehlet H. A prospective study of chronic pain after inguinal hernia repair. *Br J Surg* 1999;86:1528–1531.
10. Chung RS, Rowland DY. Meta-analyses of randomized controlled trials of laparoscopic vs conventional inguinal hernia repairs. *Surg Endosc* 1999;13:689–694.
11. Casey WF, Rice LJ, Hannallah RS, et al. A comparison between bupivacaine instillation versus ilioinguinal/iliohypogastric nerve block for postoperative analgesia following inguinal herniorrhaphy in children. *Anesthesiology* 1990;72:637–639.
12. Cunningham J, Temple WJ, Mitchel P, et al. Cooperative hernia study; pain in the postrepair patient. *Ann Surg* 1996;224:598–602.
13. Danielsson P, Isacson S, Hansen MV. Randomised study of Lichtenstein compared with Shouldice inguinal hernia repair by surgeons in training. *Eur J Surg* 1999;165:49–53.
14. Deans GT, Wilson MS, Brough WA. Controlled trial of preperitoneal local anaesthetic for reducing pain following laparoscopic hernia repair. *Br J Surg* 1998;85:1013–1014.
15. Dirksen CD, Beets GL, Go PMNYH, et al. Bassini-repair compared with laparoscopic repair for primary inguinal hernia: a randomized controlled trial. *Eur J Surg* 1998;164:439–447.
16. Dräger C, Benziger D, Gao F, et al. Prolonged intercostal nerve blockade in sheep using controlled-release of bupivacaine and dexamethasone from polymer microspheres. *Anesthesiology* 1998;89:969–979.
17. Elliott S, Eckersall S, Fligelstone L, et al. Does the addition of clonidine affect duration of analgesia of bupivacaine wound infiltration in inguinal hernia surgery? *Br J Anaesth* 1997;79:446–449.
18. Erichsen CJ, Vibits H, Dahl JB, Kehlet H. Wound infiltration with ropivacaine and bupivacaine for pain after inguinal herniotomy. *Acta Anaesthesiol Scand* 1995;39:67–70.
19. Gillion JF, Fagniez PL. Chronic pain and cutaneous sensory changes after inguinal hernia repair: comparison between open and laparoscopic techniques. *Hernia* 1999;3:75–80.
20. Johansson B, Hallenbäck B, Stubberöd A, et al. Preoperative local infiltration with ropivacaine for postoperative pain relief after inguinal hernia repair. A randomised controlled trial. *Eur J Surg* 1997;163:371–378.
21. Juul P, Christensen K. Randomized clinical trial of laparoscopic vs. open inguinal hernia repair. *Br J Surg* 1999;86:316–319.
22. Kawji R, Feichter A, Fuchsjäger N, et al. Postoperative pain and return to activity after five different types of inguinal herniorrhaphy. *Hernia* 1999;3:31–35.
23. Kehlet H, Pedersen JL. Peripheral treatment of acute pain. In: Stanley TH, Ashburn MA, Fine PG, eds. *Anesthesiology and pain management.* Amsterdam: Klüwer Academic Publishers, 1998:103–108.
24. Kehlet H, Werner M, Perkins F. Balanced analgesia—what is it and what are its advantages in postoperative pain? *Drugs* 1999;58:793–797.
25. Kissin I. Preemptive analgesia. Why its effect is not always obvious. *Anesthesiology* 1996;84:1015–1019.
26. Liem MSL, van der Graaf Y, van Steensel CJ, et al. Comparison of conventional anterior surgery and laparoscopic surgery for inguinal hernia repair. *N Engl J Med* 1997;336:1541–1547.
27. Mainiche S, Mikkelsen S, Wetterslev J, et al. A qualitative systematic review of incisional local anaesthesia for postoperative pain relief after abdominal operations. *Br J Anaesth* 1998;81:377–383.
28. Mulroy MF, Burgess FW, Emanuelsson B-M. Ropivacaine 0.25% and 0.5%, but not 0.125%, provide effective wound infiltration analgesia after outpatient hernia repair, but with sustained plasma drug levels. *Reg Anesth Pain Med* 1999;24:136–141.
29. Oakley MJ, Smith JS, Anderson JR, et al. Randomized placebo-controlled trial of local anaesthetic infusion in day-case inguinal hernia repair. *Br J Surg* 1998;85:797–799.
30. Picard PR, Tramér MR, MxQuay HJ, et al. Analgesic efficacy of peripheral opioids (all except infra-articular): a qualitative systematic review of randomised controlled trials. *Pain* 1997;72:309–318.
31. Reid MF, Harris R, Phillips PD, et al. Day-case herniotomy in children. A comparison of ilio-inguinal nerve block and wound infiltration for postoperative analgesia. *Anaesthesia* 1987;42:658–661.
32. Rosenstock C, Rasmussen H, Andersen G, et al. Incisional morphine has no analgesic effect on postoperative pain. Following inguinal herniotomy. *Reg Anesth Pain Med* 1998;23:57–63.

33. Saff GN, Marks RA, Kuroda M, et al. Analgesic effect of bupivacaine on extraperitoneal laparoscopic hernia repair. *Anesth Analg* 1998;87:377–381.

34. Schmid RL, Sandler A, Katz J. Use and efficacy of low-dose ketamine in the management of acute post-operative pain: a review of current techniques and outcomes. *Pain* 1999;82:111–125.

35. Schmitz R, Treckman J, Shah S, et al. Die "Tension-free-Technik" bei offener Leistenhernienreparation. Eine prospektive, randomisierte Studie zur postoperativen Schmerzperception ("Tension-free-Rekonstruktion" vs. Shouldice-Technik). *Chirurg* 1997; 68:259–263.

36. Tverskoy M, Oren M, Vaskovich M, et al. Ketamine enhances local anaesthetic and analgesic effects of bupivacaine by peripheral mechanism: a study in postoperative patients. *Neurosci Lett* 1996;215:5–8.

37. Tverskoy M, Braslavsky A, Mazor A, et al. The peripheral effect of fentanyl on postoperative pain. *Anesth Analg* 1998;87:1121–1124.

38. Wassef MR, Randazzo T, Ward W. The paravertebral nerve root block for inguinal herniorrhaphy—a comparison with the field block approach. *Reg Anesth Pain Med* 1998;23:451–456.

39. Zieren J, Zieren HU, Jacobi CA, et al. Prospective randomized study comparing laparoscopic and open tension-free inguinal hernia repair with Shouldice's operation. *Am J Surg* 1998;175: 330–333.

Nyhus and Condon's Hernia, Fifth Edition, edited by Robert J. Fitzgibbons, Jr. and A. Gerson Greenburg. Lippincott Williams & Wilkins, Philadelphia © 2002.

46

SCIATIC, OBTURATOR, AND PERINEAL HERNIAS: A VIEW FROM THE GYNECOLOGIST

JAMES E. CARTER

Surgeons need to be familiar with hernias of the deep pelvic structures, which can cause debilitating symptoms that are often ignored by physicians because they are not considered. As a byproduct of laparoscopic cholecystectomy, general surgeons have now developed skills in laparoscopy, and it behooves them to have a thorough knowledge of pelvic anatomy with its nooks and crannies, where pelvic and perineal hernias can hide. Otherwise, inadequate diagnostic laparoscopies will be the rule, with patients having to suffer the consequences. In this chapter, several obscure pelvic hernias that are rare and difficult to diagnose, and have symptoms that are often written off as "female trouble" are discussed.

SCIATIC HERNIA

A sciatic hernia is a protrusion of a peritoneal sac and its contents through the greater or lesser sciatic foramen. It has also been called a "sacral sciatic," "gluteal," or "ischiatic" hernia. It has been described as the rarest of all hernias (5). A search of the literature in MEDLINE for the period 1966 to 1996 generated a total of 57 cases of sciatic hernia (9). In one study, sciatic hernia was diagnosed in 20 out of 1,100 patients with chronic pelvic pain who underwent laparoscopy (9). This gives an incidence of 1.8% in women with chronic pelvic pain requiring laparoscopic intervention, which makes it seem likely that sciatic hernia has been underdiagnosed as a source of chronic pelvic pain. In 14 of the cases, the hernia was right sided, in five it was left sided, and in one it was bilateral. The mean age at diagnosis was 34.3 years (range 23 to 58), mean gravidity 1.0 (range 0 to 3), mean parity 1.0 (range 0 to 2), and mean patient weight 60 kg (range 49 to 75). All sciatic hernias contained the ipsilateral ovary alone or with its fallopian tube. Six patients also had a diagnosis of

other causes of pelvic pain: endometriosis (one patient), adhesions (two patients), endometriosis and adhesions (one patient), indirect inguinal hernia (one patient), and indirect inguinal and umbilical hernia (one patient). A total of 17 previous surgeries (mainly laparoscopies) had been performed in 14 of the 20 patients. All 20 patients reported immediate pain relief after treatment for their sciatic hernia at their initial 3-month follow-up evaluation; 14 described complete pain relief and six noted an improvement over preoperative symptoms at long-term evaluation [13-month mean follow-up (range 3 to 36 months)].

Sciatic hernias are either congenital or acquired. Approximately 20% of sciatic hernias are present in infancy and are secondary to maldevelopment of the piriformis muscle or pelvic bones (18). More commonly, adults present with an acquired weakness of the piriformis muscle. This can result from chronic increase in intraabdominal pressure. Pregnancy, severe constipation, surgery, and trauma with weakness of the pelvic muscles and tissues have been implicated (2). Atrophy of the piriformis muscle may be a predisposing factor for sciatic foramen hernias and may occur in women who have neuromuscular or hip disease (15). Tumors causing erosion or atrophy of the piriformis are also causative (5). These hernias are slightly more common in women, due to their wider pelvis and sciatic foramen.

Pertinent Anatomy

A sciatic hernia is actually a protrusion from the pelvis of a peritoneal sac through one of three openings: (a) the greater sciatic foramen, above the piriformis muscle; (b) the greater sciatic foramen, below the piriformis muscle; or (c) the lesser sciatic foramen (Fig. 46.1) (12). The piriformis muscle divides the greater sciatic foramen into a supra- and infrapiriformis area normally represented as slits between the pelvic muscle groups. The lesser sciatic foramen is bounded superiorly by the sacrospinous and inferiorly by the sacrotuberous ligaments. The suprapiriformis hernia is by far the most com-

J. E. Carter: Department of Obstetrics and Gynecology, University of California–Irvine, College of Medicine, Orange, California; Women's Health Center of South Orange County, Inc., Mission Viejo, California.

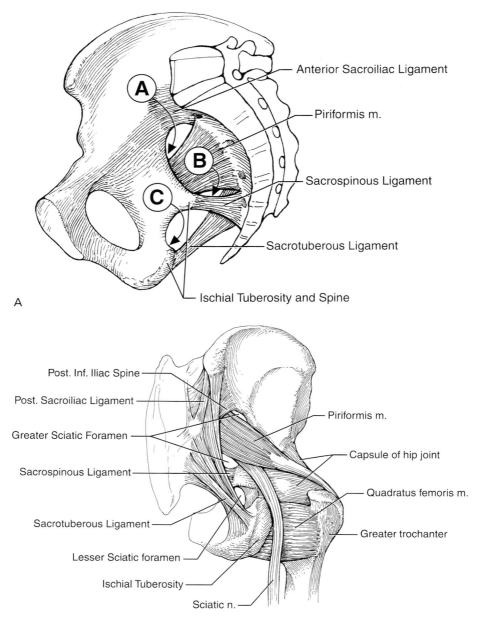

FIGURE 46.1. Sites of potential hernias through the sciatic foramina. **A:** Supra piriformis sciatic hernia. **B:** Infrapiriformis sciatic hernia. **C:** Subspinous sciatic hernia through the lesser sciatic foramen. (From Carter JE. Hernias. In: Howard FM, Perry CP, Carter JE, et al., eds. *Pelvic pain: diagnosis and management.* Philadelphia: Lippincott Williams & Wilkins, 2000:385–413, with permission.)

mon type. The hernia sac exits the pelvis above the piriformis along the course of the superior gluteal artery and nerve. The infrapiriformis hernia sac tracks a course with the inferior gluteal vessels, internal pudendal vessels, and sciatic nerve. It exits caudal to the piriformis but cephalad to the sacrospinous ligament. The subspinous hernia sac leaves the pelvis through the lesser sciatic foramen medial to the internal pudendal vessels and nerve and the sciatic nerve. It is bounded superiorly by the sacrospinous and posteriorly by

the sacrotuberous ligaments. Any hernia that exits below the sacrotuberous ligaments is considered a perineal hernia (5).

Clinical Presentation

Cases have been reported in children younger than 1 year of age, but most were found in adults between the ages of 20 and 60 years (1). Sciatic hernias present with pain originating in the pelvis, sometimes radiating to the buttocks and posterior thigh. Intermittent pain radiating to the buttocks and/or posterior thigh should raise suspicion. A reducible mass felt deep to the gluteus maximus is also one of the more important signs.

Intestinal or ureteral obstruction with or without strangulation is sometimes responsible for the first symptoms, and the diagnosis usually is established during exploratory laparotomy. Because of the large gluteal muscle overlying the sciatic foramen and the piriformis muscle, sciatic hernias are rarely evident on physical examination. Patients may report ipsilateral posterior thigh or buttocks pain, or both (9).

Thus, symptoms may range from none to those of acute strangulation. The small openings predispose the hernia to incarceration and strangulation. As it enlarges, it may present as a mass just below the inferior border of the gluteus maximus muscle (5). Compression of the sciatic nerve may occur, causing pain to radiate down the posterior thigh that is aggravated by dorsiflexion. If a palpable reducible mass is present, and symptoms are aggravated by coughing and straining, a sciatic hernia should be suspected (5). Signs of intestinal obstruction plus pain in the gluteal region suggest a sciatic hernia. The patient may complain of pain in the buttocks that radiates down the sciatic nerve or a mass, or both. The pain may be confused with intermittent claudication (1). Because of the gluteal muscle overlying the sciatic foramen and the piriformis muscle, sciatic hernias are rarely evident on physical examination (9). Sciatic hernias pass downward and may present under the lower border of the gluteus maximus muscle in the posteromedial aspect of the thigh (10). Herniations of the ureter into the sciatic foramen give rise to a pathognomonic urographic appearance of a redundant, horizontally oriented ureter within a hernia sac, which has been called a "curlicue ureter" (2). In the frontal projection on excretory urography, the knuckle of herniated ureter passes lateral to the medial wall of the bony pelvis (Fig. 46.2) (15).

Computed tomography (CT) shows the contrast-filled ureter posterior, lateral, and craniad to the ischial spine, allowing the confident diagnosis of a ureteral hernia. In adults, ureteral sciatic hernias tend to occur in women (15). It is important to differentiate the sciatic type of ureteral hernia from the inguinal herniation, in which the ureter has a vertical curlicue. Although oblique x-ray studies, CT, herniography, enterography, intravenous pyelography, and cystography have been helpful in the diagnosis of sciatic hernias, they have never been proven to be definitive. Sciatic hernias have been diagnosed most commonly and treated definitely during surgery. Laparoscopy aids in the diagnosis of hernias by providing excellent visualization of the pelvis. Intraabdominal pressure, created by insufflation, may be helpful in the detection of sciatic hernia through stretching the peritoneum to its limit of support (e.g., bone or muscle). The sciatic hernia may also be filled with the ipsilateral ovary and/or fallopian tube, leaving little room for distention of the peritoneum by intraabdominal carbon dioxide (9).

Lipoma, gluteal aneurysm, or abscess must be considered in the differential diagnosis (10). In one series, 30% of patients with sciatic hernia also had another pathologic condition, including adhesions, endometriosis, indirect inguinal hernias, and umbilical hernias (9).

Treatment

The hernia is usually approached through a lower midline abdominal incision. In women, the bowel is seen entering the hernia behind the broad ligament. Even when an intestinal obstruction is present, the bowel usually can be

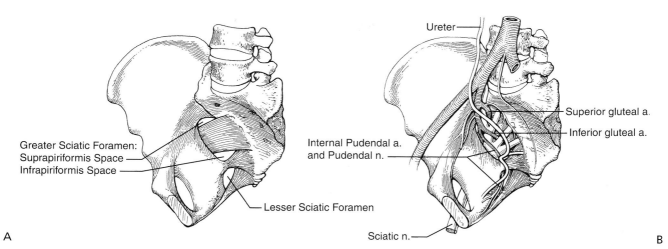

A

B

FIGURE 46.2. A: Oblique anteromedial view of the pelvis shows relation to the ischial, sacrospinous ligaments. Piriformis muscle normally fills much of the greater sciatic notch. **B:** Same view with major arteries and nerves shows course of the herniated right ureter into infrapiriformis space of the greater sciatic notch. (From Carter JE. Hernias. In: Howard FM, Perry CP, Carter JE, et al., eds. *Pelvic pain: diagnosis and management.* Philadelphia: Lippincott Williams & Wilkins, 2000:385–413, with permission.)

reduced with light traction. Where needed, the opening can be dilated with a finger, or else the piriformis muscle may be partially incised, taking great care to avoid the many nerves and vessels in the region. The sac then is everted and excised and the opening repaired by suture of the edges with monofilament polyamide or polypropylene. When this repair is not possible, the opening can be plugged with a rolled-up strip of polypropylene mesh held in place with a few stitches. Larger defects should be covered with a sheet of polypropylene mesh. A posterior or transgluteal method may be used for uncomplicated and reducible sciatic hernias diagnosed preoperatively. The gluteus maximus muscle is approached through a gluteal incision and is detached at its origin to expose the hernia. The sac is dissected free and opened. The contents are reduced and the sac is dealt with. The defect is closed using local tissues or polypropylene mesh (1).

When a sciatic hernia is approached laparoscopically, its contents are reduced and the perineal sac is transected transversely with endoscopic scissors. Using blunt dissection, the obturator internus and coccygeus muscles are identified. A 6.0 × 12.5-cm piece of mesh material is folded and placed into the space created by the atrophic piriformis muscle. A second piece of mesh is trimmed to the size of the peritoneal defect and placed over the folded mesh. This overlying mesh is secured to the obturator internus fascia laterally and the coccygeus medially with a hernia stapler. The peritoneum overlying the mesh is closed using a hernia

stapler (9). Fourteen of 20 patients reported complete pain relief and six noted improvement over preoperative symptoms with the median length of follow-up of 13 months (range 3 to 36) (9).

OBTURATOR HERNIA

An obturator hernia is an abnormal protrusion of preperitoneal fat or an intestinal loop through the obturator foramen (13). Its relation to groin hernias is seen in Fig. 46.3. On occasion, a hernia may develop through the obturator foramen alongside the obturator vessels and nerves (10). Obturator hernias are the most common of the three types of pelvic hernias (sciatic, obturator, and perineal). Over 600 cases have been reported in the literature, representing 0.073% of all hernias (4).

Obturator hernias are most commonly (more than 80%) found in thin, elderly women in the seventh or eighth decade of life. They are found on the right side in 60% of cases. The male-to-female ratio is 1:6. Bilateral obturator hernias occur in about 6% of cases, and other associated groin hernias are not uncommon (1). The age of patients in reported cases varies from 12 to 93 years, but most cases occur in patients during their seventh and eighth decades (1). Since many cases of obturator hernia are probably not reported, or possibly not diagnosed (as with sciatic hernias), it is difficult to estimate the incidence of obturator hernias

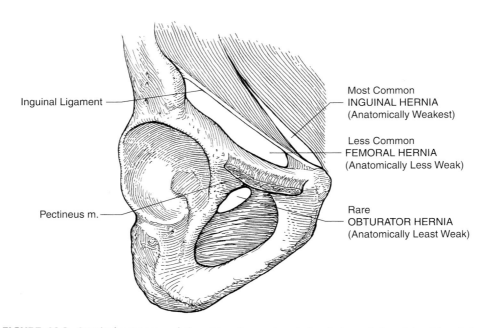

FIGURE 46.3. Surgical anatomy of the obturator region. Lateral view of the right side of the pelvis showing the sites of inguinal, femoral, and obturator hernias. (From Carter JE. Hernias. In: Howard FM, Perry CP, Carter JE, et al., eds. *Pelvic pain: diagnosis and management*. Philadelphia: Lippincott Williams & Wilkins, 2000:385–413, with permission.)

in women with chronic pelvic pain. However, as it has now been demonstrated that almost 2% of women with chronic pelvic pain in one series had sciatic hernias (9), and since obturator hernia is more common than sciatic hernias (1), it is reasonable to assume that obturator hernia may be significantly underdiagnosed in women with chronic pelvic pain, and by analogy may occur in more than 2% of patients who require surgery for chronic pelvic pain.

In one reported series, obturator hernia represented 1% (16 of 1,554) of all hernia repairs performed and 1.6% (16 of 1,000) of mechanical and intestinal obstruction encountered during the same period (8). Thus, this condition, which was first described in 1724 by Arnaud De Ronsil of France, is being diagnosed almost entirely after incarceration occurs.

Aging, loss of body weight, and chronic lung disease are associated with obturator hernia. Overall, the hernia is found more frequently on the right side than on the left. In women, it appears more often on the right side. The formation of an obturator hernia begins with a "pilot tag" of retroperitoneal fat in the first stage, followed by the appearance of a peritoneal dimple in the second stage, into which a knuckle of viscus may be partially incarcerated (Richter's hernia) in the third stage. Pilot tags of preperitoneal fat have been found in the obturator foramen in up to 64% of female cadaver dissections (11). It is not known how many of these women suffered from chronic pelvic pain. The frequency of pilot tags in cadavers and the rarity of actual obturator hernias in patients suggest that most obturator hernias do not progress beyond the first and second stages of development (1).

Parity of greater than two births is implicated as causative secondary to relaxation of pelvic tissues. The female preponderance is also attributed to the wider pelvis and more oblique obturator canals. Chronic constipation is a risk factor in the elderly.

Pertinent Anatomy

The opening of the obturator canal, located at the anterosuperior border of the foramen, is approximately 1 cm in diameter. Other than the obturator vessels and nerve, it is filled with primarily preperitoneal fat. In emaciated elderly people, loss of these fatty tissues leads to a larger space around the vessels and nerve, facilitating the formation of a hernia (6).

The obturator region is bounded superiorly by the superior horizontal ramus of the pubic bone; laterally by the hip joint and the shaft of the femur; medially by the pubic arch, the perineum, and the gracilis muscle; and inferiorly by the insertion of the adductor magnus on the adductor tubercle of the femur (13).

The obturator region is the largest bony foramen of the body. It is formed in the rami of the ischium and the pubis. It lies inferior to the acetabulum on the anterolateral wall of

the pelvis. Except for a small area, the obturator canal, the foramen is closed by the obturator membrane. Fibers of the membrane are continuous with the periosteum of the surrounding bones and with the tendons of the internal and external obturator muscles. Embryologically, the foramen and its membrane represent an area of potential bone formation that never proceeds to completion. In this sense, the obturator foramen is a lacuna and the obturator canal is the true foramen (13).

The obturator canal is a tunnel 2 to 3 cm long, beginning in the pelvis at the defect in the obturator membrane. It passes obliquely downward to end outside the pelvis in the obturator region of the thigh. The canal is bounded above and laterally by the obturator groove of the pubis, and inferiorly by the free edge of the obturator membrane and the internal and external obturator muscles. Through this canal pass the obturator artery, vein, and nerve.

The obturator nerve is usually superior to the artery and vein. The nerve separates into anterior and posterior divisions as it leaves the canal. The hernial sac may follow either division of the nerve. The obturator artery divides to form an arterial ring around the foramen (13).

The obturator hernia thus consists of a peritoneal sac and may contain small or large intestine, appendix, omentum, bladder, ovary, fallopian tube, or uterus. The sac may pass completely through the foramen and come to rest upon the obturator externus, covered by the pectineus muscle. In some instances, it may pass between the fasciculi of the obturator externus muscle or may insinuate itself between the layers of the obturator membrane (Fig. 46.4) (10).

Clinical Presentation

Needless to say, in view of the depth at which it lies, the diagnosis of an obturator hernia is extremely difficult. Pain, characterized by its distribution along the obturator nerve and known as the Howship–Romberg sign, is pathognomonic of an obturator hernia, but is by no means invariably present (10). Fifty percent of patients will complain of this characteristic pain down the inner surface of the thigh, in the knee joint, and often in the hip joint as well. This is referred pain from the cutaneous branch of the anterior division of the obturator nerve and is due to compression of the nerve in the narrow and unyielding canal. In the elderly, this pain is often misinterpreted as arthritic in origin. The nerve also contains motor fibers, and compression may lead to weakness and wasting of the adductors, and loss of the adductor reflex in the thigh. The Howship–Romberg sign is present in almost 50% of patients with obturator hernia. It is one of the four cardinal features of obturator hernia (13).

Intestinal obstruction is the most common sign and occurs in 88% of patients. It is usually in the form of acute obstruction with strangulation (13).

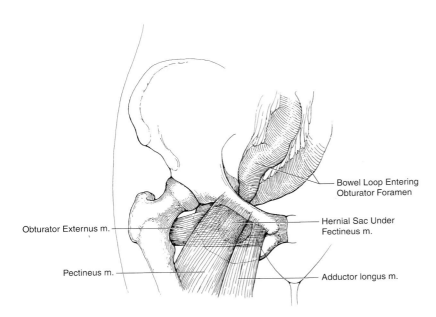

Obturator Externus m.

Pectineus m.

Bowel Loop Entering
Obturator Foramen

Hernial Sac Under
Fectineus m.

Adductor longus m.

FIGURE 46.4. Anatomic relations of obturator hernia. (From Carter JE. Hernias. In: Howard FM, Perry CP, Carter JE, et al., eds. *Pelvic pain: diagnosis and management.* Philadelphia: Lippincott Williams & Wilkins, 2000:385–413, with permission.)

The third most common point, elicited in about 30% of patients, is a history of repeated attacks of intestinal obstruction that passed spontaneously and are probably the result of intermittent compression of the small bowel in the hernia, followed by remissions (13).

The fourth cardinal manifestation of obturator hernia is a palpable mass high in the medial aspect of the thigh at the origins of the adductor muscles. It is present in only 20% of cases. The mass is best felt with the thigh flexed, adducted, and rotated outward. Patients rarely complain of a lump in the groin because large obturator hernias are unusual and many of the patients are too elderly to notice it. Also, since obturator hernia is not always thought of in cases of intestinal obstruction, examination for this palpable lump frequently does not occur. Ecchymosis in the medial part of the groin below the inguinal ligament may occur due to seeping of blood-stained effusions from an infarcted hernia and bowel. A tender mass may be palpable in the obturator area felt laterally on vaginal examination (Fig. 46.5) (1,13). Patients should be diagnosed in the dorsal position with the thigh flexed, adducted, and rotated outward so as to relax the pectineus, adductor longus, and obturator internus muscles. In this position, a slight bulge may or may not be noticeable as a tender, tense mass in the upper obturator region, the upper, inner part of the femoral (Scarpa's) triangle.

Delay in treatment is still a common feature of obturator hernias; the lack of external signs such as inguinal mass or characteristic signs that may help in early detection of obturator hernia may contribute to this delay (6). The common symptom of intestinal obstruction varies in severity. One third of the reported patients had had previous attacks of obstruction symptoms. In many cases, the initial symptoms are mild nausea, vomiting, and anorexia. At this stage,

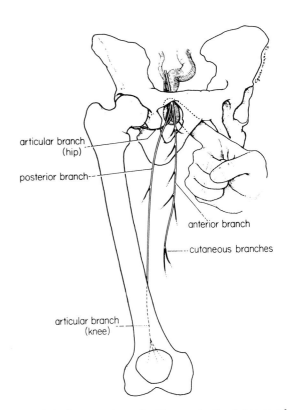

articular branch
(hip)

posterior branch

anterior branch

cutaneous branches

articular branch
(knee)

FIGURE 46.5. Compression of either or both divisions of the obturator nerve by the hernia may produce pain (Howship–Romberg sign). Palpation by vagina or rectum may confirm the presence of a hernia. (From Carter JE. Hernias. In: Howard FM, Perry CP, Carter JE, et al., eds. *Pelvic pain: diagnosis and management.* Philadelphia: Lippincott Williams & Wilkins, 2000:385–413, with permission.)

the obstruction is incomplete Richter's type, and both clinically and via imaging, diagnosis is difficult. CT correctly diagnosed eight of nine cases of surgically confirmed obturator hernia (6). In the one case where CT did not correctly diagnose obturator hernia, the scan focused on the upper abdomen and did not evaluate the pelvic area. The Howship–Romberg sign was present in six of the eight correctly diagnosed cases. CT was 100% accurate in diagnosis as long as the pelvic view was taken. The low-density mass between the obturator and pectineus muscles—containing air density in some cases and apparently different from the opposite (nonincarcerated) side—and dilated bowel in the abdomen are the common CT findings of the obturator hernia (6). Ultrasonogram has been successful in the diagnosis of some cases but has resulted in questionable diagnosis in others (6). Definite and early diagnosis is possible with awareness of the clinical courses of this hernia and by performing CT on suspected cases (6). A small-bowel series may occasionally demonstrate a knuckle of intestine in the obturator canal. Herniography has been shown to identify obturator hernias that may or may not be symptomatic (5).

Preoperative diagnosis of obturator hernia is uncommon, occurring in as few as 10% of cases (3). The differential diagnosis must take into consideration inguinal adenitis; psoas abscess; obturator neuritis; diseases of the hip joint; internal, perineal, and femoral hernias; and other causes of intestinal obstruction (6).

Treatment

For the operation of obturator hernias, the abdominal, femoral, and inguinal routes have been described. The first of these seems to be preferred because of the frequent necessity for an intestinal resection by the time the hernia has been diagnosed (10).

The midline extraperitoneal approach is the best method for dealing with an obturator hernia when the diagnosis has been made preoperatively. It allows good exposure of the internal opening of the obturator canal without interfering with the abdominal contents. An incision is made from the umbilicus to the pubis in the midline, without breaching the peritoneum, which is peeled off the bladder in the midline, and also laterally to expose the superior pubic ramus and the obturator internus muscle. The sac will be seen as a projection of peritoneum passing into the obturator canal. It is incised at its base. The contents are reduced into the peritoneal cavity, the sac is transected at the neck, and the peritoneal defect is closed. The sac is extracted from the canal by traction or by an artery forceps, which is passed down into the sac to grasp the distal end and to extract the sac by inversion. The internal opening of the obturator canal is closed with a continuous monofilament nylon suture, taking bites of the tissues around it, such as the periosteum of the superior pubic ramus and the fascia of the internal obturator muscle. Care must be exercised not to injure the obturator nerve and vessels. Alternatively, a sheet of pros-

thetic mesh may be laid down to cover the area and tack down around its edges. The peritoneum is allowed to return to the pelvic wall, and the abdominal incision is closed (1).

The midline transperitoneal approach is the most common method for repair of obturator hernia since most cases are unexpectedly encountered during laparotomy for intestinal obstruction of unknown cause. Reduction by gentle traction on the loops of bowel is often successful. This attempt may be augmented by pressure on the hernial sac over the medial aspect of the thigh. Extraction of the bowel can be made easier by carefully incising the sharp edge of the obturator membrane. Care must be taken to identify and avoid injury to the obturator nerve. Nonviable bowel is resected, and the abdomen is closed in the usual manner (1).

For cases in which obturator hernia without bowel obstruction is suspected, CT appears to be the only way to establish the diagnosis before operation (3). The general absence of preperitoneal fat and the weak supporting structures render such association not surprising (3). When the diagnosis is known, the preperitoneal approach is ideal. If necrotic bowel is suspected, a transperitoneal approach is performed (3).

After reduction of the herniated viscera, the obturator hernia defect is closed. Prosthetic mesh using large sheet prosthesis has been reported (16). Hernias in unusual locations are identified precisely from the inner hernia orifice and easily treated, including obturator hernias using preperitoneal approach and large sheet prosthesis (16). This technique utilizes mesh covering both obturator foramina and the inguinal and femoral orifices.

A laparoscopic approach to the preperitoneal prosthetic herniorrhaphy is possible (10). Seven obturator hernias were repaired laparoscopically in a series of 290 laparoscopic preperitoneal hernia repairs. However, "technical complications" affected 5.3% of the patients, and continued scrutiny and critical review was suggested before widespread acceptance of the procedure (17).

Placement of large sheet prosthetic mesh as reported (16) seems ideal for pelvic hernias of all kinds, especially in combination, because the simple procedure allows both diagnosis of all inguinal and pelvic hernias, regardless of location, and repair of all defects, actual or potential. In the case of obturator hernias, the high incidence of recurrence bilaterally and difficulty with clinical diagnosis may warrant bilateral repair, even when only a unilateral hernia is evident (3). The placement of the large sheet prosthesis can be performed either transperitoneally or preperitoneally, but the preperitoneal approach avoids the risks of intraabdominal adhesions and allows a commanding view from above of all the anatomy, with each part displayed with a satisfying clarity of a diagram (3).

Laparoscopic preperitoneal repair, whether by transabdominal or extraperitoneal approach, allows complete exposure of the myopectineal orifice, a structural window situated between the abdomen and thigh. Restoration of defects in the myopectineal orifice effects a radical or complete cure of groin herniation. At the time of laparoscopic approach to the myopectineal orifice, femoral and obturator hernias can be readily visualized and also repaired utilizing the techniques described above. Thus, the use of the laparoscopic approach for the diagnosis and repair of hernias of the groin allows the complete examination of the femoral and obturator canals as well. Through the technique of laparoscopy, the evaluation and treatment of groin hernias, including indirect inguinal, direct inguinal, and femoral, can be readily associated with evaluation and treatment of pelvic hernias, specifically sciatic and obturator hernias (7).

PERINEAL HERNIAS

A perineal hernia is the protrusion of a viscus through the floor of the pelvis (pelvic diaphragm) into the perineum. A hernial sac is present (14). Perineal hernias are also called pelvic hernias, ischiorectal hernias, pudendal hernias, posterior labial hernias, subpubic hernias, hernias of the pouch of Douglas, and vaginal hernias. Scarpa in 1821 first reported a case, but de Garengeot is supposed to have seen one in 1731 (1). The condition is considered extremely rare, and fewer than 100 cases have been reported (5). Primary perineal hernias are spontaneously occurring hernias. A secondary or postoperative hernia may occur following abdominoperineal resection of the rectum and related procedures (1).

Primary perineal hernias occur most commonly between the ages of 40 and 60 years and are five times more common in women than in men. They occur more frequently in women due to the broader female pelvis and attenuation of the pelvic floor during pregnancy. Other factors are obesity, ascites, and recurrent pelvic floor infection. Secondary perineal hernias are incisional ones through the reconstructed pelvic floor in patients who have had extensive pelvic surgery. They are seen in approximately 1% of abdominoperineal resections and 3% to 10% of pelvic exenterations, usually occurring within a year of the surgery (5).

Pertinent Anatomy

The pelvic floor is formed by the levator ani and the iliococcygeus muscles and their fascia. The circumference of the pelvic outlet is bounded anteriorly by the pubic symphysis and the subpubic ligament, laterally by the pubic rami and the ischial tuberosities, and posteriorly by the sacrotuberous ligaments and the coccyx. The transversus perinei muscles divide the space into the urogenital triangle anteriorly and the ischiorectal posteriorly. Two types of perineal hernia are described, anterior and posterior, depending on their relationship to the transversus perinei muscles (1) (Figs. 46.6 and 46.7).

A primary perineal hernia may occur anterior or posterior to the superficial transverse perineus muscle. An anterior hernia protrudes through the urogenital diaphragm

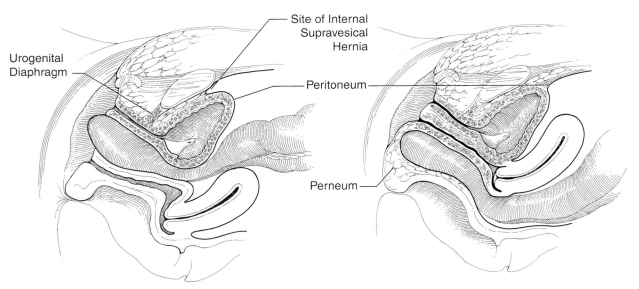

A

B

FIGURE 46.6. The course of anterior and posterior perineal hernias in women—sagittal section of the female pelvis. **A:** Course of the anterior perineal hernia. The sac passes between the urinary bladder and the vagina to reach the surface of the perineum. **B:** Course of a posterior perineal hernia. The sac passes between the vagina and rectum to reach the surface of the perineum. (From Carter JE. Hernias. In: Howard FM, Perry CP, Carter JE, et al., eds. *Pelvic pain: diagnosis and management.* Philadelphia: Lippincott Williams & Wilkins, 2000:385–413, with permission.)

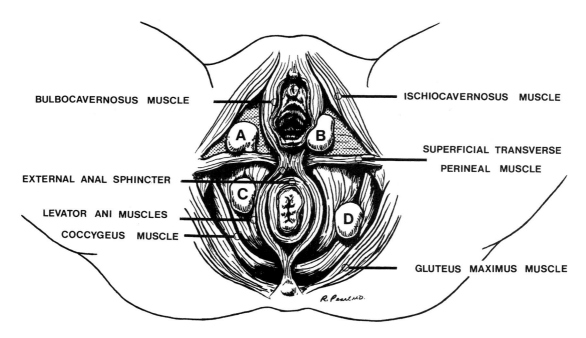

FIGURE 46.7. The female perineum showing possible sites of perineal hernias. A primary perineal hernia may occur anterior or posterior to the superficial transversus perineal muscle. An anterior hernia protrudes through the urogenital diaphragm into the triangle formed by the bulbocavernosus muscle medially, the ischial cavernosus muscle laterally, and the superficial transverse perineus muscle inferiorly. Anterior hernias occur only in women. A posterior perineal hernia may merge between component muscle, bundles of levator ani muscle or between that muscle and the coccygeus muscle, midway between the rectum and the ischial tuberosity. (From Carter JE. Hernias. In: Howard FM, Perry CP, Carter JE, et al., eds. *Pelvic pain: diagnosis and management.* Philadelphia: Lippincott Williams & Wilkins, 2000:385–413, with permission.)

into the triangle formed by the bulbocavernosus muscle medially, the ischial cavernosus muscle laterally, and the superficial transverse perineal muscle inferiorly.

A posterior perineal hernia may emerge between component muscle bundles of levator ani muscle, or between muscle and the coccygeus muscle midway between the rectum and the ischial tuberosity.

An anterior perineal hernia passes through the pelvic and urogenital diaphragms, lateral to the urinary bladder and vagina, and anterior to the urethra. It has been variously called pudendal, labial, lateral, or vaginal–labial. It is found only in women (14). Posterior perineal hernia occurs in both women and men but is more frequent in women. The hernia enters between the rectum and the uterus, and passes posterior to the broad ligament and lateral to the uterosacral ligament. It may pass through the levator ani muscle or between it and the iliococcygeus muscle, or even directly through the iliococcygeus muscle. It may remain in the midline and pass forward to press into the vaginal wall or backward into the rectum. It may also lie in the ischiorectal fossa below the lower margin of the gluteus maximus muscle and may be confused with a sciatic hernia.

Anterior perineal hernias contain intestine or bladder. Posterior perineal hernias may contain omentum, small bowel, or rectum. The hernias have a wide neck and usually soft borders with no rigid fibrous ring, so that incarceration or strangulation is rare (1).

A lateral pelvic hernia has also been described. In this case, the peritoneal sac passes through a gap in the line of origin of the levator ani muscle from the fascia of the internal obturator muscle. It passes anteriorly into the labia majus or posteriorly into the ischiorectal fossa (1).

Clinical Presentation

The patient may complain of a soft protuberance that is easily reduced when the recumbent position is assumed. Symptoms are usually mild. In cases of anterior hernia, minor urinary discomfort may have been noted. In cases of posterior hernias, in which the mass may assume a large size or even protrude below the lower edge of the gluteus maximus muscle, sitting may be difficult or impossible. A dragging sensation may be felt on standing or straining. Rarely, constipation may be attributed to the hernia. A posterior hernia protruding into the posterior wall of the vagina may interfere with labor (1).

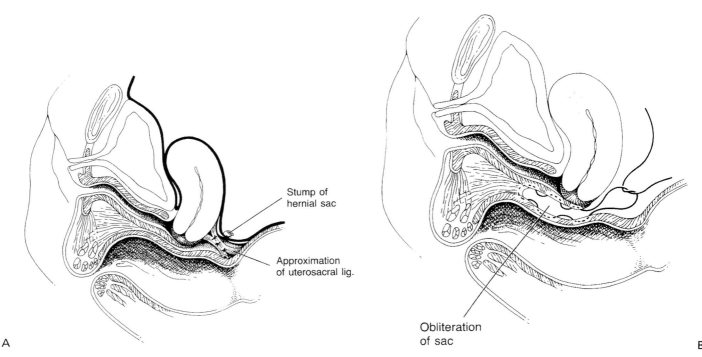

A   B

FIGURE 46.8. Repair of perineal hernia—abdominal approach. Ligate sac and approximate the uterosacral ligaments **(A)**. Alternate procedure. Obliterate the sac with continuous suture through the cervix and rectal wall **(B)**.

Physical examination may reveal a soft and easily reducible mass with a cough impulse. The direction in which it reduces indicates the anatomic nature of the hernia. Strangulation is rare since the hernial defect is usually large and bounded by soft and often atrophied muscle. If strangulation occurs, local pain, swelling, and signs of inflammation will develop, together with the signs and symptoms of intestinal obstruction. The hernia then will become tender and irreducible (1).

Bimanual rectal and vaginal examinations will help to differentiate perineal hernia from rectocele or cystocele. Plain abdominal films, or a barium enema with postevacuation views, may confirm the presence of the hernia. CT or herniography can be used to diagnose difficult cases (5).

The differential diagnosis for perineal hernia includes cystocele, rectocele, perineal abscess, lipoma, fibroma, and polyps. Rectal prolapse must sometimes be differentiated from a perineal hernia. The two may coexist, with the perineal hernia appearing anterior to the prolapsed rectum.

Treatment

Three options are available for surgical repair: abdominal, perineal, or combined abdominal–perineal approach. The abdominal approach is preferable since it allows better exposure of the anatomy of the defect and a more secure repair. With the patient under general anesthesia, the

abdomen is opened through a midline subumbilical incision. The bowel will disappear through a defect in the pelvic floor and usually can be reduced easily. Occasionally, mild traction or even outs sac is everted and excised. Small defects can be closed byide pressure on the hernia may be needed. The empty interrupted sutures of monofilament polyamide or polypropylene. Since atrophied muscle tissue is used for the repair, the recurrence rate is high. Recurrence can be avoided by using a sheet of prosthetic nonabsorbable mesh to reinforce the repair. It is laid on the pelvic floor of the region to cover the repair and is tacked down by nonabsorbable monofilament sutures. When the defect is large and the edges are thinned and friable, they cannot be approximated. In these cases, a synthetic nonabsorbable mesh prosthesis is sutured to cover the defect. The rectovesical pouch then can be eliminated by a series of sutures (Fig. 46.8) (1).

With secondary or postoperative hernias, reinforcement of the pelvic floor is often required with free fascial grafts, synthetic mesh, or tissue grafts consisting of muscle, omentum, or mesenteric leaf. Prosthetic mesh may be sutured to the sacroperiosteum posteriorly below the level of S-3. Anteriorly, it can be sutured to the vaginal apex. If possible, the defect can be obliterated by suturing the retroflexed uterus to the sacrum. Muscle flaps from the rectus abdominis, gluteus, gracilis, and bulbocavernosus muscles have also been described in the repairs of the pelvic floor (5).

REFERENCES

1. Abrahamson J. Hernias. In: Zinner MJ, Schwartz SI, Ellis H, eds. *Maingot's abdominal operations.* Stamford, CT: Appleton & Lange, 1997:479–580.
2. Beck WC, Baurys W, Brochu J, et al. Herniation of the ureter into the sciatic foramen ("curlicue ureter"). *JAMA* 1952;149:441–442.
3. Bergstein JM, Condon RE. Obturator hernia: current diagnosis and treatment. *Surgery* 1996;119:133–136.
4. Bjork KJ, Mucha P, Cahill DR. Obturator hernia. *Surg Gynecol Obstet* 1988;167:217–222.
5. Cali RL, Pitsch RM, Blatchford GJ, et al. Rare pelvic floor hernias: report of a case and review of the literature. *Dis Colon Rectum* 1991;25:604–612.
6. Ijiri R, Kanamaru H, Yokoyama H, et al. Obturator hernia: the usefulness of computed tomography in diagnosis. *Surgery* 1996; 119:137–140.
7. Kavic MS, ed. *Laparoscopic hernia repair.* The Netherlands: Harwood Academic Publishers, 1997.
8. Lo CY, Lorentz TG, Lau PWK. Obturator hernia presenting as small bowel obstruction. *Am J Surg* 1994;167:396–398.
9. Miklos JR, O'Reilly MJ, Saye WB. Sciatic hernia as a cause of chronic pelvic pain in women. *Obstet Gynecol* 1998;91:998–1001.
10. Netter FH, Iason AH, Pansky B. Hernias, section 16. In: Oppenheimer E, ed. *The CIBA collection of medical illustrations.* Vol 3. *Digestive system, part 2. Lower digestive tract.* New Jersey: CIBA, 1962:204–230.
11. Singer R, Leary PM, Hofmuyr N. Obturator hernia. *S Afr Med J* 1955;29:73–75
12. Skandalakis JE. Sciatic hernia. In: Skandalakis JE, Gray SW, Mansberger AR, et al., eds. *Hernia surgical anatomy and technique.* New York: McGraw–Hill 1989:168–173.
13. Skandalakis JE. Obturator hernia. In: Skandalakis JE, Gray SW, Mansberger AR, et al., eds. *Hernia surgical anatomy and technique.* New York: McGraw–Hill, 1989:174–184.
14. Skandalakis JE. Perineal hernia. In: Skandalakis JE, Gray SW, Mansberger AR, et al., eds. *Hernia surgical anatomy and technique.* New York: McGraw–Hill, 1989:185–206.
15. Spring DB, Vanderman F, Watson RA. Computed tomographic demonstration of ureterosciatic hernia. *AJR Am J Roentgenol* 1983;141:579–580.
16. Stoppa RE, Warlaumont CR. The preperitoneal approach and prosthetic repair of groin hernia. In: Nyhus LM, Condon RE, eds. *Hernia,* 3rd ed. Philadelphia: JB Lippincott Co, 1989:199–225.
17. Tucker JG, Wilson RA, Ramshaw BJ, et al. Laparoscopic herniorrhaphy: technical concerns in prevention of complications and early recurrence. *Am Surg* 1995;61:36–39.
18. Zimmerman LM, Anson DJ, eds. *Anatomy and surgery of hernia.* Baltimore: Williams & Wilkins, 1953;352.

EDITOR'S COMMENTS

Dr. Carter feels that these hernias may not be as unusual as most general surgeons think and, if we looked harder, we might be finding more of them. I must agree with this because, before the widespread use of laparoscopy by general surgeons, it was difficult to make the diagnosis except in situations wherein a complication such as strangulation or bowel obstruction had developed. Dr. Carter's well-written chapter is an excellent reference for surgeons when encountering these types of hernias.

Dr. Carter strongly advocates the use of prosthetic material in the repair of these hernias, making a point that the rigid structures around them do not lend themselves to primary repair. Most general surgeons have become more comfortable with prosthetic material in inguinal herniorraphy, and I think there will be little difficulty in accepting Dr. Carter's concept. It will be interesting to see over the next several years if the incidence of these hernias does not increase because of their recognition by general surgeons.

R.J.F., Jr.

Nyhus and Condon's Hernia, Fifth Edition, edited by Robert J. Fitzgibbons, Jr. and A. Gerson Greenburg. Lippincott Williams & Wilkins, Philadelphia © 2002.

47

BIOMATERIALS FOR THE REPAIR OF ABDOMINAL WALL HERNIA: STRUCTURAL AND COMPOSITIONAL CONSIDERATIONS

VOLKER SCHUMPELICK
UWE KLINGE
BERND KLOSTERHALFEN

As their crucial task, alloplastic meshes for hernia repair shall achieve a long-lasting reinforcement of the abdominal wall. For either inguinal regions or, even more, incisional hernias, the disappointing experiences of mesh-free repairs with high recurrence rates and inadequate rerecurrence rates of about 50% (28,46,66) make the additional implantation of nonabsorbable meshes favorable, with its significant decrease in recurrence rates. Unfortunately, the long-term implantation of alloplastic material initiates some side effects, mainly determined by the acute and chronic reaction of the host tissue to the foreign body. Since the selected prosthesis considerably affects the clinical results, the best suitable mesh should be chosen consciously on the basis of the mesh material, the structure of the mesh, the histologic host tissue response and its function (in particular, with regard to expected implantation times of several decades), and, not superficially, of its proper appearance during operation.

Originally, the meshes are used particularly for recurrent or incisional hernias to avoid the desperate repetition of the primarily failing technique, which results in recurrence in more than half of the patients. These disastrous results make change and improvement of surgical technique imperative. Several studies had proven that doubling of autologous fascia cannot afford a durable increased strength of the repair (55,65). As a successful alternative, the additional implantation of nonabsorbable alloplastic materials, the so-called surgical meshes, seem to fulfill all requirements almost ideally.

V. Schumpelick and **U. Klinge:** Department of Surgery, University Hospital of the RWTH Aachen, Aachen, Germany.
B. Klosterhalfen: Department of Pathology, University Hospital of the RWTH Aachen, Aachen, Germany.

HISTORY OF SURGICAL MESHES

The history of surgical meshes is an outstanding example for the progress in hernia surgery, and the possible benefit for patients from the use of biomaterials in general. The idea of strengthening the abdominal wall and, in particular, surgical hernia repair with autologous materials has been claimed in the last century, although meshes were first commercially available 40 years ago. In 1959, Usher et al. (78–80) reported the successful implantation of surgical meshes at first in 13 dogs and afterward in patients with abdominal wall hernias. In the 1970s, mainly French surgeons elaborated further technical details to cure various hernias with the help of mesh prosthesis, but it was in the 1990s that the use of meshes spread unimaginably due to the simple Lichtenstein tension-free repair (44) and the newly developed laparoscopic techniques, which are based on the obligate use of meshes. Meanwhile, about 1 million meshes are reported to be incorporated each year worldwide. In some countries, more than 90% of all hernias were routinely repaired by the aid of meshes.

It was more than 160 years ago that Belams used the air bladders of fish to close the gap of an inguinal hernia (9). He intended to provoke "an adhesive inflammation" and applied this technique on 30 dogs and afterward in three patients, always with success. In 1886, Macewen used the gathered hernial sac to seal the internal hernial ring. One year later, Trendelenburg proposed the implantation of a 4 × 4-cm^2 strip of periost; Rehn later used a strip of the fascia lata (62). It was Billroth who at the end of the last century dreamed of strengthening the repair: "If we could artificially produce tissues of the density and toughness of fascia, the secret of the radical cure of hernia would be discovered" (26). Artificial material was introduced in 1889 by

Witzel, who used a mesh of silver wire for abdominal wall hernias (86); Busse in 1901 even used meshes made of gold wire. In 1931 Fieschi proposed the implantation of rubber sponges. In 1940, Ogilvie published the use of cloth meshes to treat contaminated gunshot wounds with defects of the abdominal wall, and in 1949, Preston took meshes of metallic wire to treat hernia patients (58,59).

The triumphant progress of meshes had its beginning after World War II, with the development of synthetic polymers for medical purposes, particularly, with the construction of the polyester (PE) mesh Mersilene (Ethicon, Inc., Norderstedt, Germany) in 1954 and the polypropylene (PP) mesh Marlex (C.R. Bard, Inc., Billerica, MA U.S.A.) in 1962 (Table 47.1).

In 1973, Stoppa reported the simultaneous repair of recurrent inguinal hernias on both sides by putting a large piece of mesh in the preperitoneal space, and 1 year later, Rives combined the preperitoneal implantation of mesh with a conventional hernia repair (72). Lichtenstein published his tension-free mesh technique in 1986 (44), which was feasible even with local anesthesia and had a short learning curve. The laparoscopic repair of hernia started in 1988 with Ger and in 1989 with Bogojavalensky. Within the next few years, the transabdominal preperitoneal prosthetic (TAPP), the intraperitoneal onlay mesh (IPOM) and, finally, the totally extraperitoneal prosthetic (TEPP) repairs were developed and perfected, all of which are currently competing with the mesh-free techniques, mainly Shouldice, for the best results (49).

Principles of Mesh Repair

For considerations of structural and compositional properties of meshes, it is essential to understand the way meshes work. Both the appearance of many recurrences several years after the first repair and the high rate of rerecurrences after repeated closure by sutures indicate the importance of pathophysiologic reasons rather than technical ones. For many years, a vague disease of the connective tissue was suspected, although this never could be linked to specific defects (83,84). It was not until recently that studies of Ajabnoor (2) and Friedman et al (21). hinted at the unbalanced distribution of collagen types I (mature, high-tensile strength) and III (immature, low-tensile strength) in patients with hernia. This could be confirmed by our own studies in patients with primary inguinal hernias showing a significantly lowered ratio of collagen I:III due to an increase of collagen type III. This disorder could be detected in the skin, the fascia, and the hernial sac, underlining the presence of a systemic defect of collagen metabolism. Furthermore, similar investigations in patients with recurrent or incisional hernias revealed an even more pronounced alteration of scar formation with a much higher decreased collagen I:III ratio, as well as a distinctive expression of collagenases and proteins of the extracellular matrix (Table 47.2).

Although the pathophysiologic principles of the formation of a stable scar as the result of the normal wound healing process are unknown, the proven disorders of collagen metabolism in hernias may easily explain the high recurrence rates in all cases with a simple repetition of the previous (failing) repair technique. The disorder of the collagen metabolism might explain as well the success of surgical meshes inducing an inflammatory foreign body reaction with a consecutive, intense fibrosis resulting in a compound of nonabsorbable mesh filaments as a mechanical-sealing mechanism and an embedding collagen-rich scar tissue. Both components form the mechanical stable artificial abdominal wall. Consequently, hernia patients showing a defect in forming stable scar tissue will finally need a mesh repair.

In contrast to the use of meshes as a durable reinforcement of the abdominal wall, the meshes have to withstand the mechanical strain from the beginning in case of large

TABLE 47.1. HISTORIC OVERVIEW OF MESH REPAIR

Event	Introduction
Polyester mesh	Wolstenholme. *Arch Surg* 1956;73:1004
Polypropylene mesh	Usher. *Arch Surg* 1962;84:325
Giant prosthetic reinforcement of the visceral sac (GPRVS)	Stoppa et al., 1973 (72)
Transinguinal preperitoneal prosthesis	Rives et al. *Chirurgie* 1973;99:564
	Schumpelick et al. *Chirurg* 1996;67:419.
Subfascial prosthesis to Lichtenstein	Lichtenstein and Shulman, 1986 (44)
Preperitoneal prosthesis by extraperitoneal access	Nyhus et al. *Ann Surg* 1988;208:733
	Wantz. *Surg Gynecol Obstet* 1989;169:408
Mesh plug	Rutkow/Robbins. *Surgery* 1993; 114:3
Plug, laparoscopically	Shultz et al. *Clin Laser Mon* 1990;8:103
Intraperitoneal onlay mesh prosthesis (IPOM)	
Transabdominal preperitoneal prosthesis (TAPP)	Schultz et al. *Clin Laser Mon* 1990;8:103
	Corbitt. *Surg Laparosc Endosc* 1991;1:23
Totally extraperitoneal prosthesis (TEPP)	Ferzli et al. *J Laparoendosc Surg* 1992;2:281
	McKernan/Laws. *Surg Endosc* 1993;7:26

TABLE 47.2. IMMUNOHISTOCHEMICAL ANALYSIS OF THE COMPONENTS OF THE EXTRACELLULAR MATRIX[a]

	Control	Stable Scar	Incisional Hernia	Recurrent Incisional Hernia
Tenascin (skin)	+	++	+++	++++
Tenascin (fascia)	++++	++	−	−
Fibronectin (skin)	+++	+	++	++++
Fibronectin (fascia)	++++	+++	−	−
MMP-1 (skin)	+++	++++	++	++
MMP-1 (fascia)	+++	++++	+	−
MMP-13 (skin)	−	−	+++	++++
MMP-13 (fascia)	−	−	−	−
Collagen 1/3 (skin)	++++	+++	++	+
Collagen 1/3 (fascia)	++++	+++	++	+

MMP, matrix metalloproteinases.
Scale from absent (−) to predominant (++++)
Analysis was conducted in healthy fascial tissue (controls; n = 7), stable scars (n = 7), patients with incisional hernias (n = 7), and patients with recurrent incisional hernias (n = 5).

abdominal wall defects. To achieve an initial mechanical strength, it is necessary to fix them sufficiently.

MESH MATERIALS

Nonabsorbable meshes (Table 47.3) are knit, fabricated, net-like material with a high strength at the cut border, or almost a film-like sheet, usually made of PP, polyethylene terephthalate (polyester; PE) or expanded polytetrafluorethylene (ePTFE) (3,24). Up to now, the superiority of either material has been controversial (51). The various meshes differ largely in their basic polymers, their weight (from less than 30 g/m^2 to more than 100 g/m^2), and their pore size

(from less than 100 μm to more than 5 mm), implying considerable differences of their textile and mechanical properties. A pore size of at least 100 μm is required to permit an ingrowth of connective tissue.

The construction of a mesh made of monofilaments might reduce the attachment of bacteria, although it usually leads to an increased stiffness of the abdominal wall after implantation. In contrast, meshes made of multifilament show an elevated pliability but may cause problems in case of bacterial infection.

According to existing international textile standards (8,16,24,32,39), a complete examination of a surgical mesh consists of the description of the basic filament, weight, pore size (the measurement of the pore size is difficult, for

TABLE 47.3. NONABSORBABLE MESHES USED FOR HERNIA REPAIR

Material	Trade Name
Nonabsorbable	
Polypropylene	Marlex (heavy-weight, monofilament) (C. P. Bard, Inc.)
	Perfix plug (C. R. Bard, Inc.)
	Visilex mesh (C. R. Bard, Inc.)
	Prolene (heavy-weight, double filament) (Ethicon, Inc.)
	SurgiPro (multifilament) (Autosuture, Inc., United States Surgical, Norwalk, CT)
	Vypro (low-weight, large-pore, multifilament) (Ethicon, Inc.)
	Atrium (heavy-weight, monofilament) (Atrium Medical Corporation, Hudson, NH)
Polytetrafluorethylene	Teflon (multifilament)
	Gore-Tex (soft-tissue patch) (W. L. Gore-Tex & Associates, Flagstaff, AZ)
	Dual mesh (30- to 60-μm pores on one side) (W. L. Gore & Associates)
	Mycro mesh (2-mm perforations) (W. L. Gore & Associates)
	Composix mesh (combination of polypropylene and ePTFE) (C. R. Bard, Inc.)
Polyvinyl	Ivalon sponge
Polyamide	Nylon
Polyethylene terephtalate	Mersilene (multifilament) (Ethicon, Inc.)
	Parietex (Sofradim, Inc., Lyon, France)
Absorbable	
Polyglactin 910	Vicryl (multifilament) (Ethicon, Inc.)
Polyglycolic acid	Dexon (multifilament) (Braun–Dexon, Inc., Melsungen, Germany)

ePTFE, expanded polytetrafluoroethylene.

the complex combination of several filaments prevents a uniform pore size), pulling force at strips, subsequent tearing force, force of tearing out a seam, bending stiffness, recovery angle, and a test pressing through the stamp that reflects best the *in vivo* strain.

Polypropylene (Marlex, Prolene, Atrium, Vypro, SurgiPro)

PP (-CH2-CH(CH3)-)n) is a thermoplast based on propane with a molecular weight of 100,000. It is supposed to resist physical decay even after years of being implanted. Filaments made of PP have a similar strength to steel, although they are only one eighth the density of iron. A disadvantage is the high bending stiffness of the monofilaments, being susceptible to increase even during incorporation. Nevertheless, most of the current meshes are built of monofilaments. After implantation, this polymer initiates a (sub)acute inflammatory reaction of the host tissue with a consecutive fibrosis and high mechanical stability. Direct contact with the intestine has to be prevented very carefully because PP meshes tend to form intense adhesions and later fistulas (50,68).

As a consequence of the physiologic wound contraction, depending largely on the extent of inflammation, the PP meshes show a considerable shrinkage of about 20% in length and 40% of the original area (3,4), sometimes folding and forming sharp edges. PP regularly causes, as do many other materials, the development of edema around the implant, so that drainage for 2 to 7 days is usually advisable.

The induction of an intense fibrosis entirely embedding the mesh into a scar plate is frequently followed by a restriction of the abdominal wall mobility and complaints of the patient (48,52,81). Animal experiments and preliminary clinical experience with a low-weight, large-pore mesh indicate that both a reduction in the amount of manufactured polymer and an increase in pore size reduce the rate of side effects and, in parallel, improve the biocompatibility (67).

Predominantly PP meshes are used for several techniques of inguinal hernia repair, usually with excellent results and recurrence rates of less than 1%. For the repair of incisional hernias, recurrence rates of PP meshes are reported at a mean of less than 10%. They are implanted as onlay onto the rectus fascia or as sublay behind the rectus muscle, with a large overlap of at least 5 to 8 cm. Due to the extended preparation, the rate of hematoma for all mesh materials is reported to be significantly increased (65,76). In case of infection, it is recommended that a monofilament mesh be left in place and the infection treated with antibiotics (Fig. 47.1) (3).

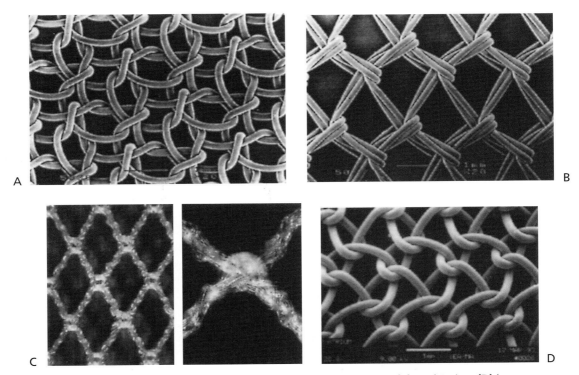

FIGURE 47.1. "Macroscopic" view of Marlex **(A)**, Prolene **(B)**, Vypro **(C)**, and Atrium **(D)** in scanning electron microscopy.

Polyethylene Terephthalate (Dacron, Mersilene, Parietex)

PE is a macromolecular compound made by polycondensation of polybasic carbonic acids usually of ethylene glycol and terephthalic acid. The resulting polymer has a high mechanical stability (73,85,87). PE meshes are based on multifilaments and, corresponding to their textile structure, permit a high pliability (e.g., Mersilene) as well as the construction of very stiff nets (e.g., Parietex). In general, PE meshes are used in the same way as PP meshes, although these mesh modifications are preferred by French surgeons. As for PP, any direct contact with the intestine has to be prevented. The rate of fibrous seroma in PE is supposed to be higher. Experimentally, Tang et al. proved in mice the importance of fibrin for the regulation of the inflammatory response, which is probably additionally influenced by the phagocyte integrin MAC-1 (CD11b/CD 18) (Fig. 47.2) (74).

A recently recognized problem of PE is the obligate degradation with an entire loss of mechanical stability, which furthermore can be considerably accelerated in the presence of an insidious infection (47,63,64,82). Meanwhile, a few cases of recurrence due to a rupture within the PE mesh have been reported (66). However, the clinical consequence of this observation is controversial. Nevertheless, a durable strength

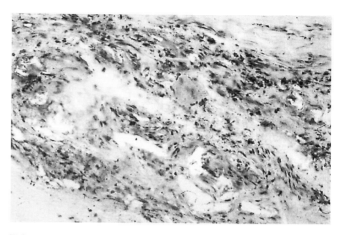

FIGURE 47.3. Mersilene (PE; multifilament) after 96-month implantation interval; only fragments of the PE filaments can be observed in light microscopy. Hematoxylin and eosin + polarized, original magnification ×400.

that will last decades seems to be questionable if PE meshes are used for hernia repair (Fig. 47.3).

Whereas significant differences in clinical results for the various mesh materials cannot statistically be proved according to some reviews (51), some groups nonetheless report significantly varying rates of recurrence, infection, and fistula formation. In 1998, Leber et al. reported a relative increase of complications for PE meshes to such an extent that they demanded abolishment of the implantation of this mesh material (43).

Polytetrafluorethylene (Gore-Tex)

Meshes made of hydrophobic ePTFE have comparatively small pores, with a size of 1 to 6 μm. In contrast to PP or PE meshes, the ePTFE material is mainly encapsulated by fibrous tissue and not embedded into a scar plate. Correspondingly, these materials show an increased rate of eventrations in animal experiments (70). Thus the achievement of a sufficiently mechanical strength requires a tight and durable fixation of the mesh in the surrounding tissue. As a consequence, several modifications have been developed either with added perforations or as a combination with a second layer with larger pores (10,12,13,15). Unfortunately, the outstanding advantage of adhesions failing to form with ePTFE in intraperitoneal applications correlates with the disadvantage that ePTFE is not integrated into the recipient tissues. Those meshes with an improved incorporation reveal an increase in adhesion formation as well (69). Recently, the long-term stability of ePTFE got to be dubious, showing a splitting up of the mesh material after long implantation (66). Furthermore, the small pore size hinders the destruction of the bacteria by macrophages, so that ePTFE meshes always have to be removed in case of infection (Figs. 47.4 and 47.5) (3).

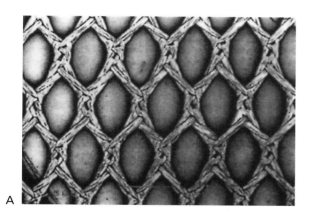

A

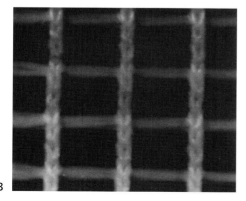

B

FIGURE 47.2. "Macroscopic" view of Mersilene **(A)** and Parietex **(B)**.

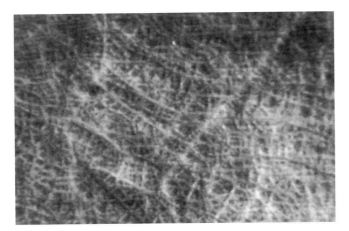

FIGURE 47.4. Expanded polytetrafluoroethylene mesh surface area in the scanning electron microscope.

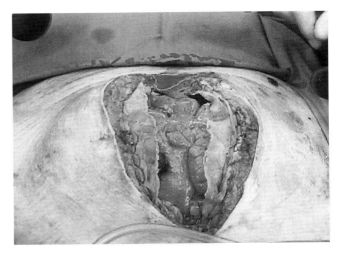

FIGURE 47.6. Marlex mesh implanted for 6 years. See Color Plate 9.

Despite all problems associated with ePTFE, there are several reports of sufficient results available both for inguinal hernia and for incisional hernia of the abdominal wall, with the reservation that the implantation time often is limited.

Absorbable Meshes (Polyglactin 910, Vicryl, Polyglycolic Acid, Dexon)

In principle, all absorbable materials—whether synthetic or natural—cannot provide a sufficient strength of the repair followed by high rates of recurrences or even implying regularly large incisional hernias as seen after the application of a laparostoma (41,77). The augmentation of a regular fascial closure by sutures with absorbable meshes cannot decrease the rate for incisional hernias, as Pans et al. demonstrated in 1998 (54). This is surprising with regard to the

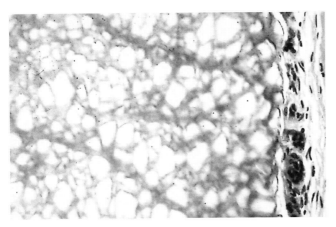

FIGURE 47.5. Expanded polytetrafluoroethylene mesh after 3 months of implantation; generally, in light microscopy the polymer reacts with the formation of a small layer of epithelioid cells and foreign body giant cells, as well as a thin layer of connective tissue. Hematoxylin and eosin, original magnification ×400.

vast amount of induced collagen fibers replacing the absorbable meshes, but might be understandable in the presence of a basic systemic collagen disease with a corresponding disorder of scar formation.

Absorbable meshes are preferred for temporary wound closure as a laparostomy in case of abdominal wall defects or peritonitis, for they show a considerably lowered risk of bowel fistulas. The temporary implantation as an inlay permits daily revision and reduces the intraabdominal pressure promoting the blood supply to the bowels, kidneys, and the abdominal wall itself. Furthermore, they are used accordingly to cover the nonabsorbable meshes to prevent direct contact with the intestine until the peritonealization is finished. Natural absorbable materials, such as skin of the pig, human cutis or fascia lata, dura mater, or bovine serosa, are increasingly being replaced—mainly due to infectious problems—by synthetic materials. These are usually made of absorbable multifilaments with a mean time of 2 to 3 weeks to halve their mechanical strength and of 6 to 8 weeks to be completely absorbed.

There is still controversy over whether the use of long-term absorbable meshes can protect the scar reaction until the collagen maturing and cross-linkage is finished, and thus provide sufficiently strong connective tissue structures to prevent a hernia recurrence (Fig. 47.6).

Structure and Textile Properties of Common Surgical Meshes

The Marlex mesh (Table 47.4), one of the most common meshes, is made of PP monofilaments characterized by a remarkable mechanical stability. Adapting the size by cutting produces some fluff and forms rather sharp edges that might favor the erosion of adjacent structures. As a consequence of its fabrication, it reveals a considerable asymme-

TABLE 47.4. TEXTILE AND MECHANICAL PROPERTIES OF COMMON SURGICAL MESHES

	Unit	Marlex	Mersilene	Prolene	Parietex	Vypro
Polymer		PP	PE	PP	PE	PP and PG
Filament		Mono	Multi	Mono	Multi	Multi
Count of bow	(Per 10 cm)	98	91	46	49	52
Fineness of yarn in g/km	(Tex)	18.9	6.1	20.6	98.0	PP 6.7
						PG[a] 8.9
Weight	(g/m^2)	95.1	39.5	108.5	129.6	54.6
						PP 26.8
Proportion of pores	(%)	85	90	84	79	91
Pore size	(mm)	0.1–0.8	0.6–1.0	1.0–1.6	1.0–1.7	2–5
Bending stiffness	(cN/cm^2)					
Vertically		34.7	0.4	6.7	10.0	6.6
Horizontally		134.4	0.1	12.9	24.2	2.0
Recovery angle 5 min	(°)					
Vertically		110	82	105	71	116
Horizontally		120	123	111	148	89
Force tearing out the seam	(N)					
Vertically[a]		57.2	15.2	57.0	68.5	29.6
Horizontally[a]		55.8	15.5	74.6	55.4	29.0
Pulling strength at stripes of 5 cm						
Maximum pulling strength	(N)					
Vertically		432	205	597	391	387
Horizontally		567	100	767	636	63
Elasticity when rupture occurred	(%)					
Vertically		145.1	31.3	80.4	51.7	49.1
Horizontally		100.3	69.1	95.8	35.0	31.4
Subsequent tearing force	(N)					
Vertically		6.6	6.4	<0.1	33.6	10.6
Horizontally		40.3	6.8	44.1	27.8	11.6
Test pressing through the stamp						
Maximum force F$_{max}$	(N)	1,656	443	2,369	2,026	718
Deformation at F$_{max}$	(mm)	51.3	36.6	44.2	36.1	39.1
Force at contact zone	(N/cm)	58.8	19.5	90.9	90.4	31.9
Deformation at 16 N	(%)	14	16	7	4	16

F$_{max}$, force at which rupture occurs; PE, polyethylene terephtalate; PG, polyglactin; PP, polypropylene.
[a]Suture = 2-0 Prolene; tensile strength: thread 36.5 N and loop 61.9 N.

try of stability in vertical and horizontal direction, particularly with regard to the pulling strength and the subsequent tearing force. The memory effect, measured by the recovery angle, is high—favorable for laparoscopic maneuvers. A high proportion of pores of 85% prove the wanted transparency; the pore size varies between 0.1 and 0.6 mm. The force for tearing out the seam exceeds the physiologic range of 16 N/cm (33,34) by a factor of 3 to 4. The deformation at this 16 N/cm reaches 14%. In summary, Marlex mesh is a heavy-weight PP mesh with small pores.

Prolene mesh (Table 47.4) is quite similar to Marlex mesh, although it is constructed of dual monofilaments with an increased weight and stability as well as a lowered elasticity, with a deformation of 7% at 16 N/cm. In the test pressing through the stamp, applied pressures of more than 400 kPa cannot destroy the textile structure. As seen for Marlex, Prolene mesh showed the same asymmetry in vertical and horizontal direction, which was even more pronounced in the test measuring the subsequent tearing force. The pore size varies between 1.0 and 1.6 mm. As with Mar-

lex, Prolene mesh represents a heavy-weight PP mesh with small pores.

In contrast, the recently developed Vypro mesh (Table 47.4) is based on braided PP to increase flexibility. Adapting the strength to the physiologic forces, the amount of nonabsorbable material can be reduced by more than 70% (compared to Marlex), increasing the elasticity to 32% at a pulling force of 16 N. To improve handling during operation, the relatively soft mesh is stiffened by combination with the absorbable polyglactin 910 covering the PP fibers. Thereby, the bending stiffness and the initial tearing force are increased considerably. The weight of the compound rises from 26 to 55 g/m^2 (28% to 57%). An optimization of the textile structure of the material increases the even distribution of the load in all directions, leading to circular rips in the mesh during the test "pressing through the stamp." The larger pores (of about 5 mm) encourage high transparency, elasticity, and easy embedding of the material into the artificial abdominal wall. In summary, the Vypro is a low-weight PP Mesh with large pores.

Unlike the other meshes, Mersilene mesh (Table 47.4) is made of braided PE. Braided materials generally are less stiff and much more flexible (extension at 16 N/cm, 16%) with a low bending stiffness (by a factor of 400 compared with Prolene and 2,000 compared with Marlex). The count of yarn is higher, the filaments are thinner, and the weight is less (42%). The force for tearing out the seam is 15 N, just below the calculated limit of 16 N. However, the maximum holding force testing the pressing through the stamp (19.5 N/cm) exceeds this critical value. Mersilene represents a low-weight PE mesh with small pores.

The Parietex mesh is another mesh of PE multifilaments but is additionally coated by bovine collagen. It has the highest weight of all mentioned meshes with a high mechanical stability comparable to that of Prolene. Due to the rigid structure of the mesh, the elasticity is low, with 4% at 16 N. The pore size measures between 1.0 and 1.7 mm. This mesh can be classified as heavy-weight PE mesh with small pores.

Mechanical Requirements to Surgical Meshes

The crucial task of meshes is providing a sufficient mechanical seal of the tissue defect with regard to the physiologic requirements. The tensile strength of a fascia closure is a function of the intraabdominal pressure ranging from 0 to 20 kPa (31,71). Measurements in patients with inguinal hernia repair reveal considerable lower pressures of 8 ± 2 kPa for coughing with a maximum of 12 kPa (57). This corresponds to published reports of Lipton, Calcagno, and Read, who always found forces of less than 10 N/cm while repairing inguinal hernias (19,45,60,61). These observations correspond as well to the forces necessary to tear out a seam measured in cadavers by Tauber and Seidel in 1974 (75).

Assuming the body to be a thin-walled cylinder, the tensile strength is the product of the tension strength according to the formula of LaPlace and the area of the cross section. The relation to the circumference allows the definition of the required tensile strength in newton per centimeter (33,34). In case of a maximum intraabdominal pressure and a circumference of 100 cm, there results a demanded force of at maximum 16 N/cm according to the following formula:

$$F = p^{*} d/4 \ (N/cm)$$

where d=diameter, p=intra-abdominal pressure, and F=tensile strength.

The comparison of the assumed physiologic strength of maximum 16 N/cm and the measured stability of common meshes reveal that these meshes are considerably oversized. The Prolene mesh, for example, would need an intraabdominal pressure of more than 1.3 bar to cause a mesh rupture. Consequently, material can be saved with a marked reduction of the surface area if the mesh strength is adapted to the physiologic requirements.

Tissue Response of the Host

The tissue response mainly determines the biocompatibility and suitability of the mesh. It should be pointed out that the appearance of a mesh intraoperatively is completely different compared to the integrated mesh only a few weeks later. The type of material, the amount, the surface area, and the mesh structure all affect the extent of inflammation and the level of the persisting foreign body reaction. Furthermore, the local reaction to the alloplastic material can differ widely both interindividually and intraindividually, making a conclusive evaluation more difficult. Although many mechanisms of the particular adjustment of the interaction of alloplastic materials and of the local cells are unknown, some principal differentiation can be made with the reservation that long-term experiences are still rare (37). Thus, the consequences of a chronic inflammatory reaction with a persisting high degree of cell proliferation and cell turnover for the risk of mesh migration or for the final extent of fibrosis with consecutive complaints of the patient cannot be appraised definitively.

However, parallel to the spread of polymer meshes in hernia surgery, the literature shows an increasing number of reports about major and minor complications after mesh implantation. Visceral erosions after implantation of PP and PE mesh modifications with subsequent formation of fistulas are well-known clinical and experimental complications. Common minor complications of these meshes are local wound disturbances including seromas in 30% to 50%, misfeelings in 10% to 20%, and restriction of abdominal wall mobility in up to 25% of all cases. In general, reasons for the failure of the implants include persistent and active inflammatory processes, irregular or low formation of scar tissues, unsatisfying integration of the mesh in the regenerative tissue area, inappropriate biomechanical properties of the implant, and improper surgical technique during implantation.

Altogether, recent morphologic studies could show that, although particular material properties of surgical meshes influence the histologic picture of the implant bed, all surgical meshes such as Marlex, Mersilene, Gore-Tex, and others generally show to various extents: first, a persisting inflammation over years after implantation (37); second, a continuous cellular stress response to the presence of polymer fibers characterized by the induction of the heat shock protein (HSP) (40); third, consistent tissue damage with features of apoptosis (TUNEL), DNA strand breaks, and necrosis; and fourth, a persistent and compensating tissue repair indicated by proliferating cells in the interface (Ki67). These parameters represent basic cellular reactions and adaptation patterns to stresses of different origin being decisive for the estimation of the inertness and biocompatibility of surgical meshes. Moreover, persistent DNA strand breaks and persistent cell proliferation indicate a chronic irritation of the recipient host tissues by the mesh.

Influence of the Mesh Weight

The long-term implantation of alloplastic material starts a (sub)acute inflammatory reaction accompanied by a moderate seroma and an infiltrate of polymorphonuclear granulocytes (PMNs) and macrophages for about 1 to 3 weeks (38). The climax occurs after 14 to 21 days, later changing to a more or less chronic inflammation sealing the foreign body into epithelioid granulomas. Simultaneously, a collagen-rich scar tissue is formed, building a three-dimensional framework around and throughout the mesh. The number of fibroblasts and the level of vascularization correlates inversely to the extent of inflammation, whereas an intense acute inflammation at the beginning directly enhances the developing amount of fibrous tissue.

In 1996, we emphasized that mechanical data of the artificial abdominal wall after mesh implantation should be adapted to physiologic values. The original stiffness and scar formation after implantation of the Marlex and Prolene meshes have been supposed to be the basis of the abdominal wall restriction. Moreover, the total amount of the manufactured PP meshes, the small size of their pores, and their large surface areas aggravate the acute and chronic inflammatory process, basically affecting the integration of the mesh fibers into the recipient tissues. On closer inspection of the material properties and morphologic data of the different PP mesh samples with different weights, pore sizes, and surface areas, the activity of inflammation and, consequently, the connective tissue formation are closely related to the amount of material implanted, the type of filament (multi- or monofilament), and the proportion of pores that define the surface or contact area with the foreign material and the recipient tissues (39). In particular, larger amounts of PP with a huge surface enlargement by processing multifilaments induce a strong and active inflammatory tissue reaction, resulting in a mesh completely embedded in a scar plate with a domination of PMNs, whereas the reduction of the material and diminishing of the plane area support a chronic, macrophage-controlled tissue response. In contrast, the construction of low-weight meshes with large pores permits the formation of fibrous tissue just around the mesh filaments with mainly fat tissue filling up the pores, preserving most of its flexibility.

Mesh-Specific Tissue Reaction

Polypropylene

Generally, heavyweight PP meshes have similar histologic patterns after implantation (6,7,11,35,38). In common, there is a predominant foreign body reaction with typical foreign body granulomas, including epithelioid cells and giant cells (51). However, and contrary to ePTFE, PE, and the reduced PP mesh, there is a persistent acute inflammation with varying amounts of CD15-positive PMN and focal fibrinoid necrosis in most cases. The inflammatory process is accompanied by pronounced perifilamentous fibrosis with an extensive amount of deposited collagen fibers. Adjacent to the mesh, the fibers are mainly oriented parallel to the PP threads. In the periphery, connective tissue with numerous collagen fibers form a thick capsule in which the whole mesh is integrated. These mesh modifications are characterized by complete penetration of connective tissue into the pores. As a result, the meshes and the newly formed connective tissues around the meshes form a complex unit. Fibroblasts are still common at the interface, whereas vascular structures are rare. After an implantation of more than a year, the inflammatory reaction is reduced but still detectable within the interface. Compared with ePTFE and PE, the heavyweight PP meshes have the most inflammatory and connective tissue cells in the interface, but the lowest amount of fat tissue and vascularization (Fig. 47.7).

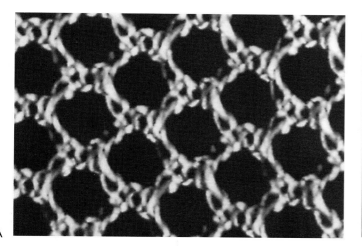 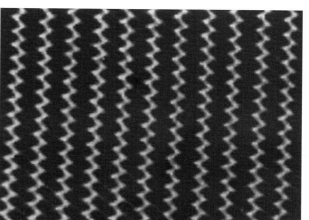

FIGURE 47.7. Macroscopic structure of Dexon **(A)** and Vicryl **(B)**.

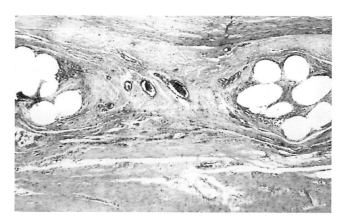

FIGURE 47.8. Marlex after long-term implantation (36 months) completely embedded in a scar plate. Hematoxylin and eosin, original magnification ×100.

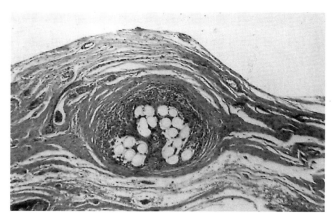

FIGURE 47.9. Vypro after 3 months of implantation with foreign body granulomas in the interface and a moderate formation of connective tissue. Hematoxylin and eosin, original magnification ×250.

In contrast, the inflammatory response of the low-weight meshes with a reduction of PP to less than 30% of Marlex is considerably reduced compared with the heavy-weight meshes (Marlex, Prolene). The tissue reaction is characterized by the formation of foreign body granuloma with a moderate number of multinuclear giant cells. Signs of acute inflammation such as infiltrates of PMNs and fibrinoid necrosis are rare. The collagen fibers form moderate capsules that are centrally and concentrically orientated around single mesh filaments, whereas in the periphery there is a thin scar plate oriented parallel to the mesh. Accordingly, the number of fibroblasts is low, in contrast to the pronounced vascularization (Fig. 47.8).

Polyester

Low-weight PE meshes show mainly chronic local inflammation characterized by the formation of typical foreign body granuloma and numerous multinucleated giant cells. Histologic signs of an acute inflammation such as CD15-positive PMNs or necrosis can be detected only in small areas or around single mesh filaments. Collagen synthesis is low compared with PP, forming a thin capsule around the mesh fibers, in which there are occasional small aggregates of CD3-positive T lymphocytes. Overall, the partial volume of all inflammatory cells is reduced compared with both PP and ePTFE meshes. Pores are filled with mainly fat tissue and only a few pores show penetrating connective tissue. The partial volume of vessels is comparatively low. Even after years, there is a persistent localized inflammatory reaction, together with incomplete integration of the mesh into the artificial abdominal wall, although at some point with signs of complete degradation of the filaments (Fig. 47.9).

As seen with the heavy-weight PP meshes, the heavy-weight PE meshes show an intense acute inflammatory reaction in the early period after implantation. As found typically with PE, the mesh fibers are embedded in copious amounts of fibrin and dense infiltrates predominantly of monocytes and polymorphous granulocytes. The picture varies considerably between inflammation, hemorrhage, and cell destruction in the transmission electron microscope (TEM) and areas with groups of fibroblasts. Later, the mesh is enclosed into a well-vascularized scar tissue, consisting of framework of extensive fibrosis. Adjacent to the mesh fibers are seen two to three layers of epithelioid cells, with signs of activation in TEM representing maturing granulomas with syntheses of connective tissue together with a persistent intense subacute inflammation.

ePTFE

The interface reaction of ePTFE meshes is characterized by inflammation dominated by macrophages (14,22,51). Light microscopy shows only poor integration of ePTFE meshes into the artificial abdominal wall. The implant is mainly surrounded by connective tissue, while penetration of cells into ePTFE pores or adherence to the surface is rare. TEM of the extracellular matrix reveals that newly formed collagen bundles were more tangled than oriented in parallel lines with little cross-linking. At the interface, PMNs are found only exceptionally, but macrophages, epithelioid cells, multinucleated foreign-body giant cells, and fibroblasts are still detectable after years. The vascularization of the mesh fiber–connective tissue interface is comparably high, whereas the total partial volume of all inflammatory cells is relatively low.

Altogether, the histologic results of the tissue response clearly demonstrate that heavy-weight meshes such as Prolene and Parietex induce an acute and active inflammatory reaction in the interface, whereas the low-weight meshes Vypro and Mersilene produce a more chronic inflammatory type. Fibrosis again directly correlates with the activity of the inflammation, indicated by the significant increase of the partial volume connective tissue in the interface mesh–recipient tissues of the heavy-weight meshes Prolene and Parietex.

Another important factor influencing the activity of inflammation in the interface is the surface or contact area between mesh and recipient tissues. Our studies demonstrated that an increase in the plane area of the mesh by using multifile filaments directly enhances the activity of the inflammatory reaction. Moreover, the pore size should be as large as possible to decrease the contact area to a minimum.

Cellular Response of the Interface Mesh–Recipient Tissues

Immunohistochemical investigations strongly indicate that the implantation of meshes leads to a permanent cell turnover at the interface, persistent cell stress, and, coincidentally, the detection of an increased level of DNA strand breaks. The cellular response is characterized by the expression of HSP70 as an inducible stress marker (40); the proliferation rate with Ki67 positively; and the rate of cell damage, apoptosis, and DNA strand breaks with TUNEL-positive cells. HSP70 expression conversely correlates to the activity of the inflammatory reaction, which could be shown by our group in a recent study. In particular, macrophages expressing high intracellular amounts of HSP70 liberate low levels of the proinflammatory cytokines TNFα and, in question, IL-1 and IL-6. This correlation may be one reason why the inflammatory reaction of the low-weight meshes Mersilene and Vypro is less active than of the heavy-weight meshes Parietex and Prolene.

In contrast to the HSP70 expression, Ki67 and TUNEL-positive cells can basically be determined in the interface of the heavy-weight meshes. Here again, the low expression of HSP70 could play a central role because HSP70 is known to influence cell maturation and proliferation, as well as exhibit a broad spectrum of cytoprotective effects with a decrease in the rate of cell damage and apoptosis.

The analyses of the cellular response in human explanted mesh samples give strong evidence for the hypothesis that all meshes are not inert and exhibit a chronic irritation of the artificial abdominal wall. If meshes were completely inert, none of the parameters of HSP70, Ki67, and TUNEL should be detected in the interface.

Risk of Foreign-Body Carcinogenesis

The absence of published cases of mesh-induced tumors should not be misinterpreted as the sure proof that surgical meshes are absolutely noncarcinogenic. Tumor development in response to the subcutaneous implantation of plastics and other inert materials, known as foreign-body (FB) carcinogenesis, was first observed over 40 years ago. It is a classic model of multistage endogenous tumor genesis that requires one half or two thirds of the rodent lifespan for sarcoma or tumor development. However, unlike chemical rodent carcinogenesis, FB carcinogenesis is generally dismissed as a phenomenon unique to the rodent. The early experimental studies demonstrated unequivocally that the physical characteristics of the implant, such as size, shape and surface morphology, but not the chemical composition were essential for FB carcinogenesis (17,29,53,56). Furthermore, a dose-response relationship was found between the implant size and tumor frequency. Materials that will induce FB tumors include films of polyester, nylon, polyethylene, polystyrene, poly(vinyl chloride), cellophane, poly(dimethylsiloxane), and PTFE. It was concluded that tumor formation was directly related to cellular events during the FB reaction and formation of the fibrotic capsule surrounding the implant. Subsequent studies have extended these observations and demonstrated that subcutaneously implanted materials of any chemical composition can cause tumors in several animal species, provided they possess a smooth and impermeable surface. In powdered, perforated, or porous form, these materials lose their tumorigenicity, confirming a primary role for the physical characteristics of the implant rather than its chemical composition. Other studies have shown that the frequency of FB tumors varies directly with the capsule thickness. Taken together, these results suggest that FB tumor initiation and progression occur in cells within the fibrotic capsule. Tumors observed have been mainly fibrosarcomas or histiocytomas (for review of FB carcinogenesis see Brand et al., 1976).

In 1997, James et al. (30) reported that the cellular response in the case of FB carcinogenesis is characterized by an accumulation of proliferating and damaged cells in the interface. Silicone foils and, as positive control, impermeable cellulose acetate filters indicated significantly elevated TUNEL-positive and proliferating cell nuclear antigen–positive cells compared to the negative control (porous cellulose acetate filters). The results of this group show direct parallels to our findings of the heavy- and low-weight meshes, which also reveal a "dose-dependent" irritation of the recipient tissues, with significantly increased cell damage and proliferating rates in the heavy-weight mesh groups compared to the low-weight mesh groups.

The legitimate question will arise of whether FB carcinogenesis is a serious topic in the case of surgical meshes. Fortunately, it has to be stated that up to now in literature no example of tumor development after mesh implantation is documented. However, there is an increasing number of case reports of FB carcinogenesis after implantation of other biomaterials, in particular vascular prosthetic devices, although the mean survival time of these patients is usually less than 10 years. In this regard, it must be remembered that these vascular devices are knit material, like surgical meshes. With a close look at the results of the animal models of tumor development after polymer implantation, sarcomas should be observed in humans after 30 to 50 years, a period of time correlating to one half or two thirds of the rodent lifespan. With regard to the fact that scientific statements like retro- or prospective investigations of the long-term effects of meshes in hernia surgery and other implants are not available, in general FB carcinogenesis cannot not be safely dismissed without continued investigation and an appropriate patient follow-up, and therefore should be regarded as a still possible risk.

MESH-RELATED COMPLICATIONS

Although the improvement of the recurrence rates after the introduction of meshes generally is accepted, the estimation of the rate of the expected side effects and their cumulative risks is discussed controversially. This is reasonable, for several complications occur with a latency sometimes of years. With regard to missing therapeutic alternatives as for incisional or recurrent hernias, this might be of minor importance, but particularly for primary inguinal hernias with available appropriate mesh-free techniques the careful consideration of mesh-related side effects and the specific risk of developing recurrence mainly determine the necessity of implanting meshes. Even though a final evaluation cannot be made, several minor and major complications—recurrence as a mainly technical problem excluded—are certainly related to meshes as a foreign body and should be regarded with special attention.

Early Complications

During the first days after implantation of meshes, almost regularly a collection of liquid around the prosthesis can be detected by ultrasound (66). These sometimes extended seroma are caused by the destruction of lymphatic vessels but reflect as well the inflammatory potency of the alloplastic material. Depending on the patient's tissue reaction, liquid amounts of several liters are rarely seen. Though a specific maximum volume is not recommended, large volumes should be drained to facilitate the ingrowth of tissue.

Simultaneously, for the first 5 days, the patient's body temperature shows a slight increase to $38.0 \pm 0.3°C$ after implantation of a larger piece of mesh. Correspondingly, a rise of C-reactive protein, indicating an acute inflammatory process, has been reported (25). The spread of the inflammation to adjacent structures is confirmed by computed tomography (CT) and ultrasound, revealing a thickened spermatic cord after implantation of meshes in the inguinal region (27). Furthermore, in about 30% of the cases, intraabdominal adhesions are found even after extraperitoneal mesh placement (20).

The clinically apparent extent of inflammatory response shows remarkable variations between patients as well, without any evident individual risk factors, although it has to be assumed that the level is affected by the amount of implanted material.

Infection

Studies have demonstrated that the implantation of meshes does not increase the risk of infection (1,5,23). With or without mesh, the infection rate varies similarly between 1% and 5%. Nevertheless, a single shot antibiosis often is recommended.

As a consequence of our own poor experiences, in any case we would avoid mesh implantation simultaneously with bowel resection. Experimental studies have shown that in the presence of biomaterials a prolonged persistence of bacteria can be observed (18), explaining the fact that sometimes an infection appears with a delay of several weeks or even months. The failure to eradicate bacteria might be due to an increased adherence to the alloplastic material, particularly in case of multifilaments or in meshes with very small pores. Only for these materials, such as ePTFE, a removal of infected meshes is obligate, whereas monofilament meshes primarily should be treated with antibiotic drugs (3,42).

Mesh Shrinkage

The extent of mesh shrinkage as the obligate consequence of the physiologic wound contraction reflects mainly the activity of the inflammatory reaction (3). Animal experiments confirmed for heavy-weight PP meshes a reduction of mesh area of about 40% after 6 weeks, whereas the shrinkage seems to be somewhat less in the case of low-weight meshes (36). This phenomenon makes understandable that an overlap of at least 5 to 8 cm has to be achieved. Otherwise, the development of a recurrence is programmed. Furthermore, this shrinkage is assumed to be responsible for a considerable mesh folding seen, with monofilament meshes sometimes even forming sharp edges

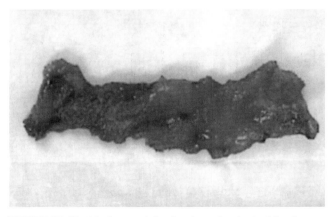

FIGURE 47.10. Marlex mesh having been implanted for 6 years.

that tend to erode adjacent structures. The corresponding extension of preparation is followed by a significant increase of the rates of bleeding complications as could be proven in many clinical studies (Fig. 47.10).

Mesh-Related Complaints

The intentional induction of an extended area of scar tissue not only strengthens the abdominal wall but sometimes leads to a considerable restriction of the abdominal wall mobility as well as to a high rate of complaints in up to 50% of all patients, particularly after implantation of a large piece of mesh. The impaired function can even make every-day activities impossible; therefore, in some cases a heavy-weight mesh has had to be replaced by a low-weight one, which up to now has shown remarkable improvement (52,65,67).

By the means of three-dimensional stereography, this restriction of the abdominal wall compliance can be qualified. Furthermore, the measured curvature reveals a significantly lowered stiffness if using a low-weight mesh with large pores in comparison to a heavy-weight mesh with small pores, directly correlating to the degree of complaints.

Mesh Migration and Fistula Formation

The migration of a mesh with the formation of fistula, mostly to bowels and bladder but sometimes even with cutting off the spermatic cord, belongs to the most serious complications of mesh surgery (43,51,68). In one third of the published cases, it appears with a delay of more than 5 years. A high level of persisting remodeling of scar tissue at the interface to the mesh might increase the risk for migration, although to date there is no experimental evidence to suggest this. However, the experience in orthopedic and gynecologic surgery, as well the experience of abdominal surgeons with the Angelchik prosthesis or with gastric banding, strongly indicates that FB migration cannot be prevented by suturing. Because of the long latency of this complication, sometimes turning the "simple" hernia repair into a life-threatening procedure, the cumulative risk for a long implantation period cannot be evaluated.

With regard to the high rate of fistula formation in case of any direct contact between a nonabsorbable mesh—except for ePTFE—and the intestine, it is strongly recommended that the mesh be covered by either hernia sac, omentum, or ePTFE, which is not known to be of danger. This high risk for fistula formation is also the reason to use absorbable meshes for the temporary closure of the abdominal wall. The reduction of adhesions is known to cause less harm and, furthermore, they are often found to be dissolved. The compulsory development of extended hernias in about 80% of the cases—a major disadvantage of absorbable meshes—necessitates a secondary reconstruction of the abdominal wall later on.

CONCLUSION

With regard to the increased recurrence rates following mesh implantation, the implantation of meshes has become essential in hernia surgery. Strengthening the abdominal wall by forming a strong scar-mesh compound for the first time, it is possible to repair even recurrent hernias with satisfactory recurrence rates. Apart from indisputable advantages, we have to face some mesh-related side effects as well, although their cumulative risk over the years cannot be calculated yet. With regard to the extended use of meshes and the limited knowledge of the late complications, surveillance of the long-term outcome seems to be imperative, particularly because one third of the mesh recipients are younger than 40 years old. However, it is evident that the clinical outcome is highly influenced by the type and amount of the implanted material. The mesh-related resulting complaints, the reports of mesh migration and fistula formation, the macroscopic appearance of shrunken and clogged meshes, and the histologic proof of persistent inflammation at the interface confirm that meshes are not incorporated inertly, leading to a chronic irritation of the recipient tissues. Optimization of meshes should be achieved to reduce the mesh-related risk. The compatibility of surgical meshes increases with low-weight, large pores and monofilament mesh constructions. The surgeon working with and implanting surgical meshes has the right to demand as much detailed information about the chosen surgical mesh as possible.

Surgical biocompatibility of any biomaterial or implant is defined as the sum total of all functional and histologic properties and, therefore, histology is an essential procedure and of immense importance for biomaterial research. Simple and descriptive histology, again, should be history in surgical mesh research. To avoid lots of unpleasant surprises after several years of implantation, we have to take special care of the long-term fate of meshes. Mesh-related complications should be recorded in special registers. The success of meshes probably is overstressed by the tendency to favor publishing excellent results instead of reporting problems (51), so that the published results cannot be reproduced in daily work. Particularly with regard to the indication of mesh techniques for primary inguinal hernias, a reliable estimation of the cumulative long-term risk of meshes is imperative.

REFERENCES

1. Abramov D, Jeroukhimov I, Yinnon A, et al. Antibiotic prophylaxis in umbilical and incisional hernia repair: a prospective randomised study. *Eur J Surg* 1996;162:945–948.
2. Ajabnoor MA, Mokhtar AM, Rafee AA, et al. Defective collagen metabolism in Saudi patients with hernia. *Ann Clin Biochem* 1992;29[Pt 4]:430–436.
3. Amid P. Classification of biomaterials and their related complications in abdominal wall hernia surgery. *Hernia* 1997;1:5–8.
4. Amid PK, Shulman AG, Lichtenstein IL, et al. Biomaterials for

abdominal wall hernia surgery and principles of their applications. *Langenbecks Arch Chir* 1994;379:168–171.

5. Avtan L, Avci C, Bulut T, et al. Mesh infections after laparoscopic inguinal hernia repair. *Surg Laparosc Endosc* 1997;7:192–195.

6. Beets G, van Mameren H, Go P. Long-term foreign body reaction to preperitoneal polypropylene mesh in the pig. *Hernia* 1998;2:153–155.

7. Beets GL, Go PM, van Mameren H. Foreign body reactions to monofilament and braided polypropylene mesh used as preperitoneal implants in pigs. *Eur J Surg* 1996;162:823–825.

8. Beets GL, van Geldere D, Baeten CG, et al. Long-term results of giant prosthetic reinforcement of the visceral sac for complex recurrent inguinal hernia [see comments]. *Br J Surg* 1996;83:203–206.

9. Belams. *Magazin für ausländische Literatur der gesamten Heilkunde und Arbeiten des ärztlichen Vereins in Hamburg*. Hamburg: Perthes und Besser, 1832. Gu J, ed.

10. Bellon JM, Bujan J, Contreras L, et al. Integration of biomaterials implanted into abdominal wall: process of scar formation and macrophage response. *Biomaterials* 1995;16:381–387.

11. Bellon JM, Bujan J, Contreras L, et al. Macrophage response to experimental implantation of polypropylene prostheses. *Eur Surg Res* 1994;26:46–53.

12. Bellon JM, Bujan J, Contreras LA, et al. Comparison of a new type of polytetrafluoroethylene patch (Mycro Mesh) and polypropylene prosthesis (Marlex) for repair of abdominal wall defects. *J Am Coll Surg* 1996;183:11–18.

13. Bellon JM, Bujan J, Contreras LA, et al. Improvement of the tissue integration of a new modified polytetrafluoroethylene prosthesis: Mycro mesh. *Biomaterials* 1996;1713:1265–1271.

14. Bellon JM, Bujan J, Contreras LA, et al. Similarity in behavior of polytetrafluoroethylene (ePTFE) prostheses implanted into different interfaces. *J Biomed Mater Res* 1996;31:1–9.

15. Bellon JM, Contreras LA, Bujan J, et al. Experimental assay of a dual mesh polytetrafluoroethylene prosthesis (non-porous on one side) in the repair of abdominal wall defects. *Biomaterials* 1996;17:2367–2372.

16. Bellon JM, Contreras LA, Bujan J, et al. Tissue response to polypropylene meshes used in the repair of abdominal wall defects. *Biomaterials* 1998;19:669–675.

17. Brand KG, Johnson KH, Buoen LC. Foreign body tumorigenesis. *CRC Crit Rev Toxicol* 1976;4:353–394.

18. Bucknall TE, Teare L, Ellis H. The choice of a suture to close abdominal incisions. *Eur Surg Res* 1983;15:59–66.

19. Calcagno D, Wantz G. Suture tension and the Shouldice repair. *Lancet* 1985;1(8443):1446.

20. Farmer L, Ayoub M, Warejcka D, et al. Adhesion formation after intraperitoneal and extraperitoneal implantation of polypropylene mesh. *Am Surg* 1998;64:144–146.

21. Friedman DW, Boyd CD, Norton P, et al. Increases in type III collagen gene expression and protein synthesis in patients with inguinal hernias [see comments]. *Ann Surg* 1993;218:754–760.

22. Galgut P, Pitrola R, Waite I, et al. Histological evaluation of biodegradable and non-degradable membranes placed transcutaneously in rats. *J Clin Periodontol* 1991;18:581–586.

23. Gilbert AI, Felton LL. Infection in inguinal hernia repair considering biomaterials and antibiotics [published erratum appears in *Surg Gynecol Obstet* 1993;177:528]. *Surg Gynecol Obstet* 1993;177:126–130.

24. Goldstein H. Selecting the right mesh. *Hernia* 1999;3:23–36.

25. Gürleyik E, Gürleyik G, Cetinkaya F, et al. The inflammatory response to open tension free inguinal hernioplasty versus conventional repairs. *Am J Surg* 1998;175:179–182.

26. Halsted W. *Surgical papers by William Stewart Halsted*. Baltimore: John Hopkins Press, 1924.

27. Hergan K, Scheyer M, Oser W, et al. [The normal CT and ultrasonic findings after a laparoscopic inguinal hernia operation.] *Rofo Fortschr Geb Rontgenstr Neuen Bildgeb Verfahr* 1995;162:29–32.

28. Hesselink V, Luijendijk RW, de Wilt JHW, et al. An evaluation of risk factors in incisional hernia recurrence. *Surg Gynecol Obstet* 1993;176:228–234.

29. Iomhair MM, Lavelle SM. Effect of film size on production of foreign body sarcoma by perforated film implants. *Technol Health Care* 1997;5:331–334.

30. James SJ, Pogribna M, Miller BJ, et al. Characterization of cellular response to silicone implants in rats: implications for foreign-body carcinogenesis. *Biomaterials* 1997;18:667–675.

31. Kirsch U. *Zu Naht und Knoten*. Melsungen: Braun-Melsungen, 1973. Medizinische Mitteilungen der Firma Braun-Melsungen.

32. Klinge U, Conze J, Klosterhalfen B, et al. [Changes in abdominal wall mechanics after mesh implantation. Experimental changes in mesh stability]. *Langenbecks Arch Chir* 1996;381:323–332.

33. Klinge U, Conze J, Limberg W, et al. [Pathophysiology of the abdominal wall]. *Chirurg* 1996;67:229–233.

34. Klinge U, Klosterhalfen B, Conze J, et al. A modified mesh for hernia repair adapted to abdominal wall physiology. *Eur J Surg* 1998;164:951–960.

35. Klinge U, Klosterhalfen B, Müller M, et al. Influence of polyglactin 910-coating on functional and morphological parameters of polypropylene-mesh modifications for abdominal wall repair. *Biomaterials* 1999;20:613–623.

36. Klinge U, Klosterhalfen B, Müller M, et al. Shrinking of polypropylene-meshes in-vivo: an experimental study in dogs. *Eur J Surg* 1998;164:965–969.

37. Klinge U, Klosterhalfen B, Müller M, et al. Foreign body reaction to meshes used for the repair of abdominal wall hernias. *Eur J Surg* 1999;165:665–673.

38. Klosterhalfen B, Klinge U, Henze U, et al. [Morphologic correlation of functional abdominal wall mechanics after mesh implantation.] *Langenbecks Arch Chir* 1997;382:87–94.

39. Klosterhalfen B, Klinge U, Schumpelick V. Functional and morphological evaluation of different polypropylene-mesh modifications for abdominal wall repair. *Biomaterials* 1998;19:2235–2246.

40. Klosterhalfen B, Klinge U, Tietze L, et al. Expression of heat shock protein 70 (HSP 70) at the interface of polymer-implants in vivo. *J Mat Sci Mat Med* 2000;11:175–181.

41. Lamb J, Vitale DL, Kaminski DL. Comparative evaluation of synthetic meshes used for abdominal wall replacement. *Surgery* 1983;93:643–648.

42. Law NW, Ellis H. A comparison of polypropylene mesh and expanded polytetrafluoroethylene patch for the repair of contaminated abdominal wall defects—an experimental study [see comments]. *Surgery* 1991;109:652–655.

43. Leber GE, Garb JL, Alexander AI, et al. Long-term complications associated with prosthetic repair of incisional hernias. *Arch Surg* 1998;133:378–382.

44. Lichtenstein IL, Shulman AG. Ambulatory outpatient hernia surgery. Including a new concept, introducing tension-free repair. *Int Surg* 1986;71:1–4.

45. Lipton S, Estrin J, Nathan I. A biomechanical study of the aponeurotic inguinal hernia repair. *J Am Coll Surg* 1994;178:595–599.

46. Luijendijk R, Lemmen MHM, Hop WCJ, et al. Incisional hernia recurrence following "vest-over-pants" or vertical Mayo repair of primary hernias of the midline. *World J Surg* 1997;21:62–66.

47. Maarek J, Guidon R, Aubin M, et al. Molecular weight characterization of virgin and explanted polyester arterial prosthesis. *J Biomed Mat Res* 1984;18:881–894.

48. McLanahan D, King LT, Weems C, et al. Retrorectus prosthetic mesh repair of midline abdominal hernia. *Am J Surg* 1997;173: 445–449.

49. Memon MA, Rice D, Donohue JH. Laparoscopic herniorrhaphy. *J Am Coll Surg* 1997;184:325–335.

50. Molloy RG, Moran KT, Waldron RP, et al. Massive incisional hernia: abdominal wall replacement with Marlex mesh. *Br J Surg* 1991;78:242–244.

51. Morris Stiff GJ, Hughes LE. The outcomes of nonabsorbable mesh placed within the abdominal cavity: literature review and clinical experience. *J Am Coll Surg* 1998;186:352–367.

52. Müller M, Klinge U, Conze J, et al. Abdominal wall compliance after Marlex mesh implantation for incisional hernia repair. *Hernia* 1998;2:113–117.

53. Ott G. [Foreign body induced sarcoma]. *Exp Med Pathol Klin* 1970;32:1–118.

54. Pans A, Elen P, Dewe W, et al. Long-term results of polyglactin mesh for the prevention of incisional hernias in obese patients. *World J Surg* 1998;22:479–482.

55. Paul A, Korenkov M, Peters S, et al. Unacceptable results of the Mayo procedure for repair of abdominal incisional hernias. *Eur J Surg* 1998;164:361–367.

56. Paulini K, Beneke G, Korner B, et al. The relationship between the latent period and animal age in the development of foreign body sarcomas. *Beitr Pathol* 1975;154:161–169.

57. Peiper C, Junge K, Füting A, et al. Intraoperative Messung der Nahtkräfte bei der Shouldice-Reparation primärer Leistenhernien. *Chirurg* 1998;69:1077–1081.

58. Poole G. Mechanical factors in abdominal wound closure: the prevention of fascial dehiscence. *Surgery* 1985;97:825–828.

59. Preston D, Richards CF. Use of wire mesh prosthesis in the treatment of hernia. *Surg Clin North Am* 1973;53:549–555.

60. Read R. Attenuation of the rectus sheath in inguinal herniation. *Am J Surg* 1970;120:610–614.

61. Read RE, McLoad P. Influence of relaxing incisions on suture tension in Basssini and McVay's repairs. *Arch Surg* 1981;116: 440–445.

62. Rehn E. *Die Operationen bei den Unterleibsbrüchen.* Leibzig: Fischer, Gohbandt, Sauerbruch, Johann Ambrosius Barth-Verlag, 1957. Bier-Braun K, ed. Chirurgische Operationslehre.

63. Riepe G, Loos J, Imig H, et al. Long-term in vivo alterations of polyester vascular grafts in humans. *Eur J Vasc Endovasc Surg* 1997;13:540–548.

64. Riepe G, Schröder A, Imig H. Degeneration von Gefäßprothesen aus Dacron. *Zentralbl Chir* 1994;119[Suppl]:148–150.

65. Schumpelick V, Conze J, Klinge U. [Preperitoneal mesh-plasty in incisional hernia repair. A comparative retrospective study of 272 operated incisional hernias]. *Chirurg* 1996;67:1028–1035.

66. Schumpelick V, Kingsnorth G. *Incisional hernia of the abdominal wall.* Berlin: Springer–Verlag, 1999.

67. Schumpelick V, Klosterhalfen B, Müller M, et al. Minimierte Polypropylen Netze zur präperitonealen Netzplastik (PNP)— eine prospektive randomisierte klinische Studie. *Chirurg* 1999; 70:422–430.

68. Seelig MH, Kasperk R, Tietze L, et al. [Enterocutaneous fistula after Marlex net implantation. A rare complication after incisional hernia repair]. *Chirurg* 1995; 66:739–741.

69. Simmermacher R, van der Lei B, Schakenraad JM, et al. Improved tissue ingrowth and anchorage of expanded polytetrafluorethylene by perforation: an experimental study in the rat. *Biomaterials* 1991;12:22–24.

70. Simmermacher RK, Schakenraad JM, Bleichrodt RP. Reherniation after repair of the abdominal wall with expanded polytetrafluoroethylene. *J Am Coll Surg* 1994;178:613–616.

71. Stelzner F. Function of the abdominal wall and development and therapy of hernias. *Langenbecks Arch Chir* 1994;379:109–119.

72. Stoppa R, Abourachid H, Duclaye C, et al. [Plastic surgery of inguinal hernia. Interposition without fixation of Dacron mesh by subperitoneal median approach.] *Nouv Presse Med* 1973;2: 1949–1951.

73. Stoppa RE, Rives JL, Warlaumont CR, et al. The use of Dacron in the repair of hernias of the groin. *Surg Clin North Am* 1984; 64:269–285.

74. Tang L, Ugarova TP, Plow EF, et al. Molecular determinants of acute inflammatory responses to biomaterials. *J Clin Invest* 1996; 97:1329–1334.

75. Tauber R, Seidel W. Bedeutung mechanischer Faktoren bei der Entstehung der abdominellen Wunddehiszenz. *Zentralbl Chir* 1975;19:1178–1182.

76. Trupka A, Hallfeldt K, Schmidbauer S, et al. [Incisional hernia repair with an underlay polypropylene mesh plasty: an excellent technique from French hernia surgeons.] *Chirurg* 1998;69: 766–772.

77. Tyrell J, Silberman H, Chandrasoma P, et al. Absorbable versus permanent mesh in abdominal operations. *Surg Gynecol Obstet* 1989;168:227–232.

78. Usher F, Fries J, Ochsner JL, et al. Marlex mesh, a new plastic mesh for replacing tissue defects: clinical studies. *Arch Surg* 1959: 138–45.

79. Usher F, Hill J, Ochsner J. Hernia repair with Marlex mesh: a comparison of techniques. *Surgery* 1959;46:718–724.

80. Usher F, Wallace S. Tissue reaction to plastics. *AMA Arch Surg* 1959;76:997–999.

81. Vestweber K, Lepique F, Haaf F, et al. [Results of recurrent abdominal wall hernia repair using polypropylene mesh]. *Zentralblatt für Chirurgie* 1997;122:885–888.

82. Vinard E, Eloy R, Descotes J, et al. Stability of performances of vascular prostheses retrospective study of 22 cases of human implanted prostheses. *J Biomed Mat Res* 1988;22:633–648.

83. Wagh P, Read R. Collagen deficiency in rectus sheath of patients with inguinal herniation. *Proc Soc Exp Biol Med* 1971;137:382–384.

84. Wagh PV, Read RC. Defective collagen synthesis in inguinal herniation. *Am J Surg* 1972;124:819–822.

85. Wantz GE. Incisional hernioplasty with polyester mesh [Letter]. *Arch Surg* 1998;133:1137.

86. Witzel O. Über den Verschluß von Bauchwunden und Bruchpforten durch versenkte Silberdrahtnetze (Einheilung von Filigranpelotten). *Zbl Chirurgie* 1900;10:257–260.

87. Yuce K. Retention mesh: an alternative to retention sutures. *Eur J Surg* 1994;160:641–642.

48

ASSESSING THE QUALITY OF HERNIA REPAIR

ERIK NILSSON
STAFFAN HAAPANIEMI

Patients undergoing herniorrhaphy have the right to assume that the repair will last for the rest of their life (1).

WHY ASSESS?

Quality control of hernia surgery is of great importance to society for a number of reasons. Hernia repair is a common procedure, with an incidence of approximately 200 operations per 100,000 inhabitants each year in the United Kingdom (8) and in Sweden (9), and an even higher incidence in the United States (14). Although specialized hernia centers exist in the industrialized world, hernia surgery is usually considered an area of general surgery often performed by nonspecialized surgeons or trainees. Reported recurrence rates following hernia repair vary ten-fold regardless of the technique used (3), implying that there is a risk that inadequate health service may be provided. New methods have been introduced in recent years, and these need validation when put into general practice. For surgical units and individual surgeons, knowledge of performance is vital, whether one is satisfied with past achievements or considers improvement necessary. Finally, quality assessment must be considered in the purchaser–provider situation.

PREREQUISITES

Five essential features of comparative audit at a national level were recently outlined. These are high-quality data collection, relevant and valid measures of outcome, appropri-

ate and valid measures of case-mix, a defined and representative population, and appropriate statistical analysis (13). These features are of great relevance also for quality assessment in general. We would like to emphasize the importance of prospective data recording using protocols with clearly defined items.

OUTCOME MEASURES

Recurrence

Proxy indicators of recurrence rate and data necessary for evaluating recurrence rates are given in Table 48.1. The percentage of operations performed for recurrent hernia in a defined population is an inverse index of quality of hernia surgery in the past, but even drastic changes in quality take a long time to identify. The percentage of operations on cohorts for recurrence at 3 to 5 years after surgery may also provide a crude indicator of recurrence rate (16). These data are readily available, and variations in this index suggest a fluctuation in recurrence rate. The cumulative incidence of reoperation has been shown to underestimate the recurrence rate, as determined by questionnaire and selective follow-up, by 40% 3 years after surgery (7). It presupposes the existence of unique identification numbers (person numbers) (11) and knowledge of the death of patients for life-table calculations. When many parallel units use the same protocol prospectively, reoperations following referrals may automatically be taken into account. Factors that have to be considered when discussing recurrence rates in a restricted sense are well known and are listed in Table 48.1. Aspects on definition of recurrence and methods of control have been discussed recently (10). The greatest obstacle to routine assessment of outcome quality in hernia surgery may be the requirement of physical examination of all operated patients several years after surgery, as this would probably exceed the resources of most surgical units.

E. Nilsson: Department of Surgery, Linköping University, Linköping, Sweden; Department of Surgery, Motala Hospital, Motala, Sweden.

S. Haapaniemi: Department of Surgery, University of Linköping; Department of Surgery, University Hospital, Linköping, Sweden.

TABLE 48.1. RECURRENCE

1. Proxy indicator	
A. Percentage of operations for recurrent hernia	
B. Reoperation rate of cohort by year	
C. Cumulative incidence of reoperation	
2. Recurrence rate	
In order to evaluate data, we need to know:	
A. Definition of recurrence	
Preoperatively	"Expansive cough impulse" (Shuttleworth and Davies. *Lancet* 1960;i:126) or "A weakness in the operation area necessitating a further operation or the provision of a truss" (Marsden. *Lancet* 1959;i:461)
Postoperatively	Recurrent groin hernia irrespective of type of hernia at the initial and subsequent operations
B. Method of control	Physical examination of all patients or questionnaire and selective follow-up
C. Time and completeness of follow-up	

Removal of Prosthesis

Since the large scale introduction of mesh prosthesis, the removal of mesh plugs due to persistent pain or dislocation has been documented (12), as well as excision of flat mesh because of chronic groin sepsis (19). Although rare, such reoperations must be accounted for in quality assessment.

Postrepair Pain

Chronic pain following hernia repair is well recognized by all hernia surgeons. In one study of 470 patients (93% response rate), 6% of the patients reported moderate or severe pain (4) more than 1 year after open hernia repair. The incidence of pain was significantly increased in patients operated on for recurrence and in patients with significant pain in the immediate postoperative period. Pain of moderate or severe intensity was also observed in 6% of 233 eligible patients with 96% follow-up 4 years after open hernia repair (S. Haapaniemi and E. Nilsson, *unpublished data* 2001). Chronic pain after open hernia repair is an important clinical problem, and hence it must be considered in quality assessment.

Postoperative Complications

In routine hernia, surgery postoperative complication rate may depend more upon the intensity of follow-up than on the quality of operations performed. Whatever method is used for quality assessment, complications observed by the operating unit should be recorded and serious adverse events should be discussed at complication conferences.

Time to Normal Activity and Time to Work

These measures have obvious economic implications for hernia repair. They are influenced by socioeconomic factors (15) and by advice given to patients, including medication for pain relief (5,18). Therefore, in order to evaluate time for convalescence as an outcome measure, one has to consider the conditions of the study under scrutiny.

OTHER QUALITY COMPONENTS

As "structure" and "process" are phrases unfamiliar to hernia surgeons, we suggest the use of other terminology for quality components that may be more appealing—patient care, education, and economic consideration. Questions in italics below are provided as a checklist for surgeons and managers.

Quality of Patient Care

We use this term to cover all aspects of treatment excluding surgery.

1. Availability and waiting lists. *Can a date for operation be offered to elective cases within reasonable time (less than 3 months) once diagnosis and indication for surgery have been settled?*
2. Information and advice to patients. *Are patients, prior to surgery, offered both oral and written information concerning surgery and advice regarding postoperative activity, return to work, and pain relief?*
3. Utilization of the experience of patients. *Are the views of patients concerning hospital stay and postoperative course regularly collected and given to surgeons in a stratified form?*

Quality of Education

1. Guidelines and description of techniques. *Are step-by-step instructions for infiltration anesthesia and repair methods used by the surgical unit readily available?*
2. Trainee program. *Does the surgical unit have an updated educational program aiming at qualifying surgeons in training for primary hernia repair?*

3. Learning from the past. Sentinel indicators such as mortality following an elective hernia operation and procedure-related complications need to be discussed openly. However, the following question may be more important in raising the overall quality of hernia surgery: *Is outcome audit of the surgical unit and of individual surgeons regularly performed, and are the results discussed among members of the unit?*

Quality of Economics

1. Cost awareness. *Is the cost of surgery (monetary unit per minute), equipment, and overnight stay known to all members of the unit?*
2. Equity, the rationing of scarce surgical resources. *Is the principle of justice (2,17) known and practiced by all surgeons, as demonstrated by a willingness to include economic considerations in hernia repair routines?*

THE SWEDISH HERNIA REGISTER

Background

In 1992, a register for inguinal and femoral hernias was established among eight Swedish hospitals (11). Each operation on patients more than 15 years of age is recorded according to a protocol in which patient characteristics, type of hernia, method of repair, anesthesia, complications, and reoperations (if applicable) are noted. By using person numbers, it is possible to adjust all calculations for death of

patients. Each year an external reviewer compares data sent to the Register center with a sample of theater logbooks and patient files from some of the aligned units in order to check validity of data.

Participating Units and Operations Registered

The number of aligned units increased from eight in 1992 to 44 in 1999, which is approximately 50% of all units performing hernia surgery in Sweden. By December 1998, the total number of hernia repairs registered was 26,929. They were performed during 25,862 operations (1,067 operations were bilateral) on 24,310 patients (92% men and 8% women). Of all operations, 4,174 or 15.5% were done for a recurrent hernia, and of these recurrences 720 followed an operation that had been registered previously.

Time Trends for Methods of Repair, Anesthesia, and Day-Case Surgery

Figure 48.1 illustrates methods of repair used from 1992 to 1998. As can be seen, great changes in the use of repair methods have taken place. In 1992, musculoaponeurotic repairs ("Bassini," "McVay," "Marcy," and other conventional open repairs) were used in 68% of all operations, the "Shouldice" technique in 26%, and mesh techniques in 6% of all procedures. In 1998, corresponding figures were 16%, 17%, and 67%, respectively. That year, mesh techniques were utilized for primary and recurrent hernias in 64% and

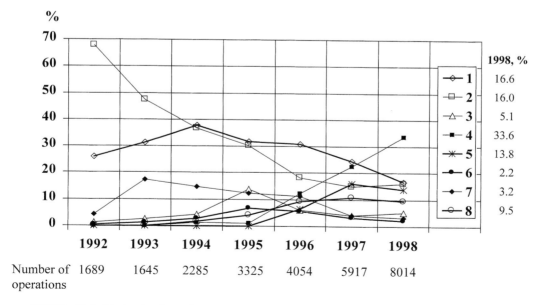

FIGURE 48.1. Methods of repair used from 1992 to 1998. *Open diamond,* "Shouldice"; *open square,* conventional open; *open triangle,* mesh, groin incision ("Lichtenstein" and mesh plug excluded; *filled square,* "Lichtenstein"; *asterisk,* mesh plug; *filled circle,* mesh, preperitoneal; *filled diamond,* transabdominal preperitoneal prosthesis; *open circle,* totally extraperitoneal prosthesis.

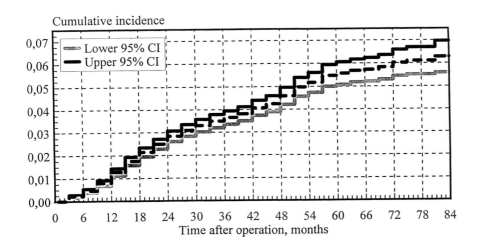

Cumulative incidence

FIGURE 48.2. Cumulative incidence of reoperation at 5 years, 5.6% (95% confidence interval, 5.1 to 6.1). Of 26,939 hernia repairs performed from 1992 through 1998, 3,253 have been followed for 5 years.

85% of cases, respectively. The use of repairs with absorbable sutures declined from 33% in 1992 to 3% in 1998. A slight increase in the use of infiltration anesthesia (as sole method of anesthesia) was noticed during the observation period, from 2% of all operations in 1992 to 9% in 1998. Day-case surgery increased from to 33% in 1992 to 54% in 1998.

Cumulative Incidence of Reoperation

The cumulative incidence of reoperation considering all 26,929 hernia repairs registered, is shown in Fig. 48.2. The risk of having had a reoperation due to a recurrent hernia 5 years after surgery was 5.6% [95% confidence interval (CI), 5.1 to 6.1]. For primary and recurrent hernia repairs, the figures are 4.9% (95% CI, 4.3 to 5.5) and 9.3% (95% CI, 7.9 to 10.7), respectively. This demonstrates a decline in reoperation rate from 7.9% (95% CI, 7.7 to 8.9) based upon all repairs performed 1992 to 1996. Further evidence for a reduction in reoperation was provided by a multivariate analysis, taking into account items given in Tables 48.2

and 48.3. The relative risk for reoperation was significantly higher for operations performed between 1992 and 1995 as compared to operations done between 1996 and 1998 (relative risk, 1.37; 95% CI, 1.14 to 1.66).

Risk Analyses

With the increasing number of hernia repairs, it is possible to perform multivariate analyses of risk for reoperation. Results of such an analysis covering 17,985 hernia repairs performed between 1996 and 1998 are shown in Fig. 48.1. The conclusions are evident. Recurrent hernias and direct hernias should be treated with extra caution due to their inherently greater risk of reoperation. Postoperative complications should be eschewed for the same reason. On the other hand, the relative risk of reoperation attached to surgical techniques varies with time and setting due to the well-known fact that two operations with the same eponym may be carried out quite differently. For this reason, all eponyms have been placed within quotation marks. Table 48.3 shows the relative risk for reoperation according to

TABLE 48.2. RELATIVE RISK FOR REOPERATION, 1996 TO 1998 (17,985 HERNIA REPAIRS)

Variable	Operations	Reoperations for Recurrence	R[a]	95% CI
Recurrent hernia vs. primary hernia	2,688	72	2.17	1.58–2.97
Postoperative complication vs. no complication	1,860	47	2.14	1.54–2.97
Direct hernia[b] vs. indirect and femoral hernia	7,915	125	1.53	1.17–2.01
Absorbable suture vs. nonabsorbable suture or mesh	839	19	1.27	0.75–1.33
In-hospital stay vs. day-case surgery	8,226	126	1.23	0.92–1.64
Older than median vs. median or younger	8,540	115	1.00	0.75–1.33

CI, confidence interval; R, relative risk.
[a]Multivariate analysis according to Cox's proportional hazards model considering all variables in Table 48.1 and methods of repair (Table 48.2).
[b]Including combined hernias and "other" groin hernias not classified in any of the three major groups.

TABLE 48.3. RELATIVE RISK FOR REOPERATION, 1996 TO 1998 (17,985 HERNIA REPAIRS)

Methods	Operations	Reoperations for Recurrence	R^a	95% CI
"Shouldice"	4,036	50	1.0	Reference
Conventional open[b]	2,895	49	1.35	0.88–2.06
Mesh, groin incision ("Lichtenstein" and mesh plug excluded)	903	13	0.99	0.53–1.85
"Lichtenstein"	4,517	22	0.50	0.30–0.83
Mesh plug	2,313	20	0.96	0.57–1.62
Mesh, preperitoneal	586	22	1.53	0.89–2.63
TAPP	954	16	0.79	0.45–1.42
TEPP	1,781	32	1.32	0.84–2.08

CI, confidence interval; R, relative risk; TAPP, transabdominal preperitoneal prosthesis; TEPP, totally extraperitoneal prosthesis.
[a]Multivariate analysis according to Cox's proportional hazards model. Adjusted for variables in Table 48.1.
[b]All open repairs excluding operations with "Shouldice" technique.

multivariate analysis for all repairs carried out between 1996 and 1998. As can be seen, the "Lichtenstein" technique carries a significantly lower risk for reoperation compared to the "Shouldice" technique. It must be emphasized that these figures represent a disequilibrium in the relative merits of methods in general surgical practice at a time when rapid changes of techniques and some improvement of outcome took place.

Register Data and Improvement Work

The Swedish Hernia Register has been driven by an ambition to provide surgeons in aligned hospitals with high-quality data for improved work (9). It provides participating hospitals with stratified information about their own achievement and aggregated data for all units. This may be used in designing pathways for the majority of hernia patients with primary hernias and for the difficult cases with very large or recurrent hernias. According to numerous reports from specialized hernia centers, infiltration anesthesia may be used almost exclusively in open groin hernia repair. This technique was, however, utilized in only 9% of all procedures registered in the Swedish Hernia Register in 1998. Therefore, a controlled clinical trial comparing infiltration anesthesia, regional anesthesia, and general anesthe-

sia in nonspecialized units has been launched within the scope of the Register.

"THE MEANING OF IT ALL"

This quotation from Richard Feynman (6) is used here to discuss whether registration and assessing serves its purpose—to benefit patients undergoing hernia repair. By analyzing variations in cumulative incidence of reoperation and day-case surgery, it was concluded that 3 years of Register work, with its associated and ongoing audit processes, improved both quality and cost-effectiveness of hernia surgery (9). Furthermore, as demonstrated in Table 48.4, the percentage of operations for recurrent hernias is lower and the percentage of day-case surgery is higher in the initially participating eight hospitals as compared to later aligned units. Such differences may be expected to disappear as the overall quality of hernia surgery increases. And improvement of Swedish hernia surgery is needed. Given that 20,000 hernia repairs are performed annually and that 15% of these are done for recurrences, 3,000 unnecessary and often complicated hernia repairs take place each year in Sweden. Resources allocated for health care may be used in better ways.

TABLE 48.4. OPERATIONS FOR RECURRENCE AND DAY-CASE SURGERY IN INITIALLY PARTICIPATING HOSPITALS AND LATER ALIGNED UNITS ACCORDING TO THE SWEDISH HERNIA REGISTER

	Initial Eight Hospitals		Later Aligned Units[a]	Total
	1992 to 1994	1995 to 1998		
No. of repairs	4,903	6,083	15,943	26,929
Recurrent hernia repair (%)	16.4[b]	13.5[b]	16.0[b]	15.5
Day-case surgery (%)	43.5[b]	60.4[b]	48.5[b]	50.3

[a]Two units started registration in 1994, 27 units in 1995 or later.
[b]Differences between groups were statistically significant ($p < 0.001$).

CONCLUSION

Quality assessment of hernia surgery is essential. It is necessary for society to ensure adequate outcome at reasonable cost. It is necessary for education and for evaluation of new methods. For surgeons and surgical units, quality assessment is necessary for improving and defending achievements. Person number is an adjunct but not an indispensable one. We have a long way to go in order to make hernia repair a "once-in-a-lifetime experience" for our patients.

ACKNOWLEDGMENTS

In 1998, the following hospitals were aligned to the Register: Eksjö, Ersta sjukhus Stockholm, Falköping, Falun, Huddinge sjukhus Stockholm, Hudiksvall, Kalix, Kalmar, Karolinska sjukhuset Stockholm, Kristianstad/Hässleholm, Lidköping, Lindesberg, Linköping, Ljungby, Ludvika, Lundby sjukhus Gothenburg, Lund/Landskrona, Lycksele, Mora, Motala, Norrköping/Finspång, Norrtälje, Piteå, Samariterhemmets sjukhus Uppsala, Skellefteå, Skene, Södertälje, S:t Görans sjukhus Stockholm, Säffle, Uddevalla/Strömstad, Varberg, Värnamo, Västervik/Oskarshamn, Västra Frölunda, and Östersund. The authors thank hernia surgeons in participating hospitals for their collaboration. The Swedish Hernia register is financially supported by the National Board of Health and Welfare and the Federation of County Councils, Sweden. Secretary Gunnel Nordberg and statistician Lennart Gustafsson, Ph.D., have provided invaluable work for the Swedish Hernia Register.

REFERENCES

1. Abrahamson J. Etiology and pathophysiology of primary and recurrent groin hernia formation. *Surg Clin North Am* 1998; 78:953–972.
2. Beauchamp TL, Childress JF, eds. *Principles of biomedical ethics.* Oxford: University Press, 1983.
3. Bendavid R. Expectations of hernia surgery (inguinal and femoral). In: Paterson-Brown S, Garden J, eds. *Principles and practice of surgical laparoscopy.* London: WB Saunders, 1994: 12.1, pp. 387–414.
4. Callesen T, Bech K, Kehlet H. Prospective study of chronic pain after hernia repair. *Br J Surg* 1999;86:1528–1531.
5. Callesen T, Klarskov B, Bech K, et al. Short convalescence after inguinal herniorrhaphy with standardised recommendations: duration and reasons for delayed return to work. *Eur J Surg* 1999;165:236–241.
6. Feynman RP. *The meaning of it all. Thoughts of a citizen–scientist.* Reading, MA: Perseus Books, Addison–Wesley, 1998.
7. Kald A, Nilsson E, Anderberg B, et al. Reoperation as surrogate endpoint in hernia surgery: a three year follow-up of 1565 herniorrhaphies. *Eur J Surg* 1998;164:45–50.
8. Nicholson S. Inguinal hernia repair. *Br J Surg* 1999;86:577–578.
9. Nilsson E, Haapaniemi S. Hernia registers and specialization. *Surg Clin North Am* 1998;78:1141–1155.
10. Nilsson E, Haapaniemi S. Quality control and scientific rigour.
In: Bendavid R, ed. *Hernias of the abdominal wall: principles and management.* New York: Springer New York Inc., 2001:122–127.
11. Nilsson E, Haapaniemi S, Gruber G, et al. Methods of repair and risk for reoperation in Swedish hernia surgery from 1992 to 1996. *Br J Surg* 1998;85:1686–1691.
12. Palot JP, Avisse C, Caillez-Tomasi JP, et al. The mesh plug repair of groin hernias: a three year experience. *Hernia* 1998;2:31–34.
13. Reeves B, Emberton M. Tackling the quality agenda in surgery: taking comparative audit into the next century. *Ann R Coll Surg Engl* 1999;81:138–143.
14. Rutkow IM. Epidemiologic, economic, and sociologic aspects of hernia surgery in the United States in the 1990s. *Surg Clin North Am* 1998;78:941–951.
15. Salcedo-Wasicek MC, Thirlby RC. Postoperative course after inguinal herniorrhaphy. A case-controlled comparison of patients receiving worker's compensation vs patients with commercial insurance. *Arch Surg* 1995;130:29–32.
16. Sandblom G, Gruber G, Kald A, et al. Audit and recurrence rate after hernia surgery. *Eur J Surg* 2000;166:154–158.
17. The Senate of Surgery of Great Britain and Ireland. Secretariat, 35-43 Lincoln's Inn Fields, London WC2A 3PN. *The surgeon's duty of care.* London: 1997.
18. Shulman AG, Amid PK, Lichtenstein IL. Returning to work after herniorrhaphy: "take it easy" is the wrong advice. *Br Med J* 1994;309:216–217.
19. Taylor SG, O'Dwyer PJ. Chronic groin sepsis following tension-free inguinal hernioplasty. *Br J Surg* 1999;86:562–565.

EDITOR'S COMMENT

Access to large data bases affords the interested investigator an opportunity to develop a unique perspective on any specific medical condition in question. This group has paved the way to a formal and complete analysis of hernia surgery, including elements of process and outcome for an entire nation. They are to be congratulated for the effort. While the data elements allow analysis to define utilization and cost, variables of interest to those providing specific financial support for the health care system, the outcome data are somewhat more sensitive as they reflect the experience of an organization or even an individual surgeon. There will always be a distribution of results for any operation or approach to disease management. To account for those differences, to identify the bases or a basis for differences requires a great deal of diligence in selecting variables and presenting data. The latter must be conducted in the least threatening fashion possible. The former must address issues that allow stratification of patient populations, so that any outcome measure is risk-adjusted to account for patient variation.

It is difficult to argue against a data-referenced system. How the data are gathered—there is often an error rate—how they are verified, and whether they are verified, how they are processed and analyzed, and how they are reported, and to whom, in what form and format are complex questions. For exercises of this sort, worthy as they are, one could predict resistance from many quarters. The ultimate impact of a less-than-satisfactory "report card," for lack of a better term, with reference to financial support, patient referrals, and eventual practice patterns must be considered in the design and implementation of such detailed systems. There is little doubt that sociopolitical structures, from hospitals to countries, play a role in how the data are to be used.

Data of this sort should be used to improve health care, however that is defined prospectively. If "adverse information" is generated, however that is defined, the root cause of observed differences—from accepted and defined reference standards— must be identified. *Once this information is in hand, a corrective action educational plan can be developed, its methods and goals defined, and its implementation secured. Only when all the participants have the same objective, quality patient care, will the plan succeed. While it is desirable to keep the process* blameless, *the very nature of cultural differences may make that aspect of the plan most difficult.*

A.G.G.

Nyhus and Condon's Hernia, Fifth Edition, edited by Robert J. Fitzgibbons, Jr. and A. Gerson Greenburg. Lippincott Williams & Wilkins, Philadelphia © 2002.

49

CLINICAL RESEARCH

JAMES O. GIBBS
DOMENIC J. REDA
WILLIAM G. HENDERSON
DOROTHY D. DUNLOP
OLGA JONASSON
LEIGH A. NEUMAYER

The efficacy of hernia operations has, in the past, been judged by clinical series, recurrence rate, and, to a lesser extent, morbidity and charges. Most of the clinical series were generated in specialty centers that had a particular interest in a certain operation. Extrapolation of results from such hernia-enthusiast centers with a vested interest toward publishing good results introduces bias. Not surprisingly, the practicing general surgeon often could not reproduce the same results. In addition, society has come to demand that surgical interventions be evaluated in terms of impact on the patient's quality of life as well as clinical outcomes. For this reason, clinical series are being replaced by impartial discharge audits, and health-related quality-of-life outcomes are being assessed. Society is now demanding accountability for its health care expenditures. Charges, which do not consider cost shifting and other factors, are no longer considered acceptable measures by which to compare treatments. The health care provider now must have a way to measure the true costs of recommended treatment modalities, including societal costs and nonfinancial costs.

A clinical trial is the "gold standard" that one might use to compare different treatments in an objective fashion with the express purpose of eliminating bias. This chapter briefly summarizes the nature of a clinical trial, discusses steps and issues in designing a trial, describes a clinical trials course

available to the surgeon investigator, and gives an overview of research funding sources. In the Appendix (page 584), the protocol for the Department of Veterans Affairs (VA) cooperative study to compare laparoscopic and open, tension-free herniorrhaphy is provided. This recently activated trial can serve as a model for the reader considering other comparative projects.

THE NATURE OF A CLINICAL TRIAL

Controlled clinical trials are randomized, prospective studies that are designed to evaluate new treatments and procedures. Patients are randomly assigned to intervention and control groups. Usually, the control group receives the standard treatment, or in some trials, a placebo. Some studies are designed to evaluate more than one experimental or alternative treatment, and patients are randomized to more than one treatment arm. After treatment is administered, the groups are compared on outcomes of interest, such as mortality, morbidity, and change in patient functional status. For example, in the hernia trial described in the Appendix, patients randomized to laparoscopic repair are compared with those who receive open tension-free repair with regard to recurrence rates and several other outcomes.

Clinical trials are *experimental* studies in which the investigator controls both the assignment of subjects to study groups and the application of the experimental treatment. In contrast, in *observational* studies, the investigator records data without interfering with the course of events. In an observational study of laparoscopic versus open hernia repair, the investigator would compare groups of patients who themselves selected one or the other the type of operation, without assurance that the groups are equivalent on all other factors that might affect outcome. The advantage of the clinical trial is that the experimental design controls

J.O. Gibbs: Institute for Health Services, Research and Policy Studies, Northwestern University, Evanston, Illinois; Cooperative Studies Program Coordinating Center, The Edward Hines, Jr. VA Hospital, Hines, Illinois.
D.J. Reda, W.G. Henderson: Cooperative Studies Program Coordinating Center, The Edward Hines, Jr. VA Hospital, Hines, Illinois.
D.D. Dunlop: Institute for Health Services, Research and Policy Studies, Northwestern University, Evanston, Illinois.
O. Jonasson: Department of Surgery, University of Illinois; American College of Surgeons, Chicago, Illinois.
L.A. Neumayer: Department of Surgery, University of Utah; Department of Surgery, Salt Lake City VA Medical Center, Salt Lake City, Utah.

for the effects of other known and unknown factors that may be related to outcome, and increases confidence that any differences found in outcomes are attributable to the experimental treatment. On the other hand, clinical trials may be more difficult to perform because subjects must consent to random assignment to treatment, and this assignment may raise ethical issues not present in observational studies.

The results of clinical trials should be distinguished from the performance measures that hospitals and group practices are increasingly using to convince third party payers and the public of their merit. These measures, although sometimes referred to as outcomes, are intended to describe the performance of the institution on selected quality indicators such as risk-adjusted mortality and morbidity and patient satisfaction. They are not based on clinical trials. They are derived from patient surveys and administrative records.

WHEN SHOULD A CLINICAL TRIAL BE DONE?

Several factors should be considered when deciding whether a clinical trial should be done. When a new surgical technique is in development, it probably is too early to conduct a large randomized trial. The technique may be in a period of rapid refinement. There is also likely to be a relatively small number of surgeons who can perform the procedure. There may not be enough preliminary safety or efficacy data to justify subjecting a large number of people to the procedure.

On the other hand, once a procedure has gained widespread acceptance, it may be too late to conduct a randomized study. Between these two extremes, a promising treatment emerges, surgeons and patients become familiar with the technique, and safety and efficacy data accumulate, usually from case reports, case series, and small studies. At some point in this process, the general perception of the usefulness of the emerging treatment is in a state of equipoise; that is, opposing viewpoints are held in balance and there is general consensus that the efficacy and safety of the new treatment in comparison with existing treatments remain an open question. At this time, justification for a randomized trial is strongest.

In practice, though, it may be difficult at this time to find surgeons whose opinion is truly in equipoise. While equipoise may exist among the community of surgeons— that is, half believing the treatment is effective, half believing it is not—individual surgeons may have a definite preference and may be unwilling to randomize patients to what they consider to be an inferior treatment. Even so, the window of time during which equipoise exists is the optimal time to conduct the randomized trial.

DESIGNING A CLINICAL TRIAL
Defining the Objectives of the Study

A research proposal for a clinical trial should begin with a concise definition of objectives. It is important to have a clear statement of the research objective(s) because (a) it helps the researcher to stay focused on the main issue(s) of the study and not be diverted by peripheral issues; (b) the remainder of the research design follows from the statement of the objectives; (c) it helps the researcher communicate the research ideas to the reviewers, which will ultimately affect approval and funding decisions; and (d) it helps define priorities for data analysis and report writing.

The number of study objectives should be limited; that is, the study should be focused and not too diffuse. The investigator should not try to cover too many issues in one study. These are better handled in multiple smaller studies. If there are several desired objectives, the researcher should divide them into primary and secondary objectives. The primary objective(s) should be limited ideally to one and at most two objectives. This is the basis for determining the study sample size. The secondary objectives are generally related to secondary outcome variables, subsets of the study sample, or research issues other than the main issue of the study. Secondary objectives are often exploratory in nature, which may require further research for definitive answers.

The following elements should be contained in the primary research objective: the population to be studied; identification of the experimental intervention; identification of the comparison group; and the primary outcome of interest. An example of a primary objective is the following:

To compare laparoscopic hernia repair (experimental intervention) to open tension-free mesh hernia repair (comparison group) on recurrence of hernia (primary outcome) in men presenting with symptomatic inguinal hernias (population).

Background and Rationale

After a statement of objectives, the investigator should provide the background and rationale for the trial. This should include (a) a description of the disease being studied and its prevalence in the population, which will convey to the reader the importance of the problem; (b) previous work on the development of the intervention(s) under evaluation; and (c) a description of the results of previous observational and randomized trials using the interventions, and how the proposed study will contribute to this body of knowledge. If enough data from previous studies are available, a metaanalysis could be done to help estimate event rates or expected treatment effects that will be useful in later sample size calculations. If new methodologies are being proposed in the conduct of the study, their backgrounds and previous studies developing the methodologies should also be described.

Patient Selection

Once the population of interest is specified in the primary research objective, most study protocols also specify certain inclusion and exclusion factors to define patient selection in more detail. Inclusion factors are generally related to the disease of interest, possibly including some qualifiers related to stage or severity of disease, and perhaps some demographic variables such as gender or age. More specific exclusion factors are also often defined. These are generally related to one of four factors: (a) medical conditions that prevent the patient from ethically being randomized to any of the treatment groups; (b) medical conditions that may prevent observation of the primary outcome; (c) conditions that result in high likelihood of the patient being lost to follow-up; or (d) patient unable or refusing to give informed consent. Exclusion criteria should be kept to a minimum, because they will limit generalizability of the study and will make it more difficult to meet recruitment targets.

It is helpful in the proposal to define the expected recruitment sources for the patients. It is also useful to define a specific population that will be screened for possible inclusion in the study. A screening form containing basic data on patient demographics (age, gender, race), disease severity, and comorbidities should be collected on all included and excluded patients. These data will be useful later for comparing included versus excluded patients to evaluate generalizability of the study, and could be used to evaluate loosening entry criteria in the middle of the study if recruitment targets are not being met. In some studies, it might be beneficial to consider collecting a minimal amount of follow-up data on excluded patients (e.g., treatment received and outcomes) to further evaluate generalizability of the study.

Defining Treatment Groups

Clinical trials in surgery typically involve comparing several different surgical techniques, or possibly one surgical technique to medical treatment, a medical device, or occasionally "watchful waiting" (i.e., no surgical intervention, with the patient carefully followed and offered treatment if his or her condition significantly worsens). It is important that the treatments given be carefully defined, so that the people conducting the trial treat patients uniformly and the readers of the study understand what treatments have been evaluated.

In drug trials, the type of drug, dosage, frequency of administration, and duration of treatment are carefully defined. Similarly, the specific techniques of the operation should be defined in a surgical trial. For example, in a hernia operation this might include anesthesia method, equipment used, location and method of incision, handling of internal structures, replacement of bowel loop in abdominal cavity, closing and reinforcement of abdominal wall using simple stitching or sterile mesh, closure of the incision, and postoperative care. Although different surgeons have their own preferences about what methods to use, all operating surgeons in a trial should agree to perform the operation in a uniform fashion.

There should be a specified level of experience required for all surgeons in the trial (e.g., 25 or more operations). Most new operations have a learning curve before the surgeon becomes proficient enough to consistently obtain good results.

A data form should be designed to collect important information about the operation. These data might include date and times of operation, surgeon, anesthesia used, surgical technique, blood loss and blood replaced, medications used, intra- and postoperative complications, postoperative vital status, and length of hospital stay.

Outcome Measures

In the planning stage, it is decided how the treatments will be compared, that is, what measures will be evaluated to determine whether the treatment effects differ or not. These are called outcome measures. An example of an outcome measure is hernia recurrence, which is the primary outcome measure in the study of laparoscopic versus open hernia repair described in the Appendix (page 584). The same study also measures other treatment effects, such as pain and time to return to normal activities.

Designating Primary and Secondary Outcome Measures

Ultimately, in the hypothesis-testing framework, the investigator seeks to make a decision regarding whether to recommend one treatment over the other. In so doing, a hierarchy might be imposed on the outcome measures, one or more being designated as primary and the remainder as secondary outcome measures. This hierarchy should result in designating as primary the outcome measure(s) that would be most influential in judging the comparative worth of the two treatments.

Once this designation is made, the study design process proceeds with estimating how many patients would be needed to be able to detect a prespecified treatment difference in the primary outcome measure with reasonable certainty.

In general, selection of a single primary outcome measure is preferred because it simplifies both the sample size estimation process and, ultimately, the evaluation of study results and recommendation about treatment selection. When there are several primary outcome measures, the required sample size estimate increases in order to control the overall likelihood of falsely concluding the two treatments are different when, in fact, no differences exist. In addition, multiple primary outcome measures complicate the decision process since one outcome measure may indicate treatment A is better than treatment B while another may indicate it to be inferior. In those cases, it is not possible to arrive at a summary conclusion about the two treatments. Occasionally, full evaluation of treatments may require designating multiple primary outcome measures, especially if one outcome measure does not fully capture the range of possible treatment effects that are considered important.

Assessment of Patient-Based Health Outcomes

The outcome of operative treatment has usually been measured by rates of mortality and morbidity accompanying the operation. These outcomes focus on the negative consequences of treatment. If the purpose of the intervention is to improve patients' health and well-being, it is also important to document improvements in quality of life. Health-related quality of life (HRQoL) refers to the ability to function physically, socially, and in one's usual role activities; freedom from pain; and perception of positive health status. It can be measured with generic instruments, allowing comparison of outcomes across conditions and procedures, and with procedure-specific measures that focus on pain and the type of functioning directly associated with a particular condition or procedure.

HRQoL is classified as a "patient-based" outcome because it is measured from the patient's point of view. Patient satisfaction is another patient-based outcome that is increasingly included in the evaluation of treatment. Measuring patient-based outcomes need not increase the number of primary outcome measures. If the primary outcome is a clinical measurement, patient-based outcomes can be included as important secondary outcomes.

Avoiding Bias in Assessing Outcomes

Well-designed clinical studies incorporate features intended to minimize bias. The potential for bias and the possible sources of bias depend on the type of outcome measure and the degree to which the assigned treatment is masked to the patient and the investigator. It is generally thought that "hard" end points such as a laboratory result are less likely to be affected by bias than "soft" end points such as a diagnosis. Such "soft" end points could be affected by both patient and investigator bias, especially when the assigned treatment intervention is known to both. For example, the patient's likelihood of seeking medical advice for a potential complication may be influenced by their knowledge of which procedure was done. The investigator may have a prior bias that one procedure is more likely to produce a certain adverse outcome and may inadvertently evaluate a patient who received that procedure more carefully.

Since personal expectations of the patient or physician regarding a treatment can influence the outcome, *blinding,*

in which the treatment assignment is masked, is widely used to eliminate this potential source of bias. When both the patient and the evaluating physician are unaware of the treatment assignment (i.e., control or intervention), the study is referred to as a double-blind study.

Blinding is often difficult in a surgical trial. Sham surgery for the control group has occasionally been done, but there are obvious ethical dilemmas with this approach. A blinded evaluator who is not part of the treatment team can sometimes be used. Also, if the clinical outcome can be evaluated by a diagnostic or laboratory test (e.g., coronary artery graft patency from an angiogram), a blinded central reading laboratory can be established.

It is important to provide clear definitions of end points and provide for objective assessment of outcomes. In the VA hernia study described in the Appendix, specific criteria for assessment of recurrence of a hernia were defined because surgeons differ in the criteria they use to diagnose a recurrence. To avoid bias in the assessment of the outcome (recurrence), a surgeon other than the one who performed the procedure and the study nurse assess recurrence. In the case of disagreement, an additional assessment is to be obtained by (a) another independent surgeon, (b) ultrasound, or (c) the reoperation report.

Selection of Site Principal Investigator and Participating Surgeons

In multisite, cooperative studies, it is important to carefully consider the qualifications of prospective site principal investigators (PIs) and participating surgeons. The site PI has overall responsibility for site performance and must be able to recruit qualified participating surgeons.

In the VA study of laparoscopic versus open hernia repair, it was necessary to determine that sites had at least one participating surgeon qualified to perform preperitoneal laparoscopic herniorrhaphy, as well as surgeons experienced in the Lichtenstein open tension-free repair. When newer surgical techniques are evaluated, it is a good idea to develop methods for assessing and monitoring surgeon performance. The VA study (see Appendix, page 584) required that prospective participating surgeons submit the outcomes of their ten most recent consecutive cases, and these cases were analyzed for early recurrence and perioperative complications; surgeons with excess (10% or more) early recurrences or excess complications were required to be assisted by an experienced surgeon, with demonstrated satisfactory outcomes, during the next ten cases. In addition, to ensure adherence to the study protocols, two surgeons with expertise in open and laparoscopic tension-free repair visited each site during the first 6 months of the study to observe operative procedures.

The site PI must also ensure timely and accurate data collection. Most studies require a site coordinator for the day-to-day administration of the project, and the site PI must be able to recruit and supervise a qualified person for this position.

Randomization and Stratification

Many extraneous factors can contribute to a person's response to an intervention (e.g., patient cooperation, patient education, physician communication). *Random assignment* of patients to treatment groups provides three key safeguards for assuring that the outcome of the study reflects differences due to the intervention rather than outside factors. First, randomization provides an objective method to assign patients to treatment groups, removing any subjective bias in the allocation of participants. Second, randomization balances uncontrollable extraneous factors (e.g., patient's diet and exercise lifestyle) between the intervention and control groups. Third, randomization provides a basis for valid statistical tests. Recognizing that people are not test tubes, it is essentially impossible to select two groups of people who are identically equal. The solution is to select patients who are probabilistically equal; that is, they have an equal chance of being assigned to the control or intervention treatment. This assumption forms the foundation for statistical testing.

Stratification is used to equalize controllable factors across the treatment groups. Strata are defined by important controllable factors that could bias the study results. Since practical logistics limit the number of stratification factors, a useful exercise is to list all factors that would threaten the validity of the study results if the treatment groups were not balanced on those factors due to an "unlucky" randomization. Those factors are then ranked, and the two or three most important factors are used to define the study strata. For example, the hernia protocol in the Appendix has three stratification factors: (a) study site; (b) hernia type: primary or recurrent; and (c) number: unilateral or bilateral. Randomization is done separately within each stratum. In the hernia study example, four separate randomization lists are maintained for *each* study site: primary unilateral, primary bilateral, recurrent unilateral, recurrent bilateral. In a multisite study, it is usually a good idea to stratify by site because of site differences in surgeons and patient populations.

A simple general rule succinctly summarizes the role of randomization and stratification for balancing controllable and uncontrollable extraneous factors across the treatment groups. Stratify what you can control. Randomize what you cannot control.

Data Collection and Entry

In bench research and small clinical studies, it is typical for the method by which data will be recorded to be decided at the time of data collection. Often data are recorded on blank sheets of paper or in a spreadsheet format. This works quite well in small studies.

In multicenter trials involving large numbers of patients with multiple protocol visits and perhaps hundreds of variables per patient, a higher level of organization is needed. The data collection instruments, traditionally paper case report forms, should be developed in advance of the start of data collection. It is often helpful to borrow well-developed instruments from previous studies. When a new instrument is needed, the proposed case report form should undergo pilot testing so that any problems with the design of the form can be corrected prior to the start of data collection.

Until the mid-1980s, the data collection format for virtually all clinical trials was the paper case report form. With the advent of the personal computer (PC) and the Internet revolution, the paper format is no longer preeminent. Several electronic technologies have emerged, including facsimile/scanning and remote data entry.

The paper case report form is generally viewed as the most convenient, because of its flexibility and ease of integration into routine clinic visits. With this approach, forms are generally completed as the study visit is conducted, and then mailed to a central site, where they are reviewed, entered into a computer, and electronically checked for errors. With this process, there can be a significant delay from the original completion of a data form until a site is informed of the results of the central review.

Facsimile/scanning technologies move the forms into the study database more quickly by eliminating the mailing step. Well-designed systems also automate the review of the scanned form for more rapid feedback to the site where the data problem originated. However, scanning works best for data in which responses can be circled or checked, such as multiple-choice questions. Open-ended types of data fields, such as a blood chemistry, in which results are entered into blank data fields, are more prone to scanning errors, especially when the entered data include alphabetic characters.

Distributed systems are divided into two types. For both, data are entered into a PC at the site. For strictly PC-based systems, the data entry screens are entirely resident on the PC; the data are stored on the PC, and then periodically transmitted to the central site either by modem or by mailing a diskette of downloaded data. The other type of system uses a PC as a gateway to the Internet. Data entry screens are accessed through the Internet connection, and data forms are sent to the central site as they are completed. The advantages of these systems are twofold. First, the data entry screens are capable of having embedded logic, which coaches the person entering the data when an invalid response is entered, thus improving data quality. Second, electronic data transmission reduces the time until the data are ready for analysis.

While electronic systems facilitate data quality and speed the data collection/review cycle, they require a technically literate staff at the sites. They also are more difficult to modify if the need for protocol modifications arises.

Because each type of system is optimized for specific situations, choice of system is often not clear-cut. The VA hernia repair trial includes a large number of case report forms that are completed by the study subjects. Because of that, the traditional paper case report form was chosen. Three concerns influenced the decision. First, it was not clear whether study subjects were familiar enough with PCs to complete electronic questionnaires. Second, some of the patient assessments involved the study subjects completing diaries at home. Third, it was thought more important to have the site staff focus their time on patient recruitment and follow-up rather than entering patient questionnaires and diaries into the computer.

Sample Size

The sample size, the number of patients to be entered into the study, is a key decision determined during the study design. An adequate sample size will provide sufficient statistical power to detect clinically meaningful differences between the treatment groups and place bounds on the likelihood of incorrectly declaring treatment group differences. The sample size is typically determined with the help of a statistician because the calculation depends on the statistical method that will be used to test the primary hypothesis. However, key components influencing the sample size require the input of the principal investigator and other central decision makers. First, the primary hypothesis must be firmly in place. Related information is usually needed on the mean and variance of the event rate of the primary outcome. A search of the literature or a pilot study may be needed to provide estimates of these quantities. Second, the magnitude of a clinically important difference between the intervention and control groups must be determined. This defines the smallest treatment difference of clinical interest that can be supported by sound rationale. Third, the minimum power of the study must be determined. Power is the probability of correctly detecting this clinically important treatment difference, if it exists, through statistical testing. Good studies are generally designed for at least 80% power. Finally, a bound is set on the probability of incorrectly concluding the treatments are different. In statistical jargon, this is the probability of a type I error or α. Generally, this error rate bound is set at $\alpha = 0.05$ or less.

Meeting Patient Recruitment Targets

Underrecruitment of patients is a significant problem in clinical trials. When significant underrecruitment occurs, the ability of the study to arrive at a definitive answer regarding treatment comparisons is compromised. The likelihood of failing to detect a treatment difference when, in fact, one exists increases as the achieved sample size decreases.

In addition, funding mechanisms for studies generally require that the total duration of intake be fixed, that is, there is no flexibility to automatically extend the study if

recruitment is slower than expected. Therefore, a realistic estimate of the recruitment rate as well as the available pool of patients is needed in order to determine how many sites are required, as well as the length of the recruitment period.

Some sources of information that may be helpful are disease prevalence and incidence rates, patient census information for sites under consideration, and recruitment patterns from previous studies in that disease area. Often, pilot studies are used to simulate the recruitment process. For the VA hernia study, discharge record files were used to determine the number of hernia patients and the number of hernia operations performed at potential sites during a prior year as a basis for selecting sites and for determining the length of the recruitment period.

Completeness of Follow-up

Although randomization eliminates systematic pretreatment differences between the groups being compared, it cannot control differences not attributable to the treatments from being introduced during the treatment/follow-up phase of the study. In order to preserve the benefits of randomization, the comparison groups should be treated identically (apart from the randomly assigned treatment) after randomization.

Missing data will invariably arise in randomized clinical trials. When possible, the reason that a data item, an entire component of an evaluation, or an entire visit is not completed should be recorded. This will aid in evaluating the potential for treatment comparisons to be biased.

When the reason for missing data is related to the outcome measures in the study, resultant analyses will be biased. For example, if patients in one treatment group feel better than patients in the other group, they may be more likely to adhere to the treatment regimen, maintain the required follow-up schedule, and complete all components of an evaluation. When this occurs, a summary of the data collected in the other group is likely to exclude the worst cases, making the inferior treatment appear to be better than it actually is.

One particularly vexing problem is the view among many clinicians that patients should no longer be evaluated as part of the study if they do not follow the study protocol, or if treatment is discontinued because it is no longer considered effective or safe for the patient. While this may seem clinically reasonable, it has the unfortunate effect of introducing the same type of biases as described above.

The preferred approach is to follow all patients for the full follow-up period, regardless of their adherence to the assigned treatment regimen. The primary analysis, designated as "intention to treat," will include all randomized patients categorized into their original randomized groups, and is considered to be the only valid statistical comparison in a randomized study. Many researchers will also prefer to do an analysis based on the subset of patients who follow the treatment protocol. Because it may be a biased analysis, this should be relegated to a secondary analysis. Typically, both types of analysis are done. If the results of both analyses are in agreement, then only the intention-to-treat analysis is reported. If they disagree, then both sets of results may be reported. In the latter case, the analysis should also include a characterization of the patients who did not follow the treatment protocol.

Analyses and Publication

As with all other aspects of the study, consideration of the analysis of the study data should be done during the planning phase of the project. This should include an analytic as well as a publication plan.

Analyses should focus on addressing the primary and secondary objectives of the study. The analytic plan should include (a) a characterization of the patients who were screened but excluded from the study, (b) baseline characteristics of the study sample, (c) whether there are any differences between the treatment groups at baseline, (d) assessment of the completeness of adherence to the study regimens, (e) ascertainment of the completeness of follow-up and reasons for early withdrawal from the study, (f) summary of major protocol deviations such as misrandomizations, (g) efficacy analyses, (h) identification of potential prognostic factors whose impact on the treatment effects will be evaluated, (i) appropriate safety analyses, and (j) how missing data will be handled.

The importance of a prespecified analytic plan cannot be overemphasized. When a statistically meaningful result emerges from an analysis that was specified in advance of data collection, the potential for attaching importance to a spurious result is reduced. In addition, the possibility of the investigator's biases influencing the direction of the analysis is also minimized.

While *post hoc* analyses will invariably be done, statistically significant relationships found in such analyses should be treated as hypothesis generating rather than definitive.

A prespecified publication plan will be easier to conceptualize once the analytic plan is devised. Publication plans should identify the primary and secondary papers that will be written to report the study results, and may include a timetable for development as well as identification of an individual to lead the development effort of each paper. Particularly for initial trials of new operative techniques, it is worthwhile to write a "methods" manuscript describing the protocol and research design of the study. Before completion of data collection, it may be appropriate to publish descriptive findings and preliminary test group comparisons on outcome measures. In addition to a primary manuscript describing the main results of the trial, secondary papers may focus on secondary outcomes or subgroups of patients. For example, the writing plan for the VA hernia study includes secondary papers on the subgroups of patients with bilateral and recurrent hernias.

It is helpful to establish a writing committee that will monitor the publication process as well as review drafts of manuscripts and requests for *post hoc* analyses. Finally, specification of rules for authorship during study planning may eliminate potential conflicts during the manuscript-writing phase of the study.

Human Rights Considerations

The research proposal should include a brief description of the procedures that will be used in the study to obtain the patient's voluntary consent to participate. This description specifies who can solicit consent, when consent can be solicited, and under what circumstances. There should be a comprehensive discussion of the ethical considerations that apply to the study. The investigator should identify all of the issues believed to be of importance from a human rights perspective. There should be some indication of the degree of risk and a description of the safeguards to protect the patients. The purpose of this discussion is to inform reviewers of potential risks as well as to facilitate review by the institutional review board (IRB). All potential funding agencies will require review of the proposal and patient consent forms by an IRB.

Study subjects indicate their willingness to participate in a study by signing a consent form. This document should describe the study in language that will be easily understood by the participant, so that a reasonable decision concerning participation can be made. It should include information about the procedures to be used, the potential risks and benefits of participation, alternate therapies in lieu of participation, and statements indicating that participation is voluntary and that the participant can withdraw from the trial at any time without prejudice. Usually, the investigator's local IRB will provide guidelines for developing informed consent forms.

Quality Control

While a well-designed protocol is essential to conduct a study that has a reasonable chance of addressing the objectives of the research, even the most thoughtfully written protocol will not achieve its goals if the conduct of the study is haphazard.

There are several strategies typically employed whose purpose is to assure that the data collected in the study are valid and reliable. During the development phase of the proposal, it is preferable to select clinical and laboratory procedures that have already been demonstrated to be valid and reliable.

A manual of operations should be written, which will be used as an instruction manual on how the participating sites should manage the day-to-day operations of the study. This manual should contain instructions on how to complete the case report forms, and how to perform the study interventions and evaluations of the patients. Additional reference materials such as coding lists (e.g., medications, adverse events, previous definition of diagnostic terms) should also be included.

Prior to study initiation, all laboratories providing study data should certify that they are using acceptable methods of analysis and that the reliability of the measurements is sufficient. Participating sites should have a study initiation visit to evaluate whether the site is ready to begin the study.

A study initiation meeting is essential to provide a thorough review of the protocol and operations manual, and training of study interventions and evaluations. In surgical trials, it may be necessary to have the study chair visit each site and observe several operations.

During the data collection phase, there should be continual interaction between the sites and the coordinating center. This office should monitor the performance of each site with regard to recruitment and retention of patients, adherence to the study protocol, and data completeness and quality. When possible, this monitoring should include periodic visits to each site to observe study operations and to check the data recorded on the case report forms with supporting documentation in the patient's medical record.

Most multicenter clinical trials have an external oversight committee whose responsibility it is to monitor the progress of the study. This data and safety monitoring board (DSMB) is the only group connected with the study that views the treatment comparison data during the data collection phase of the study. The DSMB evaluates whether the study is being conducted properly, whether any revisions to the protocol are needed, and whether the study should continue.

AMERICAN COLLEGE OF SURGEONS CLINICAL TRIALS COURSE

Starting in 1998, the American College of Surgeons (ACS) has sponsored an annual 5-day course on the design of clinical trials for beginning and midlevel surgical investigators. The course is taught by ten faculty members: five surgeons experienced in clinical research and five clinical trial biostatisticians. The course consists of 14 lecture/discussion sessions on various aspects of designing a clinical trial, interspersed with breakout sessions during which students are divided into five to six planning committees to design a clinical trial.

The lecture sessions include such topics as defining hypotheses, selection of patients, stratification and randomization, defining interventions, defining end points, statistical analysis, sample size determination, planning measurements, trial management, ethical issues, funding sources, and publication of results. The knowledge gained in the lec-

tures is then applied in the breakout sessions to design an actual clinical trial. On the last day of the course, the student groups take turns presenting their clinical trials and receiving critiques from other students and faculty in the audience. The course has been taught several times and has received excellent feedback. For more information, contact the ACS.[1]

RESEARCH FUNDING

The major source of funding for clinical research is the National Institutes of Health (NIH). The goals of NIH-supported research are to advance the understanding of biologic systems, improve the control of disease, and enhance health. NIH includes 18 institutes. The institutes are organized primarily by disease type (e.g., the National Cancer Institute) and organ systems (e.g., the National Heart, Lung, and Blood Institute). There is no separate institute for surgery, but surgery trials are relevant for most of the institutes.

The National Institutes of Health System of Review

The peer-review system for grant applications used by NIH is based on two sequential levels of review, referred to as the "dual-review system." The first level involves panels of experts established according to scientific disciplines or current research areas for the primary purpose of evaluating the scientific and technical merit of grant applications. These panels are referred to as scientific review groups (SRGs), which are commonly called study sections. Investigators can request that a grant application be assigned to a particular study section. Therefore, it is worthwhile to learn the composition and interests of the various study sections. The second level of review is performed by a national advisory board or council composed of both scientific and public representatives who are noted for their expertise, interest, or activity in matters related to the mission of the specific institute that they serve. Council recommendations are based not only on considerations of scientific merit (as judged by the SRGs), but also on the relevance of the proposed study to an institute's programs and priorities.

National Institutes of Health Grant Review Criteria

The grant review criteria used by NIH have been modified recently. The major change is that, for the first time, the criteria for evaluating grant proposals include "innovation." This may be helpful to junior investigators (those without a proven track record) because it may increase the risk that reviewers and the funding agency are willing to take in funding research. Until now, the criteria have favored established researchers and research with substantial preliminary data. The new evaluation criteria are:

1. Significance (Does the study address an important problem?)
2. Approach (Are the design and methods appropriate to address the aims?)
3. Innovation (Does the project employ novel concepts, approaches, or methods?)
4. Investigator (Is the investigator appropriately trained to carry out the study?)
5. Environment (Will the scientific environment contribute to the probability of success?)

The Young Surgical Investigator Conference

A valuable resource for new investigators is the Young Surgical Investigator Conference, convened biennially (even years) by the Surgical Research and Education Committee of the ACS. The conference is held in proximity to the NIH campus, and provides an opportunity for young surgical investigators to meet established surgical investigators and staff from NIH—from the individual institutes and from the Center for Scientific Review (the home of study sections and the center of the peer-review process). The goal of these conferences is to introduce young surgeons to the process, the content, the style, and the people involved in successful grant writing and interactions with NIH. The conference takes place over a 2-day period and is attended by approximately 200 young surgical investigators, 50 established surgical investigators who facilitate grantsmanship workshops and mock study sections, and 35 NIH staff members. This conference has been very successful, as measured by the success rate of conference attendees in obtaining grant awards from NIH and other extramural funding sources. Information about the conference can be obtained from the Education and Surgical Services Department of the ACS.[1]

Other Sources of Funding

In addition to NIH, there are other government agencies that fund clinical trials. The Cooperative Studies Program (CSP) of the Veterans Health Administration supports clinical trials that focus on medical problems that are common and relevant to the veteran population.[2] The hernia repair study described in the Appendix (page 584) is an example of a VA cooperative study. The CSP has several coordinating centers throughout the country that support the investigator in proposing and executing a multisite research project. VA's Health Services Research and Development

Program is another potential source of funding.[3] The focus of health services research includes the evaluation of the outcomes of different treatments. VA research studies require that the principal investigator be at least a five-eighths time VA employee.

The Agency for Healthcare Research and Quality (AHRQ), formerly the Agency for Health Care Policy and Research (AHCPR), a component of the U.S. Department of Health and Human Services, Public Health Service, is the federal government's focal point for research to enhance the quality, appropriateness, and effectiveness of health care services and access to those services.[4] Surgical trials that evaluate new surgical techniques or surgical versus medical management of disease are relevant to AHRQ's focus on ways to improve the effectiveness and appropriateness of clinical practice.

Many surgical specialty societies and private foundations support surgical research. A convenient compilation of research support available from the specialty societies is the ACS's Surgical Research Clearinghouse.[1]

Resources for Grant Writing

The ACS makes available a number of guides for proposal writing on its Web site.[1] "Proposal Writing: The Business of Science" provides tips on how to write each major section of a proposal. "Young Surgical Investigators' Guide to Grant Application" is a slide presentation that gives an overview of the application process and guides for writing each section of a proposal.

For personal assistance in designing a study and writing the statistical sections of a grant proposal, a good place to look is academic medical centers and allied professional schools. The medical center may have research centers with biostatisticians on staff. Departments of preventive medicine and schools of public health are good places to look for statistical consultation. Some VA medical centers have active research programs and have biostatisticians on staff.

AN EXAMPLE OF A HERNIA TRIAL

The Appendix includes the protocol for a recently activated VA cooperative study of laparoscopic versus open hernia repair. It is intended to provide an example of a clinical trial, and it should be useful as a model or template for the reader who is considering other trials. It was developed by VA surgical and research staff in collaboration with the ACS and Northwestern University researchers. Funding was awarded by VA's CSP in 1998 after review by an external scientific review committee. Patient intake began in January 1999, and the study is scheduled to be completed in 2004.

END NOTES

[1]Department of Education and Surgical Services
American College of Surgeons
633 N. Saint Clair Street
Chicago, Illinois 60601
312/202/5100
http://www.facs.org
Click on the Education and Surgical Services Department link. Then click on the Surgical Research and Education link.

[2]Office of the Chief
Cooperative Studies Program (125)

Department of Veterans Affairs
810 Vermont Avenue, NW
Washington, DC 20420

[3]Office of the Director (124)
Health Services Research and Development Service
Department of Veterans Affairs
810 Vermont Avenue, NW
Washington, DC 20420

[4]Agency for Healthcare Research and Quality
2101 E. Jefferson Street, Suite 501
Rockville, MD 20852
Telephone: (301) 594-1364

APPENDIX

PROTOCOL FOR VA COOPERATIVE STUDY NO. 456[1]
TENSION-FREE INGUINAL HERNIA REPAIR: COMPARISON OF OPEN AND LAPAROSCOPIC SURGICAL TECHNIQUES

PROTOCOL

SPECIFIC AIMS

Primary Aim

To compare open tension-free inguinal hernia repair (Lichtenstein method) with preperitoneal laparoscopic inguinal hernia repair on recurrence rates at 2 years.

Secondary Aims

1. To compare the two operative methods on the following secondary outcomes:

a. Postoperative complications
b. Pain
c. Time to return to normal activities
d. Health-related quality of life
e. Patient satisfaction
f. Caregiver burden
g. Cost

2. To determine the role of comorbidity in influencing postoperative complications, patient-centered outcomes, and cost of inguinal hernia treatment.

Chair: Leigh A. Neumayer, M.D., Chief, Surgical Service, VA Medical Center, Salt Lake City, Utah.

Cochair: Robert J. Fitzgibbons, Jr., M.D., Professor, Department of Surgery, and Chief, Division of General Surgery, Creighton University, Omaha, Nebraska.

Coordinating Center: Hines VA Cooperative Studies Program Coordinating Center, Hines, Illinois.

---

[1]This protocol was developed by Department of Veterans Affairs (VA) surgical and research staff in collaboration with the American College of Surgeons and Northwestern University researchers. Funding was awarded by VA's CSP in 1998 after review by an external scientific review committee. Patient intake began in January 1999, and the study is scheduled to be completed in 2004.

The protocol has been edited for this Appendix. Some sections have been updated to include changes made since the protocol was originally submitted for review. The following material from the original protocol is not included in this Appendix: Abstract; Investigator Experience; Budget; Curricula Vitae; Data Forms; Patient Consent Form; and Patient Instructions.

BACKGROUND AND SIGNIFICANCE

Inguinal hernia is a common condition, especially in men, appearing in all age groups with peak incidence in the newborn, young adult, and elderly populations (148). A National Health Survey on Hernia, conducted in 1960, determined that hernias occur at a rate of 15/1,000 population (32). Surgical repair of inguinal hernias represents a large component of health care effort and expenditures with approximately 700,000 herniorrhaphies performed each year in the United States (24,142), at great cost to the health care system. In the Veterans Health Administration (VHA), inguinal hernia repairs account for 10% of all general surgery procedures (10,000 per year). Costs to the economy are also large, as herniorrhaphy patients in the workforce convalesce (137). Recently developed tension-free methods have been found to be superior to traditional, tension-producing techniques, both in terms of rate of recurrence and patient-centered outcomes. The newly introduced minimal access (laparoscopic) tension-free techniques for hernia repair are controversial.

The most effective method of repair of an inguinal hernia in any given patient is not clearly defined; choice of procedure is based on the surgeon's level of familiarity and expertise with a procedure rather than on evidence that the procedure is optimal for that patient. Recurrence of the hernia, the customary indicator of failure, occurs in 1% to 10% of patients undergoing a primary repair. A study comparing "conventional" open hernia repair with laparoscopic extraperitoneal hernia repair has recently been published (100); the study found that laparoscopic repair was superior in all respects studied to conventional repair consisting primarily of tension-producing techniques. This study must be repeated in the United States, since conventional *tension-producing* hernia repair methods have now been largely supplanted by open, *tension-free* techniques using prosthetic mesh, the method we propose to compare with the laparoscopic tension-free technique. We hypothesize that the open tension-free repair is comparable or even superior in some respects (complications, convalescence, and rate of recurrence), and will achieve the same degree of patient satisfaction as the laparoscopic repair with more safety and lower cost. The open tension-free repair may prove to be the procedure of choice for repair of most inguinal hernias.

Open tension-free techniques, inserting prosthetic mesh over the defect, are now the most common method of repair of inguinal hernias in the United States (79). The main outcome measure of herniorrhaphy is the rate of recurrence; large specialty centers report rates of recurrence of less than 1% for open tension-free techniques. The recurrence rate in other practices is not known, but is thought to be 5% to 10%. Laparoscopic herniorrhaphy also has a low rate of recurrence in expert hands (1% to 5%), and proponents claim that patients recover more quickly and have less

pain. The open and laparoscopic tension-free repairs have not been compared in a randomized clinical trial of sufficient size and power to be conclusive, and the effectiveness of laparoscopic herniorrhaphy in community practices or in the Veterans Affairs (VA) system is unknown. Since the two approaches differ greatly in requirements for anesthesia and surgical facilities and in cost of the equipment and supplies needed to perform the procedure, we aim to determine whether open tension-free herniorrhaphy can achieve equal or better recurrence rates and lower costs while matching the rate of patient satisfaction with laparoscopic herniorrhaphy.

Classification

Primary inguinal hernias are classified as indirect or direct (118,164). Femoral hernia, a type of acquired inguinal hernia, is not the subject of this study. Indirect inguinal hernias occur as protrusions of bowel through the internal inguinal ring into a sac that may extend into the scrotum. Direct inguinal hernias are acquired as a result of loss of the integrity of the floor of the inguinal canal; these occur medial to the internal inguinal ring. Surgical repair is more difficult to achieve and less certain when hernias are associated with loss of integrity of the floor of the inguinal canal. Recurrent hernias, resulting from a failed attempt at repair, are even more likely to recur after a repeat repair.

Bilateral inguinal hernias occur in 17% of patients presenting to surgeons for treatment [analysis of 42 recent series in which bilateral incidence rate is documented (4,5, 10,15,16,19,25,29,41–43,45,51,64,65,71,72,80,83,87,104, 107,113,114,116,122,123,125,143,152,156,163,165,171, 173,174,176)]. Simultaneous repair of both hernias is now common practice although still somewhat controversial. Wantz (166) cautions against simultaneous repair of indirect inguinal hernias if the distal hernia sac is to be dissected from the cord, to avoid ischemic orchitis; our protocols will avoid distal sac dissection and simultaneous repair will be customary. Recent studies have documented that recurrence on either side is not more common after simultaneous repair, using either open or laparoscopic techniques (4,161). Patients with bilateral inguinal hernias are eligible for enrollment in this study.

Symptoms

Symptoms of an inguinal hernia are a feeling of heaviness, pain, or discomfort in the groin or testicle, usually accompanied by a visible bulge in the inguinal canal or scrotum. Occasionally, the hernia becomes irreducible (incarcerated, or trapped in the inguinal canal). While chronic incarceration may be minimally symptomatic, acute incarceration may cause intestinal obstruction and/or compromise of the blood supply to the entrapped intestine, leading to gangrene and bowel perforation. Patients with an acute hernia emergency will not be eligible for enrollment in this study.

Because the level of preexisting symptoms or disability influences the postoperative patient-centered outcomes (109), the level of patient symptoms related to the hernia will be recorded preoperatively, using a hernia symptom scoring instrument developed in preliminary work (see Preliminary Studies, below).

Comparison of Surgical Techniques

Bassini's classic description in 1889 provided the anatomic basis for repair: suture of the conjoined tendon (internal oblique and transversus abdominis muscles) to the shelving edge of Poupart's (inguinal) ligament, closing the anterior space in the pelvis through which herniation occurs. Modern "conventional" repairs are all variations on Bassini's technique. The two best known are the Shouldice (67,92,150) (approximating the layers of the floor of the inguinal canal in multiple layers) and Cooper ligament (119) (approximation of the conjoined tendon to Cooper's ligament with a relaxing incision in the external oblique aponeurosis above) repairs, although dozens of others have been described. The proliferation of anterior techniques indicates the prevailing unease of surgeons with the reliability of any one of them.

Table 49.1 summarizes the literature on inguinal hernia repair trials. There are few well-designed comparative trials, most reported from European centers (67,95,100); recently, the Shouldice repair was claimed to be the "gold standard" (67). All of these repairs require the approximation of tissues, under tension, which are not normally in apposition. Patients experience pain, often lasting for more than a year (28) and the recurrence rate for hernias after a first repair is 1% to 10%. Low recurrence rates have been reported from single specialized clinics, but are rarely matched in ordinary practice. In a recent study reported from an academic center in Denmark (49), direct hernias (Nyhus type III) were repaired using a Cooper ligament technique; the 2-year recurrence rate was 30%. Indirect hernias (Nyhus type II), repaired with a ringplasty and Bassini technique, recurred at a rate of 4%.

The fact that so many types of repair have been described attests to the frequency of the major complication of the surgical procedure, namely recurrence of the hernia (23,48). The rate of recurrence is generally accepted to be 1% to 10%, with least recurrence in simple, small hernias (23,63) and highest recurrence rate after repair of a recurrent hernia (23). The characteristic *tension* created by overlapping muscle and fascia is considered the root cause of late failure, and the pain and disability occurring uniformly in the postoperative period.

Tension-Free Open Hernia Repair

Newer open surgical techniques, with lower reported rates of recurrence, have avoided the creation of tension by interposition of a nonabsorbable prosthesis made of polypropylene or other material into the defect (153). The *tension-free technique* described by Lichtenstein (99) inserts the prosthesis in a traditional, open surgical procedure that can be performed using local anesthesia (4). Most patients leave the hospital or outpatient surgical center on the day of the operation; proponents of this procedure claim that patients have little pain and disability in the postoperative period because the procedure is tension free. Lichtenstein recorded a personal experience with 6,321 patients with a recurrence rate of 0.7%, including reoperations for recurrent hernias (99). The Lichtenstein tension-free repair with prosthesis is the open technique chosen for this study.

Tension-free anterior (open) repair techniques have gained wide acceptance. In an informal poll of 600 general surgeons in 1995, a tension-free repair with mesh was used alone or in combination with another technique by 70% (79). Most are performed in an ambulatory surgical setting using local anesthesia, and have given good results in terms of reported patient satisfaction and low rates of recurrence (57,99,136). Recurrence rates reported from single centers specializing in hernia repair are less than 1%, and it is claimed that patients have less pain, return to work earlier, and have greater satisfaction than after a conventional repair (long-term patient follow-up is often incomplete). A cost analysis that includes disability and time to return to work as well as operating room costs has not been done.

Tension-Free Laparoscopic Repair

With the advent of minimal access surgical procedures via video-monitored operative laparoscopic techniques, additional "tension-free" hernia repairs have been developed (26,53,54,65,77,100,117,147,158). Laparoscopic techniques are more complex, requiring an experienced surgeon, expensive instrumentation, and general anesthesia in an operating room setting (33). In a large prospective multicenter study (686 patients with 869 hernias), Fitzgibbons et al. have reported both safety and efficacy (a 4.5% recurrence rate after a minimum observation period of 15 months) of the laparoscopic technique (45). Phillips reported results in 3,229 patients, with a recurrence rate of approximately 2% (125).

The laparoscopic approach has enjoyed great popularity with patients and has recently been found, in a large randomized clinical trial, to be superior in all important respects to a variety of conventional (tension-producing) repairs (100). Laparoscopic recurrence in this study from

TABLE 49.1. RECENT PERTINENT LITERATURE CITATIONS, INGUINAL HERNIA REPAIR—COMPARATIVE TRIALS

Citation	No. of Patients	Findings
Bessell et al. (10)	104	Shouldice vs. TEPP: comparable in postop activity levels and return to work; lap required more time in OR. Pain/analgesic use less with TEPP.
Birth et al. (11)	1,000	859 patients with 1,000 hernias (14% bilateral). 117 recurrent hernias (11.7%). All done laparoscopically with TAPP. 7.6% complications and 11 early recurrences.
Davies et al. (30)	300	All laparoscopic (TAPP) 265 patients with 300 hernias (11.6% bilateral, 10.3% recurrent). Seen at 6 mo by independent observer and then annually with no late recurrence to date with two-thirds followed >1 yr.
Friis and Lindahl (49)	208	Randomized to Lichtenstein vs. Cooper's ligament (direct hernias) vs. ring-plasty (indirect hernias). 18% recurrent. Recurrence rate for primary direct hernias 7% for tension-free vs. 30% for Cooper's ligament repair. No difference in complications.
Lukaszczyk et al. (106)	157	Nonrandomized; 157 hernias in 151 patients; lap (TAPP) in 50, conventional open in 107. 72 min for lap vs. 52 min for open. No differences in return to work, driving car, getting in/out of bed comfortably.
Sandbichler et al. (144)	200	Lap repair (TAPP) of recurrent hernias only. 39% had recurred within 2 yr of original operation. Patients described postop pain as much less severe than previous (open) operation. One recurrence (0.5%) at 6 mo.
Schrenk et al. (146)	86	34 Shouldice vs. 28 TAPP and 24 TEPP. TAPP had lowest VAS on mobilization on d 0 (TEPP and Shouldice equivalent) and d 1 (TEPP); all equivalent at d 2–30. Patient satisfaction (analgesic use, return to physical activity, sexual intercourse, return to work) all equivalent.
Toy et al. (157)	441	TAPP repair in 441 hernias in 351 patients (20% bilateral, 21% recurrent). 3.8% recurrence; after 25 cases per surgeon, recurrence fell to 0.39%. Return to work in 7.7 d.
Wilson et al. (173)	242	121 TAPP vs. 121 Lichtenstein. 13% bilateral, 12% recurrent. No difference in OR time, postop VAS or analgesic use.
Lawrence et al. (95)	125	TAPP vs. darn repair of primary unilateral hernia. Primary outcome = safety (short-term complications); secondary = pain (VAS) and QOL, cost. 10% greater complications in lap, less pain on movement but not at rest for lap. Pain and some functional activity better at 10 d and 6 wk in lap, shorter time to return to work.
Barkun et al. (6)	92	Primary unilateral hernias; TEPP or TAPP vs. variety of open (35% tension-free). Duration of convalescence = primary outcome; pain, QOL, LOS, complications = secondary. No differences at 30 d; cost higher for lap.
Tschudi et al. (160)	87	TAPP vs. Shouldice, randomly assigned. Outcome measures: pain, op time, LOS, complications, return to normal activity, time to return to work. Lap had less pain and earlier return to activity and work.
Liem et al. (100)	994	487 TEPP and 507 open (3% tension-free). More wound infections in open (6 vs. 0), lap patients had more rapid recovery (resume normal activity at 6 vs. 10 d; return to work at 14 vs. 21 d, athletic activities at 24 vs. 36 d); median f/u 607 d, 6% recurrences in open and 3% in lap (half open recurrences in yr 1, half in yr 2; 14 of 17 recurrences in lap in yr 1).
Kozol et al. (91)	62	Randomized to TAPP vs. open (various repairs) under general anesthesia. Patients in lap group had less pain at 24 and 48 h than those in open group. They also used fewer analgesic tablets.
Kald et al. (81)	200	Randomized to TAPP vs. Shouldice under general anesthesia. Op time 72 min for lap, 62 for open; LOS and complications not different. Time off work was 10 d for lap, 23 d for open. Direct costs were higher for lap but more than offset by cost savings of earlier return to work for lap.
Liem et al. (101)	273	Part of larger study, prospectively recorded costs. Cost for lap was higher, savings in indirect costs did not offset direct costs for lap repairs.

f/u, follow-up; lap, laparoscopy; LOS, length of stay; op, operative; OR, operating room; postop, postoperative; QOL, quality of life; TAPP, transabdominal preperitoneal prosthesis; TEPP, totally extraperitoneal prosthesis; VAS, visual analog scale.

the Netherlands was 3%, whereas recurrence for conventional repairs was 6%; when compared to conventional tension-producing techniques, patients had less pain, fewer wound infections, and resumed normal activities sooner. Costs for the laparoscopic repair were higher than the conventional repairs and were only partially offset by savings in indirect costs (i.e., earlier return to work) (101).

Contrary to conventional repairs where recurrences tend to accumulate over time, most recurrences of the laparoscopic technique occur quickly, within the first year, and are the consequence of an error in technique; there is a pronounced learning curve (30,100). Advocates of the laparoscopic approach stress the large degree of patient satisfaction with the procedure, diminished pain and discomfort, and early return to work, implying (but not documenting) that the higher costs of laparoscopy are offset by the lower costs of convalescence (173).

An objective prospective comparison of tension-free techniques with the statistical power to be definitive has been recommended by most proponents of either surgical method (102). Without the benefit of a thorough comparison with tension-free open techniques, this new clinical information will spur interest amongst surgeons and may result in a shift from an open to laparoscopic tension-free approach as the procedure of choice. A definitive trial comparing laparoscopic herniorrhaphy with an open tension-free technique should now be done to aid surgeons and their patients in decisions regarding the optimal choice of method for repair of an inguinal hernia.

The laparoscopic technique chosen for this study is the preperitoneal procedure, in which the preperitoneal space is opened and a large sheet of prosthetic material is positioned over the hernia defect and stapled in place (5,113,125).

Complications of Herniorrhaphy

Complications can occur after open (23,132,138) or laparoscopic procedures (45,97,159); these are usually minor and transient, but can cause considerable pain and disability lasting for a year or more (28). The need for general or regional anesthesia for laparoscopic repair, rather than local anesthesia as is used for open repair, may lead to an excess of life-threatening complications such as thromboembolism or myocardial infarction (8,34,73). Intraoperative complications related to the operative technique are few. Those common to both techniques include bleeding, injury to the bowel, bladder, vas deferens, and vascular structures. Intraoperative complications seen with laparoscopic repair are mostly associated with trocar injuries and include bowel perforation or injury to major blood vessels. Immediate postoperative complications (occurring within 2 weeks of operation) are similar for both techniques and include wound infection (requiring

opening of the wound), urinary tract infection, epididymitis, urinary retention, bleeding (requiring evacuation of a hematoma or transfusion), and wound or scrotal hematoma. Early postoperative complications (occurring within 4 to 6 weeks of operation) include pain (neuralgia of groin or scrotum), persistent hematoma, seroma, and testicular swelling and pain. Those early complications specific to laparoscopic repair include infections or seroma of the trocar sites. These physician-centered outcome measures are usually reported, but the impact of surgical complications on health-related quality of life (HRQoL) has not been documented with patient self-reported data, as we propose to do in this study.

Pain Assessment and Reassessment

Quantifiable features of pain include intensity, time course, quality, impact, and personal meaning (1,127). Bodily pain will be assessed in the Short Form-36 (SF-36) questionnaire, validated in numerous test–retest trials. Impact and personal meaning are inferred from the SF-36 dimensions of general health perceptions and physical functioning (78,128). Pain directly linked to the hernia is assessed in hernia-specific items appended to the SF-36 (13,66). Numerous studies have documented that *acute* pain is more severe in the open than in laparoscopic herniorrhaphies, and most have found that these differences disappear after 1 week (7,95,100).

Two recent studies have documented the frequency of chronic postoperative pain. Liem et al. (100) found that 14% of open *tension* procedures and 2% of laparoscopic *tension-free* hernia repairs resulted in chronic pain "serious enough for the patient to mention" 6 months postoperatively. Cunningham et al. (28) studied 315 patients for 1 year and 276 for 2 years after inguinal herniorrhaphy; 63% had some groin or inguinal pain when interviewed at 1 year; 11.9% and 10.6% of patients had moderate to severe pain at 1 and 2 years postoperatively. Moderate pain was defined as pain preventing return to normal preoperative activities (i.e., inability to continue with prehernia activities such as golf, tennis, or other sports, and inability to lift objects without pain that the patient had been lifting before the hernia occurrence). Severe pain was defined as pain that incapacitated the patient at frequent intervals or interfered with activities of daily living (i.e., a pain constantly present or intermittently present but so severe as to impair normal activities, such as walking) (28). We will use these definitions in our study, comparing chronic pain and its adverse impact on physical functioning in patients managed by the two operations. Specific pain information related to the hernia is provided by our hernia-specific questionnaire, which rates average and "worst today" pain at rest and during activities, on visual analog scales of intensity and distress as described in the Agency for Health

Care Policy and Research (AHCPR) Clinical Practice Guideline No. 1, Acute Pain Management (1), as modified by Price (128–130).

Recurrence After Hernia Repair

Recurrence of a hernia after surgical repair has long been recognized as a principal cause of failure of management. Using tension-producing techniques, recurrence rates after primary repair are between 1% and more than 10% (67,92,120,150), although some single center series in hernia centers are reported to be lower, and rates as high as 30% have also been observed (49). Thirty to forty percent of recurrences are diagnosed within 2 years of operation and 90% of patients with a recurrence have returned for evaluation within 3 years of the original operation (61,144). In contrast, recurrences after laparoscopic repair are usually related to a technical error in mesh placement or fixation, and usually appear within 6 months of operation (45,100).

Diagnosis of a recurrence is not straightforward. A visible or palpable bulge may be reactive tissue and not a hernia. An impulse on cough or Valsalva, accompanied by a bulge that is reducible, is the usual accepted diagnostic criterion (133), and is the definition adopted for this study. To maintain objectivity, it is important for an independent expert observer to evaluate patients for recurrence, as is planned in follow-up visits.

Patient-Centered Outcome Measures

The outcome of treatment has usually been measured by rates of mortality and morbidity accompanying the operation. If the purpose of the intervention is to improve patient well-being, it is necessary to document that quality of life has actually been improved (17,37,47,69,70, 78,86,93,98,108,126). Combining medical with patient-centered outcome measurements provides a rigorous evaluation of clinical practice (36). Is the quality of life of patients who have had complications or recurrence of the hernia improved or was it worsened by a hernia repair, especially if the patient had minimal preoperative symptoms or severe comorbidity (62,109)?

Functional status (return to normal activities) and HRQoL are best evaluated using information reported by patients themselves, rather than through clinical ratings or interpretations of data by health professionals (12,124). Instruments have been developed in recent years that are reliable, valid, and sensitive to change in various dimensions of patient health status (9,39,52,88,112,145,167). A set of generic self-report instruments has been developed from the RAND Medical Outcomes Study (MOS) and the RAND Health Insurance Experiment (14,68,168) The most widely used of these self-report measures is the MOS SF-36

(50,112,167,168). It consists of 36 items measuring eight dimensions of health status: General Health Perceptions, Physical Functioning (PF), Physical Role Functioning, Bodily Pain, Vitality/Energy, Social Functioning (SF), Emotional Role Functioning, and Mental Health. The SF-36 will be used in our study.

Recent studies (7,78,95) have compared a variety of open and laparoscopic herniorrhaphy procedures using the SF-36 or the Nottingham Health Profile Questionnaire (NHPQ) together with pain assessment measures. Even with relatively small sample sizes, significant and clinically meaningful differences in acute end points between the two types of surgical procedures were reported. At ten days, Jenkinson et al. (78) found that the open group reported notably greater levels of dysfunction relative to the laparoscopic group; the laparoscopic group demonstrated significant improvement from baseline at 6 weeks while no differences from baseline were detected in the open group. Barkun et al. (6) found no differences between open and laparoscopic groups on the NHPQ and a Visual Analog Scale (VAS) pain measure at 7 days postoperatively, while laparoscopic patients showed significantly greater improvement on the NHPQ than open patients at 1 month postoperatively. Lawrence et al. conducted a randomized trial of open versus laparoscopic herniorrhaphy, and found that pain scores and quality of life indices credited significant benefit to the laparoscopic approach in the short term, but that return to normal activity was similar. Reductions have been reported in return-to-work time for laparoscopic patients (5.6 to 14 days versus 10.3 to 28 days for open repair patients). Fitzgibbons' group compared Lichtenstein open repair and laparoscopic preperitoneal repair in 53 patients and did not find significant differences in either pain or sickness impact profiles (44). Some of these differences occur because of individual surgeon preferences in instructions to patients. In our trial, instructions to patients will be standardized and identical for both procedures.

Important levels of detail are often missing from generic health status assessment instruments, and focused disease and treatment-specific indices can be useful in evaluating the efficacy of interventions and longer term outcomes (13,58,66,76,88,105). We will augment the SF-36 with a set of brief condition-specific measures assessing activity level, pain, and patient satisfaction with the outcome (13,58,66,76,88,105). Finding no condition-specific (hernia or general surgery) scales in surgical specialties other than orthopedics (13,58,98), we conducted individual interviews and focus groups with laparoscopic and open hernia repair patients and with surgeons to develop new items and scales for evaluating treatment outcomes in these areas (see Preliminary Studies, below).

To fully assess the impact of a medical condition or surgical procedure, it is necessary to examine the impact on others who either assist in the patient's care or who assume responsibility for certain activities that he is unable to complete (111). Evidence from studies of patients with arthritis suggests that having a supportive spouse improves coping and psychological well-being (111,134). A randomized study of patients with osteoarthritis of the knee demonstrated that when spouses were trained to assist in coping skills, patients had significantly lower levels of pain, psychological disability, and pain behavior (85). The disability of one family member may also place a burden on other family members. Allair et al. (3) found that when the wife/mother has moderate-to-severe rheumatoid arthritis, other family members spend 7 hours or more per week on household tasks. Issues related to the impact of hernia surgery on the patient's caregiver will be investigated in this study.

Functional status and HRQoL measures are relatively new in surgical research and are still uncommon (47,175). Recent studies of patient-centered outcomes have been reported in a number of the surgical specialties, however (2,21,55,82,105, 121,139,154,155,175), and in some reports, operative and nonoperative treatments have been compared.

Comorbidity

The ultimate outcome of treatment as appreciated by the patient is influenced by a number of preoperative risk factors. Among these are socioeconomic and educational level, race, age, functional status, and the burden of comorbid disease (27,40,62,109,121). While it is obvious that the total health burden of a patient with comorbidity affects operative mortality and the 30-day complication rate (20,22,31,46,60, 74,84,89), comorbidities also influence physical and social functioning and other aspects of HRQoL (151,162), negatively influencing the entire range of treatment outcomes (38). While functional declines in health may be attenuated by interventions such as cataract extraction and lens replacement (110), health status may still decline with time regardless of a single intervention (145). Through collection and analysis of demographic data, SF-36 questionnaires, and medical history, we intend to analyze the impact of these preexisting factors, individually and collectively, on the outcome of hernia management.

The same type of hernia management in patients with comorbidity may result in markedly different outcomes. Patients with the most to gain may benefit the most from an intervention, while patients with good functional status gain relatively little from the same intervention (109). We will collect data on specified preexisting diseases, selected in part based on unpublished data (56) derived from the National VA Surgical Risk Study, that were found to influence morbidity and mortality rates in herniorrhaphy patients. The direct effects of comorbidity as well as age, race, socioeconomic and educational status, and the hernia symptom score, will be evaluated as will the interaction of comorbidity with the type of hernia treatment.

PRELIMINARY STUDIES
Focus Groups

To develop condition-specific medical and patient-centered outcome measurement instruments, focus groups were convened as follows: (a) surgeons with expertise in hernia surgery and laparoscopy (to develop estimates of medical outcomes for sample size determinations); (b) general surgeons managing patients with inguinal hernias (to develop the symptom scoring system); (c) preoperative patients with inguinal hernia (to develop hernia-specific patient-centered questionnaires); (d) postoperative patients—open and laparoscopic (to develop hernia-specific questionnaires related to pain, expectations of surgical outcome, satisfaction with care, and caregiver impact assessment).

Pilot Study

A pilot study of hernia symptoms and self-reported demographic and health status was conducted in September 1996. General surgeons in the metropolitan Chicago, Dallas, Omaha, and Montreal areas and additional surgeons and primary care physicians working in the Salt Lake City, Durham, and West Los Angeles VA Medical Centers (VAMCs) received packets consisting of symptom questionnaires and self-reported assessments of functional status including hernia-specific areas and questionnaires pertaining to anticipated and realized surgical outcomes. A second distribution of preoperative questionnaires was done in August 1997 to increase sample size and verify the findings from the first pilot.

Symptom Score Assessment

A symptom scoring method was developed to determine eligibility for a companion study that compares hernia repair with "watchful waiting." Forty-four symptom score questionnaires were returned in the first and 21 in the second mailings. The patients ranged in age from 15 to 85 years. Thirty-eight percent had inguinal hernias that reduced spontaneously and 3% were incarcerated. Twenty-four percent were small (not visible when standing), 64% were large (visible), and 11% were scrotal. Sixty-four percent of the patients had no pain or pain *not* interfering with normal activities. Twenty-eight percent had pain related to the hernia that did interfere with activities, and 8% had constant pain. Two percent had a prior episode of hernia-related bowel obstruction, 62% had hernias which enlarged within the prior 6 months, 2/3 had hernias present for < 6 months, and 16% of the patients had severe comorbidities. Most patients (61%) and/or their employers (15%) insisted on repair, but their physicians felt it would be safe to delay repair for 6 months in 85% of the patients.

Self-Reported Health Assessments

Areas covered in the new self-reported hernia-specific questionnaires were: preoperative ability to perform physical activities, hernia-related pain, appearance of the hernia, and expectations for pain, appearance of the wound, recovery time, and postoperative level of functioning. Additional information was collected from patients who had undergone operation about their reactions to anesthesia, postoperative pain, appearance of the incision, surgery-related complications, physical activities, recovery time, and satisfaction with the results of the operation.

Patient-centered measures were pilot-tested by general surgeons who were asked to distribute them to their hernia patients during a 2-week time period. Packets of forms were provided corresponding to measures that were proposed to be collected at baseline, first postoperative visit, in-home follow-up, and the final assessment. Ninety-six patients returned forms. Most respondents were Caucasian (75%), 16% were African-American, 5% Hispanic, 3% Asian, and 1% other; nearly all respondents had at least a high school education (95%), 32% were college graduates, and 17% were graduates of professional or graduate school; mean age = 55.7, s.d. = 16.9.

The SF-36 was used to obtain general estimates of functional status and a means of validating the condition-specific measures. A number of hernia-specific measures of functional performance (e.g., the "Activities Assessment" and the "Pain Assessment") were developed for this pilot study to provide a potentially more sensitive method of detecting differential outcomes in patients managed by watchful waiting, open, or laparoscopic herniorrhaphy. Analysis of the psychometric characteristics of the new measures indicated that their convergent–discriminant validity was very good. A simple summative index of 12 items from the Activities Assessment was computed. The highest correlation was found between the Activity Index and the Physical Functioning scale of the SF-36 ($r = 0.75$; $p = 0.001$) with conceptually unrelated scales showing lower correlations. Average pain correlated most strongly with the SF-36 Body Pain score, as expected ($r = 0.63$; $p = 0.002$). The SF-36 demonstrated good reliability in this sample with Cronbach's alpha greater than 0.90 for the Physical Functioning, Physical Role Functioning, Vitality, and Bodily Pain scales. Mean time to complete the forms was 5 to 15 minutes, and most patients believed that the amount of information collected was "just about right" and "important" or "very important." Revisions in these forms were made based on patient feedback in the pilot study.

The symptom score was compared with the SF-36 components and with the Activities Assessment. Patients were categorized as minimally symptomatic [Symptom Score (SS) less than 5] or symptomatic (SS 5 or more). Significant differences were found between minimally symptomatic and symptomatic patients in the SF-36 dimensions of physical functioning ($p = 0.018$) and physical role functioning ($p = 0.045$). Similar differences between the minimally symptomatic and symptomatic patients on items from the Activities Assessment were in the expected direction, with the "climbing stairs" item approaching statistical significance ($p = 0.056$).

Caregiver Assessments

Preoperative data indicated that caregivers were concerned about the patient's ability to perform various activities. The proportion of caregivers who indicated that they were concerned ranged from 57% for social activities to 70% for work and recreational activities. About one third indicated that they spent additional time doing chores due to the patient's condition, ranging from 3 to 10 hours in the past week.

Recurrence Rates in the Veterans Health Administration

A retrospective review at the Salt Lake City VAMC, where 100 to 110 herniorrhaphies are performed every year, revealed recurrence rates as follows: 3% to 6% for open repair without prosthesis (Bassini or McVay), 4% for open tension-free repair (with prosthesis). In this single institution review, 16% of hernias were recurrent but the recurrence rates for primary versus recurrent hernia repairs were not different.

Rate of Laparoscopic Hernia Repair in the Veterans Health Administration

Review of the inguinal herniorrhaphies performed at the 14 VA hospitals chosen for this multicenter study reveals that 0% to 20% of the repairs in fiscal year (FY) 1997 were performed laparoscopically. The penetration of the laparoscopic repair at all VAs is presumed less than this since the VAs chosen for this study are ones in which there is known expertise in laparoscopic repair and this does not presently exist at all VAs.

SIGNIFICANCE FOR THE VETERANS HEALTH ADMINISTRATION

Inguinal hernia occurs as a congenital or acquired condition in adults of both genders but is strongly predominant in males (164). Large population studies have concluded that the rate of occurrence of inguinal hernias in adults is 15/1,000 (32). Physical examinations of 13,000,000

Selective Service Registrants in the U.S. during the years 1941–44 resulted in rejection of more than 4,000,000 registrants; of those rejected and classified as "4-F," nearly 6% were rejected because of hernias, a rate of 18/1,000 in this age group (140). Inguinal hernias are also acquired during later life as conditions appear that contribute to increased intraabdominal pressure, such as constipation and prostatism, such that inguinal hernias are commonly found in older men. Inguinal hernia repair (herniorrhaphy) is one of the most frequently performed operations in the U.S., and is one of the most common operations performed in the VA medical system. In FY 1996, approximately 10,000 herniorrhaphies were performed in the VA system, representing 10% of general surgery cases and 3% of all surgery cases (115).

The success rate for inguinal hernia repair is high; approximately 10% of repairs, however, eventually fail and often require reoperation. Repair of a recurrent hernia is less successful, with rerecurrence reported in approximately 20% of patients (75). Disability as a result of the presence of a hernia or a recurrence, or during convalescence from herniorrhaphy, leads to great expense (135) in active service populations and in military veterans. Lingering consequences of pain, neuralgias, and testicular swelling or atrophy may cause long-term disability in many patients but are not accurately defined (23).

Herniorrhaphy is the recommended treatment for essentially all inguinal hernias (18,137,169). This recommendation is based on the following observations: (a) the hernia is successfully repaired in approximately 90% of patients with very low mortality, low morbidity, and low cost; (b) a hernia "accident"(acute incarceration, obstruction, strangulation) may occur and require emergency surgical treatment, with an attendant higher risk of mortality, especially in the elderly (172). Mortality for elective and emergency herniorrhaphy is low; the most recent available data from the National VA Surgical Risk Study in 1996 is a rate of 0.38%. The morbidity of either elective or emergency herniorrhaphy has not been thoroughly documented, thus the patient's perception of the outcome of a herniorrhaphy, as contrasted with the medical assessment of recurrence or mortality, may be much less accurate due to these poorly documented and troublesome non–life-threatening complications.

Given the high frequency of inguinal hernias in the population of patients served by the VA medical system, and the high costs of surgical treatment and disability, a study of hernia management is indicated. It is important to establish whether an open operation (the tension-free repair of Lichtenstein) or a laparoscopic operation provides the best results in terms of successful repair, patient-centered outcome and functional status, and cost. The implications of these findings for the VA patient population and for the surgical services responsible for their care are meaningful.

COLLABORATION WITH THE AMERICAN COLLEGE OF SURGEONS

In the context of a new initiative in Surgical Clinical Trials in the American College of Surgeons, and with the encouragement of the Chief Research and Development Officer of the VA, the College has formed several working groups to develop clinical trials proposals in areas of disease that are of importance to the VA; these include evaluation of new surgical technology (laparoscopic and open tension-free hernia repair, deep brain stimulation, and pallidotomy in Parkinson's disease) or treatment options (prevention of leg ulcers and amputation in diabetics). The study proposed here, laparoscopic and open tension-free hernia repair, is the first of these proposals to be completely developed, and may represent a unique opportunity for collaboration of the American College of Surgeons and the VA Cooperative Studies Program (CSP). A parallel proposal, to be conducted in community health care systems, has been submitted to the National Institutes of Health (NIH); the proposal evaluates the role of watchful waiting, or open tension-free hernia repair in minimally symptomatic patients.

RESEARCH DESIGN AND METHODS
Overview of Study Design

We propose to conduct a multicenter randomized clinical trial to compare the outcomes of two methods of surgical management of inguinal hernia. Men presenting to a physician with an inguinal hernia will be considered for the trial. The study is designed to evaluate the effectiveness of open tension-free and laparoscopic preperitoneal hernia repair; the frequency of recurrence at 2 years is defined as the primary outcome measure. Subjects will be followed to the end of the study. The rate of complications, pain, time to return to normal activities, HRQoL, patient satisfaction, and cost are secondary outcome measures. The design of the trial is represented in Fig. 49.1.

Fourteen VA medical centers with the capability of enrolling 50 to 75 patients a year will be selected. Subjects will be recruited by physicians at each site and referred to the site coordinator, who will screen them for eligibility. The trial will be randomized but not blinded.

Type of hernia (primary or recurrent, unilateral or bilateral) may affect outcome measures, namely rate of recurrence, return to normal activities, and HRQoL. Therefore, subjects will be stratified on these variables prior to randomization to prevent imbalances.

The project timetable is as follows: 3 months start-up, 3 years intake, 2 years of follow-up, and 6 months for close-out and final analysis.

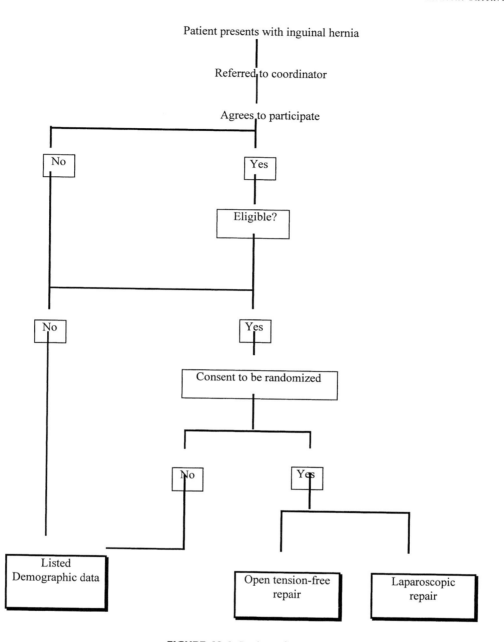

Patient presents with inguinal hernia

Referred to coordinator

Agrees to participate

No | Yes

Eligible?

No | Yes

Consent to be randomized

No | Yes

Listed Demographic data

Open tension-free repair | Laparoscopic repair

FIGURE 49.1. Design of trial.

Site Selection

Criteria for Participating Veterans Health Administration Medical Centers

1. Patient volume sufficient to enroll 50 to 75 new patients per year.
2. Prospective enrollment of qualified surgeons as participants in the study, with agreements to list all new patients encountered, regardless of eventual participation in the randomized study.

All the sites under consideration were selected for their known expertise in laparoscopic surgery and have at least one surgeon presently on staff who is qualified to perform either of the repairs (see below). Some VAMCs have chosen not to offer laparoscopic repair at this time because of the unproven outcomes; however, many VA surgeons have practices outside of the VA where they are performing these repairs. The equipment needed to perform laparoscopic hernia repair is the same as is needed for laparoscopic cholecystectomy and, therefore, any VAMC with a full general surgery program will have the needed equipment to perform laparoscopic hernia repairs. Some of the disposable supplies are somewhat different (e.g., stapler used to affix the mesh); however, these items are easily obtained.

3. Institutional review board (IRB) approval of the project at the local site.

Principal Site Investigator, Participating Surgeons

A surgeon will be appointed as principal investigator at each site (site PI), responsible for overall coordination of the study at that site, recruitment of surgeons as participants, and for timely and accurate collection of data and communication to the coordinating center. The site PI will supervise a full-time site coordinator. The site PI may be a participating surgeon.

The site PI will recruit qualified participating surgeons. The participating surgeon must have performed a minimum of 25 Lichtenstein hernia repairs to qualify to perform the Lichtenstein repair for the study and/or 25 laparoscopic preperitoneal hernia repairs to perform that procedure for the study. The minimum of 25 was chosen as this was shown previously to be a point at which the learning curve reached a plateau (103). Each site must have at least one surgeon qualified to perform each operative technique. Only surgeons experienced in the surgical technique to which the patient is randomized will perform the selected procedure; patients will be referred to the appropriate surgeon. Participating surgeons will agree to invite all men with an inguinal hernia seen by them to enroll in the study and be interviewed by the site coordinator, and to list all hernia patients who do not agree to participate, with demographic and comorbidity data.

The Site Coordinator's Responsibilities

1. Maintaining continuous communications with the participating physicians to facilitate ongoing patient accrual into the study.
2. The initial encounter with patients identified as candidates for the study by the participating surgeon.
3. Listing all other hernia patients of the participating surgeons who elect not to participate in the study.
4. Determining eligibility, collecting baseline data, and obtaining informed consent.
5. Conducting the randomization procedures by telephone call to the Hines CSP Coordinating Center (CSPCC), disclosing the treatment selected, and referring the patient to a participating surgeon.
6. Collecting data on comorbid conditions and operative data in consultation with the operating surgeon.
7. Follow-up of patients at designated intervals, collection of data on all complications, independent assessment of recurrence and other complications, obtaining patient self-report assessments at the appropriate intervals, tabulation of postoperative health care utilization patient diaries, and arranging for long-term assessment by the surgeon.

The coordinator will be trained to examine patients for hernia recurrence and to recognize the complications tracked in this trial. The coordinator will serve as an independent assessor; when the surgeon/coordinator assessments disagree, an independent surgical opinion will be obtained.

Subject Recruitment

Subjects will be recruited when they visit a participating surgeon, and an inguinal hernia is diagnosed. Participating surgeons will have agreed to notify the coordinator when such a patient is encountered and will offer the patient the opportunity to meet with the coordinator and learn more about the study. The coordinator will first determine the subject's eligibility for the study.

Inclusion Criteria

Men will be eligible for enrollment into the study if they meet the following criteria:

- Are 18 years of age or older.
- Have a diagnosis of inguinal hernia. If a patient has bilateral hernias, one of the hernias will be selected at random as the study hernia by the Hines CSPCC. However, both hernias will be treated and followed.
- Give informed consent for randomization.

Exclusion Criteria

Patients will be excluded for the following reasons:

- Hernia cannot be detected on physical examination
- Recurrent hernia was repaired previously with mesh
- American Society of Anesthesiologists (ASA) class IV or V, or contraindications to general anesthesia
- Presence of bowel obstruction, strangulation, peritonitis, or perforation
- Presence of local or systemic infection
- Presence of contraindications to pelvic laparoscopy such as previous pelvic surgical procedures (e.g., radical prostatectomy and/or pelvic irradiation)
- Participation in another clinical trial

Informed Consent Procedures

After determination of eligibility, informed consent will be obtained for randomization. Patients will be given the explanation that the trial intends to compare two procedures with similar reported recurrence rates, and the risks of each treatment will be described. Randomization is to one of the two treatment arms (open or laparoscopic herniorrhaphy). If the patient declines referral to the coordinator or refuses randomization, basic demographic information will be obtained and the patients will be listed only.

Stratification and Randomization

The purpose of stratification is to ensure that at the end of the study there will be equality between treatment groups on a few of the most important baseline variables related to outcome. (Randomization results in a high likelihood of equality between treatment groups on known and unknown factors but does not guarantee this.) The important baseline variables that will serve as stratification factors will be participating center, primary or recurrent hernia, and unilateral or bilateral hernia.

The patients will be stratified into four strata within each center:

> Primary–unilateral
> Recurrent–unilateral
> Primary–bilateral
> Recurrent–bilateral

The randomization scheme will be developed at the Hines CSPCC. The randomization will be blocked within each stratum so that after each block of "x" patients that are randomized within the stratum the treatment groups will be equally represented. This ensures that at any time the patient accrual period is stopped there will be an approximately equal number of patients in each treatment group. The blocking factor "x" will not be known to the participants so that they cannot determine the randomization scheme.

To randomize a patient, the site coordinator will call the Hines CSPCC. Staff at the CSPCC will confirm that the patient is eligible for the trial and has signed the consent form, will properly stratify the patient, and will provide the randomized treatment assignment.

Intervention

Patients randomized to open repair will undergo a standardized tension-free herniorrhaphy with prosthesis [method of Lichtenstein (99)]. Patients randomized to laparoscopic herniorrhaphy will undergo a standardized preperitoneal repair with prosthesis, using either a transperitoneal or extraperitoneal approach (45). During the implementation period of the trial, a preliminary laboratory session will be conducted with all site PIs to standardize herniorrhaphy techniques, reach consensus on all aspects of perioperative patient management (including postoperative patient instructions, follow-up schedules, definitions of recurrence, and complications), and to ensure that the site PI is thoroughly familiar with the protocol.

Each site will be visited by one of two expert surgeons (the study chair or co-chair) to observe the operative procedures and ensure that participating surgeons adhere to the protocol in all respects. The first visit will take place in the first 6 months of the study and then as needed thereafter, based on routine examination of operative records randomly selected from each site (five open and five laparoscopic herniorrhaphies, and, if appropriate, viewing of videotapes of the laparoscopic procedures).

Measurement

Table 49.2 summarizes the schedule of measurement. All enrolled patients will be assessed at baseline and followed on various measures for at least 2 years.

TABLE 49.2. SCHEDULE OF DATA COLLECTION

Data	Form No.	Baseline	Operation	Follow-up[a]				
				1–2 Wk	6 Wk	3 Mo	6 Mo	Yearly
Demographic	1	X						
Clinical								
Hernia type and symptoms	1	X						
Comorbidity and risk factors	1	X						
Operative data	2		X					
Complications	3–5, 17	X		X	X	X		X
Recurrence	16					X		X
Patient-Centered								
Time to resume activities	8				X			
Activities assessment	6, 7	X		X		X	X	X
Pain	9, 10	X		X (daily)		X	X	X
HRQoL (SF-36)	11	X		X		X	X	X
Satisfaction with care	12, 13			X		X		X
Caregiver assessment	14	X		X		X		
Cost[b]	30–35, 40–42							

HRQoL, health-related quality of life; SF-36, Medical Outcomes Study Short Form-36.
[a]Six-week and 6-month follow-up on patient-centered measures will be done by phone and mail. Three-month and yearly follow-ups will be office based.
[b]Cost data will be collected for the duration of the participants' enrollment in the study and not only at the indicated time points. Department of Veterans Affairs (VA) costs will be estimated from operative data (Form 2) and determined from local hospital and centralized VA cost and utilization files. Non–VA costs will be determined from patient diaries and Medicare files for 3 months postoperatively.

Initial Assessment

- Demographic data.
- Risk factors and comorbidities: these data will be collected by site coordinators using a checklist developed from an analysis of risk factors for hernia cases in the National VA Surgical Risk Study (56,89,90) and surgeon expert opinion.
- Hernia type, size, and symptoms: patients will be examined by the coordinator and participating surgeon to determine hernia location, unilateral or bilateral, size, and whether primary or recurrent, and their symptoms assessed.
- Preoperative activities, preoperative pain and discomfort, SF-36, and caregiver assessment will be completed by the subjects and caregiver at the time of enrollment.

Operative Data

A set of operative data items [previously validated (20)] will be collected on all hernia surgical repairs. Additional items will be collected for hernias repaired laparoscopically, and other additional items for open repairs. Included in the operative data will be the intraoperative Nyhus classification of the inguinal hernia.

Complications and Postoperative Follow-up

Intraoperative complications will be recorded on Form 3. Early postoperative complications will be determined at the 2-week postoperative visit and up until the 3-month visit if the patient presents with a complication after the first postoperative visit. Long-term complications will be assessed at 3 months and annually. Occurrence of life-threatening complications such as pulmonary embolism and myocardial infarction will be tracked for the first 30 postoperative days.

Recurrence

Recurrence is defined as a visible bulge or a palpable bulge that is reducible. Evaluation of recurrence will be done at 3 months and yearly. At the 3-month visit, the site coordinator and the operating surgeon or another surgeon should make independent assessments. At years 1 and 2, the patient must be assessed by an independent surgeon (i.e., a surgeon other than the operating surgeon) and the site coordinator. A third means of determination must be employed to resolve assessor disagreement and to confirm a recurrence. This evidence may be (a) an examination by a second surgeon, (b) an ultrasound, or (c) reoperation. If a patient has moved from the area, the evaluation of a surgeon not affiliated with the study will be sought for yearly follow-up. If reoperation has occurred, a copy of the operative report will be requested.

Patient-Centered Outcome Measures

A combination of generic and hernia-specific health status measures will be included in this study. The SF-36 serves as the generic measure of functional status and HRQoL. Hernia-specific assessments include postoperative activities, pain and discomfort, satisfaction with care, and caregiver assessments.

Pain

Postoperative pain will be measured on visual analogue pain scales at intervals indicated in Table 49.2. Based on patients' comments in the pilot study and consultation with Lawrence (96) and Price (131), we substituted 15-cm visual analogue scales with labeled end points for the 12-item instrument based on the labeled 10-point assessment scale from the AHCPR acute pain management guidelines (1).

Postoperative Activities, HRQoL, and Satisfaction with Care

Postoperative activities, HRQoL, and satisfaction with care will be obtained directly from patients by questionnaire during office visits at intervals indicated in Table 49.2, or by mail or telephone at yearly intervals if the patient is unable to return to the study site. The site coordinator will assist patients in completing the forms in the office or by phone, review the forms for completeness, and forward the completed forms to the Hines CSPCC. Form 8, "Resumption of Activities," will be completed for all operated patients by the coordinator during a phone call at 6 weeks postoperatively.

Caregiver Assessment

The caregiver questionnaire assesses the impact of the hernia and the hernia operation on the person at home who assists the patient during recuperation. This person is asked about her/his concern for the patient's ability to perform activities and the amount of assistance others are providing in tasks around the house. Impact on the caregiver is an important element of cost analysis as well as HRQoL.

Costs

Our cost analysis will be a cost-minimization analysis, conducted from a societal perspective, taking into account measures of direct medical costs, direct nonmedical costs, and indirect costs (59,141,149,170). Direct medical costs include all costs associated with the treatment; direct *nonmedical* costs are directly associated with treatment but are nonmedical in nature. Indirect costs are not directly attributable to the treatment but may be the result of the condition or treatment, such as work time and productivity lost by patient and caregiver. We have selected a cost-minimization analysis, rather than cost effectiveness, because we expect the differences in quality-adjusted life years between the two study arms to be small. In addition, we are not aware of any validated techniques for assessing hernia treatment preferences with which to "quality adjust" life years. Our focus on cost minimization, however, does not preclude us from conducting cost-effectiveness analyses if we find that the effectiveness of the two surgical techniques differs significantly. If differences are found in effectiveness measures (i.e., recurrence rates and patient-centered outcomes), we also will examine effectiveness ratios.

Data will be collected from a variety of sources (administrative data, primary data collection, and patient diary with verification) in order to provide a comprehensive measure of resource utilization and to allow for validation of reported utilization. Cost estimations will be based on national VA accounting and budgeting systems [Cost Distribution Reports (CDRs) or Decision Support Systems (DSSs)] for VA hospital utilization and outpatient clinic visits, Medicare Reimbursement rates (Average DRG rates) for non-VA hospitalization and as alternative estimation for VA hospital costs, Medicare Fee Schedules for non-VA physician and other professional services, and Medicare's Resource-Based Relative Value Scale (RBRVS) for outpatient procedures. Since our study will span a time period exceeding 1 year, costs will be adjusted to reflect societal rate of time preference and inflation, both currently 3% to 5%.

Time Frame for Data Collection

Subjects will be followed throughout the course of the study to obtain data on their health care utilization. Data collection about health care use during the first 3 months of study regarding the index operation, the index admission and subsequent inpatient and outpatient health care use, and medications will be obtained by the site coordinator through online medical record review and patient diary/interview. Beyond 3 months, data collection will be limited to hospital readmissions and outpatient visits available through VA and Medicare administrative data systems. The collection of utilization data will commence after the point of randomization; prerandomization costs are assumed to be equal across study arms.

Data Sources

Index Operation

The Operative Data Form will be used to collect detailed data on utilization that is expected to differ between open and laparoscopic repair (time of operation, anesthesia, and supplies, e.g., disposable trocars). This form will be completed by the study coordinator immediately postoperatively.

Index Stay

For all randomized subjects, we will obtain information about resource use for the index hospital stay or partial stay corresponding to the index surgical procedure using the *VA Index Admission forms*. These forms will be completed by the site coordinator immediately postdischarge, from data that are readily available in the VA medical records or the local hospital computerized record [i.e., Veterans Integrated Services Technology Architecture (VISTA), formerly the Decentralized Hospital Computing System (DHCP)].

Health Care Use up to 3 Months After Surgery

- *VA Hospital Admissions:* Study personnel will collect details about hospital readmission during the 3-month period immediately following the index admission using the *VA Index Admission forms*. Detailing will focus on the reason for the admission (i.e., whether the admission is related to the index admission), diagnostic procedures performed, medications used, specific bed sections, and length of stay.

- *VA Outpatient Care:* Study personnel will collect details about each VA outpatient visit for every study patient. Details will include specific outpatient procedures (e.g., medical supplies, laboratory testing, and radiology and other imaging procedures). These data will be collected from the patient's medical record and hospital computer records.

- *Non-VA Health Care:* The utilization of non-VA care cannot be captured with the same uniformity and precision as VA utilization, because each non-VA provider maintains its own, often distinct, accounting system, and because obtaining non-VA data cannot practically be obtained with the completeness of VA data. However, collecting such data is essential to assess whether there may be differential barriers to access to VA care between the treatment groups. We will use approaches that have been successful in other cooperative studies.

  A patient diary will be used during the 3 months after the index admission to collect self-reported data on medical care during the observation period for non-VA health care. These data will be summarized on Form 40 by the Site Coordinator. The data will be verified with providers and by requesting copies of billing data [e.g., the Uniform Hospital Billing Form (UB-92) for hospital admissions, and Health Care Financing Administration (HCFA) 1500: Detailed Professional Charges For Physician Visits]. Patients will be given the diary at the time of their enrollment and will be contacted by the coordinator at 2 weeks and 6 weeks to ensure that the patient is filling out the diary. At 3 months, the patient will mail the completed form to the coordinator in the prepaid addressed envelope or bring the completed form to the 3-month visit.

- *Medicare Claims Data:* Health care utilization data will also be obtained from Medicare Standard Analytic Files (SAFs) for all patients 65 and over for submitted claims for non-VA inpatient, outpatient, and physician care. These data will be obtained annually from the HCFA for all Medicare-eligible patients for the 3-month postdischarge period.

Health Care Use Beyond 3 Months of Index Admission:
- Use and costs of health care over the long term are expected to be comparable for the open and laparoscopic surgery groups. Also, since it is likely that the majority of health care use will be under VA auspices, data collection will focus on VA health care use only. This focus, which will make use of automated administrative information systems, will also minimize burden on study patients.
- *Inpatient Care:* All resource use beyond the 3 months after the index admission will be obtained from the Department of Veterans Affairs' main Patient Treatment File (PTF) in Austin, Texas. The PTF is a nationwide discharge data set that contains a record for each episode of inpatient care provided in VA facilities. Each episode contains data on admission and discharge diagnosis codes, procedures performed (operating room and non–operating room procedures), bed section, specific length of stay, total length of stay, and discharge information. These data will be downloaded annually for all study subjects.
- *Outpatient Care:* All VA outpatient resource use will be obtained from the Department of Veterans Affairs' main Outpatient Care Files (OPC). The OPC contains a record for each outpatient episode of care provided in VA facilities. Three files provide information about each episode regarding the specific clinic stop(s), primary care clinic, diagnostic code information, and procedure coding. In FY 1997, current procedural terminology (CPT) coding was added to the information collected in outpatient settings in VA. However, the validity and reliability of this new coding effort has not been evaluated.

Cost Estimation Methods
Direct Costs
Index Operation Costs for the specific surgery will be estimated by obtaining information from relevant services regarding the costs of specific resources used in the operating room: specific surgical equipment, medications, respiratory and anesthesia services, operating room personnel, and overhead. Since the VA cost accounting system is in transition, there is no well-validated cost accounting system to provide cost estimates at the operation procedure level. However, since we will collect detailed data about specific resources used in open and laparoscopic surgeries, we will use relevant expenditure data to estimate the costs of specific resources. For example, the cost of specific surgical supplies will be obtained from VA Surgery Service and/or Supply Service. Since costs at specific VAMCs may differ, we will obtain VAMC-specific costs. For sensitivity analyses, we will also use available market data to estimate costs for specific supplies.

Index Admission and Subsequent Veterans Health Administration Hospital Admissions Costs of inpatient care will be estimated using proxies for (a) an average room and board cost, (b) procedure costs, and (c) medication costs. Information from the VA accounting and budgeting systems (e.g., CDR

and DSS) will be used to estimate room and board costs for specific bed sections (e.g., intensive care unit versus general medicine). The Medicare Fee Schedule, based on the RBRVS, will be used to estimate the cost for procedures (those other than the hernia surgery) provided during hospital admissions. Costs for medications will be estimated using national cost data available from the Pharmacy Benefits Management (PBM) System. For sensitivity analyses, we will also use Medicare DRG reimbursement rates to estimate inpatient costs at VA hospitals.

Veterans Health Administration Outpatient Care Costs for outpatient care received at VA facilities will be estimated using information from the VA accounting and budgeting systems (e.g., CDR and DSS). For example, in the present CDR, an average cost for each clinic stop can be estimated. Costs for procedures will be estimated using Medicare's RBRVS.

Non-VA Health Care
- *Hospital Admissions:* We will use Medicare DRG rates for estimating the cost of hospital admissions to non-VA facilities (94). Although hospital billing data will be obtained for all non-VA hospital admissions, the information will only be used for purposes of tracking and validating utilization, not for estimating costs of care.
- *Outpatient Visits and Physician Costs:* We will use the Medicare Fee Schedule to "cost out" physician and other professional services. Data on national reimbursement rates will be used to construct these cost estimates.
- *Other Medical Costs:* Costs such as pharmaceuticals will be based on prevailing prices for the VA, obtained through the VA's PBM system.
- *Productivity Costs:* The Resumption of Activities form asks patients questions regarding the length of time until their return to normal daily activity, and specific counts of days lost from work or other normal activities.

Sample Size

It is fairly well established in a prospective multicenter study that the 2-year recurrence rate for laparoscopic herniorrhaphy is about 4% (45). The 2-year recurrence rate for open tension-free hernia repair is less well established, but is probably somewhere between 1% and 10%. In the Liem study (100), the 2-year recurrence rate for the open tension-producing methods was found to be about 3% higher than that for laparoscopic herniorrhaphy (6% vs. 3%). However, the surgeons on the CSP No. 456 planning committee believed that the 2-year recurrence rate for open tension-free hernia repair will be about 1%. The surgeons further believe that a clinically meaningful difference in recurrence rates would be 3%.

Accordingly, we have estimated the following sample sizes using Nquery Advisor 2.0 for a two-sided test of two

Power	Laparoscopic Recurrence Rate	Open Recurrence Rate	No.
80%	4%	7%	1,812
		6.5%	2,498
		6%	3,726
		2%	2,282
		1.5%	1,342
		1%	848
85%	4%	7%	2,072
		6.5%	2,856
		6%	4,262
		2%	2,610
		1.5%	1,534
		1%	960
90%	4%	7%	2,424
		6.5%	3,342
		6%	4,988
		2%	3,054
		1.5%	1,796
		1%	1136

proportions with alpha = 0.05, power = 80%, 85%, 90%, and various differences in recurrence rates:

A target sample size of 1,812 will be selected for this study. This will allow for at least 80% power to detect a 3% deviation from the laparoscopic herniorrhaphy 2-year recurrence rate of 4%. This sample size will be adjusted for interim monitoring and dropout (see next two sections).

Interim Statistical Monitoring

Outcomes from the study will be reviewed by the Data Monitoring Board, the Hines CSPCC Human Rights Committee, and the Hines CSPCC staff annually. The EaSt program (35) was run to obtain O'Brien–Fleming boundaries under the following assumptions: alpha = 0.05 (two sided), power = 0.80, P_1 = 0.04, P_2 = 0.07, 5 looks. The maximum sample size was estimated to be 1,988. At the end of each year, the observed Z-value will be calculated and the EaSt program will be entered. Actual patient accrual is entered into the analysis portion of the program, and the program calculates the nominal critical point and significance level. These are then compared to the observed Z-value to decide whether or not to continue the study.

Dropout

We will increase the final sample size of 1,988 to 2,200 patients to allow for a 10% dropout. We believe that we can keep the dropout rate down to 10% or less for the following reasons:

1. Dropout rates in VA cooperative studies in general tend to be low because the veterans tend to be a very compliant population.

2. The critical follow-up time is only for 2 years.
3. The study treatment is a one-time treatment occurring over a short period of time. Therefore, we do not need to keep patients compliant to a treatment over a long period of time.
4. The veterans will tend to receive most of their health care in the VA system. Central VA databases based on outpatient visits, inpatient visits, and beneficiary records can be searched for recurrences, reoperations, and health care utilization, and costs for those patients who are lost to follow-up.
5. If the veterans fail to return to the VA system, Medicare databases will be searched for recurrences, reoperations, and health care utilization, and costs for those patients over 65 years of age. The Equifax system at the Hines CSPCC can also be used to locate veterans lost to follow-up, and these people can be contacted by mail and telephone for end point data.

Statistical Analysis

Recurrence Rates

The major aim of this study is to compare two types of operative treatments (open tension-free and preperitoneal laparoscopic herniorrhaphy) in patients with inguinal hernias. The primary outcome for comparisons are the 2-year recurrence rates. The primary analysis will compare the recurrence rates sequentially with five interim analyses at annual intervals using O'Brien–Fleming boundaries for a two-tailed alpha = 0.05 level of testing. In addition, the primary outcome of recurrence will be analyzed in several ways. A chi-squared test will be used to compare 2-year recurrence rates. Logistic regression on recurrence within 2 years will be used to adjust for covariates representing stratification factors (participating center, primary/recurrent, unilateral/bilateral). Similar analyses using a Cox regression analysis will compare the two surgical treatments on time to recurrence using the stratification factors as covariates. This analysis will be tried only if we obtain adequate data on time to recurrence. Crossovers, as a consequence of conversion of a laparoscopic to an open approach because of technical problems encountered intraoperatively, are expected to occur 1% to 2% of the time and will be analyzed as intention to treat.

Secondary Outcomes

Secondary outcomes including complications, patient centered outcomes, time to return to work, and cost will be compared for the two surgical treatments. The occurrence of operative complications will be compared between treatment groups using logistic regression to adjust for stratification factors. Patient-centered outcomes (pain, functional status, satisfaction with care, caregiver assessment) will be compared between treatment groups using generalized estimating equations (GEE) to adjust for covariates representing stratification factors and to account for repeated measures. A Cox regression analysis will compare the time to return to work or regular activities of the two surgical treatments adjusting for stratification factors.

Cost Data

It is expected that the laparoscopic herniorrhaphy will cost more than open tension-free repair due to the specialized equipment and need for general anesthesia. However, these costs might be counterbalanced if patients return to work or normal activity sooner and have fewer recurrences. Costs of laparoscopic equipment will be averaged across all patients (not just study patients) receiving the service to develop an average equipment cost per patient.

In comparing average costs between two surgical techniques, because costs are not normally distributed, a log or square root transformation of the data will be calculated prior to the statistical testing. A two-sample *t*-test for independent groups will be used to compare costs. Nonparametric tests, such as Wilcoxon's rank sum test, will also be used. In addition, regression analyses on the transformed costs will be used to test for a significant treatment group effect adjusting for covariates representing stratification factors.

All VA and non-VA costs will be analyzed together. However, from past studies, we know that non-VA costs will be a small fraction of total health care costs. Cost analyses will be conducted separately for hernia-related costs alone, and all health care costs.

If differences are found in the effectiveness measures (i.e., recurrence rates, HRQoL, and patient satisfaction), we also will examine cost-effectiveness ratios. That is, we will calculate the net costs between the open and laparoscopic herniorrhaphy groups and the net effectiveness, measured as the difference in recurrence rates, HRQoL, or patient satisfaction. The ratio of net costs and net effectiveness will yield the cost-effectiveness ratio.

Duration of the Trial

The trial will consist of five phases: Implementation, Patient Intake, Patient Follow-up, Close-out of Participating Centers, and Final Analysis.

Implementation (3 Months)

The following tasks will be accomplished during this phase:

1. Funding of the chair's offices and hiring of personnel.
2. Funding of the Hines CSPCC and hiring of personnel in that center.
3. Final selection of participating centers and hiring of personnel.
4. Review and approval of the study protocol by the research committee and IRB at each participating center.
5. Development of an operations manual.
6. Finalization of data collection forms and printing of forms.
7. Development of computer data management software to edit and manage incoming study data.
8. Development of materials to advertise the study at each participating center.
9. Appointment of executive committee and data safety and monitoring board.
10. Kickoff training meeting for all participating investigators and coordinators.

Patient Intake Period (3 Years)

It is anticipated that each of 14 participating centers will randomize 50 to 75 patients per year for 3 years (at least 160 patients per center) to reach a sample size for the entire study of 2,200 patients.

Follow-up Period (2 Years)

Two years are requested to follow all patients for major outcomes of the study, including recurrence rates, pain, HRQoL, and costs. The range of follow-up times will be from 2 to 5 years (average will be 3.5 years).

Close-out of Participating Centers (3 Months)

Final Analysis (6 Months, to Run Concurrently with Close-Out of Participating Centers)

The 14 participating centers will be given 3 months of funding to close out the data collection. During this period, all final follow-up visits and data collection will be completed. Also, any outstanding missing forms or data corrections will be completed at this time.

The chair's office and the Hines CSPCC will use the final 6-month period following data collection to perform the final analyses and manuscript preparation. A provisional publication plan for the study is provided below. Many manuscripts will be written from the study data. Each of these will require extensive data analysis and continual interchanges between the study chair, writing committees, and the Hines CSPCC. The goal will be to have the major manuscripts written and submitted during the 6-month final analysis period.

Also during this period, the master data file for the study will be documented and archived at the Hines CSPCC, so that additional manuscripts, metaanalyses, and use of the data by study investigators and outside investigators can be accommodated as resources will permit.

GENDER AND MINORITY INCLUSION FOR RESEARCH INVOLVING HUMAN SUBJECTS

The subjects of this study will be adult men from all ethnic backgrounds. The participating VA hospitals are located throughout the country; therefore, a substantial population of African-American and Latino patients will be available for enrollment.

All subjects will be men. The condition of inguinal hernia in women is so unlike that in men, from anatomic and surgical treatment aspects as well as outcome, that a comparison of patient groups of mixed gender is meaningless. Inguinal hernias in adult women are infrequent (25 times less common than in men) (169) and consist of simple indirect and femoral hernias almost exclusively (119). In a recent series of 955 patients with inguinal hernias treated at the Royal Victoria Hospital in Montreal, 91% of the subjects treated were men. The infrequent rate of occurrence of inguinal hernias in women has been attributed to the observations of Nobbe, cited by Watson (169), that Nuck's canal in the female, analogous to the processus vaginalis in the male, is rarely patent after birth (8% to 10%) while the processus vaginalis in the male is patent in 30% to 40% of men. Large indirect, and direct hernias do not, for practical purposes, occur in women due to the flattened configuration and tilt of the pelvis and subsequent narrow confines of the floor of the inguinal canal. Recurrences of indirect inguinal hernias in women are very rare and are due to technical errors, since ligation and division of the round ligament (analogous to the spermatic cord in the male) can be done with impunity, assuring that the sac and the internal inguinal ring are completely closed (148). These maneuvers cannot be done in men, and the spermatic cord is relatively large, precluding complete closure of the internal ring; thus, recurrences of indirect inguinal hernias occur with regularity. Femoral hernias occur in both sexes but are much more likely to occur in older, obese women, causing acute bowel obstruction requiring emergency operation (148). Femoral hernias and emergency hernia procedures will not be included in this study.

While inguinal hernia is a major cause of disability in men, it is a minor cause of health problems in women.

ORGANIZATION AND ADMINISTRATION

The organization and administration of this cooperative study will be patterned after that of the more than 25 currently ongoing cooperative studies in the VA health care system. The overall direction of the study will be provided by the CSP in VA Headquarters. They will establish the overall policies and procedures applied to the cooperative study through the chair's office and Hines CSPCC. The protocol must be reviewed and approved by the VA Cooperative Studies Evaluation Committee prior to implementation,

and reviewed again by that committee once every 3 years. The final decisions regarding implementation and funding rests with the VA's Chief Research and Development Officer. He will be requested to fund the VA chair's office, the Hines CSPCC, and the VA participating sites.

The study chair's office and the Hines CSPCC jointly will perform the day-to-day scientific and administrative coordination of the study. They will help to develop the study protocol, operations manual, and case report forms; ensure the appropriate support for the participating centers; schedule meetings and conference calls; train participants in conducting the study; manage the study data; answer questions about the protocol from the study sites; conduct site visits; publish newsletters; prepare interim and final progress reports; prepare data analyses and manuscripts; and archive study data at the end of the study.

Representatives of the American College of Surgeons and the Northwestern University Institute for Health Services Research and Policy Studies will collaborate on protocol development, sample size calculation, conduct of the study, development and implementation of the impact study, and analysis and publication of the data. They will be instrumental in development of sample size estimates and some of the outcome measures of the study.

The study group will consist of an investigator and a nurse coordinator from each participating center, the study chair, study biostatistician, and representatives from the American College of Surgeons and Northwestern University. The investigator at each site will be responsible administratively and scientifically for the conduct of the study at that center. The investigator will be expected to attend all annual study group meetings. A nurse coordinator will be hired at each center for patient intake and management, clinical coordination, and completion of the research data forms.

The executive committee will be concerned with the overall management of the study. It will be composed of the study chair, who heads the committee, study biostatistician, three VA participating investigators, and representatives from the Hines CSPCC, the American College of Surgeons, and Northwestern University. This committee will meet every 12 months to review data not broken down by treatment group, and make decisions on changes in the study, the fate of hospitals whose performance is substandard, the initiation of any subprotocols, and publication of the study results.

Interim, independent, and unbiased review of the study's ongoing progress will be provided by the Data Monitoring Board. This committee will be composed of five members who are independent from the planning and conduct of the study: three general surgeons, a health services researcher, and a biostatistician. The study chair, study biostatistician, Hines CSPCC chief, and CSP chief, and representatives of the American College of Surgeons, and Northwestern University will be *ex officio* (nonvoting) members of the board.

The Data Monitoring Board will meet every 12 months, usually after a meeting of the study group and executive committee, to monitor the study. Its prime responsibility will be to review the progress of the study and to decide whether or not the study should continue. To help them make their assessment, the study chair and the study biostatistician will furnish the Data Monitoring Board with appropriate monitoring data at least 3 weeks before each meeting.

Part of each Data Monitoring Board meeting is a joint session held with the Hines VA CSPCC Human Rights Committee. This committee is composed primarily of lay people. Their responsibility is to ensure that the patients' rights and safety are protected during the conduct of the study. This committee initially reviews all new protocols and reviews all ongoing studies every 12 months. They also occasionally perform human rights site visits to the participating centers to determine the patients' satisfaction with participation in the study.

Prior to the entry of each participating center, the center's local research and development and human studies committees must also review and approve that center's participation in the study. These local committees may also require the investigator to submit annual reports concerning the status of the study at the medical center.

PUBLICATION POLICIES AND PLANS

It is the policy of the VA CSP that outcome data will not be revealed to the participating investigators and study chair until the data collection phase of the study is completed. This policy safeguards against possible biases affecting the data collection. The members of the Data Safety and Monitoring Board and the Hines CSPCC Human Rights Committee will be monitoring the outcome results to ensure that the study is stopped if a definitive answer is reached earlier than the scheduled end of the study.

All presentations and publications from this study will be done in accordance with the CSP policy as stated in the CSP guidelines. The presentation or publication of any data collected by participating investigators on patients entered into the cooperative study is under the direct control of the study's executive committee. This is true whether the publication or presentation is concerned with the results of the principal undertaking or is associated with the study in some other way. No individual participating investigator has any inherent right to perform analyses or interpretations or to make public presentations or seek publication of any of the data other than under the auspices and approval of the executive committee.

The executive committee has the authority to establish one or more publication committees, usually made up of subgroups of participating investigators and some members of the executive committee, for the purpose of producing manuscripts for presentation and publication. Any presentation or publication, when formulated by the executive committee or its authorized representatives, should be circulated to all participating investigators for their review, comments, and suggestions at least 4 weeks prior to submission of the manuscript to the presenting or publication body.

All publications must give proper recognition to the study's funding sources, and should list all participants in the study. If an investigator's major salary support and/or commitment is from the VA, the investigator must list the VA as his/her primary institutional affiliation. Submission of manuscripts or abstracts must follow the usual VA policy. Ideally, a subtitle is used, stating, A VA Cooperative Study or, if the study is jointly funded, a VA/(Joint Funding Source) Cooperative Study. A copy of the letter to the editor and the manuscript/abstract submitted for publication/presentation should be sent to the CSP chief, and for information purposes, to the members of the study's Data Monitoring Board. The CSP also requires that a copy of every manuscript and abstract be reviewed and approved by the Hines CSPCC director prior to submission as a last quality control step.

The following is a tentative plan for the development of manuscripts from the study:

1. Year 1
   a. Description of the protocol and design of the study; discussion of the unique collaboration between the VA, American College of Surgeons, and Northwestern University.
   b. Results of the pilot study for the development of the hernia-specific patient-centered outcome measures.
2. End of 3-Year Accrual Period
   a. Baseline characteristics of randomized patients, and short-term outcomes—postoperative pain/discomfort, HRQoL, return to work/normal activity, patient satisfaction.
   b. Operative data and complications.
      (1) For laparoscopic repair
      (2) For open repair
   c. Baseline correlations between subjective measures.
3. Months 1 and 2 of the Final Analysis Period
   a. Main clinical and patient-centered results of laparoscopic repair versus open repair recurrence rates, complications, postoperative pain and discomfort, HRQoL, patient satisfaction.
   b. Health care utilization and costs.
4. Months 3 to 6 of the Final Analysis Period
   a. Results from treatment of bilateral and recurrent hernias.
   b. Predictors of outcome for
      (1) Laparoscopic repair
      (2) Open repair
   c. Variations in treatment effects across participating centers.

REFERENCES

1. Agency for Health Care Policy and Research: Acute pain management guideline panel. *Acute pain management: operative or medical procedures and trauma.* 1992:1.
2. Albert TJ, Purtill J, Mesa J, et al. Health outcome assessment before and after adult deformity surgery. A prospective study. *Spine* 1995;20:2002–2004.
3. Allaire SH, Meenan RF, Anderson JJ. The impact of rheumatoid arthritis on the household work performance of women. *Arth Rheum* 1991;34:669–678.
4. Amid PK, Shulman AG, Lichtenstein IL. Simultaneous repair of bilateral inguinal hernias under local anesthesia. *Ann Surg* 1996;223:249–252.
5. Arregui M, Davis CJ, Yucel O, et al. Laparoscopic mesh repair of inguinal hernia using a preperitoneal approach: a preliminary report. *Surg Laparosc Endosc* 1992;2:53–58.
6. Barkun JS, Wexler MJ, Bertleff S, et al. Laparoscopic versus open inguinal herniorrhaphy: preliminary results of a randomized controlled trial. *Surgery* 1995;118:703–710.
7. Reference deleted.
8. Beck DH, Mcquillan PJ. Fatal carbon dioxide embolism and severe haemorrhage during laparoscopic salpingectomy. *Br J Anaesth* 1994;72:243–245.
9. Bergner M, Bobbitt RA, Carter WB, et al. The sickness impact profile: development and final revision of a health status measure. *Med Care* 1981;19:787–805.
10. Bessell JR, Baxter P, Riddell P, et al. A randomized controlled trial of laparoscopic extraperitoneal hernia repair as a day surgical procedure. *Surg Endosc* 1996;10:495–500.
11. Birth M, Friedman RL, Melullis M, et al. Laparoscopic transabdominal preperitoneal hernioplasty: results of 1000 consecutive cases. *J Laparoendosc Surg* 1997;6:293–300.
12. Black N, Petticrew M, Ginzler M, et al. Do doctors and patients agree? Views of the outcomes of transurethral resection of the prostate. *Int J Tech Assess Health Care* 1991;7:533–544.
13. Bombardier C, Melfi C, Paul J, et al. Comparison of a generic and a disease-specific measure of pain and physical function after knee replacement surgery. *Med Care* 1995;33[Suppl]:AS131–144.
14. Brook RH, Ware JE Jr, Davies-Avery A, et al. *Conceptualization and measurement of health for adults in the Health Insurance Study.* 1979:8.
15. Brooks DC. A prospective comparison of laparoscopic and tension-free open herniorrhaphy. *Arch Surg* 1994;129:361–366.
16. Brown RB. Laparoscopic hernia repair: a rural perspective. *Surg Laparosc Endosc* 1994;4:106–109.
17. Burney RE, Jones KR, Coon JW, et al. Outcomes assessment in common general surgical conditions. *Surg Forum* 1995;46:618–621.
18. Cameron AEP. Accuracy of clinical diagnosis of direct and indirect inguinal hernia. *Br J Surg* 1994;81:250.
19. Chan ACW, Lee TW, Ng KW, et al. Early results of laparoscopic intraperitoneal onlay mesh repair for inguinal hernia. *Br J Surg* 1994;81:1761–1762.
20. Charlson MD, Pompei P, Ales KL, et al. A new method of classifying prognostic comorbidity in longitudinal studies: development and validation. *J Chron Dis* 1996;40:373–383.
21. Cleary PD, Reilly DT, Greenfield S, et al. Using patient reports to assess health-related quality of life after total hip replacement. *Qual Life Res* 1993;2:3–11.
22. Concato J, Horwitz RI, Feinstein AR, et al. Problems of comorbidity in mortality after prostatectomy. *JAMA* 1992;267:1077–1082.
23. Condon RE. Complications of hernia. In: Nyhus LM, Condon RE, eds. *Hernia.* Philadelphia: JB Lippincott Co, 1994.

24. Conseil d'Evaluation des Technologies de la Sante. *Variations in the frequency of surgical procedures by region in the Province of Quebec.* 1993:15
25. Corbitt JD, Jr. Laparoscopic herniorrhaphy. A preperitoneal tension-free approach. *Surg Endosc* 1993;7:550–555.
26. Corbitt JD. Laparoscopic herniorrhaphy. *Surg Laparosc Endosc* 1991;1:23–25.
27. Cullen DJ, Apolone G, Greenfield S, et al. ASA physical status and age predict morbidity after three surgical procedures. *Ann Surg* 1994;220:3–9.
28. Cunningham J, Temple WJ, Mitchell P, et al. Cooperative hernia study. Pain in the postrepair patient. *Ann Surg* 1996;224:598–602.
29. Davies N, Thomas M, McIlroy B, et al. Early results with the Lichtenstein tension-free hernia repair. *Br J Surg* 1994;81:1475–1478.
30. Davies NM, Dunn D, Appleton B, et al. Experience with 300 laparoscopic inguinal hernia repairs with up to 3 years follow-up. *Ann R Coll Surg Engl* 1995;77:409–412.
31. Del Guercio LRM, Cohn JD. Monitoring operative risk in the elderly. *JAMA* 1980;243:1350–1355.
32. Department of Health Education and Welfare. *National Health Survey on Hernias, 1960.* 1960; Series B, No. 25.
33. Dorsey JH, Holtz PM, Griffiths RI, et al. Costs and charges associated with three alternative techniques of hysterectomy. *N Engl J Med* 1996;335:476–482.
34. Dripps RD, Lamount A, Eckenhoff JE. The role of anesthesia in surgical mortality. *JAMA* 1961;261:261.
35. EaSt, A Software Package for the Design and Interim Monitoring of Group Sequential Clinical Trials. Cytel Software Corporation, 1996.
36. Eddy DM. Principles for making difficult decisions in difficult times. *JAMA* 1994;271:1792–1798.
37. Editorial. Quality of life and clinical trials. *Lancet* 1995;346:1–2.
38. Ettinger WH, Davis MA, Neuhaus JM, et al. Long-term physical functioning in persons with knee osteoarthritis from NHANES. I. Effects of comorbid medical conditions. *J Clin Epidemiol* 1994;47:809–815.
39. Euroqol Group. A new facility for the measurement of health related quality of life. *Health Policy* 1990;16:199–208.
40. Feinstein AR. The pre-therapeutic classification of co-morbidity in chronic disease. *J Chron Dis* 1970;23:455–468.
41. Felix EL, Michas C. Double-buttress laparoscopic herniorrhaphy. *J Laparoendosc Surg* 1993;3:1–8.
42. Felix EL, Michas CA, McKnight RL. Laparoscopic herniorrhaphy. Transabdominal preperitoneal floor repair. *Surg Endosc* 1994;8:100–104.
43. Ferzli GS, Massaad A, Dysarz, III, et al. A study of 101 patients treated with extraperitoneal endoscopic laparoscopic herniorrhaphy. *Am Surg* 1993;59:707–708.
44. Filipi CJ, Fitzgibbons RJ Jr, McBride PJ, et al. An assessment of pain and return to normal activity: laparoscopic herniorrhaphy vs. open tension-free Lichtenstein repair. *Surg Endosc* 1996;10:983–986.
45. Fitzgibbons RJ Jr, Camps J, Cornet DA, et al. Laparoscopic inguinal herniorrhaphy. Results of a multicenter trial. *Ann Surg* 1995;221:3–13.
46. Foster ED, Davis KB, Carpenter JA, et al. Risk of noncardiac operation in patients with defined coronary disease: the coronary artery surgery study (CASS) registry experience. *Ann Thorac Surg* 1986;41:42–50.
47. Fraser SCA. Quality-of-life measurement in surgical practice. *Br J Surg* 1993;80:163–169.
48. French Associations for Surgical Research, Oberlin P, Boudet MJ, et al. Recurrence after inguinal hernia repair: prognostic facts in a prospective study of 1706 hernias. *Br J Surg* 1995;82 [Suppl 1]:65.

49. Friis E, Lindahl F. The tension-free hernioplasty in a randomized trial. *Am J Surg* 1996;172:315–319.

50. Gandek B. MOS bibliography. 1996.

51. Geis WP, Crafton WB, Novak MJ, et al. Laparoscopic herniorrhaphy: results and technical aspects in 450 consecutive patients. *Surgery* 1993;114:765–774.

52. Gelber RD, Cole BF, Goldhirsch A, et al. Adjuvant chemotherapy plus tamoxifen compared with tamoxifen alone for postmenopausal breast cancer: meta-analysis of quality-adjusted survival. *Lancet* 1996;347:1066–1071.

53. Ger R, Monroe K, Duvivier R, et al. Management of indirect inguinal hernias by laparoscopic closure of the neck of the sac. *Am J Surg* 1990;159:370.

54. Ger R, Mishrick A, Hurwitz J, et al. Management of groin hernias by laparoscopy. *World J Surg* 1993;17:46–50.

55. Gibbons GW, Burgess AM, Guadagnoli E, et al. Return to well-being and function after infrainguinal revascularization. *J Vasc Surg* 1995;21:35–44.

56. Gibbs JO. National Veterans Administration Surgical Risk Study: herniorrhaphy data. 1996.

57. Gilbert AI. Sutureless repair of inguinal hernia. *Am J Surg* 1992;163:331–335.

58. Glicklich RE, Metson R. Techniques for outcomes research in chronic sinusitis. *Laryngoscope* 1995;105:387–390.

59. Gold MR, Siegel JE, Russell LB, et al., eds. *Cost effectiveness in health and medicine.* New York: Oxford University Press, 1996.

60. Goldman L, Caldera DL, Southwick FS, et al. Cardiac risk factors and complications in non-cardiac surgery. *Medicine* 1978;57:357–370.

61. Greenburg AG. Revisiting the recurrent groin hernia. *Am J Surg* 1987;154:35–40.

62. Greenfield S, Apolone G, McNeil BJ, et al. The importance of co-existent disease in the occurrence of postoperative complications and one-year recovery in patients undergoing total hip replacement. *Med Care* 1993;31:141–154.

63. Grosfeld J. Pediatric hernia. In: Nyhus LM, Condon RC, eds. *Hernia.* Philadelphia: JB Lippincott Co, 1994.

64. Hawasli A. Laparoscopic inguinal herniorrhaphy: classification and 1 year experience. *J Laparoendosc Surg* 1992;2:137–143.

65. Hawasli A. Laparoscopic inguinal herniorrhaphy: the mushroom plug repair. *Surg Laparosc Endosc* 1992;2:111–116.

66. Hawker G, Melfi C, Paul J, et al. Comparison of a generic (SF-36) and a disease specific (WOMAC) (Western Ontario and McMaster Universities Osteoarthritis Index) instrument in the measurement of outcomes after knee replacement surgery. *J Rheumatol* 1995;22:1193–1196.

67. Hay J, Boudet M, Fingerhut A, et al. Shouldice inguinal hernia repair in the male adult: the gold standard? *Ann Surg* 1995;222:719–727.

68. Hays RD, Shapiro MF. An overview of generic health-related quality of life measures for HIV research. *Qual Life Res* 1992;1:91–97.

69. Herxheimer A. Clinical trials: two neglected ethical issues. *J Med Ethics* 1993;19:211–218.

70. Hicks NR. Some observations on attempts to measure appropriateness of care. *BMJ* 1994;309:730–733.

71. Himpens JM. Laparoscopic inguinal hernioplasty. *Surg Endosc* 1993;7:315–318.

72. Hoffman HC, Traverso ALV. Preperitoneal prosthetic herniorrhaphy. *Arch Surg* 1993;128:964–970.

73. Hugh TB. Laparoscopic hernia repair. *Med J Aust* 1993;159:151–152.

74. Iezzoni LI. Chronic conditions and risk of in-hospital death. *Health Serv Res* 1994;29:435–460.

75. Ijzermans JNM, de Wilt H, Hop WCJ, et al. Recurrent inguinal hernia treated by classical hernioplasty. *Arch Surg* 1991;126:1097–1100.

76. Jacobson AM, deGroot M, Samson JA. The evaluation of two measures of quality of life in patients with type I and type II diabetes. *Diabetes Care* 1994;17:267–274.

77. Jacoby HE, Brodie DA. Laparoscopic herniorrhaphy. Diagnostic and therapeutic technology assessment (DATTA). *JAMA* 1996;275:1075–1082.

78. Jenkinson C, Lawrence K, McWhinnie D, et al. Sensitivity to change of health status measures in a randomized controlled trial: comparison of the COOP charts and the SF-36. *Qual Life Res* 1995;4:47–52.

79. Jonasson O. Poll of general surgeons attending the 1995 Spring Meeting, American College of Surgeons, Boston. 1995.

80. Kald A, Smedh K, Anderberg B. Laparoscopic groin repair: results of 200 consecutive herniorrhaphies. *Br J Surg* 1995;82:618–620.

81. Kald A, Anderberg B, Carlsson P, et al. Surgical outcome and cost-minimisation-analyses of laparoscopic and open hernia repair: a randomised prospective trial with one year follow up. *Eur J Surg* 1997;163:505–510.

82. Katz JN, Phillips CB, Poss R, et al. The validity and reliability of a Total Hip Arthroplasty Outcome Evaluation questionnaire. *J Bone Joint Surg Am* 1995;77:1528–1534.

83. Kavic MS. Laparoscopic hernia repair. Three year experience. *Surg Endosc* 1995;9:12–15.

84. Keats AS. The estimate of anesthetic risk in medical evaluations. *Am J Cardiol* 1963;12:330–333.

85. Keefe FJ, Caldwell DS, Baucom D, et al. Spouse-assisted coping skills training in the management of osteoarthritic knee pain. *Arthritis Care Res* 1996;9:279–291.

86. Kelly MP, Anderson JR, Carey LM, et al. Some considerations for identifying quality measures of surgical outcome. *Health Serv Manage Res* 1994;7:265–270.

87. Kennedy GM, Matyas JA. Use of expanded polytetrafluoroethylene in the repair of the difficult hernia. *Am J Surg* 1994;168:304–306.

88. Keoghane SR, Lawrence KC, Jenkinson CP, et al. The Oxford laser prostate trial: sensitivity to change of three measures of outcome. *Urology* 1996;47:43–47.

89. Khuri S, Daley J, Henderson W, et al. The national Veterans Administration surgical risk study: risk adjustment for the comparative assessment of the quality of surgical care. *J Am Coll Surg* 1995;180:519–531.

90. Khuri SF, Daley J, Henderson W, et al. Risk adjustment of the postoperative mortality rate for the comparative assessment of the quality of surgical care. *J Am Coll Surg* 1997;185:315–327.

91. Kozol R, Lange PM, Kosir M, et al. A prospective, randomized study of open vs laparoscopic inguinal hernia repair. *Arch Surg* 1997;132:292–295.

92. Kux M, Fuchsjager N, Schemper M. Shouldice is superior to Bassini inguinal herniorrhaphy. *Am J Surg* 1994;168:15–18.

93. Laupacis A, Sackett DL. An assessment of clinically useful measures of the consequences of treatment. *N Engl J Med* 1988;318:1728–1733.

94. Lave JR, Pashos CL, Anderson GF, et al. Costing medical care: using Medicare administrative data. *Med Care* 1994;32[Suppl]:JS77–JS89.

95. Lawrence K, McWhinnie D, Goodwin A, et al. Randomised controlled trial of laparoscopic versus open repair of inguinal hernia: early results. *BMJ* 1995;311:981–985.

96. Lawrence, K. Personal communication to M. McCarthy. 1996.

97. LeBlanc KA, Booth WV. Avoiding complications with laparoscopic herniorrhaphy. *Surg Laparosc Endosc* 1993;3:420–424.

98. Liang MH, Fossel AH, Larson MG. Comparisons of five health

status instruments for orthopedic evaluation. *Med Care* 1990;
28:632–642.

99. Lichtenstein IL. Herniorrhaphy: a personal experience with
6,321 cases. *Am J Surg* 1987;153:553.

100. Liem MSL, van der Graaf Y, van Steensel CJ, et al. Comparison
of conventional anterior surgery and laparoscopic surgery for
inguinal hernia repair. *N Engl J Med* 1997;336:1541–1547.

101. Liem MSL, Haisema JAM, van der Graaf Y, et al. Cost-effectiveness of extraperitoneal laparoscopic inguinal hernia repair: a
randomized comparison with conventional herniorrhaphy. *Ann
Surg* 1997;226:668–676.

102. Liem MSL, van Vroonhoven TJMV. Laparoscopic inguinal hernia repair. *Br J Surg* 1996;83:1197–1204.

103. Liem MSL, van Steensel CJ, Boelhouwer RU, et al. The learning curve for totally extraperitoneal laparoscopic inguinal hernia
repair. *Am J Surg* 1996;171:281–285.

104. Lindholm A, Nilsson O, Tholin B. Inguinal and femoral hernias. Results following 238 preperitoneal radical operations.
Arch Surg 1969;98:19–23.

105. Litwin MS, Hays RD, Fink A, et al. Quality of life outcomes in
men treated for localized prostate cancer. *JAMA* 1995;273:
129–135.

106. Lukaszczyk JJ, Preletz RJ, Morrow GJ, et al. Laparoscopic
herniorrhaphy versus traditional open repair at a community
hospital. *J Laparoendosc Surg* 1996;6:209–211.

107. MacFadyen JR, Arregui M, Corbitt JR, et al. Complications of
laparoscopic herniorrhaphy. *Surg Endosc* 1993;7:155–158.

108. MacKenzie EJ, Burgess AR, McAndrew MP, et al. Patient-ori-
ented functional outcome after unilateral lower extremity fracture. *J Orthopaed Trauma* 1996;7:393–401.

109. MacWilliam CH, Ulcickas Yood M, Verner JJ, et al. Patient-
related risk factors that predict poor outcome after total hip
replacement. *Health Serv Res* 1996;31:623–637.

110. Mangione CM, Phillips RS, Lawrence MB, et al. Improved
visual function and attenuation of declines in health-related
quality of life after cataract extraction. *Arch Ophthalmol* 1994;
112:1419–1525.

111. Manne SL, Zautra AJ. Spouse criticism and support: their association with coping and psychological adjustment among
women with rheumatoid arthritis. *J Pers Soc Psychol* 1996;56:
608–617.

112. McHorney CA, Tarlov AR. Individual-patient monitoring in
clinical practice: are available health status surveys adequate?
Qual Life Res 1995;4:293–307.

113. McKernan JB, Laws HL. Laparoscopic repair of inguinal hernias using a totally extraperitoneal prosthetic approach. *Surg
Endosc* 1993;7:26–28.

114. Millikan KW, Kosik ML, Doolas A. A prospective comparison
of transabdominal preperitoneal laparoscopic hernia repair vs
traditional open hernia repair in a university setting. *Surg
Laparosc Endosc* 1994;4:247–253.

115. Neumayer L. VA Health Care Statistics. 1997.

116. Newman L III, Eubanks S, Mason E, et al. Is laparoscopic
herniorrhaphy an effective alternative to open hernia repair? *J
Laparoendosc Surg* 1993;2:121–128.

117. Nolen M, Melichar R, Jennings WC, et al. Use of a Marlex fan
in the repair of direct and indirect hernias by laparoscopy. *Surg
Laparosc Endosc* 1992;2:61–64.

118. Nyhus LM. Individualization of hernia repair: a new era.
Surgery 1993;114:1–2.

119. Nyhus LM, Condon RE, eds. *Hernia.* Philadelphia: JB Lippincott Co, 1995.

120. Nyhus LM, Condon RE, eds. The preperitoneal approach and
iliopubic tract repair of inguinal hernias. In: *Hernia.* Philadelphia: JB Lippincott Co, 1995:153–177.

121. Olsson M, Janfjall H, Orth-Gomer K, et al. Quality of life in
octogenarians after valve replacement due to aortic stenosis. A
prospective comparison with younger patients. *Eur Heart J*
1996;17:583–589.

122. Panton ONM, Panton RJ. Laparoscopic hernia repair. *Am J
Surg* 1994;167:535–537.

123. Payne JH. Laparoscopic or open inguinal herniorrhaphy? A randomized prospective trial. *Arch Surg* 1994;129:973–981.

124. Pell JP. Impact of intermittent claudication on quality of life.
The Scottish Vascular Audit Group. *Eur J Vasc Endovasc Surg*
1995;10:510–511.

125. Phillips EH, Carroll BJ, Fallas MJ. Laparoscopic preperitoneal
inguinal hernia repair without peritoneal incision. Technique
and early clinical results. *Surg Endosc* 1993;7:159–162.

126. Pickering WG. Does medical treatment mean patient benefit?
Lancet 1996;347:379–380.

127. Price DD, Bush FM, Long S, et al. A comparison of pain measurement characteristics of mechanical visual and simple
numerical rating scales. *Pain* 1994;56:217–236.

128. Price DD, Harkins SW, Barker C. Sensory-affective relationships among different types of clinical and experimental pain.
Pain 1987;28:291–299.

129. Price DD, Harkins SW. Psychological approaches to pain measurement and assessment. In: Turk DC, Melzack R, eds. *Hand-
book of pain assessment.* New York: Guilford Press, 1992.

130. Price DD, McGrath PA, Rafii A, et al. The validation of visual
analogue scales as ratio scale measures for chronic and experimental pain. *Pain* 1983;17:45–56.

131. Price DD. Personal communication to M. McCarthy, 1996.

132. Reid I, Devlin HB. Testicular atrophy as a consequence of
inguinal hernia repair. *Br J Surg* 1994;81:91–93.

133. Report of a Working Party convened by the Royal College of
Surgeons of England. Clinical Guidelines on the Management
of Groin Hernia in Adults. 1993.

134. Revenson TA, Majerovitz SD. The effects of chronic illness on
the spouse: social resources as stress buffers. *Arthritis Care Res*
1991;4:63–72.

135. Rider MA, Baker DM, Locker A, et al. Return to work after
inguinal hernia repair. *Br J Surg* 1993;80:745–746.

136. Robbins AW, Rutkow IM. The mesh-plug hernioplasty. *Surg
Clin North Am* 1993;73:501–512.

137. Robertson GSM, Haynes IG, Burton PR. How long do patients
convalesce after inguinal herniorrhaphy? Current principles and
practice. *Ann R Coll Surg Engl* 1996;75:30–33.

138. Rosario DJ, Skinner PP, Raftery AT. Transient femoral nerve
palsy complicating preoperative ilioinguinal nerve blockade for
inguinal herniorrhaphy. *Br J Surg* 1994;81:897.

139. Rose KJ, Derry PA, Wiebe S, et al. Determinants of health-
related quality of life after temporal lobe epilepsy surgery. *Qual
Life Res* 1996;5:395–402.

140. Rowntree LG. National program for physical fitness. Revealed
and developed on the basis of 13,000,000 physical examinations of selective service registrants. *JAMA* 1944;125:825–838.

141. Russell LB, Gold MR, Siegel JE, et al. The role of cost-effectiveness analysis in health and medicine. *JAMA* 1996;276:
1172–1177.

142. Rutkow IM, Robbins AW. Groin hernia. In: Cameron JL, ed.
Current surgical therapy. St. Louis: Mosby, 1995:481.

143. Rutledge RH. Cooper's ligament repair: a 25-year experience
with a single technique for all groin hernias in adults. *Surgery*
1988;103:1–10.

144. Sandbichler P, Draxi H, Gstir H, et al. Laparoscopic repair of
recurrent inguinal hernias. *Am J Surg* 1996;171:366–368.

145. Schneider JR, McHorney CA, Malenka DJ, et al. Functional
health and well being in patients with severe atherosclerotic
peripheral vascular occlusive disease. *Ann Vasc Surg* 1993;7:
419–428.

146. Schrenk P, Woisetschlager R, Rieger R, et al. Prospective randomized trial comparing postoperative pain and return to physical activity after transabdominal preperitoneal, total preperitoneal or Shouldice technique for inguinal hernia repair. *Br J Surg* 1996;83:1563–1566.

147. Schultz L, Graber J, Pietrafitta J, et al. Laser laparoscopic herniorrhaphy: a clinical trial. Preliminary results. *J Laparoendosc Surg* 1990;1:41–45.

148. Shackelford RT. Hernia of the gastrointestinal tract. In: Shackelford RT, ed. *Surgery of the alimentary tract.* Philadelphia: WB Saunders, 1955:2222.

149. Siegel JE, Weinstein MC, Russell LB, et al. Recommendations for reporting cost-effectiveness analyses. *JAMA* 1996;276:1339–1341.

150. Simons MP, Kleijnen J, van Geldere D, et al. Role of the Shouldice technique in inguinal hernia repair: a systematic review of controlled trials and a meta-analysis. *Br J Surg* 1996;83:734–738.

151. Stewart AL, Greenfield S, Hays RD, et al. Functional status and well-being of patients with chronic conditions. *JAMA* 1989;262:907–913.

152. Stoker DL, Speigelhalter DJ, Singh R, et al. Laparoscopic vs. open inguinal hernia repair: randomised prospective trial. *Lancet* 1994;343:1243–1245.

153. Stuart AE. Taking the tension out of hernia repair [Editorial]. *Lancet* 1994;343:748.

154. Stucki G, Liang MH, Fossel AH, et al. Relative responsiveness of condition-specific and generic health status measures in degenerative lumbar spinal stenosis. *J Clin Epidemiol* 1995;48:1369–1378.

155. Stucki G, Daltroy L, Liang MH, et al. Measurement properties of a self-administered outcome measure in lumbar spinal stenosis. *Spine* 1996;21:796–803.

156. Toy FK, Smoot JR. Laparoscopic hernioplasty update. *J Laparoendosc Surg* 1992;2:197–205.

157. Toy FK, Moskowitz M, Smoot JR, et al. Results of a prospective multicenter trial evaluating the ePTFE peritoneal onlay laparoscopic inguinal hernioplasty. *J Laparoendosc Surg* 1996;6:375–386.

158. Toy FK, Smoot JR. Toy-Smoot laparoscopic hernioplasty. *Del Med J* 1992;64:23–27.

159. Treacy PJ, Johnson AG. Is the laparoscopic bubble bursting? *Lancet* 1995;346[Suppl]:S23.

160. Tschudi J, Wagner M, Klaiber C, et al. Controlled multicenter trial of laparoscopic transabdominal preperitoneal hernioplasty vs Shouldice herniorrhaphy. *Surg Endosc* 1996;10:845–847.

161. Velasco JM, Gelman C, Vallina VL. Preperitoneal bilateral inguinal herniorrhaphy. *Surg Endosc* 1996;10:122–127.

162. Verbrugge LM, Lepkowski JM, Imanaka Y. Comorbidity and its impact on disability. *Milbank Quart* 1989;67:450–484.

163. Vogt DM, Curet MJ, Pitcher DE, et al. Preliminary results of a prospective randomized trial of laparoscopic onlay versus conventional inguinal herniorrhaphy. *Am J Surg* 1995;169:84–90.

164. Wantz GE. Abdominal wall hernias. In: Schwartz SI, Shires GT, Spencer FC, eds. *Principles of surgery.* New York: McGraw–Hill, 1994:1517–1543.

165. Wantz GE. Experience with the tension-free hernioplasty for primary inguinal hernias in men. *J Am Coll Surg* 1996;183:351–356.

166. Wantz GE. The Shouldice repair. In: Nyhus LM, Condon RC, eds. *Hernia.* Philadelphia: JB Lippincott Co, 1995:228.

167. Ware JE Jr, Sherbourne C. The MOS 36-item short-form health survey (SF-36): I. Conceptual framework and item selection. *Med Care* 1992;30:473–483.

168. Ware JE Jr, Kosinski M, Bayliss MS, et al. Comparison of methods for the scoring and statistical analysis of SF-36 health profile and summary measures: summary of results from the Medical Outcomes Study. *Med Care* 1995;33[Suppl]:AS264–279.

169. Watson LF, ed. *Hernia.* St. Louis: CV Mosby, 1948:1.

170. Weinstein MC, Siegel JE, Gold MR, et al. Recommendations on cost-effectiveness in health and medicine. *JAMA* 1996;276:1253–1258.

171. Wheeler KH. Laparoscopic inguinal herniorrhaphy with mesh: an 18-month experience. *J Laparoendosc Surg* 1993;3:345–350.

172. Williams JS, Hale HW. The advisability of inguinal herniorrhaphy in the elderly. *Surg Gynecol Obstet* 1966;122:100–104.

173. Wilson MS, Deans GT, Brough WA. Prospective trial comparing Lichtenstein with laparoscopic tension-free mesh repair of inguinal hernia. *Br J Surg* 1995;82:274–277.

174. Winchester DJ, Dawes LG, Modelski DD, et al. Laparoscopic inguinal hernia repair. A preliminary experience. *Arch Surg* 1993;128:781–786.

175. Wood-Dauphinee S. Quality-of-life assessment: recent trends in surgery. *Can J Surg* 1996;39:368–372.

176. Wright DM, Kennedy A, Baxter JN, et al. Early outcome after open versus extraperitoneal endoscopic tension-free hernioplasty: a randomized clinical trial. *Surgery* 1996;119:552–557.

GLOSSARY

Accident A severe complication of groin hernia, such as bowel obstruction and ischemia (gangrene)

EXTRA Extraperitoneal preperitoneal approach for repair of a groin hernia by laparoscopy

HRQoL Health-related quality of life (self-reported)

Hernia repair (herniorrhaphy, hernioplasty) Surgical procedure to cure hernia.

Hines CSPCC Hines CSPCC.

Laparoscopic herniorrhaphy Video-assisted minimal access to peritoneal cavity and preperitoneal space for herniorrhaphy

Open herniorrhaphy Conventional herniorrhaphy via an incision.

PF Physical Function (SF-36 measure)

PI Principal Investigator

Prosthesis Mesh or other synthetic sheet material

Recurrence Breakdown of hernia repair with visible and/or palpable reappearance of hernia

RR Rate of Recurrence

TAPP Transabdominal preperitoneal procedure for repair of a groin hernia by laparoscopy

TEPP Totally extra preperitoneal procedure for repair of a groin hernia by laparoscopy

APPENDIX A

HUMAN RIGHTS

CHARACTERISTICS OF THE SUBJECT POPULATION AND PLANS FOR RECRUITMENT

The fourteen sites chosen for this study are located across the country. Two thousand two hundred men coming to these institutions for appointments with a surgeon, who have a inguinal will be invited to become a participant in the study. The selected sites assure that the subjects of this study will be men from all socioeconomic and ethnic backgrounds.

Patients who agree to participate in the study will be seen by the site coordinator who will further provide oral and written descriptions of the study, verify the presence of the hernia and the patient's eligibility for the study.

The site coordinator will provide oral and written explanations of this study, including the randomization procedure for open and laparoscopic hernia assignment. The data on recurrence rates, complications, and anesthesia requirements will be provided in oral and written form. They will be further informed that operation is associated with a high degree of success, when performed by either an open or a laparoscopic preperitoneal method, and that the preferred method has not been defined. The site coordinator will then obtain written consent for randomization into either open or laparoscopic repair and will provide a copy of the signed consent forms to the clinical trial office at the Hines CSPCC for enrollment and randomization.

Patients who refuse random assignment will be dropped from the study and from further consideration or data gathering. They will be listed, only.

CONSENT PROCEDURES

Consent will be obtained from subjects after determination of their eligibility but prior to randomization. Consent will cover the following information:

a. A statement that the patient is being invited to participate in a clinical research project, the purpose of the trial, an explanation of its nature including its relationship to existing knowledge, the use to be made of the information from the trial, expected duration of the patient's participation, frequency of visits and phone contact, the nature of the self-reported patient-centered assessments, and the identification of all experimental components of the trial.

b. The procedures to be used, and restrictions on normal activities, if any.

c. Any benefits that may accrue to the patient as a result of participation in the trial, including therapeutic benefits and recognition.

d. Any alternate courses of action open to the subject in lieu of participation in the study.

e. A statement of the result to be anticipated if nothing is done.

f. A statement that the subject may decline to participate or decide to withdraw from participation at any time without prejudicing his medical care (or other VA benefits).

g. An explanation of whom to contact for answers to pertinent questions about the study and patient's rights, and whom to contact in the event of a study-related injury to the patient.

h. A statement that the provisions of the Privacy Act and Freedom of Information Act will be adhered to.

i. A statement that the patient will receive a copy of the consent form and patient information sheet.

The patient must be informed of the nature of the study and consent obtained by one of the participating surgeons or the coordinator. Signature of a witness not involved in the study is required. The Informed Consent document, plus the study information sheet must be reviewed and signed by each subject. The original copies of these consent forms must be placed in the patient's medical record at the participating institution. Copies should also be forwarded to the Hines CSPCC, the local Center's Research Office, and given to the patient.

Each patient must be allowed to read, or have the consent form read to him, and understand the document before discussing consent with the investigator. Each page of the document must be initialed by the patient.

In discussing the study with the patient, the investigator may go somewhat beyond the statements in the information sheets, but there must be no substantive addition, deletion, or modification of these statements. Local changes of the information sheets must receive prior approval by the Hines CSPCC. The consent forms are the tangible evidence of what the investigator tells the patient.

Informed consent from patients will be obtained using the Consent Form (explaining the treatment options of open and laparoscopic hernia repair).

INCLUSION, EXCLUSION CRITERIA

Subjects will be included who are 18 years of age or older, have a inguinal hernia (or bilateral inguinal hernias), and consent to participate in the study. Subjects will be excluded for the following reasons: hernia cannot be detected on physical examination; ASA Class IV or V (severe comorbid conditions) or contraindications to general anesthesia; presence of acute hernia complications such as bowel obstruction, strangulation, peritonitis, or perforation; contraindications to laparoscopy such as previous pelvic procedures (e.g., radical prostatectomy and/or pelvic irradiation); the presence of local or systemic infection; or participation in another clinical trial.

DATA TO BE COLLECTED AND CONFIDENTIALITY

The data to be gathered and the schedule for data collection are specified in Table 49.2. The data elements variously used are: demographic entry data (Form 1); documentation of comorbid conditions (Form 2); hernia size, scrotal component and bilaterality (Form 3); operative data (Form 4), herniorrhaphy complications (Forms 5A to D), recurrence (Forms 5C), return to normal activities and difficulty with activities (Forms 6 and 7); assessment of pain and discomfort (Form 8), functional status and HRQoL assessment (SF-36 Form 9); satisfaction with care (Form 10), caregiver assessment (Form 11), and costs of the medical care and of all associated medications, supplies, and scheduled or unscheduled visits to physicians, clinics, or emergency rooms (Forms 12 to 17).

Each subject will be identified by a unique number assigned sequentially at entry to the study. No individual patient will be otherwise identified and all data will be held confidential, available only to the Hines CSPCC data management personnel and Northwestern University research staff, the data monitoring board, and, at the completion of the study, to the study participants.

POTENTIAL RISKS AND REASONABLE NATURE OF THE RISKS

Risks of this study are those of routine hernia treatment by operation. Open herniorrhaphy using the Lichtenstein technique has a recurrence rate of less than 2% in single-center series. Other complications of the open method are wound infection, possibly involving the mesh used for the repair. Complications common to both the open and laparoscopic methods are scrotal hematoma or seroma, neuropathy from inguinal nerve entrapment, injury to the vas deferens, orchitis or testicular atrophy, acute urinary retention or urinary tract infection, and injury to bowel or bladder. Unique to the laparoscopic method are subcutaneous emphysema, trocar site herniation, and pneumothorax. The reported recurrence rate following laparoscopic repair varies from approximately 1% to approximately 8%. Life threatening complications such as cardiac ischemia or thromboembolism occur rarely following either procedure. Laparoscopic herniorrhaphies are routinely performed using general anesthesia; open procedures can be performed with local, regional, or general anesthesia.

APPENDIX B

BIOSTATISTICAL AND RESEARCH DATA PROCESSING

INTRODUCTION

This appendix summarizes the procedures and systems used to process the study data, monitor the study, and report the results. This includes completion of the case report forms at the participating sites, review and computerized editing at the Hines CSPCC, and production of newsletters, interim analyses and other reports.

TRAINING

An organizational meeting will be conducted before the start of data collection to review the protocol and train principal investigators and site coordinators on study procedures. An operations manual will be developed which will serve as a reference on how to conduct the study and complete the case report forms.

CASE REPORT FORMS COMPLETION

When a subject is contacted for the first time, the site coordinator at the participating site will create a patient file. It will be used to hold copies of the consent form and all completed case report forms. This file is separate from any others within the medical center that may contain information on the patient.

Blank case report forms will be printed on two-part no carbon required (NCR) paper. Once all case report forms for a patient visit examination have been completed, the site coordinator will review them for completeness, accuracy and legibility. The principal investigator will review all completed forms and sign a statement that the data are accurate and have been reviewed. A copy of each form will be retained at the participating site and the original will be mailed to the Statistical Assistant at the Hines CSPCC. Completed forms will be mailed weekly.

HINES CSPCC REVIEW

Once the forms have been received at the Hines CSPCC they will undergo a visual review and manual edit. The Statistical Assistant will log in the forms and check them for legibility and completeness. This review will also focus on reducing variability across participating sites in adherence to treatment and evaluation procedures outlined in the study protocol and operations manual. Forms for each visit will be compared with forms from previous visits to identify inconsistencies and unusual changes in measurements for that patient. If any serious errors are detected, the site coordinator at the participating site will be contacted immediately.

DATA ENTRY AND COMPUTERIZED EDIT

Once the forms have been reviewed, they will be keyed and verified by the Hines CSPCC's data entry personnel and transmitted to the Center's DEC ALPHA minicomputer. The data will be processed by a computer edit system that will check for data entry errors, missing data, values out of range, consistency between data fields, and missing forms.

The computer system will generate a data query report. Queries will be investigated by the Statistical Assistant by contacting the site coordinator at the participating site. A query will be answered by either indicating a data change or identifying the query as needing no correction. After the data changes are processed into the computerized data base, the data will be reedited by the computer program to verify that all queries were resolved. Standard procedures will be used to note data changes in the case report forms, i.e., drawing two lines through the old value, writing the new value above or next to the old value, showing the date of the change and the initials of the person making the change.

Built into the edit system will be an audit trail mechanism that will track and retain records of all errors detected and changes made to the study data base. Periodically, the site coordinator will be sent a listing of data changes with an explanation of the error associated with each change. Error analysis will be conducted to monitor unusually high error rates for a particular data item or at a particular site.

The Hines CSPCC will periodically request copies of case report forms and medical source documents such as laboratory slips, outpatient encounter forms, and hospital discharge summaries, to be compared with the study data base. These will be chosen at random. On-site auditing may be done if the Hines CSPCC determines that a participating clinic's performance warrants such a visit.

CHAIR'S OFFICE REVIEW

The Clinical Nurse Coordinator at the Salt Lake City, UT VA Medical Center will handle any questions from the participating sites regarding the medical content of the case report forms. Exceptions to the protocol needed to provide good clinical care of the patients will be resolved by the Study Chair through the Clinical Nurse Coordinator. These will be reviewed by the Data Coordinating Center to assure uniformity of adherence to the study protocol. These approvals will be documented on the Protocol Exception Approval form. The Clinical Nurse Coordinator will telefax each completed Protocol Exception Approval form to the Data Coordinating Center upon completion.

NEWSLETTERS

The Hines CSPCC will issue a quarterly newsletter to all study participants. This will include recruitment updates based on the number of patients enrolled the preceding 3 months. The newsletter will also provide information about data quality, protocol changes and clarifications, personnel changes and upcoming study events.

PROGRESS REPORTS AND MEETINGS

Interim analyses to report the progress of the study will be distributed semiannually. A complete version of the report will be distributed to the Data Monitoring Board (including the nonvoting members), and the Hines CSPCC Human Rights Committee. A blinded version, deleting summaries of outcome data reported by treatment group, will be sent to the Executive Committee and the study personnel at the participating sites.

All study personnel will meet annually in conjunction with the release of the annual progress report. The Study Group and Executive Committee will meet to review the progress of the study, discuss problems, and reinforce training. The Data Monitoring Board will meet to review the complete annual progress report, evaluate the scientific progress and operational aspects of the study, and discuss whether any changes should be made.

The following table summarizes the distribution of major reports in the study.

Reports Distribution

	Newsletters and accrual report	Treatment outcome interim analyses	Blinded interim analyses
Human rights committee		X	
Data monitoring board		X	
Executive committee	X		X
Study group	X		X

INTERIM ANALYSES

This section describes the proposed data displays that will be included in the interim progress reports.

Accrual and Follow-up

The following will be provided by participating site and by treatment group: (a) number screened, (b) number randomized, (c) number misrandomized, (d) number withdrawn for each year of follow-up, and (e) number completing each year of follow-up.

Data Received and Missing Forms

One table will present the number of forms in the study master file by form type and visit. A second table will summarize the number of missing forms by form type and participating site as well as by form type and treatment group.

Data Quality

One table will display data exception rates by site for various types of protocol violations such as misrandomization and missed visit. A second table will summarize these data by treatment group. A detailed list of misrandomized patients will be included.

Exclusions and Withdrawals

For patients excluded before randomization, a frequency listing of the exclusion reasons will be provided. For the postrandomization period, a similar table will be provided of reasons for withdrawal. These will be reported by site and then by treatment group. A detailed list of patients withdrawn from study will be included.

Description of Patient Characteristics and Comparison by the Stratification Factors and Treatment Groups at Baseline

One series of tables will report baseline patient characteristics by site and all sites combined. Baseline differences will also be reported by (a) whether the hernia is primary or recurrent and (b) whether it is unilateral or bilateral. Note that the randomization scheme includes stratification by these factors.

A second series will investigate comparability of the randomized groups at baseline. Randomization does not guarantee comparability. However, differences that do occur are assumed to be a chance occurrence rather than a result of bias. Data from these series will be perused to determine if systematic baseline differences exist. Finally, it is important to know if baseline differences exist in variables which may be associated with treatment outcomes. If so, the final analysis will need to adjust for these variables.

Outcomes

Treatment groups will be compared on recurrence, complications, cost, time to resume usual activities, and changes from baseline in pain, Health-Related Quality of Life, activity limitations. These will be reported by intention to treat.

Nyhus and Condon's Hernia, Fifth Edition, edited by Robert J. Fitzgibbons, Jr. and A. Gerson Greenburg. Lippincott Williams & Wilkins, Philadelphia © 2002.

50

UTERUS AND VAGINAL VAULT PROLAPSE, ENTEROCELES, CYSTOCELES, RECTOCELES: DEFECTS OF PELVIC SUPPORT IN WOMEN

JAMES E. CARTER

"You are correct to emphasize the reconstruction of the vaginal apex as the first step in treatment of vault prolapse with enterocele. We approach this by saying: The vagina can be thought of as a flattened fibromuscular tissue tube, lined by vaginal mucosa, that is held in place by its continuity with adjacent structures. At the apex (Delancey's level 1) it is continuous with the cardinal/uterosacral complex. Or you may want to say it is 'suspended' by the cardinal/uterosacral ligaments. Again the middle three fifths of the vagina (Delancey's level 2) is attached laterally to the pelvic sidewall. Keep in mind that the attachment of the top and the bottom of the vagina in this area is different. The distal vagina (Delancey's level 3) fuses into the urogenital diaphragm (AKA perineal membrane or perineum). All support defects present as a bulge into the vagina. A bulge indicates that there has either been a break in the integrity of the tube itself, or the tube has lost its apical suspension, lateral attachment or distal fusion. In repairing any of the bulges, you must first restore the integrity of the tube. Then and only then can you contemplate its resuspension, reattachment laterally and refusion distally."

(A.C. Richardson, *personal communications*, 2000).

In one paragraph, A. Cullen Richardson gives us the essence of pelvic support defects in women.

The loss of the upper suspensory fibers of the paracolpium and parametrium will lead to uterine prolapse and vaginal prolapse after hysterectomy. In addition, the separation of pubocervical from the rectovaginal fascia will result in apical enterocele. Defects in the pubocervical fascia result in a cystocele with the defect occurring lateral (paravaginal defects), transverse, or midline. Defects in the rectovaginal fascia result in rectocele with protrusions occurring through

splits in the rectovaginal fascia, which must be reapproximated to restore integrity. Each of these defects must be approached individually, and all defects must be repaired to ensure restoration of the integrity of the vaginal tube and its support structures. The vaginal apex in particular depends on the cardinal/uterosacral ligaments (3). An apical enterocele occurs when there is separation of the pubocervical fascia from the rectovaginal fascia and the peritoneum is in contact with the vaginal mucosa (23).

It is essential to remember that pelvic muscles relieve the tension on the endopelvic fascia and that the fascia stabilizes the organs above the pelvic floor (4). The mechanism of prolapse can then be described in this order: the pelvic floor muscles are damaged; the pelvic floor opens; the vagina now sits between high abdominal pressure and low atmospheric pressure; the ligaments can sustain this load for a short time only and then the ligaments fail and prolapse will occur. The treatment of fascial defects is surgical. The treatment of muscle injury is reeducation (4). The success of surgical intervention for vaginal vault prolapse and pelvic support defects may well be improved with the addition of pelvic floor muscle reeducation to treat pelvic floor relaxation and pelvic floor muscle injury (6).

The normal resting tone of the pubovisceral muscle squeezes the rectum, vagina, and urethra closed by compressing them against the pubic bone. Lateral to this, the flat sheet-like iliococcygeus muscle forms a horizontal shelf on which the upper pelvic organs rest. As long as the pelvic musculature functions normally, the pelvic floor is closed and the ligaments and fascia are under no tension. They simply act to stabilize the organs in their position above the levator ani muscles. When the pelvic floor muscles relax, or are damaged, the pelvic floor opens and the vagina lies between the high intraabdominal pressure and low atmospheric pressure, where it must be held in place by the ligaments. Although the ligaments can sustain these loads for

J. E. Carter: Department of Obstetrics and Gynecology, University of California–Irvine College of Medicine, Orange, California; Women's Health Center of South Orange County, Inc., Mission Viejo, California.

short periods of time, if the pelvic muscles do not close the pelvic floor, then the connective tissue will become damaged and eventually fail to hold the vagina in place (5).

The function of the levator ani muscle can be compromised either by direct injury to the muscle or by damage to the nerve supply. The neuromuscular injury occurs as a result of small nerves being torn away from their muscle fibers, resulting in a diminished ability of the muscle to contract and a loss of normal function (4).

The pelvic connective tissue is more likely to be damaged by rupture than by stretching (26). Generalized stretching or attenuation is the exception (26). However, once the vagina or uterus descends below its normal position, the constant load placed on it by the weight of the abdominal contents probably causes the same type of connective tissue elongation associated with stretching of any ligament or tendon. The failure of ligaments under this strain results not only from acute damage, but also from an inability of the connective tissue to repair itself (4).

The factors involved in pelvic organ prolapse include the inborn strength of the connective tissue and muscle; the loss of connective tissue strength, which can occur because of damage at childbirth, deterioration with age, and poor collagen repair; the loss of levator function, which can occur because of neuromuscular damage during childbirth or metabolic diseases that affect muscle function; increased loads on the supportive system, including prolonged lifting or chronic coughing from chronic pulmonary disease; and disturbance of the balance of the structural parts, such as alteration of the vaginal axis by urethral suspension or failure to reach the cardinal ligaments at hysterectomy (5).

The changes that vaginal birth causes in the pelvic floor deserve special examination. Damage to the levator ani muscles and their innervation is common during vaginal birth. Loss of the muscle's ability to support the pelvic organs and unload the ligaments may be partially responsible for the breakage and elongation of the ligaments later in life. Some damage to the connective tissue of the parametria and paracolpium occurs during childbirth and can also contribute to subsequent prolapse.

Childbirth was found to be associated with a variety of muscular and neuromuscular injuries to the pelvic floor that are linked to the development of pelvic organ prolapse. Risk factors for pelvic floor injury include forceps delivery, episiotomy, prolonged second stage of labor, and increased fetal size. Cesarean delivery appears to be protective, especially if the patient does not labor before delivery. Obstetricians may be able to reduce pelvic floor injuries by minimizing forceps deliveries and episiotomies, by allowing passive descent in the second stage, and by selectively recommending elective cesarean section (6).

The levator ani and the sphincter muscles of the pelvic floor are innervated by the anterior sacral nerve roots S2-4. Direct motor branches of these nerve roots travel over the cranial surface of the pelvic floor, where they are vulnerable to stretching and compression during parturition. During childbirth, the pelvic floor is exposed to direct compression from the fetal presenting part, as well as downward pressure from maternal expulsive efforts. These forces stretch and distend the pelvic floor, resulting in functional and anatomic alterations in the muscles, nerves, and connective tissue of the pelvic floor. Obstetricians are most familiar with muscular injuries such as lacerations to the perineum and external anal sphincter. Little is known about damage to the levator ani muscles during childbirth because these muscles are not usually visible at delivery (6).

Childbirth can affect the pelvic floor by damaging the peripheral nerves that innervate the levator ani and sphincter muscles. Childbirth causes stretching and/or compression of the pelvic nerves as they traverse the pelvic floor. The resultant injury causes partial denervation of the pelvic floor musculature. Recovery may occur as the denervated muscles are reinnervated by surrounding intact nerves (6). Denervation injuries of the pubococcygeus and external anal sphincter muscles have been demonstrated after 42% to 80% of vaginal deliveries (28,36). Denervation has not been seen after elective cesarean delivery (28), although it has been associated with cesarean deliveries performed during labor (36).

Many women demonstrate evidence of pelvic floor neuropathy in the immediate postpartum period, but most will subsequently recover neuromuscular function and only a minority experience long-term sequelae (6). Denervation injury may be cumulative with increasing parity (28).

The fascia and connective tissues of the pelvic floor may also be injured during labor and delivery. The mechanisms of connective tissue injury and repair in the pelvis are poorly understood (17). The endopelvic fascia is probably torn or ruptured (rather than stretched) during childbirth (4). Isolated breaks in the endopelvic fascia have been implicated in the genesis of cystoceles, vaginal support defects, and genuine stress incontinence (26). After an acute injury to connective tissue, new collagen is formed. Because the new collagen is never as strong as the original connective tissue, the endopelvic fascia may be weaker after childbirth (17).

The normal position of the uterus is not over the urogenital hiatus, as was believed previously, but rather over the levator plate (4). The active basal tone of the levator ani muscles helps to maintain this relationship by keeping the urogenital hiatus closed (4). The role of the endopelvic fascia may be to fix the pelvic organs in an appropriate position over the levator plate via attachments to the pelvic sidewall (4). If levator tone deteriorates, the pelvic organs become suspended over a widened urogenital hiatus by their ligaments and connective tissue supports (4). Under these circumstances, the endopelvic fascia will gradually stretch and weaken as a result of chronic tension (4). Thus, decreased levator function may be the first step in a process that ultimately causes failure of the connective tissue support of the pelvic organs (4). In addition, an inherent weakness of the endopelvic fascia may contribute to the problem. For example, fibroblasts from women with pelvic organ prolapse produce weaker types of collagen than in women with normal pelvic organ support (4).

Genital organ prolapse is a direct consequence of weakening of the pelvic floor. The pelvic floor is weaker after vaginal delivery (1,28). Childbirth is a potential cause of genital organ prolapse. Pelvic floor neuropathy associated with childbirth may also play a role in the genesis of pelvic organ prolapse. Approximately 50% of women with symptomatic pelvic organ prolapse have evidence of levator ani muscle denervation. Parous women with prolapse have more pronounced histologic and electromyographic evidence of levator denervation (6). Other factors, such as inherent variations in connective tissue quality and isolated breaks in the fascial attachments of the pelvic organs, also undoubtedly play roles (6).

Muscular injury to the pelvic floor combined with neurologic injury can result in pelvic organ prolapse. In managing parturition, the obstetrician should seek to minimize the risk of muscular and neurologic injury (6). Identified risk factors for weakening of levator ani include midline episiotomy, forceps delivery, nulliparity, birth weight, Asian race, and fetal occiput posterior position. Identified risk factors for neurologic injury include forceps delivery, prolonged second stage, third degree laceration, birth weight, and multiparity. By diminishing exposure to these risk factors, the obstetricians may reduce parturients' risk of long-term sequelae of pelvic floor injury (6).

RISK FACTORS UNDER OBSTETRICIAN'S CONTROL

Risk Factor 1: Forceps

Forceps delivery is an independent risk factor for third- and fourth-degree lacerations as well as for neurologic injury. Vacuum extraction may be less traumatic to the pelvic floor. The use of forceps should be minimized.

Risk Factor 2: Episiotomy

Midline episiotomy is associated with an increased risk of severe lacerations. The pelvic floor is not stronger after episiotomy than after spontaneous laceration. Medial lateral episiotomy may protect against sphincter lacerations, but does not appear to prevent decreased pelvic floor strength seen with vaginal delivery. Neither midline nor medial lateral episiotomy seems to fulfill its intended role of protecting the pelvic floor from injury. Obstetricians should reevaluate these procedures with respect to their long-term risks and benefits (6).

Risk Factor 3: Second Stage of Labor

A prolonged second stage has been associated with neuromuscular injury. Distinguishing between the "active" portion of the second stage (in which voluntary straining occurs) from the "passive" second stage, an active second stage greater than 1 hour was associated with a significantly higher risk of denervation injury among primigravida women. A prolongation of the passive portion of the second stage was not associated with an increased risk of denervation injury. Contemporary obstetric practice dictates that maternal pushing efforts be encouraged from the onset of complete cervical dilation. Preservation of the structure and function of the pelvic floor may best be accomplished by allowing a longer passive second stage. A prospective evaluation of these two practices on the risk of pelvic floor neuropathy has not been performed (6).

RISK FACTORS NOT UNDER OBSTETRICIAN'S CONTROL

Risk factors for pelvic floor injury not under the obstetrician's control include occiput posterior position and fetal macrosomia. The risk of damage to the pelvic floor and its long-term sequelae should be considered in the obstetric management of women with occiput posterior positions and fetal macrosomia. Because elective cesarean section appears to protect the pelvic floor, a practice of routine elective cesarean delivery might considerably reduce the prevalence of pelvic organ prolapse. The prudent use of elective cesarean delivery may be appropriate when significant risk factors for pelvic floor injury are present. Further research may identify women who would benefit from elective cesarean delivery (6).

ENTEROCELE AND VAGINAL VAULT DESCENSUS

"Anatomically, a vaginal enterocele is a condition in which there is peritoneum in contact with vaginal mucosa with no intervening fascia" (23).

Pertinent Anatomy

Enteroceles can be classified into five groups: anterior, apical, posterior, sigmoidocele, and rectal (23).

Anterior Enterocele

The anterior enterocele is very rare in patients who have had no previous surgery. It does occur in patients who have had a previous sacrospinous ligament vaginal suspension or a sacrocolpopexy. Often, the base of the bladder can be drawn down into the top of the defect. The fascial defect is in the pubocervical fascia of the anterior vaginal wall (23).

Apical Enterocele

The apical enterocele is, by definition, limited to the posthysterectomy patient. The apical enterocele occurs when the pubocervical fascia of the anterior vaginal wall separates from the rectovaginal fascia of the posterior vaginal wall. Moderate-to-marked vaginal prolapse normally accompanies the apical enterocele. Similarly, it is rare to have significant vaginal vault inversion without an accompanying enterocele (Fig. 50.1) (23).

Posterior Enterocele

A posterior enterocele can occur in a patient with the uterus in place or in a posthysterectomy patient. A posterior enterocele occurs when small intestine comes in direct contact with vaginal mucosa as a result of separation of the apical portion of the rectovaginal fascia from the pubocervical ring (uterus in place) or from the pubocervical fascia (posthysterectomy), and has descended so that the protrusion is from the posterior wall (23).

Sigmoidocele

A sigmoidocele occurs when the sigmoid adheres to vaginal mucosa and prolapses downward. Sigmoidoceles occur in patients who have had previous vaginal repairs of an enterocele. The peritoneal sac of the enterocele was dissected completely and excised. The neck of the sac was then ligated high and anchored to the anterior sigmoid. These patients present with a mass bulging in the introitus that palpably contains a loop of gut (23).

Rectal Enterocele

In this condition, the vaginal tube and its supporting tissue are intact, but the anterior rectal wall is pushed out through

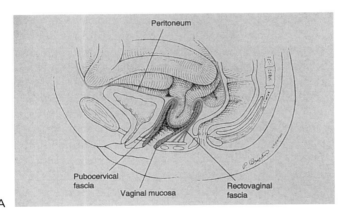
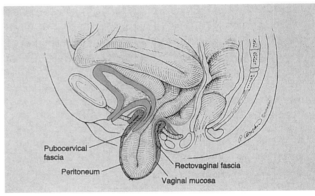
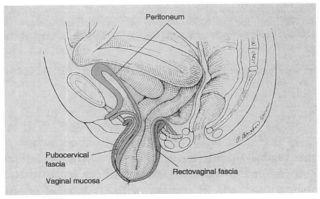
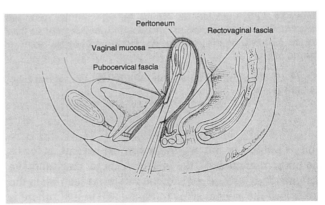

FIGURE 50.1. Apical enteroceles. Image **(A)** of a beginning enterocele. Notice the separation of the pubocervical fascia of the anterior wall from the rectovaginal fascia of the posterior vaginal wall. Further separation and further descent **(B,C)** of the vaginal apex is noted (true vaginal vault prolapse). A diagrammatic representation **(D)** of the enterocele (shown in **B** image) when pushed upward back into the abdomen before repair. (From Richardson AC. The anatomic defects in rectocele and enterocele. *Journal of Pelvic Surgery* 1995;1:214–221, with permission.)

the anus. This can be difficult to distinguish from rectal prolapse (23).

The anatomic landmarks for the enterocele and its repair are the pubocervical fascia, the rectovaginal fascia, the uterosacral ligaments, and ureter, which courses along the pelvic sidewall and is approximately 1 to 1 cm lateral to the uterosacral ligament as it passes beneath the uterine artery (19).

Clinical Presentation

All bulges into the vagina, whether anterior, posterior, or apical, represent a break in the continuity of the fibrous tissue vaginal tube and/or a loss of its suspension, attachment, or fusion to adjacent structures. Enteroceles present as bulges into the vagina. Careful vault examinations are done with the patient in the dorsal lithotomy position and in the standing position. Assessment for grading support defects is done in the maximum provocative position with strain. Vaginal defects are graded from 1 to 4 based on their relationship to the hymen (35). The vaginal cuff is grade 0 when supported at or above the level of the ischial spines. Other sites have a score of 0 if they do not descend past the imaginary plane extending from the midhymen posteriorly to the apex (midvaginal axis), with straining. The scores are as follows: past the midvaginal axis halfway to the hymen (Grade 1), to the hymen (Grade 2), halfway out of the hymen (Grade 3) and fully out of the hymen (Grade 4) (31).

The diagnosis of enterocele can be made if the prolapse has peritoneum and palpable bowel present. The presence of peritoneum can be confirmed only at the time of surgery. All patients are examined in the standing position during Valsalva's maneuver to see if bowel can be felt, to diagnose early enterocele (31).

The anterior enterocele can be difficult to distinguish from a high transverse cystocele and, in fact, involves the same fascial defect, the separation of the pubocervical fascia from the pericervical ring.

The apical enterocele is the most common of the defects in the posthysterectomy patient. The pubocervical fascia of the anterior vaginal wall is separated from the rectovaginal fascia of the posterior vaginal wall. There is moderate-to-marked vaginal prolapse accompanying the enterocele. It is rare to have significant vaginal vault inversion without an accompanying enterocele. Palpation of small bowel in the defect or visual evidence of peristalsis in the defect helps to confirm the diagnosis of an enterocele. Discrimination between an enterocele and a rectocele, however, may be clinically difficult. The "double bubble," the discreet appearance of a hernia sac on the anterior surface of a rectocele, is clinically indicative of an enterocele but generally not present. In this specific situation, examination of the patient in the standing position may allow the discrimination between an ente-

rocele and a rectocele. Since the enterocele is generally associated with vaginal vault descensus, the examiner feels for evidence of small bowel between the rectum and vagina (35).

Treatment

Anterior Enterocele

Correction of the anterior enterocele requires dissection of the vaginal mucosa to expose the defect in the pubocervical fascia. If the bladder has been drawn into the defect, the dissection must be performed to avoid entry into the bladder. Once the pubocervical fascia has been identified, it is reapproximated to the pericervical ring if the uterus is in place (which is rare) or to the rectovaginal fascia if the uterus has been previously removed. The full description of an appropriate repair for the enterocele itself will be given in the next section, Apical Enteroceles and Vault Descensus (23).

Apical Enteroceles and Vault Descensus

The apical enterocele is almost always associated with vaginal vault descensus. In addition, vaginal prolapse is very rarely present without the occurrence of an apical enterocele. Therefore, the repair of both will be described. The apical enterocele can be approached vaginally, abdominally, or laparoscopically. The laparoscopic and abdominal approaches are performed in a similar manner, but the arrival of laparoscopic techniques for pelvic vault reconstruction has resulted in the ability to clearly visualize the fascial defects that are the basis of vault prolapse. In this discussion, the laparoscopic approach is first described and then is followed by a discussion of the vaginal approach, with laparoscopic assistance. This description is based on the teachings of Richardson (23) and Saye (32).

The Laparoscopic Approach

After general endotracheal anesthesia has been induced, careful pelvic examination using the techniques of Shull (35) is performed. Insufflation with CO_2 is performed and placement of laparoscopic trocars is accomplished. A 10-mm trocar for the 10-mm laparoscope is placed at the umbilicus. If the Endo-stitch (US Surgical, Norwalk, CT, U.S.A.) is used, a 10-mm port is established on the operator's side and a 5-mm port is established on the assistant's side, both lateral to the inferior epigastric vessels with placement dependent on the individual anatomy. If 2-zero Ethibond (Ethicon, Inc., Somerville, NJ, U.S.A.) is used, 5-mm ports are established bilaterally. The patient is then placed in the Trendelenburg position and the bowel swept out of the pelvis. With use of a rectal sizer placed in the vaginal vault,

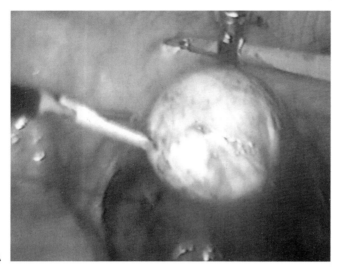
A

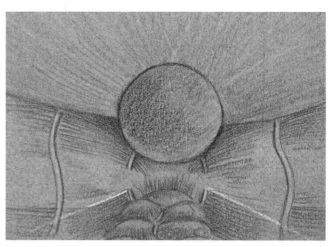
B

FIGURE 50.2. A and **B:** The vaginal vault is inverted using a rectal sizer so that it can be visualized within the pelvic cavity. The peritoneal lining overlying the rectovaginal and pubocervical fascia can be clearly seen. (Artwork by Dawn Merrill; © James E. Carter, M.D., Ph.D., F.A.C.O.G.; reprinted with permission of the Journal of the Society of Laparoendoscopic Surgeons.)

the vault is inverted so that the peritoneal lining is visible in the pelvic cavity. The peritoneal lining overlies the separated rectovaginal and pubocervical fascia (Fig. 50.2). The uterosacral ligaments are identified on both sides, with care taken to identify as well the course of the ureters lateral to the uterosacral ligaments. The uterosacral ligaments are identified as they enter into the sacrum, which is the unbroken portion of the uterosacral ligaments, and these portions are used for the reattachment to the vaginal apex. The unbroken portion of the uterosacral ligament on each side is then tagged with suture to initiate the procedure (Fig.

50.3). The peritoneum overlying the break between the pubocervical and rectovaginal fascia is then opened. The pubocervical fascia is identified ventrally between the vagina and the bladder by sharp dissection. The rectovaginal fascia is identified posteriorly (Fig. 50.4). Redundant peritoneum and excess vagina are excised. Corner stitches are then placed on each side, which approximate the edges of the pubocervical to the rectovaginal fascia overlying the vaginal mucosa.

Two-zero permanent suture (Ethibond, Ethicon, Somerville, NJ; Surgidek, US Surgical, Norwalk, CT) is

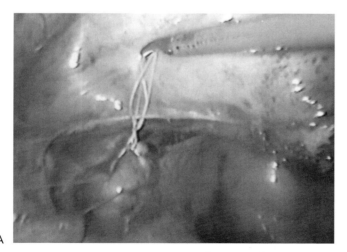
A

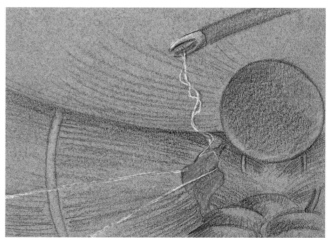
B

FIGURE 50.3. A and **B:** The left uterosacral ligament is shown here. The uterosacral ligaments are visualized as they enter into the sacrum and are tagged by suture for later identification. (Artwork by Dawn Merrill; © James E. Carter, M.D., Ph.D., F.A.C.O.G.; reprinted with permission of the Journal of the Society of Laparoendoscopic Surgeons.)

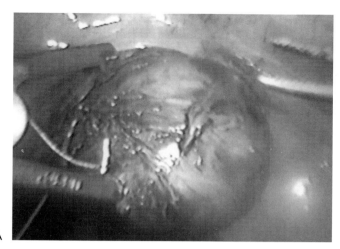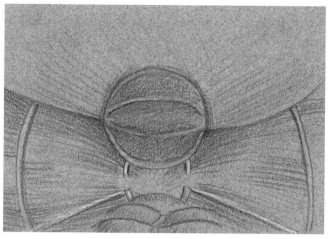

FIGURE 50.4. A and **B:** The peritoneum has been divided and with sharp dissection the pubocervical and rectovaginal fascia have been identified. The break between them is clearly visible. (Artwork by Dawn Merrill; © James E. Carter, M.D., Ph.D., F.A.C.O.G.; reprinted with permission of the Journal of the Society of Laparoendoscopic Surgeons.)

used for all aspects of the repair. This corner stitch is then incorporated into the ipsilateral uterosacral ligament, which had been previously tagged (Fig. 50.5). The now-reapproximated pubocervical and rectovaginal fascia along the edges and corner of the vaginal apex is then incorporated into the ipsilateral uterosacral ligament as it courses to the sacrum. In this way, the rectovaginal pubocervical complex is sutured to the unbroken portion of the uterosacral ligament, forming a very secure attachment of the vaginal apical corner.

This procedure is performed on both sides of the apical vault, providing very secure support of the lateral and upper corners of the vaginal vault (Fig. 50.6).

The rectovaginal fascia is then approximated to the pubocervical fascia across the center of the vaginal vault with interrupted sutures (Fig. 50.7). Reinforcing sutures from the uterosacral ligaments to the posterior rectovaginal fascia are then placed bilaterally. These sutures do not cross the midline but rather reinforce the attachment of the corner of the vaginal apex to the ipsilateral uterosacral complex, thus providing for appropriate anatomic connection to the rectovaginal septum and maintaining the maximum possible transverse dimension of the upper portion of the vagina (Fig. 50.8).

After completion of the enterocele repair and vault suspension by suture technique as described herein, additional vault defect repairs are then performed.

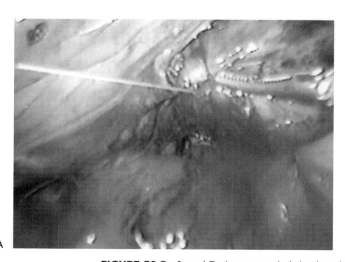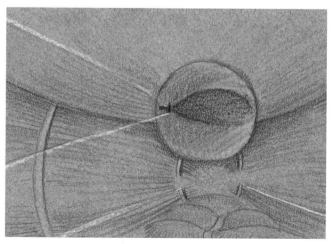

FIGURE 50.5. A and **B:** A corner stitch is placed through the pubocervical and rectovaginal fascia. (Artwork by Dawn Merrill; © James E. Carter, M.D., Ph.D., F.A.C.O.G.; reprinted with permission of the Journal of the Society of Laparoendoscopic Surgeons.)

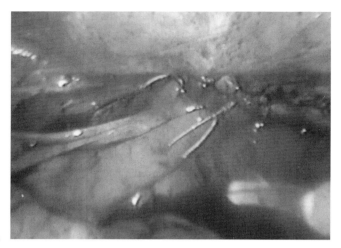
A

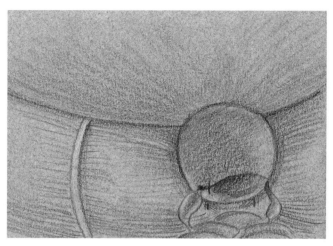
B

FIGURE 50.6. A and **B:** The lateral edges and apical corner of the vaginal vault are secured to the unbroken portion of the uterosacral ligament as it courses to the sacrum. The left apical corner is shown here. (Artwork by Dawn Merrill; © James E. Carter, M.D., Ph.D., F.A.C.O.G.; reprinted with permission of the Journal of the Society of Laparoendoscopic Surgeons.)

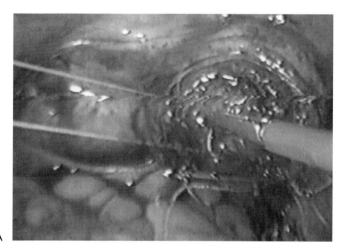
A

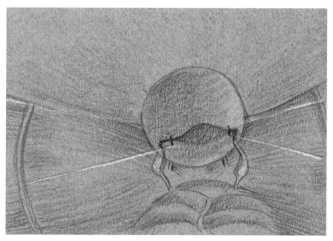
B

FIGURE 50.7. A and **B:** Interrupted sutures close the apex of the vaginal vault, restoring the integrity of the attachment of the pubocervical to the rectovaginal fascia. (Artwork by Dawn Merrill; © James E. Carter, M.D., Ph.D., F.A.C.O.G.; reprinted with permission of the Journal of the Society of Laparoendoscopic Surgeons.)

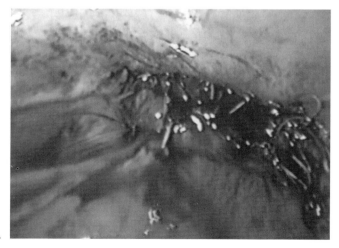
A

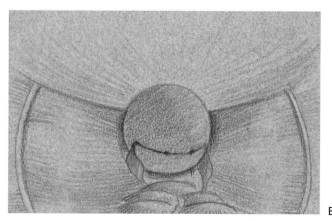
B

FIGURE 50.8. A and **B:** Completed vaginal vault apical support is visualized. (Artwork by Dawn Merrill; © James E. Carter, M.D., Ph.D., F.A.C.O.G.; reprinted with permission of the Journal of the Society of Laparoendoscopic Surgeons.)

The Vaginal Approach

The vaginal approach to the apical enterocele repair and vaginal support surgery begins with a careful intraoperative vaginal examination. The apex and posterior vaginal segments are carefully examined for loss of their lateral sulci, lack of epithelial rugation, and elongation of the vaginal apex. A rectovaginal examination is also performed to assess for rectocele and find defects in the rectovaginal septum from its normal points of attachment (15). A laparoscopic approach is used to locate and tag, with sutures, the uterosacral ligaments, and a vaginal approach is used to repair the enterocele and rectocele in a site-specific manner. In the cases described (15), open laparoscopy is performed in all cases, and accessory ports are placed under direct visualization. The pelvic cavity is examined with a sponge stick or end-to-end anastomosis sizer used to elevate the vaginal cuff. Each uterosacral ligament is found by placing the vaginal apex under tension to the contralateral side. The ureters are located bilaterally. Next, permanent 2-zero suture is used to tag each uterosacral ligament at the level of the ischial spine. The needle is cut and the suture is tied with an extracorporeal knot-tying technique, and the free end of the suture is dropped into the abdominal cavity for removal during the vaginal repairs (15).

Vaginal repair of the enterocele is performed next. A transverse incision is made through the vaginal epithelium at the posterior hymenal ring. The vaginal epithelium is incised in the midline and then dissected off the underlying rectovaginal fascia laterally and proximally with Metzenbaum scissors. As the dissection is carried toward the vaginal apex, a distinct loss of the rectovaginal fascia with a sudden protrusion of peritoneum (enterocele sac) is noted. The enterocele sac is entered and excess peritoneum is excised. Careful examination of the enterocele sac reveals it to be demarcated posteriorly by the edge of the rectovaginal septum and anteriorly by the pubocervical fascia. Dissection of the anterior vaginal mucosa from its underlying pubocervical fascia is performed, beginning at the vaginal apex and extending to the anterior vaginal segment. The edge of the pubocervical fascia is located throughout its length at the vaginal apex. The uterosacral ligaments are reattached to the vaginal apex to provide vaginal vault support by passing the previously passed uterosacral ligament sutures through the apical fascia on each side, with one end of the suture incorporating the anterior pubocervical fascia and the other end incorporating the posterior rectovaginal fascia. Next, the enterocele is repaired with closure of the fascial defect by reapproximating the pubocervical fascia anteriorly to rectovaginal fascia posteriorly with a series of four to six interrupted 2-zero permanent sutures. After closure of the enterocele defect, the uterosacral suspension sutures are tied down, resulting in suspension of the newly created vaginal apex. A laparoscopic approach is used to place an additional uterosacral ligament suspension suture on each side. The patient is given intravenous indigo carmine, and transurethral cystoscopy is performed to document bilateral ureteral patency (15).

Ross describes the apical vault repair as the cornerstone of vaginal support (30). He describes apical vault prolapse following hysterectomy as resulting from the stretch neuropathy that leads specifically to the breakdown of the endopelvic fascia. Since the neuromuscular disease is not currently treatable, the defect must be corrected with available endopelvic fascia. An important component of the endopelvic fascia is the integrity of the pericervical ring. The pubocervical, cardinal, uterosacral, paracolpial ligaments, and rectovaginal septum are all joined at this point in normal pelvic anatomy. In developing laparoscopic repairs for pelvic organ prolapse, it is clear that a good apical vault repair procedure is critical for success (30).

The ureters on both sides of the pelvic sidewall are identified and dissected out down to the cardinal tunnel to allow easy identification. With a vaginal probe in place, the left uterosacral ligament is picked up with a zero Prolene suture (Ethicon, Inc., Somerville, NJ U.S.A.) approximately 3 to 4 cm distal to the apical vaginal vault. As many parametrial and paracolpial fibers as possible are encircled with the suture. The suture passes through the left cardinal ligament close to the ureteric canal and into the posterior vaginal wall. The peritoneum has already been dissected off of the upper vaginal apex, and the proximal edges of both the rectovaginal septum and the pubocervical fascia are identified. As the suture enters the posterior vaginal wall, care is taken to include the rectovaginal septum. The suture is passed in and out of the posterior vaginal wall two to three times before taking it out into the right cardinal and uterosacral ligaments. The suture is then tied behind the vagina, using an extracorporeal knot, to start the uterosacral plication. Two to three more proximal sutures are placed in the same fashion until the vaginal apex is reached. The last suture passes along the vaginal apex and is used to incorporate the pubocervical fascia into the apical vault repair. If the pubocervical fascia is too attenuated to reach the vault apex, it is stretched out as far as possible and sutured to an anterior strip of Prolene mesh, which is included in the most apical suture. If there is a large gap between the vaginal apex and the pubocervical fascia anteriorly, or the rectovaginal septum posteriorly, a complete circular strip of Prolene mesh is sutured around the vaginal apex. The pubocervical fascia and rectovaginal septum can be sutured to this mesh to complete the support. The final step is to check the ureters bilaterally to ensure that no kinking has taken place. Undo stress on the ureters is fairly common, but simple extension of the releasing peritoneal incisions corrects this problem. At completion, the pericervical ring has been closed off and completely reestablished (30).

By closing off the top of the vaginal apex, the apical vault repair prevents transverse cystoceles in the anterior space and enteroceles in the posterior space. The uterosacral plication closes off the cul-de-sac to prevent increased posterior pressure that could lead to rectocele formation. The lateral vaginal walls are once again attached to pelvic sidewall and suspended from the sacral area, fulfilling the anatomic criteria described by Delancey (3–5).

The sacral colpopexy is also used for vaginal vault prolapse. The laparoscopic approach to the sacral colpopexy was first described by Nezhat et al. (16), and Paraiso (20) and Margossian et al. (12) have elegantly described this technique.

Laparoscopy is performed in the usual manner (12). A 5-mm trocar is inserted in the left lower quadrant and a 10-mm trocar is inserted in the right lower quadrant. Another 5-mm trocar is inserted lateral to the rectus muscle at the level of the umbilicus. The everted vaginal cuff and the enterocele sac are identified. The margins of the vaginal vault are identified with the help of a ring forceps. Dissection of the peritoneum off of the vaginal cuff is started at the apex and then extended toward the vesicouterine and rectovaginal spaces. A rectal probe identifies the rectum and helps dissect the rectovaginal space. The dissection of the posterior compartment is performed to expose 3 to 4 cm of vaginal wall. The enterocele is repaired. The rectosigmoid colon is retracted to the left side to expose the sacral area. A fan retractor, with the patient in a relatively steep Trendelenburg position with slight left lateral tilt, aids with exposure (12).

The right ureter is visualized crossing over the right common iliac artery near the bifurcation. The aortic bifurcation is easily identified. The sacral promontory, where the mesh will be sutured, is gently palpated with the laparoscopic grasping forceps. The posterior parietal peritoneum over this area is elevated and incised, then with gentle blunt dissection, the periosteum is cleaned and exposed. This is done with great care as this space is bordered by the bifurcation of the aorta, the right iliac vessel, the right ureter, the inferior mesenteric vessels, and the mesentery of the sigmoid (12).

Dissection in a lateral, rather than vertical, direction is recommended in order to prevent accidental injury to the left common iliac vein, which lies just under the aortic bifurcation. The middle sacral artery and vein are usually avoided, but may be coagulated or secured with hemoclips if damaged. The peritoneal opening is extended in the right pararectal space down to the already-dissected enterocele sac in the cul-de-sac of Douglas (12).

A 3 × 10-cm propylene mesh is rolled and introduced into the abdomen through the 10-mm right lower quadrant port. The mesh is sutured to the vaginal vault as broadly as possible to distribute the tension. The mesh is sutured to the posterior vaginal wall with three to six stitches. Another small piece of mesh is sutured to the anterior vaginal wall and secured to the posterior mesh through the apex of the vagina. This will provide an equal distribution of the supporting force on the vaginal cuff. All suturing is performed with nonresorbable Prolene sutures and tied with extracorporeal knot technique (12).

The other end of the mesh is sutured to the anterior longitudinal ligament of the sacrum at the promontory. The mesh is adjusted to hold the vaginal apex in the correct anatomic position without excessive tension. The mesh is placed retroperitoneally in the right pararectal space, and the covering peritoneum is closed with interrupted or continuous suture from the sacrum to the vagina (12).

Liu described the sacrospinous ligament suspension, which is another approach for suspending the vaginal vault. Under videolaparoscopy with a monitor, the operator places two fingers inside the vagina and palpates the right ischial spine and sacrospinous ligament. The locations of the right ischial spine and sacrospinous ligament are noted and marked through the laparoscope. A rectal probe is then placed into the rectum and the rectum is pushed toward the left side of the pelvis. A longitudinal or transverse incision is made over the peritoneum covering the sacrospinous ligament on the right side. The right pararectal space is entered, and the pararectal space is dissected toward the sacrum. The sacrospinous ligament is identified and confirmed by placing the fingers back into the vagina and palpating the ischial spine and the sacrospinous ligament. The enterocele is first repaired and the cul-de-sac obliterated prior to the vault suspension. Permanent suture is used to place suture through the sacrospinous ligament. The suture is placed at least 2 to 3 cm medially, away from the ischial spine and close to the sacrum to avoid injury to the pudendal nerve and vessels. A double bite is taken. The suture is then passed twice through the posterior wall of the vagina just below the tip of the vaginal vault, making sure the rectovaginal septum is included inside the suture while avoiding the vaginal mucosa, after which the suture is tied with the extracorporeal knot–tying technique with a knot pusher. During the knot tying, the assistant places his or her fingers, or a vaginal probe, inside the vagina, pushing the tip of the vagina to the right sacrospinous ligament. No gaps should be left between the sacrospinous ligament and the vagina (10).

Posterior Enterocele, Sigmoidocele, and Rectal Enterocele Repairs

Posterior enteroceles, sigmoidoceles, and rectal enteroceles are repaired with the same techniques as described for the enteroceles. Special attention is placed on the integrity of the entire rectovaginal fascia because these types of enteroceles are frequently accompanied by other defects.

To summarize, to surgically correct these enterocele defects, there are three tasks that must be accomplished: (a) reconstruction of the vaginal fibrous tissue tube; (b) reestablishment of the suspension and lateral attachment of the reconstructed vaginal tube; and (c) excision of the redundant peritoneum and vaginal mucosa. First, the upper edges of the pubocervical and rectovaginal fascia must be closed to reestablish the integrity of the apex of the vaginal tube. Second, both the anterior and posterior fascial layers have separated from the cardinal/uterosacral complex (loss of the suspension of Delancey's level 1) and, as they descended, their lateral attachments separated. Thus, after closing the apex of the tube, the closed tube must be resuspended from its normal support of the cardinal/uterosacral complex, or some other procedure, such as a sacrospinous ligament fixation or sacral colpopexy, will be necessary. To compensate for the loss of lateral attachment, the pubocervical fascia must be attached to the sidewall, as in a paravaginal repair, and the rectovaginal fascia must be attached to the fascia over the iliococcygeus, usually through a posterior vaginal dissection (obviously, the lower portion of the rectovaginal fascia must be evaluated for a rectocele). Excess stretched peritoneum and vaginal mucosa are excised to obtain a smooth closure. The peritoneum and vaginal mucosa have no strength, and their excision is cosmetic (23).

The traditional operations described for enterocele (such as Moskowitz's or Halban's, as usually described) will not uniformly accomplish the three listed tasks. It is possible that, with either of these, one may by chance include the two fascial margins and the uterosacral ligaments. When the anatomic defects are viewed, it seems logical to approach them directly and correct each. Usually, this is possible and appropriate (23).

There will be times when, because of multiple previous surgical attempts, it is almost impossible to identify these anatomic landmarks. In these situations, attempts must be made to compensate by the use of any of the less than truly anatomic corrections. This requires considerable surgical expertise and innovation to achieve consistent results. An accurate understanding, recognition, and identification of the anatomic defects are the proper starting point for any surgical repair procedure (23).

RECTOCELE

Rectoceles present as a bulge in the posterior vaginal wall. Rectoceles are physical findings, not anatomic entities. There are several different breaks in the supporting structures that yield a rectocele. All rectoceles involve some defect in the rectovaginal fascia. In the evaluation of the patient with a bulge in the posterior wall, the rectovaginal fascia is the structure that must be evaluated. Rectoceles are sometimes difficult to differentiate from enteroceles, and at times that differentiation can be made only at surgical intervention. Anatomically, a rectocele is a condition in which bowel muscularis is in contact with vaginal mucosa, with no intervening fascia. Normally, the rectovaginal fascia lies between the rectum and vagina. Therefore, all rectoceles represent a break in this layer that has allowed the rectal wall to push upward and impinge on the vaginal mucosa (23).

Pertinent Anatomy

The strength and integrity of the posterior walls is supplied by the rectovaginal fascia (also known as Denonvilliers' fascia). This layer of fibromuscular tissue, which lies immediately beneath the vagina mucosa, serves to separate the rectal and genital compartments in the lower pelvis. In the sagittal plain, it courses from the perineal body to the cul-de-sac. In the cul-de-sac, it merges with the fibers of the uterosacral ligaments, as well as the posterior cervix. In the area lateral to the cervix and upper vagina, it merges into the more lateral fibers of the cardinal/uterosacral complex. These represent Delancey's suspension of the posterior wall at level 1. Laterally, the rectovaginal fascia merges with parietal fascia covering the iliococcygeus and pubococcygeus muscles. This is the lateral attachment of the posterior vagina in Delancey's level 2. Distally, it merges into the perineal body at the level of the urogenital diaphragm (Delancey's fusion of level 3). The perineal body itself is suspended from the sacrum by way of this continuity of uterosacral ligaments and rectovaginal fascia. Whenever there is a break in this continuity, the perineal body becomes hypermobile (23).

Histologically, the rectovaginal fascia is similar to all of the so-called "endopelvic fascia" (which is a type of connective tissue). The endopelvic fascia differs significantly from other so-called "fascia," such as the abdominal wall fascia, fascial coverings of individual muscles, fascia lata, and so forth. The principal difference noticed immediately in microscopic sections is that its fiber content is different. In both, the usual collagen and elastin fibers are observed, but in the endopelvic fascia very prominent, long, wavy strands of smooth muscle that are unique in appearance are also seen. These smooth muscle fibers do not resemble bowel muscularis, detrusor muscle, or periarteriolar muscle. Little is known about the significance, function, or innervation of these smooth muscle fibers, but their prevalence is striking. The rectovaginal fascia contains thicker and more abundant bundles of elastin than seen in other areas of the endopelvic fascial network (23).

Clinical Presentation

A rectocele is a condition in which bowel muscularis is in contact with vaginal mucosa with no intervening fascia. Normally, the rectovaginal fascia lies between the rectum and vagina. Therefore, all rectoceles represent a break in this layer that has allowed the rectal wall to push upward and impinge upon the vaginal mucosa. These breaks can be almost anywhere in this layer. Probably the most common break is immediately above the perineal body, either transversely or in the midline; both of these will yield a low rectocele. With the low transverse break, often the break will extend laterally and up the lateral margin, yielding a hockey-stick type of defect. In some cases, it will extend up both sides, yielding a U-shaped defect. When the break is high, there can be an inverted U-shaped defect. Rarely, the break will be entirely lateral along the side of the vagina where the fascia normally attaches to the fascial covering of the iliococcygeus muscle. Preoperatively, it is not always possible to be sure where the defect will be found (23).

A helpful clinical tool is to utilize a curved ring forceps placed posteriorly and laterally in an effort to reduce the posterior defect. If there continues to be a bulge between the open arms of the forceps, the defect is midline. The forceps may be closed and used to support the midline. If there is no loss of support when the patient strains, the defect is in the midline. Loss of support at the cul-de-sac or at the perineal body is best identified intraoperatively (35).

The clinical importance of the rectovaginal septum lies in its contribution to our understanding of rectoceles. If this layer is intact, the rectum will not bulge into the vagina; that is, if it is intact, there can be no rectocele (24). Similarly, if the rectum bulges toward the introitus during Valsalva's maneuver—a true rectocele—then something has happened to destroy the integrity of this layer. In almost all patients with a rectocele, isolated tears in the rectovaginal septum can be demonstrated (24).

Treatment

It is important to emphasize that repair of a rectocele is only one part of a posterior colporrhaphy. In a complete posterior repair, there are three separate structures that must be evaluated: the rectovaginal fascia, the levator hiatus, and the perineal body with its intrinsic perineal muscles. Thus, there are three separate tasks that must be considered:

1. Determine the integrity, or lack thereof, of the rectovaginal fascia. If a true rectocele is present, correct it by closing the defect in the rectovaginal fascia.
2. Evaluate the size of the levator hiatus. Clearly, the levator muscles serve to back up the connective tissue of the endopelvic fascia. If the opening is abnormally large, there is increased stress on the overlying connective tissue. If the hiatus is markedly widened, it is desirable to bring the medial margins of the pubococcygeus muscle together in the midline to narrow the hiatus.
3. It may be necessary to reconstruct the intrinsic muscles of the perineal body if they are found to be separated by an old obstetric injury. These muscles serve to close the introital opening (23,24).

None of these individual tasks will adequately treat a defect in another area. That is, closure of a defect in the rectovaginal fascia will not affect the width of the levator hiatus, plication of the levators will not correct a rectocele, repair of the rectovaginal fascia and plication of the levator muscles will not restore normal closure of the introital opening, and reconstruction of the perineal body will not affect a rectocele or the size of the levator hiatus (23).

Standard gynecologic surgery textbooks describe several techniques used to repair rectoceles. Each is proposed to be used for any rectocele, assuming that all rectoceles are alike. All rectoceles are not alike. The specific anatomic defect(s) accounting for the rectoceles in individual patients must be corrected (24).

When the specific defects are recognized, the task of repairing them directly with a series of fine, interrupted sutures is quite simple. The main question, then, is how to recognize and identify these defects and, in turn, locate the edges of the tears in the rectovaginal septum. The following procedure is advocated (24):

1. Begin as in any standard posterior colporrhaphy. If it is necessary to resect some redundant skin and introital mucosa, the usual diamond-shaped incision at the introitus can be used.
2. It is essential that the reflection of the vaginal mucosa upward from the underlying tissue be done immediately beneath the vaginal mucosa. Sharp dissection will always be required over the area of the perineal body. Once above the perineal body (about 2 to 3 cm within the introitus), the dissection can usually be continued bluntly.
3. The dissection is extended upward in the midline to well above the bulge of the rectocele. The mucosa then is elevated laterally beyond the lateral margins of the underlying rectum, essentially to the pelvic sidewalls.
4. It is necessary at this point to achieve sufficient hemostasis to be able to view the entire dissection carefully. It is sometimes helpful to irrigate the area with warm saline, after achieving hemostasis, to see the tissue more clearly.
5. The operator should then insert a finger of the left hand in the rectum. The rectal wall then can be pushed upward to demonstrate the rectal bulge. It will then be possible to distinguish the uncovered rectal muscularis from the area in which the muscularis is covered by the smoother and semitransparent firm connective tissue of the rectovaginal septum.
6. The edges of the connective tissue should be grasped with several Babcock clamps and pulled over the area of bare rectal wall. At this point, with the finger still in the rectum, one can determine whether or not the bulge has been corrected.
7. Once the edges of the separation have been identified, they are simply sewn together with a series of interrupted sutures.

If the levator hiatus needs to be narrowed, then the necessary procedure is performed. Reconstruction of the perineal body is then done, if deemed necessary. These latter two steps, the alteration of the levator hiatus and the reconstruction of the perineal body, are familiar to all gynecologic surgeons and need not be recounted here (24).

Site-specific defect rectocele repair was evaluated in a retrospective observational study (22). Surgical correction was found at follow-up examination to have been achieved in 82% of eligible patients (73 of 89). All daily aspects of living improved significantly ($p < 0.05$), including ability to do housework (56% improvement or cure), travel (58% improvement or cure), and social activity (60% improvement or cure). Sexual function was not affected; however, reports of dyspareunia ($p < 0.04$) improved or were cured after the operation in 73% of patients (19 of 26), worsened in 19% of patients (five of 26), and arose *de novo* in three patients (12%). Bowel symptoms were assessed subjectively and were noted to have significantly improved ($p < 0.008$) after the operation. The following improvement or cure rates were obtained: stooling difficulties, 55%; pelvic pain or pressure, 73%; vaginal mass, 74%; and splinting, 65%. This study indicates that defect-specific posterior colporrhaphy is equal or superior to traditional posterior colporrhaphy. This type of repair provides durable anatomic support and is successful in restoring bowel function. It does not detrimentally affect sexual function, may aid in resumption of sexual activity, and significantly improves quality of life in social aspects of daily living (22).

A second study used standardized preoperative and postoperative assessment of vaginal topography (the Pelvic Organ Prolapse staging system of the International Continence Society, American Urogynecologic Society, and Society of Gynecologic Surgeons) and five symptoms commonly attributed to rectocele. Forty-six women who underwent rectovaginal fascia reattachment for rectocele repair were evaluated. Preoperative symptoms included the following: protrusion, 85% (n = 39); difficult defecation, 52% (n = 24); constipation, 46% (n = 21); dyspareunia, 26% (n = 12); and manual evacuation, 24% (n = 11). Posterior vaginal topography was considered abnormal in all patients with a mean Ap point (a point located in the midline of the posterior vaginal wall 3 cm proximal to the hymen) value of −0.5 cm (range, −2 to 3 cm). Postoperative symptom resolution was as follows: protrusion, 90% (35 of 39; $p < 0.0005$); difficult defecation, 54% (14 of 24; $p < 0.005$); constipation, 43% (9 of 21; $p = 0.02$); dyspareunia, 92% (11 of 12; $p = 0.01$); and manual evacuation, 36% (4 of 11; $p = 0.125$). Vaginal topography at one year was improved with a mean Ap point value of −2 cm (range −3 to 2 cm). This technique of rectocele repair improves vaginal topography and alleviates three symptoms commonly attributed to rectoceles. It is relatively ineffective for relief of manual evacuation, and constipation is variably decreased (7).

The application of the Pelvic Organ Prolapse staging system to all studies of vaginal prolapse surgery would standardize the results and allow useful comparisons for surgical techniques if uniformly applied (2).

Techniques for laparoscopic rectocele repair have been described. Lyons and Winer (11) evaluated prospectively at 3-month intervals, for 1 year, 20 patients who underwent laparoscopic rectocele repair with polyglactin mesh and concomitant reparative procedures. The mean operative time for rectocele repair was 35 minutes. Estimated blood loss was minimal, and hospital stay was less than 25 hours. Eighty percent of patients had symptomatic relief of digital defecation and prolapse at 1 year (11).

Ross reported on 13 patients who had laparoscopic rectocele repair, of whom two had grade 2 rectoceles at 1 year (31). The laparoscopic posterior vaginal repair was done by opening up the rectovaginal septum and dissecting down to the perineal body. Just proximal to the perineum, the levator ani and the rectovaginal septum were picked up on the right side of the rectum with a zero polydioxanone suture. The suture was passed out to the pelvic sidewall and through the rectovaginal septum, then brought across the rectum to the left pelvic sidewall and passed down through the rectovaginal septum. The suture was passed under the levator on the left of rectum and brought back to the midline and tied with an extracorporeal knot. This resulted in the plication of the levator ani and closure of rectovaginal septum tear over the rectum. Interrupted sutures were repeated until the entire defect was repaired. The peritoneum covering the rectum and vagina was then closed.

Paraiso et al. (20) reported a technique of laparoscopic rectocele repair. The anatomic landmarks of laparoscopic rectocele repair are the rectovaginal septum, comprising Denonvilliers' fascia and its lateral attachment to the medial aspect of the levator ani muscles. Denonvilliers' fascia is the endopelvic fascia that is attached to the uterosacral/cardinal ligament complex superiorly, the superior fascia of the levator ani muscles laterally, and the perineal body inferiorly. Rectovaginal fascia, rectovaginal septum, and Denonvilliers' are synonymous terms (20).

For the laparoscopic rectocele repair, the rectovaginal septum is opened using electrocautery, harmonic scalpel, or laser. Blunt dissection with blunt- or dolphin-tipped dissectors or hydrodissection and sharp dissection may be used to open the rectovaginal space down to the perineal body. This dissection would follow the surgical planes and be relatively bloodless. The perineal body is sutured to the rectovaginal septum and the rectovaginal fascial defects are closed with a zero nonabsorbable suture. If the rectovaginal fascia is detached from the iliococcygeus fascia, it is reattached with a zero nonabsorbable suture. The medial aspects of the levator ani muscles may also be plicated, but care should be taken to avoid creating a posterior ridge.

Cadaveric dermal allograft has been used to repair a rectovaginal fistula and may have significance for rectocele repairs where the fascial defects are extensive and the fascia is found to be irreparable (14).

CYSTOCELES/ANTERIOR SUPPORT DEFECTS

Cystoceles are classified depending on where the pubocervical fascia is disrupted as paravaginal, transverse, central, or mixed. The cystocele results from any break in the continuity of the pubocervical fascia hammock-like supports of the bladder.

Pertinent Anatomy

To understand pelvic support defects in the female, one must remember that the pathologic anatomy is a weakness in the pelvic portion of the wall of the cavity, not a problem with the displaced organs. Although some texts speak of "uterine supports" or "bladder supports" as though these organs were suspended in some way from above, in fact all of the visceral structures rest upon or are contained within the floor of the abdominopelvic cavity. They will not fall out; they are always pushed out by pressure from within. The three sites of possible defects are lateral or paravaginal defect, transverse defect, and midline defect (25).

The areas in the anterior quadrant of the pelvis in which defects were identified and the order of the frequency in which they were observed by Richardson et al. (26) are as follows:

1. Lateral or paravaginal defects. A defect is found in the fascia laterally at or near its attachment to the levator insertion in the lower margin of the superior pubic ramus. It usually results in a mild-to-moderate cystourethrocele, a loss of the urethral vesical angle, and significant stress urinary incontinence. It can be unilateral or bilateral.
2. Transverse defect. A transverse separation occurs in the pubocervical fascia from its insertion into the pericervical ring of connective tissue. It usually results in a large cystocele in which the bladder herniates beneath the mucosa of the anterior vaginal fornix. The urethra remains well supported with a good urethral vesicle angle. There is rarely, if ever, stress urinary incontinence. If this defect is repaired improperly, however, the patient can develop severe stress incontinence postoperatively.
3. Midline defect. An anteroposterior separation of the fascia occurs between the vagina and overlying bladder and/or urethra. Depending on the length of the defect, it results in a cystocele and/or urethrocele. If the defect is beneath the vesicle neck, there will be loss of the urethral vesicle angle and stress urinary incontinence. The defect is the one most easily repaired, and excellent results can be expected with the Kelly–Kennedy-type procedures.

The basic anatomy can be demonstrated. Reflecting the bladder medially shows its relationship and that of the pubocervical fascia to the lateral pelvic sidewalls and local muscles and vessels. The bladder rests on the pubocervical fascia, which incorporates the entire vagina, whose anterolateral sulci are attached to the pelvic fascia's tendinous arch (white line). The obturator vessels and nerve traverse the obturator foramen (37).

Removing all but the bladder trigone and vagina and transecting the rectum reveals the vaginal pubocervical fascia's anterolateral attachment to the white line, which is the tendinous aponeurosis of the obturator internus muscle anteriorly and of the levator ani complex posteriorly.

The pubocervical fascia incorporating the anterior vagina acts as a suspending hammock for the bladder and urethra. Childbirth trauma that avulses the vaginal fascia's anterolateral attachment to the white line can allow a collapse of one side of the vagina. If trauma is bilateral, the entire vagina collapses, thereby allowing the proximal urethra and distal bladder (urethral vesicle junction) also to collapse (37).

Removing the bladder and unroofing the vagina, including its anterolateral attachments, causes the vagina to be supported only by the levator plate and to completely lack anterolateral attachments. Avulsion of the anterolateral vaginal fascia from the arcus tendineus results in a collapse of the urethra and bladder, thereby contributing to stress urinary incontinence (37).

In the early 1970s, Richardson performed dissections of nulliparous and parous fresh cadavers. These dissections indicated that cystourethrocele was related to the three basic injuries described: (a) a transverse injury at the anterior cervix; (b) a central defect; or (c) a paravaginal defect (2,3, 24–26,37).

By far, the most common injury, occurring more than 75% to 80% of time, is the paravaginal defect. It is, in essence, an avulsion of the anterolateral sulcus from its attachment along the endopelvic fascia's arcus tendineus. Richardson noted that this defect was almost always (80%) on the right. Between 15% and 20% of the time it was either on the left or bilateral. Based on this observation, he developed the paravaginal defect repair (2,3,24–26,37). (Obviously, if one of the other defects mentioned above is found to be the problem, specific repair, rather than paravaginal defect repair, is appropriate.) For the central defect, the standard anterior colporrhaphy and Kelly plication are usually effective. The transverse defect is repaired in a manner similar to that described for the anterior enterocele.

Presentation

Defects may be identified clinically by evaluating each individual area of the anterior vaginal wall. Using a sponge forceps with the curve pointing posteriorly toward the ischial spines, the lateral aspects of the anterior vagina and pubocervical fascia can be returned to their normal point of attachment along the arcus tendineus fascia pelvis. The forceps are then placed laterally, and the patient is asked to strain maximally. If she strains and there are no evident anterior defects, she has lateral or paravaginal loss of support. If, when she strains, there is some improvement in anterior support, but she continues to have a midline bulge through the open arms of the forceps, she also has a midline defect in the pubocervical fascia. The forceps may be closed and used to support the base of the bladder centrally. When the patient strains and she has no midline descent, the support defect is midline or central.

Superior loss of support is characterized by several clinical clues. When the patient strains, if the anterior vaginal epithelium appears thin and shiny, with loss of rugae from the vaginal cuff along the base of the bladder, and the anterior vaginal wall is longer than the posterior vagina, the patient is likely to have superior loss of support of the pubocervical fascia. Superior defects frequently are associated with midline defects (35).

Presence of rugae generally indicates presence of intact fascia. Again if, with straining, a smooth vaginal bulge without vaginal rugae is present and can be corrected by placing a speculum in the vagina midline, a transverse cystocele is diagnosed (31).

Richardson et al. also identified that the major clinical problem is identification of the lateral defect as distinct from the midline defect (26). To make this distinction, they used a tongue blade placed along the vaginal axis in either side of the vagina. The tongue blades were brought up to the lower margins of the symphysis. If there was a still a cystourethrocele when the patient strained, the defect was considered to be midline. If there was no bulge, the defect was considered to be lateral. If the lateral defect was unilateral, then support on that side alone obliterated the bulge when the patient strained. In addition, if the examiner palpated carefully through the anterior vaginal wall along the posterior surface of the symphysis and the superior pubic ramus, the lateral weakness could be detected. This finding was subtle, but definite and recognizable.

Treatment

The lateral or paravaginal defect can be repaired abdominally, vaginally, or laparoscopically. For the abdominal approach, through a Pfannenstiel's incision, the retropubic space is entered in the midline and dissection is carried laterally on the affected side(s), separating the bladder entirely from the pubic ramus anteriorly and from the urethra and anterior one third of the vagina below. The dissection is carried cautiously downward until the upper 2 to 3 cm of the medial attachment of the levator muscle comes into view. At this time, a defect in the lateral expanse of the pubocervical fascia is detectable. The medial margin of the separation is usually retracted almost to, if not to, the lateral superior sulcus of the vagina. With a finger in the vagina, the superolateral sulcus of the vagina is elevated and sutures are placed through the fascia adjacent to superolateral vaginal sulcus and then into the semitendinous insertion of the levator muscle into the superior pubic ramus. Four to six such sutures are placed. Care is taken to avoid the numerous small veins in the area and also to avoid the periosteum of the pubic ramus. If hemostasis is satisfactory, no drains are inserted and the

abdomen is closed (26). The stitch opposite the vesical neck in the anterolateral vaginal sulcus, which passes through the arcus tendineus at about 1.5 to 2 cm below the obturator foramen, can be considered the "key" stitch.

Shull describes an abdominal paravaginal repair with a similar method using a step-by-step approach in a very elegant surgical technique (33).

Shull et al. also describe the technique of paravaginal repair done via the vagina (34). In this technique, marking sutures are placed at the level of the urethrovesical junction, several millimeters lateral to the normal location of the lateral sulci. In patients who have had a hysterectomy, marking sutures are also placed at the vaginal apexes. In the patient undergoing concomitant hysterectomy, a posterior colpotomy is performed and the cardinal uterosacral ligament pedicles are isolated, divided, and tagged for later use. Anterior colpotomy is performed by sharp dissection. With a cross-clamp, cut-and-tie technique, the uterus is removed. Salpingo-oophorectomy is performed if indicated. The cardinal uterosacral ligament pedicles are sewn into the ipsilateral angle of the vaginal cuff, initiating the reconstructive procedure. Several types of "culdoplasty" can be used. Regardless of the technique, nonabsorbable sutures are used and left untied until the paravaginal repair is completed. Tying the culdoplasty sutures earlier reduces the field of vision (34).

The vaginal epithelium is dissected off of the pubocervical fascia from the cut edge of the vaginal epithelium to the urethrovesical junction. The dissection is continued laterally until the index finger can be passed between the vaginal epithelium and the pubocervical fascia into the retropubic space anterior to the ischial spine. With the surgeon's index finger in the retropubic space, the dissection is continued anteriorly along the inferior ramus of the pubis and medially to the symphysis pubis. Small individual veins may require isolation and ligation. A gauze sponge is placed into the retropubic space lateral to the bladder, and a long bayonet retractor is used to displace the empty bladder and urethra medially. A right angle retractor with a fiberoptic light source is placed in the posterior aspect of the retropubic space to provide retraction and illumination. The fascia overlying the obturator internus muscle and the condensation of the arcus tendineus fascia pelvis are identified by palpation and visualization. With a long, straight needle driver and a small, round tapered needle, the first suture is placed 2 cm anterior to the ischial spine. Traction is placed on that suture, making it easier to visualize the tendinous arch and to place a series of four to six sutures from anterior to the spine to the attachment of the white line near the pubic bone. Next, the suture at the back of the pubic bone is used to penetrate the lateral edge of the pubourethral pubocervical fascia and the adjacent undersurface of the vaginal epithelium. The second suture penetrates the pubocervical fascia near the urethrovesical junction and the undersurface of the vaginal epithelium at the site of the previously placed marking suture. The third suture penetrates the perivesical fascia and the undersurface of the vaginal epithelium. This sequence is repeated until the suture placed closest to the ischial spine is used to secure the most cephalad portion of pubocervical fascia to the undersurface of the vaginal epithelium near the apex. It is important to use the lateral edges of pubocervical fascia for the repair because placement of the sutures too medially causes excessive tension on the anterior segment. It is equally important to place the sutures in vaginal epithelium several centimeters away from the cut edges of the midline incision to allow adequate tissue for midline closure. After all sutures are placed with three points of penetration (white line, pubocervical fascia, and epithelium), they are tied sequentially beginning periurethrally and ending with the stitch nearest the apex. The same procedure is repeated on the opposite side. The midline defect and pubocervical fascia are closed with a series of 2-zero interrupted nonabsorbable sutures. At that point, the bilateral paravaginal defects and the midline defect have been repaired. The culdoplasty and peritoneal sutures are tied next, providing depth and support to the posterior portion of the vaginal cuff. The permanent sutures for the culdoplasty and peritoneum are used to attach the transverse portion of pubocervical fascia to the apex of the vagina, completing the anterior fascial repair. Generally, there is no redundant anterior epithelium. The cut edges are approximated with interrupted absorbable sutures. After the repair of the anterior segment, a posterior colporrhaphy is performed.

Paravaginal defects can also be repaired laparoscopically as described by Richardson et al. (27). This technique was developed by Richardson and Saye, adhering to conventional surgical technique. In this technique, Retzius' space is accessed by a transperitoneal approach, and the pubocervical fascia is reattached to the arcus tendineus fascia and the fascia overlying the obturator internus muscle using nonabsorbable sutures. In this technique, open laparoscopy is performed using a minilaparotomy in the inferior margin of the umbilicus. A 12-mm access port is used at this site to accommodate the laparoscope. The abdomen is insufflated with 16 mm/Hg CO_2. Three other ports are placed under direct vision. Using sharp dissection with a harmonic scalpel, the retropubic space is entered through a transverse incision of the anterior peritoneum approximately 3 cm above the bladder reflection beginning along the medial border of the right obliterated umbilical ligament. The bladder has been filled with 200 to 300 mL of normal saline during the transperitoneal dissection of the retropubic space. This step helps distinguish the bladder's anterior border. Immediate identification of the loose areola tissue at the point of incision confirms a proper plane of dissection (27).

The retropubic space is developed by separating the loose areolar and fatty layers using primary blunt dissection.

Care is taken to maintain the dissection toward the superoposterior aspect of the pubic symphysis to avoid bladder injury. Once Retzius' space has been entered, the bladder is drained of its contents. Hemostasis is maintained using the harmonic scalpel and gentle dissection. Blunt dissection is performed until the pubic symphysis, bladder neck, obturator internus and neurovascular bundle, and the arcus tendineus fascial pelvis are clearly identified. The pubocervical fascia lateral to the bladder and urethra are exposed on each side with blunt dissection.

Once the lateral margin of the vagina is displayed throughout its length, from the pubic symphysis to a point about 1 to 2 cm ventral to the ischial spine, the paravaginal defect is repaired. The repair is accomplished using 2-zero nonabsorbable sutures with intracorporeal needle placement and extracorporeal knot tying. The nondominant hand or an assistant's hand is placed in the vaginal canal to elevate the anterior vaginal wall to its site of normal attachment along the arcus tendineus fascial pelvis. The first suture is placed near the apex of the vagina through the paravesical portion of the pubocervical fascia. The needle is then passed through the obturator internus fascia and muscle around the arcus tendineus fascial pelvis at a point 1 to 2 cm ventral to its origin at its ischial spine. The suture is secured using extracorporeal knot tying. Good tissue approximation is accomplished without an intervening suture bridge. The remaining sutures are placed sequentially beginning at the ischial spine and working ventrally toward the pubic symphysis. If indicated, the procedure is then performed on the opposite side. After placing the paravaginal sutures, the anterior vaginal wall is inspected using a half speculum. If lateral sulcus descensus persists, additional repair work is indicated.

After the repair is completed, the bladder is evaluated endoscopically to rule out inadvertent stitch placement in the bladder and to confirm ureteral patency. Five milliliters of indigo carmine and 10 mg of furosemide are given intravenously, and using a 30- or 70-degree cystoscope the sidewalls of the bladder are examined and the ureteral orifice are checked bilaterally for spillage of dye. The intraperitoneal pressure is reduced to 9 mm/Hg to assess hemostasis. The peritoneal defect created to access Retzius' space is closed laparoscopically using a multifire hernia stapler (27).

A similar technique is described by Liu (9), who emphasizes that the laparoscopic approach to the paravaginal defect is not a solitary procedure; rather, it is part of a larger operation in which the whole pelvic floor is reconstructed. Laparoscopy provides better visualization of pelvic floor defects, as well as greater precision in placing strategically important stitches in the repair of paravaginal defects (9).

The support of the anterior vaginal wall, bladder, and urethra is dependent on the inherent strength of the pubocervical fascia and its peripheral attachment to the pelvic sidewalls. The anterior vaginal fornix and its underlying pubocervical fascia are attached to the sidewall as described at the arcus tendineus fascia pelvis or the white line overlying the obturator internus muscle. A proximal break in this lateral attachment may result in a cystourethrocele, whereas a distal break in the area of the vesicle neck may result in bladder neck hypermobility with associated stress urinary incontinence (13). When this occurs, an approach combining the paravaginal repair with the Burch urethropexy for treatment of anterior vaginal prolapse and stress urinary incontinence associated with urethral hypermobility can be performed laparoscopically (13). The importance of utilizing two sutures on each side of the urethra during the laparoscopic Burch colposuspension portion of the procedure has been demonstrated conclusively by Persson and Wolner-Hanssen (21). They demonstrated an objective cure rate at 1 year after surgery with two sutures on either side of 83% compared to 58% with one suture on either side ($p = 0.001$). Ross (29) demonstrated that laparoscopic Burch procedure performed with sutures or mesh [as described by Ou et al. (18)] was equally effective in treating genuine stress incontinence. The cure rate at 1 year for the suture group was 91%, and the cure rate for the mesh group was 94%. If the "paravaginal plus" Burch procedure is performed, the paravaginal portion of the procedure is performed first. Then the laparoscopic urethropexy is performed using nonabsorbable zero sutures. The surgeon's nondominant hand is placed in the vagina, and a finger is used to elevate the vagina. The first suture is placed 2 cm lateral to the urethra at the level of the midurethra. A double bite, incorporating the entire thickness of the anterior vaginal wall excluding the epithelium, is taken and then the suture is passed through the ipsilateral Cooper's ligament. With an assistant's fingers in the vagina to elevate the anterior wall toward Cooper's ligament, the suture is tied down with a series of extracorporeal knots, using an endoscopic knot pusher. An additional double-bite suture is then placed in a similar fashion at the level of the urethrovesical junction approximately 2 cm lateral to the viscera, on the same side (13).

An identical procedure is performed on the contralateral side. Excessive tension on the vaginal wall is avoided when tying down the sutures, and routinely a suture bridge is left of approximately 2 to 3 cm. After completion of the Burch urethropexy, the intraabdominal pressure is reduced to 12 mm/Hg CO_2, and the retropubic space is inspected for hemostasis. After placement of the urethropexy sutures, a cotton swab is placed transurethrally to assess urethral access. If the cotton swab has a negative deflection of 20 degrees or more, the urethrovesical junction stitches are cut, replaced, and tied with less tension. If the cotton swab has a positive deflection of 10 degrees or more, the urethrovesical sutures are replaced and tied tighter (i.e., shorter suture bridge). Ideally, the cotton swab deflection should be between −20 degrees and 0 degrees. At completion of the

"paravaginal plus" Burch procedure, cystourethroscopy is performed. The patient is administered 5 mL of indigo carmine and 10 mL of furosemide intravenously and a 70-degree cystoscope is used to visualize the bladder lumen, excluding unintentional stitch penetration and confirming bilateral ureteral patency. After cystoscopy, the peritoneal defect created to access Retzius' space is closed laparoscopically using a multifire hernia stapler or other technique. After the laparoscopy has been completed and all incisions closed, a suprapubic catheter is placed and voiding trials are started on postoperative day 1 (13).

TRANSVERSE DEFECT IN PUBOCERVICAL FASCIA

The pubocervical fascia may separate from its attachment in the pericervical ring. The bladder is covered only by the vaginal mucosa. The transverse defect is repaired after completion of a vaginal hysterectomy. The peritoneum is closed. The anterior vaginal mucosa (epithelium and lamina propria) is reflected off the underling bladder and pubocervical fascia. By palpation, the demarcation of the edge of the fascia is determined. Anteroposterior sutures are placed, bringing the edge of the pubocervical fascia anteriorly to the pericervical ring of fascia posteriorly. Laterally, these sutures bring the cut ends of the cardinal and uterosacral ligaments and cut ends of the uterine vessels into this fascial closure. Then the vaginal mucosa is closed (25).

Repair of Midline Anterior Segment Defect

To repair a midline anterior segment defect, the vaginal mucosa is reflected off the underlying bladder and pubocervical fascia. The defect can be detected by careful observation and palpation. Sutures are placed to bring the separated edges of the fascia together. The pubocervical fascia is then closed. Closure of the vaginal mucosa will complete the procedure (25).

Repair of Uterine Prolapse

When uterine prolapse occurs, breaks in the pubocervical and rectovaginal layers usually accompany marked prolapse. The uterosacral ligaments are broken and retracted. After the vaginal hysterectomy is performed, the broken ends of uterosacral ligament are reattached to the rectovaginal fascia posteriorly. Sutures are placed anteroposteriorly to reestablish continuity of support from the pubocervical fascia anteriorly to the rectovaginal fascia posteriorly. The cut ends of the cardinal and uterosacral ligaments and the uterine vessels are attached to the pubocervical fascia above and the rectovaginal fascia below (25).

REFERENCES

1. Allen RE, Hosker GL, Smith ATB, et al. Pelvic floor damage and childbirth: a neurophysiological study. *Br J Obstet Gynaecol* 1990; 97:770–779.
2. Bump RC, Mattiasson A, Bo K, et al. The standardization of terminology of female pelvic organ prolapse and pelvic floor dysfunction. *Am J Obstet Gynecol* 1996;175:10–17.
3. Delancey JOL. Anatomic aspects of vaginal eversion after hysterectomy. *Am J Obstet Gynecol* 1992;166[6 Pt 1]:1717–1728.
4. Delancey JOL. Anatomy and biomechanics of genital prolapse. *Clin Obstet Gynecol* 1993;36:897–909.
5. Delancey JOL. Pelvic organ prolapse. In: Scott JR, DiSaia PJ, Hammond CP, et al., eds. *Danforth's obstetrics and gynecology,* 7th ed. Philadelphia: JB Lippincott Co, 1994:803–825.
6. Handa VL, Harris TA, Ostergard DR. Protecting the pelvic floor: obstetric management to prevent incontinence and pelvic organ prolapse. *Obstet Gynecol* 1996;88:470–478.
7. Kenton K, Shott S, Brubaker L. Outcome after rectovaginal fascia reattachment for rectocele repair. *Am J Obstet Gynecol* 1999; 181:1360–1364.
8. Laycock J. Clinical evaluation of the pelvic floor. In: Schussler B, Laycock J, Norton P, et al., eds. *Pelvic floor reeducation principles and practice,* London: Springer-Verlag, 1994:42–48.
9. Liu CY. Laparoscopic cystocele repair and paravaginal suspension. In: Liu CY, ed. *Laparoscopic hysterectomy and pelvic floor reconstruction.* Cambridge: Blackwell Science, 1996:330–340.
10. Liu CY. Laparoscopic vaginal vault suspension. In Liu CY, ed. *Laparoscopic hysterectomy and pelvic floor reconstruction.* Cambridge: Blackwell Science, 1996:349–365.
11. Lyons TL, Winer WK. Laparoscopic rectocele repair using polyglactin mesh. *J Am Assoc Gynecol Laparosc* 1997;4:381–384.
12. Margossian H, Walters M, Falcone T. Laparoscopic management of pelvic organ prolapse. *Eur J Obstet Gynecol Reprod Biol* 1995; 85:57–62.
13. Miklos JR, Kohli N. "Paravaginal plus" Burch procedure: a laparoscopic approach. *J Pelv Surg* 1998;4:297–302.
14. Miklos JR, Kohli N. Rectovaginal fistula repair using a cadaveric dermal allograft. *Int Urogynecol J* 1999;10:405–406.
15. Miklos JR, Kohli N, Lucente D, et al. Site specific fascial defects in the diagnosis and surgical management of enterocele. *Am J Obstet Gynecol* 1998;179:1418–1423.
16. Nezhat CH, Nezhat F, Nezhat C. Laparoscopic sacral colpopexy for vaginal vault prolapse. *Obstet Gynecol* 1994;84:885–888.
17. Norton PA. Pelvic floor disorders: the role of fascia and ligaments. *Clin Obstet Gynecol* 1996;36:926–938.
18. Ou CS, Presthus J, Beadle E. Laparoscopic bladder neck suspension using hernia mesh and surgical staples. *J Laparoendosc Surg* 1993;3:563–566.
19. Paraiso MFR, Falcone T, Walters MD. Laparoscopic surgery for enterocele, vaginal apex prolapse and rectocele. *Int Urogynecol J* 1999;10:223–229.
20. Paraiso MFR, Falcone T, Walters MD. Laparoscopic surgery for enterocele, vaginal apex prolapse and rectocele. *Int Urogynecol J* 1999;10:223–229.
21. Persson J, Wolner-Hanssen P. Laparoscopic Burch colposuspension for stress urinary incontinence: a randomized comparison of one or two sutures on each side of the urethra. *Obstet Gynecol* 2000;95:151–155.
22. Porter WE, Steele A, Walsh P, et al. The anatomic and functional outcomes of defect-specific rectocele repairs. *Am J Obstet Gynecol* 1999;181:1353–1359.
23. Richardson AC. The anatomic defects in rectocele and enterocele. *J Pelvic Surgery* 1995;1:214–221.
24. Richardson AC. The rectovaginal septum revisited: its relationship to rectocele and its importance in rectocele repair. *Clin Obstet Gynecol* 1993;36:976–983.
25. Richardson AC. Pelvic support defects in women (urethrocele, cystocele, uterine prolapse, enterocele and rectocele). In: Skandalakis LJ, Gadacz TRY, Mansberger AR, et al., eds. *Modern hernia repair: the embryological and anatomical basis of surgery.* New York: Parthenon Publishing Group, 1996:350–382.
26. Richardson AC, Lyon JB, Williams NL. New look at pelvic relaxation. *Am J Obstet Gynecol* 1976;126:568–573.
27. Richardson AC, Saye WB, Miklos JR. Repairing paravaginal defects laparoscopically. *Contemp OB/GYN* 1997;42:125–130.
28. Rockner G, Jonasson A, Olung A. The effect of mediolateral episiotomy at delivery on pelvic floor muscle strength evaluated with vaginal cones. *Acta Obstet Gynecol Scand* 1991;70: 51–54.
29. Ross JR. Two techniques of laparoscopic Burch repair for stress incontinence. A prospective, randomized approach. *J Am Assoc Gynecol Laparosc* 1996;3:351–357.
30. Ross JW. Apical vault repair, the cornerstone of pelvic vault reconstruction. *Int Urogynecol J* 1997;8:146–152.
31. Ross JW. Techniques of laparoscopic repair of total vault eversion after hysterectomy. *J Am Assoc Gynecol Laparosc* 1997;4:173–183.
32. Saye WB. Laparoscopic enterocele repair and vaginal vault suspension. Presented at: Society of Laparoendoscopic Surgeons postgraduate course on Laparoscopic Pelvic Floor Construction and Treatment of Stress Urinary Incontinence. December 9, 1998, San Diego, CA.
33. Shull BL. How I do the abdominal paravaginal repair. *J Pelvic Surg* 1995;1:43–46.
34. Shull BL, Benn SJ, Kuehl TJ. Surgical management of prolapse of the anterior vaginal segment: an analysis of support defects, operative morbidity, and anatomic outcome. *Am J Obstet Gynecol* 1994;171:1429–1439.
35. Shull BL. Clinical evaluation of women with pelvic support defects. *Clin Obstet Gynecol* 1993;36:939–951.
36. Snooks SJ, Swash M, Setchell M, et al. Injury to innervation of pelvic floor sphincter musculature in childbirth. *Lancet* 1984;2: 546–550.
37. Youngblood JP. Paravaginal repair for a cystourethrocele. *Clin Obstet Gynecol* 1993;36:960–966.

SUBJECT INDEX

Page numbers followed by "f" indicate figures. Page numbers followed by "t" indicate tables.

A

α₁-antitrypsin deficiency, 6, 10
Abdominal aortic aneurysms, 9
Abdominal approach
  for perineal hernias, 548, 548f
Abdominal hernia
  congenital internal. *See* Congenital
    internal abdominal hernia
  internal
    types of, 454t
Abdominal wall
  anterior. *See* Anterior abdominal wall
  computed tomography of, 92, 92f
  functional loss of, 368
  lower
    innervation of, 519t
  magnetic resonance imaging of, 92, 93f,
    94
  metastasis within, 86f
  relaxation of, 94f
    magnetic resonance imaging of, 93f
  sonography of
    relaxation of, 88, 88f
    sensitivity, specificity, and predictive
     values of, 92t
  ventral view of, 406f
  vessels of, 70f
Abdominal wall hernia
  anesthesia for, 515–527
    preoperative considerations, 515–516
  biochemical aspects of, 10–15
    collagen, 11–12
    connective tissue, 10
    wound healing, 12–13
  nonsurgical factors, 9–10
  sonography of, 81–92
    anatomy of, 81–82, 82f–83f
    criteria for, 83, 87
    differential diagnosis of, 82–83
    indications for, 81
    and preoperative examination, 83
    technique of, 81
Abdominal wall herniorrhaphy
  anesthesia for, 516–524, 517t
    epidural block, 523
    general, 524
    local, 518–523
    paravertebral block, 523
    preemptive, 518
    selection of, 518
    subarachnoid block, 523

Aberrant obturator artery, 70
Abhandlung yon der Bruchen, 22
Abscess
  perineal
    vs. perineal hernias, 548
  vs. sciatic hernia, 541
  sonography of, 90, 90f
    sensitivity, specificity, and predictive
     values of, 92t
Absorbable prosthetic mesh, 556
  commercial introduction of, 342
Absorbable sutures
  effect on wound healing, 332
Acetaminophen, 180
  for children
    after inguinal herniorrhaphy, 526
Acquaviva, Don, 199
Acquired hernias, 71–72
Acquired umbilical hernia, 72, 395
Activities of daily living (ADL)
  affected by chronic postoperative pain,
    297
  open *vs.* laparoscopic totally
    extraperitoneal herniorrhaphy, 247
Actualize
  definition of, 174
Adhesiolysis, 375f
  for ventral incisional hernia repair, 375,
    375f
Adhesions
  with intraperitoneal onlay mesh
    procedure, 276t
Adult umbilical hernia, 72
Aegineta, Paulus, 19
Aetius of Amida, 30
Afro-Caribbean infants
  vs. white infants
    umbilical hernia incidence in, 390
Age
  effect on anesthesia, 515
  effect on obturator hernias, 543
  effect on spigelian hernia, 408
  effect on type I hernias, 482
  effect on wound infection, 330–331
Aged. *See* Elderly
Agency for Healthcare Research and Quality
  (AHRQ), 583
Age of Faith and Scholasticism
  hernia treatment during, 18–19
Aggravating factors, 75–80
Air bladders

  of fish, 551
  for inguinal hernia, 165
Airway
  difficult
    anesthetic management of, 516
Albucasis, 19, 389
Alcohol
  for omphalocele and gastroschisis, 427
Alfentanil
  for inguinal herniorrhaphy, 535
Allantois
  embryology of, 389–390
Allis clamp, 143
Allodynia, 300
Al-Zahrawi, Abul Qasim, 19, 389
American College of Surgeons (ACS)
  clinical trials course of, 582
  collaboration with VA Cooperative Study
    No. 456, 592–600
  grant writing resources of, 583
American Society for Anesthesiologists
  (ASA)
  classification of physical status, 515
Amniocentesis
  for omphalocele, 425–426
A-mode techniques, 96, 96f
Anathomia, 30
Anatomic hernia repair, 181
Anatomy and Surgical Treatment of
  Abdominal Hernia, 22, 34f
Anatomy and Surgical Treatment of Hernia,
  38f
Anatomy of the Human Body, 389
Anchor knots
  effect on wound healing, 333, 334f
Ancient Hindu surgeons, 29
Ancient times
  groin hernia repair during, 17–18
  hernia treatment during, 17–18
Andrews, E., 26, 38
Andrew's operation, 110, 111f
Androgen
  for testicular descent, 436
Anemia
  with paraesophageal hiatal hernia, 497
Anesthesia
  for abdominal wall herniorrhaphy,
    515–527, 517t
    preoperative considerations, 515–516
  age effect on, 515
  balanced, 536

and pain reduction, 532
preperitoneal
    of spigelian hernia, 411
for rectocele repair, 623
reexploration
    for postoperative inguinodynia,
        311–312
for sciatic hernia, 542
for sliding hiatal hernia, 487, 487f
tension-free, 586–588
for ventral incisional hernias, 370–371,
    373–379
Laparotomy
    during nineteenth century, 35
Large bilateral prosthesis
    for preperitoneal prosthetic repair
        of groin hernias, 206–207, 207f
Large incarcerated hernia
    general anesthesia for, 518
Large umbilical hernia
    difficulties with, 397f
Laryngeal mask airway (LMA), 518, 524
Lateral femoral cutaneous nerves, 304, 304f,
    319
    course of, 319f
    origin of, 318f
    preperitoneal course of, 320f
Lateral hernia
    ultrasound examination of
        findings, 98, 98f
Lateral incisional hernia, 349–350, 350f
Lateral muscles
    of anterior abdominal wall
        blood supply of, 65
        innervation of, 65
Lateral triangle
    definition of, 174
Lateral trocars
    safe placement of, 383t
Lateral umbilical ligaments, 64–65
Laterofemoral cutaneous nerve injuries
    causing abrupt onset of inguinodynia,
        309–310
Latin Hippocrates, 18
Le Dran, Henry-Francois, 405
Leiomyosarcoma
    ultrasound examination of, 99f
Leriche's syndrome, 6
Leukotriene synthetase inhibitors
    for inguinal herniorrhaphy, 536
Levator ani muscles, 546f–547f
    innervation of, 612
    neuromuscular injury of, 612
    vaginal birth–induced injuries to, 612
Levobupivacaine
    for inguinal herniorrhaphy, 534
Lichtenstein hand-rolled polypropylene
    plug, 174
Lichtenstein patch, 51, 165–166
Lichtenstein repair, 166
    success of, 51
    sutureless version of, 40–41
    vs. TAPP, 249
Lichtenstein's cigarette plug, 155
Lichtenstein tension-free hernioplasty, 154,
    155

anesthesia for, 150
    deep subcutaneous injection, 150
    intradermal injection, 150
    subaponeurotic injection, 150
    subdermal infiltration, 150
complications of, 154
hernia recurrence after, 154, 155
for inguinal hernias, 149–157
mesh in, 151f
postoperative pain after, 154
return to work, 154
spermatic cord in, 151f
technical considerations of, 154–155
technique of, 150–154, 151f–153f
Lidocaine, 519t, 521
    adverse effects of, 522f
    for inguinal herniorrhaphy, 534
    for Lichtenstein tension-free hernioplasty,
        149–150
Lifting
    and inguinal hernias, 10
Ligamentum pubicum superius, 26
Lightheadedness
    induced by local anesthetics, 522
Linea alba, 65, 399
    fatty hernia. *See* Epigastric hernia
Linear array, 96
Linea semicircularis, 60
Linea semilunaris Spigeli, 405
Linea Spigeli, 405
Line of Douglas, 60
Lipoaponeurotic hernia theory, 51
Lipomas
    vs. perineal hernias, 548
    vs. sciatic hernia, 541
    sonography of, 87, 87f
Lister, 105
Literature
    of genitofemoral nerve neuralgia of, 321t
    historic, 27
    of inguinal hernia repair comparative
        trials, 587t
Local anesthesia
    advantages and disadvantages of, 517t
    for hernia repair
        first report of, 24
    for inguinal herniorrhaphy
        administration of, 532–535
        administration site for, 534
        anesthetic selection for, 533
        continuous wound administration of,
            533–534
        dose–response relationship of, 533
        effect of, 534t
    toxicity of
        treatment of, 522–523, 522t
Local anesthetic infiltration, 518–523
    anatomical aspect of, 518–520
    complications of, 521–523
    pharmacology of, 518
    for postoperative inguinodynia, 312
    sedation with, 521, 521t
    of soft tissues, 524
    technique of, 520–521, 520f
Locked-plug technique, 120, 124–126
    results of, 125

technique of, 124–126, 125f
Lotheissen, Georg, 26, 34, 139
Loupes, 441
Low birth weight
    contributing to umbilical hernias, 390
Lower abdominal wall
    innervation of, 519t
Lower midline syndrome, 425
Low spigelian hernia, 412
Lucas-Championniere, Justo, 34
Lumbar arteries, 65
Lumbar hernia
    sonography of, 85
Lumbar plexus, 302
    cutaneous branches of, 317, 318f
    superficial branches of, 59, 60f
Lumbosacral spine disease, 310
Lung disease
    associated with obturator hernias, 543
Lymphadenitis
    vs. childhood groin hernias, 439
Lymph nodes, 98
Lymphomas
    sonography of, 87
        sensitivity, specificity, and predictive
            values of, 92t
Lysine, 11, 12

M
Males
    groin hernias in, 438, 442
    infertility in, 45, 295–296, 447
Malformations
    associated with omphalocele, 425
Malignant disease
    causing wound dehiscence, 328
Malnourishment
    causing wound dehiscence, 328
Maloney darn, 111f
Malrotation
    associated with gastroschisis, 425
Marcaine. *See* Bupivacaine
Marcy, Henry O., 38, 38f, 129, 269
Marcy repair, 52, 108–109
    cremaster muscle removal, 109
    high ligation, 109
    internal ring, 109
    recurrence rate of, 51
    ring closure, 109, 109f
Marfan's syndrome, 6, 9
Marlex mesh, 39, 141, 160–161, 166,
    203
    in Cooper's ligament repair, 145, 146f
    development of, 552t
    electron microscopy of, 554f
    for incisional hernias, 355
    introduction of, 165
    mesh-specific tissue reaction of, 559–560,
        560f
    structure of, 556–557, 556f
Mass closure technique
    effect on wound healing, 333
Massive abdominal ventral hernia. *See*
    Incisional hernias
Massive incisional hernia
    examples, 342f

Nerve entrapment
causing abrupt onset of inguinodynia,
309–310
of genitofemoral nerve, 314
of iliohypogastric nerve, 321
of ilioinguinal nerve, 321
of obturator nerve, 308, 543
Nerve injuries
causing abrupt onset of inguinodynia,
309–310
following groin herniorrhaphy, 293
Nestor, 29
Neuralgia, 307–308, 316. *See also*
Inguinodynia
diagnosis of, 312
following Lichtenstein tension-free
hernioplasty, 154
following transabdominal preperitoneal
laparoscopic herniorrhaphy, 264
genitofemoral, 307–308, 318–319,
321*t*
Neural pathway
diagram of, 298*f*
Neuroma pain
postoperative, 302*t*
Neuropathic pain, 307–308
anatomic classification of
in postherniorrhaphy patient, 302*t*
postoperative, 301–302
Neuropraxias
following intraperitoneal onlay mesh
procedure, 274
Nicotine, 5–6
Niedhardt classification
for traumatic hernia, 73
Nineteenth century
hernia treatment during, 22–24
Nissen fundoplication, 484, 487–488
for sliding hiatal hernia, 487
Nociceptive pain
postoperative, 300–301
Nonabsorbable mesh, 553*t*
Nonprosthetic abdominal wall repair
for incisional hernias, 353–354
Nonsteroidal antiinflammatory drugs
(NSAIDs)
for inguinal herniorrhaphy, 535
Norepinephrine, 523
Normal groin
parasagittal section of, 46*f*
Nottingham Health Profile Questionnaire
(NHPQ), 589
Nursing staff
in preoperative care
for incisional hernias, 352
Nyhus classification, 187
of groin hernias, 75, 77*t*
Nyhus operation, 24
Nyhus's suprainguinal incision, 203
Nylon
foreign-body carcinogenesis risk of,
561
Nylon darn inguinale hernia repair,
110–111
Kinmonth modification of, 110–111
Nylon surgical knots

slippage of, 334*t*
Nylon sutures, 332

O
Obesity
causing epigastric hernia recurrence, 72,
404
causing hernia recurrence, 368
causing massive incisional hernia, 341
morbid
effect on anesthesia, 515
palpation difficulties in, 404
pubic tubercle identification in, 106
and Shouldice hernia repair, 129–130
symphysis pubis identification in, 106
and wound infection, 281
diagnosis of, 282–283
Obney, Nicolas, 173
Obturator artery
aberrant, 70
Obturator canal, 543
Obturator foramen, 56
Obturator hernia, 542–546
anatomical considerations of, 542*f*, 543,
544*f*
clinical presentation of, 542–544
computed tomography of, 545
preperitoneal approach to, 195
treatment of, 544–546
ultrasonography of, 545
Obturator nerve
compression of, 544*f*
entrapment of, 543
causing postoperative inguinodynia,
308
Obturator region
surgical anatomy of, 542*f*, 543
Occult recurrent hernia
causing postoperative inguinodynia, 314
Ombredanne's forceps, 2–5
Omphalocele, 71
associated malformations with, 425
complications of, 432
definition of, 424
embryology of, 423
epigastric, 423
incidence of, 425
vs. infantile umbilical hernia, 391–392
management of
in newborn, 426–427
nonoperative, 427
postoperative, 432
prenatal diagnosis and management of,
425–426
surgical treatment of, 427–431, 428*f*,
430*f*–431*f*
Omphalomesenteric duct, 392
Onlay patch
definition of, 174
On Surgery and Instruments, 19
On the Surgery, 17
Open herniorrhaphy
and pain reduction, 532
Open inguinal box, 159, 159*f*
Open laparoscopy
for pneumoperitoneum initiation, 386

Open nonmesh herniorrhaphy
ilioinguinal nerve entrapment following,
321
Open tension-free techniques, 585
Operating room set-up
for transabdominal preperitoneal
laparoscopic herniorrhaphy, 258,
258*f*
Opioids
for inguinal herniorrhaphy, 535
Orchiectomy, 146
Orchitis
following Cooper's ligament repair, 141
following inguinal hernia plug repair, 171
following transabdominal preperitoneal
laparoscopic herniorrhaphy, 265
ischemic
clinical features of, 294
incidence of, 294
management of, 294
pathophysiology of, 294
Organoaxial volvulus, 496*f*
Oribasius, 30
Osteitis pubis
in transabdominal preperitoneal
laparoscopic herniorrhaphy, 265
Osteogenesis imperfecta, 6, 9
Ottero and Fallon classification
for traumatic hernia, 73
Outcome measures
for clinical trials, 577–578
bias avoidance in, 578
for hernia repair, 567–568
for VA Cooperative Study No. 456,
595–598

P
Pain
classification of, 299*t*
definition of, 298
following herniorrhaphy
immediate onset of, 309–311
following inguinal hernia plug repair, 171
management of. *See* Anesthesia
for inguinal herniorrhaphy, 531–537.
See also Early postherniorrhaphy
pain
in obturator hernia, 543
in peristomal hernia, 416
postoperative. *See* Postoperative pain
in sciatic hernia, 541
in transmesenteric hernia, 461
in VA Cooperative Study No. 456, 596
in Winslow's foramen hernia, 459–460
Painful ejaculation syndrome, 46, 48*f*
treatment of, 48
Pancost, Joseph, 34
Panniculectomy, 368–369
Paper case report form
for clinical trials data, 579
Paracecal hernia, 463
Paraduodenal hernia
angiography of, 457, 458*f*
clinical presentation of, 456–457
computed tomography of, 456–457, 457*f*
diagnosis of, 456–457

following incisional hernias, 350
with paraesophageal hiatal hernia, 498
Stratification
of clinical trials, 579
of VA Cooperative Study No. 456,
594–595
String sign, 438
Stromayr, Kaspar, 20, 31
Subaponeurotic inguinal space
tension-free, sutureless, preshaped mesh
hernioplasty, 160
Subarachnoid block, 523
advantages and disadvantages of, 517*t*
Subaudible sounds, 95
Subchondral incisional hernias, 349
Subcostal nerve, 519*t*, 521
Subcutaneous inguinal ring, 60
Subcutaneous operation
discovery of, 34
Subdiaphragmatic fascia
vs. phrenoesophageal ligament, 490–491
Sublimaze. *See* Fentanyl
Subumbilical midline incisional hernia
massive, 349
Succinylcholine, 523
Suction drains, 398
Superficial circumflex iliac vessels, 58
Superficial epigastric vessels, 58
Superficial inguinal ring
guarded by external oblique aponeurosis
in women, 50
Superior mesenteric artery (SMA), 454,
455*f*
Superior pubic ligament
first description of, 22
Suprapiriformis hernia, 539–540
Suprapubic hernia, 348*f*
Suprapubic incisional hernia, 348
Supraumbilical herniorrhaphy
anesthesia for, 516
Supraumbilical incisional hernia, 348
Supraumbilical midline incisional hernia
massive, 349
Supravesical fossa, 66
Surfactant
for CDH, 473
Surgeons
Hindu, 181
in preoperative care
for incisional hernias, 352
selection of
for clinical trials, 578–579
Surgical knots
effect on wound healing, 333–334, 334*t*
Surgical mesh
complications of, 562–563
early, 562
infection, 562
mesh migration, 563
mesh shrinkage, 562
foreign-body carcinogenesis risk of,
561–562
historical development of, 551–553, 552*t*
interface mesh-recipient tissues
cellular response of, 561
mechanical requirements of, 558

mesh-specific tissue reaction,
559–561
mesh weight influence on, 559
properties of, 557*t*
structure of, 556–558
tissue response of host, 558
Surgical Papers, 23
Surgical technique
causing incisional hernias, 342–343
SurgiPro, 554
Suture-holding tissue
effect on wound healing, 333
Suture length (SL), 339
definition of, 337
Suture length to wound length ratio
(SL:WL ratio), 338
Sutureless preshaped mesh
in inguinal box, 160*f*
Sutureless primary inguinal hernioplasty,
162–163
external oblique aponeurosis, 163*f*
and Foley catheter, 162*f*
and Reverdin's needle, 162*f*
spermatic cord in, 163*f*
Sutureless prosthesis
for tension-free, sutureless, preshaped
mesh hernioplasty, 160–161
Sutureless repair, 166, 229
of inguinal hernia, 174
Suture line
tension on, 328
Sutures
absorbable, 332
braiding effect of, 281
causing postoperative inguinodynia, 308
comparison of, 332
continuous, 108, 131, 332, 490
effect on wound healing, 331–332
monofilament, 332
for nonprosthetic abdominal wall repair
of incisional hernias, 353
nylon, 332
polydioxanone, 332
promoting wound infection, 281
retention, 338
Suture techniques
causing incisional hernia, 337
causing wound dehiscence, 328, 337
effect on wound healing, 334–339
monitoring of, 336–338
to prevent wound complications, 339
Swallowing mechanism, 480
Swedish Hernia Register, 569–571
participating units in, 569
reoperation
cumulative incidence in, 570, 570*f*
relative risk for, 570*t*
risk analysis in, 570–571
time trends in, 569–570, 569*f*
Symphysis pubis, 106
Symptom score assessment
for VA Cooperative Study No. 456,
590–591
Synthetic mesh, 199
causing postoperative inguinodynia, 308
introduction of, 269

promoting wound infection, 281
and wound healing, 13

T
Tait, Robert Lawson, 35
Tantalum gauze, 39
Tasks of daily living
affected by chronic postoperative pain,
297
Teflon
foreign-body carcinogenesis risk of, 561
Tension-free, sutureless, preshaped mesh
hernioplasty, 159–164
circular mesh for, 161
mesh T4, 161–162
preshaped mesh for, 160
principles of, 159
results of, 164
subaponeurotic inguinal space, 160
sutureless prosthesis for, 160–161
characteristics of, 161*t*
Tension-free hernioplasty, 149
bilayer prosthesis for, 173–180
for laparoscopic hiatal hernia repair, 489,
489*f*
Lichtenstein. *See* Lichtenstein tension-free
hernioplasty
terminology for, 174
Tension-free inguinal hernia repair
open *vs.* laparoscopic techniques
protocol for, 583–602
Tension-free laparoscopic repair, 586–588
Tension-free mesh-free herniorrhaphy
for postoperative inguinodynia, 322, 322*f*
Tension-free mesh repair, 147
and pain reduction, 532
of sliding hiatal hernia, 489*f*
Tension-free open hernia repair, 586
Tension-free reconstruction, 165–166
Tension pneumothorax, 507–508
Testicles
arteries of, 290*f*, 291
atrophy of
clinical features of, 294
following childhood groin hernia
repair, 447
following Cooper's ligament repair,
141
following Lichtenstein tension-free
hernioplasty, 154
following preperitoneal prosthetic
repair, 211
following Shouldice repair, 137
following transabdominal preperitoneal
laparoscopic herniorrhaphy, 265
incidence of, 294
management of, 294
pathophysiology of, 294
blood supply to
damage of, 293
in groin herniorrhaphy, 291
descent of, 436
mediators of, 436
gangrenous-appearing, 293
pain of, 295
sonography of